THE DEVELOPING HUMAN

Twelfth Edition

THE DEVELOPING HUMAN

CLINICALLY ORIENTED EMBRYOLOGY

T.V.N. (Vid) Persaud, MD, PhD, DSc, FRCPath (Lond.), FAAA

Professor Emeritus and Former Head, Department of Human Anatomy and Cell Science
Professor of Pediatrics and Child Health, Associate Professor of Obstetrics, Gynecology, and Reproductive Sciences, Max Rady College of Medicine, Rady Faculty of Health Sciences, University of Manitoba, Winnipeg, Manitoba, Canada

Mark G. Torchia, MSc, PhD

Associate Professor, Department of Surgery; Associate Professor, Department of Human Anatomy and Cell Sciences, Max Rady College of Medicine, Rady Faculty of Health Sciences
Vice-Provost (Teaching and Learning), University of Manitoba, Winnipeg, Manitoba, Canada

For additional online content, visit ebooks.health.elsevier.com/

ELSEVIER

Edinburgh London New York Oxford Philadelphia St Louis Sydney 2020

Elsevier
1600 John F. Kennedy Blvd.
Ste 1800
Philadelphia, PA 19103-2899

THE DEVELOPING HUMAN: CLINICALLY ORIENTED EMBRYOLOGY, TWELFTH EDITION ISBN: 978-0-443-11698-8

Publisher: Jeremy Bowes
Content Development Specialist: Nicholas Henderson
Publishing Services Manager: Shereen Jameel
Project Manager: Gayathri S
Design Direction: Margaret Reid

Printed in India

Last digit is the print number: 9 8 7 6 5 4 3 2 1

For Gisela

My lovely wife and best friend, for her endless support and patience; our three children—Indrani, Sunita, and Rainer (Ren)—and grandchildren (Brian, Amy, and Lucas).

—T.V.N. (Vid) Persaud

For Eddie James, Kitt Miko, and Flynn Henryk, the "Torchia brothers,"

Our dear grandsons and little rays of sunshine; my amazing wife Barbara, our children Muriel and Erik, and their spouses Caleb and Sarah—thank you for your support, encouragement, laughs, and love.

—Mark G. Torchia

For Our Students and Their Teachers

To our students: We hope you will enjoy reading this book; increase your understanding of human embryology; pass all of your examinations; and be excited and well prepared for your careers in patient care, research, and teaching, or whatever the future holds. You will remember some of what you hear, much of what you read, more of what you see, and almost all of what you experience.

To their teachers: May this book be a helpful resource to you and your students. We appreciate the numerous constructive comments we have received over the years from both students and teachers. Your remarks have been invaluable to us in improving this book.

Contributors

David D. Eisenstat, MD, MA, FRCPC, FRACP
Professor and Head of the Department
Children's Cancer Centre
The Royal Children's Hospital
Melbourne; Group Leader
Neuro-Oncology
Stem Cell Biology Theme
Lead, Cancer Flagship
Department of Paediatrics
Murdoch Children's Research Institute
University of Melbourne
Co-Lead
Victorian Paediatric Cancer Consortium (VPCC)
Melbourne
Victoria, Australia

Alison M. Elliott, PhD, MS, CGC
Associate Professor
Department of Medical Genetics
Faculty of Medicine, University of British Columbia
Investigator
BC Children's and Women's Health Research Institutes
Lead
GenCOUNSEL
Vancouver
British Columbia, Canada

Michael Narvey, MD, FRCPC, FAAP
Section Head, Neonatal Medicine
Health Sciences Centre and St. Boniface Hospital
Associate Professor
Pediatrics and Child Health
Max Rady College of Medicine, Rady Faculty of Health Sciences, University of Manitoba, Winnipeg
Manitoba, Canada

Jeffrey T. Wigle, PhD
Principal Investigator
Institute of Cardiovascular Sciences
St. Boniface Hospital Research Centre
Professor
Department of Biochemistry and Medical Genetics
Max Rady College of Medicine
Rady Faculty of Health Sciences
University of Manitoba, Winnipeg
Manitoba, Canada

FIGURES AND IMAGES (SOURCES)

We are grateful to the following colleagues for the clinical images they have given us for this book and also for granting us permission to use figures from their published works:

Steve Ahing, DDS
(retired) Faculty of Dentistry, University of Manitoba, Winnipeg, Manitoba, Canada
Figure 19.19F

Franco Antoniazzi, MD
Department of Pediatrics, University of Verona, Verona, Italy
Figure 20.7

Edward Araujo Jr. MD
Department of Obstetrics, Paulista School of Medicine, Federal University of São Paulo, São Paulo, Brazil
Figures 6.3, 6.2B, 7.21

Dean Barringer and Marnie Danzinger
Figure 6.6

Volker Becker, MD[†]
Pathologisches Institut der Universität, Erlangen, Germany
Figure 7.19 and 7.22

J. V. Been, MD
Department of Pediatrics, Maastricht University Medical Centre, Maastricht, The Netherlands
Figure 10.7C

Beryl Benacerraf, MD
Diagnostic Ultrasound Associates, P.C., Boston, Massachusetts, USA
Figures 13.28, 13.34A, and 13.36A

David Bolender, MD
Department of Cell Biology, Neurobiology, and Anatomy, Medical College of Wisconsin, Milwaukee, Wisconsin, USA
Figure 14.15B and C

Dr. Alberto Borges Peixoto
Mario Palmerio Hospital, University of Uberaba, Uberaba, Brazil
Figures 6.3, 6.2B, 7.21

Dr. Mario João Branco Ferreira
Servico de Dermatologia, Hospital de Desterro, Lisbon, Portugal
Figure 19.5A

Albert E. Chudley, MD, FRCPC, FCCMG
Department of Pediatrics and Child Health, Section of Genetics and Metabolism, Children's Hospital, University of Manitoba, Winnipeg, Manitoba, Canada
Figures 4.6, 9.38, 11.19A and B, 11.28A, 12.24, 12.42, 12.43, 14.12, 15.6, 16.13D and E, 16.14, 16.15, 17.14, 17.33, 17.36, 18.20, 18.21, 18.23, 19.8, 20.4A and B, 20.6C, 20.8, 20.9, 20.10, 20.15, 20.17, 20.17, 20.21A, and 20.22

Blaine M. Cleghorn, DMD, MSc
Faculty of Dentistry, Dalhousie University, Halifax, Nova Scotia, Canada
Figures 19.18 and 19.19A–E

Dr. M.N. Golarz De Bourne
St. George's University Medical School, True Blue, Grenada
Figure 11.21

Heather Dean, MD, FRCPC
Department of Pediatrics and Child Health, University of Manitoba, Winnipeg, Manitoba, Canada
Figures 12.40 and 20.16

Marc Del Bigio, MD, PhD, FRCPC
Department of Pathology (Neuropathology), University of Manitoba, Winnipeg, Manitoba, Canada
Figures 17.13, 17.29 (inset), 17.30B and C, 17.32B, 17.37B, 17.38, 17.40, and 17.42B

David D. Eisenstat, MD, MA, FRCPC
Manitoba Institute of Cell Biology, Department of Human Anatomy and Cell Science, University of Manitoba, Winnipeg, Manitoba, Canada
Figure 17.2

Vassilios Fanos, MD
Department of Pediatrics, University of Verona, Verona, Italy
Figure 20.7

João Carlos Fernandes Rodrigues, MD
Servico de Dermatologia, Hospital de Desterro, Lisbon, Portugal
Figure 19.5B

Frank Gaillard, MB, BS, MMed
Department of Radiology, Royal Melbourne Hospital, Parkville, Victoria, Australia
Figures 4.16 and 9.19B

Gary Geddes, MD
Lake Oswego, Oregon, USA
Figure 14.15A

Barry H. Grayson, MD and Bruno L. Vendittelli, MD
New York University Medical Center, Institute of Reconstructive Plastic Surgery, New York, New York, USA
Figure 9.41

Christopher R. Harman, MD, FRCSC, FACOG
Department of Obstetrics, Gynecology, and Reproductive Sciences, Women's Hospital and University of Maryland, Baltimore, Maryland, USA
Figures 7.18 and 12.23

[†]Deceased.

Jean Hay, MSc†
Department of Anatomy, University of Manitoba, Winnipeg, Manitoba, Canada
Figure 17.25

Blair Henderson, MD
Department of Radiology, Health Sciences Centre, University of Manitoba, Winnipeg, Manitoba, Canada
Figure 13.6

Lyndon M. Hill, MD
Magee-Women's Hospital, Pittsburgh, Pennsylvania, USA
Figures 11.7 and 12.14

Klaus V. Hinrichsen, MD†
Medizinische Fakultät, Institut für Anatomie, Ruhr-Universität Bochum, Bochum, Germany
Figures 5.12A, 9.2, and 9.26

Dr. Jon Jackson and Mrs. Margaret Jackson
Figure 6.9B

Evelyn Jain, MD, FCFP
Breastfeeding Clinic, Calgary, Alberta, Canada
Figure 9.24

John A. Jane, Sr., MD
David D. Weaver Professor of Neurosurgery, Department of Neurological Surgery, University of Virginia Health System, Charlottesville, Virginia, USA
Figure 14.13

Robert Jordan, MD
St. George's University Medical School, True Blue, Grenada
Figures 6.5B and 7.26

Dagmar K. Kalousek, MD
Department of Pathology, University of British Columbia, Children's Hospital, Vancouver, British Columbia, Canada
Figures 8.11AB, 11.14A, 12.12B, and 12.16A

E. C. Klatt, MD
Department of Biomedical Sciences, Mercer University School of Medicine, Savannah, Georgia, USA
Figure 7.16

Wesley Lee, MD
Division of Fetal Imaging, William Beaumont Hospital, Royal Oak, Michigan, USA
Figures 13.20 and 13.29A

Deborah Levine, MD, FACR
Departments of Radiology and Obstetric & Gynecologic Ultrasound, Beth Israel Deaconess Medical Center, Boston, Massachusetts, USA
Figures 6.7 6.13 8.10, 9.38C and D, 17.35B, and cover image (magnetic resonance image of 27-week fetus)

†Deceased.

E.A. (Ted) Lyons, OC, MD, FRCPC, FACR
Departments of Radiology, Obstetrics & Gynecology, and Human Anatomy & Cell Science, Division of Ultrasound, Health Sciences Centre, University of Manitoba, Winnipeg, Manitoba, Canada
Figures 3.6 3.8, 4.1, 4.14, 5.19, 6.1, 6.8, 6.10, 6.12, 7.24 7.27 7.30, 11.19C and D, 12.45, and 13.3

Margaret Morris, MD, FRCSC, MEd
Professor of Obstetrics, Gynaecology, and Reproductive Sciences, Women's Hospital and University of Manitoba, Winnipeg, Manitoba, Canada
Figure 12.46

Stuart C. Morrison, MD
Section of Pediatric Radiology, The Children's Hospital, Cleveland Clinic, Cleveland, Ohio, USA
Figures 7.14 11.20, 17.29E, and 17.41

John B. Mulliken, MD
Children's Hospital Boston, Harvard Medical School, Boston, Massachusetts, USA
Figure 9.43

Dwight Parkinson, MD†
Departments of Surgery and Human Anatomy & Cell Science, University of Manitoba, Winnipeg, Manitoba, Canada
Figure 17.15

Maulik S. Patel, MD
Consultant Pathologist, Surat, India
Figure 4.16

Srinivasa Ramachandra, MD
Figure 9.19A

Dr. M. Ray†
Department of Human Genetics, University of Manitoba, Winnipeg, Manitoba, Canada
Figure 20.14B

Martin H. Reed, MD, FRCPC
Department of Radiology, University of Manitoba and Children's Hospital, Winnipeg, Manitoba, Canada
Figure 11.27

Gregory J. Reid, MD, FRCSC
Department of Obstetrics, Gynecology, and Reproductive Sciences, University of Manitoba, Women's Hospital, Winnipeg, Manitoba, Canada
Figures 9.38A and B, 11.18, 12.38, 13.12, and 14.10C

Michael and Michele Rice
Figure 6.9A

Dr. S. G. Robben
Department of Radiology, Maastricht University Medical Centre, Maastricht, The Netherlands
Figure 10.7C

†Deceased.

Prem S. Sahni, MD
Formerly of the Department of Radiology, Children's Hospital, Winnipeg, Manitoba, Canada
Figures 8.11C, 10.7B, 10.14, 11.4C, 11.28B, 12.16, 12.17, 12.19, 14.11D, 14.16, and 16.13C

Marcos Antonio Velasco Sanchez, MD
Centro de Estudios e Investigacion en Ultrasonido General del Estado de Guerrero, and Hospital General (S.S.A.) de Acapulco, Guerrero, Mexico
Figure 18.6

Dr. M.J. Schuurman
Department of Pediatrics, Maastricht University Medical Centre, Maastricht, The Netherlands
Figure 10.7C

P. Schwartz and H.M. Michelmann
University of Göttingen, Göttingen, Germany
Figure 2.14

Joseph R. Siebert, MD
Children's Hospital and Regional Center, Seattle, Washington, USA
Figures 16.13B, and 17.16

Bradley R. Smith, MD
University of Michigan, Ann Arbor, Michigan, USA
Figures 5.16C, 5.17C, 5.20C, 8.6B, 9.3A (inset), 14.14A and 18.17B

Gerald S. Smyser, MD
Formerly of the Altru Health System, Grand Forks, North Dakota, USA
Figures 9.12, 9.20, 13.44, 17.24, 17.32A, 17.34, 17.37A, and 18.23

Pierre Soucy, MD, FRCSC
Division of Pediatric Surgery, Children's Hospital of Eastern Ontario, Ottawa, Ontario, Canada
Figures 9.10, 9.11, and 18.21

Dr. Y. Suzuki
Achi, Japan
Figure 16.13A

R. Shane Tubbs, PhD
Children's Hospital Birmingham, Birmingham, Alabama, USA
Figure 17.42A and C

Edward O. Uthman, MD
Consultant Pathologist, Houston/Richmond, Texas, USA
Figure 3.10

Zoumpourlis Vassilis, PhD
Research Professor, Head of the Biomedical Applications Unit, Institute of Biology, Medicinal Chemistry & Biotechnology, NHRF, Athens, Greece
Figure 2.13

Jeffrey T. Wigle, PhD
Department of Biochemistry and Medical Genetics, University of Manitoba, Winnipeg, Manitoba, Canada
Figure 17.2

Nathan E. Wiseman, MD, FRCSC
Pediatric Surgeon, Children's Hospital, Winnipeg, Manitoba, Canada
Figure 11.17A

M.T. Zenzes
In Vitro Fertilization Program, Toronto Hospital, Toronto, Ontario, Canada
Figure 2.18A

Preface

The Developing Human is now 50 years in print. Dr. Keith Leon Moore was the sole author of the first four editions. We were greatly honored when Dr. Moore invited us to join him as coauthors. Sadly, Dr. Moore passed away on November 25, 2019 at the age of 94 years. A world-renowned embryologist and anatomist, Dr. Moore's lifelong scholarly contributions remain an enduring legacy.

This 12th edition of *The Developing Human* has been thoroughly revised and updated. We are thankful for the continued support and expertise of our distinguished contributors.

We have entered an era of achievement in the fields of molecular biology, genetics, and clinical embryology, perhaps like no other. The sequencing of the human genome has been achieved, and several mammalian species, as well as the human embryo, have been cloned. Scientists have created and isolated human embryonic pluripotential stem cells, and their use in treating certain intractable diseases continues to generate widespread debate. Moreover, the recently discovered CRISP-*Cas9* editing has not only become a revolutionary tool for developmental biologists but also segments of disease-associated variations can be clinically identified in human embryos, clipped out, and repaired. These remarkable scientific developments have already provided promising directions for research in human embryology, which will have an impact on the treatment of diseases in the future.

This book is written for science and biomedical students, keeping in mind those who may not have had a previous acquaintance with human anatomy or clinical embryology. This edition is logically organized and even more learner-friendly. It provides a clear and comprehensive account of the sequence of events that occur between the moment of fertilization and the time of birth. We have tried to present the text in an interesting way so that it can be easily integrated with what will be taught in more detail in other disciplines, such as human anatomy, physical diagnosis, medical rehabilitation, and surgery. We hope this new edition will serve to educate and inspire students to develop an interest in clinically oriented embryology.

The 12th edition of *The Developing Human* has been thoroughly revised to reflect current understanding of some of the molecular events that guide the development of the embryo. This book also contains more *clinically oriented material* than previous editions; these sections are set as blue boxes to differentiate them from the rest of the text. In addition to focusing on clinically relevant aspects of embryology, we have revised the Clinically Oriented Problems with brief answers that emphasize the importance of embryology in modern medical practice.

This edition follows the official international list of embryologic terms (*Terminologia Embryologica,* FIPAT. Terminologia Embryologica. 2nd ed. FIPAT.library.dal.ca. Federative International Programme for Anatomical Terminology, February 2017). It is important that physicians and scientists throughout the world use the same name for each structure.

We have added many new figures of clinical cases and new color photographs of embryos (normal and abnormal). Many of the illustrations have been improved using three-dimensional renderings and more effective use of colors. There are also many new diagnostic images (ultrasound and magnetic resonance images) of embryos and fetuses to illustrate their three-dimensional aspects. *A set of 18 animations* that will help students understand the complexities of embryologic development comes with this book. When one of the animations is especially relevant to a passage in the text, the icon has been added in the margin. Maximized animations are available to instructors who have adopted *The Developing Human* for their teaching sessions (consult your Elsevier representative).

The coverage of teratology (studies concerned with birth defects) and genetics has been increased and updated because the study of the abnormal development of embryos and fetuses is helpful in understanding risk estimation, the causes of birth defects, and how malformations may be prevented. Recent advances in the molecular aspects of developmental biology have been highlighted (in *italics*) throughout the book, especially in those areas that appear promising for clinical medicine or have the potential to make a significant impact on the direction of future research.

We have continued our attempts to provide an easy-to-read account of human development before birth and during the neonatal period. Every chapter has been thoroughly reviewed and revised to reflect new findings from research and their clinical significance.

The chapters are organized to present a systematic and logical approach to embryonic development. The first chapter introduces readers to the scope and importance of embryology, the historical background of the discipline, and the terms used to describe the stages of development. The next four chapters cover embryonic development, beginning with the formation of gametes and ending with the formation of basic organs and systems. The development of specific organs and systems is then described in a systematic manner, followed by chapters dealing with the highlights of the fetal period, the placenta and fetal membranes, the causes of human birth defects, and common signaling pathways used during development. At the end of each chapter, there are summaries of key features, which provide a convenient means of ongoing review. There are also references that contain both classic works and recent research publications.

T.V.N. (Vid) Persaud
Mark G. Torchia

Acknowledgments

The Developing Human is widely used by medical, dental, and many other students in the health sciences. The suggestions, constructive criticisms, and comments we received from instructors and students around the world have helped us improve this 12th edition.

When learning embryology, illustrations are an essential feature to facilitate both understanding of the subject and retention of the material. Many figures have been improved, and newer clinical images replace older ones.

We are indebted to the following colleagues (listed alphabetically) for either critical reviewing of chapters, making suggestions for improvement of this book or providing some of the new figures: Dr. Steve Ahing (retired), Department of Oral Pathology, Faculty of Dentistry, University of Manitoba, Winnipeg, Manitoba, Canada; Dr. David L. Bolender, Medical College of Wisconsin, Milwaukee, Wisconsin; Dr. Albert Chudley, Departments of Pediatrics and Child Health and Biochemistry and Medical Genetics, University of Manitoba, Winnipeg, Manitoba, Canada; Dr. Blaine M. Cleghorn, Department of Dental Clinical Sciences, Faculty of Dentistry, Dalhousie University, Halifax, Nova Scotia; Dr. Frank Gaillard, Department of Radiology, Royal Melbourne Hospital, Melbourne, Victoria, Australia; Dr. Boris Kablar, Department of Medical Neuroscience, Dalhousie University, Halifax, Nova Scotia; Dr. Peeyush Lala, Department of Anatomy and Cell Biology, Schulich Medicine & Dentistry, Western University, London, Ontario, Canada; Dr. Deborah Levine, Beth Israel Deaconess Medical Center, Harvard University, Boston, Massachusetts; Dr. Marios Loukas, St. George's University, Grenada; Dr. Bernard J. Moxham, Cardiff School of Biosciences, Cardiff University, Cardiff, Wales, United Kingdom; Dr. Drew Noden, Cornell University, College of Veterinary Medicine, Ithaca, New York; Dr. Shannon Perry (Retired), School of Nursing, San Francisco State University, San Francisco, California; Dr. Gregory Reid (Retired), Department of Obstetrics, Gynecology, and Reproductive Sciences, University of Manitoba, Winnipeg, Manitoba, Canada; Dr. J. Elliott Scott (Deceased), Departments of Oral Biology and Human Anatomy and Cell Science, University of Manitoba, Winnipeg, Manitoba, Canada; Dr. Brad Smith, University of Michigan, Ann Arbor, Michigan; Dr. Gerald S. Smyser, formerly of the Altru Health System, Grand Forks, North Dakota; Dr. Richard Shane Tubbs, Departments of Neurosurgery, Neurology, and Structural & Cellular Biology, Tulane University School of Medicine, New Orleans, Louisiana; Dr. Ed Uthman, Clinical Pathologist, Memorial Hermann Katy Hospital, Houston/Richmond, Texas; and Dr. Michael Wiley (Retired), Division of Anatomy, Department of Surgery, Faculty of Medicine, University of Toronto, Toronto, Ontario, Canada. A number of illustrations were prepared by Hans Neuhart.

The collection of animations of developing embryos was produced in collaboration with Dr. David L. Bolender, Professor Emeritus. Medical College of Wisconsin, Milwaukee, Wisconsin. The animations have been skillfully enhanced with narration—we thank the Elsevier St. Louis Multimedia Department.

At Elsevier, we are indebted to Mr. Jeremy Bowes, Publisher, and Mr. Nicholas Henderson, Content Development Specialist, for their invaluable insights and unstinting support in the preparation of this 12th edition of the book. Finally, we thank the entire Elsevier production team, especially Ms. Padmavathy Kannabiran (Project Manager) and Ms. Gayathri S (Senior Project Manager), for bringing this book to completion. This new edition of *The Developing Human* is the result of their dedication and technical expertise.

T.V.N. (Vid) Persaud
Mark G. Torchia

Get the most out of *The Developing Human,* 12th Edition!

Included in your purchase is a rich variety of **BONUS content** to enhance the printed book and your learning. Look out for this icon ▶ indicating where there is directly related electronic material. Benefit from:

- **18 superb animations, with expert voice-overs**—to guide you through key embryology concepts:

Animation Title	Associated Chapter(s)	Animation Title	Associated Chapter(s)
Fertilization	2	Gastrointestinal Tract	11
Blastocyst	3	Urinary System	12
Implantation	3	Reproductive System	12
Gastrulation	4	Heart	13
Folding of the Embryo	4,5	Vascular System	13
Body Cavities	4,8	Limb Development	16
Pharyngeal Apparatus	9	The Nervous System	17
Face and Palate	9	Development of the Ears	18
Respiratory System	10	Development of the Eyes	18

- **Multiple Choice Questions, with explanations**—to help check your understanding and prepare for assessments

Don't miss out on this wealth of extra content—see the inside front cover for your access instructions!

Biography

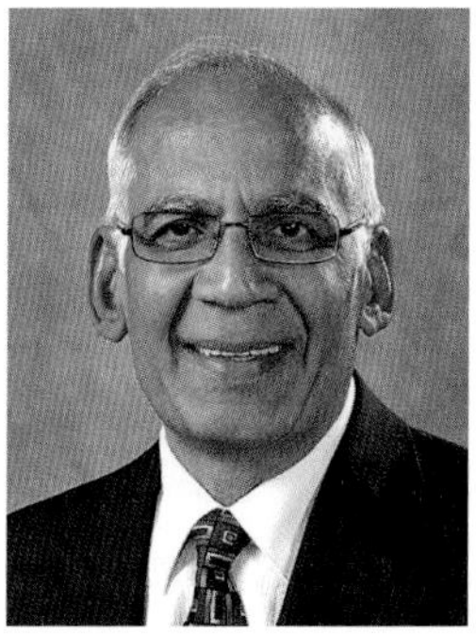

T.V.N. (VID) PERSAUD

Dr. Persaud was the recipient of the **Henry Gray/Elsevier Distinguished Educator Award in 2010**—"the American Association of Anatomists' highest honor in recognition of sustained excellence and leadership in human anatomy education"; the **Honored Member Award of the American Association of Clinical Anatomists (2008)** for "his distinguished career and significant contributions to the field of clinically relevant anatomy, embryology, and the history of anatomy"; and the **J.C.B. Grant Award of the Canadian Association of Anatomists (1991)** "in recognition of meritorious service and outstanding scholarly accomplishments in the field of anatomical sciences." In 2010 Professor Persaud was inducted as a **Fellow of the American Association of Anatomists** (AAA). The rank of Fellow honors distinguished AAA members who have demonstrated excellence in science and in their overall contributions to the medical sciences. In 2003 Dr. Persaud was a recipient of the **Queen Elizabeth II Golden Jubilee Medal**, presented by the Government of Canada for "significant contribution to the nation, the community, and fellow Canadians."

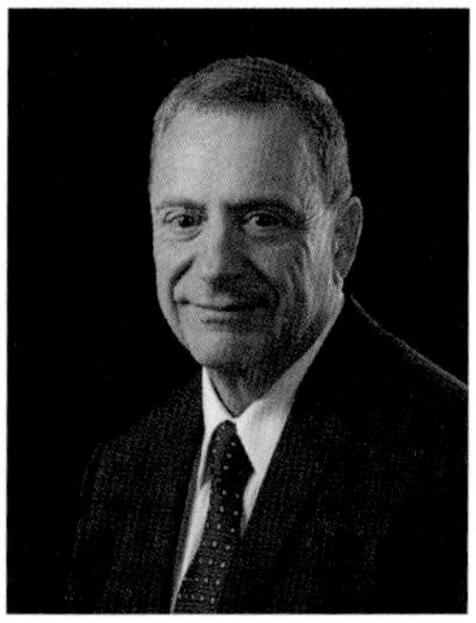

MARK G. TORCHIA

Dr. Mark G. Torchia is the recipient of the distinguished **Inaugural Governor General Award for Innovation**, which "recognize[s] and celebrate[s] outstanding Canadian individuals, teams and organizations—trailblazers and creators who contribute to our country's success, who help shape our future and who inspire the next generation." Dr. Torchia is also a **Manning Principle Prize Laureate** (2015), which recognizes "leaders and visionaries who are positively impacting the Canadian economy while improving the human experience in its various dimensions around the world." He is also a recipient of the **Norman and Marion Bright Memorial Medal and Award** for recognizing "individuals who have made an outstanding contribution to chemical technology" and the **TIMEC Medical Device Champion Award**. Dr. Torchia continues to engage learners at all levels through outreach opportunities and formal curricula. He has been nominated for Manitoba Medical Students' Association teaching awards since their initiation and was awarded the **Award for Teaching Excellence** (2016) from the Rady Faculty of Health Sciences, University of Manitoba.

Tribute to Dr. Keith Leon Moore

At the age of 94 years, Dr. Keith Leon Moore passed away. He authored several anatomy and embryology textbooks, which not only won numerous awards but were translated into many languages. Truly an international icon in the field of anatomy, Dr. Moore's books had a tremendous impact on generations of students and on medical education.

Dr. Moore had been the recipient of many prestigious awards and recognitions. He was the recipient of the **inaugural Henry Gray/Elsevier Distinguished Educator Award in 2007**—the American Association of Anatomists' (AAA) highest award for excellence in human anatomy education at the medical/dental, graduate, and undergraduate levels of teaching; the **Honored Member Award of the American Association of Clinical Anatomists (1994)** for significant contributions to the field of clinically relevant anatomy; and the **J.C.B. Grant Award of the Canadian Association of Anatomists (1984)** "in recognition of meritorious service and outstanding scholarly accomplishments in the field of anatomical sciences." In 2008 Dr. Moore was inducted as a **Fellow of the American Association of Anatomists**, which honors distinguished AAA members who have demonstrated excellence in science and in their overall contributions to the medical sciences. In 2012 Dr. Moore received an **Honorary Doctor of Science** degree from the Ohio State University and from the University of Western Ontario in 2015, as well as the **Queen Elizabeth II Diamond Jubilee Medal** honoring significant contributions and achievements by Canadians, and the **Benton Adkins Jr. Distinguished Service Award** for an outstanding record of service to the American Association of Clinical Anatomists.

Dr. Moore's lifelong contributions as a medical educator in anatomical sciences will stand as a lasting legacy.

Dr. Keith Leon Moore (1925–2019)

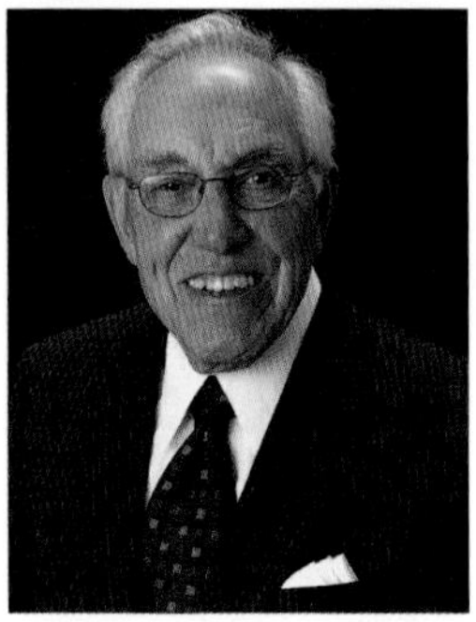

Contents

Introduction to Human Development

1

CHAPTER OUTLINE

Human development is a continuous process that begins when an **oocyte** (ovum) from a female is fertilized by a **sperm** (spermatozoon) from a male to form a single-celled **zygote** (Fig. 1.1). Cell division, cell migration, programmed cell death (apoptosis), differentiation, growth, and cell rearrangement transform the zygote, a highly specialized totipotent cell, into a multicellular human being. Most developmental changes occur during the embryonic and fetal periods; however, important changes occur during later periods of development: the neonatal period (first 4 weeks), infancy (first year), childhood (2 years to puberty), adolescence (11–19 years), and early adult (20–25 years).

DEVELOPMENTAL PERIODS

It is customary to divide human development into **prenatal** (before birth) and **postnatal** (after birth) periods. The development of a human from a zygote to birth is divided into two main periods, **embryonic** and **fetal**. The changes that occur prenatally are summarized in the timetable of human prenatal development (see Fig. 1.1). The most *visible* advances occur during the third to eighth weeks—the embryonic period. During the fetal period, differentiation and growth of tissues and organs occur, and the rate of body growth increases.

STAGES OF EMBRYONIC DEVELOPMENT

Early development is described in various stages: stage 1 begins at fertilization, and embryonic development ends at stage 23, which occurs on day 56 post fertilization (see Fig. 1.1). The fetal period follows the embryonic period, ending at the time of birth.

POSTNATAL PERIOD

This is the period occurring after birth. Explanations of frequently used postnatal developmental terms and periods follow.

INFANCY AND CHILDHOOD

Infancy is roughly the first year after birth. An **infant** aged 1 month or younger is called a **neonate (newborn)**. The transition from intrauterine to extrauterine existence requires many critical changes, especially in the cardiovascular and respiratory systems. The body grows rapidly during infancy; total length increases by approximately 50%, and weight is usually tripled. **Childhood** is the period between infancy and puberty. During early childhood, there is continued rapid growth and active ossification (formation of bone); the primary (deciduous) teeth continue to appear and are later replaced by the secondary (permanent) teeth. As the child grows older, the rate of body growth slows down. However, just before puberty, growth accelerates—the prepubertal growth spurt.

PUBERTY AND ADULTHOOD

Puberty is the period when humans become functionally capable of reproduction. In females, the first signs of puberty may begin after age 8; in males, puberty commonly begins at age 9. Attainment of full growth and maturity is generally reached between 18 and 21 years. Ossification and growth are virtually completed during early adulthood (21–25 years). Brain development continues into early adulthood, including changes in gray matter volume.

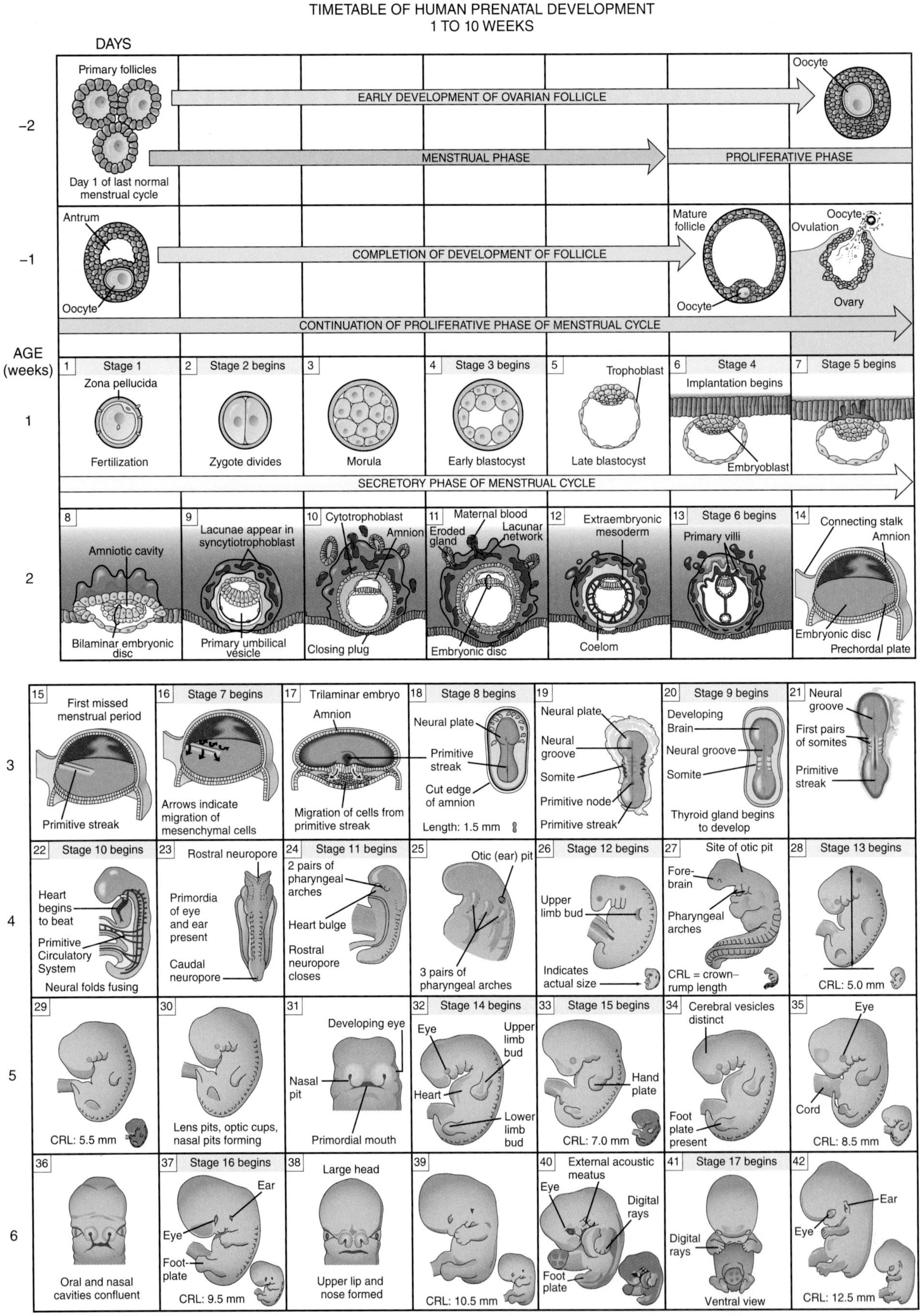

Fig. 1.1 Early stages of development. Development of an ovarian follicle containing an oocyte, ovulation, and the phases of the menstrual cycle are illustrated. Human development begins at fertilization, approximately 14 days after the onset of the last normal menstrual period. Cleavage of the zygote in the uterine tube, implantation of the blastocyst in the endometrium (lining) of the uterus, and early development of the embryo are also shown. The alternative term for the umbilical vesicle is the yolk sac; this is an inappropriate term because the human vesicle does not contain a yolk.

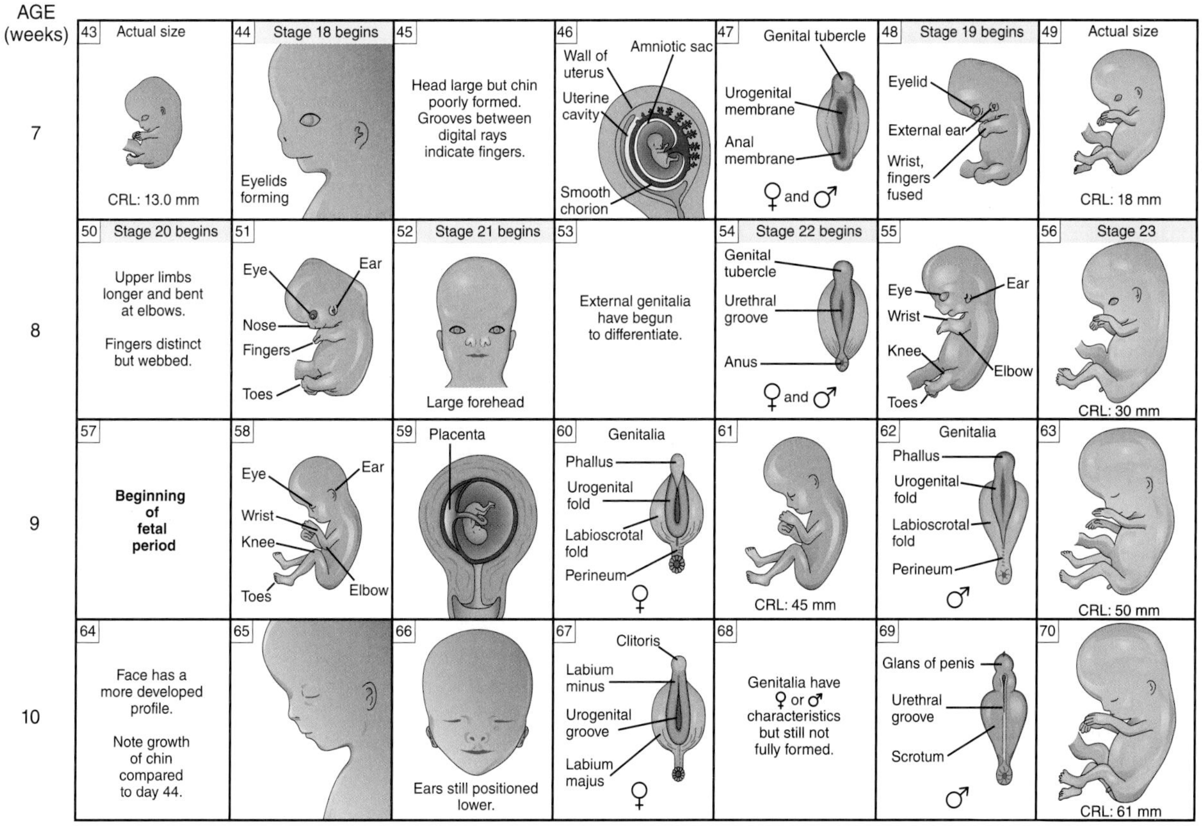

Fig. 1.1 cont'd

SIGNIFICANCE OF EMBRYOLOGY

Clinically oriented embryology refers to the study of embryos but generally means the prenatal development of embryos, fetuses, and neonates. **Developmental anatomy** refers to the structural changes of a human from fertilization to adulthood; it includes embryology, fetology, and postnatal development. **Teratology** is the division of embryology and pathology that deals with various genetic and/or environmental factors that disturb normal development and produce birth defects (see Chapter 20).

Clinically oriented embryology is a critical science as it:

- Bridges the gap between prenatal development and obstetrics, perinatal medicine, pediatrics, and clinical anatomy
- Develops knowledge concerning the beginning of life and the changes occurring during prenatal development
- Builds an understanding of the causes of variations in human structure
- Illuminates clinically oriented anatomy and explains how normal and abnormal relations develop
- Supports the research and application of stem cells for the treatment of certain chronic diseases.

Much of the modern practice of obstetrics involves **applied embryology**. Embryologic topics of special interest to obstetricians are oocyte and sperm transport, ovulation, fertilization, implantation, fetal-maternal interactions, fetal circulation, critical periods of development, and causes of birth defects.

In addition to caring for the mother, physicians guard the health of the embryo and fetus. The significance of embryology is readily apparent to pediatricians because some of their patients have birth defects resulting from maldevelopment, such as congenital heart disease.

Birth defects cause most deaths during infancy. Knowledge of the development of structure and function is essential for understanding the physiologic changes that occur during the neonatal period and helping fetuses and neonates in distress. Progress in surgery, especially in the fetal, perinatal, and pediatric age groups, has made knowledge of human development even more clinically significant. Surgical treatment of fetuses is now possible in some situations. Understanding and correcting most defects depend on knowledge of normal development and the deviations that may occur. Understanding common congenital birth defects and their causes also enables healthcare providers to explain the developmental basis of birth defects, often dispelling parental feelings of guilt. (*Note that throughout this book, we provide data related to the incidence or prevalence of specific birth defects. It is important for the reader to appreciate that these are estimates based on the best available data at the time, and the data may vary across sex, race, geography, age of the mother or father, and many other variables. Unless otherwise specific, the values for incidence are shown as rates per live birth.*)

HISTORICAL GLEANINGS

If I have seen further, it is by standing on the shoulders of giants.
—SIR ISAAC NEWTON, ENGLISH MATHEMATICIAN, 1643–1727

This statement, made more than 300 years ago, emphasizes that each new study of a problem rests on a knowledge base established by earlier investigators. The theories of every age offer explanations based on the knowledge and experience of investigators of the period. People have always been interested in knowing how they developed and were born and why some embryos and fetuses develop abnormally. Ancient people developed many answers to the reasons for these birth defects.

ANCIENT VIEWS OF HUMAN EMBRYOLOGY

Egyptians of the Old Kingdom, approximately 3000 BCE, knew of methods for incubating birds' eggs. **Akhnaton** (Amenophis IV) praised the sun god Aton as the creator of the germ in a woman, maker of the seed in man, and giver of life to the son in the body of his mother. The ancient Egyptians believed that the soul entered the infant at birth through the placenta.

A brief Sanskrit treatise on **ancient Indian embryology** is thought to have been written in 1416 BCE. This scripture of the Hindus, called **Garbha Upanishad**, describes ancient views concerning the embryo. It states:

From the conjugation of blood and semen [seed], the embryo comes into existence. During the period favorable for conception, after the sexual intercourse, [it] becomes a Kalada [one-day-old embryo]. After remaining seven nights, it becomes a vesicle. After a fortnight it becomes a spherical mass. After a month it becomes a firm mass. After two months the head is formed. After three months the limb regions appear.

Greek scholars made many important contributions to the science of embryology. The first recorded embryologic studies are in the books of **Hippocrates of Cos**, the famous Greek physician (c.460–377 BCE) who is regarded as the "father of medicine." To understand how the human embryo develops, he recommended this experiment:

Take twenty or more eggs and let them be incubated by two or more hens. Then each day from the second to that of hatching, remove an egg, break it, and examine it. You will find exactly as I say, for the nature of the bird can be likened to that of man.

Aristotle of Stagira (c.384–322 BCE), a Greek philosopher and scientist, wrote a treatise on embryology in which he described the development of the chick and other embryos. Aristotle promoted the idea that the embryo developed from a formless mass, which he described as a "less fully concocted seed with a nutritive soul and all bodily parts." This embryo, he thought, arose from menstrual blood after activation by male semen.

Claudius Galen (c. CE 130–201), a Greek physician and medical scientist in Rome, wrote a book, *On the Formation of the Foetus*, in which he described the development and nutrition of fetuses and the structures that we now call the allantois, amnion, and placenta.

The **Talmud** contains references to the formation of the embryo. The Jewish physician **Samuel-el-Yehudi**, who lived during the second century AD, described six stages in the formation of the embryo, from a "formless, rolled-up thing" to a "child whose months have been completed." Talmud scholars believed that the bones and tendons, the nails, the marrow in the head, and the white of the eyes were derived from the father, "who sows the white," but the skin, flesh, blood, and hair were derived from the mother, "who sows the red." These views were based on the teachings of both Aristotle and Galen.

EMBRYOLOGY IN THE MIDDLE AGES

The growth of science was slow during the medieval period, but a few high points of embryologic investigation undertaken during this time are known to us. It is cited in the **Quran** (CE seventh century), the holy book of Islam, that human beings are produced from a mixture of secretions from the male and female. Several references are made to the creation of a human being from a *nutfa* ("small drop"). Reference is made to the leech-like appearance of the early embryo. Later, the embryo is said to resemble a "chewed substance."

Constantinus Africanus of Salerno (c. CE 1020–87) wrote a concise treatise entitled *De Humana Natura*. Africanus described the composition and sequential development of the embryo in relation to the planets and each month during pregnancy, a concept unknown in antiquity. Medieval scholars hardly deviated from the **Theory of Aristotle**, which stated that the embryo was derived from menstrual blood and semen. Because of a lack of knowledge, drawings of the fetus in the uterus often showed a fully developed infant frolicking in the womb (Fig. 1.2).

THE RENAISSANCE

Leonardo da Vinci (1452–1519) made accurate drawings of dissections of pregnant uteri containing fetuses (Fig. 1.3). He introduced the quantitative approach to embryology by making measurements of prenatal growth.

It has been stated that the embryologic revolution began with the publication of William Harvey's book *De Generatione Animalium* in 1651. **Harvey** (1578–1657) believed that the male seed or sperm, after entering the womb or uterus, became metamorphosed into an egg-like substance from which the embryo developed. Harvey was greatly influenced by one of his professors at the University of Padua, **Fabricius of Acquapendente**, an Italian anatomist and embryologist who was the first to study embryos from different species of animals. Harvey examined chick embryos with simple lenses and made many new observations. He also studied the development of the fallow deer; however, when unable to observe early developmental stages, he concluded that embryos were secreted by the uterus. **Girolamo Fabricius** (1537–1619) wrote two major embryologic treatises, including one entitled *De Formato Foetu* (The Formed Fetus), which contained many illustrations of embryos and fetuses at different stages of development.

Early microscopes were simple, but they opened an exciting new field of observation. In 1672 **Regnier de Graaf** observed small chambers in the rabbit's uterus and concluded that they could not have been secreted by the uterus. He stated that they must have come from organs that he

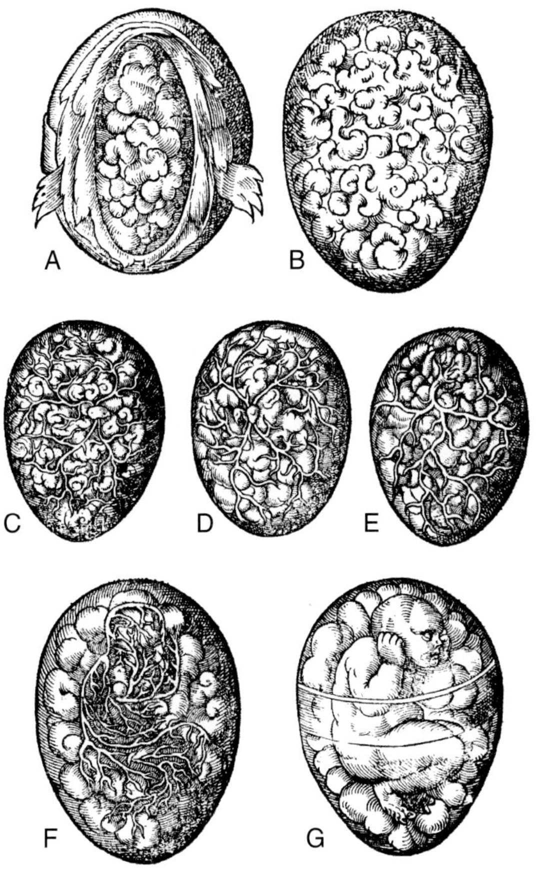

Fig. 1.2 (A–G) Illustrations from Jacob Rueff's *De Conceptu et Generatione Hominis* (1554) showing the fetus developing from a coagulum of blood and semen in the uterus. This theory was based on the teachings of Aristotle, and it survived until the late 18th century. (From Needham J: *A history of embryology*, ed 2, Cambridge, UK, 1934, Cambridge University Press, with permission of Cambridge University Press, England.)

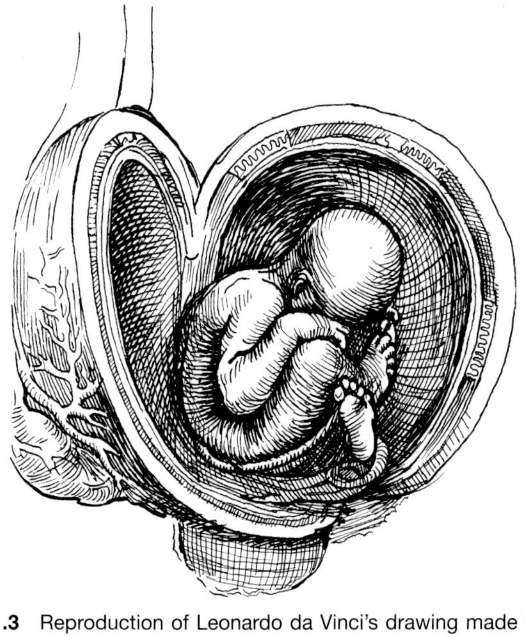

Fig. 1.3 Reproduction of Leonardo da Vinci's drawing made in the 15th century showing a fetus in a uterus that has been incised and opened.

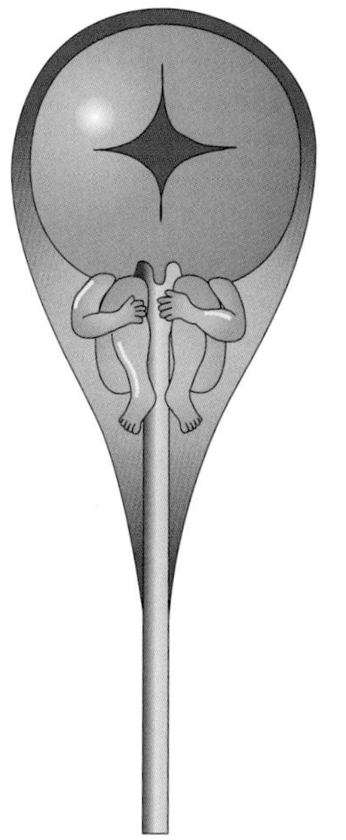

Fig. 1.4 Copy of a 17th-century drawing of a sperm by Hartsoeker. The miniature human being within it was thought to enlarge after the sperm entered an ovum. Other embryologists at this time thought the oocyte contained a miniature human being that enlarged when it was stimulated by a sperm.

called ovaries. Undoubtedly, the small chambers that de Graaf described were blastocysts (see Fig. 1.1). He also described follicles, which were called graafian follicles (now referred to as vesicular ovarian follicles.)

Marcello Malpighi, studying what he believed were unfertilized hen's eggs in 1675, observed early chick embryos. As a result, he thought the egg contained a miniature chick. A young medical student in Leiden, **Johan Ham van Arnhem**, and his countryman, **Anton van Leeuwenhoek**, using an improved microscope in 1677, first observed human sperm. However, they misunderstood the sperm's role in fertilization. They thought the sperm contained a miniature preformed human being that enlarged when it was deposited in the female genital tract (Fig. 1.4).

Caspar Friedrich Wolff refuted both versions of the preformation theory in 1759 after observing that parts of the embryo develop from "globules" (small spherical bodies). He examined unincubated eggs but could not see the embryos described by Malpighi. He proposed the layer concept, whereby the division of what we call the zygote produces layers of cells (now called the **embryonic disc**) from which the embryo develops. His ideas formed the basis of the theory of **epigenesis**, which states that "development results from growth and differentiation of specialized cells." These important discoveries first appeared in Wolff's doctoral dissertation, *Theoria Generationis.* He also observed embryonic masses of tissue that partly contribute to the development of the urinary and genital systems—wolffian bodies and wolffian ducts—now called the mesonephros and mesonephric ducts, respectively (see Chapter 12).

The preformation controversy ended in 1775 when **Lazzaro Spallanzani** showed that both the oocyte and sperm were necessary for initiating the development of a new individual. From his experiments, including artificial insemination in dogs, he concluded that the sperm was the fertilizing agent that initiated the developmental processes. **Heinrich Christian Pander** discovered the three germ layers of the embryo, which he named the blastoderm. He reported this discovery in 1817 in his doctoral dissertation.

Etienne Saint Hilaire and his son, **Isidore Saint Hilaire**, made the first significant studies of abnormal development in 1818. They performed experiments on animals that were designed to produce birth defects, initiating what we now know as the science of teratology.

Karl Ernst von Baer described the oocyte in the ovarian follicle of a dog in 1827, approximately 150 years after the discovery of sperm. He also observed cleaving zygotes in the uterine tube and blastocysts in the uterus. He contributed new knowledge about the origin of tissues and organs from the layers described earlier by Malpighi and Pander. Von Baer formulated two important embryologic concepts, namely, that there are distinct stages of embryonic development and that general characteristics precede specific ones. His significant and far-reaching contributions resulted in him being regarded as the "father of modern embryology."

Matthias Schleiden and **Theodor Schwann** were responsible for the great advances being made in embryology when they formulated the cell theory in 1839. This concept states that the body is composed of cells and cell products. The cell theory soon led to the realization that the embryo developed from a single cell, the zygote, which underwent many cell divisions as the tissues and organs formed.

Wilhelm His, Sr. (1831–1904), a Swiss anatomist and embryologist, developed improved techniques for fixation, embedded with paraffin wax, serial sectioning, and staining of tissues and for reconstruction of embryos. His method of graphic reconstruction paved the way for the current production of three-dimensional (3D), stereoscopic, and computer-generated images of embryos. Wilhelm His, Sr., was twice nominated for the Nobel Prize in Medicine.

Franklin P. Mall (1862–1917), inspired by the work of Wilhelm His, began to collect human embryos for scientific study. Mall's collection forms a part of the **Carnegie Collection of Embryos**, which is known throughout the world. It is now in the National Museum of Health and Medicine at the Armed Forces Institute of Pathology in Washington, DC.

Wilhelm Roux (1850–1924) pioneered analytic experimental studies on the physiology of development in amphibia, which was pursued further by **Hans Spemann** (1869–1941). For his discovery of the phenomenon of primary induction—how one tissue determines the fate of another—Spemann received the Nobel Prize in 1935. Over the decades, scientists have been isolating the substances that are transmitted from one tissue to another, causing induction.

Robert G. Edwards (1925–2013) and **Patrick Steptoe** (1913–88) pioneered one of the most revolutionary developments in the history of human reproduction: the technique of **in vitro fertilization**. These studies resulted in the birth of Louise Brown, the first "test tube baby," in 1978. Since then, many millions of couples throughout the world, who were considered infertile, have experienced the birth of their children because of this new reproductive technology. Edwards was awarded the 2010 Nobel Prize in Physiology and Medicine for the development of in vitro fertilization.

John Gurdon (1933–) and **Shinya Yamanaka** (1962–) were awarded the 2012 Nobel Prize in Physiology and Medicine for the discovery that mature cells can be reprogrammed to become pluripotent. Gurdon and Yamanaka showed that the genome can be conserved during differentiation and can be reprogrammed to an immature stage. Their discovery led to a better understanding of development and paved the way for therapeutic cloning and the use of stem cells in treating specific clinical conditions.

GENETICS AND HUMAN DEVELOPMENT

In 1859 **Charles Darwin** (1809–82), an English biologist and evolutionist, published his book *On the Origin of Species*, in which he emphasized the hereditary nature of variability among members of a species as an important factor in evolution. **Gregor Mendel**, an Austrian monk, developed the principles of heredity in 1865, but medical scientists and biologists did not understand the significance of these principles in the study of mammalian development for many years.

Walter Flemming observed chromosomes in 1878 and suggested their probable role in fertilization. In 1883 **Edouard van Beneden** observed that mature germ cells have a reduced number of chromosomes. He also described some features of meiosis, the process whereby the chromosome number is reduced in germ cells.

Walter Sutton (1877–1916) and **Theodor Boveri** (1862–1915) declared independently in 1902 that the behavior of chromosomes during germ cell formation and fertilization agreed with Mendel's principles of inheritance. In the same year, **Sir Archibald Garrod** (1857–1936) reported alcaptonuria (a genetic disorder of phenylalanine-tyrosine metabolism) as the first example of mendelian inheritance in human beings. Many geneticists consider Garrod the "father of medical genetics." It was soon realized that the zygote contains all the genetic information necessary for directing the development of a new human being.

Felix von Winiwarter reported the first observations on human chromosomes in 1912, stating that there were 47 chromosomes in body cells. **Theophilus Shickel Painter** concluded in 1923 that 48 was the number, a conclusion that was widely accepted until 1956, when **Joe Hin Tjio** and **Albert Levan** correctly reported finding only 46 chromosomes in embryonic cells.

James Watson and **Francis Crick** deciphered the molecular structure of DNA in 1953, and in 2021 the human genome was finally completely sequenced and officially published in 2022. The biochemical nature of the genes on the 46 human chromosomes has been decoded. Chromosome studies were soon used in medicine in several ways, including clinical diagnosis, chromosome mapping, and prenatal diagnosis.

Once the normal chromosomal pattern was firmly established, it soon became evident that some people with congenital birth defects had an abnormal number of chromosomes. A new era in medical genetics resulted from the demonstration by **Jérôme Jean Louis Marie Lejeune** and associates in 1959 that infants with **Down syndrome (trisomy 21)** have 47 chromosomes instead of the usual 46 in their body cells. It is now known that chromosomal aberrations are a significant cause of birth defects and embryonic death (see Chapter 20).

In 1941 **Sir Norman Gregg** reported an "unusual number of cases of cataracts" and other birth defects in infants whose mothers had contracted rubella in early pregnancy. For the first time, concrete evidence was presented showing that the development of the human embryo could be adversely affected by an environmental factor (**rubella virus**). Twenty years later **Widukind Lenz** and **William McBride** reported rare limb deficiencies and other severe birth defects, induced by the sedative **thalidomide**, in the infants of mothers who had ingested the drug. The **thalidomide tragedy** alerted the public and health-care providers to the potential hazards of drugs, chemicals, and other environmental factors during pregnancy (see Chapter 20).

Sex chromatin was discovered in 1949 by **Dr. Murray Barr** and his graduate student **Ewart (Mike) Bertram**. Their research revealed that the nuclei of nerve cells in female cats had sex chromatin and that male cats did not. The next step was to determine whether a similar phenomenon existed in human neurons. **Keith L. Moore**, who joined Dr. Barr's research group in 1950, discovered that sex chromatin patterns existed in the somatic cells of humans and many representatives of the animal kingdom. He also developed a **buccal smear sex chromatin test**.

MOLECULAR BIOLOGY OF HUMAN DEVELOPMENT

Rapid advances in molecular biology have led to the application of sophisticated techniques (e.g., recombinant DNA technology, genomic sequencing, RNA genomic hybridization, chimeric models, transgenic mice, stem cell manipulation, and gene therapy). These techniques are now widely used in research laboratories to address such diverse problems as the genetic regulation of morphogenesis, the temporal and regional expression of specific genes, and how cells are committed to form the various parts of the embryo. We continue to expand our understanding of how, when, and where selected genes are activated and expressed in the embryo during normal and abnormal development (see Chapter 21).

The first mammal, a sheep named **Dolly**, was cloned in 1997 by **Ian Wilmut** and his colleagues using the technique of somatic cell nuclear transfer. Since then, other animals have been successfully cloned from cultured differentiated adult cells. Interest in human cloning has generated considerable debate because of its social, ethical, and legal implications. Moreover, there is concern that cloning may result in neonates with birth defects and serious diseases.

Human embryonic stem cells are pluripotential, capable of self-renewal, and able to differentiate into specialized cell types, including artificial gametes. The isolation and reprogrammed culture of human embryonic stem cells hold great potential for the treatment of chronic diseases, including spinal cord injuries, age-related macular degeneration, amyotrophic lateral sclerosis, Alzheimer disease, and Parkinson disease, as well as other degenerative, malignant, and genetic disorders (see the National Institutes of Health web page "NIH Stem Cell Information" [2022] and the International Society for Stem Cell Research [ISSCR] Guidelines for Stem Cell Research and Clinical Translation: 2021 update).

Culturing human stem cells is an invaluable tool in biomedical research. This technology was used to produce small 3D structures from human pluripotent and tissue stem cells (synthetic embryology). The resulting 3D models of human organoids are now used for investigating fundamental developmental processes and diseases (see Chapter 21).

DESCRIPTIVE TERMS IN EMBRYOLOGY

In anatomy and embryology, several terms relating to position and direction are used, and reference is made to various planes of the body. All descriptions of the adult are based on the assumption that the body is erect, with the upper limbs by the sides and the palms directed anteriorly (Fig. 1.5A). This is the **anatomical position**.

The terms **anterior** or **ventral** and **posterior** or **dorsal** are used to describe the front or back, respectively, of the body or limbs and the relations of structures within the body to one another. When describing embryos, the terms ventral and dorsal are used (see Fig. 1.5B). Superior and inferior are used to indicate the relative levels of different structures (see Fig. 1.5A). For embryos, the terms **cranial** (or **rostral**) and **caudal** are used to denote relationships to the head and caudal eminence, respectively (see Fig. 1.5B). Distances from the center of the body or the source or attachment of a structure are designated as **proximal** (nearest) or **distal** (farthest). In the lower limb, for example, the knee is proximal to the ankle and distal to the hip.

The **median plane** is an imaginary vertical plane of section that passes longitudinally through the body. Median sections divide the body into right and left halves (see Fig. 1.5C). The terms **lateral** and **medial** refer to structures that are, respectively, farther from or nearer to the median plane of the body. A **sagittal plane** is any vertical plane passing through the body that is parallel to the median plane (see Fig. 1.5C). A **frontal (coronal) plane** is any vertical plane that intersects the median plane at a right angle (see Fig. 1.5E) and divides the body into anterior or ventral and posterior or dorsal parts. A **transverse (axial) plane** refers to any plane that is at right angles to both the median and coronal planes (see Fig. 1.5D).

CLINICALLY ORIENTED PROBLEMS

1. What sequence of events occurs during puberty? Are the events the same for males and females? At what age does presumptive puberty occur in males and females?
2. How do the terms *embryology* and *teratology* differ?
3. What is the difference between the terms *egg*, *ovum*, *ovule*, *gamete*, and *oocyte*?

Discussion of these problems appears in the Appendix at the back of the book.

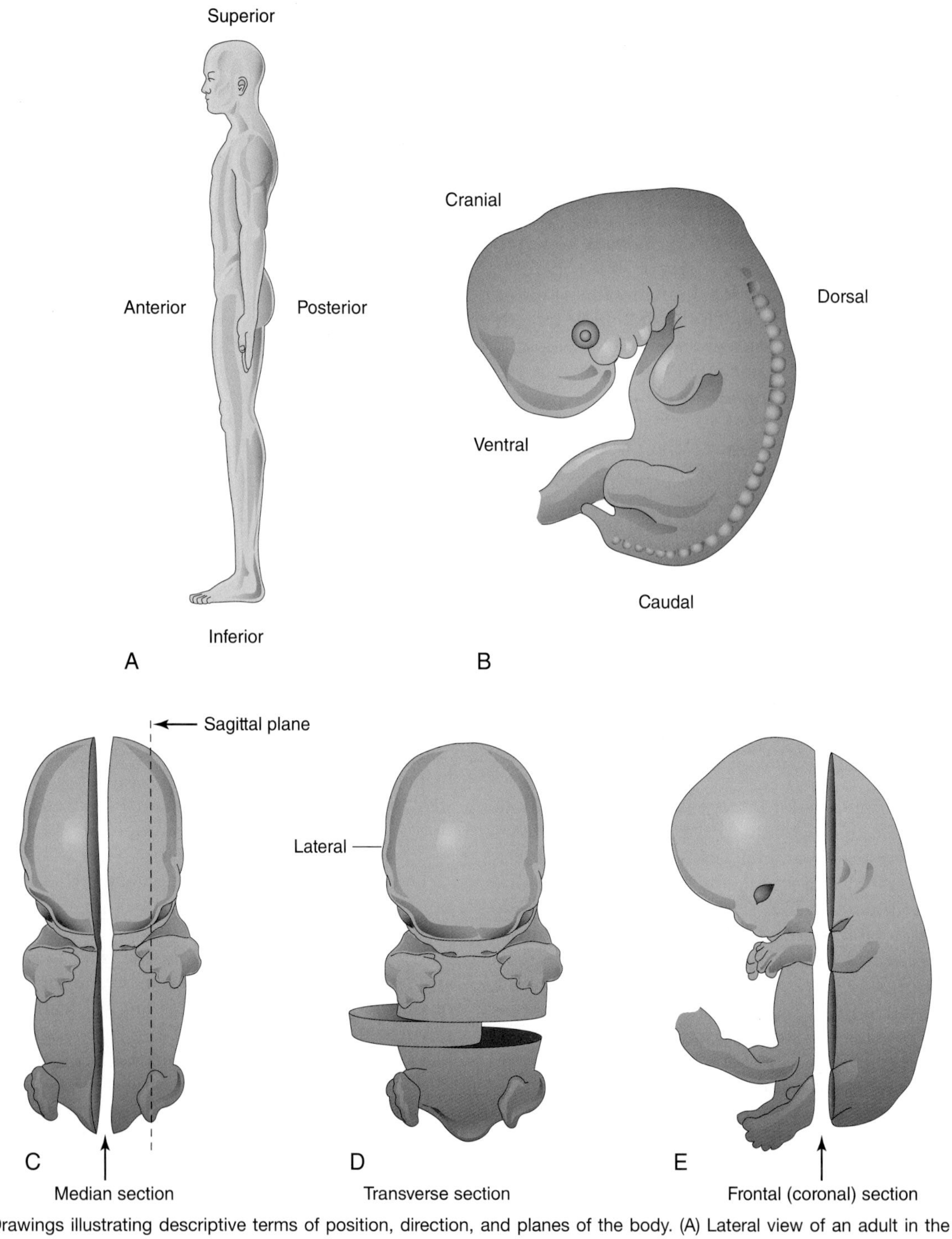

Fig. 1.5 Drawings illustrating descriptive terms of position, direction, and planes of the body. (A) Lateral view of an adult in the anatomical position. (B) Lateral view of a 5-week embryo. (C and D) Ventral views of a 6-week embryo. (E) Lateral view of a 7-week embryo. In describing development, it is necessary to use words denoting the position of one part to another or to the body as a whole. For example, the vertebral column (spine) develops in the dorsal part of the embryo, and the sternum (breastbone) develops in the ventral part of the embryo.

BIBLIOGRAPHY AND SUGGESTED READING

Allen GE: Inducers and "organizers": Hans Spemann and experimental embryology, *Hist Philos Life Sci* 15:229, 1993.

Astarăstoae V., Ioan B.G., Rogozea L.M. et al: Advances in genetic editing of the human embryo. *Am J Ther*, 30, (2), 2023, e126–e133. https://doi.org/10.1097/MJT.0000000000001604.

Bao M, Cornwall-Scoones J, Zernicka-Goetz M: Stem-cell-based human and mouse embryo models, *Cur Opin Gen Dev* 76:101970, 2022.

Churchill FB: The rise of classical descriptive embryology, *Dev Biol (N Y)* 7:1, 1991.

Corsini NS, Knoblich JA: Human organoids: new strategies and methods for analyzing human development and disease, *Cell* 185:2756, 2022.

Craft AM, Johnson M: From stem cells to human development: a distinctly human perspective on early embryology, cellular differentiation and translational research, *Development* 144:12, 2017.

Dunstan GR, editor: *The human embryo: Aristotle and the Arabic and European traditions*, Exeter, UK, 1990, University of Exeter Press.

Gasser R: *Atlas of human embryos*, Hagerstown, MD, 1975, Harper & Row.

Horder TJ, Witkowski JA, Wylie CC, editors: *A history of embryology,* Cambridge, UK, 1986, Cambridge University Press.
Kohl F, von Baer KE: 1792–1876. Zum 200. Geburtstag des "Vaters der Embryologie", *Dtsch Med Wochenschr* 117:1976, 1992.
Lovell-Badge R, Anthony E, Barker RA, et al: ISSCR guidelines for stem cell research and clinical translation: the 2021 update, *Stem Cell Rep* 16(6):1398–1408, 2021. https:/doi.org/10.1016/j stemcr.2021.05.012
Meyer AW: *The rise of embryology,* Stanford, CA, 1939, Stanford University Press.
Moore KL, Persaud TVN, Shiota K: *Color atlas of clinical embryology,* ed 2, Philadelphia, PA, 2000, Saunders.
Neaves W: The status of the human embryo in various religions, *Development* 144:2541, 2017.
Needham J: *A history of embryology,* ed 2, Cambridge, UK, 1959, Cambridge University Press.
Nurk S, Koren S, Rhie A, et al: The complete sequence of a human genome, *Science* 37(6):44–53, 2022.
Nusslein-Volhard C: *Coming to life: how genes drive development,* Carlsbad, CA, 2006, Kales Press.
O'Rahilly R: One hundred years of human embryology. In Kalter H, editor: *Issues and reviews in teratology,* vol 4, New York, 1988, Plenum Press.
O'Rahilly R, Müller F: *Developmental stages in human embryos,* Washington, DC, 1987, Carnegie Institution of Washington.
Pedroza M., Gassaloglu S.I., Dias N. et al: Self-patterning of human stem cells into post-implantation lineages. *Nature* 622(7983), 574–583, 2023. https://doi.org/10.1038/s41586-023-06354-4.
Persaud TVN, Tubbs RS, Loukas M: *A history of human anatomy,* ed 2, Springfield, IL, 2014, Charles C. Thomas.
Pinto-Correia C: *The ovary of Eve: egg and sperm and preformation,* Chicago, IL, 1997, University of Chicago Press.
Rossant J: Why study human embryo development? *Dev Biol* 509:43–50, 2024. https://doi.org/10.1016/j.ydbio.2024.02.001.
Richardson MK, Keuck G: The revolutionary developmental biology of Wilhelm His, *Sr. Biol Rev Camb Philos Soc* 97:1131–1160, 2022.
Rugg-Gunn PJ, Moris N, Tam PPL: Technical challenges of studying early human development, *Development* 150(11):dev201797, 2023. https://doi.org/10.1242/dev.201797 Epub 2023 Jun 1. PMID: 37260362.10163788
Stern CD: Reflections on the past, present and future of developmental biology, *Dev Biol* 488:30–34, 2022.
Streeter GL: Developmental horizons in human embryos: description of age group XI, 13 to 20 somites, and age group XII, 21 to 29 somites, *Contrib Embryol Carnegie Inst* 30:211, 1942.
Tang X-Y, Wu S, Wang D, et al: Human organoids in basic research and clinical applications, *Signal Transduct Target Ther* 7(1):168, 2022. https://doi.org/10.1038/s41398/s41392-022-01024-9
Van Winkle LJ: Molecular and Clinical Advances in Understanding Early Embryo Development. *Cells* 12(8),1171, 2023. https://doi.org/10.3390/cells12081171.

First Week of Human Development

2

CHAPTER OUTLINE

He who sees things grow from the beginning will have the finest view of them.
—ARISTOTLE, 384–322 BCE

Human development begins at fertilization when a sperm fuses with an oocyte to form a single cell, the **zygote**. This highly specialized *totipotent cell* (capable of giving rise to any cell type) marks the beginning of each of us as a unique individual. The zygote, just visible to the unaided eye, contains chromosomes and genes that are derived from the mother and father. The zygote divides many times and becomes progressively transformed into a multicellular human being through cell division, migration, growth, and differentiation.

GAMETOGENESIS

Gametogenesis is the process of formation and development of specialized generative cells, **gametes** (oocytes/sperms), from bipotential **primordial germ cells**. This development, involving the **chromosomes** and **cytoplasm** of the gametes, prepares these sex cells for fertilization. During **gametogenesis**, the chromosome number is reduced by half (haploid) during meiosis, and the shape of the cells is altered (Fig. 2.1). A chromosome is defined by the presence of a **centromere**, the constricted portion of a chromosome. Before DNA replication in the S phase of the cell cycle, chromosomes exist as single-chromatid chromosomes (Fig. 2.2). A **chromatid** (one of a pair of chromosome strands) consists of parallel DNA strands. After DNA replication, chromosomes are double-chromatid chromosomes.

MEIOSIS

Meiosis is a special type of cell division that occurs only during gametogenesis and involves two meiotic cell divisions (see Fig. 2.2); diploid germ cells give rise to **haploid** gametes (sperms and oocytes).

The **first meiotic division** is a reduction division because the chromosome number is reduced from diploid to haploid by pairing of homologous chromosomes in **prophase** (first stage of meiosis) and their segregation at **anaphase** (the stage when the chromosomes move from the equatorial plate). Homologous chromosomes, or **homologs** (one from each parent), pair during prophase and separate during anaphase, with one representative of each pair randomly going to each pole of the meiotic spindle (see Fig. 2.2A–D). The spindle connects to the chromosome at the centromere

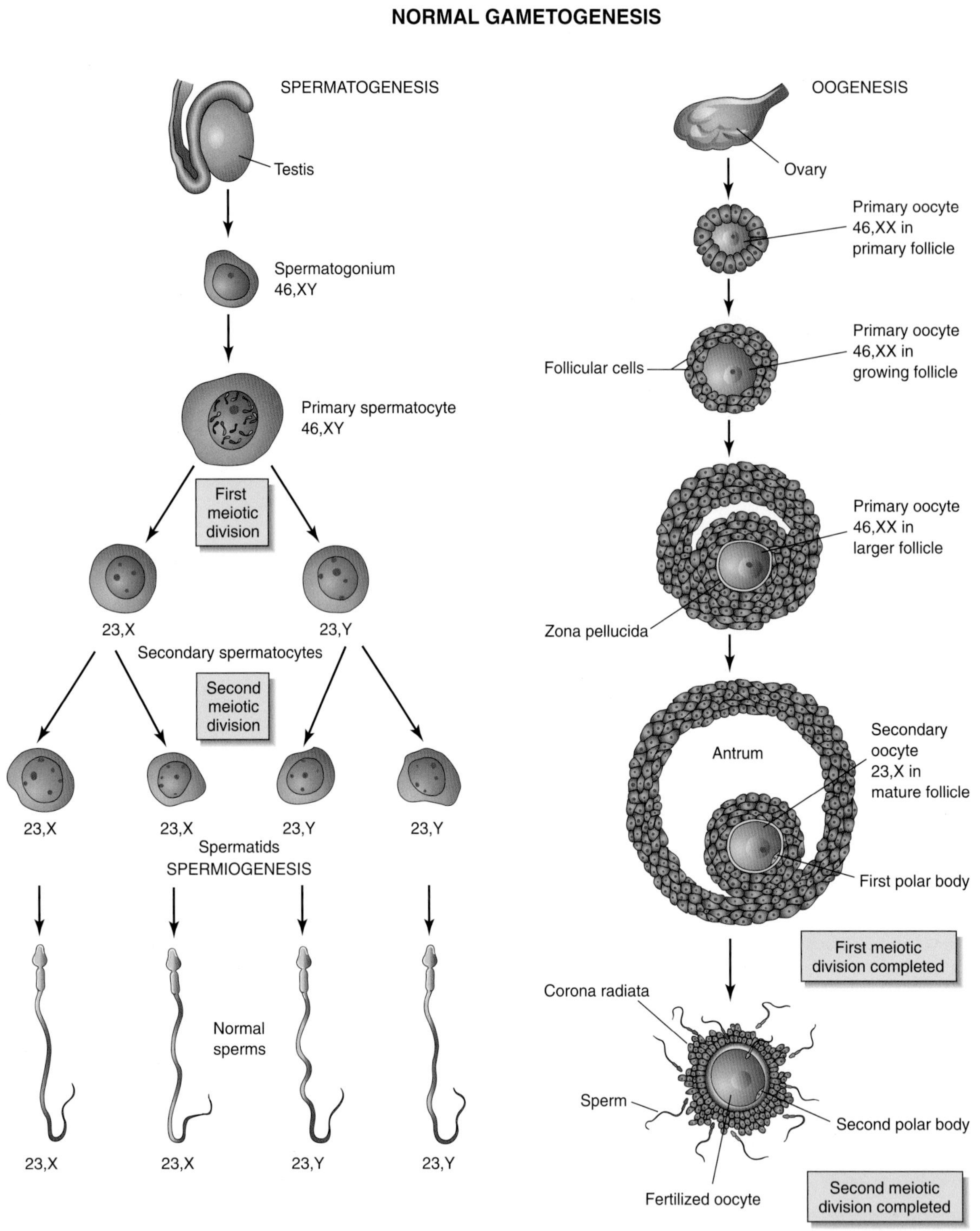

Fig. 2.1 Simplified diagram demonstrating normal gametogenesis: conversion of germ cells into gametes (sex cells). The drawings compare spermatogenesis and oogenesis. Oogonia are not shown in this figure because they differentiate into primary oocytes before birth. The chromosome complement of the germ cells is shown at each stage. The number designates the total number of chromosomes, including the sex chromosome(s) shown after the comma. ***Notes:*** *(1) Following the two meiotic divisions, the diploid number of chromosomes, 46, is reduced to the haploid number, 23. (2) Four sperms form from one primary spermatocyte, whereas only one mature oocyte results from maturation of a primary oocyte. (3) The cytoplasm is conserved during oogenesis to form one large cell, the mature oocyte (see Fig. 2.5C). The polar bodies are small nonfunctional cells that eventually degenerate.*

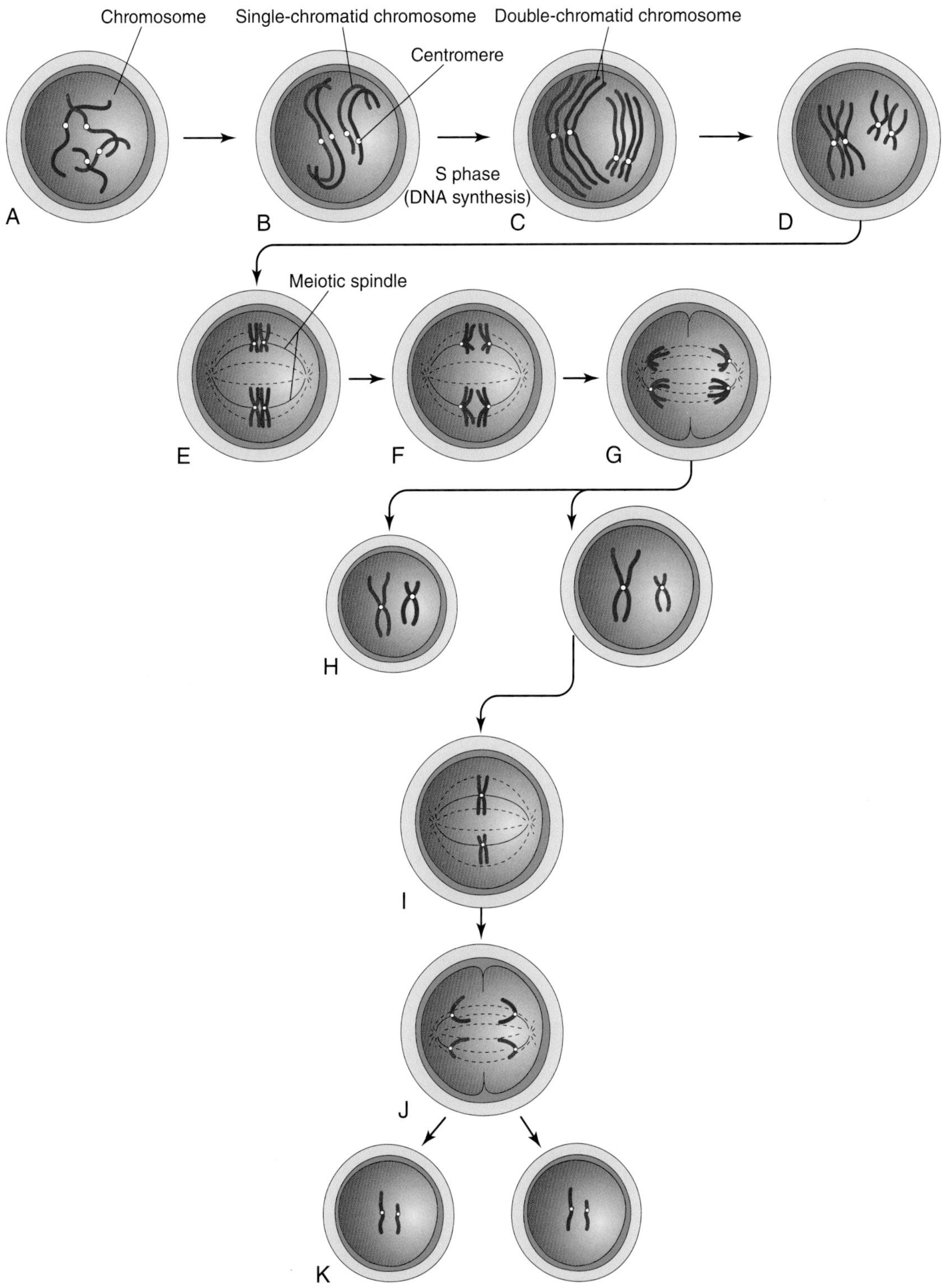

Fig. 2.2 Diagrammatic representation of meiosis. Two chromosome pairs are shown. (A–D) Stages of prophase of the first meiotic division. The homologous chromosomes approach each other and pair; each member of the pair consists of two chromatids. Observe the single crossover in one pair of chromosomes, resulting in the interchange of chromatid segments. (E) Metaphase. The two members of each pair become oriented on the meiotic spindle. (F) Anaphase. (G) Telophase. The chromosomes migrate to opposite poles. (H) Distribution of parental chromosome pairs at the end of the first meiotic division. (I–K) Second meiotic division. It is similar to mitosis, except that the cells are haploid.

(the constricted part of the chromosome) (see Fig. 2.2B). At this stage, they are double-chromatid chromosomes.

The X and Y chromosomes are not homologs, but they have homologous segments at the tips of their short arms. They pair in these regions only. By the end of the first meiotic division, each new cell formed **(secondary oocyte or spermatocyte)** has the haploid chromosome number. This separation or disjunction of paired homologous chromosomes is the physical basis of segregation, the separation of **allelic genes** (occupy the same locus on a specific chromosome) during meiosis.

The **second meiotic division** (see Fig. 2.1) follows the first division without a normal interphase (i.e., without an intervening step of DNA replication). Each double-chromatid chromosome divides, and each half, or chromatid, is drawn to a different pole. Thus the haploid number of chromosomes (23) is retained, and each daughter cell formed by meiosis has one representative of each chromosome pair (now a single-chromatid chromosome). The second meiotic division is similar to an ordinary mitosis except that the chromosome number of the cell entering the second meiotic division is haploid.

Meiosis:

- Provides constancy of the chromosome number from generation to generation by reducing the chromosome number from diploid to haploid, thereby producing haploid gametes
- Allows random assortment of maternal and paternal chromosomes between the gametes
- Relocates segments of maternal and paternal chromosomes by crossing over chromosome segments, which "shuffles" the genes and produces a recombination of genetic material

Abnormal Gametogenesis

Disturbances of meiosis during gametogenesis, such as nondisjunction (Fig. 2.3), result in the formation of chromosomally abnormal gametes. If involved in fertilization, these gametes with numeric chromosome abnormalities cause abnormal development, as occurs in infants with trisomy 21 (Down syndrome, see Chapter 21).

SPERMATOGENESIS

Spermatogenesis (a summary is presented here) is the sequence of events by which **spermatogonia** (primordial germ cells) are transformed into mature sperms; this maturation process begins at puberty and is regulated by testosterone signaling through androgen receptors in the Sertoli cells (see Fig. 2.1). Spermatogonia are dormant in the seminiferous tubules of the testes during the fetal and postnatal periods (see Fig. 2.12). They increase in number during puberty. After several **mitotic** divisions, the spermatogonia grow and undergo changes.

Spermatogonia are transformed into **primary spermatocytes**, the largest germ cells in the seminiferous tubules of the testes (see Fig. 2.1). Each primary spermatocyte subsequently undergoes a reduction division—the first meiotic division—to form two haploid **secondary spermatocytes**, which are approximately half the size of primary spermatocytes. Subsequently, the secondary spermatocytes undergo a second meiotic division to form four haploid **spermatids**, which are approximately half the size of secondary spermatocytes (see Fig. 2.1). The spermatids are gradually transformed into four **mature sperms** by a process known as **spermiogenesis** (Fig. 2.4). The entire process, which includes spermiogenesis, takes approximately 2 months. *MicroRNAs in the germ cells and androgens trigger the signals for the differentiation of spermatogonia. Moreover, several regulatory proteins and signaling pathways, including mTORCH1/rpS6 and p-FAK-Y407, are involved in the transformation.* When spermiogenesis is complete, the sperms enter the lumina of the **seminiferous tubules** (see Fig. 2.12).

Sertoli cells lining the seminiferous tubules support and nurture the developing male germ cells and are involved in the regulation of spermatogenesis. Testosterone produced by the Leydig (interstitial) cells is an essential factor that promotes spermatogenesis. Sperms are transported passively from the seminiferous tubules to the epididymis, where they are stored and become functionally mature during puberty. The **epididymis** is an elongated coiled duct (see Fig. 2.12) and is continuous with the **ductus deferens** which transports sperms to the urethra (see Fig. 2.12).

Mature sperms are free-swimming, actively motile cells consisting of a **head** and a **tail** (Fig. 2.5A). The head of the sperm forms most of the bulk of the sperm and contains the nucleus. The anterior two-thirds of the head is covered by the **acrosome**, a cap-like saccular organelle containing several enzymes (see Figs. 2.4 and 2.5A). When released, the enzymes facilitate the dispersion of follicular cells of the **corona radiata** and sperm penetration of the **zona pellucida** during fertilization (see Fig. 2.5C).

The tail of the sperm consists of three segments: Fig. 2.5A *middle piece* **middle piece, principal piece**, and **end piece** (see Fig. 2.5A). The tail provides the motility of the sperm, which assists its transport to the site of fertilization. The middle piece contains **mitochondria**, which provides **adenosine triphosphate** (ATP), necessary to support the energy required for motility.

Many genes, mitochondrial fusion proteins, such as MFN2, nuage-associated proteins, and molecular factors (microRNAs) are essential in the regulation of spermatogenesis. For example, recent studies indicate that retinoic acid and proteins of the Bcl-2 family are involved in the maturation of germ cells, as well as their survival at different stages. At the molecular level, HOX genes influence microtubule dynamics, shaping of the head of the sperm, and formation of the tail. For normal spermatogenesis, the Y chromosome is essential; microdeletions result in defective spermatogenesis and infertility.

OOGENESIS

Oogenesis is the sequence of events by which **oogonia** (primordial germ cells) are transformed into mature oocytes. Oogenesis continues until **menopause**, which is the permanent cessation of the menstrual cycle (see Figs. 2.7 and 2.11).

PRENATAL MATURATION OF OOCYTES

During early fetal life, oogonia proliferate by **mitosis**. Oogonia enlarge to form **primary oocytes** only before birth; for this reason, no oogonia are shown in Figs. 2.1 and 2.3. As the oocytes form, connective tissue cells surround them and

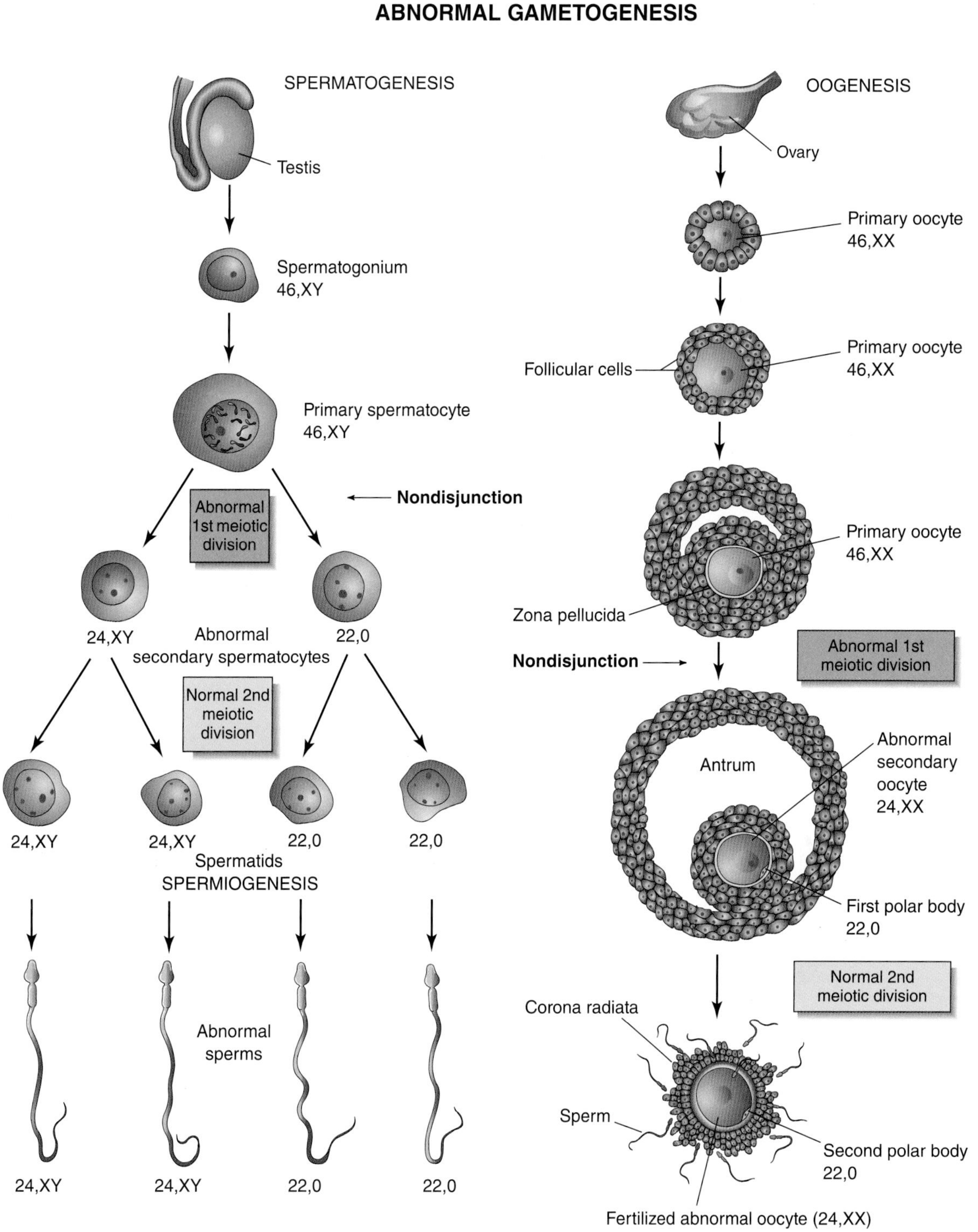

Fig. 2.3 Abnormal gametogenesis. The drawings show how nondisjunction (failure of one or more pairs of chromosomes to separate at the meiotic stage) results in an abnormal chromosome distribution in gametes. Although nondisjunction of sex chromosomes is illustrated, a similar defect may occur in autosomes (any chromosomes other than sex chromosomes). When nondisjunction occurs during the first meiotic division of spermatogenesis, one secondary spermatocyte contains 22 autosomes plus an X and a Y chromosome, and the other one contains 22 autosomes and no sex chromosome. Similarly, nondisjunction during oogenesis may give rise to an oocyte with 22 autosomes and 2 X chromosomes (as shown), or it may result in one with 22 autosomes and no sex chromosome.

form a single layer of flattened, **follicular cells** (see Fig. 2.8). As the primary oocyte enlarges during puberty, the follicular epithelial cells become cuboidal in shape and then columnar, forming a **primary follicle** (see Figs. 2.1 and 2.9A).

The primary oocyte is surrounded by an extracellular matrix, the **zona pellucida** (see Figs. 2.8 and 2.9B), comprised of three glycoproteins (ZPA, ZPB, and ZPC). Scanning electron microscopy of the surface of the zona pellucida reveals

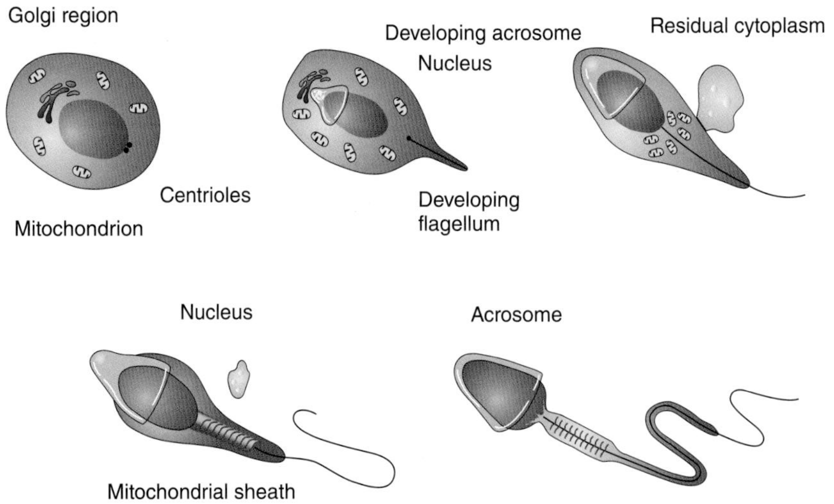

Fig. 2.4 Illustrations of spermiogenesis, the last phase of spermatogenesis. During this process, the rounded spermatid is transformed into an elongated sperm. Note the loss of cytoplasm (see Fig. 2.5C), development of the tail, and formation of the acrosome. The acrosome, derived from the Golgi region (first drawing) of the spermatid, contains enzymes that are released at the beginning of fertilization to assist the sperm in penetrating the corona radiata and zona pellucida surrounding the secondary oocyte.

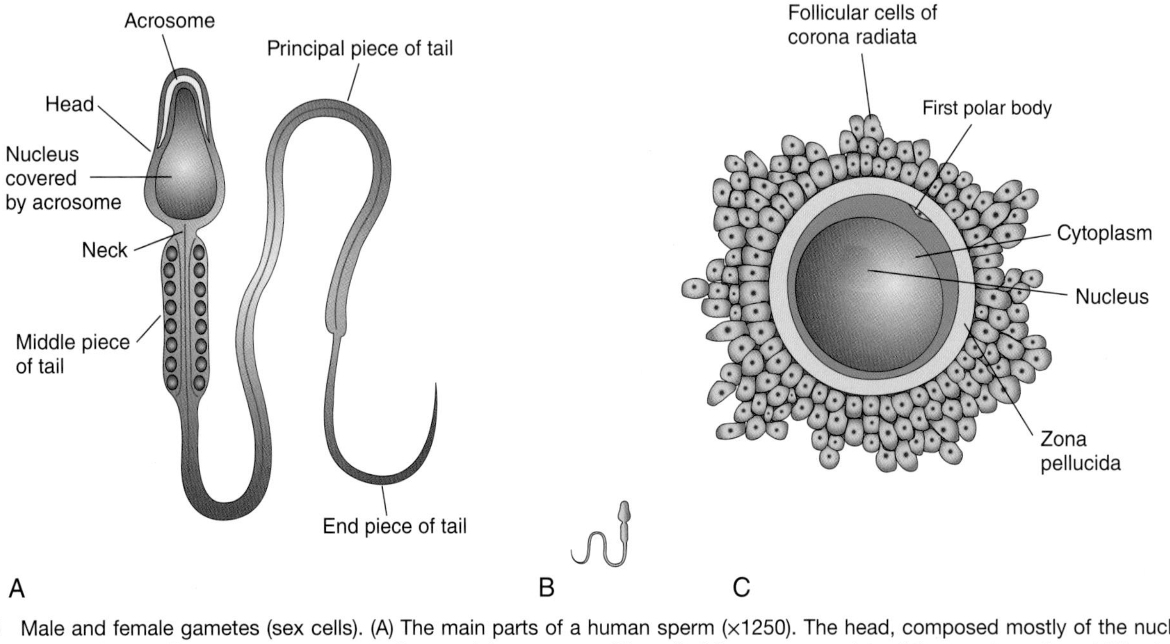

Fig. 2.5 Male and female gametes (sex cells). (A) The main parts of a human sperm (×1250). The head, composed mostly of the nucleus, is partly covered by the cap-like acrosome, an organelle containing enzymes. The tail of the sperm consists of three regions, the middle piece, the principal piece, and the end piece. (B) A sperm drawn to approximately the same scale as the oocyte. (C) A human secondary oocyte (×200), surrounded by the zona pellucida and corona radiata.

a regular mesh-like appearance with intricate fenestrations. Primary oocytes begin the first meiotic divisions before birth (see Fig. 2.3), but completion of **prophase** (see Fig. 2.2A–D) does not occur until puberty. The follicular cells surrounding the primary oocytes secrete **oocyte maturation inhibitor**, which arrests the meiotic process of the oocyte.

POSTNATAL MATURATION OF OOCYTES

Beginning during puberty, one ovarian follicle usually matures each month and **ovulation** (release of oocyte from the ovarian follicle) occurs (see Fig. 2.7), except when hormonal contraceptives are used.

The primary oocytes remain dormant in ovarian follicles until puberty (see Fig. 2.8). As a follicle matures, the primary oocyte increases in size, and shortly before ovulation, the primary oocyte completes the first meiotic division to give rise to a **secondary oocyte** (see Fig. 2.10A and B) and the first polar body. Unlike the corresponding stage of spermatogenesis, however, the division of **cytoplasm** is unequal. The secondary oocyte receives almost all the cytoplasm (see Fig. 2.1), and the **first polar body** receives very little, and this cell is destined for degeneration.

At ovulation, the nucleus of the secondary oocyte begins the second meiotic division but is arrested at metaphase (see Fig. 2.2E). If a sperm penetrates the secondary oocyte, the second meiotic division is completed, and most cytoplasm is again retained by one cell, the fertilized oocyte (see Fig. 2.1). The other cell formed, the **second polar body**, will degenerate. As soon as the polar bodies are extruded, maturation of the oocyte is considered complete.

There are approximately 2 million primary oocytes in the ovaries of a neonate, but most of them regress during childhood so that by adolescence, no more than 40,000 primary oocytes remain. Of these, only approximately 400 become secondary oocytes and are expelled at ovulation during the reproductive period. Very few of these oocytes, if any, are fertilized.

The long duration of the first meiotic division, from puberty to before menopause (up to 45 years) may account in part for the relatively high frequency of **meiotic errors**, such as nondisjunction (failure of paired chromatids of a chromosome to dissociate), that occur with increasing maternal age. The primary oocytes in suspended prophase (dictyotene) are vulnerable to environmental agents such as radiation.

COMPARISON OF GAMETES

Gametes are **haploid** cells that can undergo **karyogamy** (fusion of nuclei of two sex cells). The oocyte is a massive cell compared with the sperm, and it is immotile, whereas the much smaller sperm is highly motile (see Fig. 2.5A). The oocyte is surrounded by the **zona pellucida** and a layer of follicular cells, the **corona radiata** (see Figs. 2.5C and 2.8).

With respect to **sex chromosome constitution**, there are two kinds of sperms, 23,X and 23,Y, whereas there is only one kind of secondary oocyte, 23,X (see Fig. 2.1). By convention, the number 23 is followed by a comma and an X or Y to indicate the sex chromosome constitution; for example, 23,X indicates that there are 23 chromosomes in the complement, consisting of 22 **autosomes** (chromosomes other than sex chromosomes) and 1 sex chromosome (X in this case). The difference in the sex chromosome complement of sperm forms the basis of the primary sex determination of the embryo.

Abnormal Gametes

The ideal biological maternal age for reproduction is from 20 to 35 years. Mothers younger than 20 years are at increased risk of anomalies in their offspring, such as gastroschisis (a defect in the abdominal wall allowing the bowels to develop outside the abdomen), although the reasons for this are not readily apparent. Conversely, the likelihood of chromosomal abnormalities in an embryo gradually increases as the mother ages. In older mothers, there is an appreciable risk of Down syndrome (trisomy 21) or other forms of trisomy in the infant (see Chapter 20). The likelihood of a fresh pathogenic variant (mutation) in a gene (change in DNA) also increases with age. Sperm quality and testicular function decline with age, and advanced paternal age increases pathogenic variants, which can lead to a higher incidence of offspring with severe genetic abnormalities. Therefore the older the parents are at the time of conception, the more likely they are to have accumulated pathogenic variants that the embryo might inherit.

During gametogenesis, homologous chromosomes sometimes fail to separate, a pathogenic process called **nondisjunction**; as a result, some gametes have 24 chromosomes and others only 22 (see Fig. 2.3). If a gamete with 24 chromosomes unites with a normal one with 23 chromosomes during fertilization, a zygote with 47 chromosomes forms (see Fig. 20.2). This condition is called **trisomy** because of the presence of three representatives of a particular chromosome instead of the usual two. If a gamete with only 22 chromosomes unites with a normal one, a zygote with 45 chromosomes forms. This condition is called **monosomy** because only one representative of the particular chromosome pair is present. For a description of the clinical conditions associated with numeric disorders of chromosomes (see Chapter 20).

Having between 4% and 14% sperm with normal morphology in the ejaculate is considered adequate to achieve pregnancy. Typical gross abnormalities include defects of the head (e.g., elongated or double), midpiece (e.g., thin or irregular), and/or tail (e.g., short or double tail). Most morphologically abnormal sperms lack normal motility and are unable to pass through the mucus in the cervical canal. Although some oocytes have two or three nuclei, these cells die before they reach maturity. Similarly, some ovarian follicles contain two or more oocytes, but this phenomenon is rare.

UTERUS, UTERINE TUBES, AND OVARIES

A brief description of the structure of the uterus, uterine tubes, and ovaries is presented for understanding reproductive ovarian cycles and the implantation of blastocysts (Figs. 2.6 and 2.7 and see Fig. 2.20).

UTERUS

The uterus is a thick-walled, pear-shaped muscular organ. It consists of two major parts (see Fig. 2.6A and B): the **body**, the superior two-thirds, and the **cervix**, the inferior one-third.

The **body of the uterus** narrows from the **fundus**, the rounded superior part of the body, to the **isthmus**, the 1-cm-long constricted region between the body and cervix (see Fig. 2.6A). The **cervix** of the uterus is its tapered vaginal end. The lumen of the cervix, the **cervical canal**, has a constricted opening at each end. The **internal os** (opening) of the uterus communicates with the cavity of the uterine body, and the **external os** communicates with the vagina (see Fig. 2.6A and B).

The walls of the body of the uterus consist of three layers (see Fig. 2.6B):

- **Perimetrium**, the thin external peritoneal layer attached to the myometrium
- **Myometrium**, the thick smooth muscle layer
- **Endometrium**, the thin internal layer

During the **luteal (secretory) phase** of the menstrual cycle, three layers of the **endometrium** can be distinguished microscopically (see Fig. 2.6C):

- A thin **compact layer** consisting of densely packed connective tissue containing the necks of the uterine glands
- A thick **spongy layer** composed of edematous connective tissue containing the dilated, tortuous bodies of the uterine glands
- A thin **basal layer** containing the blind ends of the uterine glands

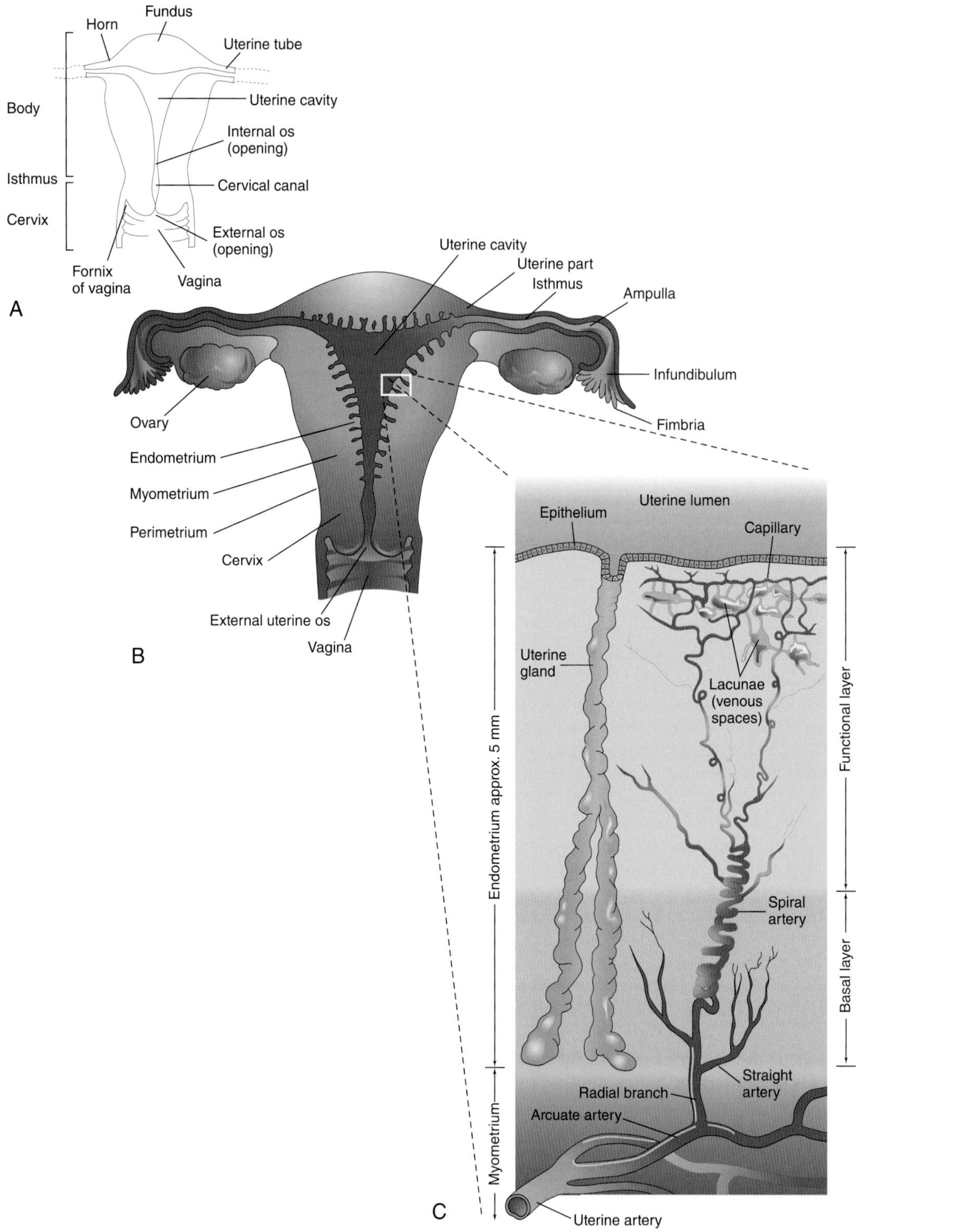

Fig. 2.6 (A) Parts of the uterus and vagina. (B) Diagrammatic frontal section of the uterus, uterine tubes, and vagina. The ovaries are also shown. (C) Enlargement of the area outlined in (B). The functional layer of the endometrium is sloughed off during menstruation.

At the peak of its development, the **endometrium** is 4- to 5-mm thick (see Fig. 2.6B and C). The compact and spongy layers, known collectively as the **functional layer**, disintegrate and are shed during menstruation and after **parturition** (delivery of a fetus). The basal layer of the endometrium has its own blood supply and is not sloughed off during **menstruation** (see Fig. 2.7).

UTERINE TUBES

The **uterine tubes**, approximately 10 cm long and 1 cm in diameter, extend laterally from the horns of the uterus (see Fig. 2.6A and B). Each tube opens at its proximal end into the horn of the uterus and into the peritoneal cavity at its distal end. The uterine tube is divided into four parts:

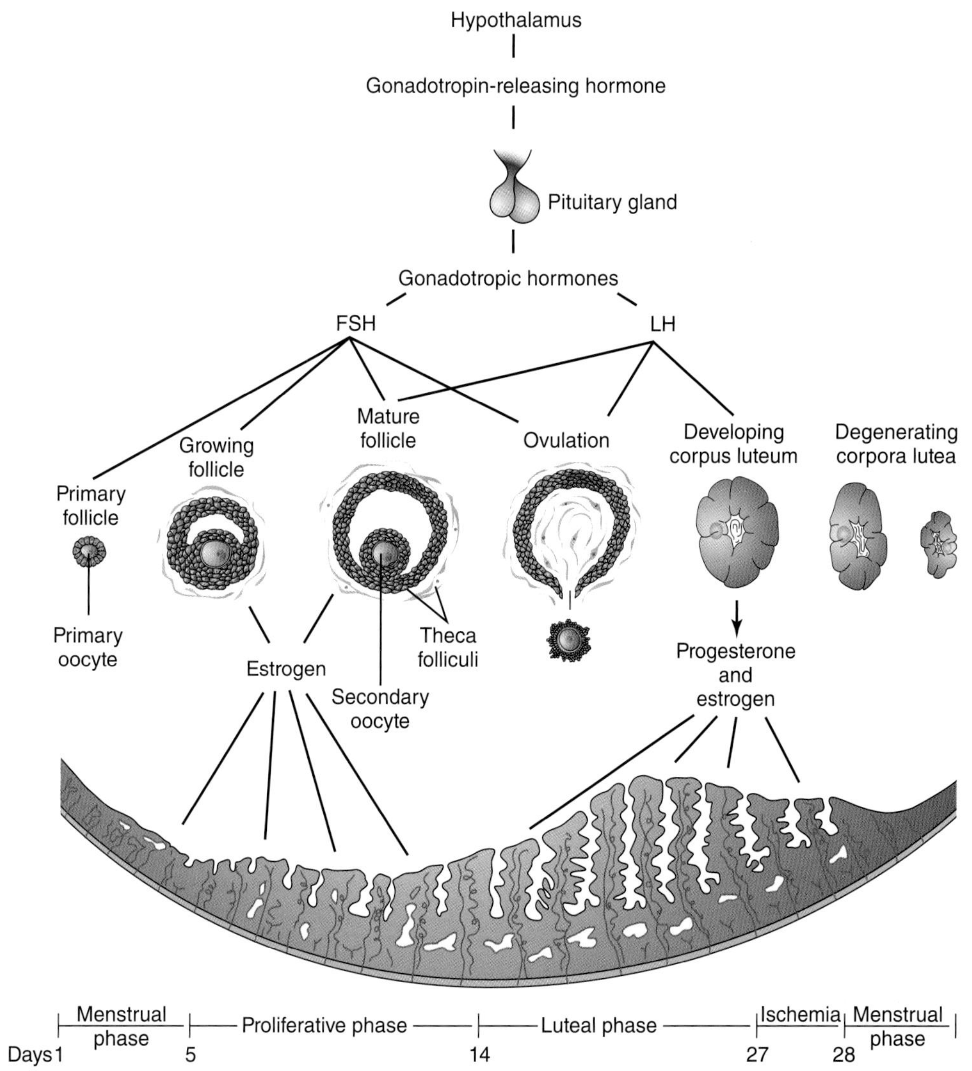

Fig. 2.7 Schematic drawings illustrating the interrelations of the hypothalamus of the brain, pituitary gland, ovaries, and endometrium. One complete menstrual cycle and the beginning of another are shown. Changes in the ovaries, the *ovarian cycle*, are induced by the gonadotropic hormones (*FSH* and *LH*). Hormones from the ovaries (estrogens and progesterone) then promote cyclic changes in the structure and function of the endometrium, the *menstrual cycle*. Thus the cyclic activity of the ovary is intimately linked with changes in the uterus. The ovarian cycles are under the rhythmic endocrine control of the pituitary gland, which in turn is controlled by the gonadotropin-releasing hormone produced by neurosecretory cells in the hypothalamus. *FSH*, Follicle-stimulating hormone; *LH*, luteinizing hormone.

infundibulum, **ampulla**, **isthmus**, and **uterine part** (see Fig. 2.6B). One of the uterine tubes collects and transports an oocyte from one of the ovaries to the fertilization site, the **ampulla** (see Fig. 2.6A). The uterine tube is lined with cilia and, together with muscular contractions by the tube, conveys the cleaving zygote to the uterine cavity.

OVARIES

The **ovaries** are almond shaped and located close to the lateral pelvic walls on each side of the uterus. The ovaries produce oocytes (see Fig. 2.6B) and estrogen and progesterone, the hormones responsible for the development of secondary sex characteristics and regulation of pregnancy.

FEMALE REPRODUCTIVE CYCLES

Commencing at puberty, females undergo menstrual cycles, involving activities of the **hypothalamus** of the brain, pituitary gland, ovaries, uterus, uterine tubes, vagina, and mammary glands (see Fig. 2.7). These monthly cycles prepare the reproductive system for pregnancy.

Gonadotropin-releasing hormone (GnRH) is synthesized by neurosecretory cells in the hypothalamus. GnRH is carried by a capillary network, the **hypothalamic-hypophyseal portal system**, to the anterior lobe of the pituitary gland. The hormone stimulates the release of two hormones produced by the pituitary gland that act on the ovaries:

- **Follicle-stimulating hormone** (FSH) stimulates the development of ovarian follicles and the production of estrogen by the follicular cells.
- **Luteinizing hormone** (LH) serves as the "trigger" for ovulation (release of a secondary oocyte) and stimulates the follicular cells and corpus luteum to produce progesterone.

These two hormones also induce the growth of the ovarian follicles and the endometrium.

1

OVARIAN CYCLE

FSH and LH produce cyclic changes in the ovaries—the **ovarian cycle** (see Fig. 2.7)—development of follicles (Fig. 2.8), **ovulation**, and **corpus luteum formation**. During each cycle, FSH promotes the growth of several primordial follicles into 5 to 12 primary follicles (Fig. 2.9A); however, only one primary follicle usually develops into a **mature follicle** and ruptures through the surface of the ovary, expelling its oocyte (Fig. 2.10). *Early oocyte differentiation and ovarian reserve are regulated by the TATA box–binding protein associated factor 4b (TAF4b) transcription genetic pathways.*

FOLLICULAR DEVELOPMENT

Development of an ovarian follicle (see Figs. 2.8 and 2.9) is characterized by:

- Growth and differentiation of a primary oocyte
- Proliferation of follicular cells
- Formation of the zona pellucida
- Development of the theca folliculi

As the **primary follicle** increases in size, the adjacent connective tissue organizes into a capsule, the **theca folliculi** (see Fig. 2.7). This theca soon differentiates into two layers, an internal vascular and glandular layer, the **theca interna**, and a capsule-like layer, the **theca externa** (Fig. 2.8). The follicular cells divide actively, producing a stratified layer around the oocyte (see Fig. 2.9B). Thecal cells are thought to produce an **angiogenesis factor** that promotes the growth of blood vessels in the theca interna, which provide nutritive support for follicular development. The ovarian follicle soon becomes oval and the oocyte eccentric in position. Subsequently, fluid-filled spaces appear around the follicular cells, which coalesce to form a single large cavity, the **antrum**, which contains**follicular fluid** (see Figs. 2.8 and 2.9B). After the antrum forms, the ovarian follicle is called a vesicular or **secondary follicle**.

The primary oocyte is pushed to one side of the follicle, where it is surrounded by a mound of follicular cells, the **cumulus oophorus**, that projects into the antrum (see Fig. 2.9B). The follicle continues to enlarge until it reaches maturity and produces a swelling (**follicular stigma**) on the surface of the ovary (see Fig. 2.10A).

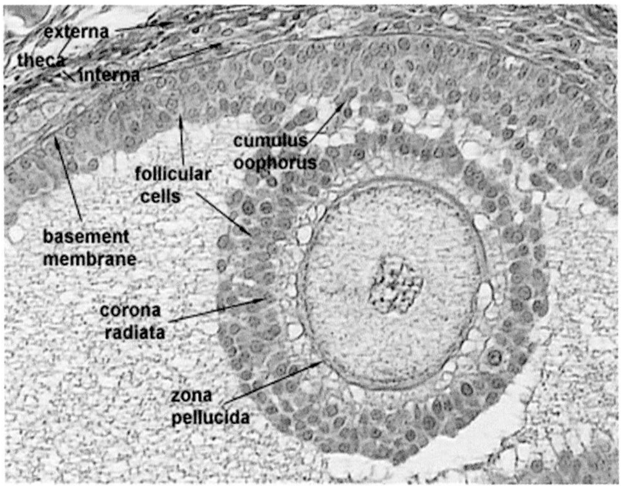

Fig. 2.8 Photomicrograph of a region from a mammalian tertiary follicle showing the oocyte surrounded by follicular (granulosa) cells. The top of the photo shows some cells of the theca.(From Jones RE, Lopez KH: *Human reproductive biology*, ed 4, London, 2014, Elsevier.)

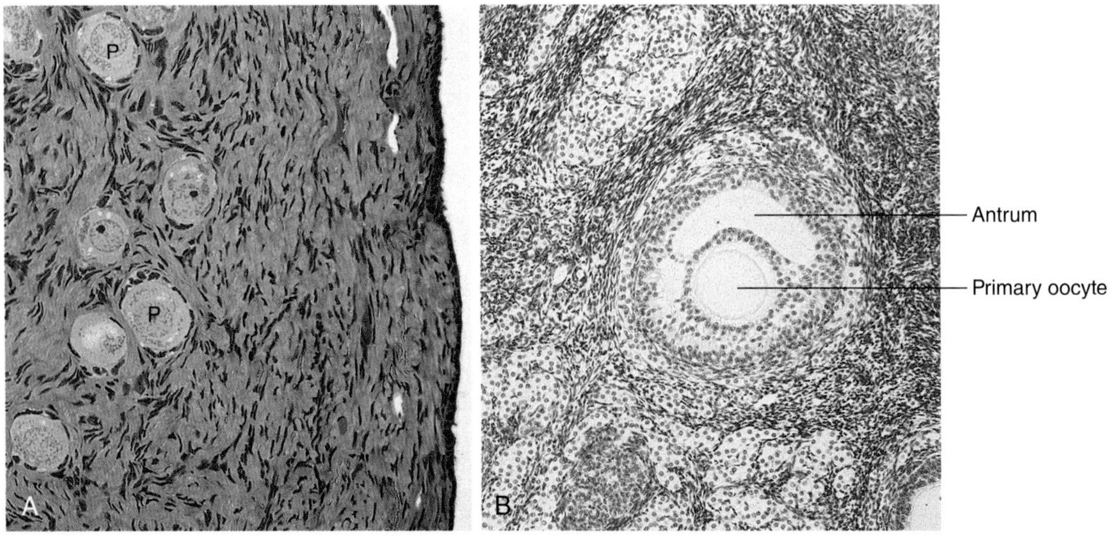

Fig. 2.9 Micrographs of the ovarian cortex. (A) Several primordial follicles *(P)* are visible (×270). Observe that the primary oocytes are surrounded by follicular cells. (B) Secondary ovarian follicle. The oocyte is surrounded by granulosa cells of the cumulus oophorus (×132). The antrum can be clearly seen.(From Gartner LP, Hiatt JL: *Color textbook of histology*, ed 2, Philadelphia, 2001, Saunders.)

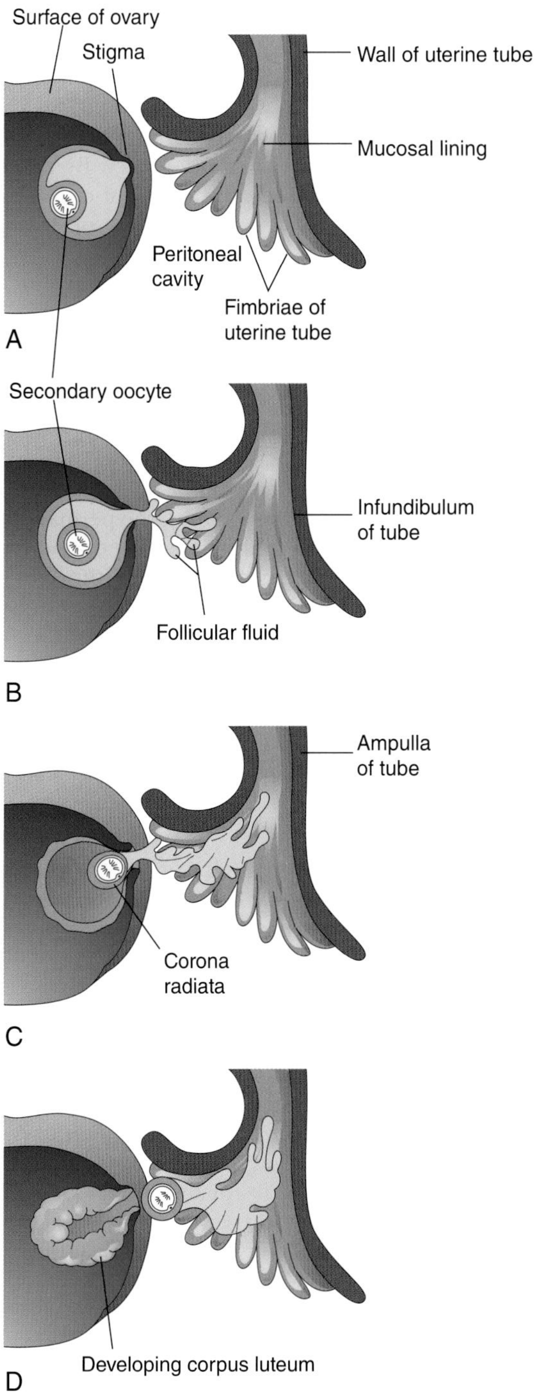

Fig. 2.10 (A–D) Illustrations of ovulation. Note that fimbriae of the infundibulum of the uterine tube are closely applied to the ovary. The finger-like fimbriae move back and forth over the ovary and "sweep" the oocyte into the infundibulum. When the stigma (swelling) ruptures, the secondary oocyte is expelled from the ovarian follicle with the follicular fluid. After ovulation, the wall of the follicle collapses and is thrown into folds. The follicle is transformed into a glandular structure, the corpus luteum.

The early development of ovarian follicles is induced by FSH, but the final stages of maturation require LH as well. Growing follicles produce **estrogen**, a hormone that regulates the development and function of the reproductive organs. The theca interna produces **follicular fluid** and some estrogen (see Fig. 2.10B). Its cells also secrete androgens that pass to the follicular cells (see Fig. 2.8), which, in turn, convert them into estrogen.

OVULATION

Around the middle of the ovarian cycle, the ovarian follicle, under the influence of FSH and LH, undergoes a sudden growth spurt, producing a cystic swelling or bulge on the surface of the ovary. A small avascular spot, the stigma, soon appears on this swelling (see Fig. 2.10A). Before ovulation, the secondary oocyte and some cells of the cumulus oophorus detach from the interior of the distended follicle (see Fig. 2.10B).

Ovulation is triggered by a **surge in LH production** (Fig. 2.11). Ovulation usually follows the LH peak by 24 to 36 hours. The LH surge, elicited by the high estrogen level in the blood, appears to cause the stigma to balloon out, forming a vesicle (see Fig. 2.10A). The stigma soon ruptures, expelling the secondary oocyte with the follicular fluid (see Fig. 2.10B–D). Expulsion of the oocyte is the result of intrafollicular pressure, and possibly by the contraction of smooth muscle in the theca externa (sheath) owing to stimulation by prostaglandins. *Mitogen-activated protein kinases 3 and 1 (MAPK 3/1), also known as extracellular signal–regulated kinases 1 and 2 (ERK1/2), in ovarian follicular cells, seem to regulate signaling pathways that control ovulation. Plasmins and matrix metalloproteins also appear to play a role in controlling the rupture of the follicle.* The expelled secondary oocyte is surrounded by the **zona pellucida** (see Fig. 2.8) and one or more layers of follicular cells, which are radially arranged as the **corona radiata** (see Fig. 2.10C), forming the oocyte-cumulus complex. The LH surge also seems to induce the resumption of the first meiotic division of the primary oocyte. Hence, mature ovarian follicles contain secondary oocytes (see Fig. 2.10A and B). The binding of the sperm to the zona pellucida (sperm-oocyte interactions) is a complex and critical event during fertilization (see Fig. 2.14A and B).

Mittelschmerz and Ovulation

A variable amount of pelvic and lower abdominal pain, **mittelschmerz** (German *mittel*, mid + *schmerz*, pain), accompanies ovulation in some females. Ovulation normally results in slight bleeding into the peritoneal cavity, which may cause pain, as can the enlargement of the oocyte just before ovulation. Mittelschmerz may be used as a secondary indicator of ovulation, but there are better primary indicators, such as elevation of basal body temperature.

Anovulation

Some females do not ovulate (**anovulation**) because of an inadequate release of gonadotropins. Ovulation can be induced by the administration of gonadotropins or an ovulatory agent such as clomiphene citrate. The latter stimulates the release of pituitary gonadotropins (FSH and LH), resulting in the maturation of several ovarian follicles and multiple ovulations. The incidence of multiple pregnancy increases significantly when ovulation is induced.

CORPUS LUTEUM

Shortly after ovulation, the walls of the ovarian follicle and theca folliculi collapse and are thrown into folds (see Fig. 2.10D). Under LH influence, they develop into a glandular structure, the **corpus luteum**, which secretes progesterone and some estrogen, causing the endometrial glands to secrete and prepare the endometrium for implantation of the blastocyst (see Figs. 2.7 and 2.10).

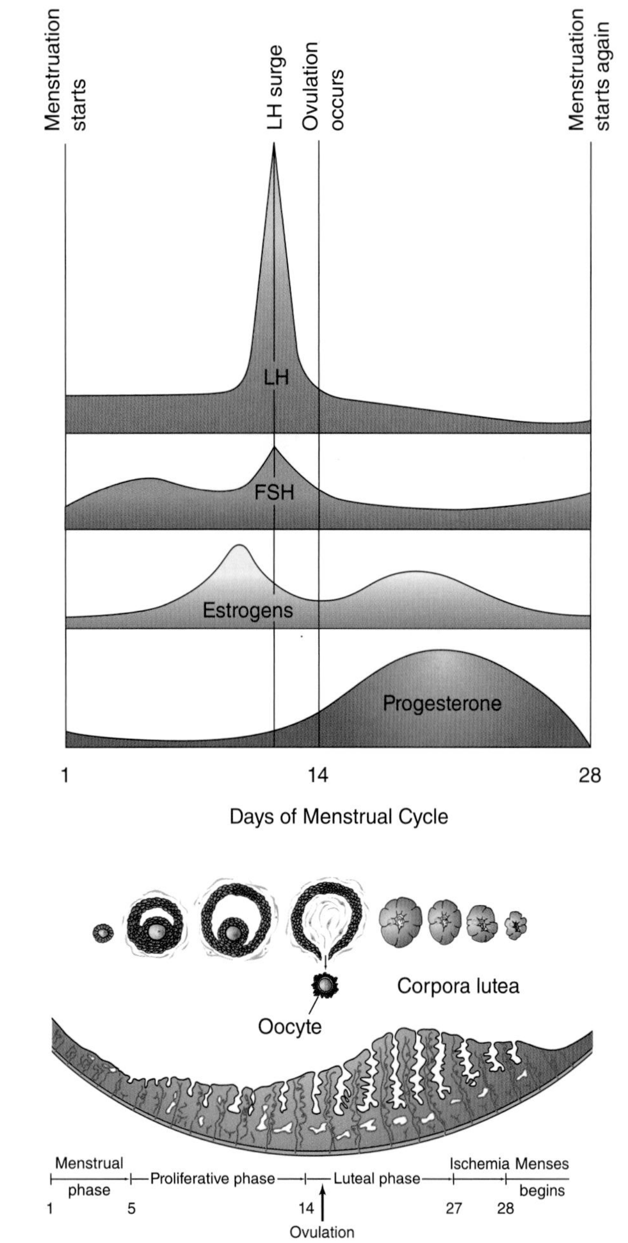

Fig. 2.11 Illustration of the blood levels of various hormones during the menstrual cycle. *FSH* stimulates the ovarian follicles to develop and produce estrogens. The level of estrogen rises to a peak just before the *LH* surge. Ovulation normally occurs 24–36 hours after the LH surge. If fertilization does not occur, the blood levels of circulating estrogens and progesterone fall which causes the endometrium to regress and menstruation to start again. *FSH*, Follicle-stimulating hormone; *LH*, luteinizing hormone.

If the oocyte is fertilized, the corpus luteum enlarges to form a **corpus luteum of pregnancy** and increases its hormone production. Degeneration of the corpus luteum is prevented by **human chorionic gonadotropin** (hCG), a hormone secreted by the syncytiotrophoblast of the blastocyst (see Fig. 2.20B). The corpus luteum of pregnancy remains functionally active throughout the first 20 weeks of pregnancy. By this time, the placenta has assumed the production of estrogen and progesterone necessary for the maintenance of pregnancy (see Chapter 7).

If the oocyte is not fertilized, the corpus luteum involutes and degenerates 10 to 12 days after ovulation (see Fig. 2.7). It is then called **corpus luteum of menstruation**. The corpus luteum is subsequently transformed into white scar tissue in the ovary, called **corpus albicans**.

MENOPAUSE

Ovarian cycles terminate at **menopause**, the permanent cessation of menstruation due to the depletion of oocytes and follicles. Menopause usually occurs between the ages of 48 and 55 years. The endocrine, somatic (body), and psychological changes occurring at the termination of the reproductive period are called the **climacteric**.

MENSTRUAL CYCLE

The **menstrual cycle** is the time during which the oocyte matures, ovulates, and enters the uterine tube. The hormones produced by the ovarian follicles and corpus luteum (estrogen and progesterone) produce continuous cyclic changes in the endometrium (see Fig. 2.11)—the **endometrial cycle**, commonly referred to as the menstrual cycle because menstruation (menses; "period"; flow of blood from the uterus) is an obvious event.

The endometrium is a "mirror" of the ovarian cycle because it responds consistently to the fluctuating concentrations of gonadotropic and ovarian hormones (see Figs. 2.7 and 2.11). The average menstrual cycle is 28 days, with day 1 of the cycle designated as the day on which menstrual flow begins. Menstrual cycles normally vary in length by several days. In 90% of females, the length of the cycles ranges between 23 and 35 days. Almost all these variations result

Anovulatory Menstrual Cycles

The typical menstrual cycle, illustrated in Fig. 2.11, is not always realized because the ovary may not produce a mature follicle, in which case ovulation does not occur. In anovulatory cycles, the endometrial changes are minimal; the proliferative endometrium develops as usual, but ovulation does not occur, and no corpus luteum forms. Consequently, the endometrium does not progress to the luteal phase; it remains in the proliferative phase until menstruation begins. Anovulatory cycles may result from ovarian hypofunction. The estrogen, with or without progesterone, in oral contraceptives, acts on the hypothalamus and pituitary gland, resulting in the inhibition of the secretion of GnRH, FSH, and LH, the secretion of which is essential for ovulation to occur.

from alterations in the duration of the proliferative phase of the menstrual cycle (see Fig. 2.11).

PHASES OF MENSTRUAL CYCLE

MENSTRUAL PHASE

The functional layer of the uterine wall (see Fig. 2.6C) is sloughed off and discarded with the **menses**, which usually lasts for 4 to 5 days. The blood discharged from the vagina is combined with small pieces of endometrial tissue. After menstruation, the eroded endometrium is thin (see Fig. 2.11).

PROLIFERATIVE PHASE

This phase, lasting approximately 9 days, coincides with the growth of ovarian follicles and is controlled by estrogen secreted by the follicles. There is a two- to threefold increase in the thickness of the endometrium and its water content during this phase of repair and proliferation (see Fig. 2.11). Early during this phase, the surface epithelium reforms and covers the endometrium. The uterine glands increase in number and length, and the spiral arteries elongate (see Fig. 2.6).

LUTEAL PHASE

The luteal phase (secretory phase), lasting approximately 13 days, coincides with the formation, functioning, and growth of the corpus luteum. The progesterone produced by the corpus luteum stimulates the uterine glandular epithelium to secrete a glycogen-rich material. The glands become wide, tortuous, and saccular, and the endometrium thickens because of the influence of progesterone and estrogen from the corpus luteum (see Figs. 2.7 and 2.11) and because of increased fluid in the connective tissue. As the **spiral arteries** grow into the superficial compact layer, they become increasingly coiled (see Fig. 2.6C). The venous network becomes complex, and large **lacunae** (venous spaces) develop. Direct arteriovenous anastomoses are prominent features of this stage.

If fertilization occurs:

- Cleavage of the zygote (formation of a blastocyst) begins.
- The blastocyst begins to implant in the endometrium on approximately the sixth day of the luteal phase (see Fig. 2.20A).
- Human chorionic gonadotropin, a hormone produced by the syncytiotrophoblast (see Fig. 2.20B), keeps the corpora lutea secreting estrogens and progesterone.
- The luteal phase continues, and menstruation does not occur.

If fertilization does not occur:

- The corpora lutea degenerate.
- Estrogen and progesterone levels fall, and the secretory endometrium enters an ischemic phase.
- Menstruation occurs (see Fig. 2.7).

ISCHEMIA

Ischemia occurs when the oocyte is not fertilized; spiral arteries constrict (see Fig. 2.6C), giving the endometrium a pale appearance. This results from the decreasing secretion of hormones, primarily progesterone, by the degenerating corpora lutea (see Fig. 2.11). In addition to vascular changes, hormone withdrawal results in the stoppage of glandular secretion, a loss of interstitial fluid, and a marked shrinking of the endometrium. Toward the end of the ischemic phase, the spiral arteries become constricted for longer periods. This results in **venous stasis** (congestion and slowing of circulation in veins) and patchy **ischemic necrosis** in the superficial tissues. Eventually, rupture of damaged vessel walls follows, and blood seeps into the surrounding connective tissue. Small pools of blood form and break through the endometrial surface, resulting in bleeding into the uterine cavity and through the vagina. As small pieces of the endometrium detach and pass into the uterine cavity, the torn ends of the arteries bleed into the cavity, resulting in a loss of 20 to 80 mL of blood. Eventually, over 3 to 5 days, the entire compact layer and most of the spongy layer of the endometrium are discarded in the menses (see Fig. 2.11). Remnants of the spongy and basal layers remain to undergo regeneration during the subsequent proliferative phase of the endometrium.

PREGNANCY

If pregnancy occurs, the menstrual cycles cease, and the endometrium passes into a pregnancy phase. With the termination of pregnancy, the ovarian and menstrual cycles resume after a variable period (usually 6 to 10 weeks if the female is not breast-feeding). Except during pregnancy, the reproductive cycles continue normally until menopause.

TRANSPORTATION OF GAMETES

1

OOCYTE TRANSPORT

The secondary oocyte is expelled at ovulation from the ovarian follicle with the escaping follicular fluid (see Fig. 2.10C and D). During ovulation, the fimbriated end of the uterine tube becomes closely applied to the ovary. The finger-like processes of the tube, **fimbriae**, move back and forth over the ovary. The motion of the fimbriae and fluid currents produced by the cilia of the mucosal cells of the fimbriae "sweep" the secondary oocyte into the funnel-shaped **infundibulum** of the uterine tube (see Fig. 2.10B). The oocyte then passes into the **ampulla** of the tube (see Fig. 2.10C), mainly as the result of **peristalsis** (movements of the wall of the tube characterized by alternate contraction and relaxation), which causes the oocyte to pass toward the uterus.

FEMALE INFERTILITY

Infertility occurs in approximately 9% of females aged 15 to 49 years old. This is most commonly due to ovulation dysfunction and tubal disease (25% of diagnosed infertility).

SPERM TRANSPORT

The reflex ejaculation of semen may be divided into two phases:

- **Emission**: Semen passes to the prostatic part of the urethra through the ejaculatory ducts due to motility of the active tail flagellum and after peristaltic contractions of

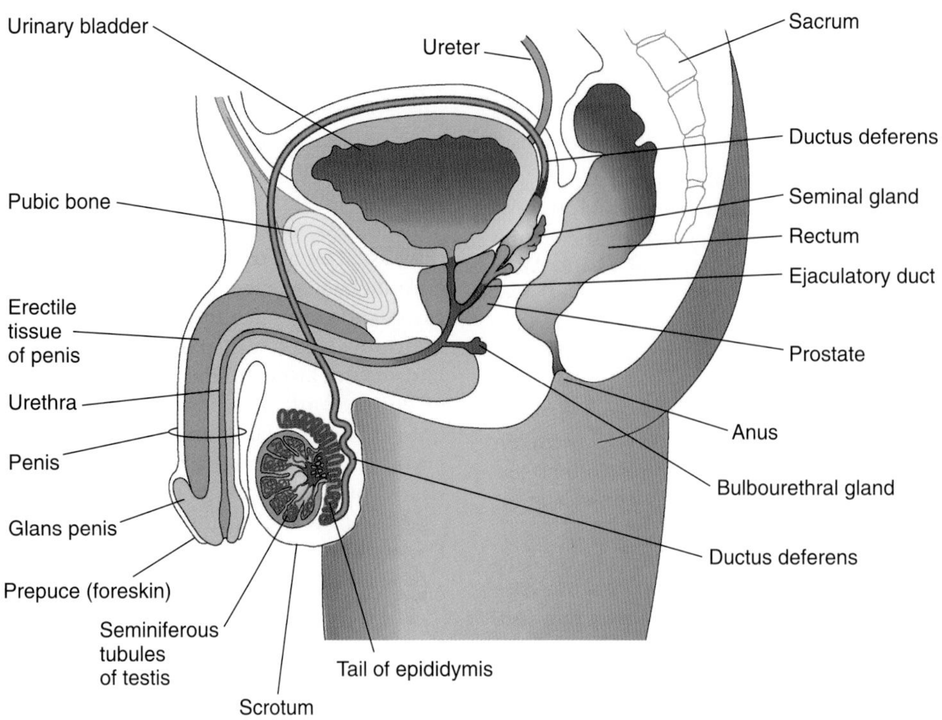

Fig. 2.12 Sagittal section of the male pelvis shows the parts of the male reproductive system.

the muscular coat of the ductus deferens (Fig. 2.12); emission is a sympathetic response. The accessory sex glands, that is, the **seminal glands** (vesicles), **prostate**, and **bulbourethral glands**, produce secretions that are added to the sperm-containing fluid in the ductus deferens and urethra.

- **Ejaculation**: Semen is expelled from the urethra through the external urethral orifice; this results from the closure of the vesical sphincter at the neck of the bladder, contraction of the urethral muscle, and contraction of the bulbospongiosus muscles.

From 200 to 600 million sperms are deposited around the external os of the uterus and in the fornix of the vagina during intercourse (see Fig. 2.6A and B). The sperms pass through the cervical canal by movements of their tails (see Fig. 2.5A). The enzyme **vesiculase**, produced by the prostate gland, assists with reducing the viscosity (liquification) of a seminal fluid coagulum that forms shortly after ejaculation. When ovulation occurs, the cervical mucus increases in amount and becomes less viscid (sticky), making it more favorable for sperm transport.

Passage of sperm through the uterus into the uterine tubes results mainly from muscular contractions of the walls of these organs. Sperm motility, facilitated by movement of the tail (flagellum), is also essential. **Prostaglandins** in the semen are thought to stimulate uterine motility at the time of intercourse and assist in the movement of sperm to the site of fertilization. **Fructose**, secreted by the seminal glands, is an energy source for the sperms in the semen.

The volume of **ejaculate** (sperms mixed with secretions from the accessory sex glands) averages 3.5 mL, with a range of 2 to 6 mL. The sperms are nonmotile during storage in the epididymis (see Fig. 2.12) but become motile in the ejaculate. The sperms move 2 to 3 mm/min, but the speed varies with the pH of the environment. They move slowly in the acidic environment of the vagina but more rapidly in the alkaline environment of the uterus. It is not known how long it takes sperm to reach the fertilization site in the ampulla of the uterine tube (see Figs. 2.10C and 2.21). **Motile sperms** have been recovered from the ampulla 5 minutes after their deposition near the external uterine os (see Fig. 2.6B). Some sperms, however, take as long as 45 minutes. Approximately 200 sperms reach the fertilization site; however, most sperms degenerate and are absorbed in the female genital tract.

MATURATION OF SPERMS

Freshly ejaculated sperms are unable to fertilize an oocyte. Sperms must undergo a period of conditioning, or **capacitation**, lasting approximately 7 hours. During this period, a glycoprotein coat and seminal proteins are removed from the surface of the sperm **acrosome** (see Figs. 2.4 and 2.5A). The membrane of the sperm is extensively altered. **Capacitated sperms** show no morphologic changes, but they are more active. Sperms are capacitated while in the uterus or uterine tubes by substances secreted by these parts of the female genital tract. During **in vitro fertilization (IVF)**, capacitation is induced by incubating the sperms in a defined medium for several hours (see Fig. 2.16). Completion of capacitation permits the acrosome reaction to occur.

The **acrosome** of the capacitated sperm binds to a glycoprotein (ZP3) on the zona pellucida (Fig. 2.14A and B). Studies have shown that the sperm plasma membrane, bicarbonate for cAMP generation, calcium ions, prostaglandins, and progesterone play a critical role in the **acrosome reaction**. This reaction of sperms must be completed before the sperms can fuse with the oocyte. When capacitated sperms come into contact with the corona radiata surrounding a secondary oocyte (see Fig. 2.14A and B), they undergo complex molecular changes that result in the development of perforations in the acrosome. Multiple point fusions of the **plasma membrane** of the sperm and the external **acrosomal membrane** occur. Breakdown of the membranes at these sites produces apertures (openings). The changes induced by acrosome reaction are associated with the release of enzymes, including hyaluronidase and acrosin, from the acrosome that facilitate fertilization. *Capacitation and acrosome reaction appear to be regulated by a tyrosine kinase, src kinase.* The acrosome reaction also prepares the sperm cell membrane for sperm-oocyte fusion.

Male Fertility

During the evaluation of male fertility, an analysis of semen is made. Sperms account for less than 10% of the semen. The remainder of the ejaculate consists of secretions of the seminal glands, prostate, and bulbourethral glands. There are usually more than 100 million sperms per milliliter of semen in the ejaculate of normal males. Males whose semen contains 20 million sperms per milliliter, or 50 million in the total specimen, are more likely to be fertile. A male with fewer than 10 million sperms per milliliter of semen is less likely to be fertile, especially when the specimen contains immotile and abnormal sperms. Male infertility may result from a low sperm count, poor sperm motility, medications and drugs, endocrine disorders, exposure to environmental pollutants, cigarette smoking, abnormal sperms, altered genome, or obstruction of a genital duct, as in the ductus deferens (see Fig. 2.12). Between 10% and 15% of couples are unable to conceive a child. Low sperm count and low testosterone levels contribute to about 35% of infertility in couples. Computer-assisted sperm morphometric analysis and fluorescence probes now provide a more objective and rapid assessment of the ejaculate. Guidelines for sperm vitality assessment (basic semen analysis) are provided in the *World Health Organization Laboratory Manual for the Examination and Processing of Human Semen*, 6th edition, 2021.

Vasectomy

The most effective method of permanent contraception in males is vasectomy, the surgical removal of all or part of the ductus deferens (vas deferens). The success rate of vasectomy is high (99%); complications are few. Following vasectomy, there are no sperms in the semen or ejaculate, but the volume is essentially the same. Reversal of vasectomy is technically feasible by microsurgical techniques; however, the success rate is variable.

Dispermy and Triploidy

Although several sperms penetrate the corona radiata and zona pellucida (Fig. 2.15A), usually only one sperm enters the oocyte and fertilizes it. Two sperms may participate in fertilization during an abnormal process known as **dispermy**, resulting in a triploid zygote with an extra set of chromosomes. **Triploid conceptions** occur in 1% to 3% of pregnancies and account for approximately 20% of chromosomally abnormal spontaneous abortions. There are two forms of triploidy: *diandric* (two sperms fertilize a normal oocyte or a sperm with two sets of chromosomes fertilizes a normal oocyte) and *digynic* (a normal sperm fertilizes an oocyte with two sets of chromosomes). Triploid embryos (69) are nearly always aborted or the newborn dies shortly after birth.

VIABILITY OF GAMETES

Studies on early stages of development indicate that human oocytes are usually fertilized within 12 hours after ovulation. In vitro observations have shown that the oocyte cannot be fertilized after 24 hours and that it degenerates shortly thereafter. Most human sperms probably do not survive for more than 48 hours in the female genital tract. After ejaculation, sperms that pass through the cervix enter the uterus. Some sperm are stored in folds of the **cervical crypts** and are gradually released and passed along the body of the uterus into the uterine tubes. The short-term storage of sperms in the crypts provides a gradual release of sperms and thereby increases the chances of fertilization. Sperms (semen) and oocytes can be frozen and stored for decades and can be used for *IVF*.

SEQUENCE OF FERTILIZATION

1

The usual site of fertilization is in the ampulla of the uterine tube (see Figs. 2.6B and 2.21). If the oocyte is not fertilized here, it slowly passes along the tube to the body of the uterus, where it degenerates and is resorbed. Although fertilization may occur in other parts of the tube, it does not occur in the body of the uterus. Gene activation occurs in the fertilized oocyte as it traverses through the uterine tube. Chemical signals (attractants), secreted by the oocyte and surrounding follicular cells, guide (chemotaxis) the capacitated sperms to the oocyte.

Fertilization is a complex sequence of coordinated molecular (Fig. 2.13) and physical events that begin with contact between a sperm and an oocyte (Fig. 2.14A and B) and end with the intermingling of maternal and paternal chromosomes at metaphase of the first mitotic division of the zygote (see Fig. 2.15E).

The fertilization process takes approximately 24 hours. Transgenic and gene knockout studies in animals have shown that carbohydrate-binding molecules and gamete-specific proteins on the surface of the sperms are involved in sperm-egg recognition and union.

PHASES OF FERTILIZATION

As it has been stated, fertilization is a sequence of coordinated events (see Figs. 2.14 and 2.15):

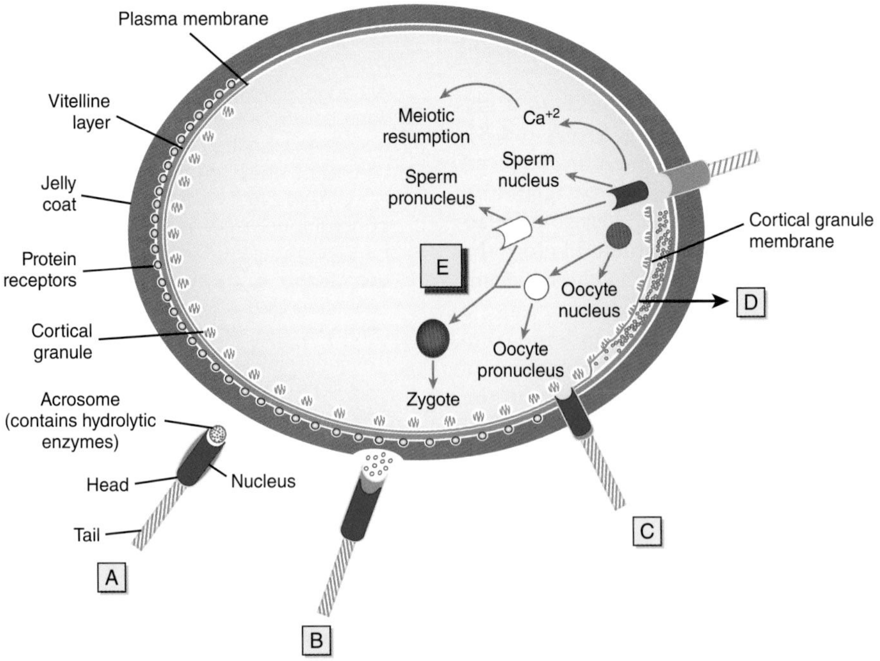

Fig. 2.13 The events taking place in fertilization. (A) Sperm preparation-capacitation: molecules (resact, speract) secreted from the oocyte orient and stimulate sperm (guanylate cyclase). (B) Acrosome reaction: release of hydrolytic enzymes. The sperm via the SED1 protein is connected to ZP3. (C) Fusion of sperm with the plasma membrane of the oocyte: sperm pre-acrosin binds to ZP2. Proteins of sperm IZUMO, ADAMs 1, ADAMs 2, ADAMs 3, and CRISP1 bind to receptors on the oocyte (Juno, integrins, CD9, CD81). Other molecules identified as playing a role in gamete fusion are trypsin-like acrosin, spermosin, SPAM1, HYAL5, and ACE3. (D) Cortical reaction: Ca^{2+} release/wave of Ca^{2+} and formation of fertilization cone. Enzymes released by cortical granules digest sperm receptors ZP2 and ZP3 (block of polyspermy). (E) Sperm chromatin decondensation to form male pronucleus: the oocyte nucleus completes the second meiosis and eliminates the second polar body.(From Georgadaki K, Khoury N, Spandidos D, Zoumpourlis V: The molecular basis of fertilization [review]. *Int J Mol Med* 38:979–986, 2016.)

- **Passage of a sperm through the corona radiata.** Dispersal of the follicular cells of the corona radiata surrounding the oocyte and zona pellucida appears to result mainly from the action of the enzyme *hyaluronidase* released from the acrosome of the sperm (see Fig. 2.5A). Tubal mucosal enzymes and movements of the tail of the sperm are also important in the dispersal and penetration of the corona radiata (see Fig. 2.14A).
- **Penetration of the zona pellucida.** The formation of a pathway for the sperm through the zona pellucida also results from the action of enzymes released from the acrosome. The enzymes esterase, acrosin, and neuraminidase appear to cause lysis of the zona pellucida, thereby forming a path for the sperm to enter the oocyte. The most important of these enzymes is **acrosin**, a proteolytic enzyme.
- **Zona reaction.** Once the sperm penetrates the zona pellucida, a change in the properties of the zona pellucida (zona reaction) occurs that makes it impermeable to other sperms. The zona reaction is believed to result from the action of lysosomal enzymes released by cortical granules near the plasma membrane of the oocyte. The contents of these granules, which are released into the **perivitelline space** (see Fig. 2.14A), also cause changes in the oocyte plasma membrane that make it impermeable to other sperms.
- **Fusion of cell membranes of the oocyte and sperm.** The plasma or cell membranes of the oocyte and sperm fuse and break down in the area of fusion. The head and tail of the sperm enter the cytoplasm of the oocyte (see Fig. 2.14A and B), but the sperm cell membrane and mitochondria remain behind. Phospholipase C-zeta from the sperm causes changes in calcium concentration that, in turn, reactivate cell cycling in the oocyte.
- **Completion of the oocyte second meiotic division.** Penetration of the oocyte by a sperm activates the oocyte into completing the second meiotic division and forming a **mature oocyte** and a second polar body (see Fig. 2.15B). Following the decondensation of the maternal chromosomes, the nucleus of the mature oocyte becomes the **female pronucleus.**
- **Formation of the male pronucleus.** Within the cytoplasm of the oocyte, the nucleus of the sperm enlarges to form the male pronucleus (see Fig. 2.15C), and the tail degenerates. Morphologically, the male and female pronuclei are indistinguishable. During the growth of the pronuclei, they replicate their DNA-1 n (haploid), and 2 c (two chromatids). The oocyte containing the two haploid pronuclei is called an **ootid** (see Fig. 2.15C).
- **Fusion of the pronuclei.** As the pronuclei fuse into a single diploid aggregation of chromosomes, the **ootid becomes a zygote.** The chromosomes in the zygote become arranged on a cleavage spindle (see Fig. 2.15E) in preparation for cleavage of the zygote (see Fig. 2.17).

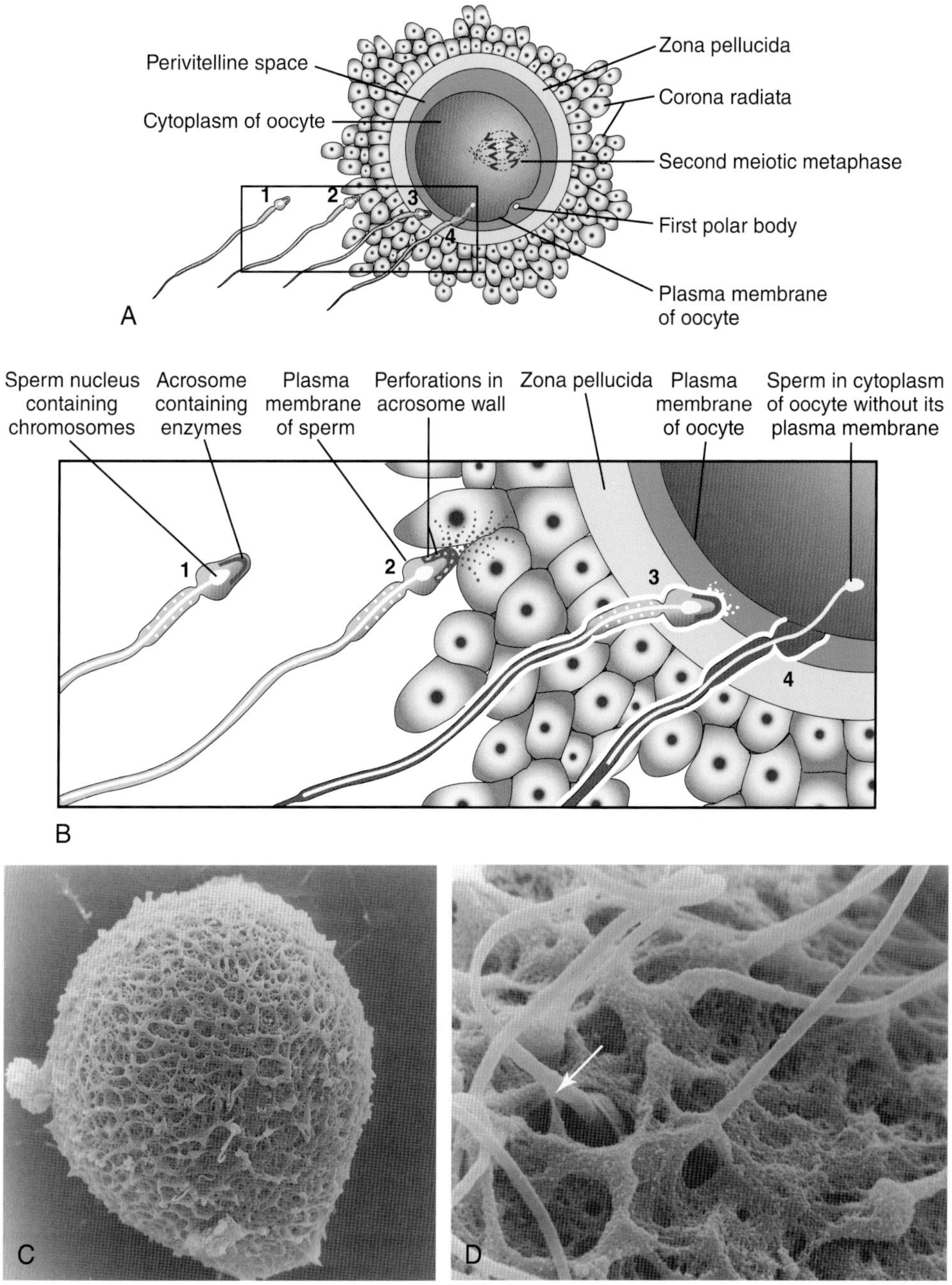

Fig. 2.14 Acrosome reaction and sperm penetrating an oocyte. The detail of the area outlined in (A) is given in (B). (*1*) Sperm during capacitation, a period of conditioning that occurs in the female reproductive tract. (*2*) Sperm undergoing the acrosome reaction, during which perforations form in the acrosome. (*3*) Sperm digesting a path through the zona pellucida by the action of enzymes released from the acrosome. *(4)* Sperm after entering the cytoplasm of the oocyte. Note that the plasma membranes of the sperm and oocyte have fused and that the head and tail of the sperm enter the oocyte, leaving the sperm's plasma membrane attached to the oocyte's plasma membrane. (C) Scanning electron microscopy of an unfertilized human oocyte showing relatively few sperms attached to the zona pellucida. (D) Scanning electron microscopy of a human oocyte showing penetration of the sperm (*arrow*) into the zona pellucida.(Courtesy P. Schwartz and H.M. Michelmann, University of Goettingen, Goettingen, Germany.)

The zygote is genetically unique because half of its chromosomes come from the mother and half from the father. The zygote contains a new combination of chromosomes that is different from those in the cells of either of the parents. This mechanism forms the basis of **biparental inheritance** and variation of the human species. Meiosis allows an independent assortment of maternal and paternal chromosomes among the germ cells (see Fig. 2.2). **Crossing over of chromosomes**, by relocating segments of the maternal and paternal chromosomes, "shuffles" the genes, thereby producing a recombination of genetic material. *The embryo's chromosomal sex is determined at fertilization.* Fertilization by an X-bearing sperm produces a 46,XX zygote, which develops into a female, whereas fertilization

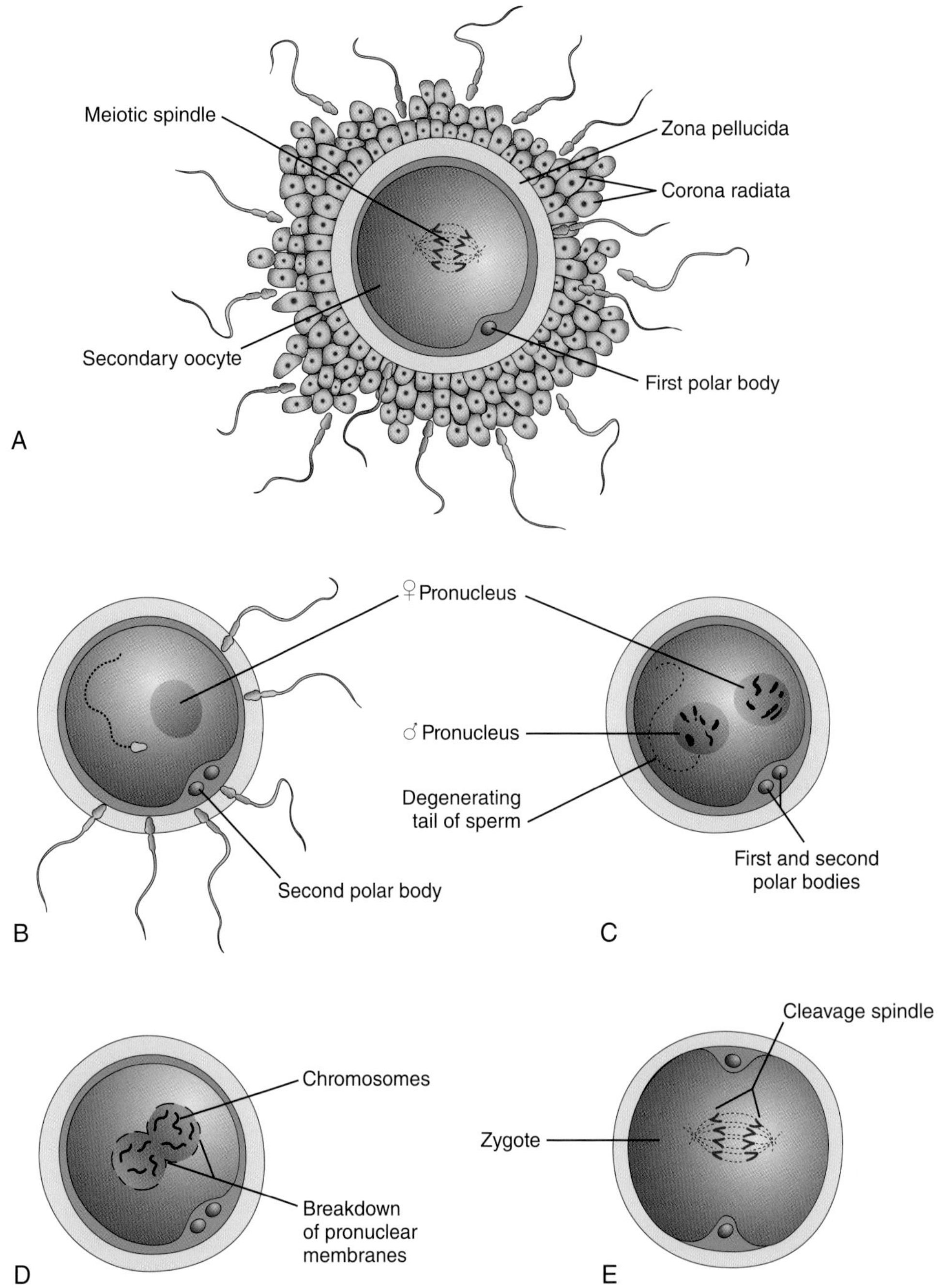

Fig. 2.15 Illustrations of fertilization, the procession of events beginning when the sperm contacts the secondary oocyte's plasma membrane and ending with the intermingling of maternal and paternal chromosomes at the metaphase of the first mitotic division of the zygote. (A) Secondary oocyte surrounded by several sperms, two of which have penetrated the corona radiata. (Only 4 of the 23 chromosome pairs are shown.) (B) The corona radiata is not shown. A sperm has entered the oocyte, and the second meiotic division has occurred, causing a mature oocyte to form. The nucleus of the oocyte is now the female pronucleus. (C) The sperm head has enlarged to form the male pronucleus. This cell, now called an ootid, contains the male and female pronuclei. (D) The pronuclei are fusing. (E) The zygote has formed; it contains 46 chromosomes, the diploid number.

by a Y-bearing sperm produces a 46,XY zygote, which develops into a male.

OUTCOMES OF FERTILIZATION

- Stimulates the penetrated oocyte to complete the second meiotic division
- Restores the normal diploid number of chromosomes (46) in the zygote
- Results in variation of the human species through the mingling of maternal and paternal chromosomes
- Determines the chromosomal sex of the embryo
- Causes metabolic activation of the ootid and initiates cleavage of the zygote

Preselection of Embryo's Sex

Because X and Y sperms are formed in equal numbers, the expectation is that the sex ratio at fertilization (primary sex ratio) would be 1.00 (100 males per 100 females). However, that there are more male neonates than female neonates born in all countries. In North America, for example, the sex ratio at birth (secondary sex ratio) is approximately 1.05 (105 males per 100 females). Various microscopic techniques, particularly flow cytometric and cell-sorting, have been developed in an attempt to separate X and Y sperms (sex selection) using:

- The differential swimming abilities of the X and Y sperms
- Different speed of migration of sperms in an electric field
- Differences in the appearance of X and Y sperms
- DNA difference between X (2.8% more DNA) and Y sperms

The use of a selected sperm sample during IVF may produce the chosen sex.

Assisted Reproductive Technologies

IN VITRO FERTILIZATION AND EMBRYO TRANSFER

It has been reported that one in eight females and one in 10 males may be infertile. **In vitro fertilization (IVF)** of oocytes and transfer of cleaving zygotes into the uterus have provided an opportunity for many women who are infertile (e.g., owing to tubal occlusion). In 1978 Robert G. Edwards and Patrick Steptoe pioneered IVF, one of the most revolutionary developments in the history of human reproduction. Their studies resulted in the birth of the first "test tube baby," Louise Brown. Since then, globally, more than 10 million children have been born after IVF. In the United States, 2% of infants born annually are conceived using assisted reproductive technology.

The steps involved during IVF and embryo transfer are as follows (Fig. 2.16):

- Ovarian follicles are stimulated to grow and mature by the administration of clomiphene citrate or gonadotropin (superovulation).
- Several mature oocytes are aspirated from mature ovarian follicles using ultrasound-guided transvaginal needle aspiration.
- The oocytes are placed in a Petri dish containing a special culture medium and capacitated sperms.
- Fertilization of the oocytes and cleavage of the zygotes are monitored microscopically for 3 to 5 days.
- Depending on the mother's age, one to three of the resulting embryos (four-cell to eight-cell stage, or early blastocysts) are transferred by introducing a catheter through the vagina and cervical canal into the uterus. Any remaining embryos are stored in liquid nitrogen for later use.
- The patient lies supine (face upward) for several hours. The chances of multiple pregnancies are higher following IVF, as is the incidence of spontaneous abortion.

Several studies have reported an increased risk of preterm birth and low birth weight, and a higher incidence of birth defects, including embryonal tumors and chromosomal (molecular) changes (pathogenic variants in genes [mutations]), in children conceived as a result of assisted reproductive technologies. Long-term follow-up and evaluation of these children will guide parents and physicians.

CRYOPRESERVATION OF EMBRYOS

Early embryos resulting from IVF can be preserved for decades by freezing them in liquid nitrogen with a cryoprotectant (e.g., glycerol or dimethyl sulfoxide). Successful transfer of four- to eight-cell embryos and blastocysts to the uterus after thawing is now a common practice. The longest period of sperm cryopreservation that resulted in a live birth was reported to be 40 years.

INTRACYTOPLASMIC SPERM INJECTION

A sperm can be injected directly into the cytoplasm of a mature oocyte. This technique has been successfully used for the treatment of couples for whom IVF failed or in cases where there are too few sperms available.

ASSISTED IN VIVO FERTILIZATION

A technique enabling fertilization to occur in the uterine tube is called **gamete intrafallopian (intratubal) transfer**. It involves superovulation (similar to that used for IVF), oocyte retrieval, sperm collection, and laparoscopic placement of several oocytes and sperm into the uterine tubes. Using this technique, fertilization occurs in the ampulla, its usual location.

SURROGATE MOTHERS

Some females produce mature oocytes but are unable to become pregnant Also, a female may have a serious medical problem, such as heart disease or had her uterus excised **(hysterectomy)**. In these cases, IVF may be performed, and the embryos transferred to a surrogacy mother—another female's uterus, for fetal development and delivery.

CLEAVAGE OF ZYGOTE

Cleavage consists of repeated mitotic divisions of the zygote, resulting in a rapid increase in the number of cells (blastomeres) (Figs. 2.17 and 2.18). Cleavage occurs as the zygote passes along the uterine tube toward the uterus (see Fig. 2.21). During cleavage, the zygote is contained within the zona pellucida (see Fig. 2.18A). Division of the zygote into blastomeres begins approximately 30 hours after fertilization. Subsequent cleavage divisions follow one another, forming progressively smaller blastomeres (see Fig. 2.17D–F). After the nine-cell stage, the blastomeres change their shape and tightly align themselves against each other (see Fig. 2.17D). This phenomenon, **compaction**, is mediated by cell surface–adhesion glycoproteins including the E-cadherin-catenin complex (adherens junctions). Compaction results in changes to the cell membrane cytoskeleton, permits greater cell-to-cell interaction, and is a prerequisite for segregation of the internal cells that form the **embryoblast (inner cell mass)** of the blastocyst (see Fig. 2.17E and F). Cellular disturbances in compaction at the morula stage may affect the normal development of the blastocyst. Polarization of the blastomere (apical versus basolateral domains) also occurs. *Hippo signaling plays an essential role in segregating the embryoblast from the trophoblast.* When there are 12 to 32 blastomeres, the developing human is called a **morula**. Internal cells of the morula are surrounded by **trophoblastic cells**. The morula forms approximately 3 days after fertilization as it enters the uterus (see Fig. 2.21).

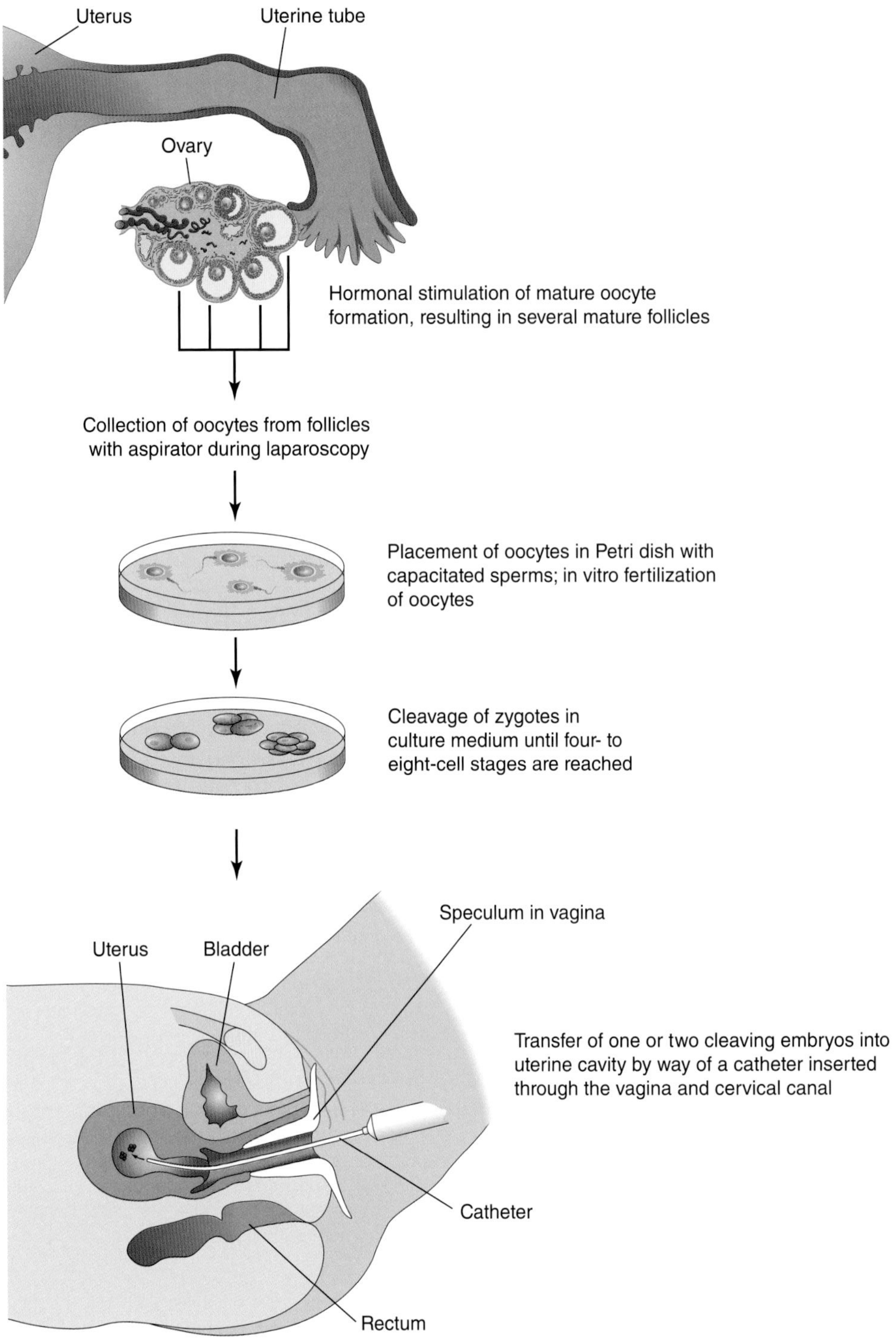

Fig. 2.16 In vitro fertilization and embryo transfer procedures.

Mosaicism

Nondisjunction is relatively common in cleavage-stage embryos due to a lack of coordination of chromosome segregation and, as such, these early embryos are naturally aneuploid mosaic (an embryo with two or more cell lines with different chromosome complements.) However, embryos at this early stage also have cell mechanisms that can eliminate abnormal lineage cells. If the mosaicism is not eliminated, some cells of the embryo would have a normal chromosome complement, and others would have an additional chromosome, e.g., chromosome 21 in trisomy 21 syndrome). In general, individuals who are mosaic for a given trisomy, such as mosaic trisomy 21 syndrome, are less severely affected than those with the usual nonmosaic condition.

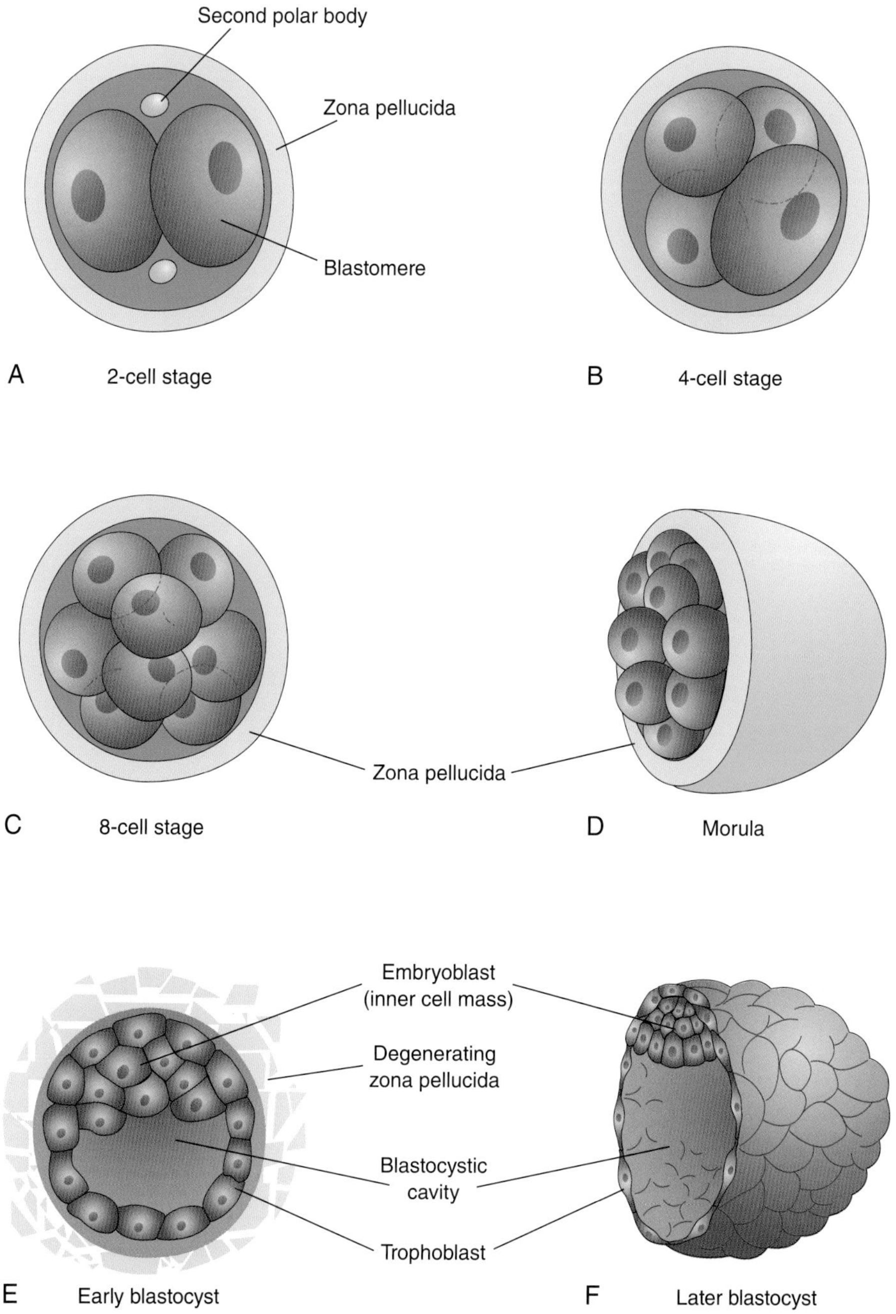

Fig. 2.17 Illustrations of a cleaving zygote and formation of the blastocyst. (A–D) Various stages of cleavage of the zygote. The period of the morula begins at the 12-cell to 16-cell stage and ends when the blastocyst forms. (E and F) Sections of blastocysts. The zona pellucida has disappeared by the late blastocyst stage (5 days). The second polar bodies shown in (A) are small, nonfunctional cells. Cleavage of the zygote and formation of the morula occur as the dividing zygote passes along the uterine tube. Blastocyst formation occurs in the uterus. Although cleavage increases the number of blastomeres, note that each of the daughter cells is smaller than the parent cells. As a result, there is no increase in the size of the developing embryo until the zona pellucida degenerates. The blastocyst then enlarges considerably (F).

FORMATION OF BLASTOCYST

Shortly after the morula enters the uterus (approximately 4 days after fertilization), a fluid-filled space, the **blastocystic cavity**, appears inside the morula (see Fig. 2.17E). Fluid from the uterine cavity passes through the zona pellucida to form this space. The blastomeres begin to separate into two parts:

- A thin outer cell layer, the **trophoblast**, gives rise to the embryonic part of the placenta (see Fig. 2.19).
- A group of centrally located blastomeres, the **embryoblast**, gives rise to the embryo (see Figs. 2.17F and 2.19 and B).

Early pregnancy factor (EPF), an immunosuppressant glycoprotein, is secreted by the trophoblastic cells and appears in the maternal serum within 24 to 48 hours after

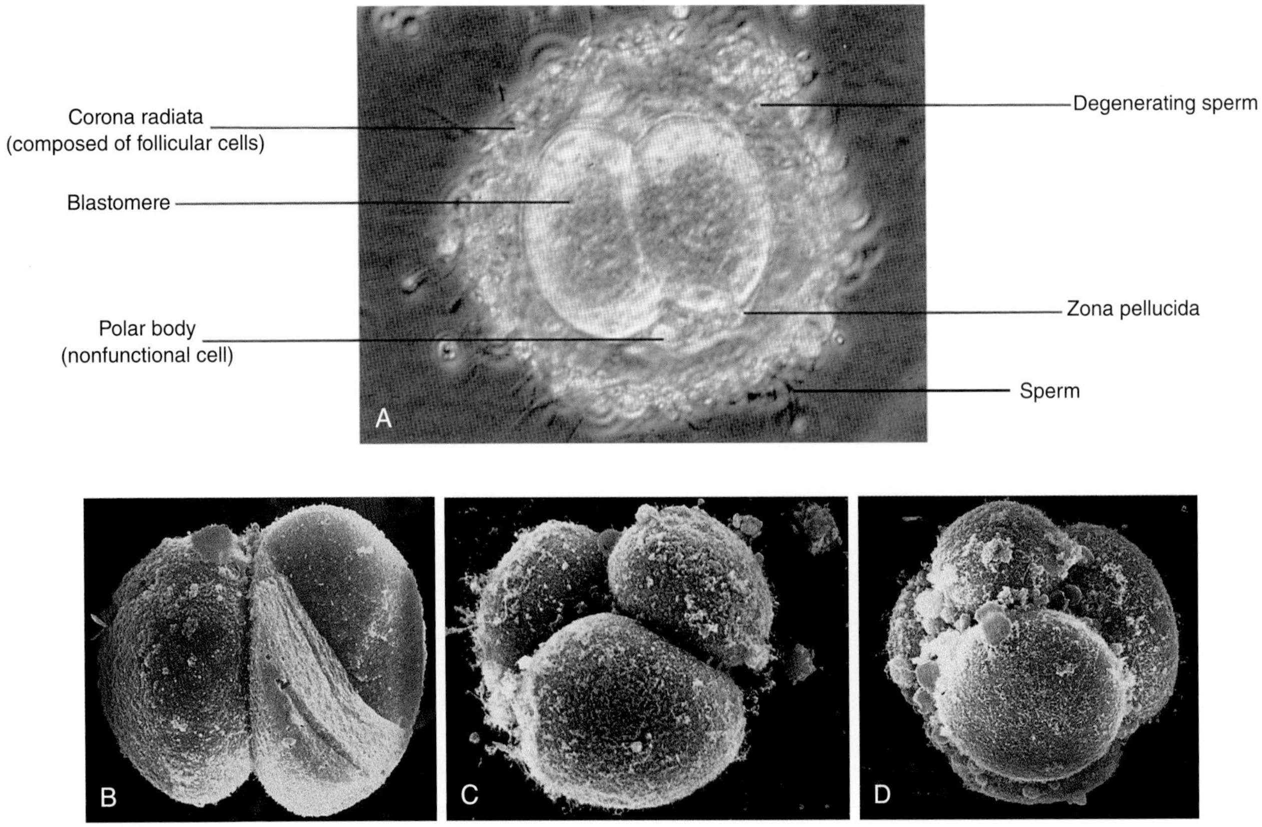

Fig. 2.18 (A) Two-cell stage of a cleaving zygote developing in vitro. Observe that it is surrounded by many sperms. (B) In vitro fertilization, the two-cell-stage human embryo. The zona pellucida has been removed. A small rounded polar body *(pink)* is still present on the surface of a blastomere (artificially colored, scanning electron microscopy, ×1000). (C) Three-cell-stage human embryo, in vitro fertilization (scanning electron microscopy, ×1300). (D) Eight-cell-stage human embryo, in vitro fertilization (scanning electron microscopy, ×1100). Note the rounded large blastomeres with several sperms attached.(A, Courtesy M.T. Zenzes, In Vitro Fertilization Program, Toronto Hospital, Toronto, Ontario, Canada. D, From Makabe S, Naguro T, Motta PM: Three-dimensional features of human cleaving embryo by ODO method and field emission scanning electron microscopy. In Motta PM, editor: *Microscopy of reproduction and development: a dynamic approach*, Rome, 1997, Antonio Delfino Editore.)

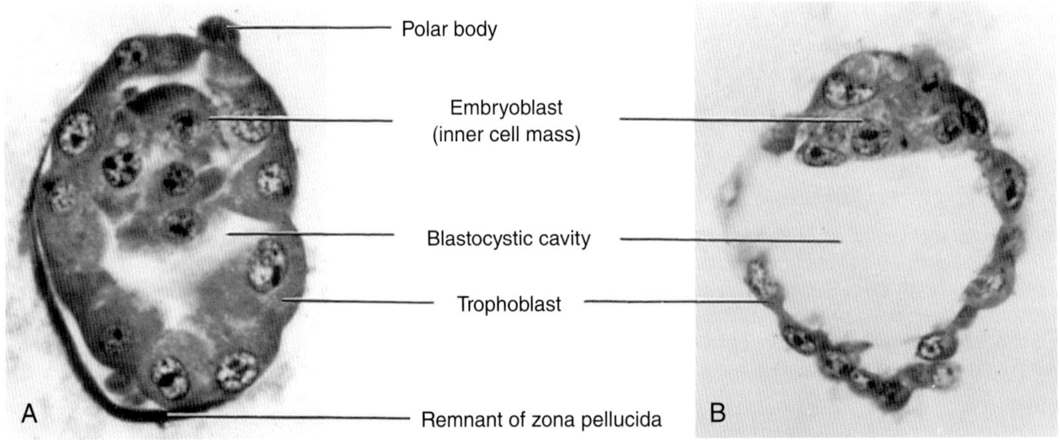

Fig. 2.19 Photomicrographs of sections of human blastocysts recovered from the uterine cavity (×600). (A) At 4 days, the blastocystic cavity is just beginning to form, and the zona pellucida is deficient over part of the blastocyst. (B) At 4.5 days, the blastocystic cavity has enlarged, and the embryoblast and trophoblast are clearly defined. The zona pellucida has disappeared.(From Hertig AT, Rock J, Adams EC: A description of 34 human ova within the first seventeen days of development, *Am J Anat* 98:435, 1956. Courtesy the Carnegie Institution of Washington.)

fertilization. EPF forms the basis of a pregnancy test during the first 10 days of development.

During this stage of development, the **conceptus** (embryo and its membranes) is called a **blastocyst** (Fig. 2.19). The embryoblast now projects into the blastocystic cavity, and the trophoblast forms the wall of the blastocyst. After the blastocyst has floated in the uterine secretions for approximately 2 days, the **zona pellucida** gradually degenerates and disappears (see Figs. 2.17E and F and 2.19A). **Shedding of the zona pellucida**, which has been observed in vitro, permits the blastocyst to increase rapidly in size. While in the uterus, the embryo derives nourishment from secretions of the uterine glands (see Fig. 2.6C).

Approximately 6 days after fertilization (approximately day 20 of the menstrual cycle), the blastocyst attaches to the endometrial epithelium (Fig. 2.20A). As soon as it attaches to the **endometrial epithelium**, the trophoblast proliferates rapidly and differentiates into two layers (see Fig. 2.20B):

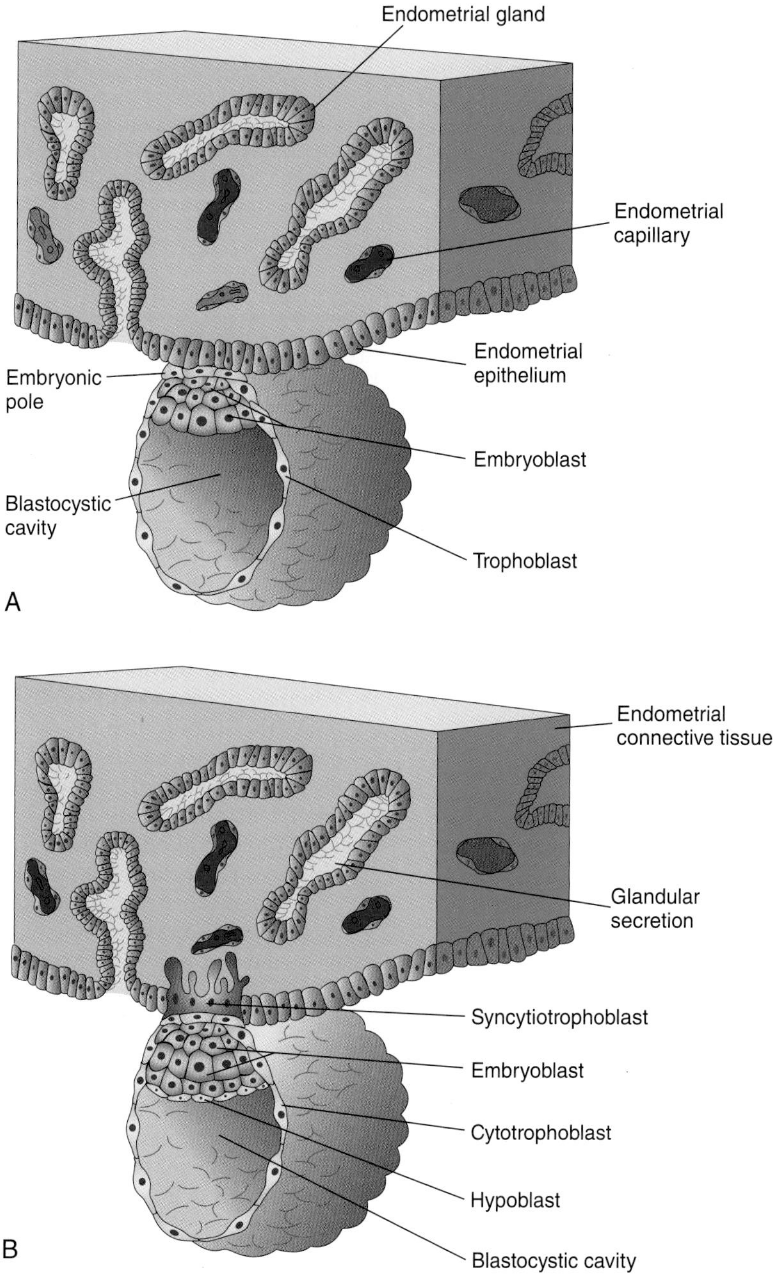

Fig. 2.20 Attachment of the blastocyst to the endometrial epithelium during the early stages of implantation. (A) At 6 days, the trophoblast is attached to the endometrial epithelium at the embryonic pole of the blastocyst. (B) At 7 days, the syncytiotrophoblast has penetrated the epithelium and has started to invade the endometrial connective tissue. ***Note:*** *In embryologic studies, the embryo is usually shown with its dorsal surface upward. Because the embryo implants on its future dorsal surface, it would appear upside down if the histologic convention (epithelium upward) were followed. In this book, the histologic convention is followed when the endometrium is the dominant consideration (e.g., Fig. 2.6C), and the embryologic convention is used when the embryo is the center of interest, as in the adjacent illustrations.*

- An inner layer, the **cytotrophoblast**, is mitotically active (i.e., mitotic figures are visible) and forms new mononuclear cells that migrate into the increasing mass of **syncytiotrophoblast**, where they fuse and lose their cell membranes; trophoblast fusion is regulated by the cyclic adenosine monophosphate (AMP) pathway.
- The **syncytiotrophoblast**, a rapidly expanding multinucleated mass in which no cell boundaries are discernible.

In carefully timed sequences, the intrinsic and extracellular matrix factors modulate the differentiation of the trophoblast. *Transforming growth factor-β regulates the proliferation and differentiation of the trophoblast by interaction of the ligand with type I and type II receptors and serine/threonine protein kinases.* In addition, it appears that microvesicles released by the inner cell mass also have an influence on the trophoblast during implantation. The finger-like processes of syncytiotrophoblast extend through the endometrial epithelium and invade the connective tissue. By the end of the first week, the blastocyst is superficially implanted in the compact layer of the endometrium and is deriving its nourishment from the eroded maternal tissues (see Fig. 2.20B). The highly invasive syncytiotrophoblast expands quickly adjacent to the **embryonic pole** (see Fig. 2.20A). The syncytiotrophoblast produces enzymes that erode the maternal tissues, enabling the blastocyst to "burrow" into the endometrium. Endometrial cells also assist in controlling the depth of penetration of the syncytiotrophoblast. At approximately 7 days, a layer of cells, the **hypoblast** (primary endoderm), appears on the surface of the embryoblast facing the blastocystic cavity (see Fig. 2.20B). Comparative embryologic data suggest that the hypoblast arises by delamination of blastomeres from the embryoblast.

Preimplantation Genetic Diagnosis

In couples with inherited genetic disorders and using IVF, preimplantation genetic diagnosis is carried out to determine the genotype of the embryo to select a chromosomally healthy embryo for transfer to the mother. The indications for preimplantation genetic diagnosis include single-gene disorders, single mutations, translocations, subchromosomal, and other genetic abnormalities. Preimplantation genetic screening of all 24 chromosomes in older or infertile patients is carried out to secure an embryo with a normal karyotype that can be transferred. The discovery of the presence of cell-free fetal DNA in the maternal plasma of pregnant females, advances in genomic medicine, and newly introduced technologies have transformed the practice of preimplantation genetic diagnosis.

A preimplantation genetic diagnosis can be carried out 3 to 5 days after IVF of the oocyte (see Fig. 2.16). One or two blastomeres are removed from the embryo and analyzed before transfer into the uterus. The sex of the embryo can also be determined from one blastomere taken from a six- to eight-cell dividing zygote, then analyzed by polymerase chain reaction and fluorescence in situ hybridization techniques. This procedure has been used to detect female embryos during IVF in cases in which a male embryo would be at risk of a serious X-linked disorder. The polar body may also be tested for diseases where the mother is the carrier (see Fig. 2.15A).

Abnormal Embryos and Spontaneous Abortions

Early implantation of the blastocyst is a critical period of development that may fail owing to inadequate production of progesterone and estrogen by the corpus luteum (see Fig. 2.7) or disturbed immune *(HLA class Ib-receptor)* interactions between the blastocyst trophoblast and endometrial immune cells. Occasionally, a patient states that her last menstrual period was delayed by several days and that her last menstrual flow was unusually profuse—very likely the patient has had an early spontaneous abortion. The overall early **spontaneous abortion rate** is thought to be 50% to 70%. Early spontaneous abortions occur for a variety of reasons, including genetic mutations and chromosomal abnormalities. More than 50% of all *known* spontaneous abortions occur because of such abnormalities. Early spontaneous abortion appears to represent a removal of abnormal conceptuses that could not have developed normally; that is, a natural screening process of embryos, without which the incidence of fetuses with significant birth defects would be far greater.

SUMMARY OF FIRST WEEK

- Oocytes are produced by the ovaries **(oogenesis)** and expelled from them during ovulation (Fig. 2.21). The fimbriae of the uterine tubes sweep the oocyte into the ampulla, where it may be fertilized. Usually, only one oocyte is expelled at ovulation.
- Sperms are produced in the testes (spermatogenesis) and stored in the epididymis (see Fig. 2.12). Ejaculation of semen results in the deposit of millions of sperm in the vagina. Several hundred sperm pass through the uterus and enter the uterine tubes.
- When an oocyte is contacted by a sperm, the oocyte completes the second meiotic division (see Fig. 2.1), forming a mature oocyte and a second polar body. The nucleus of the mature oocyte constitutes the female pronucleus (see Fig. 2.15B and C).
- After the sperm enters the oocyte, the head of the sperm separates from the tail and enlarges to become the male pronucleus (see Figs. 2.14 and 2.15C). Fertilization is complete when the male and female pronuclei unite and the maternal and paternal chromosomes intermingle during metaphase of the first mitotic division of the zygote (see Fig. 2.15D and C).
- As the zygote passes along the uterine tube toward the uterus, it undergoes cleavage into several blastomeres. Approximately 3 days after fertilization, a ball of 12 or more blastomeres (a morula) enters the uterus (see Fig. 2.21).
- A cavity forms in the morula, converting it into a blastocyst consisting of the embryoblast, a blastocystic cavity, and the trophoblast (see Fig. 2.17D–F). The trophoblast encloses the embryoblast and blastocystic cavity and later forms extraembryonic structures and the embryonic part of the placenta.
- At 4 to 5 days after fertilization, the zona pellucida is shed, and the trophoblast adjacent to the embryoblast attaches to the endometrial epithelium (see Fig. 2.17E).

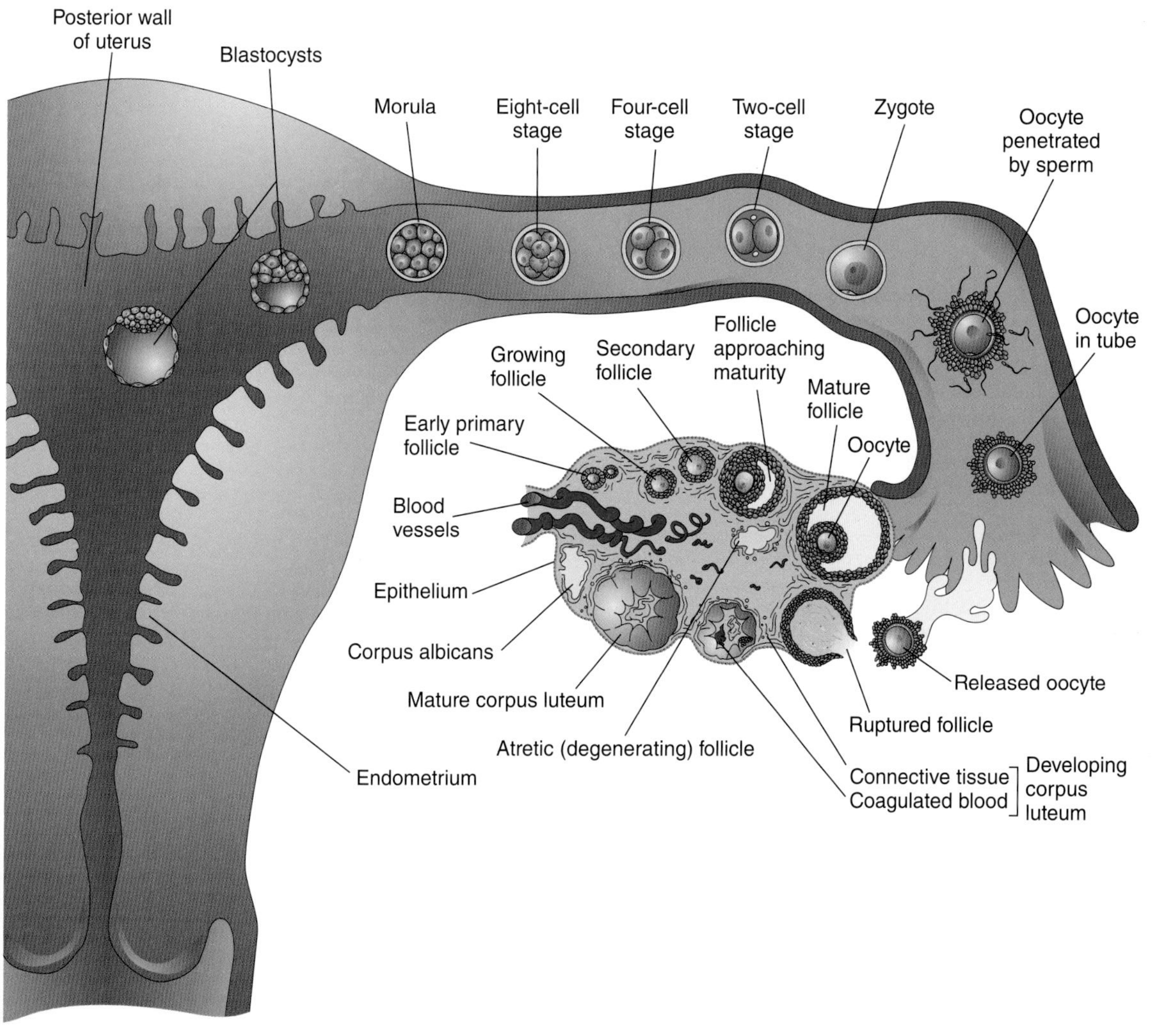

Fig. 2.21 Summary of the ovarian cycle, fertilization, and human development during the first week. Stage 1 of development begins with fertilization in the ampulla of the uterine tube and ends when the zygote forms. Stage 2 (days 2–3) comprises the early cleavage stages (from 2 to approximately 32 cells, the morula). Stage 3 (days 4–5) consists of the free (unattached) blastocyst. Stage 4 (days 5–6) is represented by the blastocyst attaching to the posterior wall of the uterus, the usual site of implantation. The blastocysts have been sectioned to show their internal structure.

- The trophoblast at the embryonic pole differentiates into two layers: an outer syncytiotrophoblast and an inner cytotrophoblast (see Fig. 2.20B). The syncytiotrophoblast invades the endometrial epithelium and underlying connective tissue. Concurrently, a cuboidal layer of hypoblast forms on the deep surface of the embryoblast. By the end of the first week, the blastocyst is superficially implanted in the endometrium (see Fig. 2.20B).

CLINICALLY ORIENTED PROBLEMS

1. What is the main cause of numeric aberrations of chromosomes? Define this process. What is the usual result of this chromosomal abnormality?
2. During the in vitro cleavage of a zygote, all blastomeres of a morula were found to have an extra set of chromosomes. Explain how this could happen. Can such a morula develop into a viable fetus?
3. What is a major cause of (a) female infertility and (b) male infertility?
4. Some people have a mixture of cells, some with 46 chromosomes and others with 47 chromosomes (e.g., some persons with Down syndrome (trisomy 21)). How do mosaics form? Would children with mosaicism and Down syndrome have the same stigmata as other infants with Down syndrome (trisomy 21)? At what stage of development does mosaicism develop? Can this chromosomal abnormality be diagnosed before birth?
5. A young female asked you about "morning-after pills" (postcoital oral contraceptives). How would you explain to her the action of such medication?
6. What is the most common abnormality in early spontaneously aborted embryos?
7. Mary, 26 years old and in good health, is unable to conceive after 4 years of marriage. Her husband, Jerry, 32 years old, also appears to be in good health. Mary and Jerry consulted their family physician, who referred them to an infertility clinic. How common is infertility in couples? What do you think are the likely causes of possible infertility in this couple? What investigation(s) would you recommend first?

Discussion of these problems appears in the Appendix at the back of the book.

BIBLIOGRAPHY AND SUGGESTED READING

Agarwal A, Sharma RK, Gupta S, et al: Sperm vitality and necrozoospermia: diagnosis, management, and results of a global survey of clinical practice, *World J Men's Health* 40:228–242, 2022.

Cameron S: The normal menstrual cycle. In Magowan BA, Owen P, Thomson A, editors: *Obstetrics and gynaecology*, ed 3, Philadelphia, 2014, Saunders, pp 57–62.

Carlson LM, Vora NL: Prenatal diagnosis. Screening and diagnostic tools, *Obstet Gynecol Clin N Am* 44:245, 2017.

Carson SA, Kallen AN: Diagnosis and management of infertility: a review, *JAMA* 326:65, 2021.

Clermont Y, Trott M: Kinetics of spermatogenesis in mammals: seminiferous epithelium cycle and spermatogonial renewal, *Physiol Rev* 52:198, 1972.

Coticchio G, Langella C, Sturmey R, et al: The enigmatic morula: mechanisms of development, cell fate determination, self-correction and implication for ART, *Human Reprod Update* 25:422, 2019.

Coticchio G, Ezoe K, Lagalla C, et al: Perturbations of morphogenesis at the compaction stage affect blastocyst implantation and live birth rates, *Human Reprod* 36:918–928, 2021.https://doi.org/10.1093/humrep/deab011.

Datta J, Palmer MJ, Tanton C, et al: Prevalence of infertility and help seeking among 15000 women and me, *Human Reprod* 31:2108, 2016.

Fauser BCJM: Towards the global coverage of a unified registry of IVF outcomes, *Reprod Biomed* 38:133, 2019.

Garcia-Herrero S, Cervero A, Mateu E, et al: Genetic analysis of human preimplantation embryos, *Curr Top Dev Biol* 120:421, 2016.

Georgadaki K, Khoury N, Spandios DA, Zoumpourlis V: The molecular basis of fertilization (review), *Int J Mol Med* 38:979, 2016.

Gleicher N, Albertini DF, Patrizio P, Orvieto R, Adashi EY: The uncertain science of preimplantation and prenatal genetic testing, *Nat Med* 28:436, 2022.

Gura Ma, Relovska S, Abt KAM, et al: TAFb transcription networks regulating early oocyte development, *Development*:dev.200074, 2022.https://doi.org/10.1242/dev.200074.

Hertig AT, Rock J, Adams EC, et al: Thirty-four fertilized human ova, good, bad, and indifferent, recovered from 210 women of known fertility, *Pediatrics* 23:202, 1959.

Jenardhanan P, Panneerselvam M, Mathur PP: Effect of environmental contaminants on spermatogenesis, *Semin Cell Dev Biol* 59:126, 2016.

Jequier AM: *Male infertility: a clinical guide*, , ed 2Cambridge, UK, 2011, Cambridge University Press.

Kolle S, Hughes B, Steele H: Early embryo-maternal communication in the oviduct, *Mol Reprod Dev*:1–13, 2020.https://doi.org/10.1002/mrd.23352.

Litscher ES, Wasserman PM: Zona pellucida genes and proteins and human fertility, *Trends Dev Biol* 13:21, 2020.

Liss J, Chromik I, Szczyglinska J, et al: Current methods for preimplantation genetic diagnosis, *Ginekol Pol* 87:522, 2016.

Madero JI, Manotas MC, Garcia-Acero M, et al: Preimplantation genetic testing in assisted reproduction, *Minerva Obstet Gynecol*, 2021.https://doi.org/10.23736/S2724-606X.21.04805-3.

Masson E, Zou WB, Génin E, et al: Expanding ACMG variant classification guidelines into a general framework, *Hum Genomics* 16(1):31, 2022.https://doi.org/10.1186/s40246-022-00407-x.

Nusbaum RL, McInnes RR, Willard HF: *Thompson and Thompson genetics in medicine*, , ed 8Philadelphia, 2016, Elsevier.

Richards S, Aziz N, Bale S, et al: ACMG Laboratory Quality Assurance Committee. Standards and guidelines for the interpretation of sequence variants: a joint consensus recommendation of the American College of Medical Genetics and Genomics and the Association for Molecular Pathology, *Genet Med* 17(5):405–424, 2015. Epub 2015 Mar 5. https://doi.org/10.1038/gim.2015.30

Pedroza M, Gassaloglu SI, Dias N, et al: Self-patterning of human stem cells into post-implantation lineages, *Nature* 622(7983):574–583, 2023.

Rock J, Hertig AT: The human conceptus during the first two weeks of gestation, *Am J Obstet Gynecol* 55:6, 1948.

Simpson JL: Birth defects and assisted reproductive technology, *Semin Fetal Neonatal Med* 19:177, 2014.

Siu KK, Serrao VHB, Ziyyat A, Lee JE: The cell biology of fertilization: Gamte attachment and fusion, *JCB* 220:1, 2021.

Smith LB, Walker WH: The regulation of spermatogenesis by androgens, *Semin Cell Dev Biol*, 2014.https://doi.org/10.1016/j.semcdb.2014.02.012.

Steptoe PC, Edwards RG: Birth after implantation of a human embryo, *Lancet* 2:36, 1978.

Solovova OA, Chernykh VB: Genetics of oocyte maturation defects and early embryo development arrest, *Genes (Basel)* 13(11), 2022.

Szell AZ, Bierbaum Rc, Hazelrigg WB, Chetkowski RJ: Live births from frozen human semen stored for 40 years, *J Assist Reprod Genet* 30(6):743–744, 2013.https://doi.org/10.1007/s10815-013-9998-9.

Szuszkiewicz J, Nitkiewicz A, Drzewiecka K, Kaczmarek MM: miR-26a-5p and miR-125b-5p affect trophoblast genes and cell functions important during early pregnancy†, *Biol Reprod* 107(2):590–604, 2022.https://doi.org/10.1093/biolre/ioac071. PMID: 35416938.

Teletin M, Vernet N, Ghyselinck NB, et al: Roles of retinoic acid in germ cell differentiation, *Curr Top Dev Biol* 125:191, 2017.

Walker WH: Regulation of mammalian spermatogenesis by MiRNAs, *Semin Cell Dev Biol* 121:24, 2022.https://doi.org/10.1016/j.semcdb.2021.05.009.

Wang X, Wen Y, Zhang J, et al: MNF2 interacts with nauge-associated proteins and is essential for male germ cell development by controlling mRNA fate during spermatogenesis, *Development* 148(7):dev196295, 2021.https://doi.org/10.1242/dev.196295.

Wei Y, Wang J, Qu R, et al: Genetic mechanisms of fertilization failure and early embryonic arrest: a comprehensive review, *Hum Reprod Update* 30:48–90, 2024.https://doi.org/10.1093/humupd/dmad026.

Wilmut I, Schnieke AE, McWhir J, Kind AJ, Campbell KH: Viable offspring derived from fetal and adult mammalian cells, *Nature* 385:810, 1997.

World Health Organization: *WHO Laboratory Manual for the Examination and Processing of Human Semen*, , ed 6.Geneva, 2021, World Health Organization.

Zhang L, Zhang W, Xu H, et al: Birth defects surveillance after assisted reproductive technology in Beijing: a whole of population-based cohort study, *BMJ Open* 11:e044385, 2021.https://doi.org/10.1136/bmjopen-2020-044385.

Second Week of Human Development

3

CHAPTER OUTLINE

As implantation of the blastocyst occurs, molecular and cellular changes in the embryoblast produce a bilaminar **embryonic disc** composed of epiblast and hypoblast (Fig. 3.1A). The embryonic disc gives rise to the germ layers that form all the tissues and organs of the embryo. Extraembryonic structures that form during the second week are the amniotic cavity, amnion, umbilical vesicle connecting stalk, and chorionic sac.

COMPLETION OF IMPLANTATION OF BLASTOCYST

3

Implantation of the blastocyst is completed during the second week, and the trophectoderm of the blastocyst becomes closely attached to the now receptive endometrium.

Implantation of blastocysts usually occurs in the uterine endometrium in the superior part of the body of the uterus, slightly more often on the posterior wall than on the anterior wall of the uterus (see Fig. 3.9). Implantation of a blastocyst can be detected by **ultrasonography** and highly sensitive **immunoassays** of **human chorionic gonadotropin (hCG)** before the end of the second week (see Fig. 3.8).

As the blastocyst implants (see Fig. 3.1), the syncytiotrophoblast enters the endometrial connective tissue through the process of interstitial invasion. The endometrium ceases to proliferate (Fig. 3.2), and syncytiotrophoblastic cells displace endometrial cells at the implantation site. The endometrial cells undergo **apoptosis** (a type of programmed cell death), which facilitates the invasion.

The molecular mechanisms of implantation involve synchronization between the invading blastocyst and a receptive endometrium. The window of implantation is relatively brief, 2 to 3 days, during which bone morphogenetic proteins (BMPs), which are essential for fertilization, are expressed in the endometrium. The microvilli of endometrial cells, cell adhesion molecules (integrins), cytokines, prostaglandins, hormones (hCG and progesterone), growth factors, cell-cell and cell-extracellular matrix communication enzymes (matrix metalloproteinase and protein kinase A), and Wnt signaling pathways play a role in making the endometrium receptive. Implantation is also modulated by tumor necrosis factor-alpha, an inflammatory cytokine, secreted by endometrial cells. These endometrial cells help to modulate the depth of penetration of the syncytiotrophoblast that reaches a maximum at 9 to 12 weeks.

The connective tissue cells around the implantation site accumulate glycogen and lipids and assume a polyhedral appearance. Some of these cells, **decidual cells**, degenerate adjacent to the penetrating syncytiotrophoblast. The syncytiotrophoblast engulfs the decidual cells, providing a rich source of embryonic nutrition. The syncytiotrophoblast produces a glycoprotein hormone, hCG, which enters the maternal blood via isolated cavities **(lacunae)** in the syncytiotrophoblast (see Fig. 3.1B); hCG maintains the hormonal activity (estrogen and progesterone) of the corpus luteum in the ovary during pregnancy (see Fig. 2.11). Immunoassays for detecting hCG in the blood or urine form the basis for pregnancy tests. Enough hCG is produced by the syncytiotrophoblast to give a positive pregnancy test as early as 10 days after conception, even though the individual is probably unaware of the pregnancy.

FORMATION OF AMNIOTIC CAVITY, EMBRYONIC DISC, AND UMBILICAL VESICLE

2

Morphologic changes occur in the **embryoblast** that result in the formation of a flat, almost circular bilaminar plate

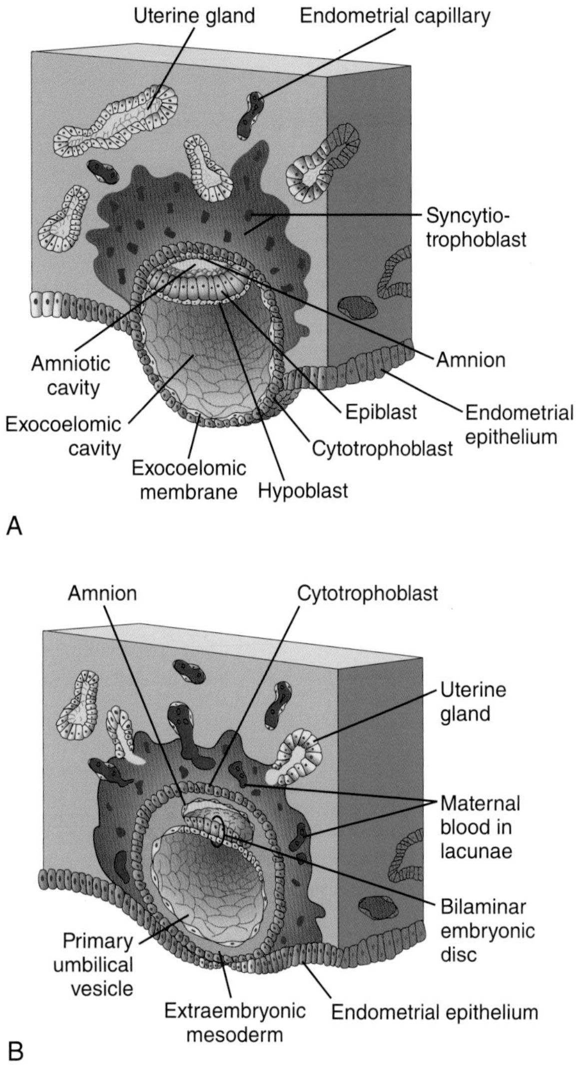

Fig. 3.1 Implantation of a blastocyst in the endometrium. The actual size of the **conceptus** is 0.1 mm, approximately the size of the period at the end of this sentence. (A) Drawing of a section through a blastocyst partially embedded in the uterine endometrium (approximately 8 days). Note the slit-like amniotic cavity. (B) Drawing of a section through a blastocyst of approximately 9 days implanted in the endometrium. Note the lacunae appearing in the syncytiotrophoblast.

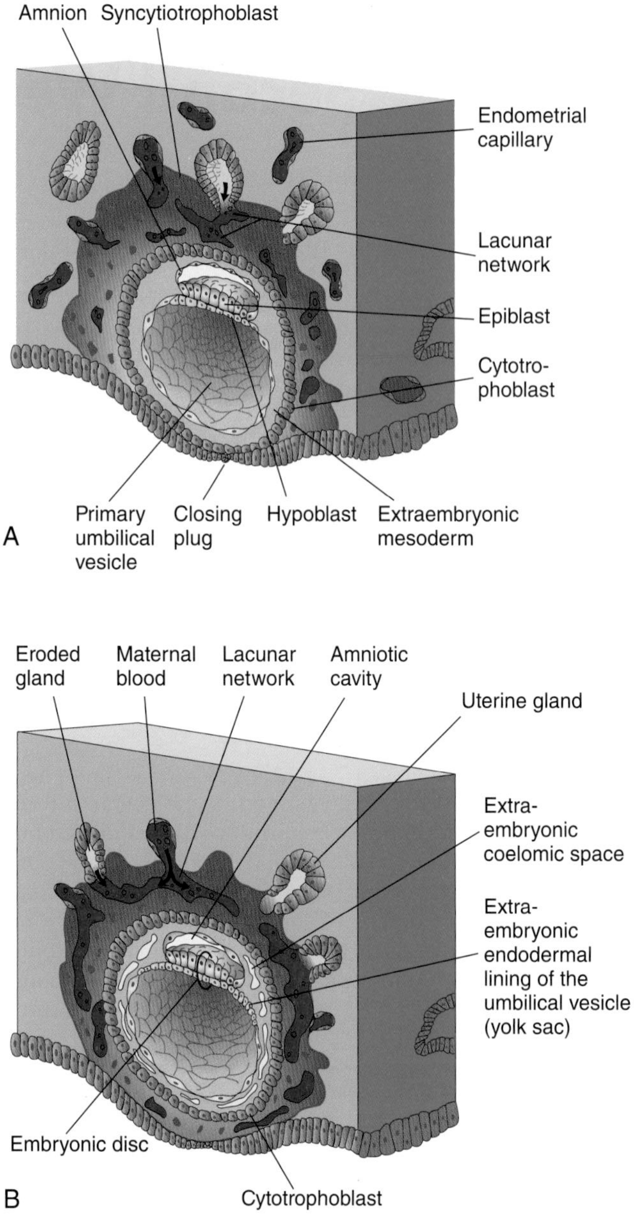

Fig. 3.2 Embedded blastocysts: (A) 10 days; (B) 12 days. This stage of development is characterized by communication of the blood-filled lacunar networks. Note in (B) that **coelomic spaces** have appeared in the **extraembryonic mesoderm**, forming the beginning of the **extra-embryonic coelom** (cavity).

of cells, the **embryonic disc**, consisting of two layers (see Fig. 3.2A and B):

- **Epiblast**, the thicker layer, consisting of high columnar cells adjacent to the amniotic cavity
- **Hypoblast**, consisting of small cuboidal cells adjacent to the exocoelomic cavity

As implantation of the blastocyst progresses, early epiblast cells become polarized through changes in cell shape and density and arrange themselves in a rosette pattern, forming an inner lumen. The cells adjacent to the implantation site undergo transformation to **amnioblasts** (amnion cells), forming the primordium of the **amniotic sac** (see Figs. 3.1A and 3.2B).

The hypoblast forms the roof of the exocoelomic cavity (see Fig. 3.1A) and is continuous with the thin **exocoelomic membrane**. This membrane, together with the hypoblast, lines the **primary umbilical vesicle**. The embryonic disc now lies between the amniotic cavity and the vesicle (see Fig. 3.1B). Cells from the vesicle endoderm form a layer of connective tissue, the **extraembryonic mesoderm** (see Fig. 3.2A), which surrounds the amnion and umbilical vesicle. This vesicle and amniotic cavity make possible morphogenetic movements of the cells of the embryonic disc.

As the amnion, embryonic disc, and umbilical vesicle form, **lacunae** (small spaces) appear in the syncytiotrophoblast (see Figs. 3.1A and 3.2). The lacunae are filled with a mixture of maternal blood from ruptured endometrial

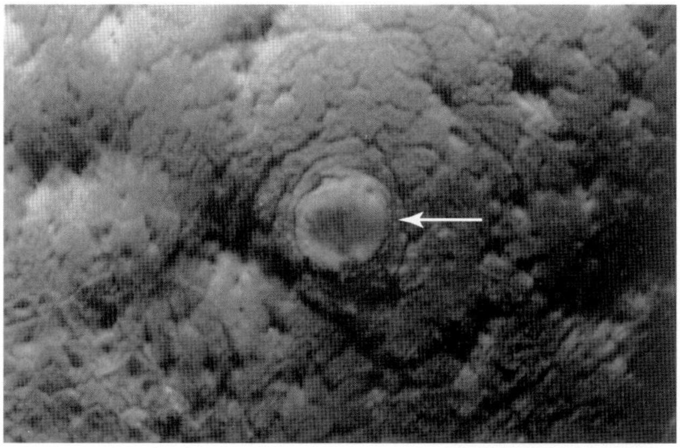

Fig. 3.3 Photograph of the endometrial surface of the body of the uterus, showing the implantation site of the 12-day embryo shown in Fig. 3.4. The implanted **conceptus** produces a small elevation *(arrow)* (×8).(From Hertig AT, Rock J: Two human ova of the pre-villous stage, having an ovulation age of about eleven and twelve days respectively, *Contrib Embryol Carnegie Inst* 29:127, 1941. Courtesy Carnegie Institution of Washington, DC.)

capillaries and cellular debris from eroded uterine glands (see Fig. 2.6C). The fluid in the lacunar spaces, **embryotroph**, passes to the embryonic disc by diffusion and provides nutritive material to the embryo.

The communication of the eroded endometrial capillaries with the lacunae in the syncytiotrophoblast establishes the **primordial uteroplacental circulation**. When maternal blood flows into the **lacunar networks** (see Fig. 3.2A and B), oxygen and nutritive substances pass to the embryo. Oxygenated blood passes into the lacunae from the spiral endometrial arteries (see Fig. 2.6C), and poorly oxygenated blood is removed from them through the endometrial veins.

The 10-day conceptus is completely embedded in the uterine endometrium (see Fig. 3.2A). Initially, there is a surface defect in the endometrial epithelium that is soon closed by a **closing plug** of a fibrin coagulum of blood (see Fig. 3.2A). By day 12, the closing plug is covered an almost completely regenerated uterine epithelium (Fig. 3.3; see Fig. 3.2B), that partially results from signaling by cyclic adenosine monophosphate and progesterone. As the conceptus implants, the endometrial connective tissue cells continue to undergo a transformation, the **decidual reaction**. The cells swell because of the accumulation of glycogen and lipid in their cytoplasm. The primary function of the decidual reaction is to provide nutrition to the early embryo and an immunologically privileged site for the conceptus.

In a 12-day embryo, adjacent syncytiotrophoblastic lacunae (small spaces) have fused to form **lacunar networks** (Fig. 3.4B; see Fig. 3.2B), giving the syncytiotrophoblast a sponge-like appearance. The networks, particularly obvious around the embryonic pole, are the primordia of the **intervillous spaces of the placenta** (see Fig. 7.5). The endometrial capillaries around the implanted embryo become congested and dilated to form **maternal sinusoids**, thin-walled terminal vessels that are larger than ordinary capillaries (Fig 3.5). The formation of blood vessels in the endometrial **stroma** (framework of connective tissue) is under the influence of estrogen and progesterone. *The expression of connexin 43 (Cx43), a gap junction protein, plays a critical role in angiogenesis at the implantation site and in the maintenance of pregnancy.*

The syncytiotrophoblast erodes the sinusoids, and maternal blood flows freely into the lacunar networks (see Figs. 3.4B and 3.7B). The trophoblast absorbs nutritive fluid from the lacunar networks, which is transferred to the embryo. The ***growth of the bilaminar embryonic disc is slow*** compared with the growth of the trophoblast (see Figs. 3.1, 3.2, and 3.7B). The implanted 12-day embryo produces a minute elevation on the endometrial surface that protrudes into the uterine cavity (see Figs. 3.3 and 3.4).

As changes occur in the trophoblast and endometrium, the extraembryonic mesoderm increases and isolated **extraembryonic coelomic spaces** appear within it (see Figs. 3.2B and 3.4B). These spaces rapidly fuse to form a large, isolated cavity, the **extraembryonic coelom** (see Fig. 3.5A). This fluid-filled cavity surrounds the amnion and umbilical vesicle, except where they are attached to the **chorion** (outermost fetal membrane) by the **connecting stalk** (see Fig. 3.7A and B). As the extraembryonic coelom forms, the primary umbilical vesicle decreases in size and a smaller **secondary umbilical vesicle** forms (see Fig. 3.5B). This smaller vesicle is formed by extraembryonic endodermal cells that migrate from the hypoblast inside the primary umbilical vesicle (Fig. 3.5C). During the formation of the secondary umbilical vesicle, a large part of the primary umbilical vesicle is pinched off, leaving a remnant of the vesicle (see Fig. 3.5B). The umbilical vesicle has important functions—for example, it is the site of origin of primordial germ cells (see Chapter 12) and may also have a role in the selective processing and transfer of nutrients from the coelomic cavity to the embryonic disc.

DEVELOPMENT OF CHORIONIC SAC

2

The end of the second week is characterized by the appearance of **primary chorionic villi** (see Fig. 3.5A and B). The villi, vascular processes of the chorion, form columns with syncytial coverings. These cellular extensions grow into the syncytiotrophoblast, which is thought to be induced by the underlying **extraembryonic somatic mesoderm**. The primary chorionic villi (see Fig. 3.5A and B) are the first stage in the development of the chorionic villi of the **placenta**, the fetomaternal organ of metabolic interchange between the embryo and mother.

The extraembryonic coelom splits the extraembryonic mesoderm into two layers (see Fig. 3.5A and B):

- Extraembryonic somatic mesoderm, lining the trophoblast and covering the amnion
- Extraembryonic splanchnic mesoderm, surrounding the umbilical vesicle

The extraembryonic somatic mesoderm and the two layers of trophoblast form the chorion, which forms the wall of the **chorionic sac** (see Fig. 3.5A and B). The embryo, amniotic sac, and umbilical vesicle are suspended in this sac by the connecting stalk. The extraembryonic coelom is the primordium of the **chorionic cavity**.

Transvaginal (endovaginal) ultrasonography is used for measuring the diameter of the chorionic sac (Fig. 3.6), which is valuable for evaluating early embryonic development and pregnancy outcome.

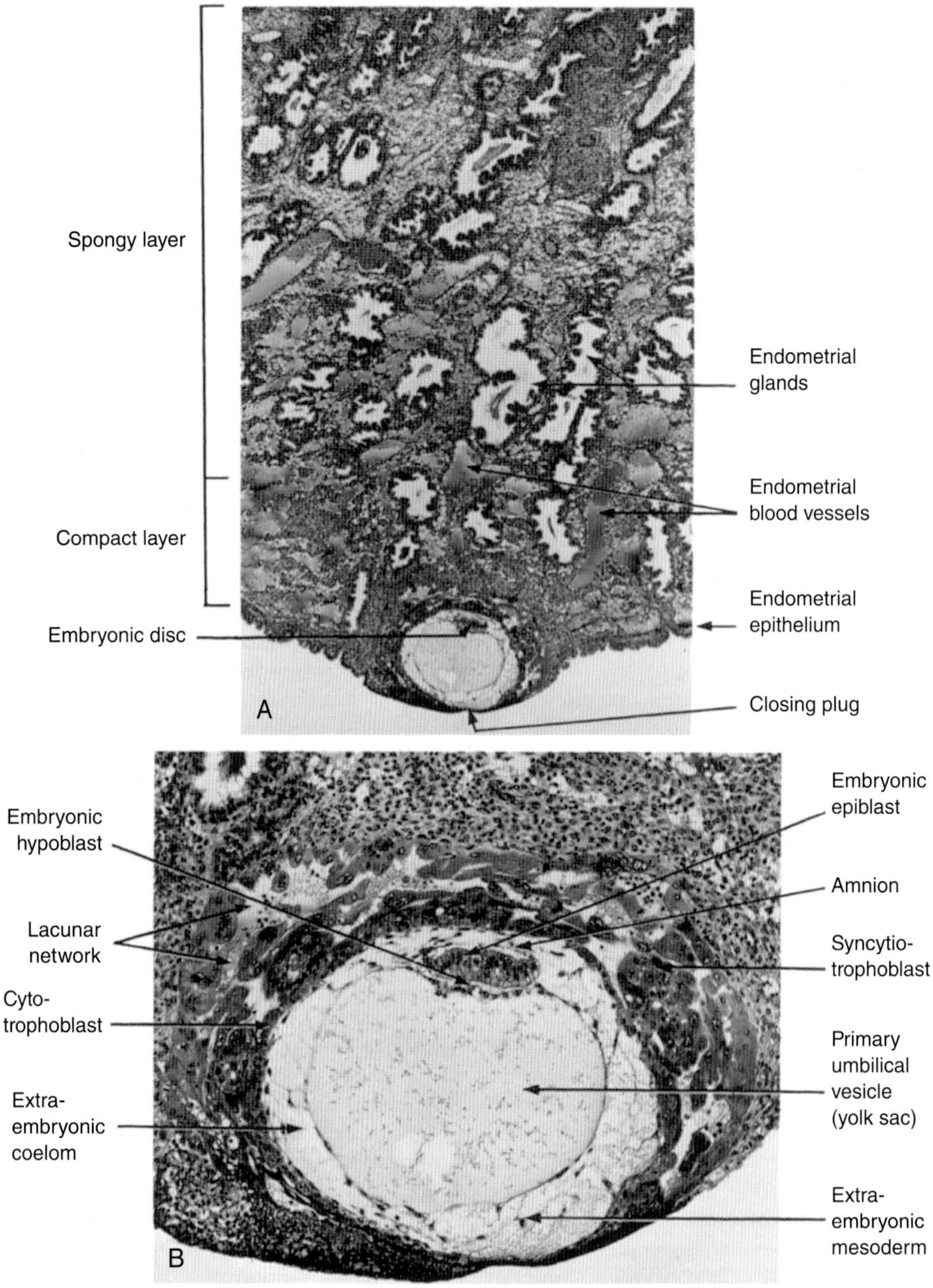

Fig. 3.4 Embedded blastocyst. (A) Section through the implantation site of the 12-day embryo described in Fig. 3.3. The embryo is embedded superficially in the compact layer of the endometrium (×30). (B) Higher magnification of the conceptus and uterine endometrium surrounding it (×100). Lacunae (small cavities) containing maternal blood are visible in the syncytiotrophoblast.(From Hertig AT, Rock J: Two human ova of the pre-villous stage, having an ovulation age of about eleven and twelve days respectively, *Contrib Embryol Carnegie Inst* 29:127, 1941. Courtesy Carnegie Institution of Washington, DC.)

A 14-day embryo still has the form of a flat **bilaminar embryonic disc** (Fig. 3.7B; see Fig. 3.5C), but the **hypoblastic endodermal cells** in a localized area are now columnar and form a uniquely thickened circular area, the **prechordal plate** (see Fig. 3.5B and C). This plate indicates the site of the primordial mouth and is an important organizer of the head region.

(simultaneous intrauterine and extrauterine pregnancies) are unusual, occurring in less than 1 in 30,000 naturally conceived pregnancies. The incidence is much higher (approximately 5%) in females treated with **ovulation induction drugs** as part of assisted reproductive technologies. The ectopic pregnancy is masked initially by the presence of the uterine pregnancy. Usually, the ectopic pregnancy can be terminated by surgical removal of the involved uterine tube without interfering with the intrauterine pregnancy (see Fig. 3.10).

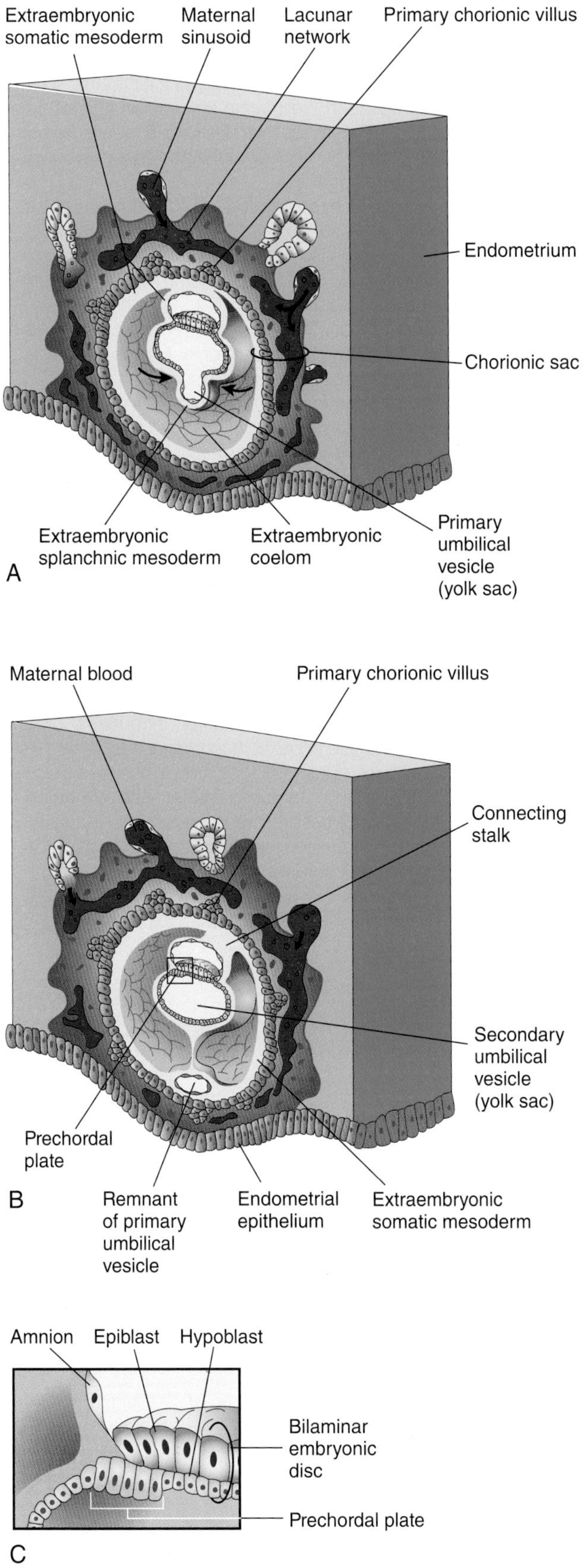

Fig. 3.5 Drawings of sections of implanted human embryos, based mainly on the studies of Hertig and colleagues (1956). Observe that (1) the defect in the endometrial epithelium has disappeared; (2) a small secondary umbilical vesicle has formed; (3) a large cavity, the extraembryonic coelom, now surrounds the umbilical vesicle and amnion, except where the amnion is attached to the chorion by the connecting stalk; and (4) the extraembryonic coelom splits the extraembryonic mesoderm into two layers: the extraembryonic somatic mesoderm lining the trophoblast and covering the amnion and the extraembryonic splanchnic mesoderm around the umbilical vesicle. (A) A 13-day embryo, illustrating the decrease in the relative size of the primary umbilical vesicle and the early appearance of primary chorionic villi. (B) A 14-day embryo, showing the newly formed secondary umbilical vesicle and the location of the prechordal plate in its roof. (C) Detail of the prechordal plate outlined in (B).

Extrauterine Implantations

Blastocysts sometimes implant outside the uterus resulting in **ectopic pregnancies**; 95% to 98% of ectopic implantations occur in the uterine tubes, *most often in the ampulla and isthmus* (Figs. 3.8, 3.9, and 3.10; see Fig. 2.6B). The incidence of ectopic pregnancy has increased in most countries, ranging from 1 in 80 to 1 in 250 pregnancies, depending partly on the socioeconomic level of the population. In the United States, the frequency of ectopic pregnancy is approximately 2% of all pregnancies; *tubal pregnancy is responsible for about 9% of pregnancy-related maternal deaths*.

A female with a **tubal pregnancy** has signs and symptoms of pregnancy. They may also experience abdominal pain and tenderness because of distention of the uterine tube, abnormal bleeding, and irritation of the pelvic peritoneum **(peritonitis)**. *The pain may be confused with appendicitis if the pregnancy is in the right uterine tube*. Ectopic pregnancies produce β-hCG at a slower rate than normal pregnancies; consequently, β-hCG assays may give false-negative results if performed too early. **Transvaginal ultrasonography** is valuable in the early detection of ectopic tubal pregnancies (see Fig. 3.8).

There are several causes of tubal pregnancy. They are often related to factors that delay or prevent the transport of the cleaving zygote into the uterus, including mucosal adhesions in the uterine tube or blockage of the tube resulting from **pelvic inflammatory disease**. Ectopic tubal pregnancies usually result in rupture of the uterine tube and hemorrhage into the peritoneal cavity during the first 8 weeks, followed by death of the embryo. *Tubal rupture and hemorrhage constitute a threat to the mother's life*. Surgical treatment may include salpingostomy (and pushing the conceptus out of the tube) or resection of the affected tube and conceptus (see Fig. 3.10). However, in some specific clinical circumstances, expectant management can be used effectively.

When blastocysts implant in the **isthmus of the uterine tube** (see Fig. 3.9D; Fig. 2.6B), the tube tends to rupture early because this narrow part of the tube is relatively unexpandable, and there is often extensive bleeding, probably because of the rich anastomoses between ovarian and uterine vessels in this area. When blastocysts implant in the uterine (intramural) part of the tube (see Fig. 3.9E), they may develop beyond 8 weeks before expulsion occurs. When an intramural uterine tubal pregnancy ruptures, it usually bleeds profusely.

Blastocysts that implant in the ampulla or on the fimbriae of the uterine tube (see Fig. 3.9A and Fig. 2.10A) may be expelled into the peritoneal cavity, where they usually implant in the **rectouterine pouch** (a pocket formed by the deflection of the peritoneum from the rectum to the uterus). In very exceptional cases, an **abdominal pregnancy** may continue to full term, and the fetus may be delivered alive through a laparotomy. Usually, however, the placenta attaches to abdominal organs (see Fig. 3.9G), which causes considerable intraperitoneal bleeding. *An abdominal pregnancy increases the risk of maternal death from hemorrhage* by a factor of 90 compared with an intrauterine pregnancy and seven times more than that for tubal pregnancy. In rare cases, an abdominal conceptus (embryo/fetus and membranes) dies and is not detected; the fetus becomes calcified, forming a **lithopedion** ("stone fetus").

Cervical implantations are unusual (less than 1% of all ectopic pregnancies) (see Fig. 3.9); in some cases, the placenta becomes firmly attached to the fibrous and muscular tissues of the cervix, often resulting in bleeding. Cervical ectopic pregnancy, in many cases, can be managed conservatively but may require surgical intervention, such as **hysterectomy** (excision of the uterus).

Heterotopic pregnancies (simultaneous intrauterine and extrauterine pregnancies) are unusual, occurring in less than 1 in 30,000 naturally conceived pregnancies. The incidence is much higher (approximately 5%) in females treated with **ovulation induction drugs** as part of assisted reproductive technologies. The ectopic pregnancy is masked initially by the presence of the uterine pregnancy. Usually, the ectopic pregnancy can be terminated by surgical removal of the involved uterine tube without interfering with the intrauterine pregnancy (see Fig. 3.10).

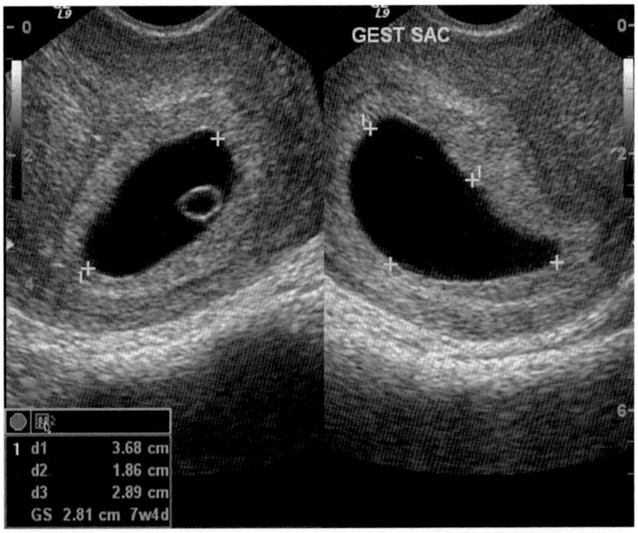

Fig. 3.6 Transvaginal sonogram (sagittal and axial) of an early chorionic sac (5 weeks) (+). The mean chorionic sac diameter is calculated from the three orthogonal measurements (*d1*, *d2*, *d3*). The secondary umbilical vesicle can also be seen in the left image.(Courtesy E.A. Lyons, MD, Professor of Radiology, Obstetrics, and Gynecology and of Anatomy, Health Sciences Centre and University of Manitoba, Winnipeg, Manitoba, Canada.)

SUMMARY OF IMPLANTATION

Implantation of the blastocyst in the uterine endometrium begins at the end of the first week (see Fig. 2.19B) and is completed by the end of the second week (see Fig. 3.2B). The cellular and molecular events relating to implantation are complex. Implantation may be summarized as follows:

- The zona pellucida degenerates (day 5). Its disappearance results from the enlargement of the blastocyst and degeneration caused by enzymatic lysis. The lytic enzymes are released from the acrosomes of sperms that surround and partially penetrate the extracellular matrix of the zona pellucida.
- The blastocyst adheres to the endometrial epithelium (day 6).
- The trophoblast differentiates into two layers, the syncytiotrophoblast and the cytotrophoblast (day 7).
- The syncytiotrophoblast erodes endometrial tissues, and the blastocyst begins to embed in the endometrium (day 8).

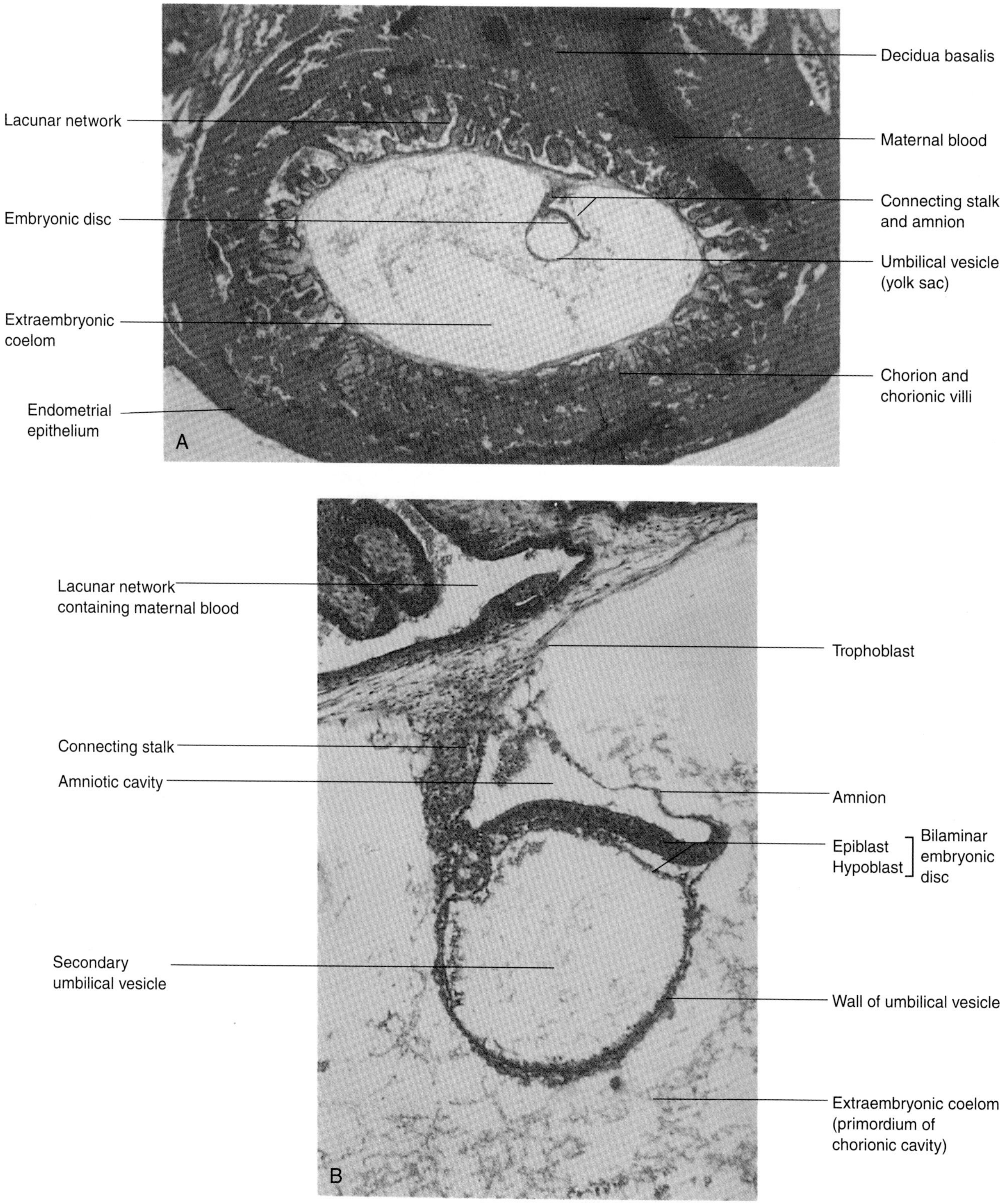

Fig. 3.7 Photomicrographs of longitudinal sections of an embedded 14-day embryo. Note the large size of the extraembryonic coelom. (A) Low-power view (×18). (B) High-power view (×95). Note the bilaminar embryonic disc composed of epiblast and hypoblast.(From Nishimura H, editor: *Atlas of human prenatal histology*, Tokyo, Igaku-Shoin, 1983.)

- Blood-filled lacunae appear in the syncytiotrophoblast (day 9).
- The blastocyst sinks beneath the endometrial epithelium, and the defect is filled by a closing plug (day 10).
- Lacunar networks form by fusion of adjacent lacunae (days 10 and 11).
- The syncytiotrophoblast erodes endometrial blood vessels, allowing maternal blood to seep in and out of lacunar

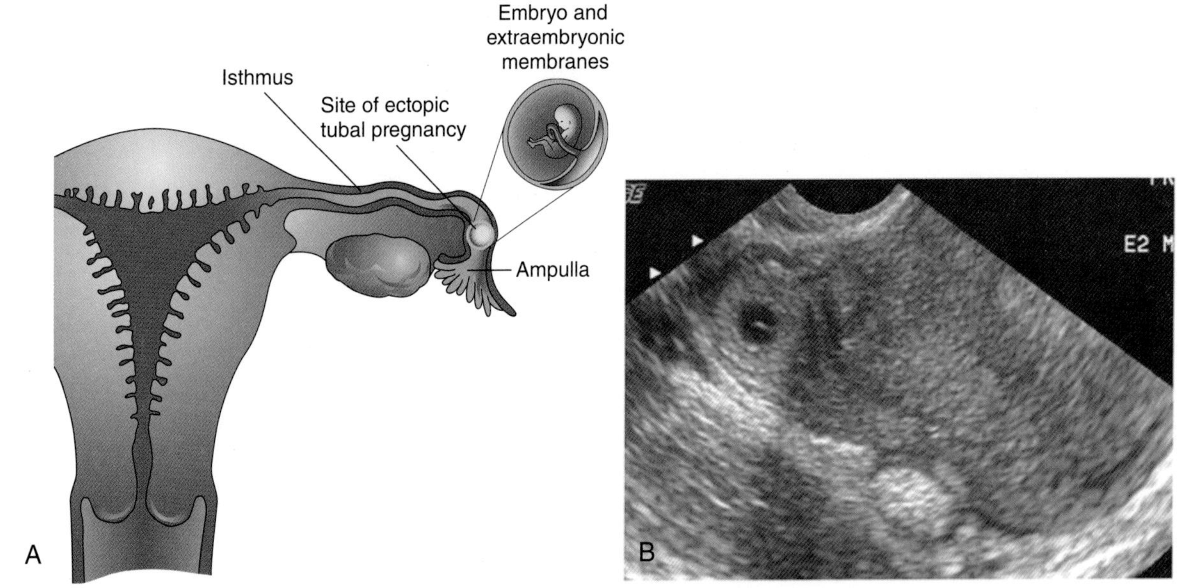

Fig. 3.8 (A) Frontal section of the uterus and left uterine tube, illustrating an ectopic pregnancy in the ampulla of the tube. (B) Ectopic tubal pregnancy. Transvaginal axial sonogram of the uterine fundus and isthmic portion of the right uterine tube. The dark ring-like mass is a 4-week ectopic chorionic sac in the tube.(Courtesy E.A. Lyons, MD, Professor of Radiology, Obstetrics, and Gynecology and of Anatomy, Health Sciences Centre and University of Manitoba, Winnipeg, Manitoba, Canada.)

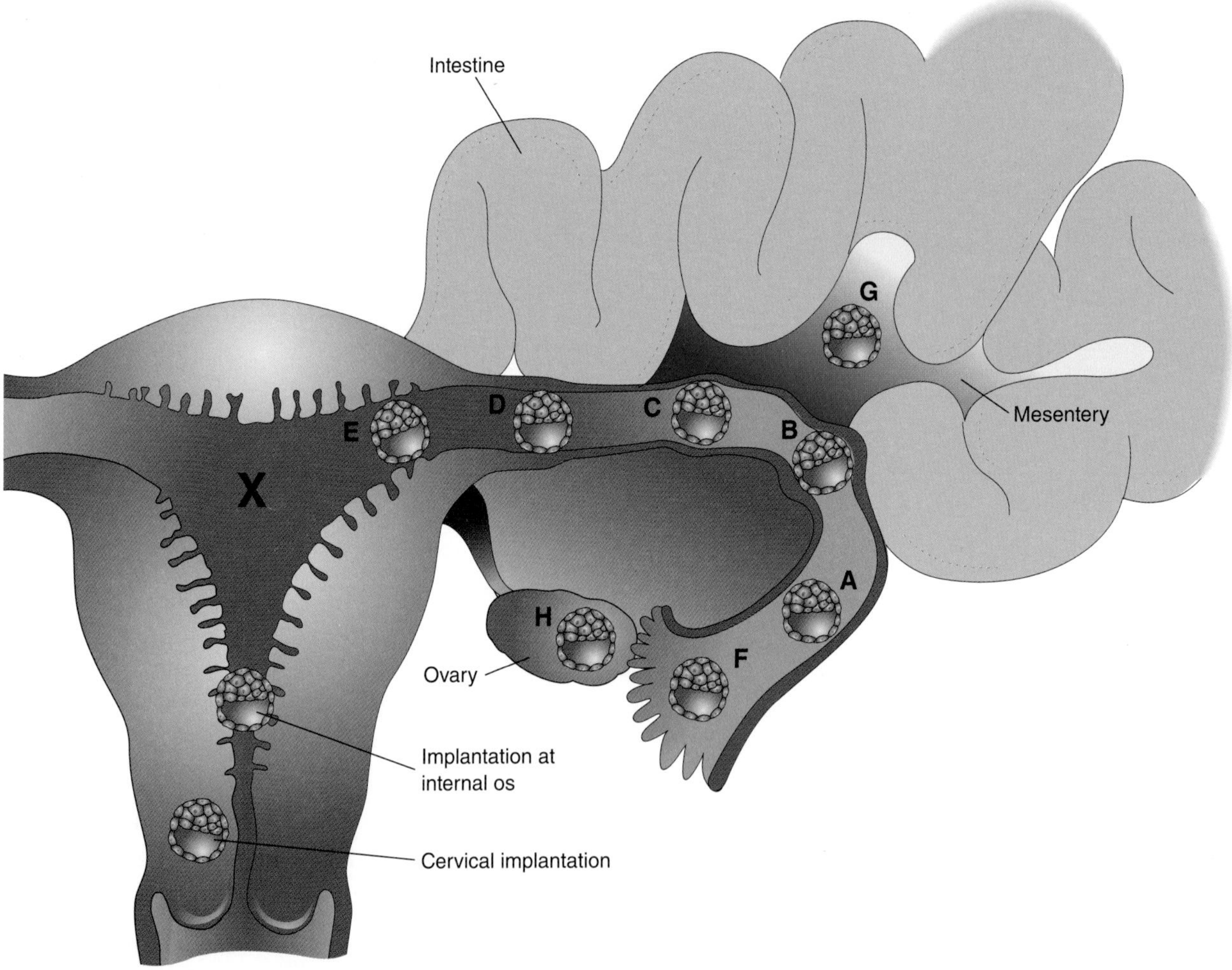

Fig. 3.9 Implantation sites of blastocysts. The usual site in the posterior wall of the body of the uterus is indicated by an X. The approximate order of frequency of ectopic implantations is indicated alphabetically (*A*, most common; *H*, least common). (*A* to *F*) Tubal pregnancies; (*G*) abdominal pregnancy; (*H*) ovarian pregnancy. Tubal pregnancies are the most common type of ectopic pregnancy. Although appropriately included with uterine pregnancy sites, a cervical pregnancy is often considered to be an ectopic pregnancy.

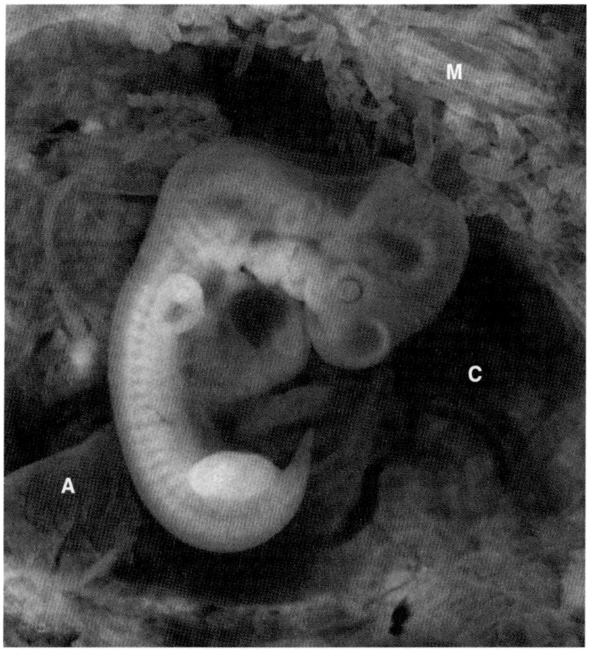

Fig. 3.10 Tubal pregnancy. The uterine tube has been surgically removed and sectioned to show the 5-week-old embryo (10-mm crown–rump length) within the opened chorionic sac (*C*). *Note the fragments of the amnion (A) and the thin mucosal folds (M) of the uterine tube projecting into the lumen of the tube.*(Courtesy Ed Uthman, MD, Pathologist, Houston/Richmond, Texas.)

Placenta Previa

Implantation of a blastocyst in the inferior segment of the uterus near the internal os (opening) of the cervix results in placenta previa, a placenta that partially or completely covers the os (see Fig. 3.9). Placenta previa may cause bleeding because of premature separation of the placenta during pregnancy or at the time of delivery of the fetus (see Chapter 7).

Abortion

Abortion is a premature stoppage of the development and expulsion of a conceptus from the uterus or the expulsion of an embryo or fetus before it is viable (capable of living outside the uterus). An abortus is any or all the products of an abortion. There are several different types of abortion:

- **Threatened abortion** (bleeding with the possibility of abortion) is a complication in approximately 25% of clinically apparent pregnancies. Despite every effort to prevent an abortion, approximately half of these embryos ultimately abort.
- **Spontaneous abortion (miscarriage)** is pregnancy loss that occurs naturally before the 20th week of gestation. It is most common during the third week after fertilization. Approximately 25% to 30% of recognized pregnancies end in spontaneous abortion, usually during the first 12 weeks. (**Early pregnancy loss** is a term used to describe pregnancy loss before the 13th week).
- **Habitual abortion** is the spontaneous expulsion of a dead or nonviable embryo or fetus in three or more consecutive pregnancies.
- **Induced abortion** is the medical termination of a pregnancy.
- **Complete abortion** is the one in which all products of conception (embryo and its membranes) are expelled from the uterus.
- **Missed abortion** is the retention of a conceptus in the uterus after the death of the embryo or fetus.

Spontaneous Abortion of Embryos and Fetuses

Spontaneous abortions (miscarriages) are the most common complication of pregnancy. It has been reported that about 30% of all pregnancies terminate in a miscarriage. Clinically, spontaneous abortions occur within the first 12 completed weeks of pregnancy, with a frequency of 25% to 30%. Moreover, 80% of embryos are spontaneously aborted during the first trimester. **Sporadic and recurrent spontaneous abortions** are two of the most common gynecologic problems. The frequency of early spontaneous abortions is difficult to establish because they often occur before a female is aware that she is pregnant, but rates of 50% to 80% have been reported. A spontaneous abortion occurring several days after the first missed period is very likely to be mistaken for delayed menstruation.

More than 50% of all known spontaneous abortions result from chromosomal abnormalities. The higher incidence of early spontaneous abortions in older females probably results from the increasing frequency of **nondisjunction during oogenesis** (see Chapter 2). In addition, events during mitosis in the first cell cycle due to DNA replication stress (e.g., double-strand breaks) may also result in aneuploidies and loss of the embryo. Failure of blastocysts to implant may result from a poorly developed endometrium and immune intolerance; however, in many cases, there are probably lethal chromosomal abnormalities in the embryo. There is a higher incidence of spontaneous abortion of fetuses with neural tube defects, cleft lip, and cleft palate. After 10 gestational weeks, 25% to 40% of spontaneous abortions are related to fetal causes, 25% to 35% to placental causes, and 5% to 10% to maternal causes, with the remainder unexplained. Recent studies indicate that increasing paternal age is also a risk factor for spontaneous abortion. Critical genetic changes include point mutations, DNA breaks and damage, genetic imprinting, and chromosomal defects with increasing age.

Inhibition of Implantation

The administration of progestins or antiprogestins (morning-after pills) for several days, beginning shortly after unprotected sexual intercourse, inhibits ovulation but may also inhibit implantation of the blastocyst.

An **intrauterine device (IUD)** usually interferes with implantation by causing a local inflammatory reaction. An IUD is typically a primary contraceptive, but copper IUDs may also be used for emergency contraception. Some IUDs contain progesterone, which is slowly released and interferes with the development of the endometrium so that implantation does not usually occur. Other IUDs have a wrap of copper wire. Copper is directly toxic to sperms and also causes uterine endothelial cells to produce substances that are toxic to sperms.

networks, thereby establishing uteroplacental circulation (days 11 and 12).

- The defect in the endometrial epithelium is repaired (days 12 and 13).
- Primary chorionic villi develop (days 13 and 14).

SUMMARY OF SECOND WEEK

- **Rapid proliferation and differentiation of the trophoblast** occur as the blastocyst completes implantation in the uterine endometrium.
- The endometrial changes resulting from the adaptation of these tissues in preparation for implantation are known as the **decidual reaction**.
- Concurrently, the **primary umbilical vesicle forms** and **extraembryonic mesoderm** develops. The extraembryonic coelom (cavity) forms from spaces that develop in the extraembryonic mesoderm. The coelom later becomes the **chorionic cavity**.
- The primary umbilical vesicle becomes smaller and gradually disappears as the **secondary umbilical vesicle develops**.
- The **amniotic cavity** appears between the cytotrophoblast and embryoblast.
- The **embryoblast differentiates** into a bilaminar embryonic disc consisting of **epiblast**, related to the amniotic cavity, and **hypoblast**, adjacent to the blastocystic cavity.
- The **prechordal plate develops** as a localized thickening of the hypoblast, which indicates the future cranial region of the embryo and the future site of the mouth; the prechordal plate is also an important organizer of the head region.

CLINICALLY ORIENTED PROBLEMS

CASE 3-1

A 22-year-old female who complained of a severe "chest cold" was sent for a radiograph of her thorax.

- Is it advisable to examine a healthy female's chest radiographically during the last week of her menstrual cycle?
- Are birth defects likely to develop in her embryo if she happens to be pregnant?

CASE 3-2

A female was given a large dose of estrogen (twice over 1 day) to interrupt a possible pregnancy.

- If fertilization had occurred, what do you think would be the mechanism of action of this hormone?
- What do laypeople commonly call this type of medical treatment? Is this what the media refer to as the "abortion pill?" If not, explain the method of action of the hormone treatment.
- How early can a pregnancy be detected?

CASE 3-3

A 23-year-old female consulted her physician about severe right lower abdominal pain. She said that she had missed two menstrual periods. A diagnosis of ectopic pregnancy was made.

- What techniques might be used to confirm this diagnosis?
- What is the most likely site of the extrauterine implantation?
- How do you think the physician would likely treat the condition?

CASE 3-4

A 30-year-old female had an appendectomy toward the end of her menstrual cycle; 8.5 months later, she had a child with a congenital anomaly of the brain.

- Could the surgery have produced this child's congenital anomaly? Explain.

CASE 3-5

A 42-year-old female became pregnant after many years of trying to conceive. She was concerned about the healthy development of her baby.

- What would the physician likely tell her?
- Can females over the age of 40 years have normal babies?
- What tests and diagnostic techniques would likely be performed?

Discussion of these problems appears in the Appendix at the back of the book.

BIBLIOGRAPHY AND SUGGESTED READING

Bianchi DW, Wilkins-Haug LE, Enders AC, et al: Origin of extraembryonic mesoderm in experimental animals: relevance to chorionic mosaicism in humans, *Am J Med Genet* 46:542, 1993.

Brosens JJ, Bennett PR, Abrahams VM, et al: Maternal selection of human embryos in early gestation: insights from recurrent miscarriage, *Semin Cell Dev Biol*, 2022.https://doi.org/10.1016/j.semcdb.2022.01.007.

Carleton AE, Duncan MC, Taniguchi K: Human epiblast lumenogenesis: From a cell aggregate to a luminal cyst, *Sem Cell Dev Biol* 131:117, 2022.

Dickey RP, Gasser R, Olar TT, et al: Relationship of initial chorionic sac diameter to abortion and abortus karyotype based on new growth curves for the 16 to 49 post-ovulation day, *Hum Reprod* 9:559, 1994.

du Fosse NA, van der Hoorn MP, Van Lith JMM, et al: Advanced paternal age is associated with an increased risk of spontaneous miscarriage: a systematic review and meta-analysis, *Hum Reprod Update* 26:650, 2020.

Enders AC, King BF: Formation and differentiation of extraembryonic mesoderm in the rhesus monkey, *Am J Anat* 181:327, 1988.

Firmin J, Maitre J-L: Morphogenesis of the human preimplantation embryo: bringing mechanics to the clinic, *Semin Cell Dev Biol* 120:22–31, 2021.https://doi.org/10.1016/j.semcdb.2021.07.005.

FitzPatrick DR: Human embryogenesis. In Magowan BA, Owen P, Thomson A, editors: *Clinical obstetrics and gynaecology*, ed 3, Philadelphia, 2014, Saunders.

Gaillard F, Bandura P: Ectopic pregnancy. https://radiopaedia.org; https://doi.org/10.53347/rID-1258

Galliano D, Pellicer A: MicroRNA and implantation, *Fertil Steril* 101:1531, 2014.

Gauster M, Wernitznig M, Moser S, et al: Early human trophoblast development: from morphology to function, *Cell Mol Life Sci* 79(6):345, 2022.https://doi.org/10.1007/s00018-022-04377-0.

Hendriks E, Rosenberg R, Prine L: Ectopic pregnancy: diagnosis and management, *Am Fam Phys* 101(10):599–606, 2020.

Hertig AT, Rock J: Two human ova of the pre-villous stage, having a development age of about seven and nine days respectively, *Contrib Embryol Carnegie Inst* 31:65, 1945.

Hertig AT, Rock J: Two human ova of the pre-villous stage, having a developmental age of about eight and nine days, respectively, *Contrib Embryol Carnegie Inst* 33:169, 1949.

Hertig AT, Rock J, Adams EC: A description of 34 human ova within the first seventeen days of development, *Am J Anat* 98:435, 1956.

Hertig AT, Rock J, Adams EC, et al: Thirty-four fertilized human ova, good, bad, and indifferent, recovered from 210 women of known fertility, *Pediatrics* 23:202, 1959.

Levine D: Ectopic pregnancy. In Callen PW, editor: *Ultrasonography in obstetrics and gynecology*, ed 5, Philadelphia, 2008, Saunders.

Lindsay DJ, Lovett IS, Lyons EA, et al: Endovaginal sonography: yolk sac diameter and shape as a predictor of pregnancy outcome in the first trimester, *Radiology* 183:115, 1992.
Luckett WP: Origin and differentiation of the yolk sac and extraembryonic mesoderm in presomite human and rhesus monkey embryos, *Am J Anat* 152:59, 1978.
Madero JI, Manotas MC, García-Acero M, et al: Preimplantation genetic testing in assisted reproduction, *Minerva Obstet Gynecol*, 2021.https://doi.org/10.23736/S2724-606X.21.04805-3.
Monsivais D, Clementi C, Peng J, et al: BMP7 induces uterine receptivity and blastocyst attachment, *Endocrinology* 158:979, 2017.
Muter J, Lynch VJ, McCoy RC, Brosens JJ: Human embryo implantation, *Development* 150(10):dev201507, 2023.https://doi.org/10.1242/dev.201507. Epub 2023 May 31. PMID: 37254877.oted.
Nogales FF, editor: *The human yolk sac and yolk sac tumors*, New York, 1993, Springer-Verlag.
Palmerola KL, Amrane S, De Los Angeles A, et al: Replication stress impairs chromosome segregation and preimplantation development on human embryos, *Cell* 185:1, 2022.
Rossant J, Tam PPL: Early human embryonic development: blastocyst formation to gastrulation, *Develop Cell* 57:152, 2022.
Saravelos SH, Regan L: Unexplained recurrent pregnancy loss, *Obstet Gynecol Clin North Am* 41:157, 2014.
Streeter GL: Developmental horizons in human embryos. Description of age group XI, 13 to 20 somites, and age group XII, 21 to 29 somites, *Contrib Embryol Carnegie Inst* 30:211, 1942.
Tulandi T: Ectopic pregnancy: clinical manifestations and diagnosis. https://www.wolterskluwer.com/en/know/clinical-effectiveness-terms; ©2022 *UpTo Date.*
You Y, Stelzl P, Joseph DN, et al: THF-alpha regulate endometrial soma secretome promotes trophoblast invasion, *Front Immunol* 12(12):737401, 2021.https://doi.org/10.3389/fimmu.2021.737401.
Zhai J, Xiao Z, Wang Y, Wang H: Human embryonic development: from peri-implantation to gastrulation, *Trends Cell Biol* 32(1):18–29, 2022.

Third Week of Human Development

4

CHAPTER OUTLINE

The rapid development of the embryo from the **trilaminar embryonic disc** during the third week (see Fig. 4.3H) is characterized by:

- Appearance of primitive streak
- Development of notochord
- Differentiation of three germ layers

The third week of development coincides with the week after the first missed menstrual period, that is, 5 weeks after the first day of the last normal menstrual period. *Cessation of menstruation is often the first indication that a female may be pregnant.* At this time, a normal pregnancy can be detected with ultrasonography (Fig. 4.1).

Pregnancy Symptoms

Frequent symptoms of pregnancy are nausea and vomiting, which may occur by the end of the third week; however, the time of onset of these symptoms varies. Vaginal bleeding at the expected time of menstruation does not rule out pregnancy—**implantation bleeding** results from leakage of blood from the closing plug into the uterine cavity from disrupted **lacunar networks** in the implanted blastocyst (see Figs. 3.2A and 3.5A). When bleeding is interpreted as menstruation, an error occurs in determining the expected delivery date of the fetus.

4

GASTRULATION: FORMATION OF GERM LAYERS

Gastrulation is a formative process by which the three germ layers, which are precursors of all embryonic tissues, and the axial orientation are established in embryos. During gastrulation, the bilaminar embryonic disc is transformed into a **trilaminar embryonic disc** (see Fig. 4.3H). Extensive cell-shape changes, rearrangement, morphogenetic movement, and alterations in the extracellular matrix and adhesive properties contribute to the process of gastrulation.

Gastrulation is the beginning of **morphogenesis** (development of body form) and is the most significant event occurring during the third week. The molecular events that are critical in human gastrulation remain largely unknown. Because of ethical and legal reasons, early human embryos are not been readily available for research purposes. Some insights have been gained from utilizing pluripotent stem cell model systems, aborted embryos, embryonic tissues cultured, and donated embryos from others remaining after successful in vitro fertilization. The protein-coding genes *TBXT (Brachury), CDH (cadherin 1), FST (follistatin), BMPs (bone morphogenetic proteins), SOX 17 (CRY-box transcription factor), FGF (fibroblast growth factor), SNAI2 (spherical nucleic acid nanoparticle 12)* have been detected in the embryonic germ layers and play a critical role in gastrulation.

Each of the three germ layers (ectoderm, mesoderm, and endoderm) (Fig. 4.2) gives rise to specific tissues and organs:

- **Embryonic ectoderm** gives rise to the epidermis, central and peripheral nervous systems, eyes and internal ears, neural crest cells, and many connective tissues of the head.

- **Embryonic mesoderm** gives rise to all skeletal muscles, blood cells, the lining of blood vessels, all visceral smooth muscular coats, serosal linings of all body cavities, ducts and organs of the reproductive and excretory systems, and most of the cardiovascular system. In the body (trunk), excluding the head and limbs, it is the source of all connective tissues, including cartilage, bones, tendons, ligaments, dermis, and stroma (connective tissue) of internal organs.

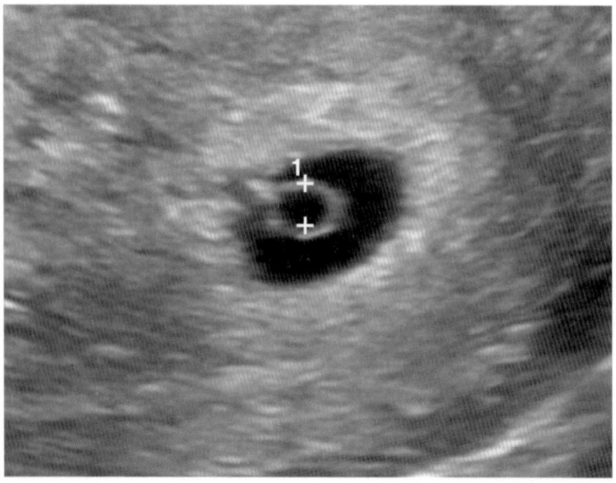

Fig. 4.1 Ultrasonograph sonogram of a 3.5-week conceptus. Note the secondary umbilical vesicle *(calipers)* and the surrounding trophoblast *(1, bright ring of tissue)*. (Courtesy E.A. Lyons, MD, Professor of Radiology and Obstetrics and Gynecology, Health Sciences Centre and University of Manitoba, Winnipeg, Manitoba, Canada.)

- **Embryonic endoderm** is the source of the epithelial linings of the respiratory and alimentary (digestive) tracts, including the glands opening into the gastrointestinal tract, and glandular cells of associated organs such as the liver and pancreas. *Transcription factors X17, GATA6, FOXA2, and TTR appear to be essential for the development of the endoderm.*

PRIMITIVE STREAK

4

Gastrulation begins with the formation of the **primitive streak** on the surface of the **epiblast** of the bilaminar embryonic disc (Fig. 4.3A–C). By the beginning of the third week, this thickened linear band of epiblast appears caudally in the median plane of the dorsal aspect of the embryonic disc (Fig. 4.4A and B and see Fig. 4.3C). The primitive streak results from the proliferation and convergence of cells of the epiblast to the median plane (midline) of the embryonic disc. As the primitive streak appears, it extends to the anterior region of the embryonic disc. At this stage, it is possible to identify the embryo's craniocaudal axis, cranial and caudal ends, dorsal and ventral surfaces, and right and left sides. As the streak elongates by the addition of cells to its caudal end, its cranial end proliferates to form the **primitive node** (see Figs. 4.3E and F and 4.4A and B).

Concurrently, the **primitive groove** (Figs. 4.4B and 4.5D) develops in the primitive streak; the groove is continuous with a small depression in the primitive node, the **primitive pit**. The primitive groove and pit result from the invagination of epiblastic cells (indicated by arrows in Fig. 4.3E).

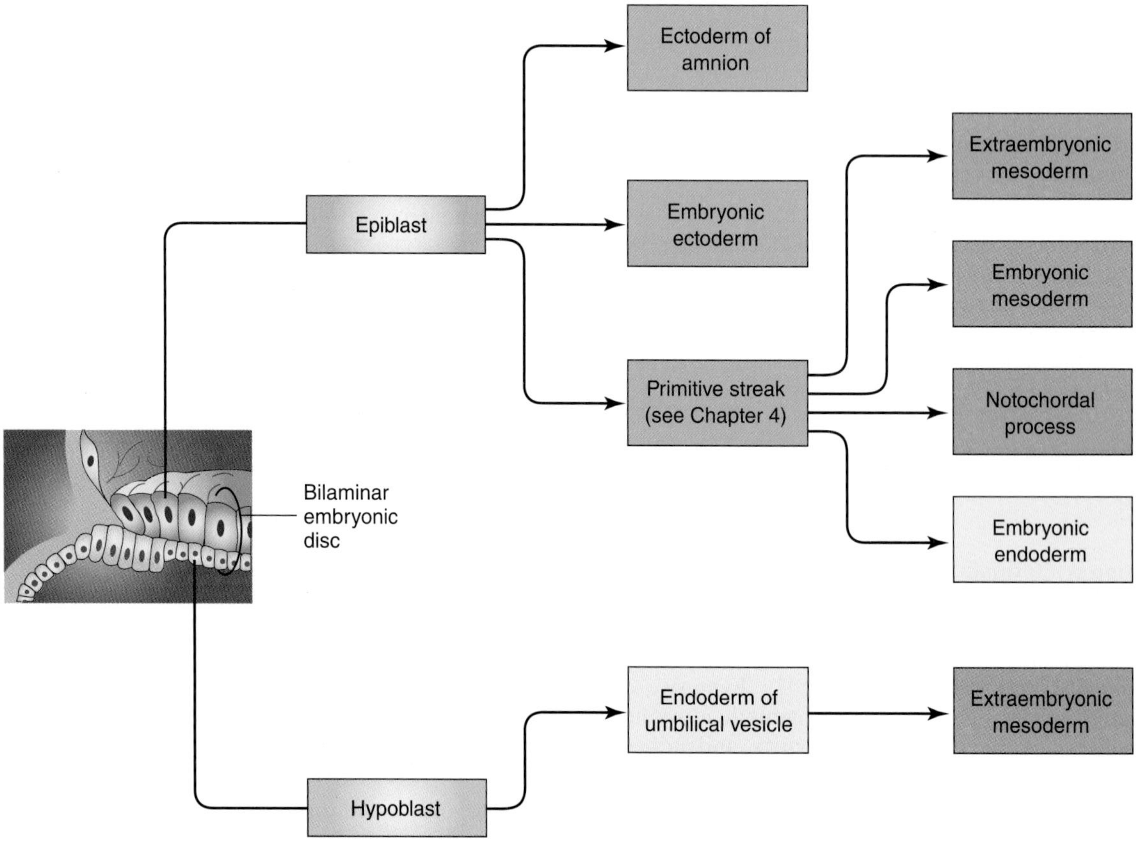

Fig. 4.2 Origin of embryonic tissues. The colors in the boxes are used in drawings of sections of embryos.

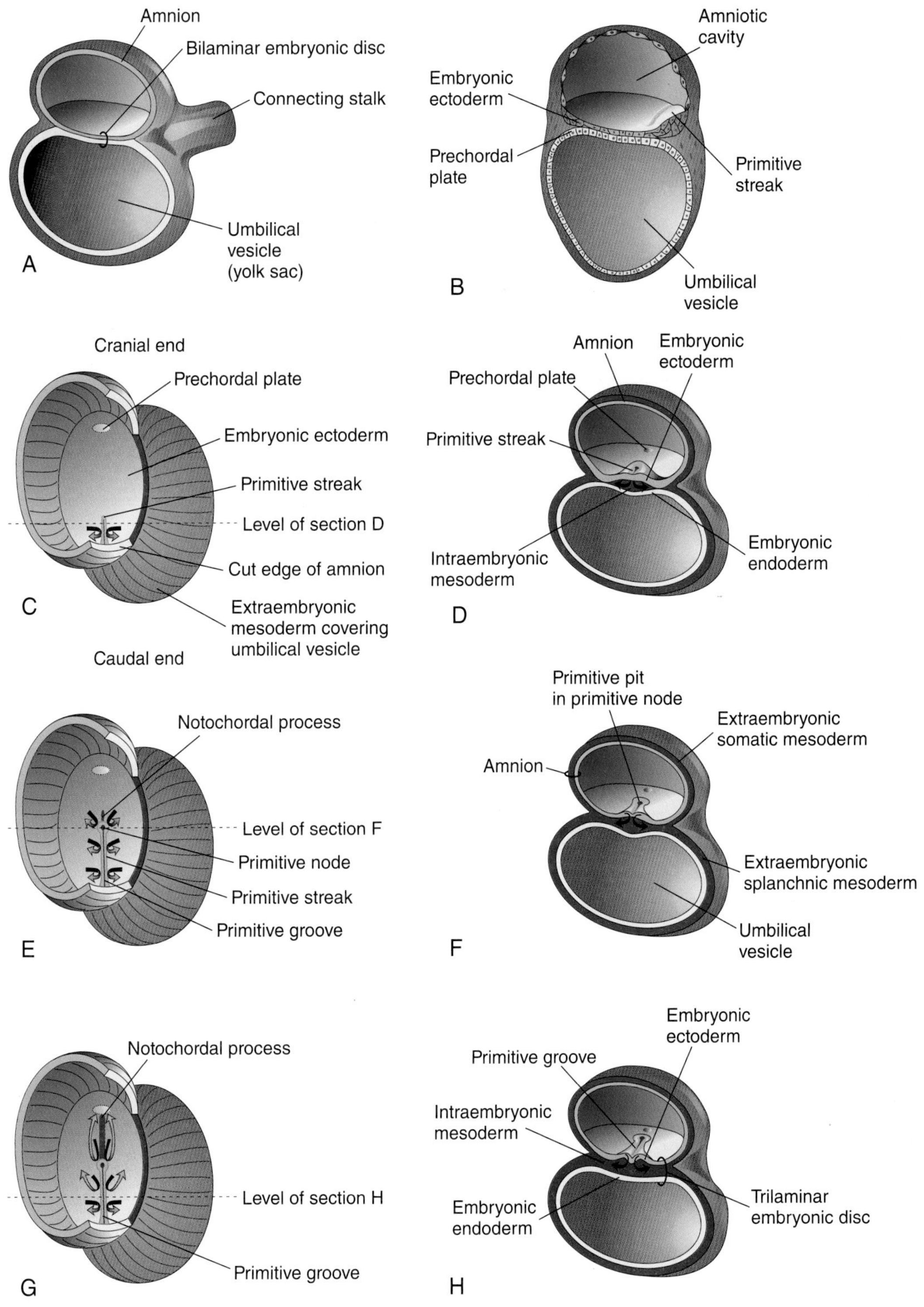

Fig. 4.3 Illustrations of the formation of the trilaminar embryonic disc (days 15–16). The *arrows* indicate the invagination and migration of mesenchymal cells from the primitive streak between the ectoderm and endoderm. (C, E, and G) Dorsal views of the trilaminar embryonic disc early in the third week, exposed by removal of the amnion. (A, B, D, F, and H) Transverse sections through the embryonic disc. The levels of the sections are indicated in (C, E, and G). The prechordal plate, indicating the head region in (C), is indicated by a light blue oval because this thickening of endoderm cannot be seen from the dorsal surface.

Shortly after the primitive streak appears, cells leave its deep surface and form **mesenchyme**, an embryonic connective tissue consisting of small, spindle-shaped cells loosely arranged in an extracellular matrix of sparse collagen (reticular) fibers (Fig. 4.5B). Mesenchyme forms the supporting tissues of the embryo, such as most of the connective tissues of the body and the framework of glands. Some mesenchyme forms **mesoblast** (undifferentiated mesoderm), which forms intraembryonic mesoderm (see Fig. 4.3D).

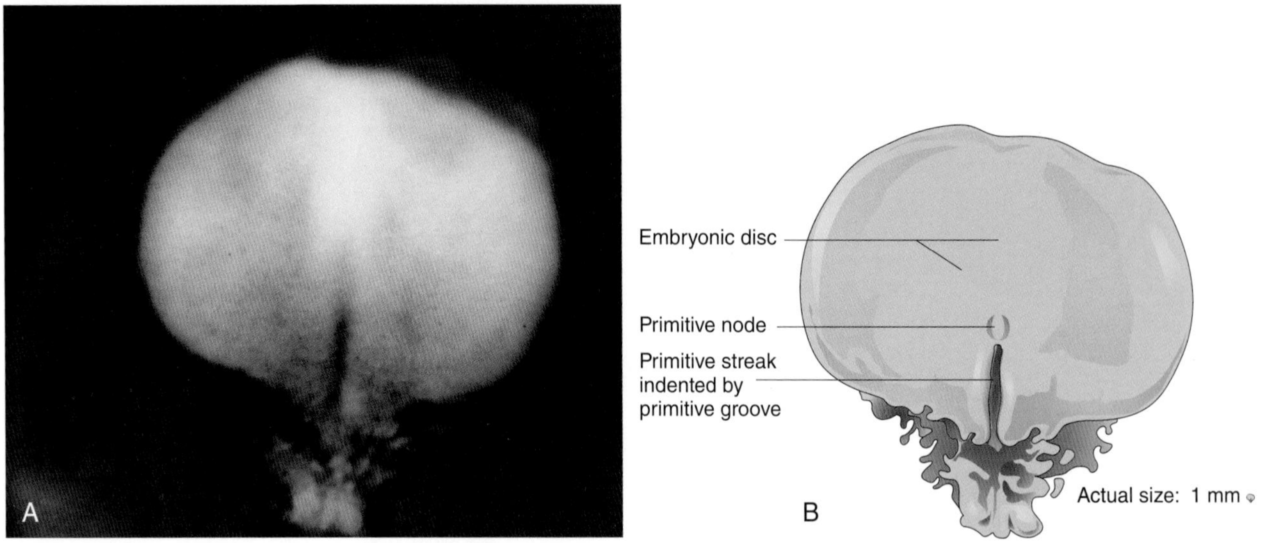

Fig. 4.4 (A) Dorsal view of an embryo approximately 16 days old. (B) Drawing of structures shown in (A). (A) From Moore KL, Persaud TVN, Shiota K: *Color atlas of clinical embryology*, ed 2, Philadelphia, 2000, Saunders.)

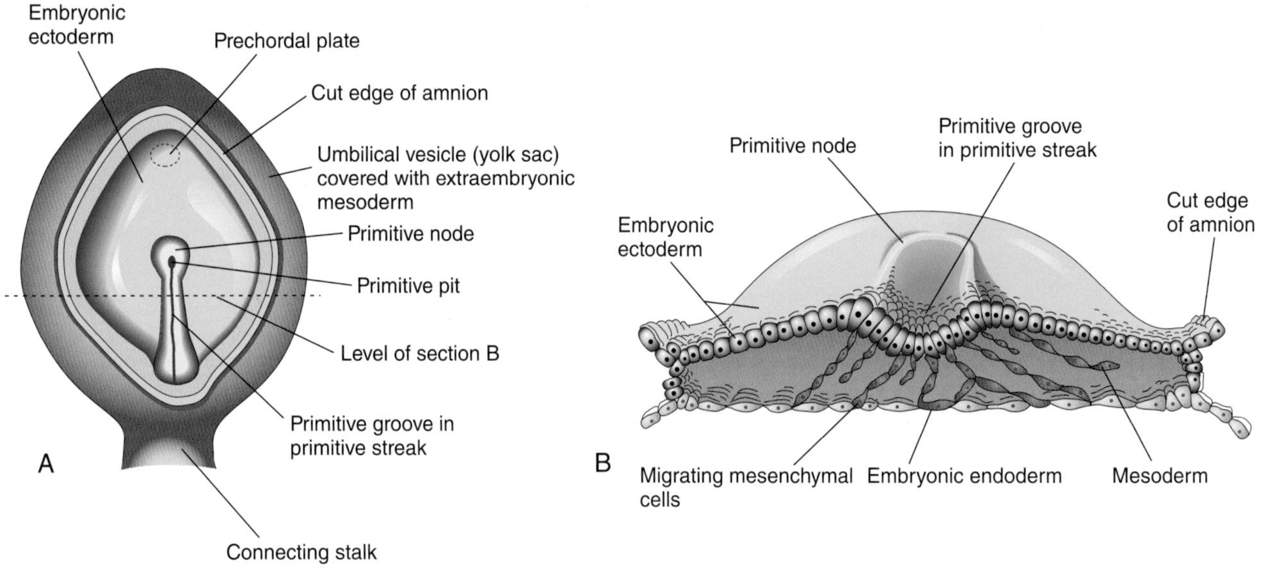

Fig. 4.5 (A) Drawing of a dorsal view of a 16-day embryo. The amnion has been removed to expose the primitive node, primitive pit, and primitive streak. (B) Drawing of the cranial half of the embryonic disc. The trilaminar embryonic disc has been cut transversely to show the migration of mesenchymal cells from the primitive streak to form a mesoblast that soon organizes to form the intraembryonic mesoderm. This illustration also shows that most of the embryonic endoderm also arises from the epiblast. Most of the hypoblastic cells are displaced to extraembryonic regions, such as the wall of the umbilical vesicle.

Cells from the epiblast, as well as from the primitive node and other parts of the primitive streak, displace and intercalate with the hypoblast, forming an **embryonic endoderm** in the roof of the umbilical vesicle (see Fig. 4.3H). The cells remaining in the epiblast form the **embryonic ectoderm**.

Research data suggest that signaling molecules (nodal factors) of the transforming growth factor-β superfamily induce the formation of mesoderm. The concerted action of other signaling molecules (e.g., Wnt3a, Wnt5a, and FGFs) also participates in specifying the fates of the germ cell layers. Moreover, transforming growth factor-β (nodal), a T-box transcription factor (veg T), and the Wnt signaling pathway appear to be involved in the specification of the endoderm

Mesenchymal cells derived from the primitive streak migrate widely. These pluripotential cells differentiate into diverse types of cells, such as fibroblasts, chondroblasts, and osteoblasts (see Chapter 5).

FATE OF PRIMITIVE STREAK

The primitive streak actively forms mesoderm until the early part of the fourth week; thereafter, production of mesoderm slows down. The primitive streak diminishes in relative size and becomes an insignificant structure in the sacrococcygeal region of the embryo (Fig. 4.6). Normally, the primitive streak undergoes degenerative changes and disappears by the end of the fourth week.

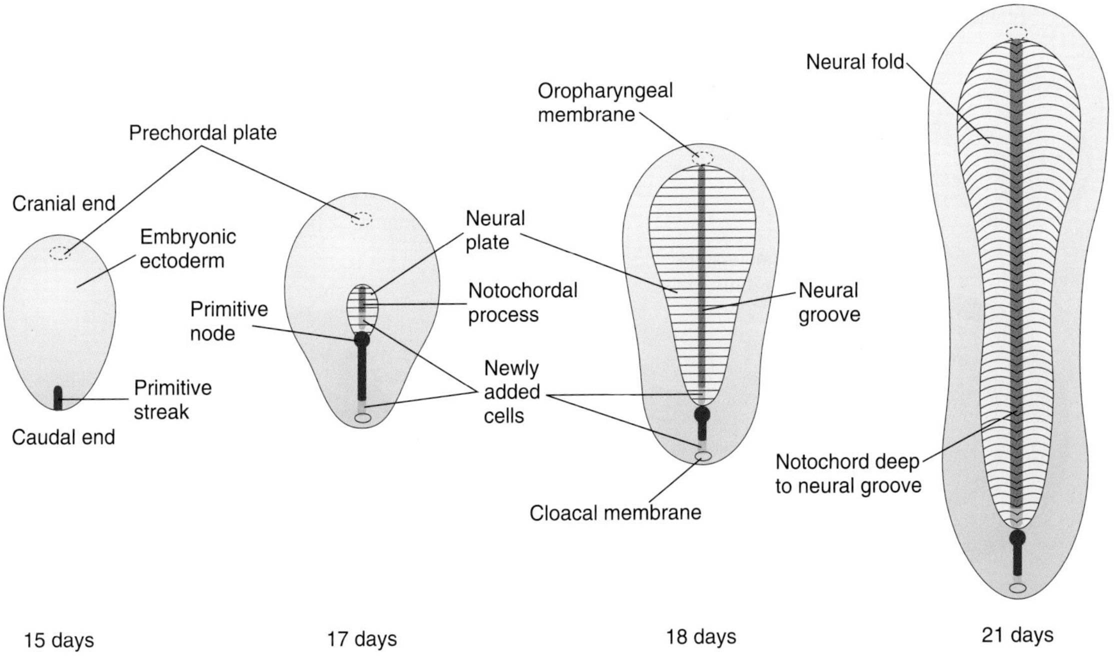

Fig. 4.6 Diagrammatic sketches of dorsal views of the embryonic disc, showing how it lengthens and changes shape during the third week. The primitive streak lengthens by the addition of cells at its caudal end, and the notochordal process lengthens by the migration of cells from the primitive node. The notochordal process and adjacent mesoderm induce the overlying embryonic ectoderm to form the neural plate, the primordium of the central nervous system. Observe that as the notochordal process elongates, the primitive streak shortens. At the end of the third week, the notochordal process is transformed into the notochord.

Sacrococcygeal Teratoma

Remnants of the primitive streak may persist and give rise to a **sacrococcygeal teratoma** (Fig 4.7). A teratoma is a germ cell tumor that may be benign or malignant. Because they are derived from pluripotent primitive streak cells, the tumors contain tissues derived from all three germ layers at varying stages of differentiation. These teratomas are the most common tumors in neonates and have an incidence of approximately 1 in 35,000. Most affected infants (80%) are females. Typically, cases of sacrococcygeal teratomas (50%–82%) are diagnosed during the first trimester on routine ultrasonography. Magnetic resonance imaging may also be used to determine the important features of the tumor. These tumors are typically benign and are usually surgically excised because the final neonatal outcome is dependent on other factors. The mortality of fetuses diagnosed antenatally with sacrococcygeal teratoma is relatively high (>32%) because of pregnancy termination.

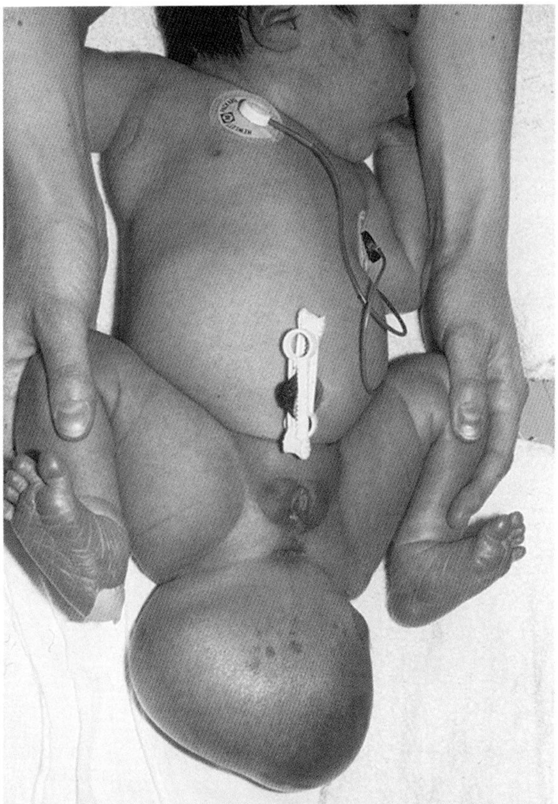

Fig. 4.7 Female infant with a large sacrococcygealteratoma that developed from remnants of the primitive streak. The tumor, a neoplasm made up of several different types of tissue, was surgically removed. (Courtesy A. E. Chudley, MD, Section of Genetics and Metabolism, Department of Pediatrics and Child Health, Children's Hospital and University of Manitoba, Winnipeg, Manitoba, Canada.)

4

NOTOCHORDAL PROCESS AND NOTOCHORD

Some mesenchymal cells migrate through the primitive streak and, as a consequence, acquire mesodermal cell fates. These cells migrate cranially from the primitive node and pit, forming a median cellular cord, the **notochordal process,** which soon acquires a lumen, the **notochordal canal** (Fig. 4.8C–E). The notochordal process grows cranially between the ectoderm and endoderm until it reaches the **prechordal plate** (see Fig. 4.8A and C), a small circular area of thickened columnar endodermal cells where the ectoderm and

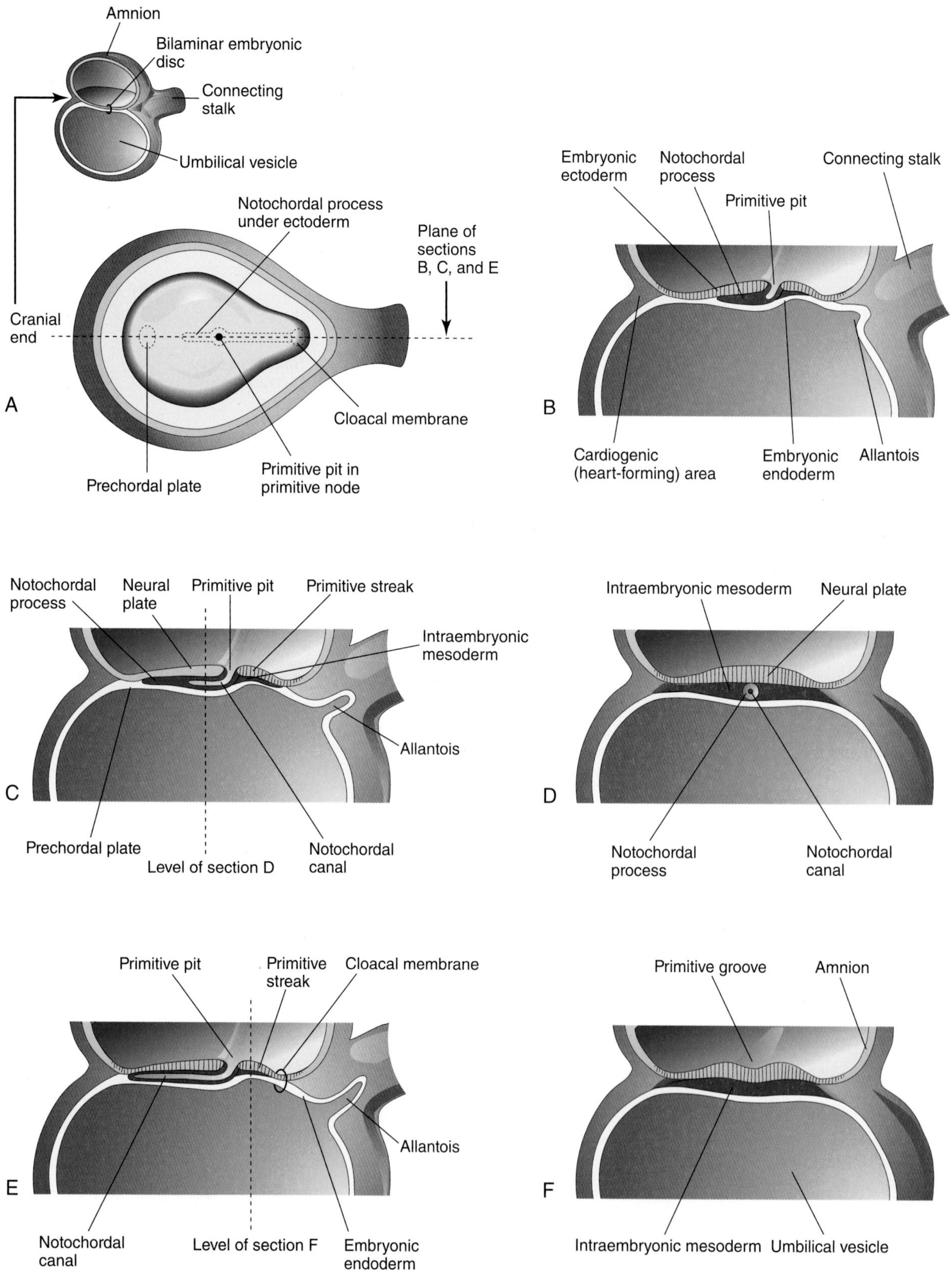

Fig. 4.8 Illustrations of developing notochordal process. The small sketch at the upper left is for orientation. (A) Dorsal view of the embryonic disc (approximately 16 days) exposed by removal of the amnion. The notochordal process is shown as if it were visible through the embryonic ectoderm. (B, C, and E) Median sections at the plane shown in (A) illustrating successive stages in the development of the notochordal process and canal. The stages shown in (C and E) occur at approximately 18 days. (D and F) Transverse sections through the embryonic disc at the levels shown in (C and E).

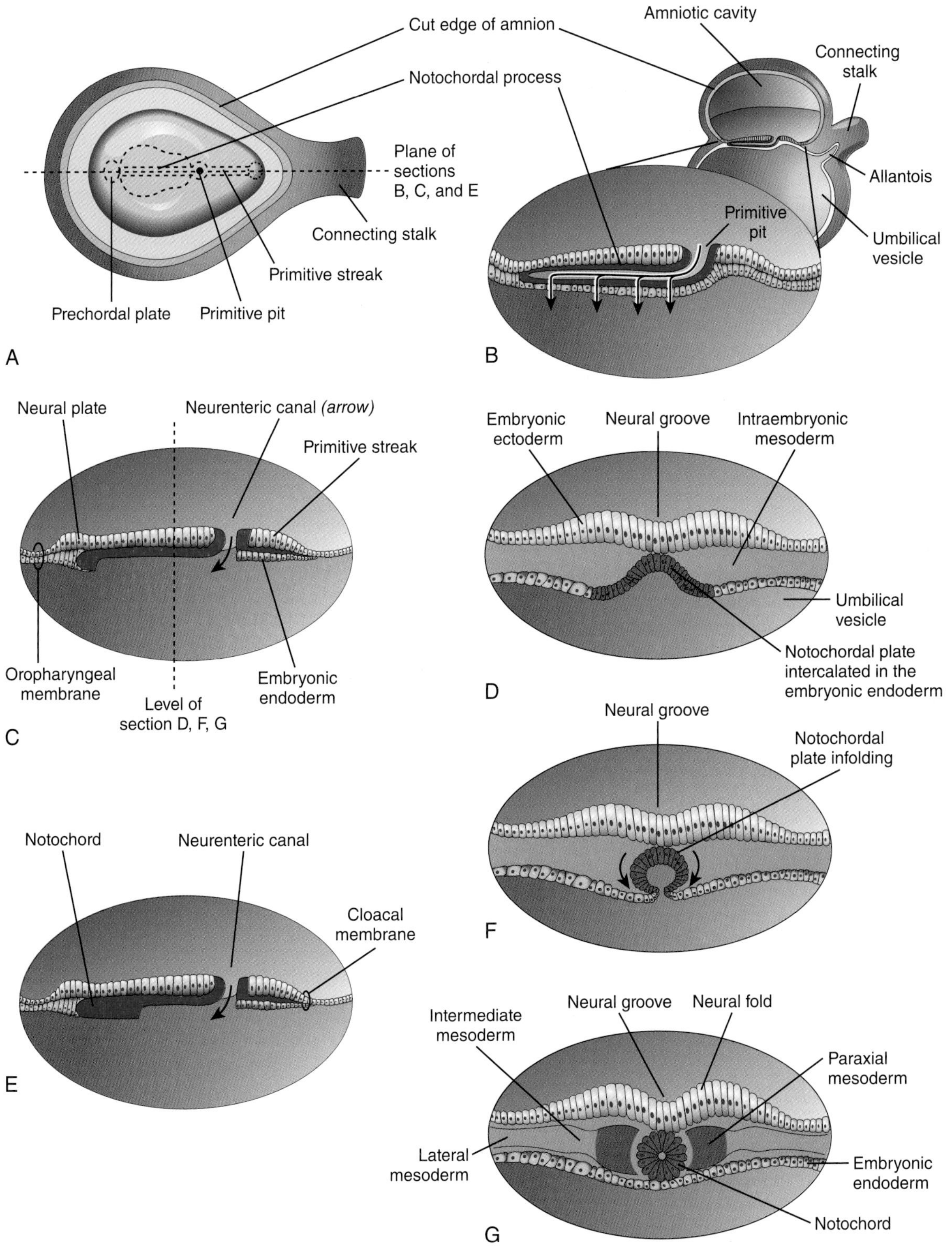

Fig. 4.9 Illustrations of notochord development by transformation of the notochordal process. (A) Dorsal view of the bilaminar embryonic disc at 18 days, exposed by removing the amnion. (B) Three-dimensional median section of the embryo. (C and E) Similar sections of slightly older embryos. (D, F, and G) Transverse sections of the trilaminar embryonic disc at the levels shown in (C and E).

endoderm are fused. The **prechordal plate** gives rise to the endoderm of the **oropharyngeal membrane**, located at the future site of the oral cavity (Fig. 4.9C). *The prechordal plate serves as a signaling center (Shh and PAX6) for controlling the development of cranial structures, including the forebrain and eyes.*

Mesenchymal cells from the primitive streak and notochordal process migrate laterally and cranially, among other mesodermal cells between the ectoderm and endoderm, until they reach the margins of the embryonic disc. These cells are continuous with the extraembryonic mesoderm covering the amnion and umbilical vesicle (Fig. 4.3). Some mesenchymal cells from the primitive streak that have mesodermal fates migrate cranially on each side of the notochordal process and around the prechordal plate (see Fig. 4.5A and C). Here they meet cranially to form the cardiogenic mesoderm in the **cardiogenic area**, where the **heart primordium** begins to develop at the end of the third week (see Figs. 4.8B and 4.12B).

Caudal to the primitive streak is a circular area, the **cloacal membrane**, which indicates the future site of the anus (see Fig. 4.8E). The embryonic disc remains bilaminar here because the embryonic ectoderm and endoderm are fused, thereby preventing the migration of mesenchymal cells between them (see Fig. 4.9C). By the middle of the third week, intraembryonic mesoderm separates the ectoderm and endoderm (see Fig. 4.9D and G) everywhere except:

- At the oropharyngeal membrane cranially (see Fig. 4.9C)
- In the median plane cranial to the primitive node (see Fig. 4.5A and B), where the notochordal process is located (see Fig. 4.6)
- At the cloacal membrane caudally (see Fig. 4.8A and E)

Signals from the primitive streak region induce notochordal precursor cells. *The molecular mechanism that induces these cells involves (at least) Shh signaling from the floor plate of the neural tube.* Initially, the **notochordal process** elongates by invagination of cells from the primitive pit. The primitive pit extends into the notochordal process, forming a **notochordal canal** (see Fig. 4.8C). The notochordal process now becomes a cellular tube that extends cranially from the primitive node to the prechordal plate (see Figs. 4.6 and 4.8A–D). Later, the floor of the notochordal process fuses with the underlying embryonic endoderm (see Fig. 4.8E). These fused layers gradually undergo degeneration, resulting in the formation of openings in the floor of the notochordal process, which brings the notochordal canal into a transient communication with the umbilical vesicle (see Fig. 4.9B). As these openings become confluent, the floor of the notochordal canal disappears (see Fig. 4.9C), and the remains of the notochordal process form the flattened, grooved **notochordal plate** (see Fig. 4.9D). Beginning at the cranial end of the embryo, the notochordal plate cells proliferate and undergo infolding, which creates the **notochord**, a cellular rod-like structure (see Fig. 4.9E–G). The **notochord** defines the primordial longitudinal axis of the embryo and gives it some rigidity. The proximal part of the notochordal canal persists temporarily as the **neurenteric canal** (see Fig. 4.9C and E), forming a transitory communication between the amniotic and umbilical vesicle cavities. When the development of the notochord is complete, the neurenteric canal normally is obliterated.

The notochord is detached from the endoderm of the umbilical vesicle, the latter once again becoming a continuous layer (see Fig. 4.9G).

The notochord extends from the oropharyngeal membrane to the primitive node (see Fig. 4.6B and D). It degenerates as the bodies of the vertebrae form, but small portions of it persist as the **nucleus pulposus** of each intervertebral disc (see Chapter 14).

The notochord functions as the primary inductor (signaling center) in the early embryo. The developing notochord induces the overlying embryonic ectoderm to thicken and form the **neural plate** (see Fig. 4.9C), the primordium of the central nervous system (CNS).

Remnants of Notochordal Tissue

Both benign and malignant tumors **(chordomas)** may form from vestigial remnants of notochordal tissue anywhere along the vertebral column. Approximately one-third of chordomas occur at the base of the cranium and extend to the nasopharynx. Chordomas grow slowly, and malignant forms can infiltrate adjacent bone. Surgical resection of chordomas gives the patient the best chance of survival.

ALLANTOIS

The allantois appears on approximately day 16 as a small diverticulum from the caudal wall of the umbilical vesicle, which extends into the connecting stalk (see Figs. 4.8B, C, and E and 4.9B). The allantois remains very small, but the allantoic mesoderm expands beneath the chorion and forms blood vessels that will serve the placenta. The proximal part of the original allantoic diverticulum persists throughout development as a stalk, the **urachus**, which extends from the bladder to the umbilical region (see Chapter 12). The urachus is represented in adults by the **median umbilical ligament**. The blood vessels of the allantoic stalk become **umbilical arteries** (see Fig. 4.13). The intraembryonic part of the umbilical veins has a separate origin.

Allantoic Cysts

Allantoic cysts, remnants of the extraembryonic portion of the allantois, are usually found between the fetal umbilical vessels; they can be detected by computed tomography. They are most commonly found in the proximal part of the umbilical cord, near its attachment to the anterior abdominal wall. The cysts are generally asymptomatic until childhood or adolescence when they may become infected and inflamed. Infected urachal cysts are surgically excised.

NEURULATION: FORMATION OF NEURAL TUBE

Formation of the neural plate and neural folds and closure of the folds to form the neural tube constitute **neurulation**. Neurulation is completed by the end of the fourth week, when the closure of the **caudal neuropore** occurs (see Fig. 5.9A and B).

NEURAL PLATE AND NEURAL TUBE

As the notochord develops, it induces the overlying embryonic ectoderm, located at the midline, to thicken and form an elongated **neural plate** of thickened epithelial cells (see Fig. 4.8C and D). The neuroectoderm of the plate gives rise to the **CNS**, the brain, and the spinal cord. **Neuroectoderm** also gives rise to various other structures such as the retina. At first, the neural plate corresponds in length to the underlying notochord. It appears rostral to the primitive node and dorsal to the notochord and mesoderm adjacent to it (see Fig. 4.6B). As the notochord elongates, the neural plate broadens and eventually extends cranially as far as the **oropharyngeal membrane** (see Figs. 4.6C and 4.9C). Eventually, the neural plate extends beyond the notochord.

On approximately the 18th day, the neural plate invaginates along its central axis to form a longitudinal median **neural groove**, which has **neural folds** on each side (see Fig. 4.9G). The neural folds become particularly prominent at the cranial end of the embryo and are the first signs of brain development. By the end of the third week, the neural folds have begun to converge and fuse, converting the neural plate into the **neural tube**, the primordium of the brain vesicles and spinal cord (Figs. 4.10 and 4.11). The neural tube soon separates from the surface ectoderm as the neural folds meet.

Neural crest cells undergo an epithelial-to-mesenchymal transition and migrate away as the neural folds meet, and the free edges of the surface ectoderm (nonneural ectoderm) fuse so that this layer becomes continuous over the neural tube and the back of the embryo (see Fig. 4.11E and F). Subsequently, the surface ectoderm differentiates into the epidermis. Neurulation is completed during the fourth week. Neural tube formation is a complex cellular and multifactorial process involving a cascade of molecular mechanisms and extrinsic factors (see Chapter 17).

NEURAL CREST FORMATION

As the neural folds fuse to form the neural tube, some neuroectodermal cells lying along the inner margin of each neural fold lose their epithelial affinities and attachments to neighboring cells (see Fig. 4.11). As the neural tube separates from the surface ectoderm, **neural crest cells** form a flattened irregular mass, the **neural crest**, between the neural tube and the overlying surface ectoderm (see Fig. 4.11E). *Wnt/β-catenin signaling activates the* GBX2 *homeobox gene, which is essential for the development of the neural crest.* The neural crest soon separates into right and left parts that shift to the dorsolateral aspects of the neural tube.

Special tracer techniques have revealed that neural crest cells disseminate widely but usually along predefined pathways. *Differentiation and migration of neural crest cells are regulated by molecular interactions of specific genes (e.g.,* FOXD3, SNAIL2, SOX9, *and* SOX10*), signaling molecules, and transcription factors.*

Neural crest cells give rise to the spinal ganglia (dorsal root ganglia) and ganglia of the autonomic nervous system. The ganglia of cranial nerves V, VII, IX, and X are also partly derived from neural crest cells. In addition, neural crest cells form the neurolemma sheaths of peripheral nerves and contribute to the formation of the **leptomeninges**, the arachnoid mater, and pia mater (see Fig. 17.10). Neural crest cells also contribute to the formation of pigment cells, the suprarenal medulla, and many other tissues and organs.

Laboratory studies indicate that cell interactions both within the surface epithelium and between it and the underlying mesoderm are required to establish the boundaries of the neural plate and specify the sites where epithelial-mesenchymal transformation will occur. *These are mediated by BMP expression and Wnt, Nrg, Notch, and FGF signaling systems. Also, signaling molecules such as ephrins are important in guiding specific streams of migrating neural crest cells. The pathways for transformation and specification of the pluripotential neural crest cells and their precursors are unclear.* Many human syndromes and diseases (neurocristopathies) result from defective migration and/or differentiation of neural crest cells.

Birth Defects Resulting From Abnormal Neurulation

The neural plate, the primordium of the CNS, appears during the third week and gives rise to the neural folds and the beginning of the neural tube. Disturbance of neurulation may result in severe birth defects of the brain and spinal cord (see Chapter 17). **Neural tube defects** are among the most common congenital anomalies (see Fig. 17.12). Available evidence suggests that a primary disturbance (e.g., a teratogenic drug; see Chapter 20) affects cell fates, cell adhesion, and the molecular mechanisms of neural tube closure. This results in the failure of the neural folds to fuse and form the neural tube.

DEVELOPMENT OF SOMITES

5

In addition to the notochord, cells derived from the primitive node form the **paraxial mesoderm** (see Figs. 4.10B and 4.11A). Close to the primitive node, this cell population appears as a thick, longitudinal column of cells (see Figs. 4.9G and 4.10B). Each column is continuous laterally with the **intermediate mesoderm**, which gradually thins into a layer of lateral mesoderm. The **lateral mesoderm** is continuous with the extraembryonic mesoderm covering the umbilical vesicle and amnion. Toward the end of the third week, the paraxial mesoderm differentiates, condenses, and begins to divide into paired cuboidal bodies, the **somites**, which form in a craniocaudal sequence.

Somites are located on each side of the developing neural tube (see Fig. 4.10C–F). Between approximately day 26 and day 32, 38 or 39 pairs of somites develop—the somite period of human development. The size and shape of the somites are determined by cell-cell interactions. By day 42 (fifth week), 42 to 44 pairs of somites are present. The somites form distinct surface elevations on the embryo and are somewhat triangular in transverse sections (see Fig. 4.11A–F). Because the somites are so prominent during the fourth and fifth weeks, they are used as one of several criteria for determining an embryo's age (see Table 5.1).

Somites first appear in the future occipital region of the head of the embryo (see Fig. 4.10C–F). The first pair of somites appear a short distance caudal to the site at which the otic placode forms (see Fig. 4.10C). They soon develop craniocaudally and give rise to most of the **axial skeleton** and associated musculature, as well as to the adjacent dermis of the

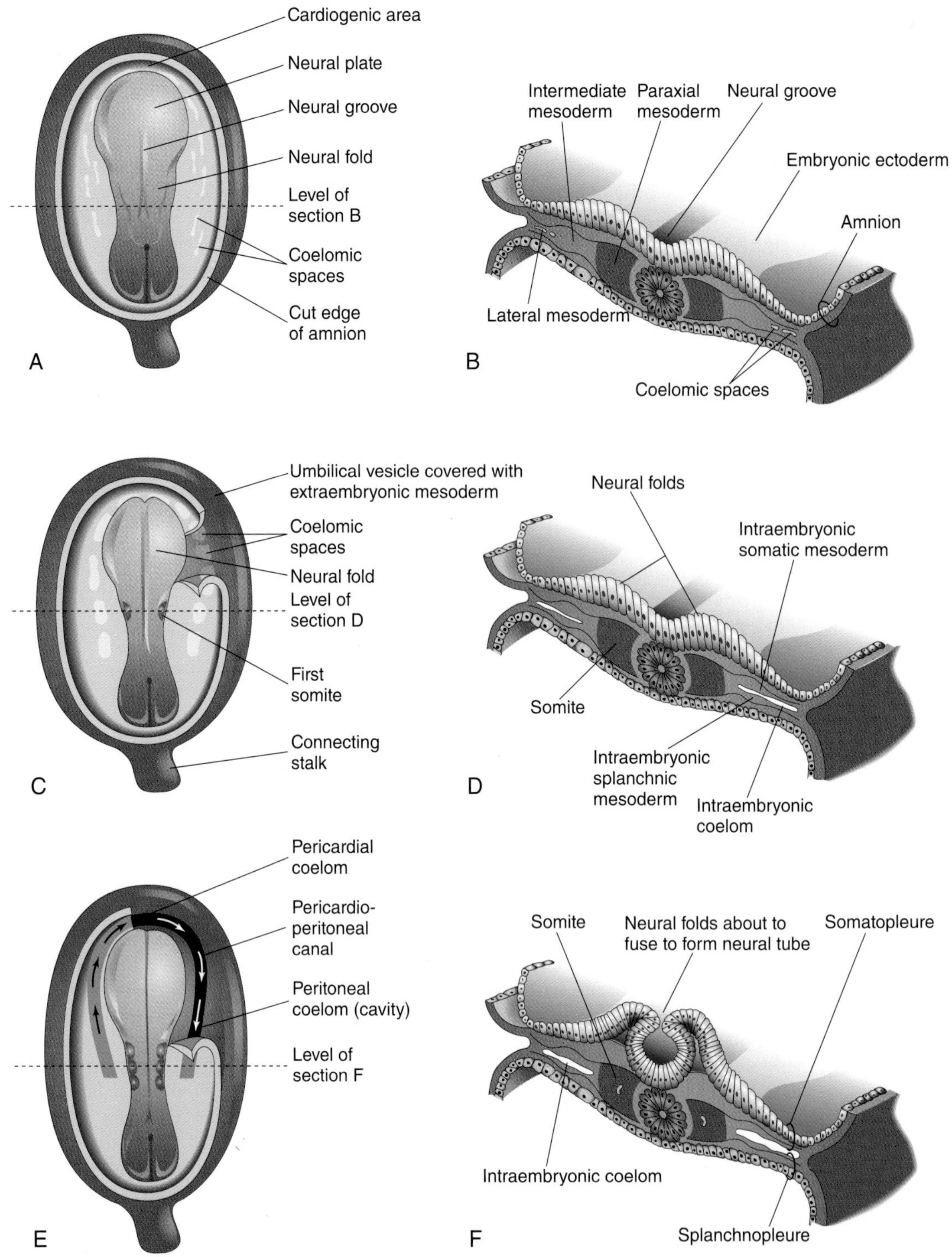

Fig. 4.10 Drawings of embryos at 19 to 21 days illustrating the development of the somites and intraembryonic coelom. (A, C, and E) Dorsal views of the embryo, exposed by removal of the amnion. (B, D, and F) Transverse sections through the trilaminar embryonic disc at the levels shown. (A) Presomite embryo of approximately 18 days. (C) An embryo of approximately 20 days showing the first pair of somites. Part of the somatopleure on the right has been removed to show the coelomic spaces in the lateral mesoderm. (E) A three-somite embryo (approximately 21 days) showing the horseshoe-shaped intraembryonic coelom, exposed on the right by removal of part of the somatopleure.

skin. Motor axons from the spinal cord innervate muscle cells in the somites, a process that requires the correct guidance of axons from the spinal cord to the appropriate target cells.

Formation of somites from the paraxial mesoderm involves the expression of WNT, FGF, and NOTCH pathway genes (Notch signaling pathway), Apelin gene (Aplnr) signaling, HOX genes, and other signaling factors. Moreover, somite formation from paraxial mesoderm is preceded by the expression of the forkhead transcription factors FoxC1 and FoxC2. The craniocaudal segmental pattern of the somites is regulated by the Delta-Notch signaling. A molecular oscillator or clock has been proposed as the mechanism

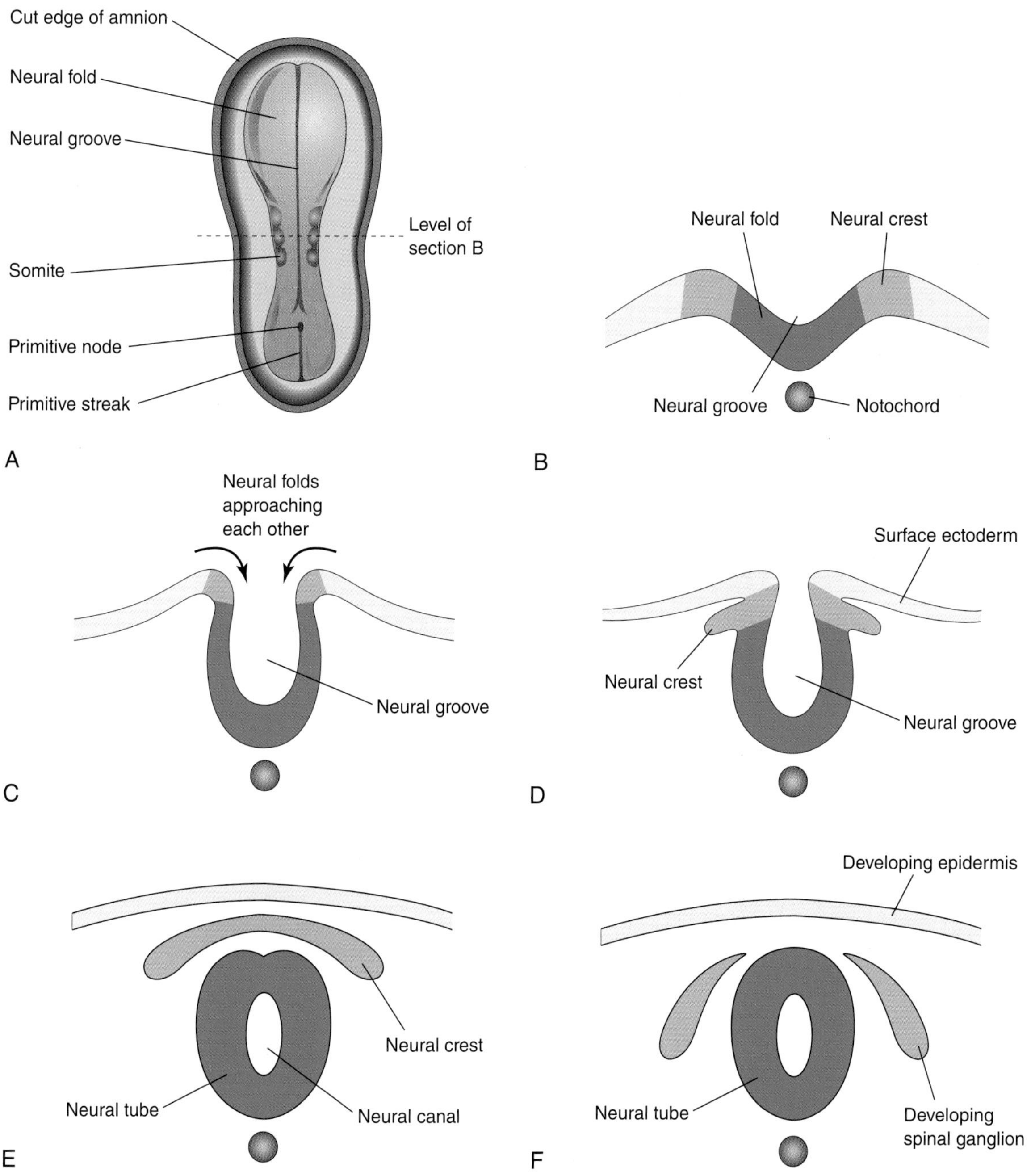

Fig. 4.11 (A–F) Diagrammatic drawings of transverse sections through progressively older embryos, illustrating the formation of the neural groove, neural folds, neural tube, and neural crest. (A) Dorsal view of an embryo at approximately 21 days.

responsible for the orderly sequencing of somites. Tbx6, a member of the T-box gene family, plays an important role in somitogenesis.

DEVELOPMENT OF INTRAEMBRYONIC COELOM

6

The intraembryonic coelom (embryonic body cavity) appears as isolated **coelomic spaces** in the lateral intraembryonic mesoderm and cardiogenic mesoderm (see Fig. 4.10A and C). These spaces coalesce to form a single horseshoe-shaped cavity, the **intraembryonic coelom** (see Fig. 4.10D and E), which divides the lateral mesoderm into two layers:

- A somatic or parietal layer of lateral mesoderm located beneath the ectodermal epithelium, which is continuous with the extraembryonic mesoderm covering the amnion
- A splanchnic or visceral layer of lateral mesoderm located adjacent to the endoderm, which is continuous with the extraembryonic mesoderm covering the umbilical vesicle

The **somatic mesoderm** and overlying embryonic ectoderm form the embryonic body wall, or **somatopleure** (see Fig. 4.10F), whereas the **splanchnic mesoderm** and underlying embryonic endoderm form the embryonic gut, or **splanchnopleure**. During the second month, the intraembryonic coelom is divided into three body cavities: **pericardial cavity**, **pleural cavities**, and **peritoneal cavity**. For a description of these divisions of the intraembryonic coelom, see Chapter 8.

EARLY DEVELOPMENT OF CARDIOVASCULAR SYSTEM

By the end of the second week, embryonic nutrition is obtained from the maternal blood by diffusion through the extraembryonic coelom and umbilical vesicle. At the beginning of the third week, blood vessel formation begins in the extraembryonic mesoderm of the umbilical vesicle, connecting stalk, and chorion (Fig. 4.12). **Embryonic blood vessels** develop approximately 2 days later. The early formation of the cardiovascular system is correlated with the urgent need for blood vessels to bring oxygen and nourishment to the embryo from the maternal circulation through the placenta. During the third week, a primordial uteroplacental circulation develops (Fig. 4.13).

VASCULOGENESIS AND ANGIOGENESIS

The formation of the embryonic vascular system involves two processes: vasculogenesis and angiogenesis. **Vasculogenesis** is the formation of new vascular channels by the assembly of individual cell precursors **(angioblasts)**. **Angiogenesis** is the formation of new vessels by budding and branching from

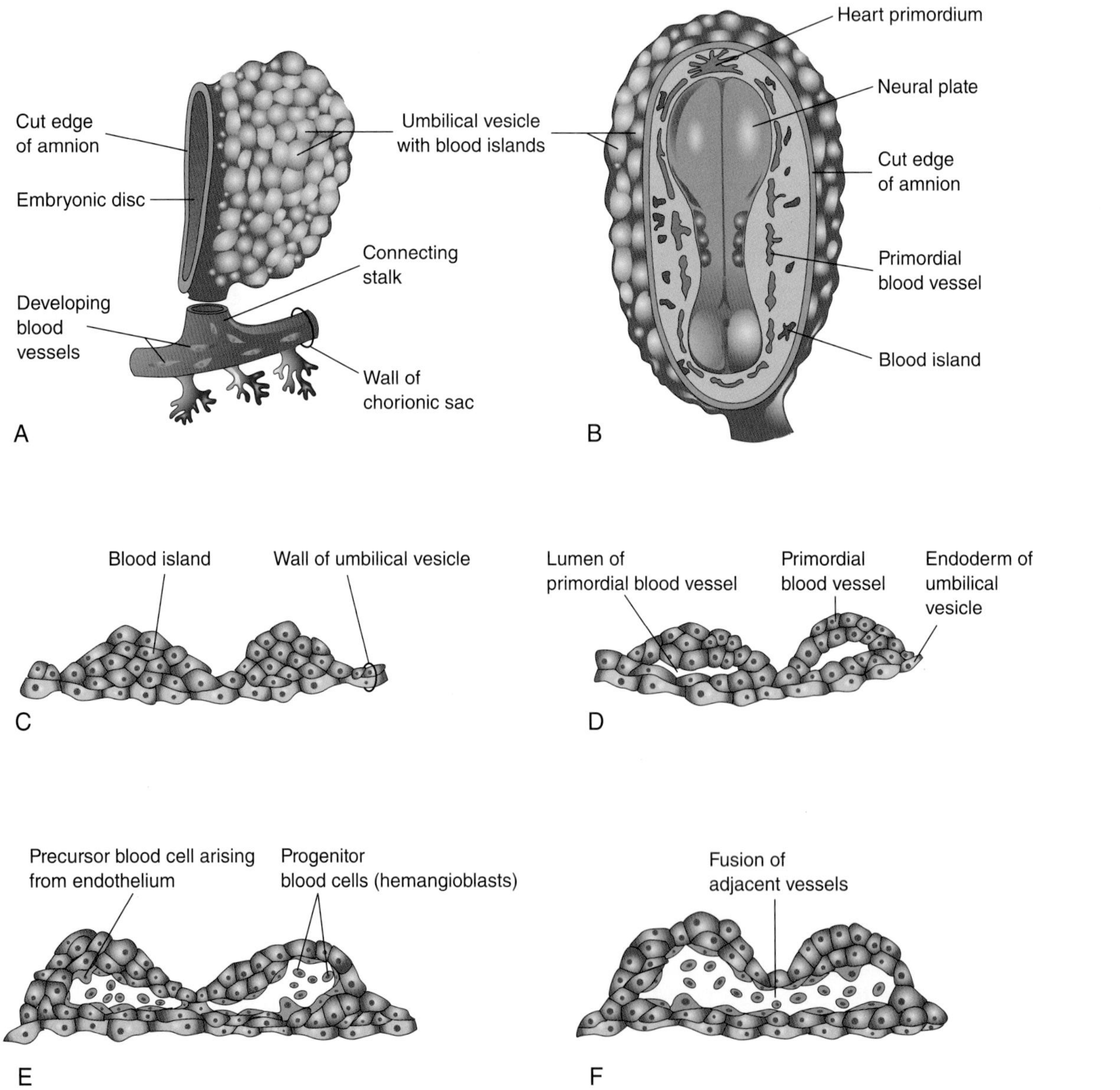

Fig. 4.12 Successive stages in the development of blood and blood vessels. (A) Lateral view of the umbilical vesicle and part of the chorionic sac (approximately 18 days). (B) Dorsal view of the embryo exposed by removing the amnion (approximately 20 days). (C–F) Sections of blood islands showing progressive stages in the development of blood and blood vessels.

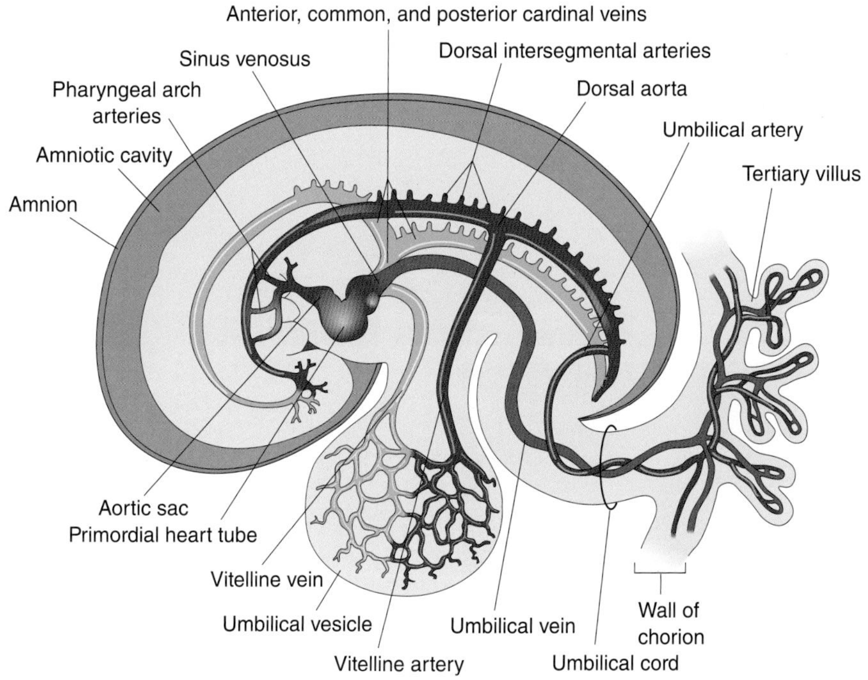

Fig. 4.13 Diagram of the primordial cardiovascular system in an embryo of approximately 21 days, viewed from the left side. Observe the transitory stage of the paired symmetric vessels. Each heart tube continues dorsally into a dorsal aorta that passes caudally. Branches of the aortae are (1) umbilical arteries establishing connections with vessels in the chorion, (2) vitelline arteries to the umbilical vesicle, and (3) dorsal intersegmental arteries to the body of the embryo. Vessels on the umbilical vesicle form a vascular plexus that is connected to the heart tubes by vitelline veins. The cardinal veins return blood from the body of the embryo. The umbilical vein carries oxygenated blood and nutrients to the chorion, which, in turn, provides nourishment to the embryo. The arteries carry poorly oxygenated blood and waste products to the chorionic villi for transfer to the mother's blood.

preexisting vessels. Blood vessel formation in the embryo and extraembryonic membranes during the third week (see Fig. 4.12) begins when mesenchymal cells differentiate into endothelial cell precursors, or angioblasts (vessel-forming cells). Angioblasts aggregate to form isolated angiogenic cell clusters, or blood islands (see Fig 4.12A and B) which are associated with the umbilical vesicle or endothelial cords within the embryo. Small cavities appear within the blood islands and **endothelial cords** by the confluence of intercellular clefts.

The angioblasts flatten to form endothelial cells that arrange themselves around the cavities in the blood islands to form the endothelium. Many of these endothelium-lined cavities soon fuse to form networks of endothelial channels (vasculogenesis). Additional vessels sprout into adjacent areas by endothelial budding (angiogenesis) and fuse with other vessels forming communicating channels (See Fig 4.12F). The mesenchymal cells surrounding the primordial **endothelial blood vessels** differentiate into the muscular and connective tissue elements of the vessels. *Anastomosis of these primordial blood vessels is spatially regulated by Fit1 (VEGFR1).*

Initially, **blood cells** develop from specialized endothelial cells (**hemangiogenic epithelium**) of vessels as they grow on the umbilical vesicle and allantois at the end of the third week (see Fig. 4.12E and F) and later in specialized sites along the dorsal aorta. Progenitor blood cells also arise directly from hemangiopoietic stem cells. **Hematogenesis** (blood formation) does not begin in the embryo until the fifth week. It occurs first along the aorta and then in various parts of the embryonic mesenchyme, mainly the liver and later in the spleen, bone marrow, and lymph nodes. Fetal and adult erythrocytes are derived from **hematopoietic progenitor cells**.

PRIMORDIAL CARDIOVASCULAR SYSTEM

The heart and great vessels form from mesenchymal cells in the **cardiogenic area** (see Figs. 4.10A and 4.12B). Paired, longitudinal endothelial-lined channels, or **endocardial heart tubes**, develop during the third week and fuse to form a **primordial heart tube** (see Fig. 4.13). The tubular heart joins with blood vessels in the embryo, connecting the stalk, chorion, and umbilical vesicle to form a **primordial cardiovascular system**. By the end of the third week, the blood is circulating, and *the heart begins to beat during the fourth week after fertilization;* the *earliest reported is between day 20 and day 23 after fertilization (34–37 gestational days).*

The cardiovascular system is the first organ system to reach a functional state. The embryonic heartbeat can be detected using **Doppler ultrasonography** during the fourth week, approximately 6 weeks after the last normal menstrual period (Fig. 4.14).

DEVELOPMENT OF CHORIONIC VILLI

Shortly after **primary chorionic villi** appear at the end of the second week, they begin to branch. Early in the third week,

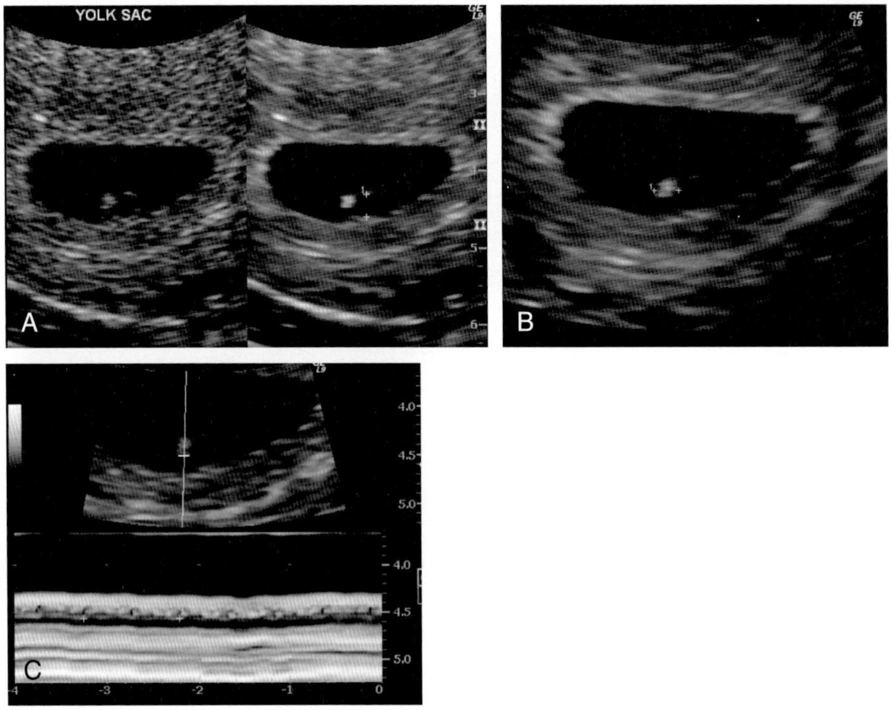

Fig. 4.14 Transvaginal ultrasonogram of a 4-week embryo. (A) Secondary umbilical vesicle (*calipers*, 2 mm). (B) Bright (echogenic) 4-week embryo (*calipers*, 2.4 mm). (C) Cardiac activity of 116 beats/min demonstrated with motion mode. The calipers are used to encompass two beats. (Courtesy E.A. Lyons, MD, Professor of Radiology and Obstetrics and Gynecology, Health Sciences Centre and University of Manitoba, Winnipeg, Manitoba, Canada.)

mesenchyme grows into these villi, forming a core of mesenchymal tissue. The villi at this stage, **secondary chorionic villi**, cover the entire surface of the chorionic sac (Fig. 4.15A and B). Some mesenchymal cells in the villi soon differentiate into capillaries and blood cells (see Fig. 4.15C and D). Villi are called **tertiary chorionic villi** when blood vessels are present.

The capillaries in the chorionic villi fuse to form **arteriocapillary networks**, which soon become connected with the embryonic heart through vessels that differentiate in the mesenchyme of the chorion and connecting stalk (see Fig. 4.13). By the end of the third week, embryonic blood begins to flow slowly through the capillaries in the chorionic villi. Oxygen and nutrients in the maternal plasma in the **intervillous space** diffuse through the walls of the villi and enter the embryo's blood (see Fig. 4.15C and D). Carbon dioxide and waste products diffuse from blood in the fetal capillaries through the wall of the chorionic villi into the maternal blood. Concurrently, cytotrophoblastic cells of the chorionic villi proliferate and extend through the syncytiotrophoblast to form an extravillous **cytotrophoblastic shell** (see Fig. 4.15C), which gradually surrounds the chorionic sac and attaches it to the endometrium.

Villi that attach to the maternal tissues through the cytotrophoblastic shell are **stem villi** (anchoring villi). The villi that grow from the sides of the stem villi are **branch villi**. It is through the walls of the branch villi that the main exchange of material between the blood of the mother and embryo takes place. The branch villi (see Fig. 7.5) are bathed in continually changing maternal blood in the intervillous space (see Fig. 4.15C). *The transcriptional coactivator WWETR1, Hippo signaling cofactor, is involved in the molecular pathway of cytotrophoblast self-renewal, syncytiotrophoblast fate, and formation of the extravillous trophoblast.*

Abnormal Growth of Trophoblast

Sometimes the embryo dies, and the chorionic villi (see Fig. 4.15A) do not complete their development; that is, they do not become vascularized to form **tertiary villi** (see Fig. 4.15C). These degenerating villi form cystic swellings, **hydatidiform moles**, which resemble a cluster of grapes (Fig. 4.16). The moles exhibit variable degrees of trophoblastic proliferation and produce excessive amounts of β-hCG. Moles can develop into malignant trophoblastic lesions, **choriocarcinomas** (3%–5% of cases) which can metastasize through the bloodstream to various sites, such as the lungs, bowel, liver, brain, and brain. Choriocarcinomas are generally sensitive to chemotherapy with survival over 90%.

The main mechanisms for the development of ***complete* hydatidiform moles** are as follows:

- Fertilization of an empty oocyte (absent or inactive pronucleus) by a sperm, followed by duplication **(monospermic mole)**—the genetic origin of the nuclear DNA is paternal. Most complete hydatidiform moles are monospermic.
- Fertilization of an empty oocyte by two sperms **(dispermic mole)**.

A ***partial* hydatidiform mole** usually results from fertilization of a normal oocyte by two sperms **(dispermy)**.

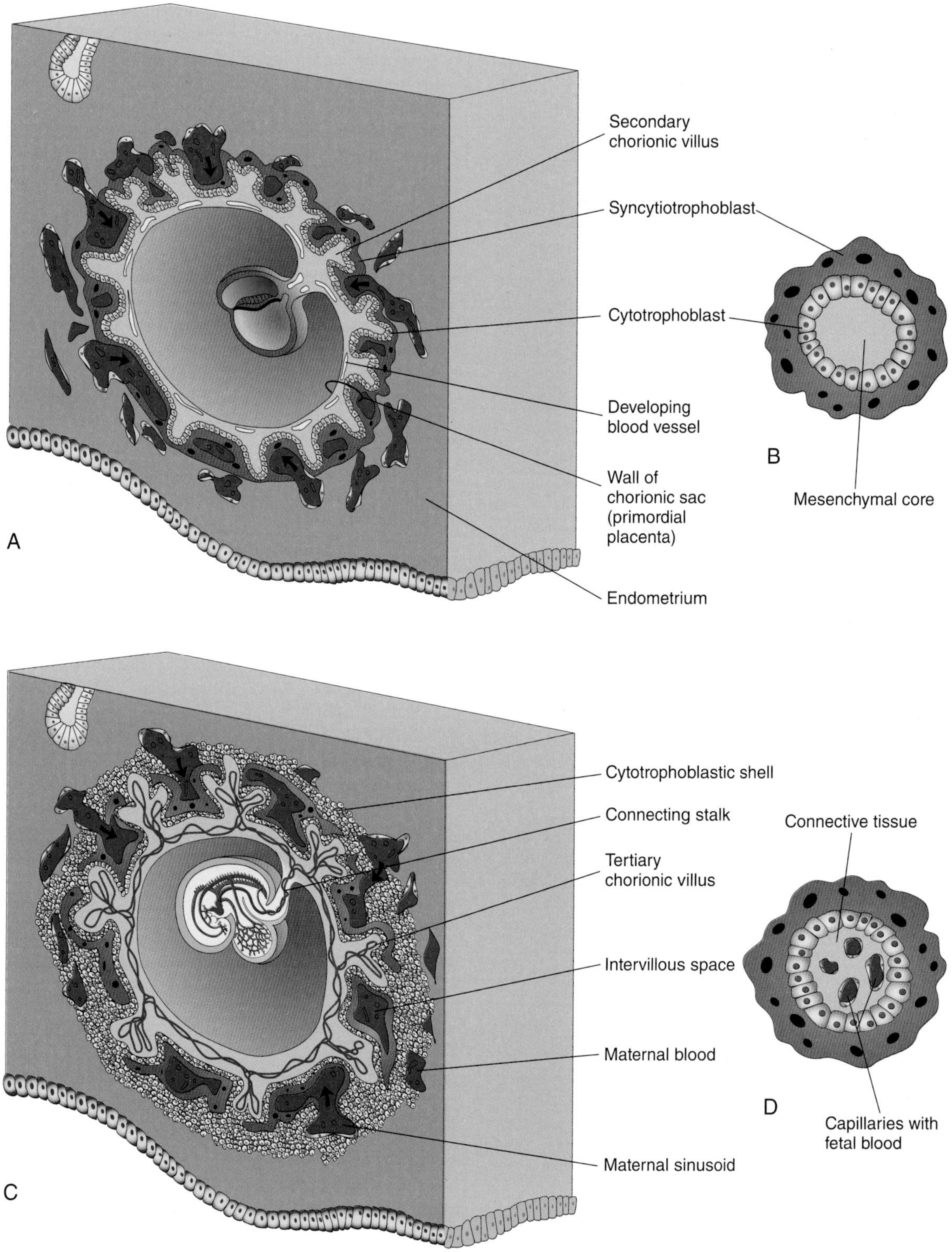

Fig. 4.15 Diagrams illustrating development of secondary chorionic villi into tertiary chorionic villi. Early formation of the placenta is also shown. (A) Sagittal section of an embryo (approximately 16 days). (B) Section of a secondary chorionic villus. (C) Section of an implanted embryo (approximately 21 days). (D) Section of a tertiary chorionic villus. The fetal blood in the capillaries is separated from the maternal blood surrounding the villus by the endothelium of the capillaries, embryonic connective tissue, cytotrophoblast, and syncytiotrophoblast.

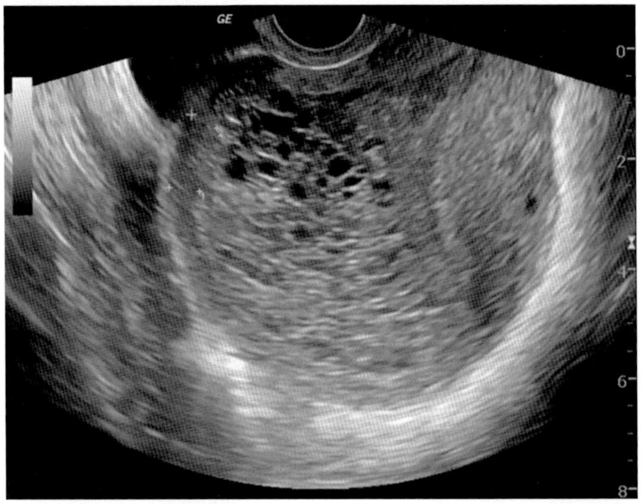

Fig. 4.16 Ultrasound image demonstrating a complete hydatidiform mole. Note numerous small cystic spaces. The "cluster of grapes sign" is a typical feature of a molar pregnancy. (Courtesy Dr. Maulik S. Patel and Dr. Frank Gaillard, Radiopaedia.com.)

SUMMARY OF THIRD WEEK

- The **bilaminar embryonic disc** is converted into a **trilaminar embryonic disc** during **gastrulation**. These changes begin with the appearance of the **primitive streak**, which appears at the beginning of the third week as a thickening of the epiblast at the caudal end of the embryonic disc (Fig. 4.4 A and B).
- The **primitive streak** results from the migration of epiblastic cells to the median plane of the disc. Invagination of epiblastic cells from the primitive streak gives rise to mesenchymal cells that migrate ventrally, laterally, and cranially between the **epiblast** and **hypoblast**.
- As soon as the primitive streak begins to produce mesenchymal cells, the epiblast is called the **embryonic ectoderm**. Some cells of the epiblast displace the hypoblast and form the **embryonic endoderm**. Mesenchymal cells produced by the primitive streak soon organize into a third germ layer, the **intraembryonic (embryonic) mesoderm**, occupying the area between the former hypoblast and cells in the epiblast. Cells of the mesoderm migrate to the edges of the embryonic disc, where they join the **extraembryonic mesoderm** covering the amnion and umbilical vesicle (Fig. 4.3).
- At the end of the third week, the embryo is a flat ovoid embryonic disc (see Fig. 4.3H). Mesoderm exists between the ectoderm and endoderm of the disc everywhere except at the **oropharyngeal membrane**, in the median plane occupied by the notochord, and at the **cloacal membrane** (see Fig. 4.9E).
- Early in the third week, mesenchymal cells from the primitive streak form the **notochordal process** between the embryonic ectoderm and endoderm. The notochordal process extends from the primitive node to the **prechordal plate**. Openings develop in the floor of the **notochordal canal**, and they soon coalesce, leaving a **notochordal plate**. This plate infolds to form the **notochord**, the primordial axis of the embryo around which the **axial skeleton** forms (e.g., vertebral column).
- The **neural plate** appears as a thickening of embryonic ectoderm, induced by the developing notochord. A longitudinal **neural groove** develops in the neural plate, which is flanked by **neural folds**. Fusion of the folds forms the **neural tube**, the primordium of the **CNS** (see Figs. 4.10A and 4.11).
- As the neural folds fuse to form the neural tube, neuroectodermal cells form a **neural crest** between the surface ectoderm and the neural tube.
- The mesoderm on each side of the notochord condenses to form longitudinal columns of paraxial mesoderm, which, by the end of the third week, give rise to **somites(see Fig. 4.10D and F).**
- The **coelom** (cavity) within the embryo arises as isolated spaces in the lateral mesoderm and cardiogenic mesoderm. The **coelomic vesicles** subsequently coalesce to form a single, horseshoe-shaped cavity that eventually gives rise to **body cavities** (see Fig. 4.10E).
- **Blood vessels** first appear in the wall of the umbilical vesicle, allantois, and chorion. They develop within the embryo shortly thereafter. Fetal erythrocytes develop from different hematopoietic precursors.
- The **primordial heart** is represented by **paired endocardial heart tubes**. By the end of the third week, the heart tubes have fused to form a **tubular heart** that is joined to vessels in the embryo, umbilical vesicle, chorion, and connecting stalk to form a **primordial cardiovascular system** (see Fig. 4.13).
- **Primary chorionic villi** become **secondary chorionic villi** as they acquire mesenchymal cores. Before the end of the third week, capillaries develop in the secondary chorionic villi, transforming them into **tertiary chorionic villi** (see Fig. 4.15C). Cytotrophoblastic extensions from the stem villi join to form a **cytotrophoblastic shell** that anchors the chorionic sac to the endometrium.

CLINICALLY ORIENTED PROBLEMS

CASE 4-1

A 30-year-old female became pregnant 2 months after discontinuing the use of oral contraceptives. Approximately 3 weeks later, she had a spontaneous abortion.

- How do the hormones in these contraceptives affect the ovarian and menstrual cycles?
- What might have caused the spontaneous abortion?

CASE 4-2

A 25-year-old female with a history of regular menstrual cycles was 5 days overdue on menses. A menstrual extraction (uterine evacuation) was performed. The tissue removed was examined for evidence of a pregnancy.

- Would a radioimmune assay have detected pregnancy at this early stage?
- What clinical findings would indicate an early pregnancy?
- What would be the age of the conceptus?

CASE 4-3

A female who had just missed her menstrual period was concerned that a glass of wine she had consumed the week before might have harmed her embryo.

- What major organ systems undergo early development during the third week?
- What severe congenital anomaly might result from teratogenic factors (see Chapter 20) acting during this period of development?
- What information might you discuss with the patient?

CASE 4-4

A female infant had a large tumor situated between her anus and sacrum. A diagnosis of sacrococcygeal teratoma was made, and the mass was surgically removed.

- What is the probable embryologic origin of this tumor?
- Explain why these tumors often contain various types of tissue derived from all three germ layers.

CASE 4-5

A female with a history of early spontaneous abortions had an ultrasound examination to determine whether her embryo was still implanted.

- Is ultrasonography helpful in assessing pregnancy during the third week? If so, do special ultrasonographic techniques need to be used?
- What structures might be recognizable?
- If a pregnancy test is negative, is it correct to assume that the female is not pregnant? Explain.
- Could an extrauterine gestation be present?

Discussion of these problems appears in the Appendix at the back of the book.

BIBLIOGRAPHY AND SUGGESTED READING

Al-Wassia H, Bamanie H, Rahbini H, Alghamdi N, Alotaibi R, Alnagrani W: Neural tube defects from antenatal diagnosis to discharge – a tertiary academic centre experience, *Med Arch* 77(1):40–43, 2023.10.5455/medarh.2023.77.40-43 PMID: 36919133; PMCID: PMC10008259

Applebaum M, Kalcheim C: Mechanisms of myogenic specification and patterning, *Results Probl Cell Differ* 56:77, 2015.

Azagury M., Buganim Y. Unlocking trophectoderm mysteries: in vivo and in vitro perspectives on human and mouse trophoblast fate induction. *Dev Cell* 59(8):941–960, 2024.

Betz C, Lenard A, Belting H-G, et al: Cell behaviors and dynamics during angiogenesis, *Development* 143:2249, 2016.

Dawes JHP, Kelsh RN: Cell fate decisions in the neural crest, from pigment to neural development, *Int J Mol Sci* 22:13531, 2021.

De Val S: Key transcriptional regulators of early vascular development, *Arterioscler Thromb Vasc Biol* 31:1469, 2011.

Dias AS, de Almeida I, Belmonte JM: Somites without a clock, *Science* 343:791, 2014.

Erickson AG, Kameneva P, Adameyko I: The transcriptional portraits of the neural crest at the individual cell level, *Sem Cell Develop Biol* 138:68–80, 2022.10.1016/j.semcdb.222.02.017

Ghimere S, Mantziou V, Moris N, et al: Human gastrulation: the embryo and its models, *Develop Biol* 474:100, 2021.

Gucciardo L, Uyttebroek A, De Wever I, et al: Prenatal assessment and management of sacrococcygealteratoma, *Prenat Diagn* 31:678, 2011.

Hall BK: *Bones and cartilage: developmental skeletal biology*, ed 2Philadelphia, 2015, Elsevier.

Kalcheim C: Epithelial-mesenchymal transitions during neural crest and somite development, *J Clin Med* 5(1):E1, 2015.

Liu W, Komiya Y, Mezzacappa C, et al: MIM regulates vertebrate neural tube closure, *Development* 138:2035, 2011.

Männer J: When does the human embryonic heart start beating? A review of contemporary and historical sources of knowledge about the onset of blood circulation in man, *J Cardiovasc Dev Dis* 9(6):187, 2022. PMID: 35735816; PMCID: PMC9225347. https://doi.org/10.3390/jcdd9060187

Mekonen HK, Hikspoors JP, Mommen G, et al: Development of the ventral body wall in the human embryo, *J Anat* 227:673, 2016.

Mukhopadhyay M: Resolving human gastrulation, *Nat Methods* 19:34, 2022. https://doi.org/10.1038/s41592-021-01384-0

Nesmith JE, Chappell JC, Cluceru JG, et al: Blood vessel anastomosis is spatially regulated by fit1 during angiogenesis, *Development* 144:889, 2017.

Payumo AY, McQuade LE, Walker WJ, et al: Tbx16 regulates *HOX* gene activation in mesodermal progenitor cells, *Nat Chem Biol* 12:694, 2016.

Ramesh T, Nagula SV, Tardieu GG, et al: Update on the notochord including its embryology, molecular development, and pathology: a primer for the clinician, *Cureus* 9(4):e1137, 2017.

Ray S, Saha A, Ghosh A, et al: Hippo signaling cofactor, WWTR1, at the crossroads of human trophoblast progenitor self-renewal and differentiation, *Proc Natl Acad Sci USA* 119(36), 2022. e 2204069119. https://doi.org/10.1073/pnas.2204069119

Savage P: Gestational trophoblastic disease. In Magowan BA, Owen P, Thomson A, editors: *Clinical obstetrics and gynaecology*, ed 3, Philadelphia, 2014, Saunders.

Tyser RCV, Mahammadov E, Nakanoh S, et al: Single-cell transcriptomic characterization of a gastrulating human embryo, *Nature* 600:285–289, 2021. https://doi.org/10.1038/s41586-021-04158-y

Van Heurn LJ, Coumans ABC, Derikx JPM, et al: Factors associated with poor outcome in fetuses prenatally diagnosed with sacrococcygeal teratoma, *Prenat Diagn* 41:1430, 2021. https://doi.org/10.1002/pd.6026

Xiao Z., Cui L.,Yuan Y. et al.: 3D reconstruction of a gastrulating human embryo, *Cell* 2024.

Yame T: Cellular basis of embryonic hematopoiesis and its implications in prenatal erythropoiesis, *Int J Mol Sci* 21(24):9346, 2020. https://doi.org/10.3390/ijms21249346

Yin J, Heutschi D, Belting HG, et al: Building the complex architectures of vascular networks:where to branch, where to connect and where to remodel, *Curr Top Dev Biol* 143:281–297, 2021.

Zhai J., Xiao Z.,Wang Y., Wang H.: Human embryonic development: from peri-implantation to gastrulation. *Trends Cell Biol* 32(1):18–29, 2022.

Fourth to Eighth Weeks of Human Development

5

CHAPTER OUTLINE

All major external and internal structures are established during the fourth to eighth weeks. By the end of this embryonic period, the main organ systems have started to develop, and the embryo has a distinctly human appearance. Because the tissues and organs are differentiating rapidly, exposure of embryos to teratogens during this period may cause major birth defects. **Teratogens** are agents (such as some drugs and viruses) that produce or increase the incidence of major birth defects (see Chapter 20).

PHASES OF EMBRYONIC DEVELOPMENT

Human development is divided into three interrelated phases:

- The first phase is **growth**, which involves cell division and elaboration of cell products.
- The second phase is **morphogenesis**, the development of shape, size, and other features of a particular organ, part, or the whole body. Morphogenesis involves cellular and molecular processes controlled by the expression and regulation of specific genes in an orderly sequence. Changes in cell fate, cell shape, and cell movement allow the cells to interact at a molecular level with each other during the formation of tissues and organs.
- The third phase is **differentiation**, during which cells are organized in a precise pattern of tissues and organs that are capable of performing specialized functions.

FOLDING OF EMBRYO

5

A significant event in the establishment of body form is the folding of the flat trilaminar embryonic disc into a somewhat cylindric-shaped embryo (Fig. 5.1). Folding occurs in the median and horizontal planes and results from the rapid growth of the embryo. The growth rate at the sides of the embryonic disc is slower than the rate of growth in the long axis as the embryo increases rapidly in length. Folding at the cranial and caudal ends and sides of the embryo occurs simultaneously. Concurrently, there is relative constriction at the junction of the embryo and umbilical vesicle.

FOLDING OF EMBRYO IN THE MEDIAN PLANE

Folding of the ends of the embryo produces **head and tail folds** that result in the cranial and caudal regions moving ventrally as the embryo elongates cranially and caudally (see Fig. 5.1A_2–D_2).

HEAD FOLD

At the beginning of the fourth week, the neural folds in the cranial region form the **primordium of the brain** (see Fig. 5.1A_2 and B_2). Initially, the developing brain projects dorsally into the amniotic cavity, the fluid-filled cavity containing the embryo. Later, the developing forebrain grows cranially beyond the **oropharyngeal membrane** and overhangs the developing heart (Fig. 5.2B and C). At the same time, the **septum transversum**, primordial heart, pericardial coelom,

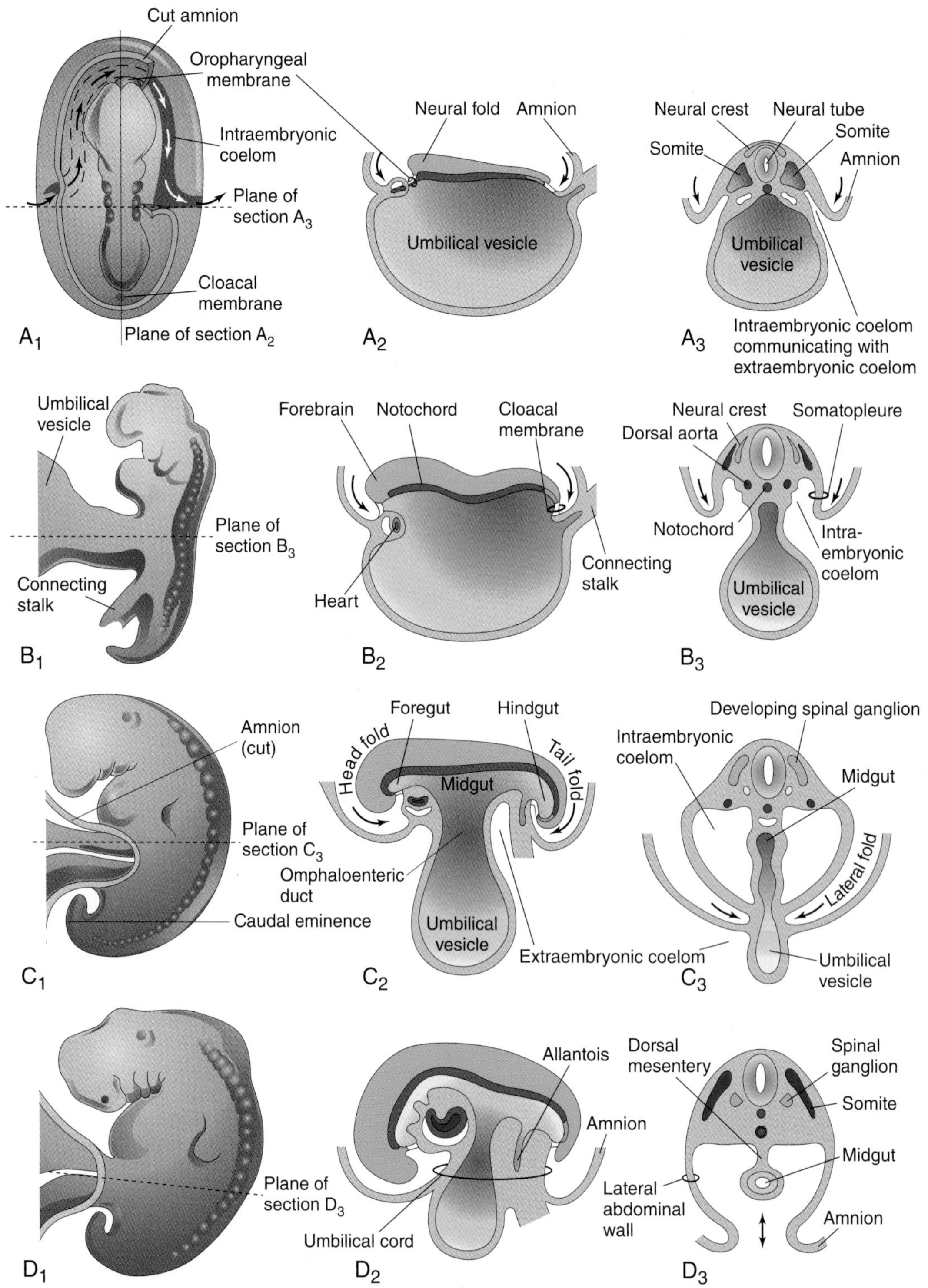

Fig. 5.1 Drawings of folding of embryos during the fourth week. (A_1) Dorsal view of an embryo early in the fourth week. Three pairs of somites are visible. The continuity of the intraembryonic coelom and extraembryonic coelom is illustrated on the right side by the removal of a part of the embryonic ectoderm and mesoderm. (B_1, C_1, and D_1) Lateral views of embryos at 22, 26, and 28 days, respectively. (A_2–D_2) Sagittal sections at the plane shown in (A_1). (A_3–D_3) Transverse sections at the levels indicated in (A_1–D_1).

and oropharyngeal membrane move onto the ventral surface of the embryo. During folding, part of the endoderm of the umbilical vesicle is incorporated into the embryo as the **foregut** (primordium of the pharynx, esophagus, and lower respiratory system) (see Fig. 5.2C and also see Chapter 11). The foregut lies between the forebrain and primordial heart, and the oropharyngeal membrane separates the foregut from the **stomodeum**, the primordial mouth (Fig. 5.3B and see Fig. 5.2C).

After folding of the head, the **septum transversum** lies caudal to the heart, where it subsequently develops into the **central tendon of the diaphragm**, the partition between

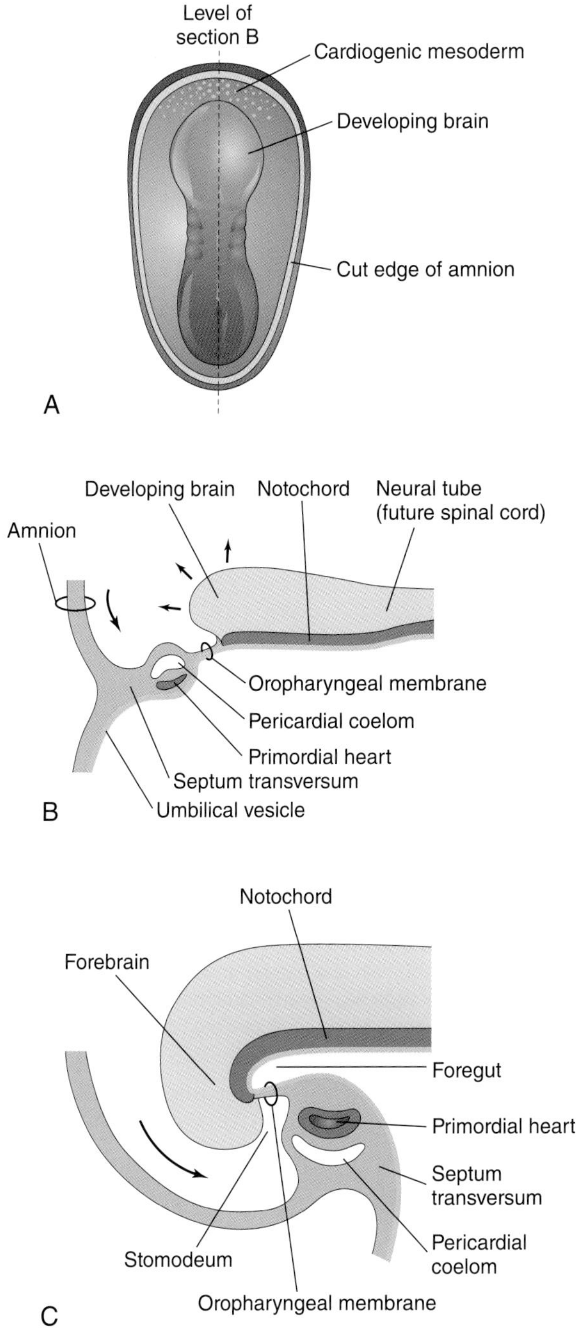

Fig. 5.2 Folding of the cranial end of the embryo. (A) Dorsal view of an embryo at 21 days. (B) Sagittal section of the cranial part of the embryo at the plane shown in (A). Observe the ventral movement of the heart in (B and C). (C) Sagittal section of an embryo at 26 days. Note that the septum transversum, primordial heart, pericardial coelom, and oropharyngeal membrane have moved onto the ventral surface of the embryo. Observe also that part of the umbilical vesicle is incorporated into the embryo as the foregut.

the abdominal and thoracic cavities (see Fig. 5.3B, and also see Chapter 8). The head fold also affects the arrangement of the **embryonic coelom** (primordium of the body cavity). Before folding, the coelom consists of a flattened, horseshoe-shaped cavity (see Fig. 5.1A_1). After folding, the **pericardial coelom** lies ventral to the heart and cranial to the septum transversum (see Fig. 5.2B and C). At this stage, the **intraembryonic coelom** communicates widely on each side with the **extraembryonic coelom** (see Figs. 5.1A_3 and 5.3A and B).

TAIL FOLD

Folding of the caudal end of the embryo results primarily from the growth of the distal part of the neural tube, the primordium of the spinal cord (Fig. 5.4A and B). As the embryo grows, the **caudal eminence** (tail region) projects over the **cloacal membrane**, the future site of the anus (see Figs. 5.3A and 5.4B). During folding, part of the endodermal germ layer is incorporated into the embryo as the **hindgut** (see Fig. 5.4B and also Chapter 11).

The terminal part of the hindgut soon dilates slightly to form the **cloaca**, the rudiment of the urinary bladder and rectum (see Fig. 5.4B, and also see Chapters 11 and 12). Before folding, the primitive streak lies cranial to the cloacal membrane (see Fig. 5.4A); after folding, it lies caudal to it (see Fig. 5.4B). The connecting stalk (primordium of the umbilical cord) is now attached to the ventral surface of the embryo (see Fig. 5.4A), and the allantois, or the diverticulum of the umbilical vesicle, is partially incorporated into the embryo (see Fig. 5.4A and B).

FOLDING OF EMBRYO IN THE HORIZONTAL PLANE

Folding of the sides of the developing embryo produces right and left **lateral folds** (see Fig. 5.1A_3 to D_3). Lateral folding is produced by the rapidly growing spinal cord and somites. The primordia of the ventrolateral abdominal wall folds toward the median plane, rolling the edges of the **embryonic disc** ventrally and forming a roughly cylindric embryo (see Fig. 5.6A). As the **abdominal wall** forms, part of the endoderm is incorporated into the embryo as the **midgut**, the primordium of the small intestine, and a portion of the large intestine (see Fig. 5.1C_2, and also see Chapter 11).

Initially, there is a wide connection between the midgut and umbilical vesicle (see Fig. 5.1A_2); however, after lateral folding, the connection is reduced, forming an **omphaloenteric duct** (see Fig. 5.1C_2). The region of attachment of the amnion to the ventral surface of the embryo is also reduced to a relatively narrow umbilical region (see Fig. 5.1D_2 and D_3). As the **umbilical cord** forms from the connecting stalk (see Fig. 5.1B_2 and D_2), ventral fusion of the lateral folds reduces the region of communication between the intraembryonic and extraembryonic coelomic cavities to a narrow communication (see Fig. 5.1C_2). As the amniotic cavity expands and obliterates most of the extraembryonic coelom, the amnion forms the epithelial covering of the umbilical cord (see Fig. 5.1D_2).

GERM LAYER DERIVATIVES

The three germ layers (ectoderm, mesoderm, and endoderm) formed during gastrulation (Fig. 5.5) give rise to the primordia of all tissues and organs. The specificity of the germ layers, however, is not rigidly fixed. The cells of each germ layer divide, migrate, aggregate, and differentiate in patterns as they form the various organ systems. The main germ layer derivatives are as follows (see Fig. 5.5):

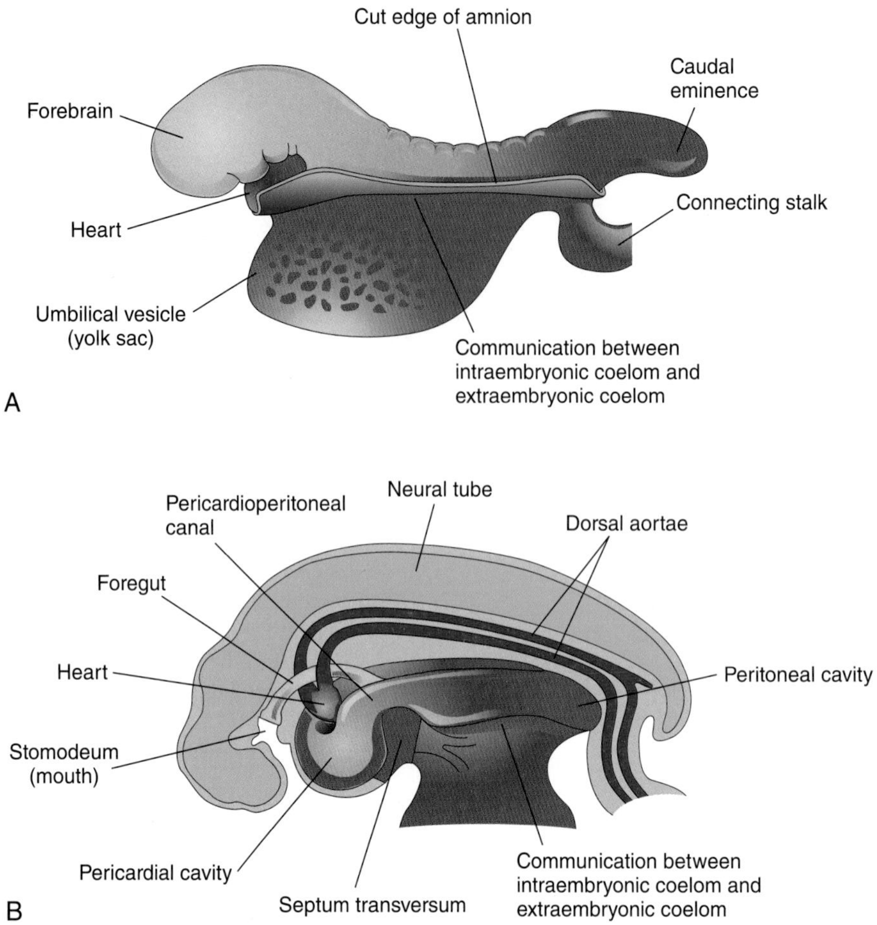

Fig. 5.3 Drawings of the effect of the head fold on the intraembryonic coelom. (A) Lateral view of an embryo (24–25 days) during folding, showing the large forebrain, ventral position of the heart, and communication between the intraembryonic and extraembryonic parts of the coelom. (B) Schematic drawing of an embryo (26–27 days) after folding, showing the pericardial cavity ventrally, the pericardioperitoneal canals running dorsally on each side of the foregut, and the intraembryonic coelom in communication with the extraembryonic coelom.

- **Ectoderm** gives rise to the central nervous system; peripheral nervous system; sensory epithelia of the eyes, ears, and nose; epidermis and its appendages (hair and nails); mammary glands; pituitary gland; subcutaneous glands; and enamel of the teeth. Neural crest cells, derived from **neuroectoderm**, the central region of early ectoderm, eventually give rise to or participate in the formation of many cell types and organs, including cells of the spinal cord, cranial nerves (V, VII, IX, and X), and autonomic ganglia; ensheathing cells of the peripheral nervous system; pigment cells of the dermis; muscles, connective tissues, and bones of pharyngeal arch origin; suprarenal medulla; and meninges (coverings) of the brain and spinal cord.
- **Mesoderm** gives rise to connective tissue, cartilage, bone, striated and smooth muscles, heart, blood, and lymphatic vessels; kidneys; ovaries; testes; genital ducts; serous membranes lining the body cavities (pericardial, pleural, and peritoneal membranes); spleen; and cortex of the suprarenal glands.
- **Endoderm** gives rise to the epithelial lining of the digestive and respiratory tracts; parenchyma (connective tissue framework) of the tonsils; thyroid and parathyroid glands; thymus, liver, and pancreas; epithelial lining of the urinary bladder and most of the urethra; and epithelial lining of the tympanic cavity, tympanic antrum, and pharyngotympanic tube (see Fig. 5.5).

CONTROL OF EMBRYONIC DEVELOPMENT

Embryonic development results from genetic plans in the chromosomes. Knowledge of the genes that control human development is increasing (see Chapter 21). Most information about developmental processes has come from studies of other organisms, especially zebrafish, chickens, and mice, because of the ethics associated with using human embryos for laboratory studies.

Most developmental processes depend on a precisely coordinated interaction of genetic and environmental factors. Several control mechanisms guide differentiation and ensure synchronized development, such as tissue interactions, regulated migration of cells and cell colonies, controlled proliferation, and programmed cell death (e.g., apoptosis). Each system of the body has its own developmental pattern.

Embryonic development is essentially a process of growth and increasing complexity of structure and function. Growth is achieved by mitosis together with the production of extracellular matrices (surrounding substances), whereas

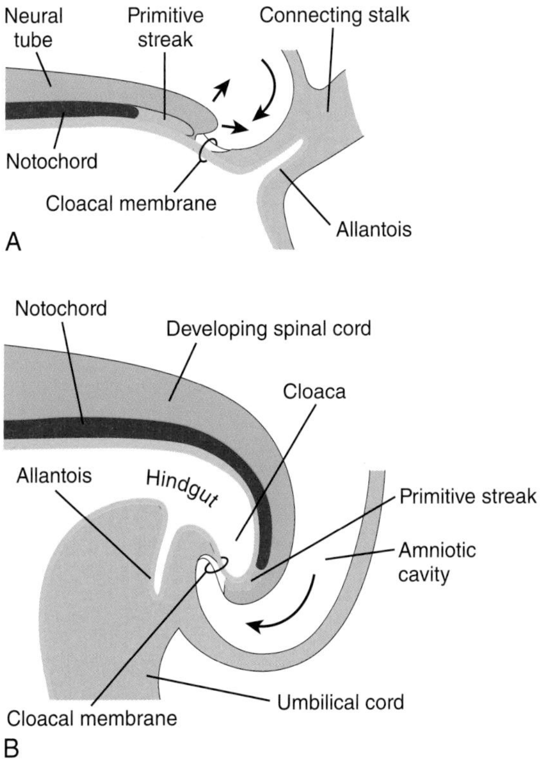

Fig. 5.4 Folding of the caudal end of the embryo. (A) Sagittal section of the caudal part of the embryo at the beginning of the fourth week. (B) Similar section at the end of the fourth week. Note that part of the umbilical vesicle is incorporated into the embryo as the hindgut and that the terminal part of the hindgut has dilated to form the cloaca. Observe also the change in position of the primitive streak, allantois, cloacal membrane, and connecting stalk.

complexity is achieved through morphogenesis and differentiation. The cells that make up the tissues of very early embryos are pluripotential which, under different circumstances, can follow more than one pathway of development. This broad developmental potential becomes progressively restricted as tissues acquire the specialized features necessary for increasing their sophistication of structure and function. Such restriction presumes that choices must be made to achieve tissue diversification.

Most evidence indicates that these choices are determined not as a consequence of cell lineage but rather in response to cues from immediate surroundings, including the adjacent tissues. As a result, the architectural precision and coordination that are often required for the normal function of an organ appear to be achieved by the interaction of the organ's constituent parts during development.

The cellular and molecular interaction of tissues during development is a recurring theme in embryology. The interactions that lead to a change in the course of development of at least one of the interactants are called **inductions**. Numerous examples of such inductive interactions can be found; for example, during the development of the eye, the optic vesicle induces the development of the lens from the surface ectoderm of the head. When the optic vesicle is absent, the eye fails to develop. Moreover, if the optic vesicle is removed and placed in association with a surface ectoderm that is not usually involved in eye development, lens formation can be induced.

Then, the development of a lens is dependent on the ectoderm acquiring an association with a second tissue. In the presence of neuroectoderm of the optic vesicle, the surface ectoderm of the head adopts a pathway of development that it would not otherwise have taken. Similarly, many of the morphogenetic tissue movements that play such important roles in shaping the embryo also provide for the changing tissue associations that are fundamental to **inductive tissue interactions**.

The fact that one tissue can influence the developmental pathway adopted by another tissue presumes that a signal passes between the two interactants. Analysis of the molecular defects in mutant animal strains shows that abnormal tissue interactions occur during embryonic development, and studies of the development of animal embryos with targeted gene mutations have begun to reveal the molecular mechanisms of induction. The mechanism of signal transfer can vary with the specific tissues involved. In some cases, the signal appears to take the form of a diffusible molecule, such as a **sonic hedgehog (Shh)**, that passes from the inductor to the reacting tissue. In others, the message appears to be mediated through a nondiffusible extracellular matrix that is secreted by the inductor and with which the reacting tissue comes into contact. In still other cases, the signal appears to require that physical contact occur between the inducing and responding tissues. Regardless of the mechanism of intercellular transfer involved, the signal is translated into an intracellular message that influences the genetic activity of the responding cells.

The signal can be relatively nonspecific in some interactions. The role of the natural inductor in a variety of interactions has been shown to be mimicked by several heterologous tissue sources and, in some instances, even by a variety of cell-free preparations. Studies suggest that the specificity of a given induction is a property of the reacting tissue rather than of the inductor. Inductions should not be thought of as isolated phenomena. They often occur in a sequential fashion that results in the orderly development of a complex structure; for example, following induction of the lens by the optic vesicle, the lens induces the development of the cornea from the surface ectoderm and adjacent mesenchyme. This ensures the formation of parts that are appropriate in size and relationship for the function of the organ. In other systems, there is evidence that the interactions between tissues are reciprocal. During the development of the kidney, for instance, the ureteric bud (metanephric diverticulum) induces the formation of tubules in the metanephric mesoderm (see Chapter 12). This mesoderm, in turn, induces the branching of the diverticulum, which results in the development of the collecting tubules and calices of the kidney.

To be competent to respond to an inducing stimulus, the cells of the reacting system must express the appropriate receptor for the specific inducing-signal molecule, the components of the particular **intracellular signal transduction pathway**, and the **transcription factors** that will mediate the particular response (see Chapter 21). Experimental evidence suggests that the acquisition of competence by the responding tissue is often dependent on its previous interactions with other tissues. For example, the lens-forming response of the head ectoderm to the stimulus provided by the optic vesicle appears to be dependent on a previous association of the head ectoderm with the anterior neural plate.

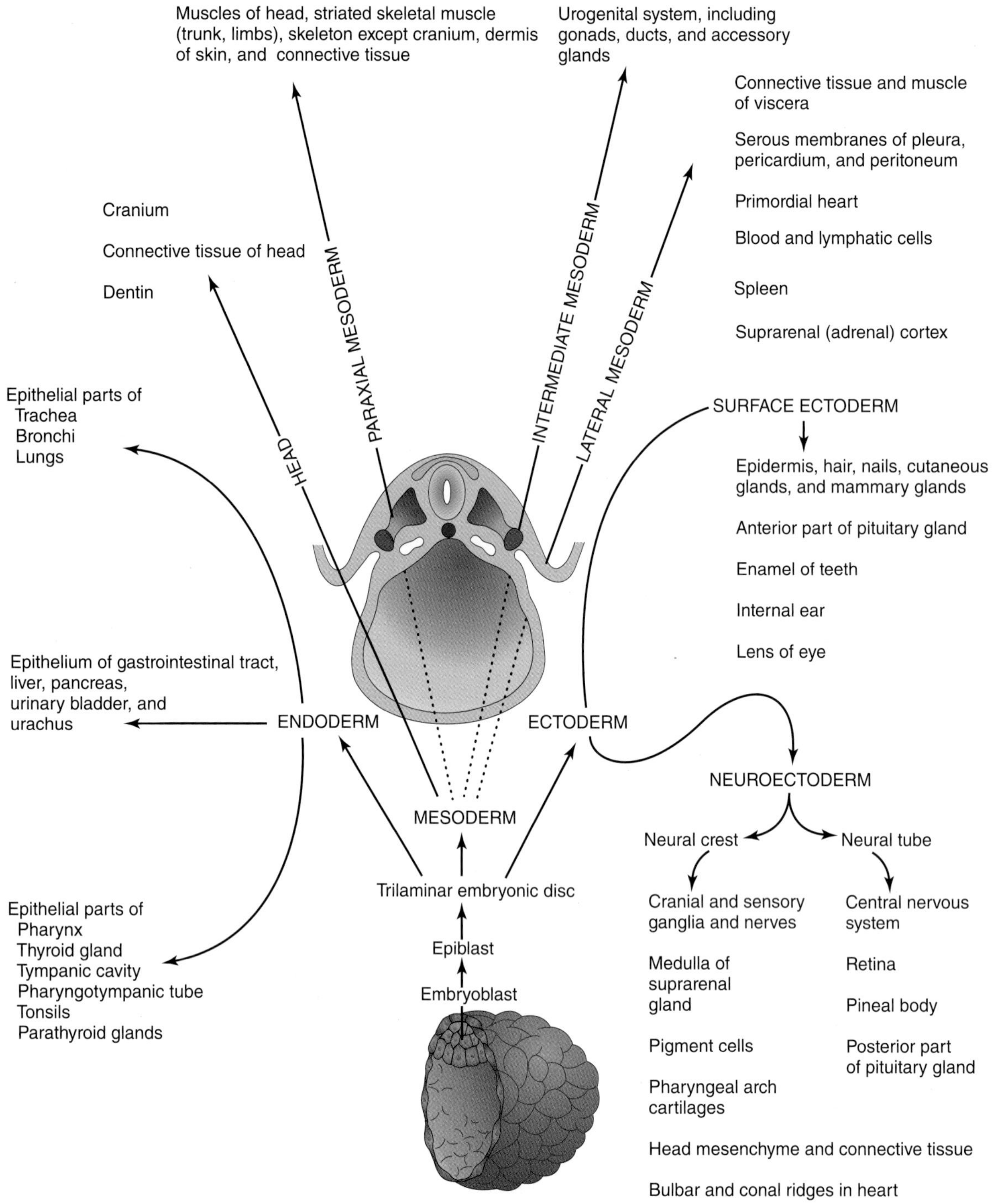

Fig. 5.5 Schematic drawing of derivatives of the three germ layers: ectoderm, endoderm, and mesoderm. Cells from these layers contribute to the formation of different tissues and organs.

The ability of the reacting system to respond to an inducing stimulus is not unlimited. Most inducible tissues appear to pass through a transient but more or less sharply delimited physiologic state in which they are competent to respond to an inductive signal from the neighboring tissue. Because this state of receptiveness is limited in time, a delay in the development of one or more components in an interacting system may lead to the failure of an inductive interaction. Regardless of the signal mechanism employed, inductive systems seem to have the common feature of proximity between the interacting tissues. Experimental evidence has demonstrated that interactions may fail if the interactants are too widely separated. Consequently, inductive processes appear to be limited in space as well as by time. Because tissue induction plays such a fundamental role in ensuring the orderly formation of precise structures, failed interactions can be expected to have drastic developmental consequences (e.g., birth defects).

HIGHLIGHTS OF THE FOURTH TO EIGHTH WEEKS

The following descriptions summarize the main developmental events and changes in the external form of the embryo during the fourth to eighth weeks. The main criteria for estimating developmental stages in human embryos are listed in Table 5.1.

FOURTH WEEK

Major changes in body form occur during the fourth week. At the beginning, the embryo is almost straight and has 4 to 12 somites that produce conspicuous surface elevations (Fig. 5.6A–D). The neural tube is formed opposite the somites, but it is widely open at the rostral and caudal **neuropores** (see Fig. 5.6C and D). By 24 days, the first pharyngeal arches are visible. The **first pharyngeal arch** (mandibular

Table 5.1 Criteria for Estimating Developmental Stages in Human Embryos

Age (Days)	Figure Reference	Carnegie Stage	Number of Somites	Length (mm)[a]	Main External Characteristics[b]
20–21		9	1–3	1.5–3.0	Flat embryonic disc. Deep neural groove and prominent neural folds. One to three pairs of somites present. Head fold evident.
22–23	5-6	10	4–12	1.0–3.5	The embryo is straight or slightly curved. Neural tube forming or formed opposite somites but widely open at rostral and caudal neuropores. First and second pairs of pharyngeal arches visible.
24–25	5-7	11	13–20	2.5–4.5	Embryo curved owing to head and tail folds. Rostral neuropore closing. Otic placodes present. Optic vesicles formed.
26–27	5-8	12	21–29	3.0–5.0	Upper limb buds appear. Rostral neuropore closed. Caudal neuropore closing. Three pairs of pharyngeal arches visible. Heart prominence distinct. Otic pits present.
28–30	5-9 5-11	13	30–35	4.0–6.0	The embryo has a C-shaped curve. Caudal neuropore closed. Four pairs of pharyngeal arches visible. Lower limb buds appear. Otic vesicles present. Lens placodes distinct. Tail-like caudal eminence present.
31–32	5-12 5-13	14	[c]	5.0–7.0	Lens pits and nasal pits visible. Optic cups present.
33–36		15		7.0–9.0	Hand plates formed; digital rays visible. Lens vesicles present. Nasal pits prominent. Cervical sinuses visible.
37–40		16		8.0–11.0	Foot plates formed. Pigment visible in the retina. Auricular hillocks developing.
41–43	5-14	17		11.0–14.0	Digital rays clearly visible in hand plates. Auricular hillocks outline the future auricle of the external ear. The trunk beginning to straighten. Cerebral vesicles prominent.
44–46		18		13.0–17.0	Digital rays clearly visible in foot plates. Elbow region visible. Eyelids forming. Notches between digital rays in the hands. Nipples visible.
47–48	5-15	19		16.0–18.0	Limbs extend ventrally. Trunk elongating and straightening. Midgut herniation prominent.
49–51		20		18.0–22.0	Upper limbs longer and bent at the elbows. Fingers distinct but webbed. Notches between digital rays in the feet. Scalp vascular plexus appears.
52–53	5-16	21		22.0–24.0	Hands and feet approach each other. Fingers are free and longer. Toes distinct but webbed.
54–55		22		23.0–28.0	Toes free and longer. Eyelids and auricles of external ears more developed.
56		23		27.0–31.0	Head is more rounded and shows human characteristics. External genitalia still have an indistinct appearance. Distinct bulge still present in the umbilical cord, caused by herniation of the intestines. Caudal eminence (tail) has disappeared.

[a]The embryonic lengths indicate the usual range. In stages 9 and 10, the measurement is the greatest length; in subsequent stages, crown-rump length measurements are given (see Fig. 5.20).

[b]At this and subsequent stages, the number of somites is difficult to determine and so is not a useful criterion.

[c]Based on Nishimura et al (1974), O'Rahilly and Müller (1987), Shiota (1991), and the Virtual Human Embryo Project (Project Leaders: Dr. Raymond Gasser and Dr. John Cork [https://www.ehd.org/virtual-human-embryo/]).

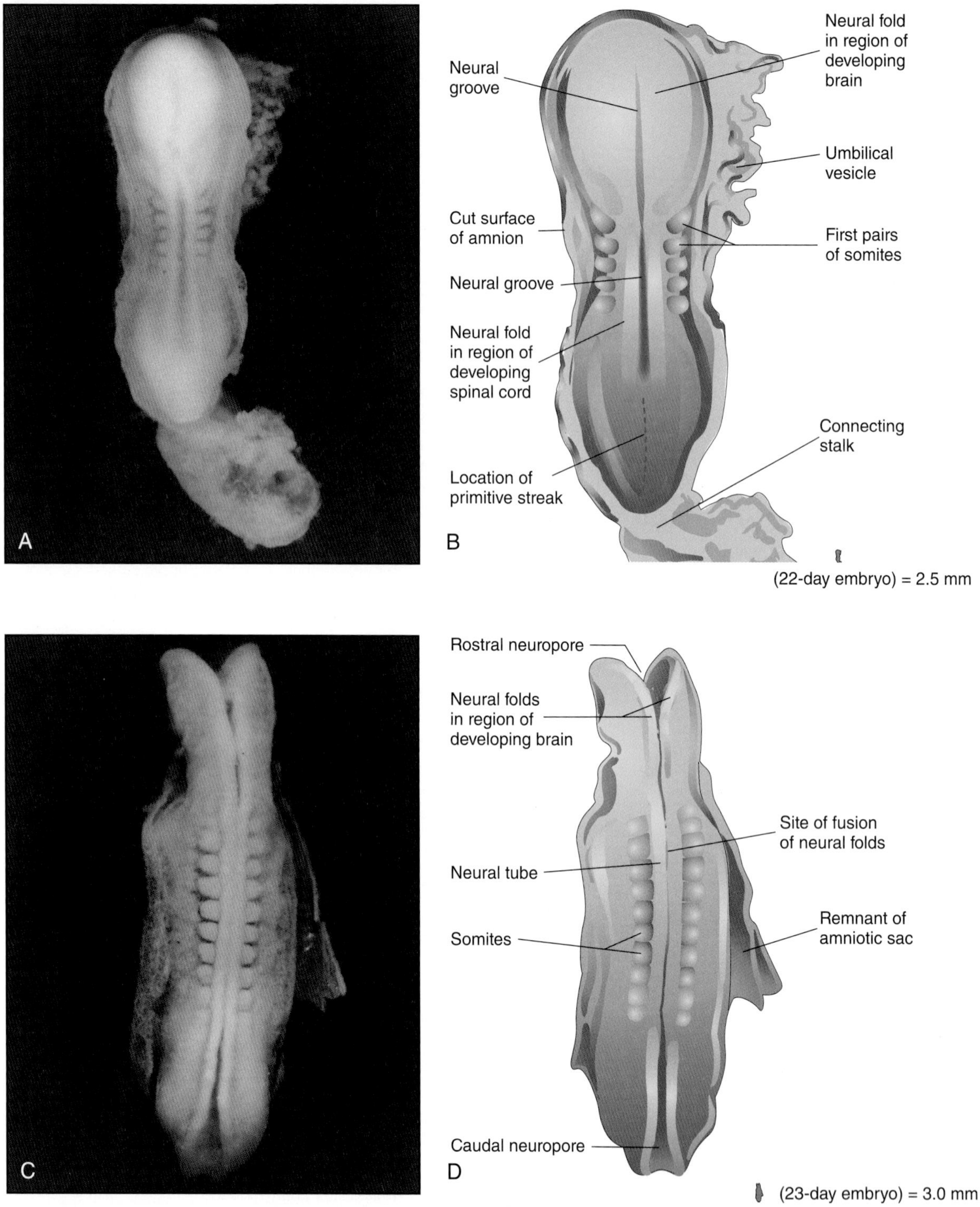

Fig. 5.6 (A) Dorsal view of a five-somite embryo at Carnegie stage 10, approximately 22 days. Observe the neural folds and deep neural grooves. The neural folds in the cranial region have thickened to form the primordium of the brain. (B) Drawing of structures shown in (A). Most of the amniotic and chorionic sacs have been cut away to expose the embryo. (C) Dorsal view of an older eight-somite embryo at Carnegie stage 10. The neural tube is in open communication with the amniotic cavity at the cranial and caudal ends through the rostral and caudal neuropores, respectively. (D) Diagram of structures shown in (C). The neural folds have fused opposite the somites to form the neural tube (primordium of the spinal cord in this region). ((A and C) From Moore KL, Persaud TVN, Shiota K: *Color atlas of clinical embryology*, ed 2, Philadelphia, 2000, Saunders.)

arch) is distinct (Fig. 5.7). The major part of the first arch gives rise to the mandible, and a rostral extension of the arch, the **maxillary prominence**, contributes to the maxilla. The embryo is now slightly curved because of the head and tail folds. The heart produces a large ventral **heart prominence** and pumps blood (see Fig. 5.7). The rostral neuropore is closing.

Three pairs of **pharyngeal arches** are visible at 26 days (Fig. 5.8), and the rostral neuropore is closed. The **forebrain** produces a prominent elevation of the head, and the folding of the embryo has given the embryo a C-shaped curvature. **Upper limb buds** are recognizable at day 26 or 27 as small swellings on the ventrolateral body walls (Fig. 5.9). The **otic pits** (primordia of the internal ears) are also visible. Ectodermal thickenings **(lens placodes)**, indicating the primordia of the future lenses of the eyes, are visible on the sides of the head (see Fig. 5.9B). The fourth pair of pharyngeal arches and lower limb buds are visible by the end of the fourth week. A long, tail-like **caudal eminence** is also a characteristic feature (Fig. 5.10 and see also Figs. 5.8 and 5.9). Rudiments of many of the organ systems, especially the **cardiovascular system**, are established (Fig. 5.11). By the end of the fourth week, the caudal neuropore is usually closed.

FIFTH WEEK

Changes in body form are minor during the fifth week compared with those that occurred during the fourth week, but the growth of the head exceeds that of other regions (Figs. 5.12 and 5.13). and results mainly from the rapid development of the brain and facial prominences. The face soon contacts the heart prominence. The rapidly growing second pharyngeal arch overgrows the third and fourth arches, forming a lateral depression on each side, the **cervical sinus**. Internally, mesonephric ridges indicate the site of the developing mesonephric kidneys (see Fig. 5.13B), which, in humans, are interim excretory organs.

SIXTH WEEK

Embryos in the sixth week show **spontaneous movements**, such as twitching of the trunk and developing limbs. It has been reported that embryos at this stage show **reflex responses to touch**. The upper limbs begin to show regional differentiation as the elbows and large **hand plates** develop (Fig. 5.14). The primordia of the digits or **digital rays**, begin to develop in the hand plates.

Development of the lower limbs occurs during the sixth week, 4 to 5 days later than that of the upper limbs. Several small swellings, **auricular hillocks**, develop around the **pharyngeal groove** between the first two pharyngeal arches (see Figs. 5.13 and 5.14B). This groove becomes the **external acoustic meatus** (external ear canal). The auricular hillocks contribute to the formation of the auricle (pinna), the shell-shaped part of the external ear. Largely because the retinal pigment has formed, the eyes are now obvious (see Fig.

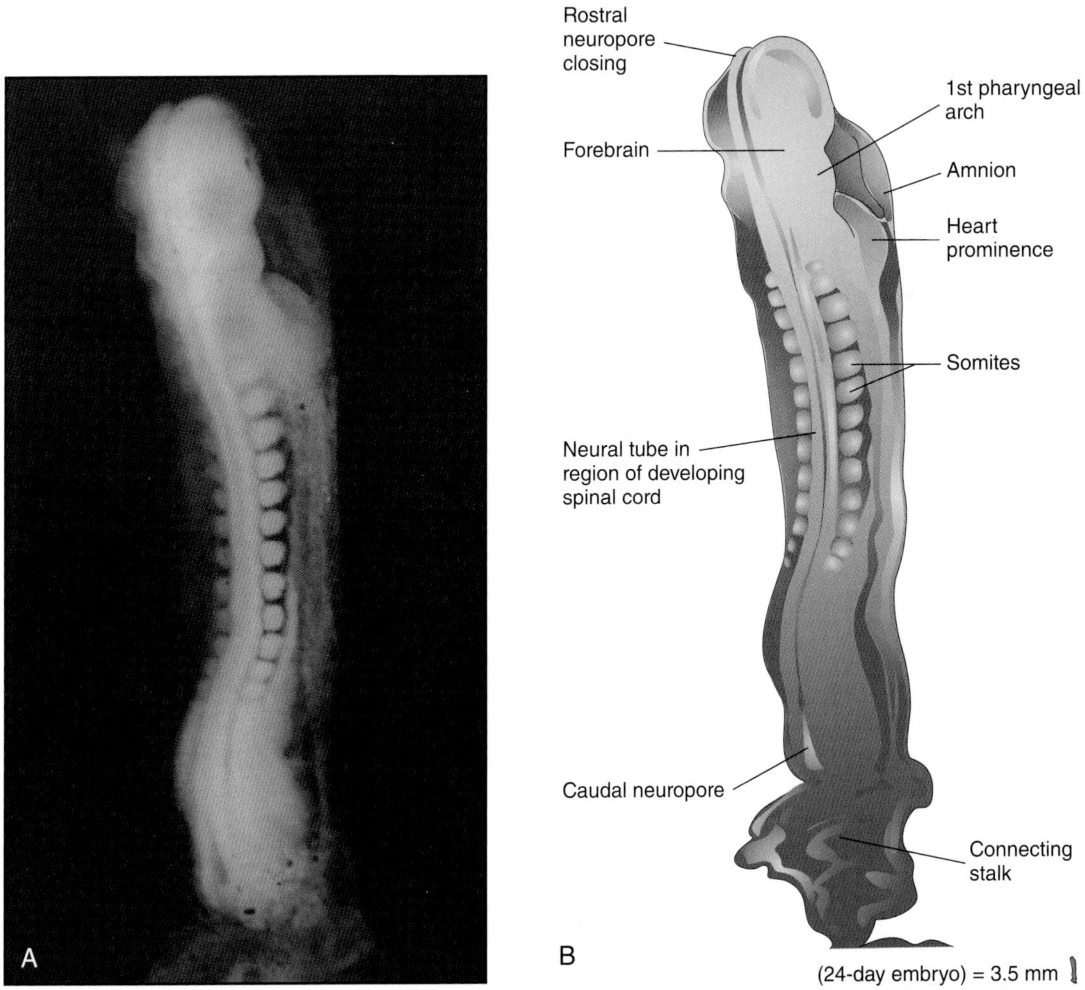

Fig. 5.7 (A) Dorsal view of a 13-somite embryo at Carnegie stage 11, approximately 24 days. The rostral neuropore is closing, but the caudal neuropore is wide open. (B) Illustration of the structures shown in (A). The embryo is lightly curved because of folding at the cranial and caudal ends. ((A) From Moore KL, Persaud TVN, Shiota K: *Color atlas of clinical embryology*, ed 2, Philadelphia, 2000, Saunders.)

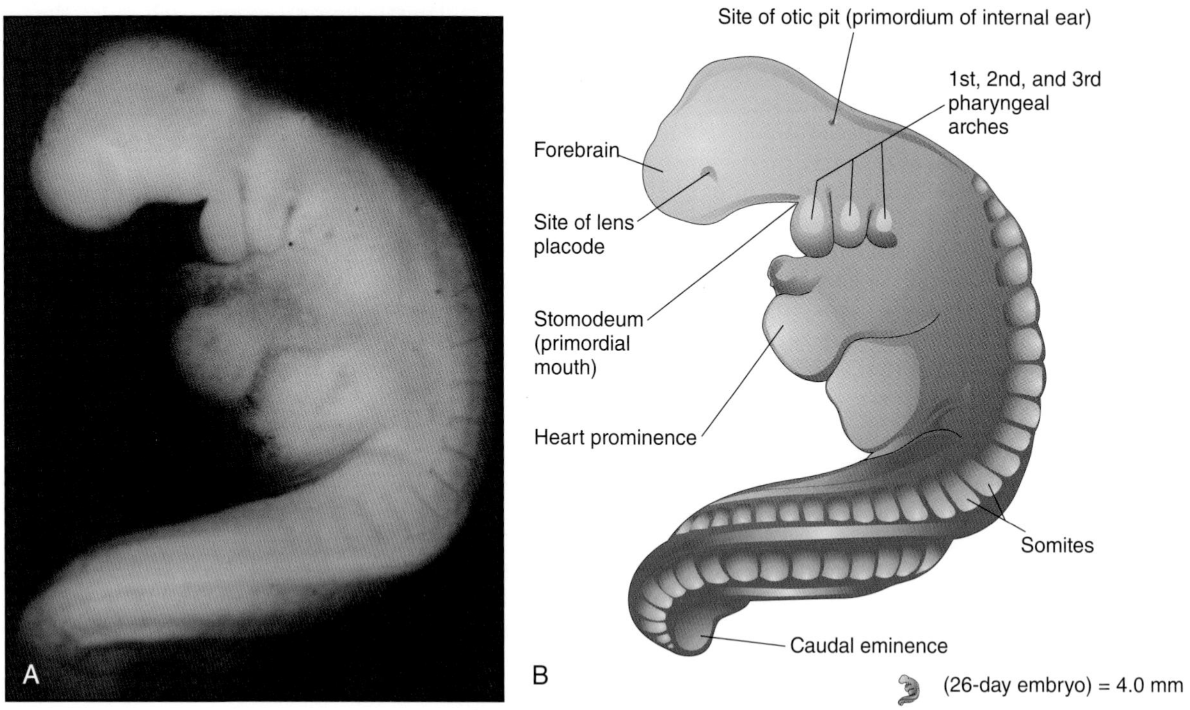

Fig. 5.8 (A) Lateral view of a 27-somite embryo at Carnegie stage 12, approximately 26 days. The embryo is curved, especially its tail-like caudal eminence. Observe the lens placode (primordium of the lens of the eye) and the otic pit, indicating early development of the internal ear. (B) Illustration of structures shown in (A). The rostral neuropore is closed, and three pairs of pharyngeal arches are present. ((A) From Nishimura H, Semba R, Tanimura T, Tanaka O: *Prenatal development of the human with special reference to craniofacial structures: an atlas*, Washington, DC, 1977, National Institutes of Health.)

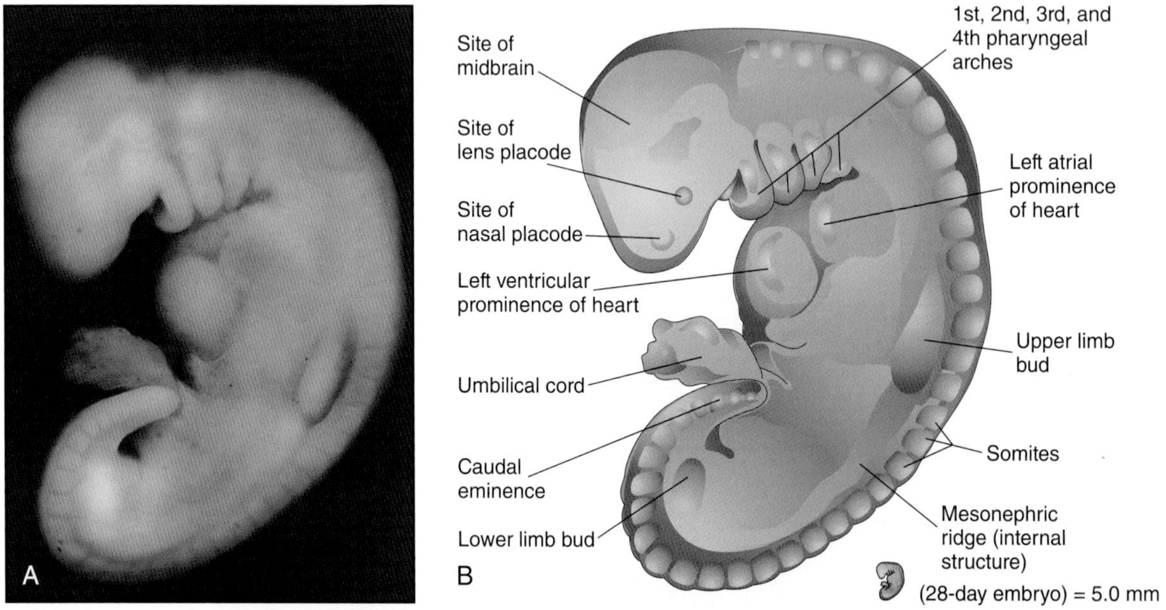

Fig. 5.9 (A) Lateral view of an embryo at Carnegie stage 13, approximately 28 days. The primordial heart is large and divided into a primordial atrium and ventricle. The rostral and caudal neuropores are closed. (B) Drawing indicating the structures shown in (A). The embryo has a characteristic C-shaped curvature, four pharyngeal arches, and upper and lower limb buds. ((A) From Nishimura H, Semba R, Tanimura T, Tanaka O: *Prenatal development of the human with special reference to craniofacial structures: an atlas*, Washington, DC, 1977, National Institutes of Health.)

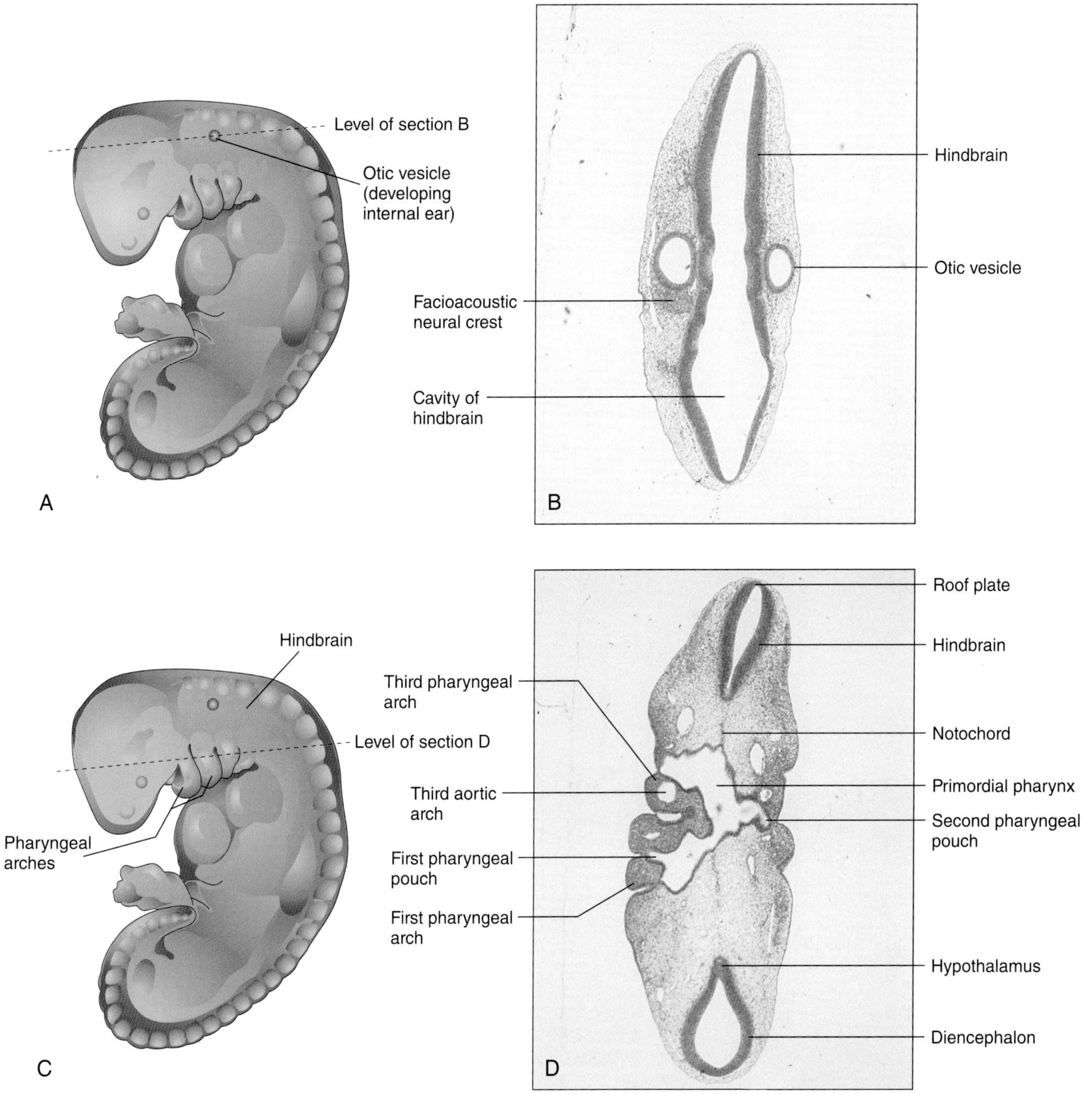

Fig. 5.10 (A) Drawing of an embryo at Carnegie stage 13, approximately 28 days. (B) Photomicrograph of a section of the embryo at the level shown in (A). Observe the hindbrain and otic vesicle (primordium of the internal ear). (C) Drawing of the same embryo showing the level of the section in (D). Observe the primordial pharynx and pharyngeal arches. (B and D, From Moore KL, Persaud TVN, Shiota K: *Color atlas of clinical embryology*, ed 2, Philadelphia, 2000, Saunders.)

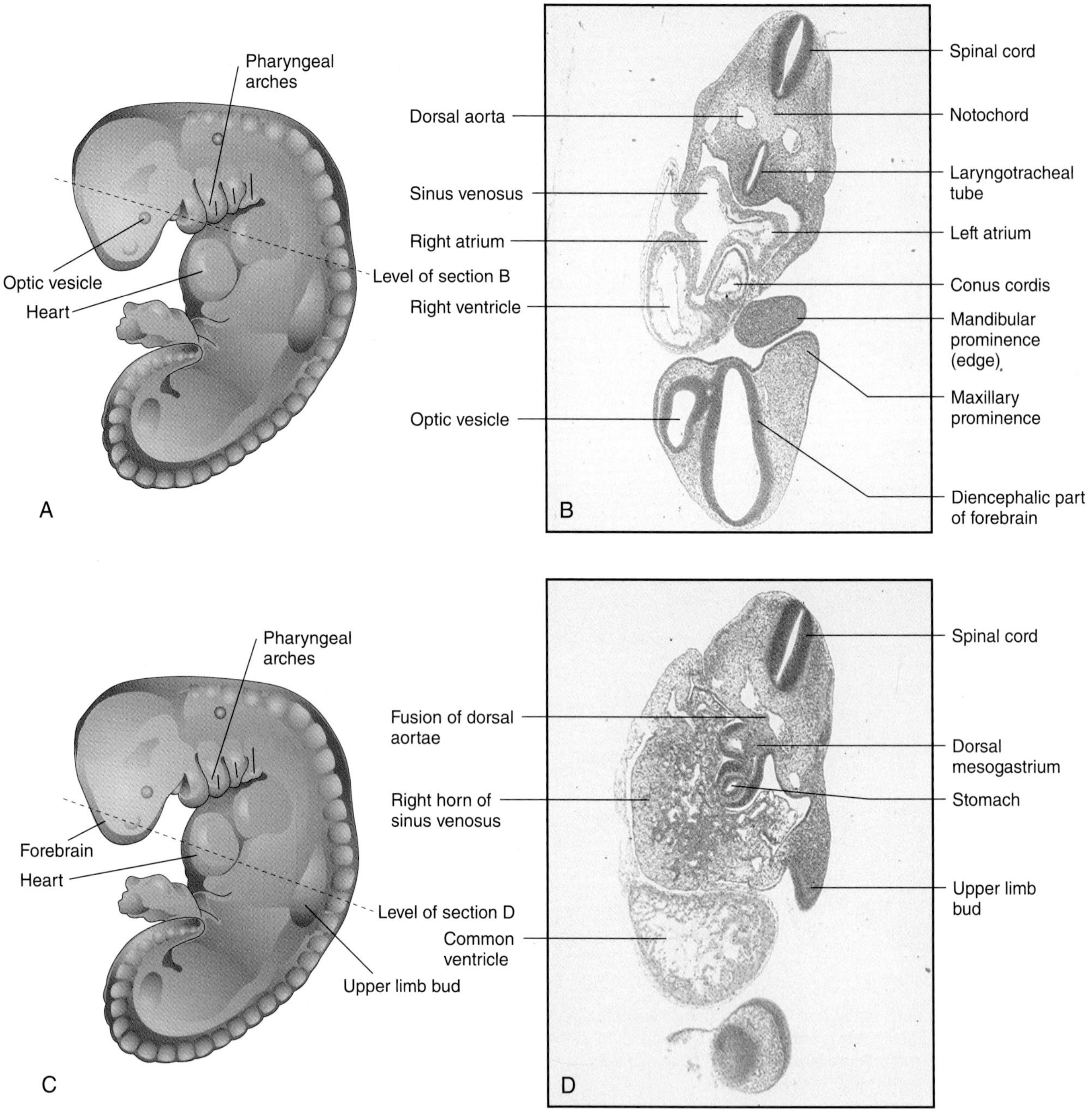

Fig. 5.11 (A) Drawing of an embryo at Carnegie stage 13, approximately 28 days. (B) Photomicrograph of a section of the embryo at the level shown in (A). Observe the parts of the primordial heart. (C) Drawing of the same embryo showing the level of the section in (D). Observe the primordial heart and stomach. (B and D) From Moore KL, Persaud TVN, Shiota K: *Color atlas of clinical embryology*, ed 2, Philadelphia, 2000, Saunders.

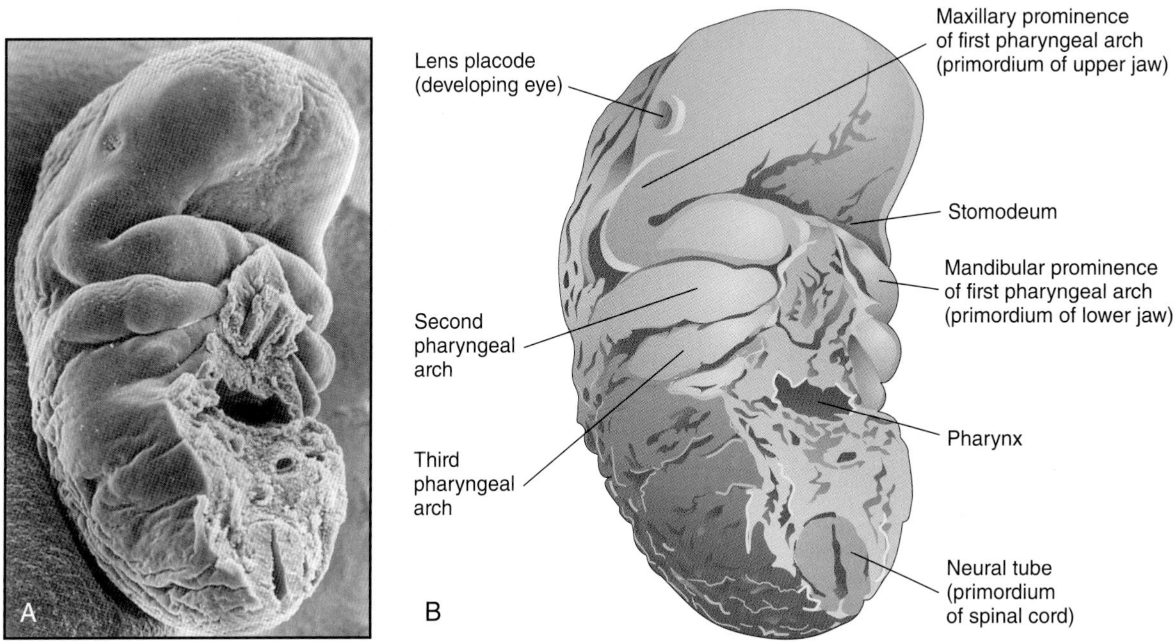

Fig. 5.12 (A) Scanning electron micrograph of the craniofacial region of a human embryo of approximately 32 days (Carnegie stage 14, 6.8 mm). Three pairs of pharyngeal arches are present. The maxillary and mandibular prominences of the first arch are delineated. Observe the large stomodeum (mouth) located between the maxillary prominences and fused mandibular prominences. (B) Drawing of the scanning electron micrograph illustrating the structures shown in (A). (A, Courtesy the late Professor K. Hinrichsen, Ruhr-Universität Bochum, Bochum, Germany.)

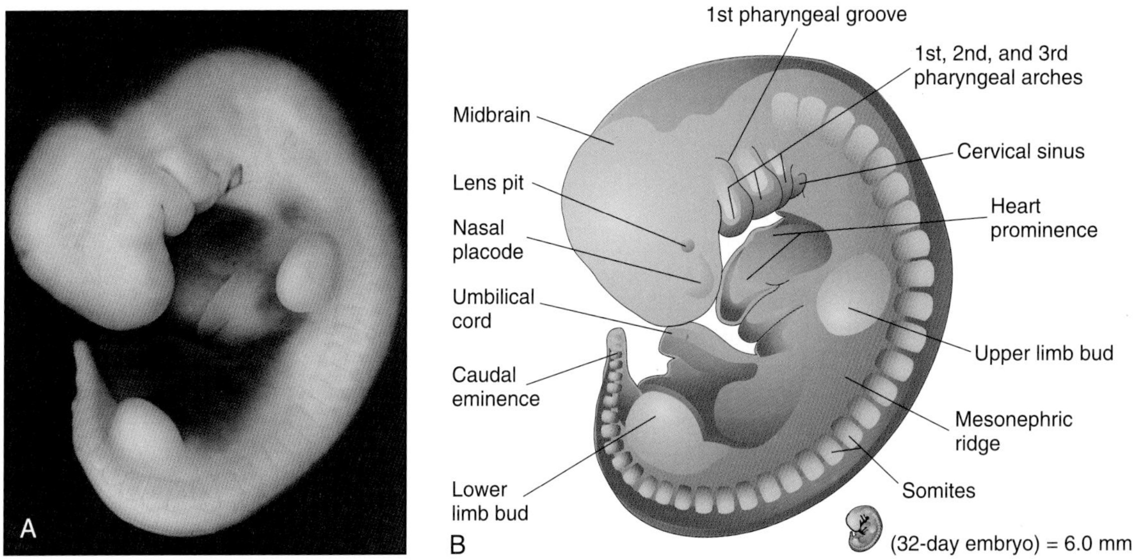

Fig. 5.13 (A) Lateral view of an embryo at Carnegie stage 14, approximately 32 days. The second pharyngeal arch has overgrown the third arch, forming the **cervical sinus**. The mesonephric ridge indicates the site of the mesonephric kidney, an interim kidney (see Chapter 12). (B) Illustration of structures shown in (A). (A) From Nishimura H, Semba R, Tanimura T, Tanaka O: *Prenatal development of the human with special reference to craniofacial structures: an atlas*, Washington, DC, 1977, National Institutes of Health.

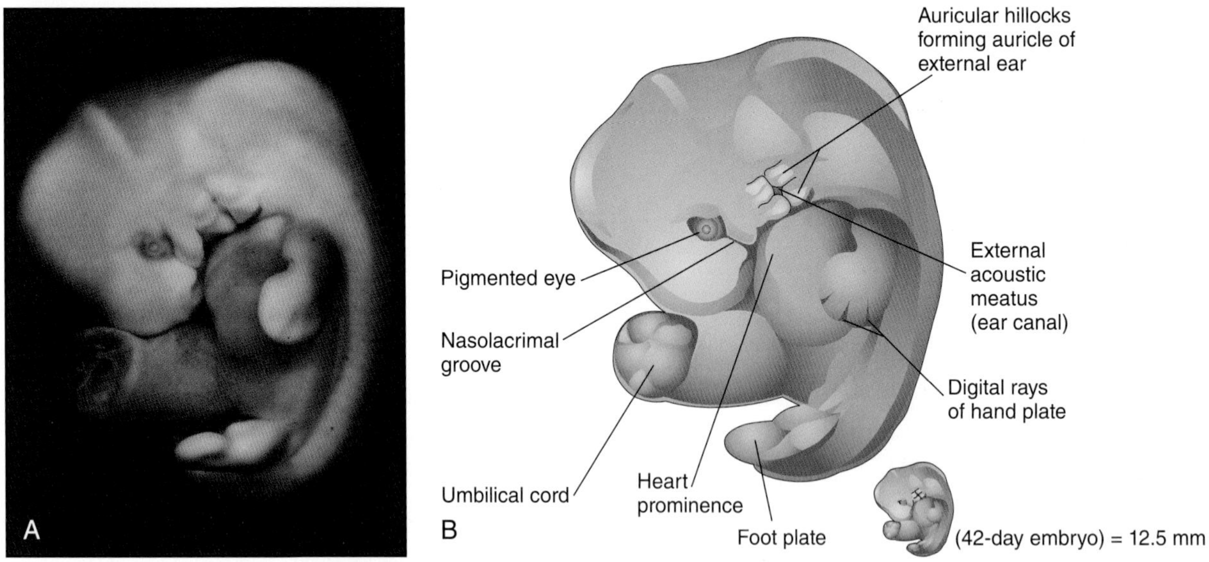

Fig. 5.14 (A) Lateral view of an embryo at Carnegie stage 17, approximately 42 days. Digital rays are visible in the hand plate, indicating the future site of the digits (fingers). (B) Drawing illustrating structures shown in (A). The eye, auricular hillocks, and external acoustic meatus are now obvious. ((A) From Moore KL, Persaud TVN, Shiota K: *Color atlas of clinical embryology*, ed 2, Philadelphia, 2000, Saunders.)

5.14). The head is now much larger relative to the trunk and is bent over the **heart prominence**. This head position results from bending in the cervical (neck) region. The trunk and neck have begun to straighten, and the intestines enter the extraembryonic coelom in the proximal part of the umbilical cord (see Fig. 5.18). This umbilical herniation is a normal event. The herniation occurs because the abdominal cavity is too small at this age to accommodate the rapidly growing intestine.

SEVENTH WEEK

The limbs undergo considerable change during the seventh week. Notches appear between the **digital rays**, separating the areas of the hand and foot plates and indicating the digits (Fig. 5.15). Communication between the primordial gut and umbilical vesicle is now reduced to the **omphaloenteric duct** (see Fig. 5.1C_2). By the end of the seventh week, **primary ossification** of the bones of the upper limbs has begun.

EIGHTH WEEK

At the beginning of this final week of the embryonic period, the digits of the hand are separated but noticeably webbed (Fig. 5.16A and B). Notches are also clearly visible between the digital rays of the feet. The **caudal eminence** is still present but stubby. The **scalp vascular plexus** has appeared and forms a characteristic band around the head. At the end of the eighth week, all regions of the limbs are apparent, and the digits have lengthened and are completely separated (Fig. 5.17).

Purposeful limb movements first occur during the eighth week. Primary ossification begins in the **femurs**. All evidence of the caudal eminence has disappeared, and both hands and feet approach each other ventrally. At the end of this week, the embryo has distinct human characteristics (Fig. 5.18); however, the head is still disproportionately large, constituting almost half of the embryo. The neck is established, and the eyelids are more obvious. The eyelids are closing, and by the end of the eighth week, they begin to unite by epithelial fusion. The intestines are still in the proximal portion of the umbilical cord (see Fig. 5.18). Although there are slight sex differences in the appearance of the external genitalia, they are not distinctive enough to permit accurate sexual identification.

ESTIMATION OF EMBRYONIC AGE

Estimates of the age of embryos, recovered after a spontaneous abortion, for example, are determined from their external characteristics and measurements of their length (Figs. 5.19 and 5.20, and also see Table 5.1). However, size alone may be an unreliable criterion because some embryos undergo a progressively slower rate of growth before death. Embryos of the third and early fourth weeks are straight (see Fig. 5.20A), so measurements indicate the greatest length. The **crown-rump length** (CRL) is most frequently used for older embryos (14–18 weeks) (see Fig. 5.20B). Because no anatomic marker indicates the CRL, one assumes that the longest CRL is the most accurate. Standing height, or **crown-heel length**, is sometimes measured. The length of an embryo is only one criterion for establishing age. The **Carnegie Embryonic Staging System** is used internationally; its staging is based on the development of structures (internal and external) in the first 9 weeks, and its use enables comparisons to be made between the findings of one person and those of another (see Table 5.1) or even between species. During the first trimester ultrasonography provides the most accurate estimation of embryonic age.

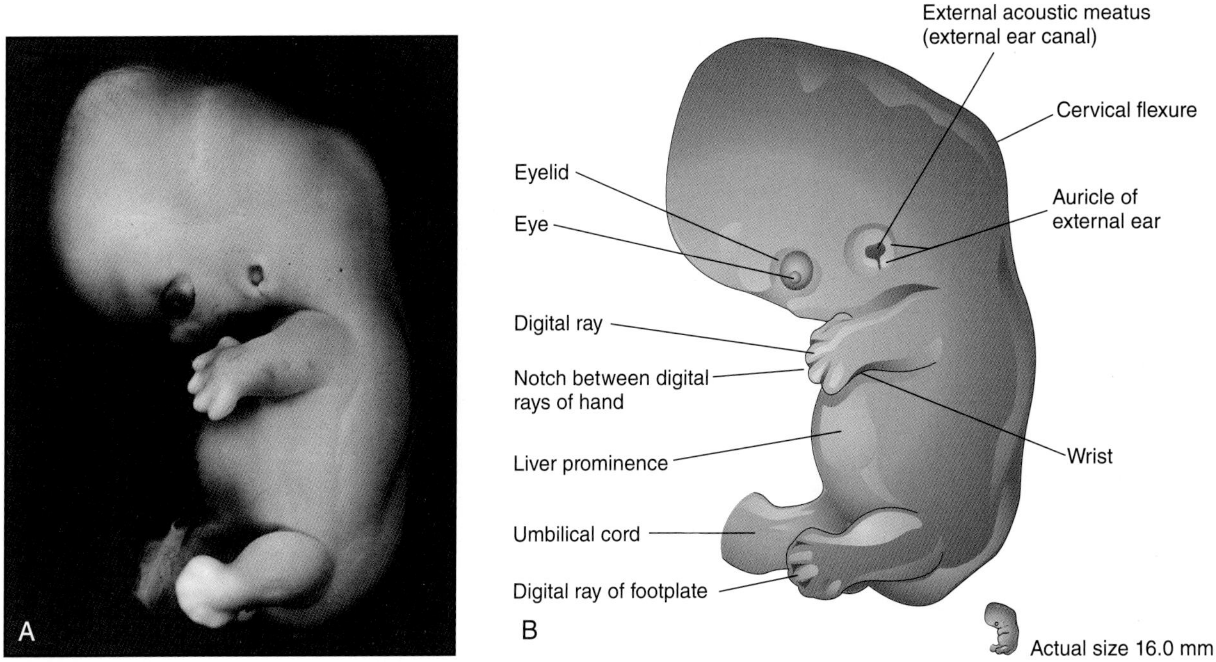

Fig. 5.15 (A) Lateral view of an embryo at Carnegie stage 19, about 48 days. The auricle and external acoustic meatus are now clearly visible. Note the relatively low position of the developing ear at this stage. Digital rays are now visible in the footplate. The prominence of the abdomen is caused mainly by the large size of the liver. (B) Drawing indicating structures shown in (A). Observe the large hand and notches between the digital rays, which indicate the developing digits (fingers). ((A) From Moore KL, Persaud TVN, Shiota K: *Color atlas of clinical embryology*, ed 2, Philadelphia, 2000, Saunders.)

Estimation of Gestational and Embryonic Age

Obstetricians date pregnancy from the presumed first day of the **last normal menstrual period (LNMP)**. This is the **gestational age**, which in embryology is superfluous because *gestation* does not begin until fertilization of an oocyte occurs. **Embryonic age** begins at fertilization, approximately 2 weeks after the **LNMP** (see Fig. 1.1). **Fertilization age** is used in patients who have undergone in vitro fertilization or artificial insemination (see Fig. 2.15).

Knowledge of embryonic age is important because it affects clinical management, especially when invasive procedures such as chorionic villus sampling and amniocentesis are necessary (see Chapter 6). In some females, the estimation of their gestational age from their menstrual history alone may be unreliable. The probability of error in establishing the LNMP is highest in females who become pregnant after cessation of oral contraception because the interval between discontinuance of hormones and the onset of ovulation is highly variable. In other females, slight uterine bleeding (spotting), which sometimes occurs during implantation of the blastocyst, may be incorrectly regarded by a female as light menstruation.

Other contributing factors to LNMP unreliability may include poor recall of menstruation, **oligomenorrhea** (scanty menstruation), pregnancy in the postpartum period (i.e., several weeks after childbirth), and use of intrauterine devices. Despite possible sources of error, the LNMP is a useful criterion in most cases. Ultrasound assessment of the size of the embryo and chorionic cavity enables clinicians to obtain an accurate estimate of the date of conception (see Fig. 5.19).

All statements about embryonic age should indicate the reference point used, that is, days after LNMP or after the estimated time of fertilization.

Ultrasound Examination of Embryos

Most females seeking obstetric care have at least one ultrasound examination during their pregnancy for one or more of the following reasons:

- Estimation of gestational age for confirmation of clinical dating
- Evaluation of embryonic growth when intrauterine growth restriction is suspected
- Guidance during chorionic villus or amniotic fluid sampling (see Chapter 6)
- Verification of fetal heartbeat
- Examination of a clinically detected pelvic mass
- Suspected ectopic pregnancy (see Fig. 3.9)
- Possible uterine birth defects (see Fig. 12.44)
- Detection of birth defects

Current data indicate that there are no confirmed biologic effects of diagnostic ultrasonography or magnetic resonance imaging evaluation on embryos or fetuses (see Figs. 5.16C, 5.17C, and 5.19).

The size of an embryo in utero can be estimated using ultrasound measurements. **Transvaginal sonography** permits an earlier and more accurate measurement of CRL in early pregnancy (see Fig. 5.19). The gestational sac can be detected early in the fifth week, and the embryo is 4 to 7 mm long (see Fig. 5.13). During the sixth and seventh weeks, discrete embryonic structures can be visualized (e.g., parts of limbs), and CRL measurements are predictive of embryonic age with an accuracy of 1 to 4 days. Furthermore, after the sixth week, the dimensions of the head and trunk can be obtained and used for the assessment of embryonic age. There is, however, considerable variability in early embryonic growth and development. Differences are greatest before the end of the first 4 weeks of development but less so by the end of the embryonic period.

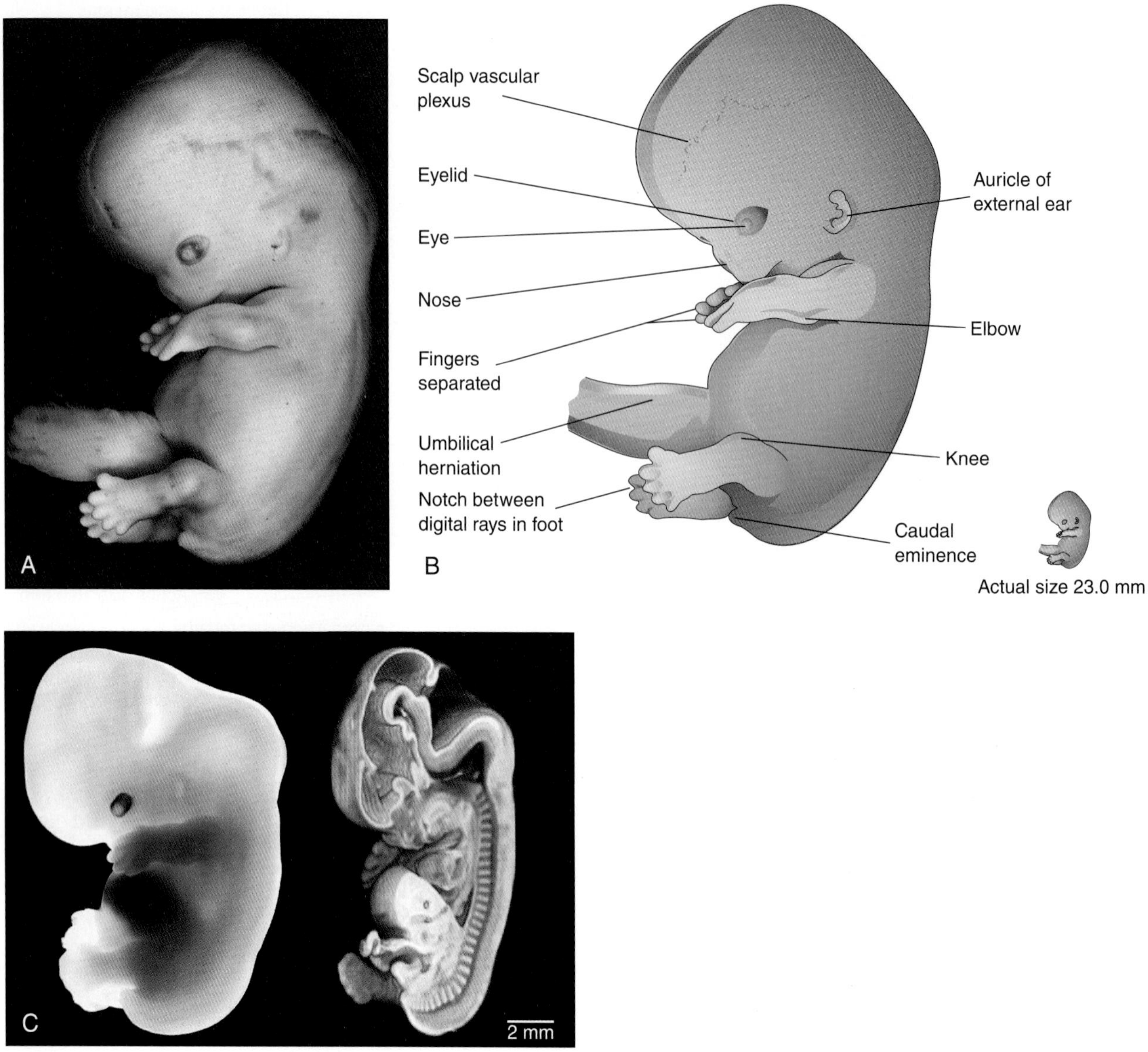

Fig. 5.16 (A) Lateral view of an embryo at Carnegie stage 21, approximately 52 days. Note that the scalp vascular plexus now forms a characteristic band across the head. The nose is stubby, and the eye is heavily pigmented. (B) Illustration of structures shown in (A). The fingers are separated, and the toes are beginning to separate. (C) A Carnegie stage 20 human embryo, approximately 50 days after ovulation, imaged with optical microscopy (*left*) and magnetic resonance microscopy (*right*). The three-dimensional data set from magnetic resonance microscopy has been edited to reveal anatomic detail from a midsagittal plane. ((A) From Nishimura H, Semba R, Tanimura T, Tanaka O: *Prenatal development of the human with special reference to craniofacial structures: an atlas*, Washington, DC, 1977, National Institutes of Health. (B) From Moore KL, Persaud TVN, Shiota K: *Color atlas of clinical embryology*, ed 2, Philadelphia, 2000, Saunders. (C) Courtesy Dr. Bradley R. Smith, University of Michigan, Ann Arbor, Michigan.)

SUMMARY OF FOURTH TO EIGHTH WEEKS

- At the beginning of the fourth week, folding in the median and horizontal planes converts the flat trilaminar embryonic disc into a C-shaped, cylindric embryo. The formation of the head region, caudal eminence, and lateral folds is a continuous sequence of events that results in a constriction between the embryo and umbilical vesicle.
- As the head region folds ventrally, part of the endodermal layer is incorporated into the developing embryonic head region as the **foregut**. Folding of the head region also results in the oropharyngeal membrane and heart being carried ventrally and the developing brain becoming the most cranial part of the embryo.
- As the caudal eminence folds ventrally, part of the endodermal germ layer is incorporated into the caudal end of the embryo as the **hindgut**. The terminal part of the hindgut expands to form the **cloaca**. Folding of the caudal region also results in the cloacal membrane, **allantois**, and connecting stalk being carried to the ventral surface of the embryo.
- Folding of the embryo in the horizontal plane incorporates part of the endoderm into the embryo as the **midgut**.
- The **umbilical vesicle** remains attached to the midgut by a narrow **omphaloenteric duct**. During the folding of

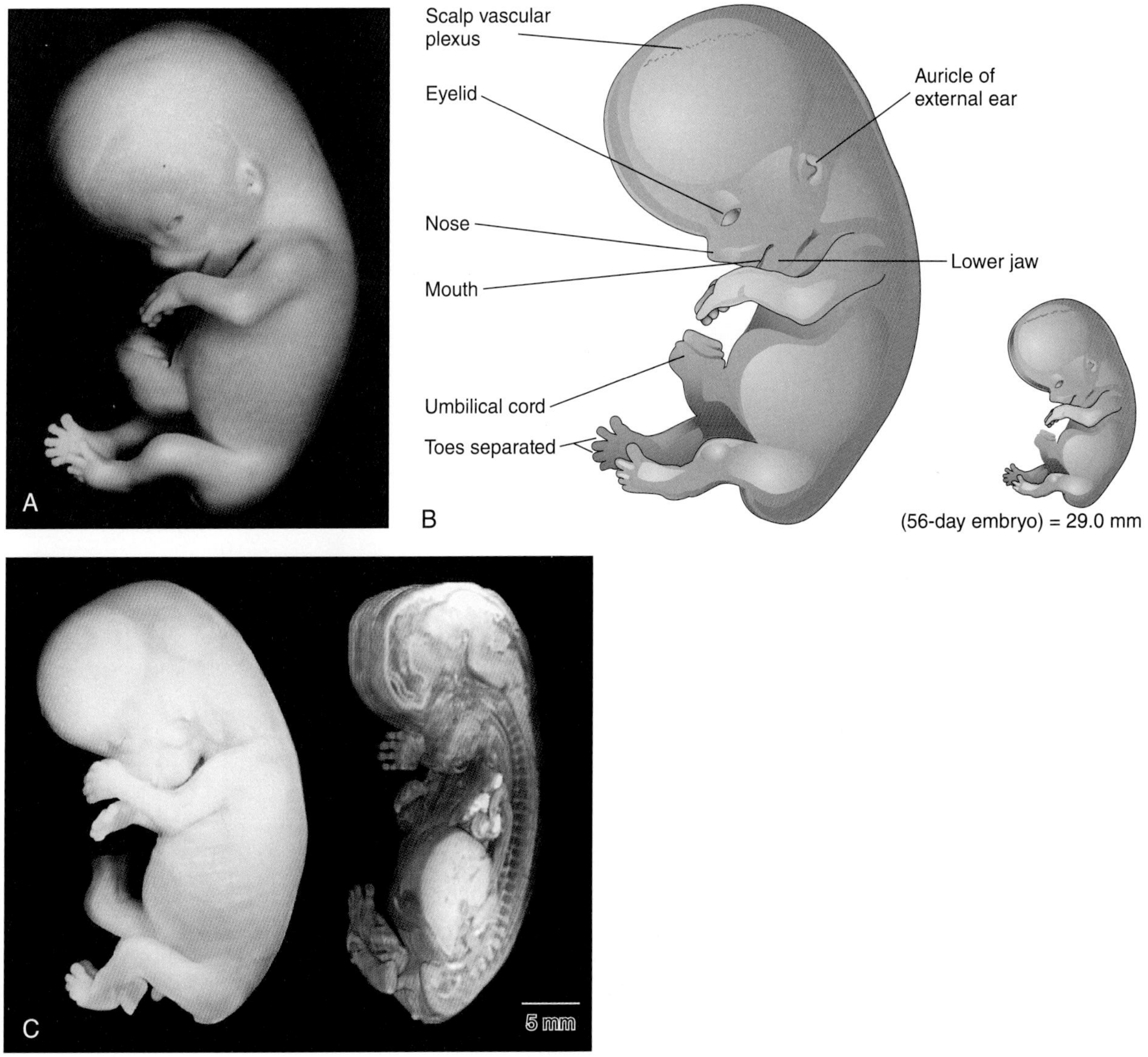

Fig. 5.17 (A) Lateral view of an embryo at Carnegie stage 23, approximately 56 days (end of embryonic period). The embryo has a distinctly human appearance. (B) Illustration of structures shown in (A). (C) A Carnegie stage 23 embryo, approximately 56 days after ovulation, imaged with optical microscopy *(left)* and magnetic resonance microscopy *(right)*. ((A) From Nishimura H, Semba R, Tanimura T, Tanaka O: *Prenatal development of the human with special reference to craniofacial structures: an atlas*, Washington, DC, 1977, National Institutes of Health. (B) From Moore KL, Persaud TVN, Shiota K: *Color atlas of clinical embryology*, ed 2, Philadelphia, 2000, Saunders. (C) Courtesy Dr. Bradley R. Smith, University of Michigan, Ann Arbor, Michigan.)

the embryo in the horizontal plane, the primordia of the lateral and ventral body walls are formed. As the **amnion** expands, it envelops the connecting stalk, omphaloenteric duct, and allantois, thereby forming an epithelial covering for the umbilical cord.
- The three germ layers differentiate into various tissues and organs so that by the end of the embryonic period, the beginnings of the main organ systems have been established.
- The external appearance of the embryo is greatly affected by the formation of the brain, heart, liver, somites, limbs, ears, nose, and eyes.
- Because the beginnings of the most essential external and internal structures are formed during the fourth to eighth weeks, this is the most critical period of development. Developmental disturbances during this period may give rise to major birth defects.
- Reasonable estimates of the age of embryos can be determined from the day of onset of the LNMP. Further refinement of gestational age can be made through ultrasound measurements of the chorionic sac and embryo.

CLINICALLY ORIENTED PROBLEMS

CASE 5-1

A 28-year-old female who has been a heavy cigarette smoker since her teens was informed that she was in the second month of pregnancy.

- What would the doctor likely tell the patient about her smoking habit and its possible impacts on the embryo and fetal health?

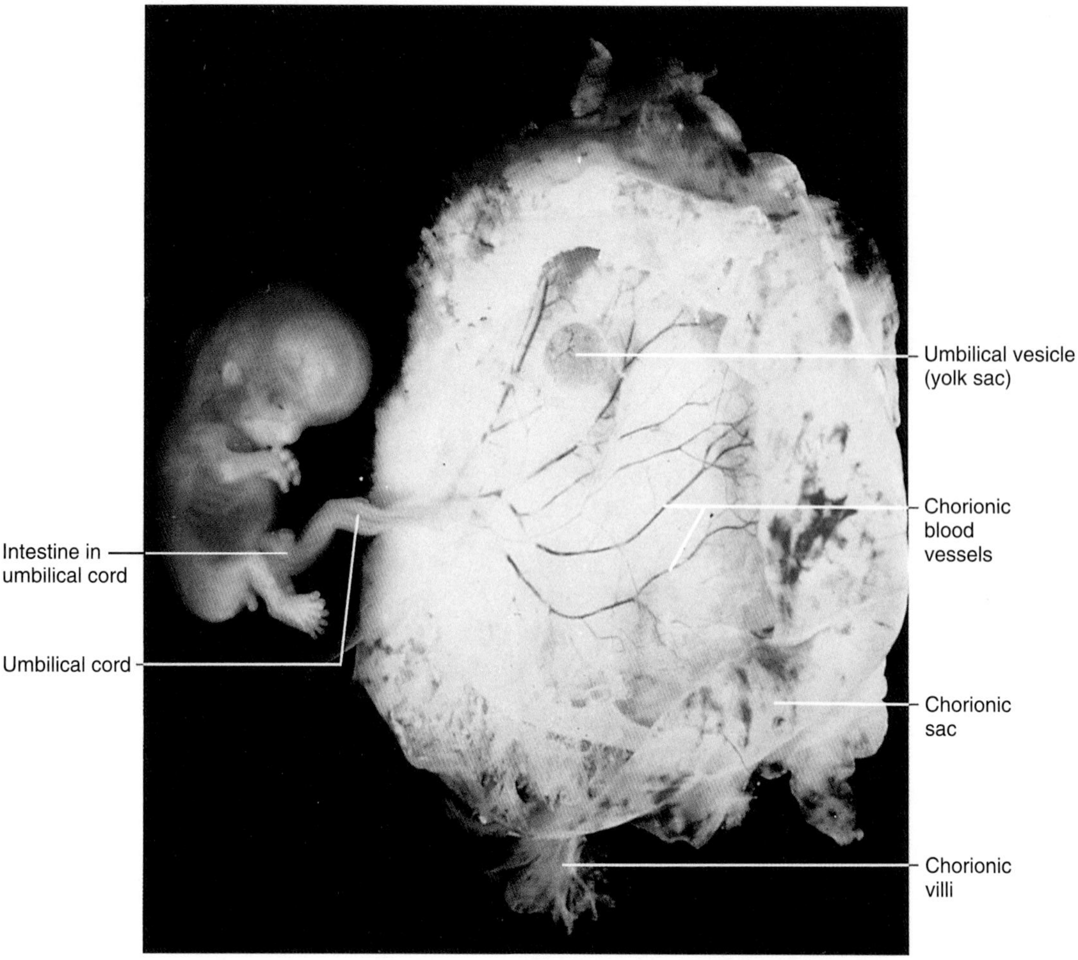

Fig. 5.18 Lateral view of an embryo and its chorionic sac at Carnegie stage 23, approximately 56 days. Observe the human appearance of the embryo. Although it may appear to be a male, it may not be possible to estimate sex because the external genitalia of males and females are similar at this stage of the embryonic period (see Fig. 1.1). (From Nishimura H, Semba R, Tanimura T, Tanaka O: *Prenatal development of the human with special reference to craniofacial structures: an atlas*, Washington, DC, 1977, National Institutes of Health.)

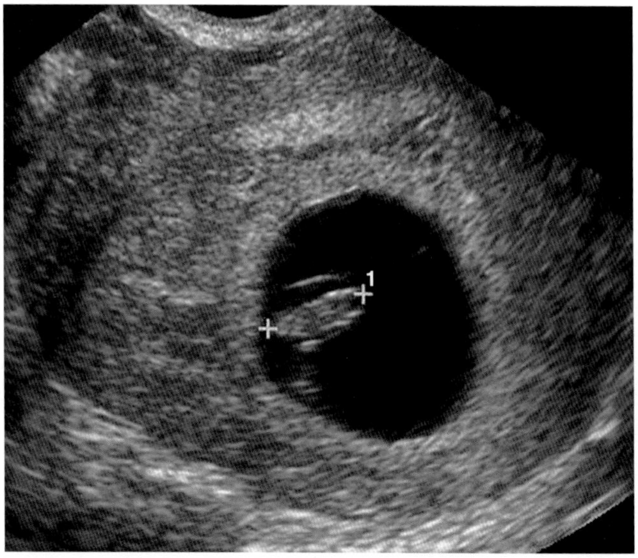

Fig. 5.19 Transvaginal sonogram of a 7-week embryo (*calipers*, crown-rump length 10 mm) surrounded by the amniotic membrane within the chorionic cavity *(dark region)*. (Courtesy Dr. E. A. Lyons, Professor of Radiology, Obstetrics, and Gynecology and Anatomy, Health Sciences Centre and University of Manitoba, Winnipeg, Manitoba, Canada.)

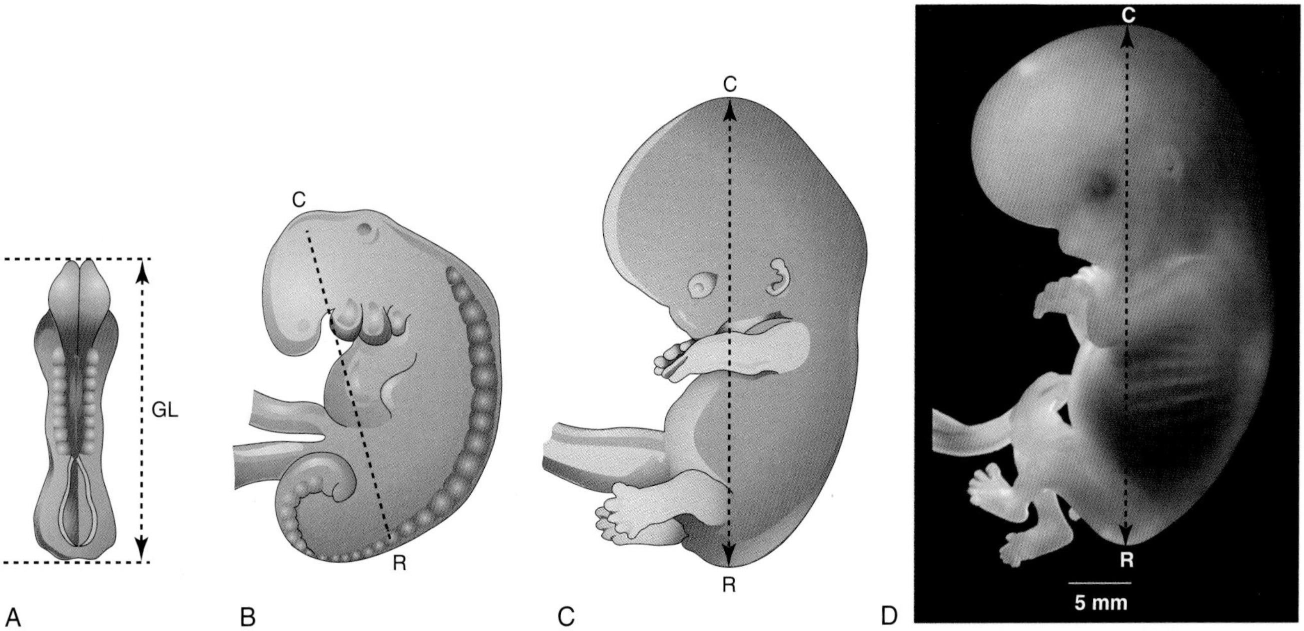

Fig. 5.20 Illustrations of methods used to measure the length of embryos. (A) GL. (B, C, and D) CR length. (D) Photograph of an 8-week-old embryo at Carnegie stage 23. *CR*, Crown-rump; *GL*, greatest length. ((D) Courtesy Dr. Bradley R. Smith, University of Michigan, Ann Arbor, Michigan.)

CASE 5-2

A pregnant patient was concerned about what she had read in the newspaper about the teratogenic effects of drugs on laboratory animals.

- Can one predict the possible harmful effects of drugs on the human embryo from studies performed on laboratory animals? Explain.

CASE 5-3

A 30-year-old female was unsure when her LNMP had occurred. She stated that her periods were irregular.

- What clinical techniques could be used for evaluating embryonic age in this pregnancy?

CASE 5-4

A female who had just become pregnant told her doctor that she had taken a sleeping pill given to her by a friend. She wondered whether it could harm the development of her baby's limbs.

- Would a drug known to cause severe limb defects be likely to cause these birth defects if it were taken during the second week? Sixth week? Eighth week?

Discussion of these problems appears in the Appendix at the back of the book.

BIBLIOGRAPHY AND SUGGESTED READING

American College of Obstetricians and Gynecologists' Committee on Obstetric Practice: Methods for estimating the due date. Committee opinion 700, *Obstet Gynecol* 129:e150, 2017.

Barnea ER, Hustin J, Jauniaux E, editors: *The first twelve weeks of gestation,* Berlin, 1992, Springer-Verlag.

Blechschmidt E, Gasser RF: Biokinetics and biodynamics of human differentiation: principles and applications, Reprint edition 2012, North Atlantic Books: Berkeley.

Briscoe J, Small S: Morphogen rules: design principles of gradient-mediated embryo patterning, *Development* 142:3996, 2015.

Butt K, Lim K: Determination of gestational age by ultrasound, *J Obstet Gynaecol Can* 36:171, 2014.

Chekrouni N, Kleipool R, De Bakker BS: The impact of using three-dimensional digital models of human embryos in the biomedical curriculum, *Ann Anat* 227:151430, 2020. https://doi.org/10.1016/j.aanat.2019.151430.

De Bakker BS, de Jong KH, Hagoort J, et al: An interactive three-dimensional digital atlas and quantitative database of human development, *Science* 354(6315), 2016.

Dhombres F, Maurice P, Guilbaud L, et al: A novel intelligent scan assistant system for early pregnancy diagnosis by ultrasound: clinical decision support system evaluation study, *J Med Internet Res*:21e14286, 2019. https://doi.org/10.2196/14286 PMID: 31271152.

Doubilet PM, Benson CB: Ultrasound of the early first trimester. In Norton ME, editor: *Callen's ultrasonography in obstetrics and gynecology,* ed 6, Philadelphia, 2017, Elsevier, pp 82–97.

Gasser RF: *Atlas of human embryos,* Baltimore, 1975, Lippincott Williams & Wilkins.

Iber D, Vetter R: Relationship between epithelial organization and morphogen interpretation, *Curr Opin Genet Dev* 75:101916, 2022. https://doi.org/10.1016/j.gde.2022.101916.

Iffy L, Shepard TH, Jakobovits A, et al: The rate of growth in young human embryos of Streeter's horizons XIII and XXIII, *Acta Anat (Basel)* 66:178, 1967.

Jirásek JE: *An atlas of human prenatal developmental mechanics: anatomy and staging,* London, 2004, Taylor and Francis.

Moore KL, Persaud TVN, Shiota K: *Color atlas of clinical embryology,* ed 2, Philadelphia, 2000, Saunders.

Nishimura H, Tanimura T, Semba R, et al: Normal development of early human embryos: observation of 90 specimens at carnegie stages 7 to 13, *Teratology* 10:1, 1974.

O'Rahilly R, Müller F: *Developmental stages in human embryos,* Washington, DC, 1987, Carnegie Institute of Washington.

O'Shea TM, Register HM, Yi JX: ELGAN-ECHO Pulmonary/Obesity Group: Growth during infancy after extremely preterm birth: Associations with later neurodevelopmental and health outcomes, *J Pediatr* 252:40–47.e.5, 2022.10.1016/j.jpeds.2022.08.015.

Pechriggl E, Blumer M, Tubbs RS, et al: Embryology of the abdominal wall and associated malformations – a review, *Front Surg* 9:891–896, 2022.10.3389/fsurg.2022.891896.

Persaud TVN, Hay JC: Normal embryonic and fetal development. In Reece EA, Hobbins JC, editors: *Clinical obstetrics: the fetus and mother,* ed 3, Oxford, 2006, Blackwell, pp 19–33.

Pooh RK, Shiota K, Kurjak A: Imaging of the human embryo with magnetic resonance imaging microscopy and high-resolution transvaginal 3-dimensional sonography: human embryology in the 21st century, *Am J Obstet Gynecol* 204:77.e1, 2011.

Rossant J, Why study human embryo development?. *Dev Biol,* 509, 2024, 43–50.

Sagner A, Briscoe J: Morphogen interpretation: concentration, time, competence, and signaling dynamics, *Wiley Interdiscip Rev Dev Biol* 6(4), 2017.

Shiota K: Development and intrauterine fate of normal and abnormal human conceptuses, *Congenital Anomalies* 31(2):67–80, 1991.

Steding G: *The anatomy of the human embryo: a scanning electron-microscopic atlas,* Basel, 2009, Karger.

Streeter GL: Developmental horizons in human embryos: description of age group XI, 13 to 20 somites, and age group XII, 21 to 29 somites, *Contrib Embryol Carnegie Inst* 30:211, 1942.

Streeter GL: Developmental horizons in human embryos: description of age group XIII, embryos of 4 or 5 millimeters long, and age group XIV, period of identification of the lens vesicle, *Contrib Embryol Carnegie Inst* 31:27, 1945.

Streeter GL: Developmental horizons in human embryos: description of age groups XV, XVI, XVII, and XVIII, *Contrib Embryol Carnegie Inst* 32:133, 1948.

Streeter GL, Heuser CH, Corner GW: Developmental horizons in human embryos: description of age groups XIX, XX, XXI, XXII, and XXIII, *Contrib Embryol Carnegie Inst* 34:165, 1951.

Stooke-Vaughan GA, Campas O: Physical control of tissue and morphogenesis across scales, *Curr Opin Genet Dev* 51:111, 2018.

Van Winkle LJ. Molecular and clinical advances in understanding early embryo development, *Cells,* 12. https://doi.org/10.3390/cells12081171.

Whitworth M., Bricker L., Mullan C. Ultrasound for fetal assessment in early pregnancy. *Cochrane Database Syst Rev.* 2015;2015(7):CD007058. https://doi.org/10.1002/14651858.CD007058.

Yamada S, Samtani RR, Lee ES, et al: Developmental atlas of the early first trimester human embryo, *Dev Dyn* 239:1585, 2010.

Fetal Period: Ninth Week to Birth

6

CHAPTER OUTLINE

The transformation of an embryo to a fetus is gradual, but the name change is meaningful because it signifies that the primordia of all major systems have formed. Development during the fetal period is primarily concerned with rapid body growth and differentiation of tissues, organs, and systems. A notable change occurring during the fetal period is the relative slowdown in the growth of the head compared with the rest of the body. The rate of body growth during the fetal period is very rapid (Table 6.1), and fetal weight gain is remarkable during the final weeks. Periods of normal continuous growth alternate with prolonged intervals of absent growth.

ESTIMATION OF FETAL AGE

Ultrasound measurements of the **crown–rump length (CRL)** of the fetus are taken to determine its size and probable age and to provide a prediction of the **expected date of delivery**. Fetal head measurements and femur length are also used to evaluate age.

The **intrauterine period** may be divided into days, weeks, or months (Table 6.2), but confusion arises if it is not stated whether the age is calculated from the onset of the last normal menstrual period (LNMP) or the estimated day of fertilization of the oocyte. Uncertainty about age arises when months are used, particularly when it is not stated whether calendar months (28–31 days) or lunar months (28 days) are meant. **Unless otherwise stated, embryologic or fetal age in this book is calculated from the estimated time of fertilization.**

TRIMESTERS OF PREGNANCY

Clinically, the gestational period is divided into three trimesters, each lasting 3 months. By the end of the first trimester, major systems have been developed (see Table 6.1). In the second trimester, the fetus grows sufficiently in size so

Viability of Fetuses

Viability is defined as the ability of fetuses to survive in the extrauterine environment. Most fetuses of less than 500 g at birth do not usually survive. In recent years, survival at gestational ages of 22 to 23 weeks has been increasingly reported, blurring the line at which the edge of viability is declared. If given expert postnatal care, many fetuses born at less than 1000 g may survive and some fetuses weighing less than 500 g may survive; such infants are referred to as extremely low-birth-weight infants. Many full-term, low-birth-weight infants result from **intrauterine growth restriction (IUGR)**. Most fetuses weighing between 750 and 1500 g usually survive, but complications may occur.

Each year, approximately 500,000 **preterm** infants (<37 weeks) are born in the United States. Many of these infants suffer from severe medical complications or early **mortality** (death). The use of antenatal steroids and the postnatal administration of endotracheal surfactant have greatly lowered the rates of acute and long-term morbidity. *Prematurity is one of the most common causes of morbidity and perinatal death.*

Table 6.1 Criteria for Estimating Fertilization Age During the Fetal Period

Age (Weeks)	Crown-Rump Length (mm)[a]	Foot Length (mm)[a]	Fetal Weight (g)[b]	Main External Characteristics
Previable Fetuses				
9	50	7	8	*Eyelids closing or closed.* Head large and more rounded. External genitalia are not distinguishable as male or female. Some of the small intestines are in the proximal part of the umbilical cord. The ears are low set.
10	61	9	14	*Intestines in the abdomen.* Early fingernail development.
12	87	14	45	*Sex is distinguishable externally.* Well-defined neck.
14	120	20	110	*Head erect.* Eyes face anteriorly. Ears are close to their definitive position. Lower limbs are well developed. Early toenail development.
16	140	27	200	*External ears stand out from the head.*
18	160	33	320	Vernix caseosa covers skin. Quickening (first movements) felt by mother.
20	190	39	460	*Head and body hair (lanugo) visible.*
Viable Fetuses[c]				
22	210	45	630	*Skin wrinkled, translucent, and pink to red.*
24	230	50	820	*Fingernails present.* Lean body.
26	250	55	1000	*Eyelids are partially open.* Eyelashes present.
28	270	59	1300	*Eyes wide open.* Considerable scalp hair is sometimes present. Skin slightly wrinkled.
30	280	63	1700	*Toenails present.* Body filling out. Testes descending.
32	300	68	2100	*Fingernails reach fingertips.* Skin smooth.
36	340	79	2900	*Body is usually plump.* Lanugo (hairs) almost absent. Toenails reach toe tips. Flexed limbs; firm grasp.
38	360	83	3400	*Prominent chest; breasts protrude.* Testes in scrotum or palpable in inguinal canals. Fingernails extend beyond fingertips.

[a]These measurements are averages and so may not apply to specific cases; dimensional variations increase with age.

[b]These weights refer to fetuses that have been fixed for approximately 2 weeks in 10% formalin. Fresh specimens usually weigh approximately 5% less.

[c]There is no sharp limit of development, age, or weight at which a fetus automatically becomes viable or beyond which survival is ensured, but experience has shown that it is rare for a baby to survive whose weight is less than 500 g or whose fertilization age is less than 22 weeks. Even fetuses born between 26 and 28 weeks have difficulty surviving, mainly because the respiratory system and the central nervous system are not completely differentiated.

Table 6.2 Comparison of Gestational Time Units and Date of Birth[a]

Reference Point	Days	Weeks	Calendar Months	Lunar Months
Fertilization	266	38	8.75	9.5
Last normal menstrual period	280	40	9.25	10

[a]The common delivery date rule (Nägele's rule) for estimating the expected date of delivery is to count back 3 months from the first day of the last normal menstrual period and add a year and 7 days.

that good anatomical and most major birth defects can be detected using high-resolution real-time ultrasonography. By the beginning of the third trimester, the fetus may survive if born prematurely. The fetus reaches a major developmental landmark at 35 weeks and weighs approximately 2500 g and usually survives if born prematurely.

MEASUREMENTS AND CHARACTERISTICS OF FETUSES

Various measurements and external characteristics are useful for estimating fetal age (see Table 6.1). CRL is the method of choice for estimating fetal age until the end of the first trimester because there is very little variability in fetal size during this period. In the second and third trimesters, several structures can be identified and measured by ultrasonographic methods, but the most common measurements are **biparietal diameter** (diameter of the head between the two parietal eminences), **head circumference**, abdominal circumference, femur length, and foot length.

Weight of a spontaneously aborted fetus is often a useful criterion for estimating age, but there may be a discrepancy between age and weight, particularly when the mother has had metabolic disturbances such as diabetes mellitus during pregnancy. In these cases, the weight often exceeds values considered normal for the corresponding CRL. Fetal dimensions obtained from ultrasound measurements closely approximate CRL measurements obtained from spontaneously aborted fetuses. Determination of the size of a fetus, especially its head circumference, is helpful to the obstetrician for the management of patients.

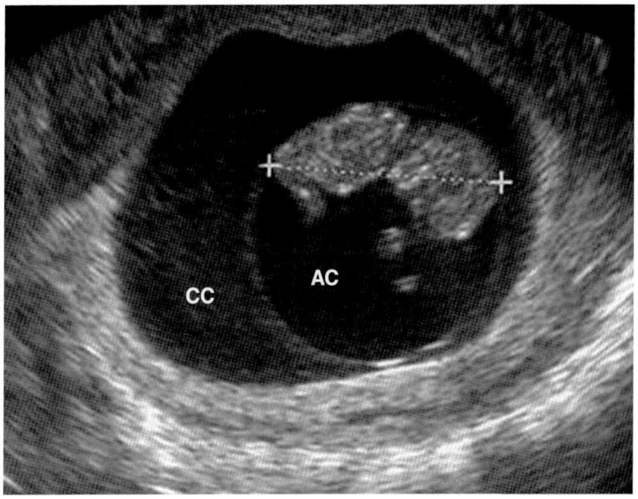

Fig. 6.1 Ultrasound image of 9-week fetus (11 weeks' gestational age). Note the amnion, *AC*, and *CC*. Crown-rump length, 4.2 cm (*calipers*). *AC*, Amniotic cavity; *CC*, chorionic cavity. (Courtesy Dr. E. A. Lyons, Professor of Radiology and Obstetrics and Gynecology and of Anatomy, Health Sciences Centre and University of Manitoba, Winnipeg, Manitoba, Canada.)

HIGHLIGHTS OF THE FETAL PERIOD

There is no formal staging system for the fetal period; however, it is helpful to describe the changes that occur in periods of 4 to 5 weeks.

NINE TO TWELVE WEEKS

At the beginning of the fetal period (ninth week), the head constitutes approximately half of the CRL of the fetus (Figs. 6.1 and 6.2A). Subsequently, growth in body length accelerates rapidly, so that by the end of 12 weeks, the CRL has almost doubled (Fig. 6.2B, and see Table 6.1). Although growth of the head slows down considerably by this time, the head is still disproportionately large compared with the rest of the body (Fig. 6.3).

At 9 weeks, the face is broad, the eyes are widely separated, the ears are low set, and the eyelids are fused (see Fig. 6.2B). By the end of 12 weeks, **primary ossification centers** appear in the skeleton, especially in the cranium (skull) and long bones. Ossification begins in the cranium between 9 and 11 weeks, first in the complex occipital bone. Early in the ninth week, the legs are short, and the thighs are relatively small (see Fig. 6.2). By the end of 12 weeks, the upper limbs have almost reached their final relative lengths, but the lower limbs are slightly shorter than their final relative lengths.

The **external genitalia** of males and females appear similar until the end of the ninth week. Their mature form is not established until the 12th week. Intestinal coils are visible in the proximal end of the umbilical cord until the middle of the 10th week (see Fig. 6.2B). By the 11th week, the intestines have returned to the abdomen (see Fig. 6.3).

At 9 weeks, the beginning of the fetal period, the liver is the major site of **erythropoiesis**, the formation of red blood cells from multipotent hematopoietic stem and progenitor cells. By the end of 12 weeks, this activity has decreased in the liver and has begun in the spleen and later in fetal bone marrow from hematopoietic mesenchymal stem cells. Urine formation begins between the 9th and 12th weeks, and urine is discharged through the urethra into the amniotic fluid. The

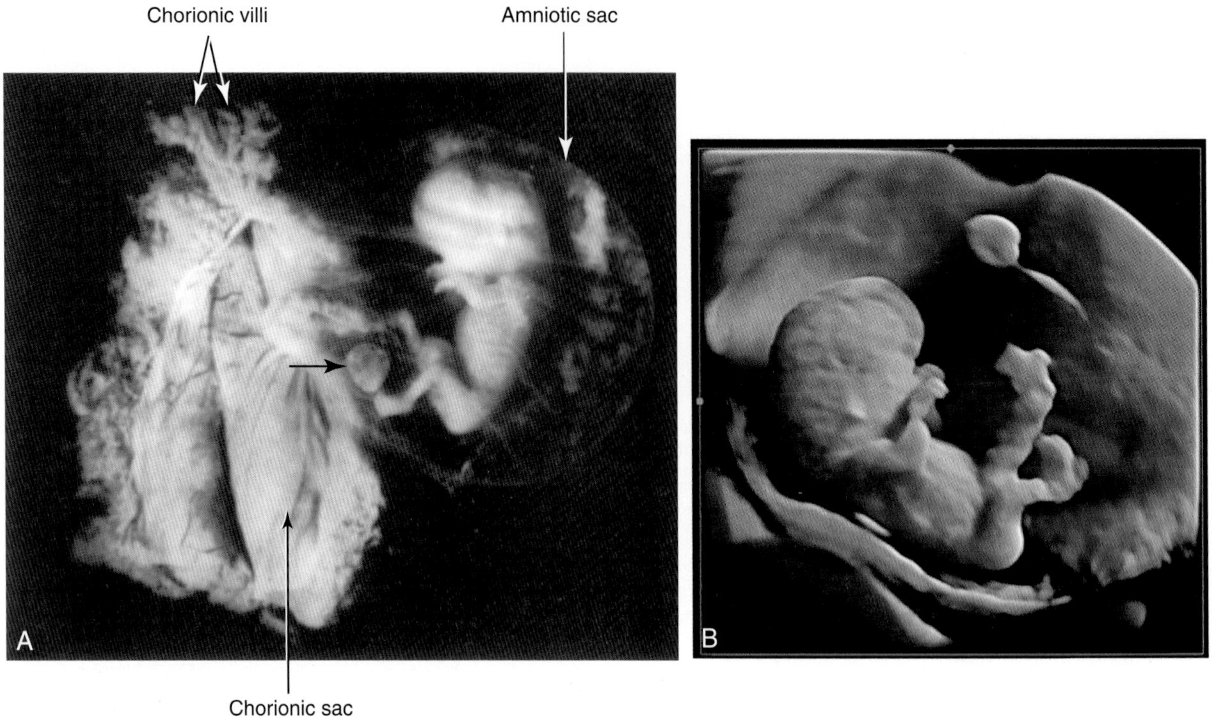

Fig. 6.2 A 9-week fetus in the amniotic sac exposed by removal from the chorionic sac. (A) Actual size. The remnant of the umbilical vesicle is indicated by an *arrow*. (B) A transabdominal 3D ultrasound of a fetus at 10 weeks + 2 days. The umbilical cord insertion can be observed on the abdomen. The amniotic membrane is seen surrounding the fetus. The small umbilical vesicle (yolk sac) remnant can be seen in the upper portion of the image close to the amniotic membrane.

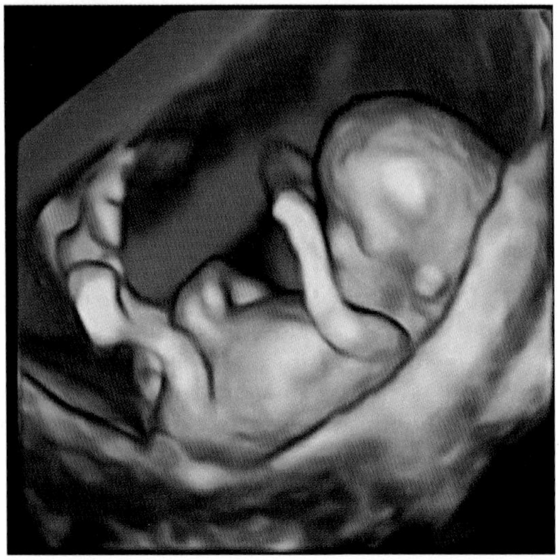

Fig. 6.3 A transvaginal 3D ultrasound (with superficial rendering) of an 11-week fetus. Note its relatively large head. The limbs are fully developed. An auricle can also be observed on the left lateral aspect of the head.

fetus reabsorbs some amniotic fluid after swallowing it. Fetal waste products are transferred to the maternal circulation by passage across the **placental membrane** (see Fig. 7.7).

THIRTEEN TO SIXTEEN WEEKS

Growth is very rapid during this period (Fig. 6.4, and see Table 6.1). By 16 weeks, the head is relatively smaller than the head of a 12-week fetus, and the lower limbs have lengthened (Fig. 6.5A). **Limb movements** first occur involuntarily by the end of the embryonic period. More coordinated movements, such as kicking, occur by the 14th week as a result of further neuromuscular development. These early fetal movements are visible during ultrasonographic examinations and can be felt by the mother.

Ossification of the fetal skeleton is active during this period, and the developing bones are visible on ultrasound images by the beginning of the 16th week. **Slow eye movements** occur at 14 weeks. Scalp hair patterning is also determined during this period. By 16 weeks, the ovaries are differentiated and contain **primordial ovarian follicles**, which contain **oogonia**, or primordial germ cells (see Fig. 12.31).

The differences in the genitalia of male and female fetuses can be recognized by 12 to 14 weeks. By 16 weeks, the eyes face anteriorly rather than anterolaterally. In addition, the external ears are close to their definitive positions on the sides of the head.

SEVENTEEN TO TWENTY WEEKS

Growth slows down during this period, but the fetus still increases its CRL by approximately 50 mm (see Fig. 6.5, 6.8A, and Table 6.1). Fetal movements **(quickening)** are commonly felt by the mother. The skin is now covered with a greasy material, the **vernix caseosa**. It consists of a mixture of dead epidermal cells and a fatty substance from the fetal sebaceous glands. The vernix protects the delicate fetal skin from abrasions, chapping, and hardening that result from exposure to the amniotic fluid. Fetuses are covered with fine, downy hair, **lanugo**, which helps the vernix adhere to the skin.

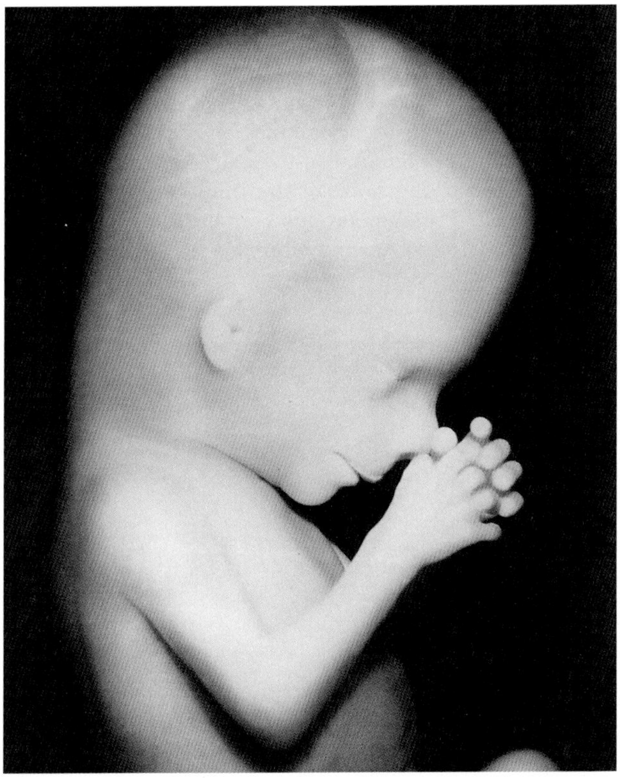

Fig. 6.4 Enlarged photograph of the head and superior part of the trunk of a 13-week fetus.

Eyebrows and head hair are visible at 20 weeks. **Brown fat** forms during this period and is the site of heat production. This specialized **adipose tissue** is connective tissue that consists chiefly of fat cells; it is found mostly at the root of the neck, posterior to the sternum, and in the perirenal area. The brown fat produces heat by oxidizing fatty acids.

By 18 weeks, the fetal uterus is formed, and canalization of the vagina has begun. Many primordial ovarian follicles containing oogonia are also visible. By 20 weeks, the testes have begun to descend, but they are still located on the posterior abdominal wall, as are the ovaries.

TWENTY-ONE TO TWENTY-FIVE WEEKS

Substantial weight gain occurs during this period, and the fetus is better proportioned (Fig. 6.6). The skin is usually wrinkled and more translucent, particularly during the early part of this period. The skin is pink to red because blood in the capillaries is visible. At 21 weeks, rapid eye movements begin, and **blink-startle responses** have been reported at 22 to 23 weeks. The secretory epithelial cells (type II pneumocytes) in the interalveolar walls of the lung have begun to secrete **surfactant**, a surface-active lipid that maintains the patency of the developing alveoli of the lungs (see Chapter 10).

Fingernails are present by 24 weeks. Although a 22- to 25-week fetus born prematurely may survive if given intensive care (see Fig. 6.6), there is also a chance that it may die because its respiratory system is still immature. The risk for **neurodevelopmental disability** is high in fetuses born before 26 weeks.

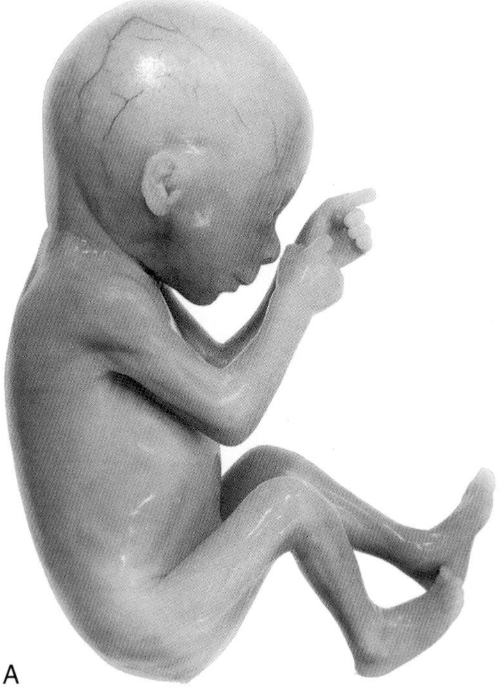

A

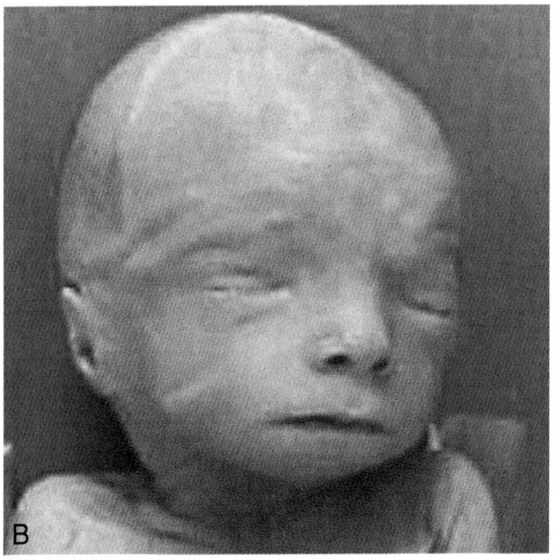

B

Fig. 6.5 (A) A 17-week fetus. Because there is little subcutaneous tissue and the skin is thin, the blood vessels of the scalp are visible. Fetuses at this age are unable to survive if born prematurely, mainly because their respiratory systems are immature. (B) A frontal view of a 17-week fetus. Note that the eyes are closed at this stage. (A, From Moore KL, Persaud TVN, Shiota K: *Color atlas of clinical embryology*, ed 2, Philadelphia, 2000, Saunders. B, Courtesy Dr. Robert Jordan, St. George's University Medical School, Grenada.)

TWENTY-SIX TO TWENTY-NINE WEEKS

During this period, fetuses usually survive if they are born prematurely and given intensive care (Fig. 6.7B and C). The **lungs and pulmonary vasculature** have developed sufficiently to provide adequate gas exchange. In addition, the central nervous system has matured to the stage where it can direct rhythmic **breathing movements** and control body temperature. The highest rate of neonatal mortality occurs in infants classified as low birth weight ($\leq$2500 g) and very low birth weight ($\leq$1500 g).

The **eyelids** are open at 26 weeks and head hair is well developed. Toenails are visible, and considerable subcutaneous fat is under the skin, smoothing out many wrinkles. During this period, the quantity of white fat increases to approximately 3.5% of the body weight. The fetal spleen has been an important site of **erythropoiesis** (formation of red blood cells). This ends at 28 weeks; by this time bone marrow has become the major site of erythropoiesis.

THIRTY TO THIRTY-FOUR WEEKS

The **pupillary reflex** (response to stimuli from light) can be elicited at 30 weeks. Usually by the end of this period, the skin is pink and smooth and the upper and lower limbs have a chubby appearance. At this age, the quantity of white fat is approximately 8% of the body weight. Fetuses 32 weeks and older usually survive if born prematurely.

THIRTY-FIVE TO THIRTY-EIGHT WEEKS

Fetuses born at 35 weeks have a firm grasp and exhibit a spontaneous orientation to light. The pupillary light reflex is present in neonates at 35 weeks. As the term approaches, the nervous system is sufficiently mature to carry out some integrative functions. Most fetuses during this "finishing period" are plump. By 36 weeks, the circumferences of the head and abdomen are approximately equal. After this, the circumference of the abdomen may be greater than that of the head. The **foot length** is usually slightly larger than the femoral length (long bone of the thigh) at 37 weeks and is an alternative parameter for confirmation of fetal age (Fig. 6.8). There is a slowing of growth as the time of birth approaches.

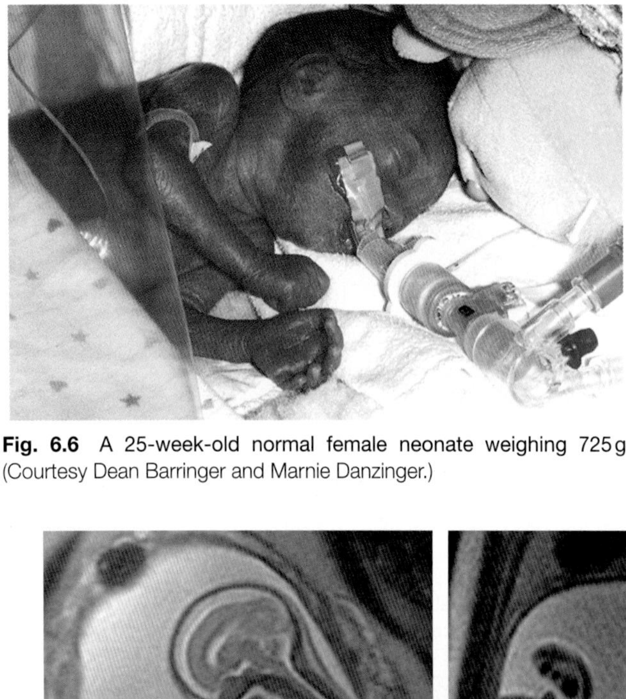

Fig. 6.6 A 25-week-old normal female neonate weighing 725 g. (Courtesy Dean Barringer and Marnie Danzinger.)

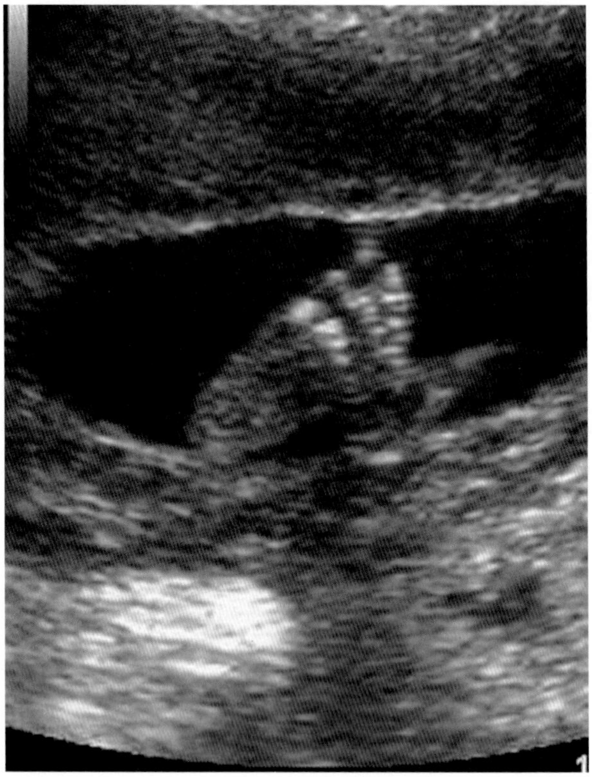

Fig. 6.8 Ultrasound scan of the foot of a fetus at 19 weeks. (Courtesy Dr. E. A. Lyons, Professor of Radiology and Obstetrics, and Gynecology and of Anatomy, Health Sciences Centre and University of Manitoba, Winnipeg, Manitoba, Canada.)

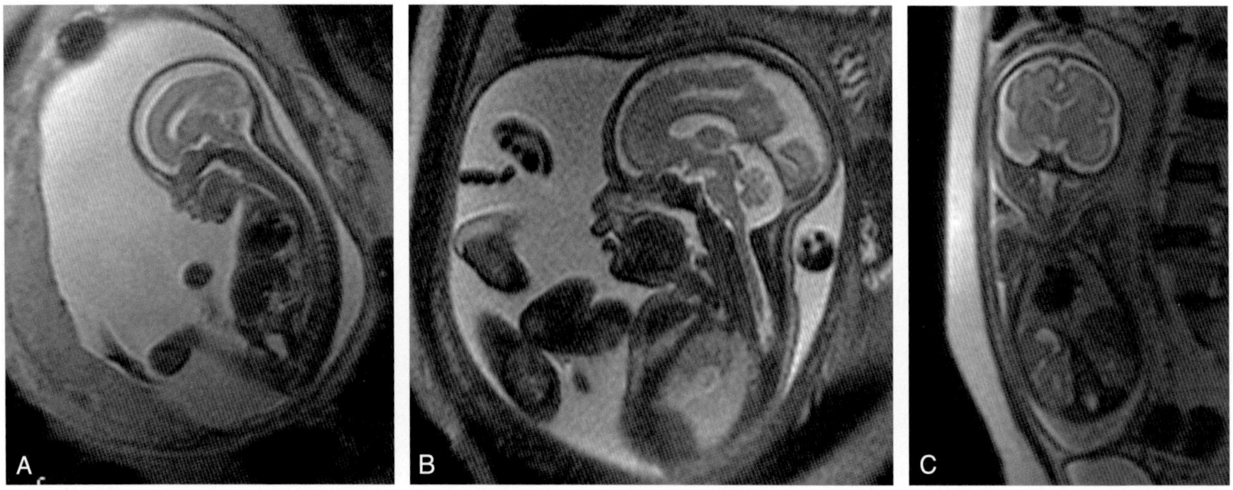

Fig. 6.7 Magnetic resonance images of normal fetuses at (A) 18 weeks, (B) 26 weeks, and (C) 28 weeks. (Courtesy Dr. Deborah Levine, Director of Obstetric and Gynecologic Ultrasound, Beth Israel Deaconess Medical Center, Boston, MA.)

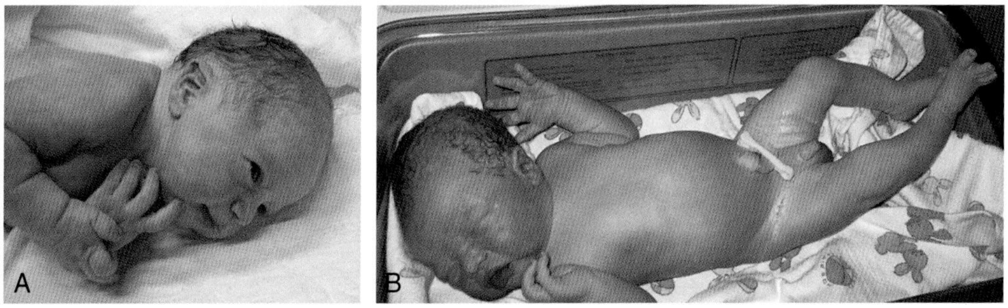

Fig. 6.9 Healthy neonates. (A) At 38 weeks. (B) At 34 weeks. (A, Courtesy Michael and Michele Rice. B, Courtesy Dr. Jon Jackson and Mrs. Margaret Jackson.)

At full term (38 weeks) (Fig. 6.9A), most fetuses usually reach a CRL of 360 mm and weigh approximately 3400 g. The amount of white fat is approximately 16% of the body weight. A fetus adds approximately 14 g of fat per day during these last weeks. The thorax (chest) is prominent, and the breasts often protrude slightly in both sexes. The testes are usually in the scrotum in full-term male neonates; premature male neonates commonly have undescended testes. Although the head is smaller at full term in relation to the rest of the body than it was earlier in fetal life, it is still one of the largest regions of the fetus. In general, male fetuses are longer and weigh more at birth than females.

Low Birth Weight

Not all low-birth-weight babies are premature. Approximately one-third of those with a birth weight of 2500 g or less are actually small for gestational age (SGA). These "small-for-date" infants may be underweight because of **placental insufficiency** (see Chapter 7). The placentas are often small or poorly attached and/or have undergone degenerative changes that progressively reduce the oxygen supply and nourishment to the fetus.

It is important to distinguish between **full-term neonates** who have a low birth weight because of IUGR and **preterm neonates** who are underweight because of a shortened gestation (i.e., premature by date). IUGR may be caused by **preeclampsia** (hypertension), smoking or some illicit drugs, multiple gestations (e.g., triplets), infectious diseases, cardiovascular defects, inadequate maternal nutrition, and maternal and fetal hormones. **Teratogens** and genetic factors are also known to cause IUGR (see Chapter 20). Infants with asymmetrical forms of IUGR who have a large head circumference relative to the infant's weight and length show a characteristic lack of subcutaneous fat, and their skin is wrinkled, suggesting that white fat has been lost.

EXPECTED DATE OF DELIVERY

The expected date of delivery of a fetus is 266 days or 38 weeks after fertilization, that is, 280 days or 40 weeks after the LNMP (see Table 6.2). Approximately 12% of fetuses are born 1 to 2 weeks after the expected time of birth.

Postmaturity Syndrome

Prolongation of pregnancy for 3 or several weeks beyond the expected date of delivery occurs in 5% to 6% of females. Some infants in such pregnancies develop the **postmaturity syndrome**, which may be associated with **fetal dysmaturity**: absence of subcutaneous fat, wrinkling of the skin, or **meconium** (greenish-colored feces) **staining of the skin**, and, often, excessive weight. Fetuses with this syndrome have an increased risk of mortality. Labor is usually induced when the fetus is postmature.

FACTORS INFLUENCING FETAL GROWTH

Fetuses require substrates (nutrients) for the growth and the production of energy. Nutrients pass freely to the fetus from the mother through the placental membrane (see Fig. 7.7). **Glucose** is a primary source of energy for fetal metabolism and growth; **amino acids** are also required. **Insulin** required for the metabolism of glucose is secreted by the fetal pancreas; no significant quantities of maternal insulin reach the fetus because the placental membrane is relatively impermeable to this hormone. Insulin, insulin-like growth factors, human growth hormone, and some small polypeptides (such as somatomedin C) are believed to stimulate fetal growth.

Many factors may affect prenatal growth; they may be maternal, fetal, or environmental factors (see Chapter 20). Some factors operating throughout pregnancy, such as maternal vascular disease, intrauterine infection, cigarette smoking, and consumption of alcohol, tend to produce infants with IUGR or SGA infants, whereas factors operating during the last trimester, such as maternal malnutrition, usually produce underweight infants with normal length and head size.

The terms *IUGR* and *SGA* are related, but they are not synonymous. IUGR refers to a process that causes a reduction in the expected pattern of fetal growth as well as fetal growth potential. Constitutionally SGA infants have a birth weight that is lower than a predetermined cutoff value for a particular gestational age (<2 standard deviations below the mean or less than the third percentile). **Severe maternal malnutrition** resulting from a poor-quality diet is known to cause restricted fetal growth.

Low birth weight is a risk factor for many adult conditions, including hypertension, diabetes, and cardiovascular disease. High birth weight due to maternal gestational diabetes is associated with later obesity and diabetes in the offspring.

CIGARETTE SMOKING

Smoking is a well-established cause of IUGR. The growth rate for fetuses of mothers who smoke cigarettes is less than normal during the last 6 to 8 weeks of pregnancy. On average, the birth weight of infants whose mothers smoked heavily during pregnancy is 200 g less than normal, and the rate of **perinatal morbidity** is increased when adequate medical care is unavailable. The effect of maternal smoking is greater on fetuses whose mothers also receive inadequate nutrition. Cigarette smoking has been implicated as a major cause of cleft lip and palate. It is also considered a risk factor for preterm birth and sudden infant death syndrome.

MULTIPLE PREGNANCY

Individuals of multiple births usually weigh considerably less than infants resulting from a single pregnancy. The total metabolic requirements of two or more fetuses exceed the nutritional supply available from the placenta during the third trimester.

ALCOHOL AND ILLICIT DRUGS

Infants born to mothers who drink alcohol often exhibit IUGR as part of the **fetal alcohol syndrome** (see Fig. 20.17). Similarly, the use of marijuana and other illicit drugs (e.g., cocaine) can cause IUGR and other obstetric complications.

IMPAIRED UTEROPLACENTAL AND FETOPLACENTAL BLOOD FLOW

The maternal placental circulation may be reduced by conditions that decrease uterine blood flow (e.g., small chorionic vessels, severe maternal hypotension, and renal disease). Chronic reduction of uterine blood flow can cause fetal starvation resulting in IUGR. Placental dysfunction (e.g., infarction; see Chapter 7) can also cause IUGR.

The net effect of these placental abnormalities is a reduction of the total area for the exchange of nutrients between the fetal and maternal bloodstreams. It is very difficult to separate the effect of these placental changes from the effect of reduced maternal blood flow to the placenta. In some instances of chronic maternal disease, the maternal vascular changes in the uterus are primary, and placental defects are secondary.

GENETIC FACTORS AND GROWTH RETARDATION

It is well established that genetic factors can cause IUGR. Repeated cases of IUGR in one family indicate that recessive genes may be the cause of the abnormal growth. Structural and numeric chromosomal aberrations have also been shown to be associated with cases of retarded fetal growth. IUGR is pronounced in infants with trisomy 21 syndrome and is very characteristic of fetuses with trisomy 18 syndrome (see Chapter 20).

PROCEDURES FOR ASSESSING FETAL STATUS

Perinatology is concerned with the well-being of the fetus and neonate, generally covering the period from approximately 26 weeks after fertilization to 4 weeks after birth. This subspecialty of medicine combines aspects of obstetrics and pediatrics.

ULTRASONOGRAPHY

Ultrasonography is the primary imaging modality in the evaluation of fetuses because of its wide availability, low cost, quality of images, and lack of known adverse effects. The chorionic sac and its contents may be visualized by ultrasonography during the embryonic and fetal periods. Placental and fetal size, multiple births, abnormalities of placental shape, and abnormal presentations can also be determined.

Ultrasound imaging gives accurate measurements of the biparietal diameter of the fetal cranium (skull), from which close estimates of fetal age and length can be made. Figs. 6.8 and 6.10 illustrate how details of the fetus can be observed in these scans. Ultrasound examinations are also helpful for diagnosing abnormal pregnancies at a very early stage. Rapid advances in imaging technology, including three-dimensional (3D) ultrasound, have made this technique a major tool for prenatal diagnosis of fetal abnormalities in early pregnancy (11–14 weeks' gestational age). Biopsy of fetal tissues, such as the skin, liver, kidney, and muscle, can be performed with ultrasound guidance.

DIAGNOSTIC AMNIOCENTESIS

This is a relatively common invasive prenatal diagnostic procedure. **Amniotic fluid** is sampled by inserting a needle through the mother's anterior abdominal, uterine wall, the chorion and the amnion, into the amniotic cavity (Fig. 6.9A). Because there is relatively little amniotic fluid before the 14th week, amniocentesis is difficult to perform before this time. Amniocentesis can be performed starting at ≥15 weeks when 15 to 20 mL of amniotic fluid can be safely withdrawn. Amniocentesis carries a relatively small risk to the fetus (a pregnancy loss of 0.5%–1.0%), especially when the procedure is performed by an experienced physician using real-time ultrasonography guidance to outline the position of the fetus and placenta.

Diagnostic Value of Amniocentesis

Amniocentesis is a technique for detecting genetic disorders (e.g., Down syndrome). The common indications for amniocentesis are:

- Advanced maternal age (≥38 years)
- Previous birth of a child with trisomy 21 (see Fig. 20.6B)
- Chromosome abnormality in either parent
- Females who are carriers of X-linked recessive disorders (e.g., *hemophilia*)
- History of neural tube defects in the family (e.g., spina bifida cystica; see Fig. 17.15)
- Carriers of inborn errors of metabolism

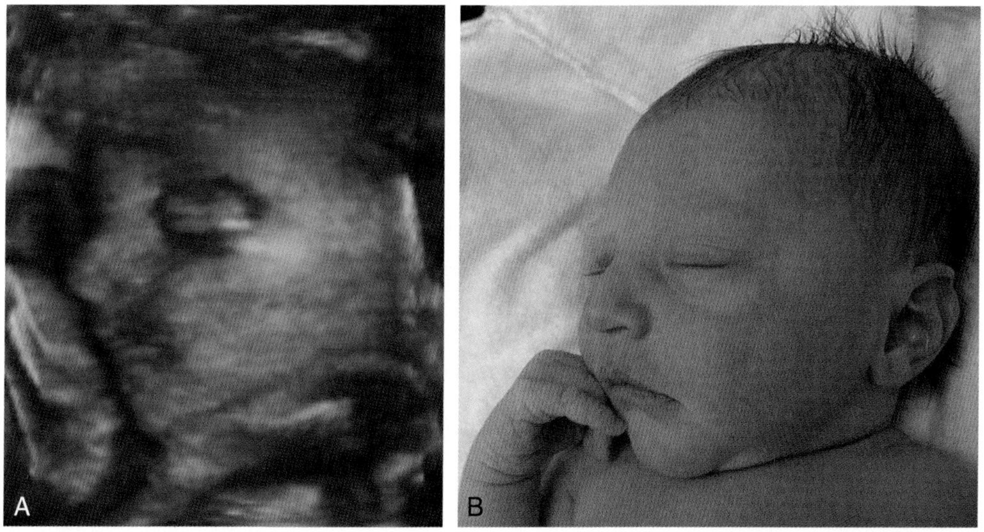

Fig. 6.10 (A) Three-dimensional ultrasound (sonogram) of a 28-week fetus showing the face. The surface features are clearly recognizable. (B) Photograph of the same neonate, 3 hours after birth. (Courtesy Dr. E. A. Lyons, Professor of Radiology and Obstetrics and Gynecology and of Anatomy, Health Sciences Centre and University of Manitoba, Winnipeg, Manitoba, Canada.)

ALPHA-FETOPROTEIN ASSAY

Alpha-fetoprotein (AFP) is a glycoprotein that is synthesized in the fetal liver, umbilical vesicle, and gut. AFP is found in high concentrations in fetal serum, with levels peaking at 14 weeks after the LNMP. Only small amounts of AFP normally enter the amniotic fluid.

Alpha-Fetoprotein and Fetal Anomalies

The concentration of AFP is high in the amniotic fluid surrounding fetuses with severe defects of the central nervous system and ventral abdominal wall. The amniotic fluid AFP concentration is measured by immunoassay; when the concentration is known and ultrasonographic scanning is performed, approximately 99% of fetuses with these severe defects can be diagnosed prenatally. When a fetus has an open neural tube defect, the concentration of AFP is also likely to be higher than normal in the maternal serum. The maternal serum AFP concentration is lower than normal when the fetus has trisomy 21 syndrome, Edward syndrome (trisomy 18), or other chromosome defects.

SPECTROPHOTOMETRIC STUDIES

Examination of amniotic fluid by spectrophotometric studies may be used for assessing the degree of **erythroblastosis fetalis**, also called **hemolytic disease of the neonate**. This disease results from the destruction of fetal red blood cells by maternal antibodies (see Chapter 7, blue box titled "Hemolytic Disease of the Neonate"). The concentration of bilirubin (and other related pigments) is correlated with the degree of hemolytic disease.

CHORIONIC VILLUS SAMPLING

Starting at 10 to 12 weeks' gestation, biopsies of trophoblastic tissue (5–20 mg) may be obtained by inserting a needle, guided by ultrasonography, through the mother's abdominal and uterine walls (transabdominal insertion) into the uterine cavity (see Fig. 6.11B). Chorionic villus sampling (CVS) can also be performed transcervically by passing a catheter through the cervix under the guidance of real-time ultrasonography. The rate of fetal loss is approximately 0.5% to 1%, comparable to amniocentesis. CVS can be used to study the **fetal karyotype** (chromosome characteristics) for detecting abnormalities including inborn errors of metabolism, and X-linked disorders. Using CVS, a diagnosis can be made weeks earlier than would be possible with amniocentesis.

CELL CULTURES AND CHROMOSOMAL ANALYSIS

The prevalence of chromosomal disorders is approximately 1 in 120 neonates. Fetal sex and chromosomal aberrations can be determined by studying the chromosomes in cultured fetal cells obtained during amniocentesis and chorionic villus sampling. Compared with conventional cytogenetic techniques, chromosomal microarray analysis has a higher resolution and is widely used for detecting chromosomal abnormalities. If conception occurs by means of assisted reproductive technologies, it is possible to obtain fetal cells by performing a biopsy of the maturing blastocyst (Fig. 6.12A and B) and culturing the cells. These cultures are commonly done when an autosomal abnormality, such as occurs in Down syndrome, is suspected. Knowledge of fetal sex can be useful in diagnosing the presence of severe sex-linked hereditary diseases, such as **hemophilia** (an inherited disorder of blood coagulation) and **muscular dystrophy** (a hereditary progressive degenerative disorder affecting skeletal muscles). Moreover, microdeletions and microduplications, as well as subtelomeric rearrangements, can now be detected with fluorescence in situ hybridization technology (see Fig. 6.12C and D). **Inborn errors of metabolism in fetuses** can also be detected by studying cell cultures. Enzyme deficiencies can be determined by incubating cells recovered from amniotic fluid and then detecting the specific enzyme deficiency in the cells.

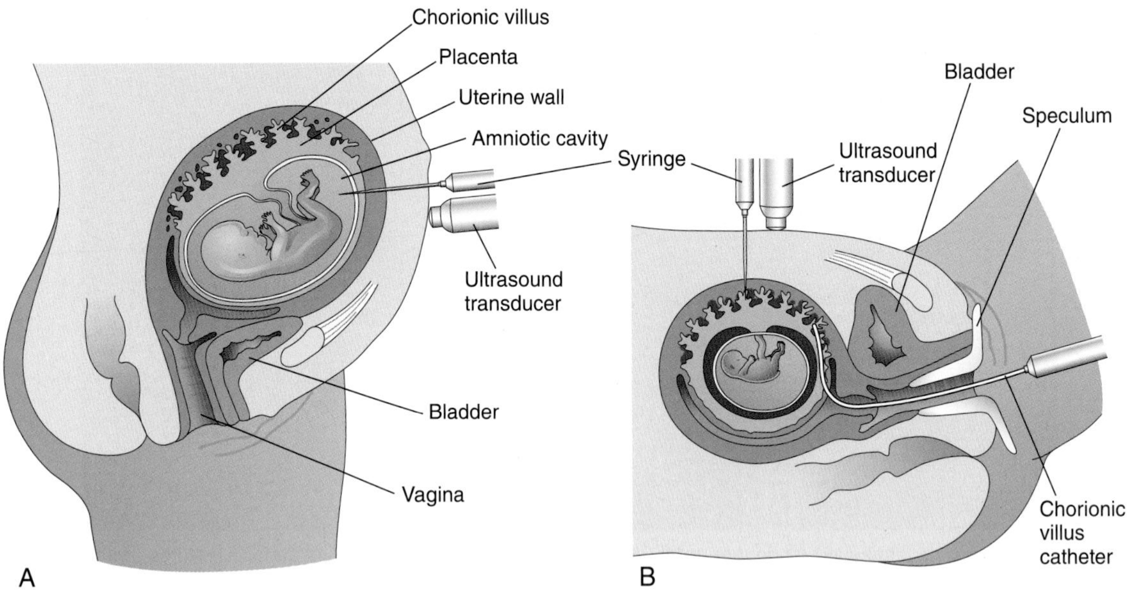

Fig. 6.11 (A) Illustration of amniocentesis. A needle is inserted through the lower abdominal and uterine walls into the amniotic cavity. A syringe is attached, and amniotic fluid is withdrawn for diagnostic purposes. (B) Drawing illustrating chorionic villus sampling. Two sampling approaches are illustrated: through the maternal anterior abdominal wall with a needle and through the vagina and cervical canal using a malleable catheter. A speculum is an instrument for exposing the vagina.

NONINVASIVE PRENATAL DIAGNOSIS

Noninvasive screening for trisomy 21 (see Chapter 20) is based on the isolation of fetal cells in maternal blood and the detection of cell-free fetal DNA and RNA. DNA-based prenatal diagnostic testing and sequencing of maternal plasma are reliable for the early detection of fetal aneuploidies. Recent technologies, such as whole-exome sequencing, have led to new opportunities in advancing prenatal diagnosis and screening for genetic abnormalities.

FETAL TRANSFUSION

Fetuses with **hemolytic disease of the neonate** can be treated by intrauterine blood transfusions. The blood is injected through a needle inserted into the fetal peritoneal cavity. With recent advances in **percutaneous umbilical cord blood sampling**, blood, and packed red blood cells can be transfused directly into the umbilical vein for the treatment of fetal anemia due to isoimmunization. The need for fetal blood transfusions is reduced nowadays owing to the treatment of Rh-negative mothers of Rh-positive fetuses with anti-Rh immunoglobulin, which in many cases prevents the development of this disease. Fetal transfusion of platelets directly into the umbilical cord vein is carried out for the treatment of **alloimmune thrombocytopenia**. Also, fetal infusion of drugs in a similar manner for the treatment of a few medical conditions in the fetus has been reported.

FETOSCOPY

Using fiberoptic instruments, external parts of the fetal body may be directly observed. The **fetoscope** is introduced percutaneously through the mother's abdominal and uterine walls into the amniotic cavity. Fetoscopy is usually carried out beginning at 16 to 20 weeks of gestation and can be performed for many weeks after that. Fetoscopy now makes it possible, for instance, to repair open spina bifida in utero, most typically at 26 weeks of gestation. With newer approaches, such as **transabdominal thin-gauge embryo fetoscopy**, it is possible to detect certain defects in the embryo or fetus during the first trimester. Because of the higher risk to the fetus compared with other prenatal diagnostic procedures, fetoscopy has few indications for routine prenatal diagnosis and the surgical management of fetuses with anomalies. Fetoscopy combined with laser coagulation is used to treat fetal conditions such as **twin-twin transfusion syndrome**. Fetoscopy has also been used for the release of amniotic bands (see Fig. 7.21).

PERCUTANEOUS UMBILICAL CORD BLOOD SAMPLING

Fetal blood samples may be obtained directly from the umbilical vein by percutaneous umbilical cord blood sampling, or cordocentesis, for the diagnosis of many fetal abnormal conditions, including aneuploidy, fetal growth restriction, fetal infection, and fetal anemia. Percutaneous umbilical cord blood sampling is usually performed after 18 weeks of gestation under continuous direct ultrasound guidance, which is used to locate the umbilical cord and its vessels. The risk of pregnancy loss is approximately 1.3% in normal fetuses, but the risk increases with fetal anomalies or other conditions. The procedure also permits treating the fetus directly, including transfusion of packed red blood cells for the management of fetal anemia resulting from isoimmunization.

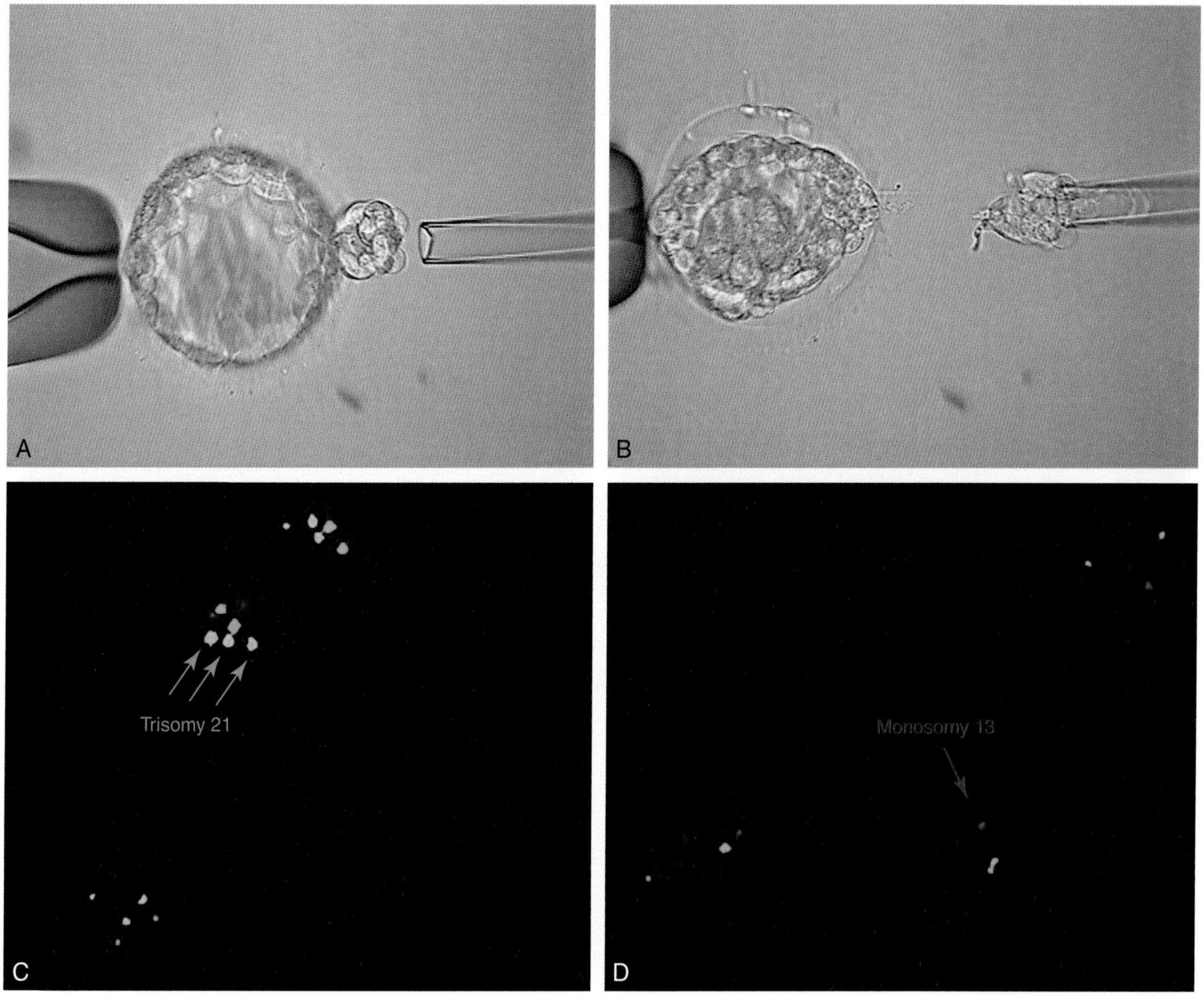

Fig. 6.12 (A) Microscopic images of the human blastocyst with trophectoderm cells (which will form extraembryonic tissues) starting to hatch. (B) The trophectoderm cells biopsied with assisted laser cutting. (C and D) Fluorescence in situ hybridization images in aneuploidy blastocysts. (C) Three dots that have stained green in (C) indicate the presence of three chromosomes 21 in the sample (46,XX, +21). (D) One dot that has stained red in (D) indicates the presence of only one chromosome 13 in the sample (45,XX, −13.) (From Liang L, Wang CT, Sun X, et al: Identification of chromosomal errors in human preimplantation embryos with oligonucleotide DNA microarray, *PLoS ONE* 8:4, 2013.)

MAGNETIC RESONANCE IMAGING

Magnetic resonance imaging (MRI) of the fetus from the surface of the abdominal wall is a noninvasive technique that provides cross-sectional images of the developing fetus in the uterus. MR images of the fetus are evaluated for suspected fetal anomalies. Important advantages of MRI are that like ultrasound, it does not use ionizing radiation, but it has higher soft tissue contrast and resolution (Fig. 6.13).

FETAL MONITORING

Continuous fetal heart rate monitoring in high-risk pregnancies is routine and provides information about the oxygenation of the fetus. There are various causes of prenatal **fetal distress**, such as maternal diseases that reduce oxygen transport to the fetus (e.g., cyanotic heart disease). Fetal distress (e.g., indicated by an abnormal heart rate or rhythm) suggests that the fetus is in jeopardy. A noninvasive method of monitoring uses transducers placed on the mother's abdomen.

SUMMARY OF FETAL PERIOD

- The fetal period begins 8 weeks after fertilization (10 weeks after the LNMP) and ends at birth. It is characterized by rapid body growth and differentiation of tissues and organ systems. An obvious change in the fetal period is the relative slowing of head growth compared with that of the rest of the body.
- At the beginning of the 20th week, **lanugo** (fine downy hair) and head hair appear, and the skin is coated with **vernix caseosa** (a waxy substance). The eyelids are closed during most of the fetal period, but they begin to reopen at approximately 26 weeks. At this time, the fetus is usually

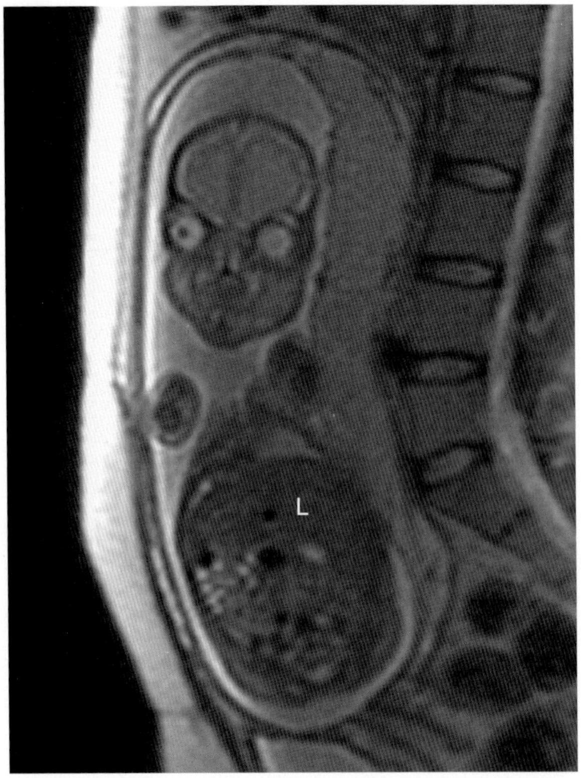

Fig. 6.13 Sagittal magnetic resonance image of the pelvis of a pregnant female. The fetus is in the breech presentation. Note the brain, eyes, and liver (L). (Courtesy Dr. Deborah Levine, Director of Obstetric and Gynecologic Ultrasound, Beth Israel Deaconess Medical Center, Boston, MA.)

capable of **extrauterine existence**, mainly because of the maturity of its respiratory system.

- Up to 30 weeks, the fetus appears reddish and wizened (wrinkled) because of the thinness of its skin and the relative absence of subcutaneous fat. Fat usually develops rapidly at 26 to 29 weeks, giving the fetus a smooth, healthy appearance (see Fig. 6.9).
- The fetus is less vulnerable than the embryo to the teratogenic effects of drugs, viruses, and radiation, but these agents may interfere with growth and normal functional development, especially of the brain and eyes.
- The physician can determine whether a fetus has a particular disease or birth defect by using various diagnostic techniques, such as amniocentesis, CVS, ultrasonography, and MRI.
- In selected cases, treatments can be given to the fetus, such as drugs to correct **cardiac arrhythmia** or thyroid disorders. Surgical correction of some birth defects in utero (Fig. 6.14) is also possible (e.g., ureters that do not open into the bladder can be surgically corrected).

CLINICALLY ORIENTED PROBLEMS

CASE 6-1

A female in the 20th week of a high-risk pregnancy was scheduled for a repeat cesarean section. Her physician wanted to establish an expected date of delivery.

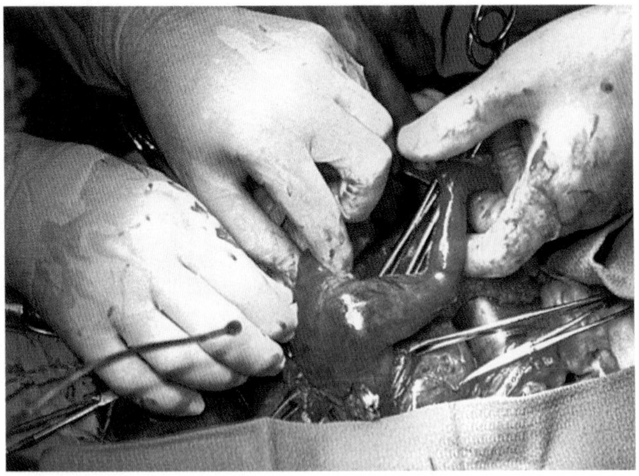

Fig. 6.14 Fetus at 21 weeks undergoing bilateral ureterostomies, the establishment of openings of the ureters into the bladder. (From Harrison MR, Globus MS, Filly RA, editors: *The unborn patient: prenatal diagnosis and treatment*, ed 2, Philadelphia, 1994, Saunders.)

- How would an expected date of delivery be established?
- When would labor likely be induced?
- How could this be accomplished?

CASE 6-2

A 44-year-old pregnant female was worried that her fetus may have major birth defects.

- How could the status of her fetus be determined?
- What chromosomal abnormality would be most likely?
- What other chromosomal aberrations might be detected?

CASE 6-3

A 19-year-old female in the second trimester of pregnancy asked a physician whether her fetus was vulnerable to over-the-counter drugs and street drugs. She also wondered about the effect of her heavy drinking and cigarette smoking on her fetus.

- What would the physician likely tell her?

CASE 6-4

An ultrasound examination of a pregnant female revealed that her fetus had IUGR.

- What factors may cause IUGR? Discuss how these factors might influence fetal growth.
- Which factors can the mother eliminate? Would removing these factors result in a reversal of IUGR?

CASE 6-5

A female in the first trimester of pregnancy who was to undergo amniocentesis expressed concerns about a miscarriage and the possibility of injury to her fetus.

- What are the risks of these complications?
- What procedures are used to minimize these risks?
- What other technique might be used for obtaining cells for a chromosomal study?

CASE 6-6

A pregnant female is told that she is going to have an AFP test to determine whether there are any birth defects.

- What is AFP, and where can it be found?
- What types of fetal defects can be detected by an AFP assay of maternal serum?
- What is the significance of high and low levels of AFP?

Discussion of these problems appears in the Appendix at the back of the book.

BIBLIOGRAPHY AND SUGGESTED READING

Benson CB, Doubilet PM: Fetal biometry and growth. Obstetric ultrasound examination 29125628; PMCID: PMC6486016. In Norton ME, editor: *Callen's ultrasonography in obstetrics and gynecology,* ed 6, Philadelphia, 2017, Elsevier.

Badeau M, Lindsay C, Blais J, et al: Genomics-based non-invasive prenatal testing for detection of fetal chromosomal aneuploidy in pregnant women, *Cochrane Database Syst Rev* 11(11):CD011767, 2017. https://doi.org/10.1002/14651858.CD011767.

Butt K, Lim K: Determination of gestational age by ultrasound, *J Obstet Gynaecol* 36:171, 2014.

Carlson LM, Vora NL: Prenatal diagnosis—screening and diagnostic tools, *Obstet Gynecol Clin N Am* 44:245, 2017.

David AL, Spencer RN: Clinical assessment of fetal wellbeing and fetal safety indications, *J Clin Pharmacol* 62(Suppl 1):567–578, 2022. https://doi.org/10.1002/jcph.2126.

De Bakker BS, de Jong KH, Hagoort J, et al: An interactive three-dimensional digital atlas and quantitative database of human development, *Science* 354, 2016.

Duan J, Wang J-C, Li H-X, et al: 1.5T magnetic resonance imaging in evaluating fetal head and abdominal malformations: a preliminary study, *Am J Transl Res* 13:9063, 2021.

Evans LL, Harrison MR: Modern fetal surgery – a historical review of the happenings that shaped modern fetal surgery and its practices, *Transl Pediatr* 10:1401, 2021. https://doi.org/10.21037/tp-20-114.

Hinrichsen KV, editor: *Human embryologie,* Berlin, 1990, Springer-Verlag.

Huang H, Wang Y, Zhang M, et al: Diagnostic accuracy and value of chromosomal microarray analysis for chromosomal abnormalities in prenatal detection: a prospective clinical study, *Medicine (Baltimore)* 100(20):e25999, 2021. https://doi.org/10.1097/MD.000 0000000025999.

Jirásel JE: *An atlas of human prenatal developmental mechanics: anatomy and staging,* London and New York, 2004, Taylor and Francis.

Khambalia AZ, Roberts CL, Nguyen M, et al: Predicting date of birth and examining the best time to date a pregnancy, *Int J Gynaecol Obstet* 123:105, 2013.

Liu Y, Xuan R, He Y, et al: Computation of fetal kicking in various fetal health examinations: a systematic review, *Int J Environ Res Public Health,* 2022. - 04. https://doi.org/10.3390/ijerph19074366.

Lapa DA, Chmait RH, Gielchinsky Y, et al: Percutaneous fetoscopic spina bifida repair: effect on ambulation and need for postnatal cerebrospinal fluid diversion and bladder catheterization, *Ultrasound Obstet Gynecol* 58(4):582–589, 2021. https://doi.org/10.1002/uog.23658.

Magann EF, Sandin AI: Amniotic fluid volume in fetal health and disease. In Norton ME, editor: *Callen's ultrasonography in obstetrics and gynecology,* ed 6, Philadelphia, 2017, Elsevier.

Margiotti K., Fabiani M., Cima A., Libotte F., Mesoraca A., Giorlandino C.: Prenatal diagnosis by trio clinical exome sequencing: single center experience. *Curr Issues Mol Biol.* 2024;46(4):3209–3217.

Morgan TA, Feldstein VA, Filly PA: Ultrasound evaluation of normal fetal anatomy. In Norton ME, editor: *Callen's ultrasonography in obstetrics and gynecology,* ed 6, Philadelphia, 2017, Elsevier.

Norton ME, Rink BD: Genetics and prenatal genetic testing. In Norton ME, editor: *Callen's ultrasonography in obstetrics and gynecology,* ed 6, Philadelphia, 2017, Elsevier.

O'Rahilly R, Müller F: Publication 637 *Development stages in human embryos,* Washington, DC, 1987, Carnegie Institution of Washington.

Peretz-Machluf R, Rabinowitz T, Shamron N: Genome-wide noninvasive prenatal diagnosis of de novo mutations, *Methods Mol Biol* 2243:2449, 2021.

Persaud TVN, Hay JC: Normal embryonic and fetal development. In Reece EA, Hobbins JC, editors: *Clinical obstetrics: the fetus and mother,* ed 3, Malden, Mass, 2006, Blackwell, pp 19–32.

Pooh RK, Shiota K, Kurjak A: Imaging of the human embryo with magnetic resonance imaging microscopy and high-resolution transvaginal 3-dimensional sonography: human embryology in the 21st century, *Am J Obstet Gynecol* 204:77.e1–77.e16, 2011.

Poon LCY, Musci T, Song K: Maternal plasma cell-free fetal and maternal DNA at 11-13 weeks' gestation: relation to fetal and maternal characteristics and pregnancy outcomes, *Fetal Diagn Ther* 33:215, 2013.

Rabinowitz T, Shomron N: Genome-wide noninvasive prenatal diagnosis of monogenic disorders: Current and future trends, *Comput Struct Biotechnol J* 18:2463–2470, 2020. https://doi.org/10.1016/j.csbj.2020.09.003.

Rao R, Platt LD: Ultrasound screening: status of markers and efficacy of screening for structural abnormalities, *Semin Perinatal* 40:67, 2016.

Rozance PJ, Brown LP, Thorn SR: Intrauterine growth restriction and the small-for-gestational-age infant. In MacDonald MG, Seshia MMK, editors: *Avery's neonatology: pathophysiology and management of the newborn,* ed 7, Philadelphia, 2016, Lippincott Williams and Wilkins.

Salihu HM, Miranda S, Hill L, et al: Survival of pre-viable preterm infants in the United States: a systematic review and meta-analysis, *Semin Perinatol* 37:389, 2013.

Streeter GL: Weight, sitting height, head size, foot length and menstrual age of the human embryo, *Contrib Embryol Carnegie Inst* 11:143, 1920.

Vermeesch JR, Voet T, Devriendt K: Prenatal and pre-implantation genetic diagnosis, *Nat Rev Genet* 17:643, 2016.

Wilson RD, Gagnon A, Audibert F: et al: Prenatal diagnosis procedures and techniques to obtain a diagnostic fetal specimen or tissue: maternal and fetal risks and benefits, *J Obstet Gynaecol Can* 37:656, 2015. (SOGC Clinical Practice Guideline No. 326, Society for Obstetrics and Gynecology of Canada, July 2015.)

Placenta and Fetal Membranes

7

CHAPTER OUTLINE

The placenta and fetal membranes separate the fetus from the **endometrium**, the inner layer of the uterine wall. An interchange of substances, such as nutrients and oxygen, occurs between the maternal and fetal bloodstreams through the placenta. The vessels in the umbilical cord connect the placental circulation with the fetal circulation. The **fetal membranes** include the **chorion**, **amnion**, **umbilical vesicle**, and **allantois**.

PLACENTA

The placenta is a **fetomaternal organ** that has two components (Fig. 7.1):

- A **fetal part** that develops from the chorionic sac
- A **maternal part** that is derived from the endometrium

The placenta and umbilical cord form a transport system for substances passing between the mother and embryo/fetus. Nutrients and oxygen pass from the maternal blood through the placenta to the embryo/fetal blood, and waste materials and carbon dioxide pass from the fetal blood through the placenta to the maternal blood. The placenta and fetal membranes perform the following functions and activities: protection, immune response, nutrition, respiration, excretion of waste products, and hormone production. Shortly after birth, the placenta and membranes are expelled from the uterus as the **afterbirth**.

DECIDUA

The **decidua** is the endometrium of the uterus in a pregnant female. It is the functional layer of the endometrium that separates from the remainder of the uterus after **parturition** (childbirth). The **three regions of the decidua** are named according to their relation to the implantation site (see Fig. 7.1):

- The **decidua basalis** is the part of the decidua deep to the conceptus which forms the maternal part of the placenta.
- The **decidua capsularis** is the superficial part of the decidua overlying the conceptus.
- The **decidua parietalis** represents the remaining parts of the decidua.

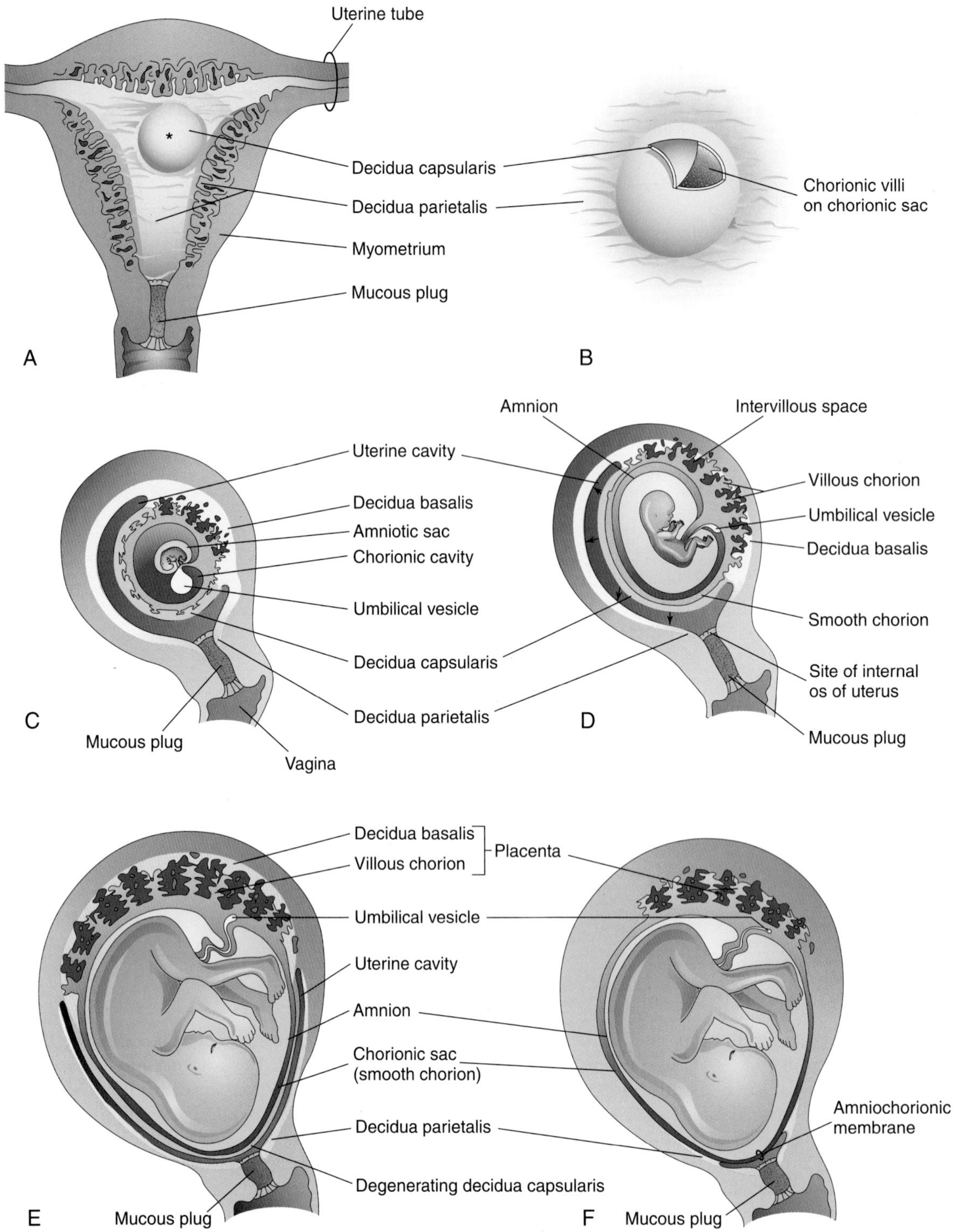

Fig. 7.1 Development of the placenta and fetal membranes. (A) Frontal section of the uterus showing elevation of the decidua capsularis by the expanding chorionic sac of a 4-week-old embryo implanted in the endometrium on the posterior wall (*asterisk*). (B) Enlarged drawing of the implantation site. The chorionic villi were exposed by cutting an opening in the decidua capsularis. (C–F) Sagittal sections of the gravid (pregnant) uterus from weeks 5 to 22 showing the changing relations of the fetal membranes to the decidua. In (F) the amnion and chorion are fused and the decidua parietalis, obliterating the uterine cavity. Note in (D–F) that the chorionic villi persist only where the chorion is associated with the decidua basalis.

In response to increasing progesterone levels in maternal blood, the connective tissue cells of the decidua enlarge to form **decidual cells**. These cells enlarge as glycogen and lipid accumulate in their cytoplasm.

The cellular and vascular changes occurring in the endometrium as the blastocyst implants constitute the **decidual reaction**. Many decidual cells degenerate near the chorionic sac in the region of the syncytiotrophoblast, and together with maternal blood and uterine secretions, they provide a rich source of nutrition for the embryo/fetus. These cells also appear to protect the maternal tissue against uncontrolled invasion by the syncytiotrophoblast and may be involved in hormone production. During early pregnancy, decidual Natural Killer (dNK) cells and gamma/delta T cells accumulate in the decidua basalis and play an essential role in the maternal immune response, tolerance of the allogeneic embryo, and protection from infections.

Decidual regions, clearly recognizable during ultrasonography, can be important in diagnosing early pregnancy (see Fig. 3.7).

DEVELOPMENT OF PLACENTA

Early development is characterized by rapid proliferation of the trophoblast and development of the chorionic sac and chorionic villi (see Chapters 3 and 4). *Homeobox genes (*HLX, MSX2, *and* DLX3*) expressed in the trophoblast and its blood vessels induce trophoblastic invasion and regulate placental development. Some trophoblastic cells (approximately 15% of trophoblastic cells in the first trimester) have primary cilia that appear to function as mediators of signaling related to migration and invasion (EG-VEGF, ERK1/2, MMP cascade). In addition, somatic mutations and mosaicism appear to be common in trophoblastic placental tissues.*

TROPHOBLAST STEM CELLS AND THEIR DIFFERENTIATION

It has long been recognized that the most primitive progenitors of trophoblast cells are contained within the "outer cell mass" or the trophoblast layer of the preimplantation blastocyst. Subsequently, when chorionic villi are formed, bipotent stem cells are contained within the cytotrophoblast layer of the villi, which differentiate into two distinct pathways: the villous pathway, in which cells proliferate and fuse, giving rise to the villous syncytiotrophoblast layer facing the maternal sinusoids, engaged primarily in exchange and endocrine functions, and the extravillous (EVT) pathway in which cells break out of the villi as discrete cell columns which proliferate at their base, migrate, and invade the decidua, endometrial glands, blood vessels, and lymphatic vessels (see Fig 7.2).

EVT cells reside within the decidua as three distinct populations: (1) **endovascular trophoblast** which adopts an endothelial phenotype to "remodel" the spiral arteries from low-flow, high-resistance tubes into high-flow, low-resistance tubes that ensure adequate supply of maternal arterial blood to the placenta for fetal nourishment; (2) invasive **Interstitial trophoblasts** dispersed within the decidua which can migrate and invade the spiral arteries from the exterior; (3) noninvasive **placental bed giant cells** (PBC), which can produce human placental lactogen (hPL). PBCs have two phenotypes—single large trophoblast cells containing one or more nuclear profiles in a voluminous cytoplasm (resulting from endomitosis or cell fusion), and cell aggregates comprising mononuclear trophoblast cells in close apposition separated by narrow intercellular spaces. The cells within the aggregates are attached by desmosomes and also possess gap junctions.

While mouse trophoblast stem cell lines were produced long ago, derivation of human trophoblast stem cell lines has been achieved only recently by Okae et al. (2018) both from the first-trimester chorionic villous cytotrophoblast and preimplantation blastocyst, having identical phenotypes, transcriptomes, and longevity. *Maintenance of the stem cell state required the activation of Wingless/Integrated (Wnt) and EGF, and inhibition of TGFβ, histone deacetylase (HDAC), and Rho-associated protein kinase (ROCK). The resulting cell lines could self-renew as CTB and differentiate into STB and EVT pathways under specific culture conditions. Transcription factor TEAD4 promotes TS cell self-renewal by inducing the expression of genes associated with the cell cycle and preventing the expression of differentiation markers. Two key transcription factors- glial cells missing-1 (GCM1) and OVO-Like 1(OVOL1) are critical for HTS cell differentiation. GCM1 regulates HTS cell differentiation into both STB and EVT. GCM1 also coordinates the development and function of EVTs by regulating the expression of the EVT regulator ASCL2 and the WNT antagonist NOTUM. OVOL1 is also implicated in HTS differentiation. OVOL1 binds upstream of several CTB-associated genes MYC, ID1, and TP63 to mediate STB differentiation. Accordingly, depletion of OVOL1 in human CTBs inhibits fusion and STB differentiation, indicating that OVOL1 mediates trophoblast differentiation by repressing the progenitor state. OVOL1 represses gene expression, at least in part, by recruiting histone deacetylases (HDACs) to selected genomic regions.*

By the end of the third week, the anatomical arrangements necessary for physiologic exchanges between the mother and embryo/fetus are established. A complex **vascular network** is established in the placenta by the end of the fourth week, which facilitates maternal-embryonic exchanges of gases, nutrients, and metabolic waste products.

Chorionic villi cover the entire chorionic sac until the beginning of the eighth week (Figs. 7.3 and 7.4; see also Fig. 7.1C). As the chorionic sac grows, the villi associated with the decidua capsularis become compressed, and the blood supply is reduced; hence, they soon degenerate (see Figs. 7.1D and 7.3B). This produces a relatively avascular bare area, the **smooth chorion** (chorion laeve). As those villi disappear, the villi associated with the decidua basalis rapidly increase, branch profusely, and enlarge. This forms the "bushy" area of the chorionic sac, the **villous chorion** (chorion frondosum).

The uterus, chorionic sac, and placenta enlarge as the embryo/fetus grows. Growth in the size and thickness of the placenta continues rapidly until the fetus is approximately 18 weeks old. The fully developed placenta covers 15% to 30% of the decidua of the endometrium and weighs approximately one-sixth as much as the fetus. At term for its own metabolic requirements, the placenta uses 40% to 60% of the oxygen and glucose that reaches the uterus.

Ultrasonography of Chorionic Sac

The size of the chorionic sac is useful in determining the gestational age of the embryo/fetus in patients with uncertain menstrual histories. The growth of the chorionic sac is extremely rapid between weeks 5 and 10. Ultrasound machines equipped with endovaginal transducers enable ultrasonographers to view the chorionic sac when it has a median sac diameter of 2 to 3 mm (see Fig. 3.7). Chorionic sacs with this diameter indicate that the gestational age is 31 to 32 days, which is approximately 18 days after fertilization.

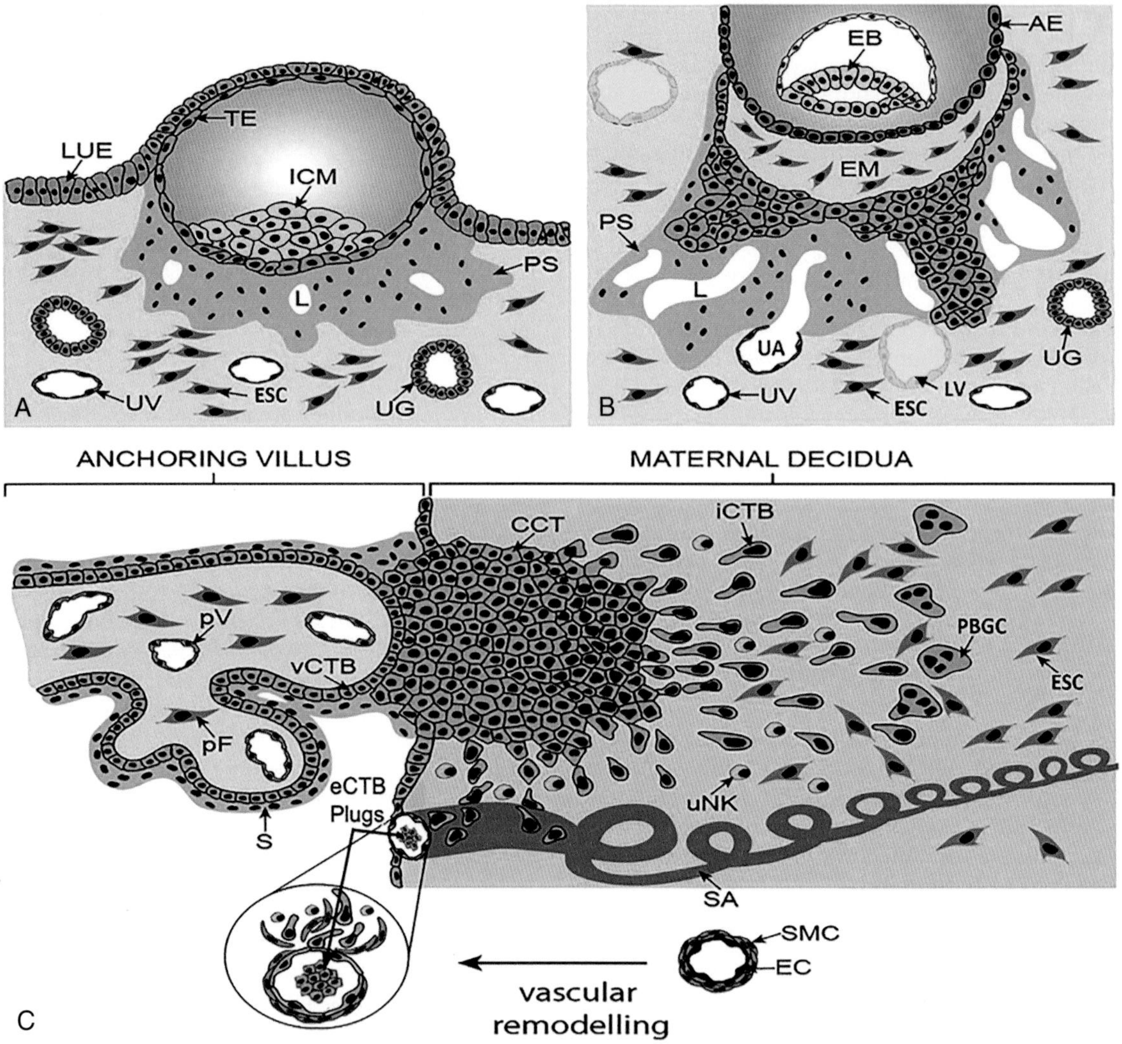

Fig. 7.2 (A) Shortly after implantation (end of the first week), the stem cells of the trophectoderm give rise to the PS by cell fusion. Lacunae (L) develop in the PS, as the precursor of the intervillous space. Invasion of the PS into uterine glands allows "uterine milk" to fill up the lacunae (histotrophic nutrition). Later, with the invasion of the PS into uterine vessels (UV/UA) maternal blood fills the lacunae (hemotrophic nutrition). Lymphatics (LL) are also invaded. (B) During the end of the second week, proliferative cytotrophoblasts (CTBs), break through the PS forming primary villi. (C) During the third week, tertiary villi are formed by migration of extraembryonic mesoderm followed by vascularization. At the base of the anchoring villi, proliferative cytotrophoblasts migrate towards the decidua as cell columns, which give rise to different invasive EVT subtypes. iCTBs migrate into the decidual stroma and differentiate into PBGC. Endovascular trophoblasts migrate into spiral arteries and contribute to uNK cell-initiated remodeling of SA. *AE*, Amniotic epithelium; *CCT*, cell column trophoblast; *EB*, embryoblast; *eCTB*, endovascular cytotrophoblast; *EM*, extraembryonic mesoderm; *ESC*, endometrial stromal cell; *EVT*, extravillous trophoblast; *ICM*, inner cell mass; *iCTB*, interstitial cytotrophoblast; *L*, lacunae; *LL*, lymphatic lumen; *LUE*, luminal uterine epithelium; *PBGC*, placental-bed giant cell; *pF*, placental fibroblast; *PS*, primitive syncytium; *pV*, placental vessel; *S*, syncytium; *SA*, spiral arteries; *TE*, trophectoderm; *UA*, Uterine artery; *UG*, uterine gland; *uNK*, uterine natural killer; *UV*, uterine vein; *vCTB*, villous cytotrophoblast. (From Lala PK, Nandi P, Hadi A, Halari C: A crossroad between placental and tumor biology: what have we learnt? *Placenta* 116:12–30, 2021.)

The placenta has two parts (Fig. 7.5; see Fig. 7.1E and F):

- The **fetal part** is formed by the **villous chorion**. The chorionic villi that arise from the chorion project into the **intervillous space** containing maternal blood (see Fig. 7.1D).
- The **maternal part** is formed by the decidua basalis, the part of the decidua related to the fetal component of the placenta (see also Fig. 7.1C–F). By the end of the fourth month, the decidua basalis is almost entirely replaced by the fetal part of the placenta.

The fetal part is attached to the maternal part of the placenta by the **cytotrophoblastic shell**, the external layer of trophoblastic cells on the maternal surface of the placenta (Fig. 7.6). The chorionic villi attach firmly to the decidua basalis through the cytotrophoblastic shell, which anchors the chorionic sac to the decidua basalis.

The shape of the placenta is determined by the persistent area of the chorionic villi (see Fig. 7.1F). Usually, this is a circular area, giving the placenta a discoid shape. As the chorionic villi invade the decidua basalis, decidual tissue is eroded to enlarge the intervillous space (see Fig. 7.5). This

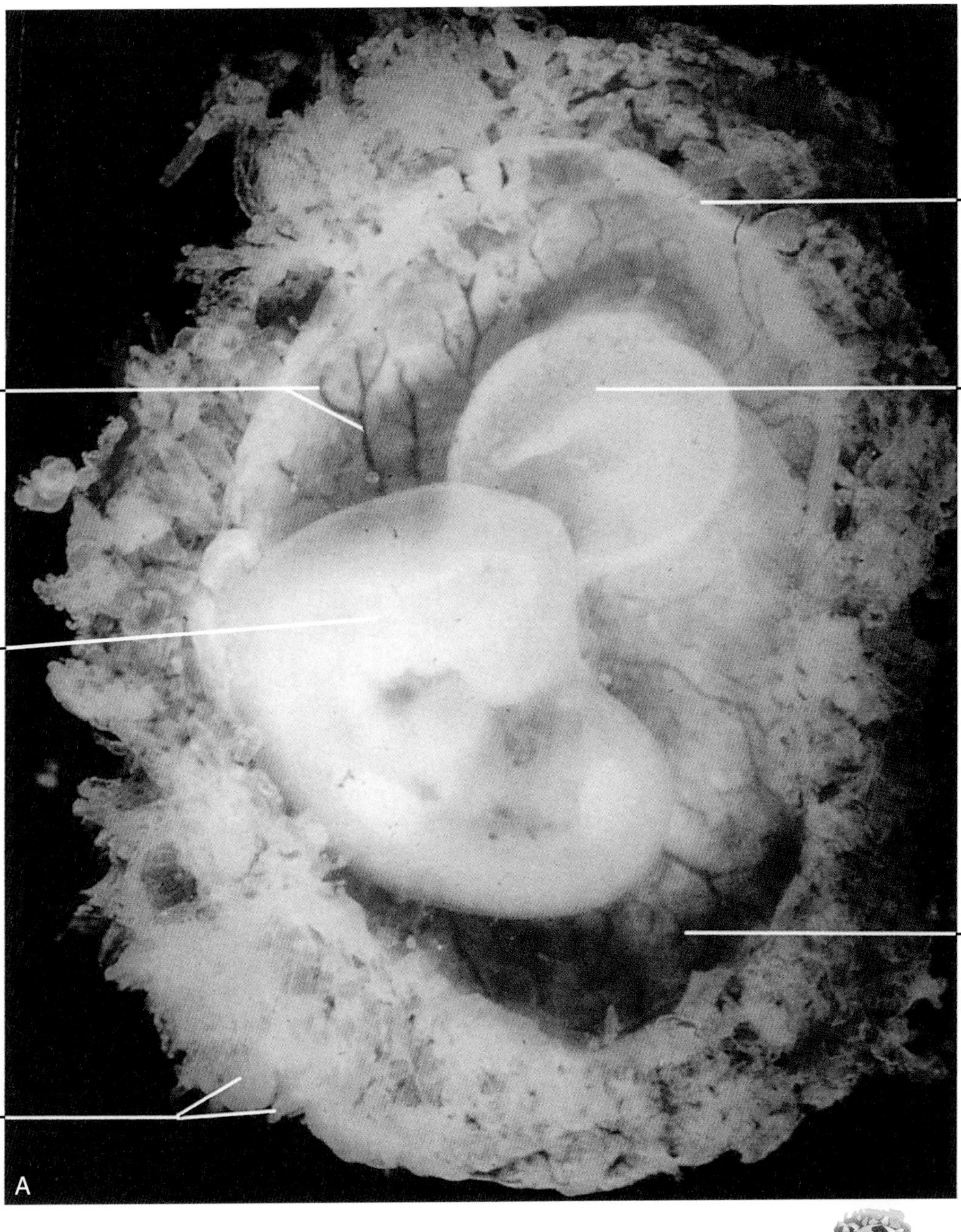

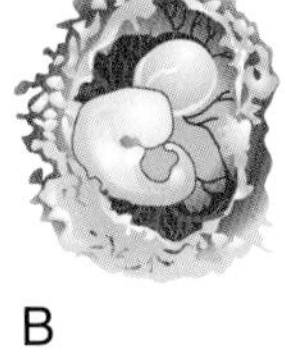

Fig. 7.3 (A) Lateral view of a spontaneously aborted embryo at Carnegie stage 14, approximately 32 days. The chorionic and amniotic sacs have been opened to show the embryo. Note the large size of the umbilical vesicle. (B) The sketch shows the actual size of the embryo and its membranes. (A, From Moore KL, Persaud TVN, Shiota K: *Color atlas of clinical embryology*, ed 2, Philadelphia, 2000, Saunders.)

erosion produces several wedge-shaped areas of decidua, the **placental septa**, which project toward the **chorionic plate**, the part of the chorionic wall related to the placenta (Fig. 7.6). The septa divide the fetal part of the placenta into irregular convex areas, or **cotyledons**. Each cotyledon consists of two or more **stem villi** and many **branch villi** (Fig. 7.7A; see also Fig. 7.6). By the end of the fourth month, the decidua basalis is almost entirely replaced by cotyledons (see Fig. 7.12). *Expression of the Wingless and Notch developmental pathways, CDX2, TEAD4, HAND1, MAZ, NFE2LE, TFAP2C, NR2F2, CTNNB1, kinase genes (*MAP2K1 *and* MAP2K2*) and the transcription factor Gcm1 (glial cells missing-1) in trophoblast*

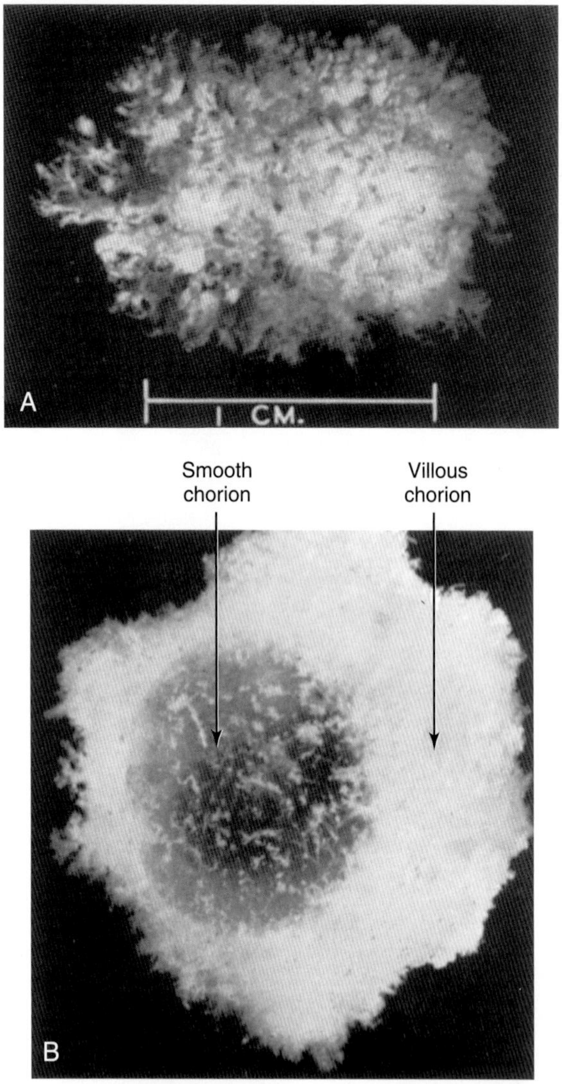

Fig. 7.4 Spontaneously aborted human chorionic sacs. (A) At 21 days. The sac is covered with chorionic villi (×4). (B) At 8 weeks. Some of the chorionic villi have degenerated, causing the smooth chorion to form. (From Potter EL, Craig JM: *Pathology of the fetus and the infant*, ed 3, Chicago, 1975, Book Medical Publishers.)

stem cells are involved in regulating the branching process of the stem villi to form the vascular network in the placenta.

The decidua capsularis, the layer of decidua overlying the chorionic sac, forms a capsule over the external surface of the sac (see Fig. 7.1A–D). As the conceptus enlarges, the decidua capsularis bulges into the uterine cavity and becomes greatly attenuated. Eventually the decidua capsularis contacts and fuses with the decidua parietalis on the opposite wall; thereby, slowly obliterating the uterine cavity (see Fig. 7.1E and F). By 22 to 24 weeks, the reduced blood supply to the decidua capsularis causes it to degenerate and disappear.

After the disappearance of the decidua capsularis, the smooth part of the chorionic sac (smooth chorion) fuses with the decidua parietalis (see Fig. 7.1F). This fusion can be separated and typically occurs if blood escapes from the intervillous space (see Fig. 7.5). The collection of blood **(hematoma)** pushes the chorionic membrane away from the decidua parietalis, thereby reestablishing the potential space of the uterine cavity.

Initially, when trophoblastic cells invade and remodel the spiral arteries, these cells create plugs within the arteries. These plugs allow only maternal plasma to enter the intervillous space. As a result, a net negative oxygen gradient is created; it has been shown that elevated oxygen levels during the early stages of development can be detrimental to the embryo and fetus. However, by 11 to 14 weeks, the plugs begin to break down, maternal whole blood begins to flow, and oxygen concentrations increase.

The **intervillous space** of the placenta, which by 11 to 14 weeks contains maternal blood, is derived from the **lacuna**e that developed in the syncytiotrophoblast during the second week of development (see Fig. 3.2A and B). This large blood-filled space results from the coalescence and enlargement of the **lacunar networks**. The intervillous space is divided into compartments by placental septa; however, there is free communication between the compartments because the septa do not reach the chorionic plate (see Fig. 7.6).

Maternal blood enters the intervillous space from the **spiral endometrial arteries** in the decidua basalis (see Figs. 7.5 and 7.6). The spiral arteries pass through gaps in the cytotrophoblastic shell and discharge blood into the intervillous space. This large space is drained by **endometrial veins** (also invaded by trophoblastic cells), which also penetrate the cytotrophoblastic shell. These veins are found over the entire surface of the decidua basalis.

The **numerous branch villi**, arising from **stem villi**, are continuously showered with maternal blood that circulates through the intervillous space (see Figs. 7.5 and 7.6). The blood in this space carries oxygen and nutritional materials that are necessary for fetal growth and development. The maternal blood also contains fetal waste, carbon dioxide, salts, and products of protein metabolism.

The amniotic sac enlarges faster than the chorionic sac. As a result, the amnion and smooth chorion fuse to form the **amniochorionic membrane** (see Figs. 7.5 and 7.6). This composite membrane fuses with the decidua capsularis and, after the disappearance of the latter, adheres to the decidua parietalis (see Figs. 7.1F, 7.5, and 7.6). It is the amniochorionic membrane that ruptures during labor. Preterm membrane rupture (i.e., at less than 37 weeks' gestation) is the most common event leading to premature labor. Membrane rupture allows amniotic fluid to escape through the vagina.

PLACENTAL CIRCULATION

The branch chorionic villi of the placenta provide a large surface area where materials may be exchanged across the very thin **placental membrane** interposed between the fetal and maternal circulations (see Figs. 7.6 and 7.7). It is through the branch villi, which arise from stem villi, that the main exchange of material between the mother and fetus takes place. Fetal and maternal circulations are separated by the placental membrane consisting of extrafetal tissues (Fig. 7.8; see also Fig. 7.7B and C).

FETAL PLACENTAL CIRCULATION

Poorly oxygenated blood passes through the **umbilical arteries** to the placenta. At the site of attachment of the umbilical cord to the placenta, the arteries divide into several radially

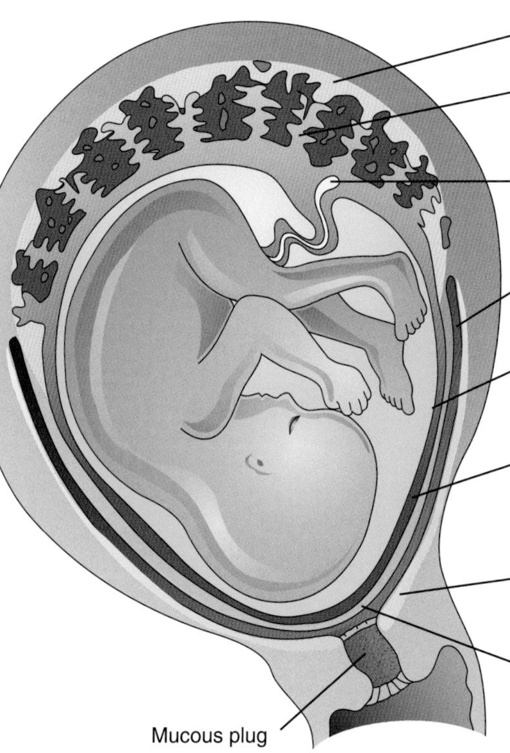

Fig. 7.5 Drawing of a sagittal section of a uterus at 16 weeks showing the relation of the fetal membranes to each other and the decidua and embryo.

disposed **chorionic arteries** that branch freely in the chorionic plate before entering the chorionic villi (see Figs. 7.6 and 7.7). The blood vessels form an extensive **arteriocapillary-venous system** within the chorionic villi (see Fig. 7.7A), which brings the fetal blood extremely close to the maternal blood (see Fig. 7.8). This system provides a large surface area for the exchange of metabolic and gaseous products between the maternal and fetal bloodstreams.

Normally, there is no intermingling of fetal and maternal blood; however, very small amounts of fetal blood may enter the maternal circulation when minute defects develop in the placental membrane (see Fig. 7.7B and C). The **well-oxygenated fetal blood** in the fetal capillaries passes into thin-walled veins that follow the chorionic arteries to the site of attachment of the umbilical cord. They converge here to form the **umbilical vein** (see Figs. 7.6 and 7.8). This large vessel carries oxygen-rich blood to the fetus.

MATERNAL PLACENTAL CIRCULATION

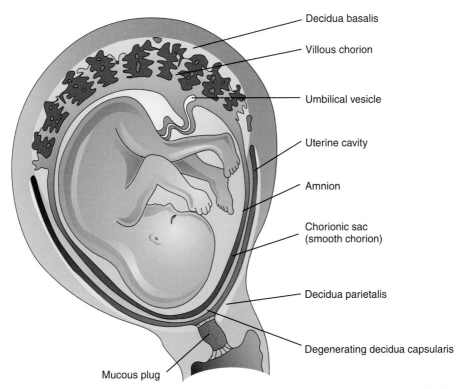

The maternal blood in the intervillous space is temporarily outside the maternal circulatory system. It enters the intervillous space through 80 to 100 spiral endometrial arteries in the decidua basalis (see Fig. 7.6). The blood flow from the spiral arteries is pulsatile.

The entering blood is at a considerably higher pressure than that in the intervillous space, and therefore blood spurts toward the **chorionic plate**, which forms the "roof" of the intervillous space. As pressure dissipates, the blood flows slowly over the branch villi, allowing an exchange of metabolic and gaseous products with the fetal blood. The blood eventually returns through the **endometrial veins** to the maternal circulation.

The welfare of the embryo/fetus depends more on the adequate bathing of the branch villi with maternal blood than any other factor. Reductions of uteroplacental circulation result in **fetal hypoxia** and **intrauterine growth restriction (IUGR)**. Severe reductions in circulation may result in embryo/fetal death. The intervillous space of the mature placenta contains approximately 150 mL of blood, which is replenished three or four times per minute.

PLACENTAL MEMBRANE

The **placental membrane** is a composite structure that consists of extrafetal tissues separating the maternal and fetal blood. Until approximately 20 weeks, the placental membrane consists of four layers (see Figs. 7.7 and 7.8): syncytiotrophoblast, cytotrophoblast, connective tissue of the villi, and endothelium of fetal capillaries. After the 20th week, cellular changes occur in the branch villi that result in the cytotrophoblast, in many of the villi, becoming attenuated.

Eventually, cytotrophoblastic cells disappear over large areas of the villi, leaving only thin patches of syncytiotrophoblast. As a result, the placental membrane consists of three layers in most places (see Fig. 7.7C). In some areas, the placental membrane becomes markedly thinned and attenuated. At these sites, the syncytiotrophoblast comes into direct contact with the endothelium of the fetal capillaries to form a **vasculosyncytial placental membrane**.

Sometimes the placental membrane is called the placental barrier; this is an inappropriate term because there are only a few substances, endogenous or exogenous, that are unable to pass through the membrane in detectable amounts. The placental membrane acts as a barrier only when a molecule

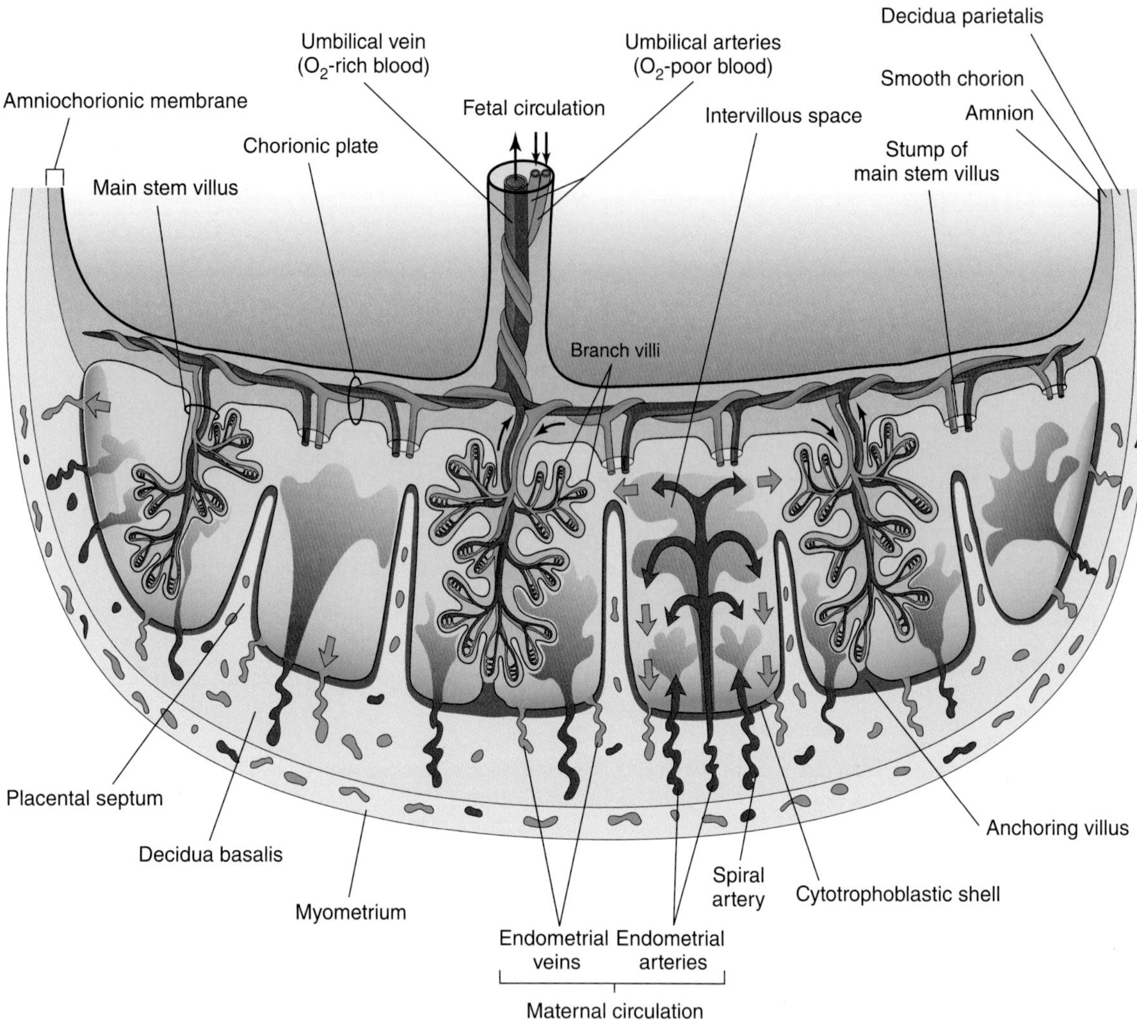

Fig. 7.6 Schematic drawing of a transverse section through a full-term placenta, showing (1) the relation of the villous chorion (fetal part of the placenta) to the decidua basalis (maternal part of the placenta), (2) the fetal placental circulation, and (3) the maternal placental circulation. Maternal blood flows into the intervillous spaces in spurts from the spiral arteries. Note that the umbilical arteries carry poorly oxygenated fetal blood (shown in *blue*) to the placenta and that the umbilical vein carries oxygenated blood (shown in *red*) to the fetus. Note that the cotyledons are separated by placental septa, projections of the decidua basalis. Each cotyledon consists of two or more main-stem villi and many branch villi. In this drawing, only one stem villus is shown in each cotyledon, but the stumps of those that have been removed are indicated.

is of a certain size, configuration, and charge, such as that of **heparin** (a compound produced in the liver, lungs, and mast cells that inhibits blood coagulation). Some metabolites, toxins, and hormones, although present in the maternal circulation, do not pass through the placental membrane in sufficient concentrations to affect the embryo/fetus. Most drugs and other substances in the maternal blood plasma pass through the placental membrane and enter the fetal blood plasma (see Fig. 7.8). The syncytiotrophoblast-free surface has many microvilli that increase the surface area for exchange between the maternal and fetal circulations. As pregnancy advances, the placental membrane becomes progressively thinner, and thus blood in many fetal capillaries is extremely close to the maternal blood in the intervillous space (see Figs. 7.6C and 7.7).

During the third trimester, numerous nuclei in the syncytiotrophoblast aggregate to form multinucleated protrusions, **syncytial knots** (see Fig. 7.7C). These aggregations regularly break off and are carried from the intervillous space into the maternal circulation. Some knots lodge in the capillaries of the maternal lungs, where they are rapidly destroyed by local enzyme action. Toward the end of pregnancy, eosinophilic **fibrinoid material** thickens on the surfaces of the villi (see Fig. 7.7C), which appears to reduce placental transfer.

FUNCTIONS OF PLACENTA

The placenta has several main functions:

- **Metabolism** (e.g., synthesis of glycogen)
- **Transport** of gases and nutrients
- **Endocrine secretion** (e.g., human chorionic gonadotropin [hCG])
- **Protection of the fetus from maternal infection and maternal immune attack**
- **Excretion** (fetal waste products)

These comprehensive activities are essential for maintaining pregnancy and promoting normal fetal development.

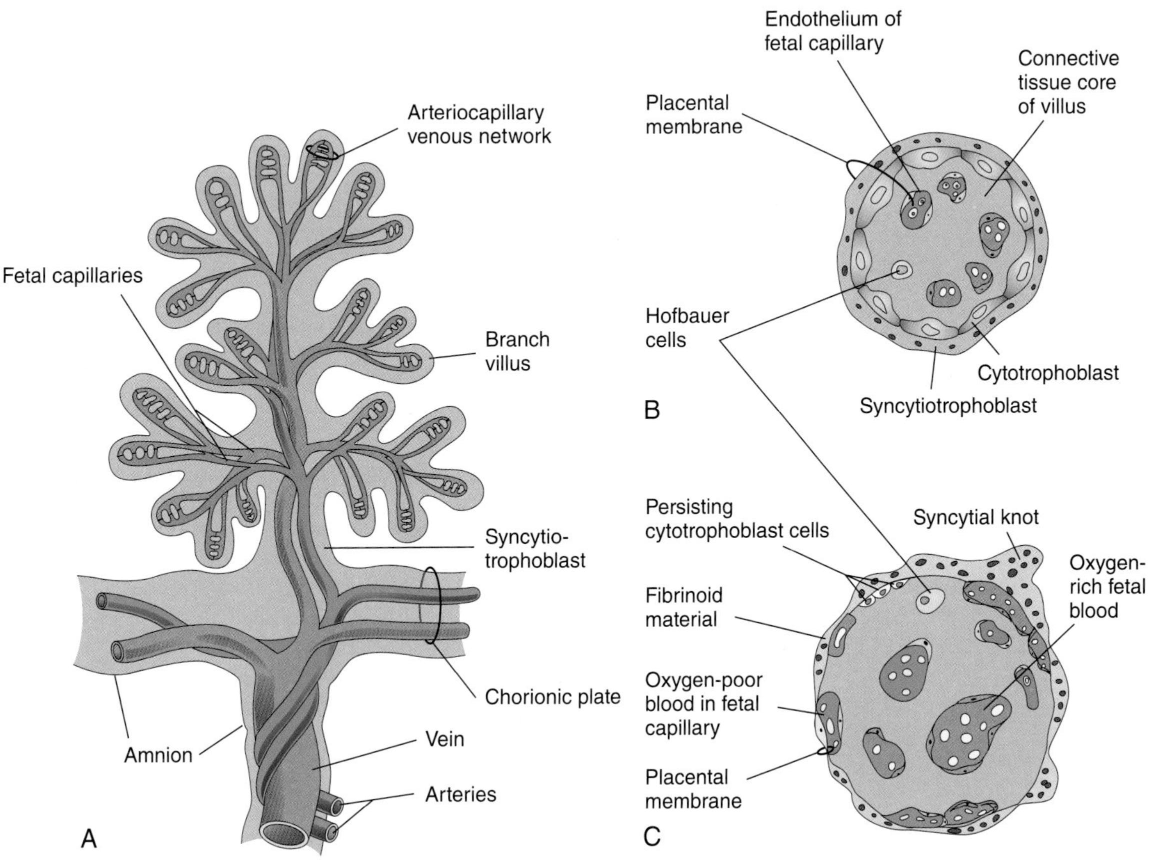

Fig. 7.7 (A) Drawing of a stem chorionic villus showing its arteriocapillary–venous system. The arteries carry poorly oxygenated fetal blood and waste products from the fetus, whereas the vein carries oxygenated blood and nutrients to the fetus. (B and C) Drawings of sections through a branch villus at 10 weeks and full term, respectively. The placental membrane, composed of extrafetal tissues, separates the maternal blood in the intervillous space from the fetal blood in the capillaries in the villi. Note that the placental membrane is very thin at full term. Fetal macrophages (Hofbauer cells) are present in the chorionic villi from early pregnancy. These phagocytic cells are involved in the development of the placenta.

PLACENTAL METABOLISM

The placenta, particularly during early pregnancy, synthesizes glycogen, cholesterol, and fatty acids, which serve as sources of nutrients and energy for the embryo/fetus. Many of its metabolic activities are undoubtedly critical for its other two major placental activities (transport and endocrine secretion). The placenta has several mechanisms that allow it to minimize the impact on the fetus from the various environmental situations (e.g., hypoxia) that may occur.

PLACENTAL TRANSFER

The transport of substances in both directions between the fetal and maternal blood is facilitated by the great surface area of the placental membrane. Almost all materials are transported across this membrane by one of the four main transport mechanisms: simple diffusion, facilitated diffusion, active transport, and pinocytosis.

Passive transport by simple diffusion is usually characteristic of substances moving from the areas of higher to lower concentration until equilibrium is established. In **facilitated diffusion**, there is transport through electrical gradients. Facilitated diffusion requires a transporter but no energy. Such systems may involve carrier molecules that temporarily combine with the substances to be transported. **Active transport** is the passage of ions or molecules across a cell membrane against a gradient and requires energy. **Pinocytosis** is a form of **endocytosis** (which brings substances into cells) in which the material is engulfed in a small amount of extracellular fluid. This method of transport is usually reserved for large molecules. Some proteins are transferred very slowly through the placenta by pinocytosis.

Other Placental Transfers

There are three other methods of transfer across the placental membrane. In the first method, fetal red blood cells pass into the maternal circulation, particularly during **parturition** (childbirth), through microscopic breaks in the placental membrane. Labeled maternal red blood cells have also been found in the fetal circulation. Consequently, red blood cells may pass in either direction through very small defects in the placental membrane.

In the second method, cells cross the placental membrane under their own power, for example, maternal leukocytes, which are involved in counteracting foreign substances and disease, and cells of *Treponema pallidum*, the organism that causes syphilis.

In the third method, some bacteria and protozoa such as *Toxoplasma gondii* infect the placenta by creating lesions and then cross the placental membrane through the defects that are thus created.

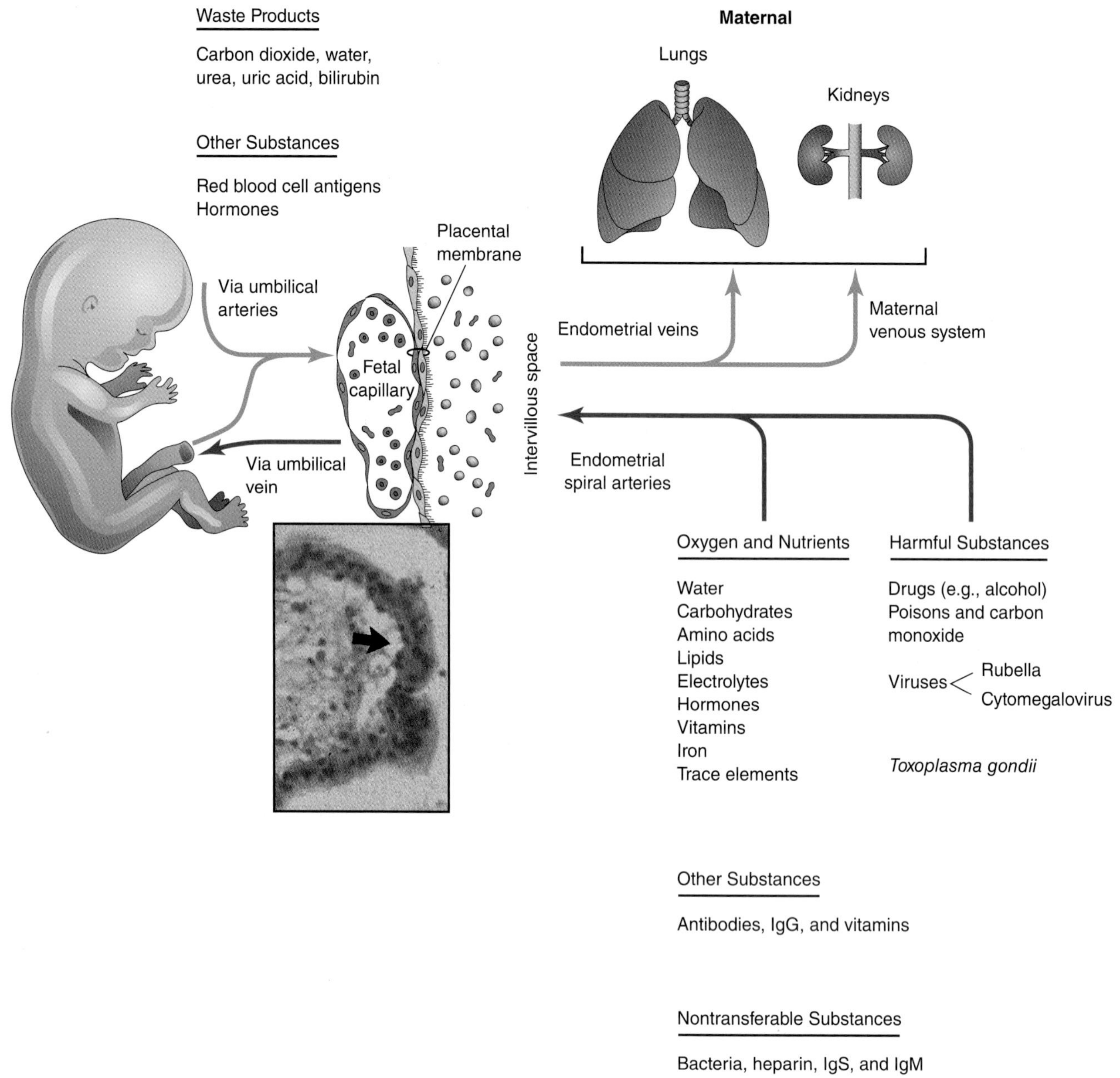

Fig. 7.8 Diagrammatic illustration of transfer across the placental membrane. The extrafetal tissues, across which transport of substances between the mother and fetus occurs, collectively constitute the placental membrane. *Inset*, Light micrograph of chorionic villus showing a fetal capillary and placental membrane (*arrow*).

TRANSFER OF GASES

Oxygen, carbon dioxide, and carbon monoxide cross the placental membrane by **simple diffusion**. The interruption of oxygen transport for several minutes endangers the survival of the embryo/fetus. The placental membrane approaches the efficiency of the lungs for gas exchange. The quantity of oxygen reaching the fetus is primarily flow limited rather than diffusion limited; hence, **fetal hypoxia** results primarily from factors that diminish either the uterine blood flow or the embryo/fetal blood flow. **Maternal respiratory failure** (e.g., from pneumonia) will also reduce oxygen transport to the embryo/fetus.

NUTRITIONAL SUBSTANCES

Nutrients constitute the bulk of substances transferred from the mother to the embryo/fetus. Water is rapidly exchanged by simple diffusion and in increasing amounts as pregnancy advances. **Glucose** produced by the mother and the placenta is quickly transferred to the embryo/fetus by facilitated (active) diffusion mediated primarily by **glucose transporter 1 (GLUT-1)**, an insulin-independent glucose carrier. Maternal cholesterol, triglycerides, and phospholipids are transferred. Although there is transport of free fatty acids (FFAs), the amount transferred appears to be relatively small, with long-chain polyunsaturated fatty acids being the FFA transported in the highest amounts.

Amino acids are actively transported across the placental membrane and are essential for fetal growth. For most amino acids, the plasma concentrations in the embryo/fetus are higher than in the mother. **Vitamins** cross the placental membrane and are essential for normal development.

Water-soluble vitamins cross the placental membrane more quickly than fat-soluble vitamins.

HORMONES

Protein hormones (e.g., insulin or pituitary hormone) do not reach the embryo/fetus in significant amounts, except thyroxine and triiodothyronine by a slow transfer. Unconjugated steroid hormones cross the placental membrane rather freely. Testosterone and certain synthetic progestins cross the placental membrane, and elevated concentrations of testosterone may cause masculinization of female fetuses (see Fig. 20.41).

ELECTROLYTES

Electrolytes are freely exchanged across the placental membrane in significant quantities, each type at its own rate. When a mother receives intravenous fluids with electrolytes, they also pass to the embryo/fetus and affect the status of water and electrolytes.

MATERNAL ANTIBODIES AND PROTEINS

The embryo/fetus produces only small amounts of antibodies because of its **immature immune system**. Some passive immunity is conferred on the fetus by the placental transfer of maternal antibodies. Immunoglobulin G (IgG) is readily transported to the fetus by **endocytosis** beginning at 16 weeks and reaching a peak by 26 weeks. At birth, fetal concentrations of IgG are higher than maternal concentrations. Maternal antibodies confer fetal immunity to some diseases, such as diphtheria, smallpox, and measles; however, no immunity is acquired to **pertussis** or **varicella**. A maternal protein, **transferrin**, crosses the placental membrane and carries iron to the embryo/fetus. The placental surface contains special receptors for this protein.

WASTE PRODUCTS

Urea and uric acid pass through the placental membrane by simple diffusion. Conjugated bilirubin (which is fat soluble) is easily transported by the placenta for rapid clearance.

Hemolytic Disease of the Neonate

Small amounts of fetal blood may pass to the maternal blood through microscopic breaks in the placental membrane. If the fetus is Rh positive and the mother is Rh negative, the fetal blood cells may stimulate the formation of anti-Rh antibodies by the immune system of the mother. These antibodies pass to the fetal blood and cause hemolysis (destruction) of the fetal Rh-positive blood cells and jaundice and anemia in the fetus.

Some fetuses with hemolytic disease of the neonate, or **fetal erythroblastosis**, fail to make a satisfactory intrauterine adjustment. They may die unless delivered early or given intrauterine, intraperitoneal, or intravenous transfusions of packed Rh-negative blood cells until after birth. Hemolytic disease of the neonate due to Rh incompatibility is relatively uncommon now because **Rh(D) immunoglobulin** given to the mother usually prevents the development of this disease in the fetus. Fetal anemia and consequent hyperbilirubinemia due to blood group incompatibility may still occur, although they are due to differences in other minor blood group antigens such as the Kell or Duffy group.

DRUGS AND DRUG METABOLITES

Drugs taken by the mother can affect the embryo/fetus directly or indirectly by interfering with maternal or placental metabolism. Some drugs cause major birth defects (see Table 20.1). The amount of drug or metabolite reaching the placenta is controlled by the maternal blood level and blood flow through the placenta. Most drugs and drug metabolites cross the placenta by simple diffusion, the exception being those with structural similarity to amino acids, such as methyldopa and some antimetabolites.

Most drugs used for the management of labor readily cross the placental membrane. Depending on the dose and timing in relation to parturition, these drugs may cause respiratory depression in the neonate. All sedatives and analgesics affect the fetus to some degree. **Neuromuscular blocking agents** given to the mother during operative obstetrics cross the placenta in only small amounts. **Inhaled anesthetics** can also cross the placental membrane and affect fetal breathing if given during parturition.

The illicit use of drugs such as opioids (e.g., fentanyl) has become widespread in North America and is of alarming concern. In utero exposure to opioids may result in poor fetal growth, preterm birth, fetal anomalies, and neonatal abstinence syndrome.

INFECTIOUS AGENTS

Cytomegalovirus, rubella virus, coxsackieviruses, and viruses associated with variola, varicella, measles, herpes, and poliomyelitis may pass through the placental membrane and cause fetal infection. In some cases, such as the **rubella virus infection**, severe birth defects such as **cataracts** may be produced. Infection with Zika virus, a mosquito-borne infection in the mother can cause severe brain and eye defects in the newborn including microcephaly and neural tube defects. **Microorganisms** such as *Treponema pallidum*, which causes **syphilis**, and *Toxoplasma gondii*, which causes **toxoplasmosis,** cross the placental membrane, often causing severe birth defects and/or death of the embryo/fetus (see Table 20.1).

PLACENTAL ENDOCRINE SYNTHESIS AND SECRETION

Using precursors derived from the fetus and/or the mother, the syncytiotrophoblast synthesizes proteins and steroid hormones. The protein hormones synthesized by the placenta include:

- Human chorionic gonadotropin (hCG)
- Human chorionic somatomammotropin (hCS) (hPL)
- Human chorionic thyrotropin (hCT)

The glycoprotein **hCG**, similar to luteinizing hormone, is first secreted by the syncytiotrophoblast during the second week; hCG maintains the corpus luteum, preventing the onset of menstrual periods. The concentration of hCG in the maternal blood and urine increases to a maximum by the eighth week and then declines. **hCS** causes decreased glucose utilization and increased free fatty acids (FFAs) in the mother. **hCT** appears to function similarly to thyroid-stimulating hormone.

The **steroid hormones** synthesized by the placenta are **progesterone** and **estrogens**. Progesterone can be found in the placenta at all stages of gestation, indicating that progesterone is essential for pregnancy. The placenta forms progesterone from maternal cholesterol or pregnenolone. The ovaries of a pregnant female can be removed after the first trimester without causing abortion because the placenta takes over the production of progesterone from the corpus luteum. Estrogens are also produced in large quantities by the syncytiotrophoblast.

THE PLACENTA AS AN ALLOGRAFT

The placenta can be regarded as an allograft (a graft transplanted between genetically nonidentical individuals) with respect to the mother. The fetal part of the placenta is a derivative of the conceptus, which inherits both paternal and maternal histocompatibility genes. What protects the placenta from rejection by the mother's immune system?

This question remains a major biologic enigma. The syncytiotrophoblast of the chorionic villi, although exposed to maternal immune cells within the blood sinusoids, lacks major histocompatibility (MHC) antigens and thus does not evoke rejection responses. However, extravillous trophoblast (EVT) cells, which invade the uterine decidua and its vasculature (spiral arteries), express class I MHC antigens. These antigens include HLA-G, which, being nonpolymorphic (class Ib), is poorly recognizable by T lymphocytes as an alloantigen, as well as HLA-C, which, being polymorphic (class Ia), is recognizable by T cells. In addition to averting T cells, EVT cells must also shield themselves from potential attack by natural killer (NK) lymphocytes and injury inflicted by activation of complement. Maternal lymphocytes within the pregnancy-associated decidua include a high proportion (65%–70%) of NK cells and a low proportion (10%–12%) of T cells. Decidual or uterine NK (named as dNK or uNK) cells are distinct from peripheral blood NK cells in phenotype (CD56 high, CD94/NKG2 high) and function in having poor cytotoxicity for EVT cells.

Multiple mechanisms appear to be in place to guard the placenta against immune rejection. None of them in isolation appears to be adequate in averting various forms of immune attack. Systemic immuno-suppression such as transient T-cell and B-cell tolerance to fetal antigens suggested by some authors is not a viable mechanism, since fetoplacental tissues grafted under the skin are promptly rejected by the mother. Thus the mechanisms must be local. Some of the postulates are listed here.

- Expression of HLA-G is restricted to a few tissues, including placental EVT cells. Its strategic location in the placenta is postulated to provide a dual immunoprotective role: (1) evasion of T-cell recognition owing to its nonpolymorphic nature and (2) recognition by the "killer-inhibitory receptors" on NK cells, thus turning off their killer function. The inadequacy of this hypothesis is suggested by several observations: (1) healthy individuals showing biallelic loss of HLA-G1 have been identified, indicating that HLA-G is not essential for fetoplacental survival; (2) this hypothesis does not explain why HLA-C, a polymorphic antigen, also expressed by EVT cells, does not evoke a rejection response in situ. Because both HLA-G and HLA-C were shown to have the unique ability to resist human cytomegalovirus-mediated MHC class I degradation, it is speculated that a selective location of these two antigens at the fetomaternal interface may help to withstand viral assault.
- Three additional roles of HLA-G have been proposed during pregnancy. HLA-G interacts with ILT2 and KIR2DL4 on macrophages and NK cells to enhance the production of proangiogenic cytokines and to enhance the EVT invasion of decidua, thereby promoting spiral artery remodeling. In addition, HLA-G binds to ILT2, ILT4, and KIR2DL4 on NK cells, T cells, and macrophages, inhibits the cytotoxicity of NK cells and $CD8^+$ T cells, and causes an increase in the percentage of T-regulatory (Treg) cells in the population, and thereby contributes to immune tolerance. Furthermore, HLA-G on EVTs could induce the production of growth-promoting factors by decidual NK cells, thereby regulating fetal growth.
- HLA-C expression by EVT has a unique and dual role in maternal-fetal immune tolerance and immunity to placental infections. High HLA-C expression levels on the cell surface may enhance detrimental inflammatory and CTL responses to maternal-fetal HLA-C mismatches in pregnancy. However, high HLA-C levels in pregnancy can also be beneficial and contribute to immune protection to a wide variety of infections and diminish infection-related pregnancy complications.
- Immunoprotection is provided locally by certain decidua-derived immunosuppressor molecules, such as prostaglandin E_2, transforming growth factor (TGF)-β, and interleukin-10. Prostaglandin E_2 derived from the decidua was shown to block the activation of maternal T cells as well as NK cells in situ by blocking the development of the IL-2 receptors on T cells and IL-2 production by T-helper cells.
- Trafficking of activated maternal leukocytes into the placenta or fetus is prevented by the deletion of these cells triggered by apoptosis-inducing ligands such as PD-L1 present on the trophoblast.
- Several immune checkpoint molecules present at the fetal-maternal interface are closely associated with pregnancy success via multiple inhibitory mechanisms. Multiple immune checkpoint molecules, including CTLA-4, PD-1, Tim-3, LAG-3, and TIGIT, either in membrane or soluble form, can influence the functions of decidual and peripheral Treg cells during pregnancy.
- Based on genetic manipulation in mice, it was shown that the presence of complement regulatory proteins (Crry in the mouse, membrane cofactor protein or CD46 in the human), which can block activation of the third component of complement (C3) in the complement cascade, protects the placenta from complement-mediated destruction, which may happen otherwise because of residual C3 activation remaining after defending against pathogens. Crry gene knockout mice died in utero because of complement-mediated placental damage, which could be averted by additional knockout of the *C3* gene.
- Experiments in mice revealed that the presence of the enzyme indoleamine 2, 3-deoxygenase (IDO) in trophoblast cells was critical for the immunoprotection of the allogeneic conceptus. It suppresses T-cell–driven

local inflammatory responses, including complement activation. Treatment of pregnant mice with an indoleamine 2, 3-deoxygenase inhibitor, 1-methyltryptophan caused selective death of allogeneic (but not syngeneic) conceptuses because of massive deposition of complement and hemorrhagic necrosis at the placental sites.

- Numerous chemokines produced by decidual stromal cells are known to attract T-cell immigration. In mouse pregnancy models, it was shown that T-cell immigration within the decidua was averted by epigenetic silencing of key T-cell–attracting inflammatory chemokine genes in decidual stromal cells. The epigenetic mechanism was evidenced by promoter accrual of repressive histone marks in the murine decidua.

THE PLACENTA AS AN INVASIVE TUMOR-LIKE STRUCTURE

The placenta in many species, including humans, is a highly invasive tumor-like structure that invades the uterus to tap into its blood supply and establish an adequate exchange of key molecules between the mother and the embryo/fetus. What protects the uterus from placental over-invasion? After the development of chorionic villi, the invasive function of the placenta is provided by the extravillous trophoblast (EVT) cells, which are produced by proliferation and differentiation of stem cells located in the cytotrophoblastic layer of the anchoring villi (see Fig. 7.6). They break out of the villous confines and migrate as cell columns to invade the decidua, where they reorganize as distinct subsets: a nearly continuous cell layer (cytotrophoblastic shell) separating the decidua from maternal blood sinusoids; cells dispersed within the decidua (interstitial trophoblast); multinucleate placental-bed giant cells produced by EVT-cell fusion; and endovascular trophoblast, which adopts an endothelial phenotype and invades and remodels the uteroplacental (spiral) arteries within the endometrium and a part of the myometrium. Optimal arterial remodeling (loss of tunica media and replacement of endothelium by the endovascular trophoblast) transforms them into low-resistance, high-flow tubes that facilitate steady placental perfusion with maternal arterial blood unhindered by the presence of vasoactive molecules. Inadequate EVT-cell invasion leading to poor placental perfusion underlies the pathogenesis of preeclampsia (a major hypertensive disorder associated with pregnancy in the mother) and certain forms of fetal growth restriction (FGR), whereas excessive invasion is a hallmark of hyper-invasive placentas (see Fig. 7.15 and the box entitled "Placental Abnormalities").

The invasive function of trophoblast cells has been examined with two *in vitro* models: Normal human EVT-cell lines have been successfully propagated from the first-trimester human placenta. First-trimester chorionic villus explants when placed on matrigel (the equivalent of basement membrane), promote sprouting of EVT cells, which invade the matrigel. Using both cell systems for invasion assays, it was shown that the molecular mechanisms responsible for their invasiveness are identical to those of cancer cells, whereas, unlike tumors, their proliferation, migration, and invasiveness are stringently regulated in situ by a variety of locally produced molecules: growth factors, growth factor–binding proteins, proteoglycans, and components of the extracellular matrix. *Numerous growth factors produced at the fetal-maternal interface, such as epidermal growth factor (EGF), TGF-α, amphiregulin, colony-stimulating factor (CSF)-1, hepatocyte growth factor (HGF), vascular endothelial growth factor (VEGF)-2, and placental growth factor (PlGF), were shown to stimulate EVT-cell proliferation, migration, and invasiveness, whereas insulin-like growth factor II and insulin-like growth factor-binding protein, IGFBP-1, were shown to stimulate EVT-cell migration and invasiveness without affecting proliferation. Two decidua-derived molecules, TGF-β and a TGF-β–binding leucine-rich proteoglycan decorin (DCN), were shown to restrain EVT-cell proliferation, migration, and invasiveness independent of each other, whereas trophoblastic cancer (choriocarcinoma) cells were shown to be resistant to the inhibitory signals of both TGF-β and DCN. The pro-inflammatory cytokine TNF-α produced by decidual macrophages is also shown to be anti-invasive.* Factors promoting trophoblast migration and invasion are both autocrine (trophoblast-derived) and paracrine (decidua-derived), whereas those restraining these functions are paracrine.

In summary, decidua plays a dual role in uteroplacental homeostasis by providing immunoprotection of the placenta and also protection of the uterus from placental over-invasion.

Preeclampsia

Preeclampsia (PE) is a critical pregnancy-associated disorder, usually occurring after the 20th week of gestation. It is the second leading cause of maternal morbidity and deaths during pregnancy. **Maternal hypertension**, **proteinuria**, and **edema** are essential features of this condition. PE can lead to **eclampsia** (one or more convulsions), resulting in miscarriage and maternal death. The origin of PE appears to be multifactorial. The primary pathology is a hypoinvasive placenta and compromised uterine angiogenesis, leading to poor placental perfusion, and a placenta that makes toxic molecules that attack the maternal vasculature, in particular the renal glomeruli. Overproduction of several anti-angiogenic molecules by the placenta/decidua, such as soluble Flt-1 (VEGF receptor-1), endoglin, and decorin (which also compromises EVT invasion and endovascular differentiation), have been associated with preeclampsia; elevated levels of these molecules have been identified as predictive biomarkers for preeclampsia. MSX2 (Msh Homeobox 2) plays a critical role in trophoblastic invasion and the development of the placenta. It has been reported that disruption in the expression of MSX2 may cause preeclampsia. Recent studies have implicated the **renin-angiotensin system** in the development of high blood pressure and edema. In eclampsia, extensive placental infarcts are present that reduce the uteroplacental circulation. This may lead to fetal malnutrition, fetal growth restriction, miscarriage, or fetal death. Moreover, the estrogen-related receptor gamma (*ESRRG*) is highly expressed in normal placenta, but it is less so in cases of fetal growth restriction and preeclampsia, likely due to altered placental function.

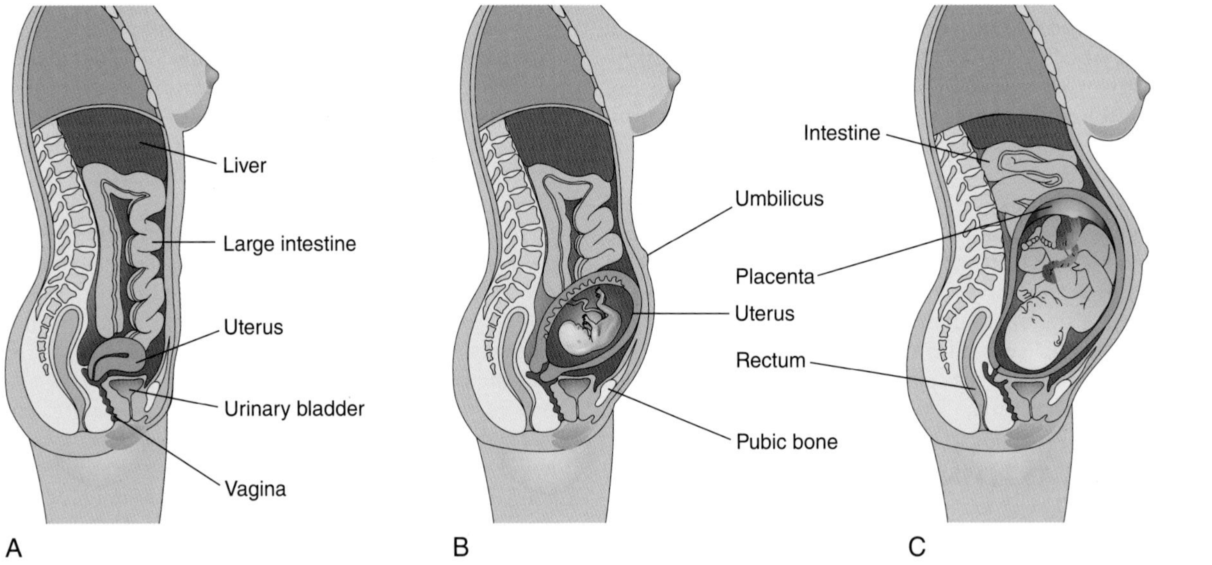

Fig. 7.9 Drawings of median sections of a female's body. (A) Not pregnant. (B) Twenty weeks pregnant. (C) Thirty weeks pregnant. Note that as the conceptus enlarges, the uterus increases in size to accommodate the rapidly growing fetus. By 20 weeks, the uterus and fetus reach the level of the umbilicus, and by 30 weeks, they reach the epigastric region. The mother's abdominal viscera are displaced and compressed, and the skin and muscles of her anterior abdominal wall are stretched.

THE PLACENTA AND ADULT DISEASES

Placental dysfunctions that lead to PE and fetal growth restriction (FGR) are implicated in the origin of several adult diseases. Studies have shown a strong association between low birth weight and increased risk for cardiovascular diseases and type 2 diabetes later in life. Low birth weight followed by rapid catch-up weight gain during infancy has been shown to further increase the risk for these diseases. A complex of placental disorders, including preeclampsia, IUGR, preterm delivery, placental abruption, and miscarriage, have been described as placental syndromes, and are attributed to levels of angiogenic biomarkers and impaired expression of angiogenic factors.

UTERINE GROWTH DURING PREGNANCY

The uterus of a nonpregnant female is in the pelvis (Fig. 7.9A). To accommodate the growing conceptus, the uterus increases in size. It also increases in weight, and its walls become thinner (see Fig. 7.9B and C). During the first trimester, the uterus extends out of the pelvis, and by 20 weeks, it extends to the level of the umbilicus. By 28 to 30 weeks, the uterus reaches the epigastric region between the xiphoid process of the sternum and the umbilicus. The increase in the size of the uterus largely results from **hypertrophy** of preexisting smooth muscular fibers and partly from the development of new fibers.

PARTURITION

Parturition is the process during which the fetus, placenta, and fetal membranes are expelled from the mother's reproductive tract (Fig. 7.10A–E). **Labor** is a sequence of involuntary **uterine contractions**, which result in dilation of the uterine cervix and expulsion of the fetus and placenta from the uterus (see Fig. 7.10F–H). The factors that trigger labor are not completely understood; however, several hormones, including **relaxin**, are related to the initiation of contractions. Relaxin is produced by the corpus luteum and placenta.

The **fetal hypothalamus** secretes **corticotropin-releasing hormone**, which stimulates the anterior **hypophysis** (pituitary) to produce **adrenocorticotropin**. This hormone causes the secretion of **cortisol** from the suprarenal (adrenal) cortex, which is involved in the synthesis of estrogens that are formed by the ovaries, placenta, testes, and, possibly, adrenal cortex.

Estrogens also increase myometrial contractile activity and stimulate the release of oxytocin and prostaglandins. From studies carried out in sheep and nonhuman primates, it seems that the duration of pregnancy and process of birth are under the direct control of the fetus.

Peristaltic contractions of uterine smooth muscle are elicited by **oxytocin**, a hormone released by the neurohypophysis of the pituitary gland. This hormone is administered clinically when it is necessary to induce labor. Oxytocin also stimulates the release of **prostaglandins** (promoters of uterine contractions) from the decidua, increasing myometrial contractility by sensitizing the myometrial cells to oxytocin.

STAGES OF LABOR

Labor is a continuous process; however, for clinical purposes, it is usually divided into three stages:

- **Dilation** begins with progressive dilation of the cervix (see Fig. 7.10A and B) and ends when the cervix is completely dilated. During this **first stage**, regular strong contractions of the uterus occur less than 10 minutes apart. The average duration of the first stage is approximately 12 hours for first pregnancies **(primipara)** and approximately 7 hours for females who have previously given birth **(multiparous)**.

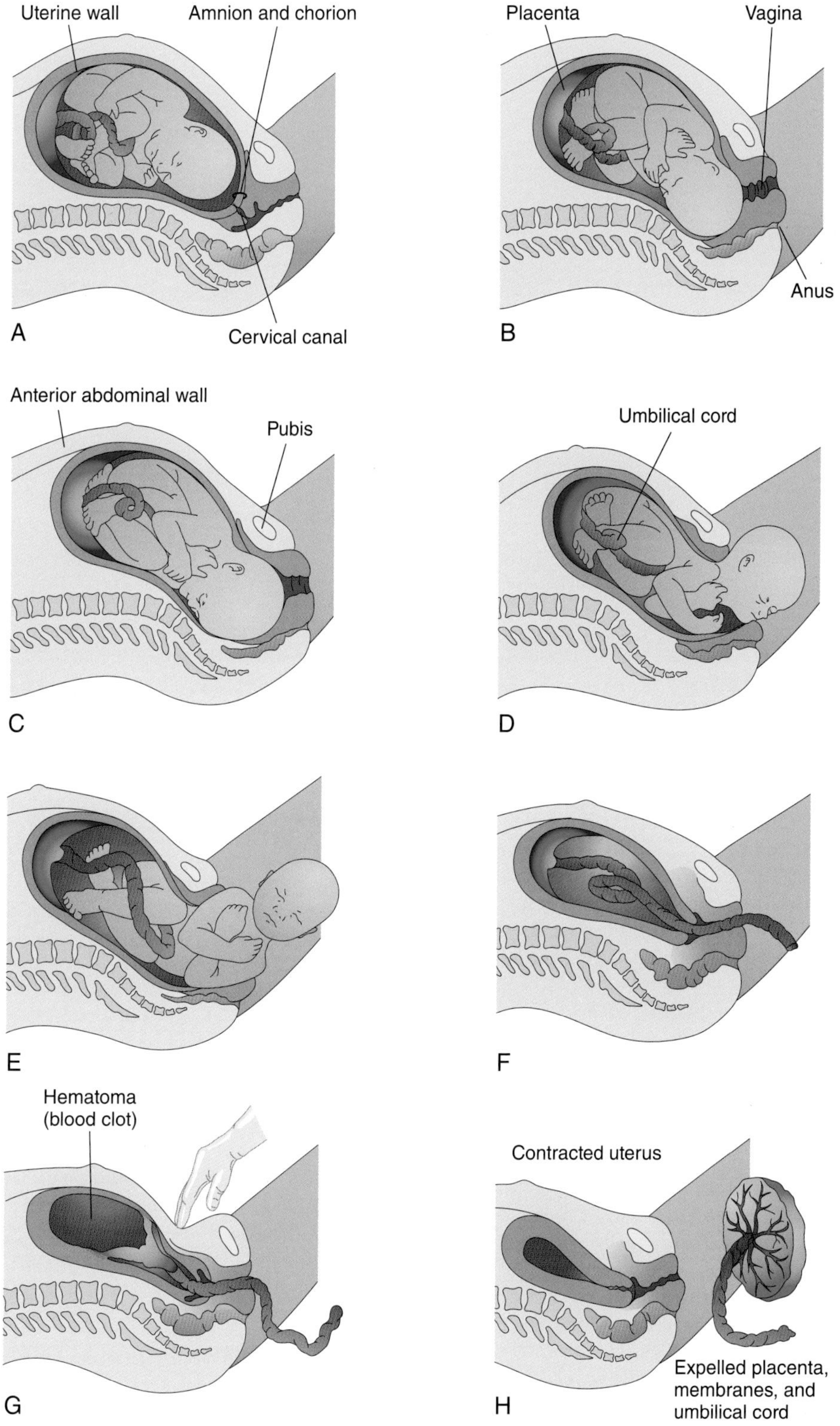

Fig. 7.10 Drawings illustrating parturition (childbirth). (A and B) The cervix is dilating during the first stage of labor. (C–E) The fetus is passing through the cervix and vagina during the second stage of labor. (F and G) As the uterus contracts during the third stage of labor, the placenta folds and pulls away from the uterine wall. Separation of the placenta results in bleeding and the formation of a large hematoma (mass of blood). Pressure on the abdomen facilitates placental separation. (H) The placenta is expelled, and the uterus contracts.

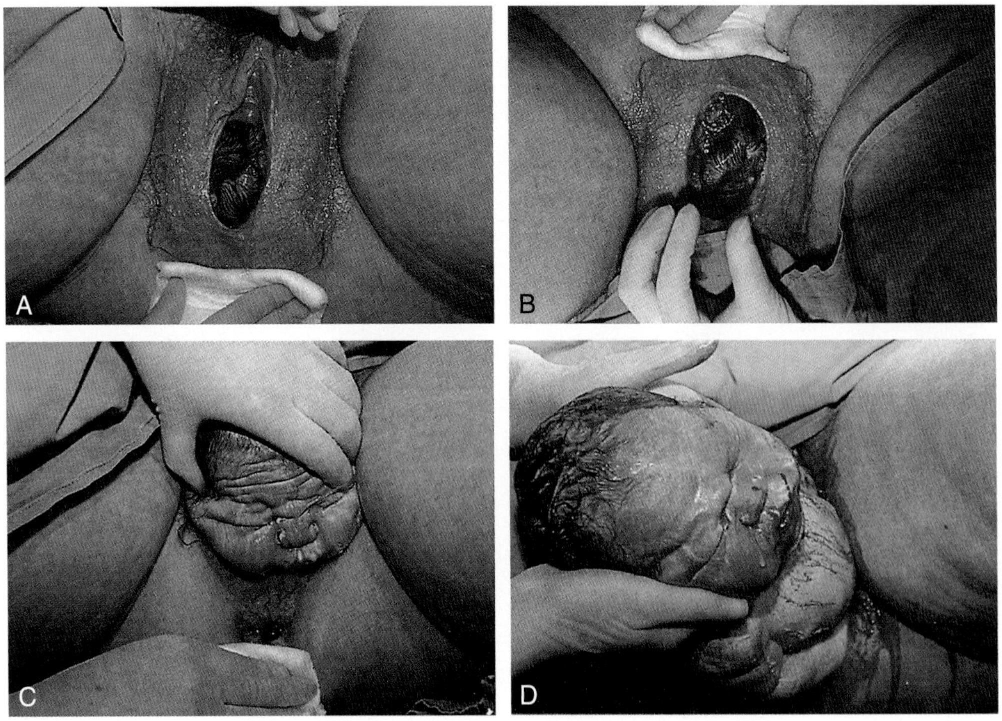

Fig. 7.11 Spontaneous vaginal delivery. (A) The second stage of labor; the scalp becomes visible with contractions and expulsive efforts by the mother. (B) Crowning of the head. (C) At delivery, the head is in the anteroposterior position. (D) Delivery of the head and shoulders. (From Symonds I, Arulkumaran S: *Essential obstetrics and gynaecology*, ed 5, Edinburgh, 2013, Elsevier, pp 183–198.)

- **Expulsion**, the **second stage of labor**, begins when the cervix is completely dilated and ends with the delivery of the fetus (Fig. 7.11; see also Fig. 7.10C–E). During the second stage of labor, the fetus descends through the cervix and vagina. When the fetus is outside the mother, it is called a **neonate**. The average duration of the second stage is 50 minutes for primigravidas and 20 minutes for multigravidas.
- The **third** or **placental stage** begins as soon as the **fetus** is born and ends with the expulsion of the placenta and membranes (the afterbirth). The duration of this third stage of labor is 15 minutes in approximately 90% of pregnancies. A **retained placenta** is one that is not expelled within 60 minutes of delivery.

Retraction of the uterus reduces the area of placental attachment (Fig. 7.10G). A **hematoma** soon forms deep in the placenta and separates it from the uterine wall. The placenta separates through the spongy layer of the decidua basalis. After delivery of the fetus, the uterus continues to contract (see Fig. 7.10H). The **myometrial contractions** of the uterus constrict the spiral arteries that supply blood to the intervillous space (see Fig. 7.6). These contractions prevent excessive uterine bleeding.

Gestational Choriocarcinoma

Abnormal proliferation of the trophoblast results in **gestational trophoblastic disease**, a spectrum of lesions including highly malignant tumors. The cells invade the decidua basalis, penetrate its blood vessels and lymphatics, and may metastasize (spread) to the maternal lungs, bone marrow, liver, and other organs. *Gestational choriocarcinomas are highly sensitive to chemotherapy, and cures are usually achieved.*

PLACENTA AND FETAL MEMBRANES AFTER BIRTH

The placenta usually has a discoid shape, with a diameter of 15 to 20 cm and a thickness of 2 to 3 cm (Fig. 7.12). It weighs 500 to 600 g, which is approximately one-sixth the weight of the average fetus. The margins of the placenta are continuous with the ruptured amniotic and chorionic sacs.

When chorionic villi persist on the entire surface of the chorionic sac (1:30000), a thin layer of the placenta attaches to a large area of the uterus. This type of placenta is a **membranous placenta**. When villi persist elsewhere, several variations in placental shape may occur: **accessory placenta** (Fig. 7.13), **bidiscoid placenta**, and **horseshoe placenta**. Although there are variations in the size and shape of the placenta, most of them are of little physiologic or clinical significance.

MATERNAL SURFACE OF PLACENTA

The characteristic cobblestone appearance of the maternal surface is produced by slightly bulging villous areas, or **cotyledons**, which are separated by grooves that were formerly occupied by placental septa (see Figs. 7.6 and 7.12A). The surface of the cotyledons is covered by thin, grayish shreds of decidua basalis that separated from the uterine wall when the placenta was extruded. Most of the decidua is temporarily retained in the uterus and is shed with the uterine bleeding after delivery of the fetus.

Examination of the placenta prenatally by ultrasonography or magnetic resonance imaging (Fig. 7.14), or postnatally by

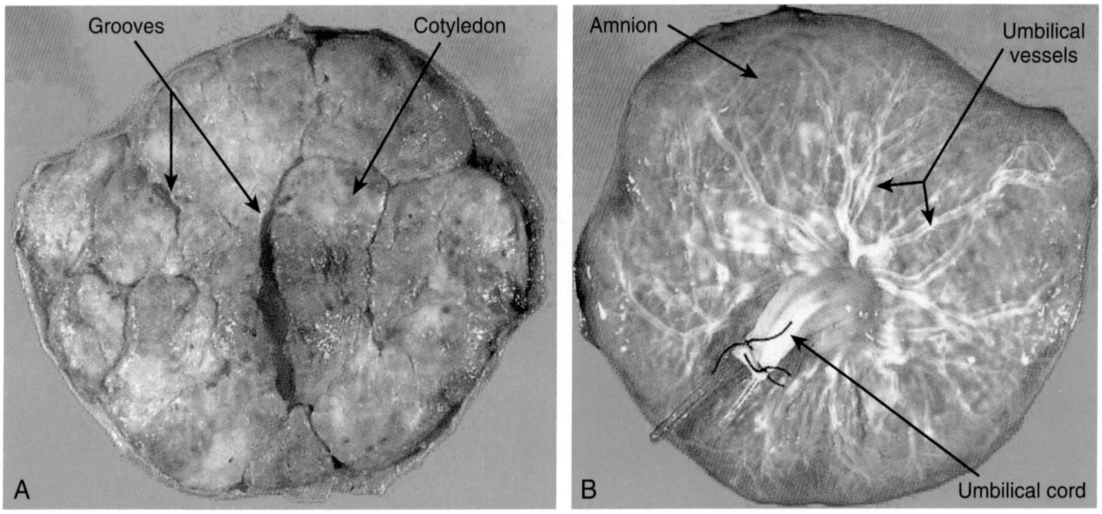

Fig. 7.12 Placentas and fetal membranes after birth, shown approximately one-third of their actual size. (A) Maternal surface, showing cotyledons and grooves around them. Each convex cotyledon consists of several main-stem villi with their many branch villi. The grooves were occupied by the placental septa when the maternal and fetal parts of the placenta were together. (B) Fetal surface showing blood vessels running in the chorionic plate deep to the amnion and converging to form the umbilical vessels at the attachment of the umbilical cord.

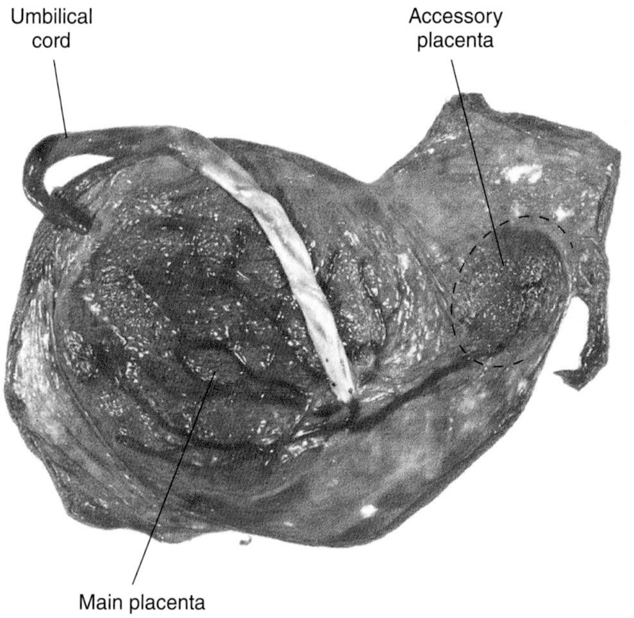

Fig. 7.13 A full-term placenta and an accessory placenta. The accessory placenta developed from a patch of chorionic villi that persisted a short distance from the main placenta.

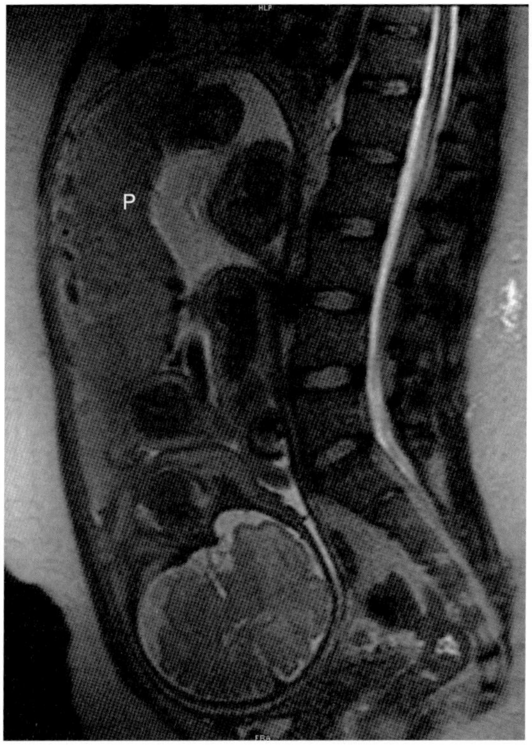

Fig. 7.14 Sagittal magnetic resonance image of the pelvis of a pregnant female. The vertebral column and pelvis of the mother are visible, as are the fetal brain, limbs, and placenta *(P)*. (Courtesy Stuart C. Morrison, Section of Pediatric Radiology, the Children's Hospital, Cleveland Clinic, Cleveland, Ohio.)

gross and microscopic study, may provide clinical information about the causes of IUGR, placental dysfunction, fetal distress and death, and neonatal illness. Placental studies can also determine whether the expelled placenta is complete. Retention of a cotyledon, or **accessory placenta**, in the uterus may cause severe uterine hemorrhage (see Fig. 7.13).

FETAL SURFACE OF PLACENTA

The umbilical cord usually attaches to the fetal surface of the placenta, and its epithelium is continuous with the amnion adhering to the fetal surface (see Figs. 7.6 and 7.12B). The fetal surface of a freshly delivered placenta is smooth and shiny because it is covered by the amnion. The chorionic vessels radiating to and from the umbilical cord are clearly visible through the transparent amnion. The umbilical vessels branch on the fetal surface to form **chorionic vessels**, which enter the chorionic villi and form the **arteriocapillary-venous system** (see Fig. 7.7A).

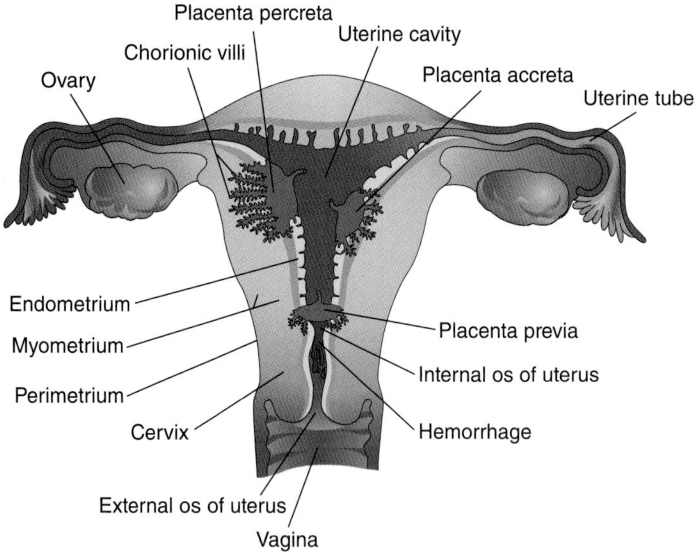

Fig. 7.15 Placental abnormalities. In placenta accreta, there is abnormal adherence of the placenta to the myometrium. In placenta percreta, the placenta has penetrated the full thickness of the myometrium. In this example of placenta previa, the placenta overlies the internal os of the uterus and blocks the cervical canal.

Placental Abnormalities

Abnormal adherence of chorionic villi to the myometrium is called **placenta accreta** (Fig. 7.15) and occurs in approximately 0.2% of all pregnancies. When chorionic villi penetrate the full thickness of the **myometrium** (muscular wall of the uterus) to or through the perimetrium (peritoneal covering), the abnormality is called **placenta percreta**. Third-trimester bleeding is the common presenting sign of these placental abnormalities. For delivery, a planned preterm cesarean hysterectomy is the recommended approach, leaving the placenta in place to prevent massive bleeding. In exceptional circumstances, alternative approaches may preserve reproductive function, but this may carry significant risk.

When the blastocyst implants close to or overlying the internal os of the uterus, the abnormality is called **placenta previa** (see Fig. 7.15). Late-pregnancy bleeding may result from this placental abnormality. The fetus has to be delivered by cesarean section when the placenta completely obstructs the internal uterine os.

Ultrasound scanning of the placenta is invaluable for clinical diagnosis of placental abnormalities.

UMBILICAL CORD

The attachment of the umbilical cord to the placenta is usually near the center of the fetal surface (see Fig. 7.12B). Abnormal insertion points are often associated with adverse perinatal outcomes (IUGR, premature rupture of membranes, hemorrhage, cord compression, and preeclampsia) as a result of umbilical cord vessel weakness. Insertion of the cord near the placental margin (**battledore placenta**) occurs in about 7% of singleton pregnancies. The attachment of the cord to the fetal membranes is termed a **velamentous insertion of the cord** (Fig. 7.16) and occurs in approximately 1% to 2%.

Doppler ultrasonography may be used for prenatal diagnosis of the position and structural abnormalities of the umbilical cord and its vessels, as well as blood flow (see Fig. 7.18). The cord is usually 1 to 2 cm in diameter and 30 to 90 cm in length (average, 55 cm). Long cords (>90th percentile for length) tend to prolapse and/or coil around the fetus and may lead to a cord knot or entanglement (see Fig. 7.20B). Prompt recognition of prolapse of the cord is important because the cord may be compressed between the presenting body part of the fetus and the mother's bony pelvis, causing fetal hypoxia or anoxia. If the deficiency of oxygen persists for more than 5 minutes, the neonate's brain may be damaged. A very short cord is associated with a small placenta and a risk of fetal complications. It may also cause premature separation of the placenta from the wall of the uterus during delivery.

The umbilical cord usually has two arteries and one large vein, which are surrounded by mucoid connective tissue **(Wharton jelly)**. Because the umbilical vessels are longer than the cord, twisting and bending of the vessels are common. They frequently form loops, producing **false knots** that are of no significance. However, in approximately 1% of pregnancies, **true knots** form in the cord, which may tighten and cause fetal death resulting from anoxia (Fig. 7.17). In most cases, the knots form during labor as a result of the

Umbilical Artery Doppler Velocimetry

As gestation and trophoblastic invasion of the decidua basalis progress, there is a corresponding increase in the diastolic flow velocity in the umbilical arteries. Doppler velocimetry of the uteroplacental and fetoplacental circulation is used to investigate complications of pregnancy, such as IUGR and fetal distress resulting from fetal hypoxia and asphyxia (Fig. 7.18). For example, there is a statistically significant association between IUGR and abnormally increased resistance in an umbilical artery.

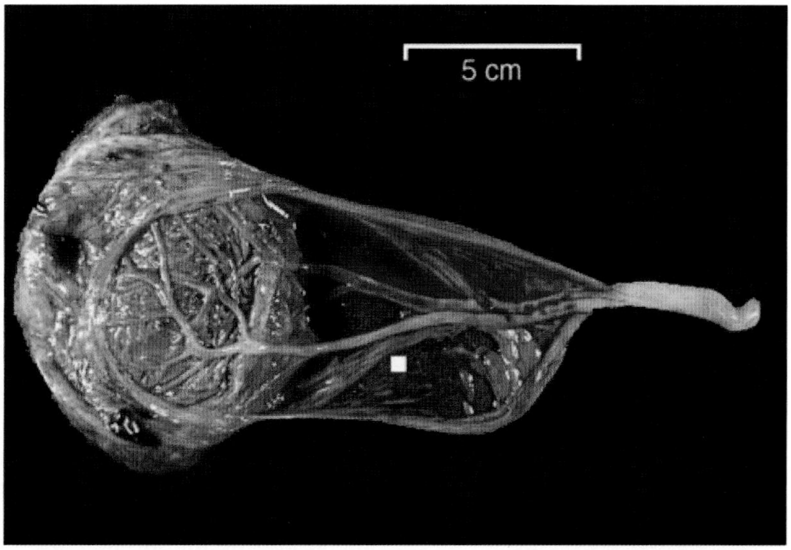

Fig. 7.16 Placenta, velamentous insertion; gross velamentous insertion of the umbilical cord occurs when the three major umbilical vessels separate within the fetal membranes before reaching the placental disc. Such a condition is usually of no major consequence in utero, but it could lead to a greater chance for cord trauma with tearing of one of the vessels and bleeding during the delivery process. (From Klatt E: *Robbins and Cotran atlas of pathology*, ed 3, Philadelphia, 2015, Elsevier, pp. 325–370.)

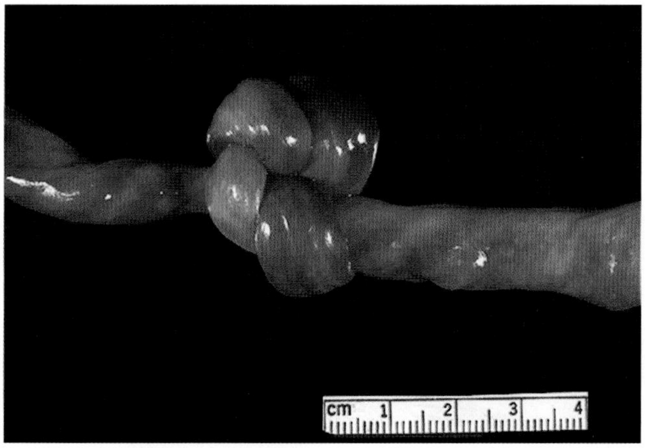

Fig. 7.17 Photograph of an umbilical cord showing a true knot. Such a knot will cause severe anoxia (decreased oxygen in fetal tissues and organs). (Courtesy Dr. E. C. Klatt, Department of Biomedical Sciences, Mercer University School of Medicine, Savannah, Georgia.)

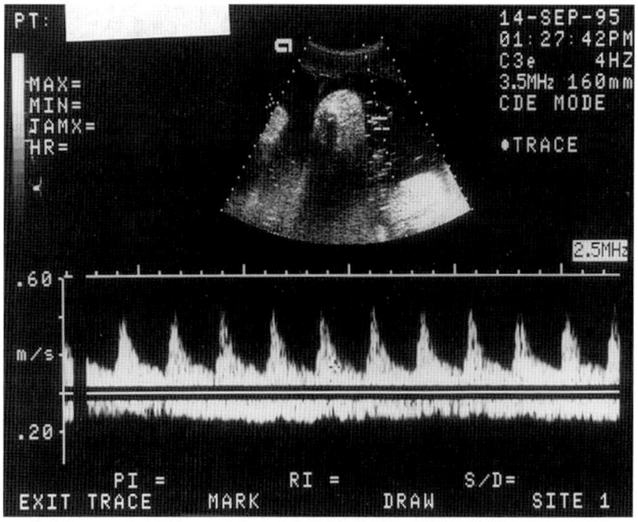

Fig. 7.18 Doppler velocimetry of the umbilical cord. The arterial waveform (*arrow*) illustrates pulsatile forward flow, with high peaks and low velocities during diastole. This combination suggests high resistance in the placenta to placental blood flow. Because this index changes over gestation, it is important to know that the pregnancy was 18 weeks' gestation. For this period, the flow pattern is normal. The nonpulsatile flow in the opposite, negative direction (*arrowhead*) represents venous return from the placenta. Both waveforms are normal for this gestational age. (Courtesy Dr. C. R. Harman, Department of Obstetrics, Gynecology and Reproductive Sciences, University of Maryland, Baltimore, Maryland.)

Absence of Umbilical Artery

In approximately 0.63 to 1 in 100 neonates, only one umbilical artery is present (Fig. 7.19), a condition that may be associated with chromosomal and fetal abnormalities. The absence of an umbilical artery is accompanied by a 15% to 20% incidence of cardiovascular defects in the fetus. The absence of an artery results from either agenesis or degeneration of one of the two umbilical arteries. A **single umbilical artery** and the defects associated with it can be detected before birth by ultrasonography.

fetus passing through a loop in the cord. Simple looping of the cord around the fetus (e.g., around the ankle) occasionally occurs (see Fig. 7.20B). If the coil is tight, then blood circulation can be affected. In approximately one-fifth of deliveries, the cord is loosely looped around the neck, without increased fetal risk.

AMNION AND AMNIOTIC FLUID

The thin but tough **amnion** forms a fluid-filled, membranous **amniotic sac** that surrounds the embryo and later the fetus. The sac contains **amniotic fluid** (Figs. 7.20 and 7.21). As the amnion enlarges, it gradually obliterates the chorionic cavity and forms the epithelial covering of the umbilical cord (see Figs. 7.19 and 7.21C and D).

AMNIOTIC FLUID

Amniotic fluid increases with the growth of the fetus and plays a major role in fetal growth and embryo/fetal development. Initially, some amniotic fluid is secreted by cells of the amnion. Most fluid is derived from maternal tissue and interstitial fluid by diffusion across the amniochorionic membrane from the decidua parietalis (see Fig. 7.6). Later there is diffusion of fluid through the chorionic plate from blood in the intervillous space of the placenta.

Before **keratinization** of the skin occurs, a major pathway for the passage of water and solutes in tissue fluid from the fetus to the amniotic cavity is through the skin; thus, amniotic fluid is similar to fetal tissue fluid. Fluid is also secreted by the fetal respiratory and gastrointestinal tracts and enters the amniotic cavity. The daily rate of contribution of fluid to the amniotic cavity from the respiratory tract is 300 mL to 400 mL.

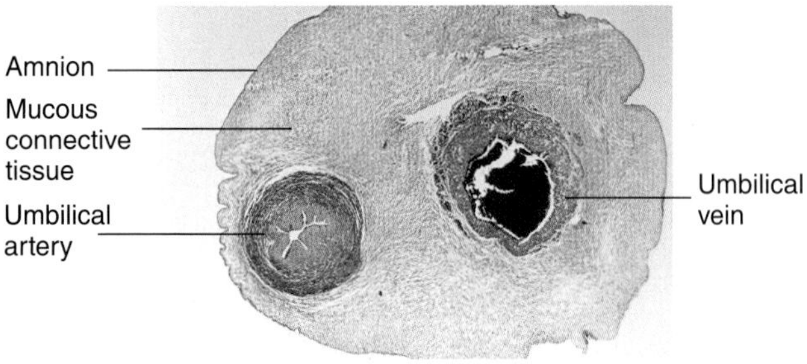

Fig. 7.19 Transverse section of an umbilical cord. Observe that the cord is covered by epithelium derived from the enveloping amnion. It has a core of mucous connective tissue (Wharton jelly). Observe also that the cord has one vein and only one umbilical artery instead of the normal two arteries. (Courtesy Professor V. Becker, Pathologisches Institut der Universität, Erlangen, Germany.)

Beginning in the 11th week, the fetus contributes to the amniotic fluid by excreting urine into the amniotic cavity. By late pregnancy, approximately 500 mL of urine is added daily. The volume of amniotic fluid normally increases slowly, reaching approximately 30 mL at 10 weeks, 350 mL at 20 weeks, and 800 to 1000 mL by 37 weeks. By 19 to 20 weeks, the fetal skin becomes keratinized and no longer supports diffusion.

CIRCULATION OF AMNIOTIC FLUID

The water content of amniotic fluid changes every 3 hours. Large amounts of water pass through the amniochorionic membrane (see Fig. 7.6) into the maternal tissue fluid and enter the uterine capillaries. An exchange of fluid with fetal blood also occurs through the umbilical cord where the amnion adheres to the chorionic plate on the fetal surface of the placenta (see Figs. 7.6 and 7.12B); thus amniotic fluid is in balance with the fetal circulation.

Amniotic fluid is swallowed by the fetus and absorbed by the fetus's respiratory and digestive tracts. It has been estimated that during the final stages of pregnancy, the fetus swallows up to 400 mL of amniotic fluid per day. The fluid passes into the fetal bloodstream, and the waste products in it cross the placental membrane and enter the maternal blood in the intervillous space. Excess water in the fetal blood is excreted by the fetal kidneys and returned to the amniotic sac through the fetal urinary tract.

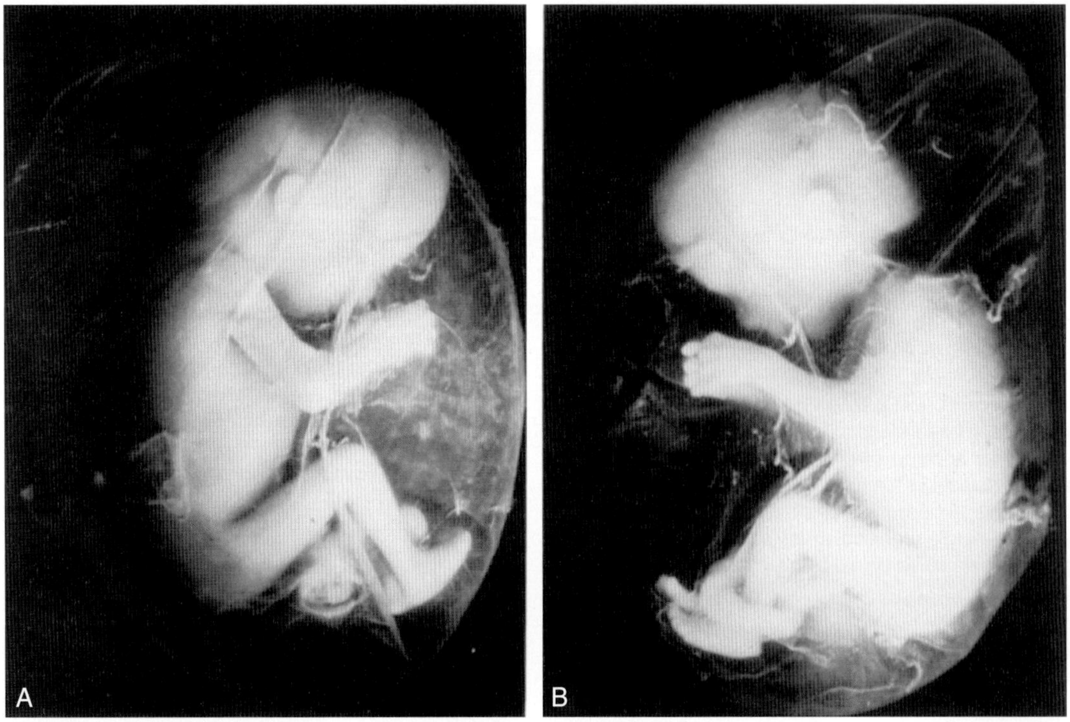

Fig. 7.20 (A) A 12-week fetus in its amniotic sac. The fetus and its membranes aborted spontaneously. It was removed from its chorionic sac with its amniotic sac intact. Actual size. (B) Note that the umbilical cord is looped around the left ankle of the fetus. Coiling of the cord around parts of the fetus affects development when the coils are so tight that the circulation to the parts is affected.

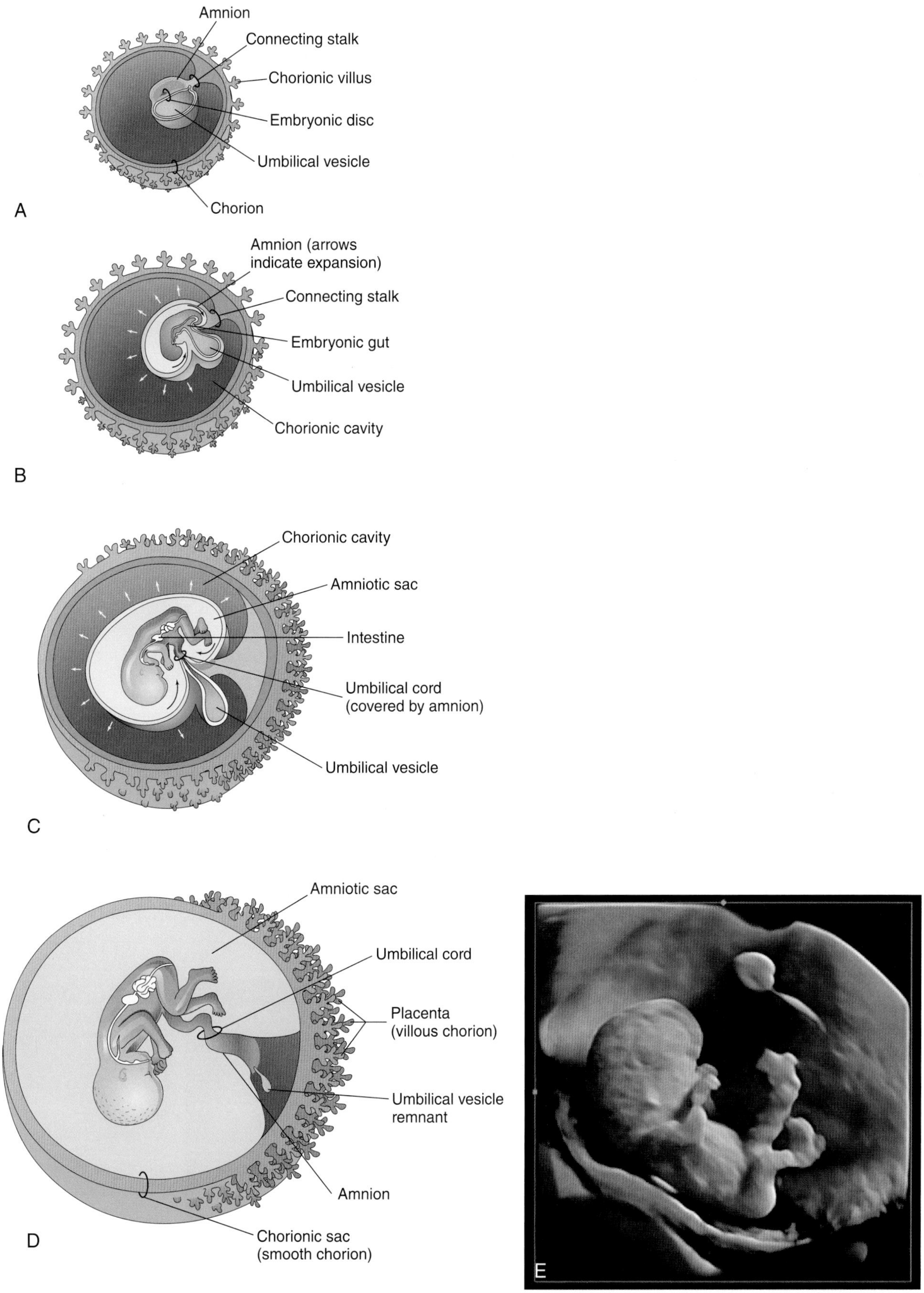

Fig. 7.21 Illustrations showing how the amnion enlarges, obliterates the chorionic cavity, and envelops the umbilical cord. Observe that part of the umbilical vesicle is incorporated into the embryo as the primordial gut. Formation of the fetal part of the placenta and degeneration of chorionic villi are also shown: (A) at 3 weeks, (B) at 4 weeks, (C) at 10 weeks, and (D) at 20 weeks. (E) 3D ultrasound image of a fetus at 10 weeks + 2 days. The umbilical cord insertion can be observed on the abdomen. The umbilical vesicle is inside the coelomic space close to the amniotic sac membrane.

COMPOSITION OF AMNIOTIC FLUID

Amniotic fluid is an aqueous solution in which undissolved material (e.g., desquamated fetal epithelial cells) is suspended. Amniotic fluid contains approximately equal portions of organic compounds and inorganic salts. Half the organic constituents are proteins; the other half consists of carbohydrates, fats, enzymes, hormones, and pigments. As pregnancy advances, the composition of the amniotic fluid changes.

Disorders of Amniotic Fluid Volume

A condition in which a low volume of amniotic fluid is present for a given gestational age, **oligohydramnios**, results in many cases from placental insufficiency with diminished placental blood flow. Preterm rupture of the amniochorionic membrane occurs in approximately 10% of pregnancies and is the most common cause of oligohydramnios.

When there is **renal agenesis** (failure of kidney formation), the absence of fetal urine contribution to the amniotic fluid is the main cause of oligohydramnios. A similar decrease in fluid occurs when there is obstructive uropathy (urinary tract obstruction). Complications of oligohydramnios include fetal birth defects (pulmonary hypoplasia and facial and limb defects) that are caused by fetal compression by the uterine wall. In extreme cases, as in renal agenesis, **Potter sequence** results from lethal pulmonary hypoplasia due to severe oligohydramnios. Compression of the umbilical cord is also a potential complication of severe oligohydramnios.

Most cases (60%) of **polyhydramnios**, or a large volume of amniotic fluid for a given gestational age, are idiopathic (or of unknown cause), 20% are caused by maternal factors, and 20% are fetal in origin. Polyhydramnios may be associated with severe defects of the central nervous system, such as **meroencephaly**. When there are other defects, such as **esophageal atresia** (blockage), amniotic fluid accumulates because it is unable to pass to the fetal stomach and intestines for absorption.

Ultrasonography has become the technique of choice for diagnosing oligohydramnios and polyhydramnios. Premature rupture of the amniochorionic membrane is the most common event leading to premature labor and delivery and the most common complication resulting in oligohydramnios. Loss of amniotic fluid removes the major protection that the fetus has against infection.

Because fetal urine enters the amniotic fluid, studies of fetal enzyme systems, amino acids, hormones, and other substances can be conducted on fluid removed by amniocentesis (see Fig. 6.13A). Studies of cells in the amniotic fluid permit diagnosis of chromosomal abnormalities such as trisomy 21 (Down syndrome). High levels of alpha-fetoprotein usually indicate the presence of a severe neural tube defect. Low levels of alpha-fetoprotein may indicate chromosomal aberrations such as trisomy 21.

SIGNIFICANCE OF AMNIOTIC FLUID

The embryo, suspended in amniotic fluid by the umbilical cord, floats freely. Amniotic fluid has critical and protective functions in the normal development of the fetus:

- Permits symmetric external growth of the embryo/fetus.
- Acts as a barrier to infection.
- Permits normal fetal lung development.
- Prevents adherence of the amnion to the embryo/fetus.
- Cushions the embryo/fetus against injuries by distributing impacts the mother receives.
- Helps control the embryo/fetus's body temperature by maintaining a relatively constant temperature.
- Enables the fetus to move freely, thereby aiding muscular development (e.g., by movements of the limbs).
- Assists in maintaining homeostasis of fluid and electrolytes.

Amniotic Band Syndrome

Amniotic band syndrome (ABS), or **amniotic band disruption complex**, may result in a variety of fetal birth defects (Fig. 7.22). The incidence of ABS is approximately 1 in every 1200 live births. The defects caused by ABS vary from simple digital constriction to major scalp, craniofacial, and visceral defects. Prenatal ultrasound diagnosis of ABS is possible. **There appear to be two possible causes of these defects**: exogenous causes, which result from delamination of the amnion due to rupturing or tearing, causing an encircling amniotic band (see Figs. 7.20 and 7.22), and endogenous causes, which result from vascular disruption.

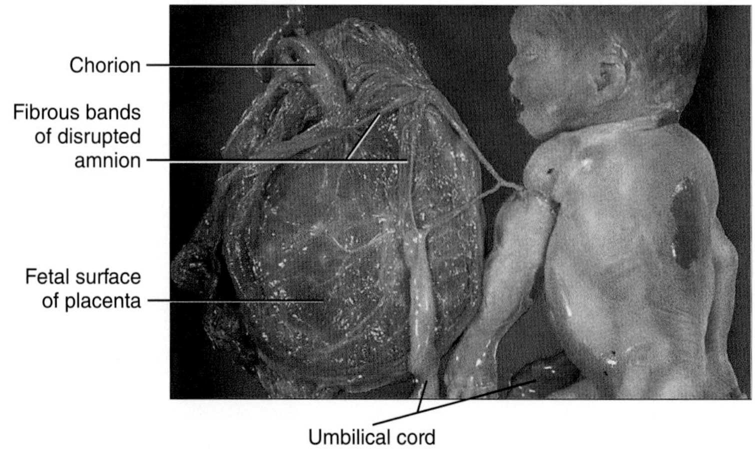

Fig. 7.22 A fetus with amniotic band syndrome showing amniotic bands constricting the left arm. (Courtesy Professor V. Becker, Pathologisches Institut der Universität, Erlangen, Germany.)

UMBILICAL VESICLE

5

The umbilical vesicle can be observed with ultrasound early in the fifth week. Early development of the umbilical vesicle is described in Chapters 3 and 5. At 32 days, the umbilical vesicle is large (see Figs. 7.1C and 7.2). By 10 weeks, the umbilical vesicle has shrunk to a pear-shaped remnant approximately 5 mm in diameter (see Fig. 7.21E) and is connected to the midgut by a narrow **omphaloenteric duct** (yolk stalk). By 20 weeks, the umbilical vesicle is very small (see Fig. 7.21D); thereafter, it is usually not visible. The presence of the amniotic sac and umbilical vesicle enables early recognition and measurement of the embryo. The umbilical vesicle is recognizable in ultrasound examinations until the end of the first trimester.

SIGNIFICANCE OF UMBILICAL VESICLE

The umbilical vesicle is essential for several reasons:

- It has a role in the **transfer of nutrients** to the embryo during the second and third weeks when the uteroplacental circulation is being established.
- **Blood cell development** first occurs in the well-vascularized extraembryonic mesoderm covering the wall of the umbilical vesicle beginning in the third week (see Chapter 4) and continues to form there until hemopoietic activity begins in the liver during the sixth week.
- During the fourth week, the endoderm of the umbilical vesicle is incorporated into the embryo as the **primordial gut** (see Fig. $5.1C_2$). Its endoderm, derived from the epiblast, gives rise to the epithelium of the trachea, bronchi, lungs, and alimentary canal.
- **Primordial germ cells** appear in the endodermal lining of the wall of the umbilical vesicle in the third week and subsequently migrate to the developing gonads (see Fig. 12.31). The cells differentiate into spermatogonia in males and oogonia in females.

FATE OF UMBILICAL VESICLE

At 10 weeks, the small vesicle lies in the chorionic cavity between the amniotic and chorionic sacs (see Fig. 7.21C). It atrophies as pregnancy advances, eventually becoming very small (Fig. 7.21D). In very unusual cases, the umbilical vesicle persists throughout pregnancy and appears under the amnion as a small structure on the fetal surface of the placenta near the attachment of the umbilical cord. The persistence of the umbilical vesicle is of no significance. The omphaloenteric duct usually detaches from the midgut loop by the end of the sixth week. In approximately 2% of adults, the proximal intra-abdominal part of the omphaloenteric duct persists as an **ileal diverticulum (Meckel diverticulum**; see Fig. 11.21).

ALLANTOIS

5

The early development of the allantois is described in Chapter 4. In the third week, it appears as a diverticulum from the caudal wall of the umbilical vesicle that extends into the connecting stalk (Fig. 7.23A). During the second month, the extraembryonic part of the allantois degenerates (see Fig. 7.23B). Although the allantois is not functional in human embryos, it is important for three reasons:

- Blood cell formation occurs in its wall during the third to fifth weeks.
- Its blood vessels persist as the umbilical vein and arteries.
- The intraembryonic part of the allantois passes from the umbilicus to the urinary bladder, with which it is continuous. As the bladder enlarges, the allantois involutes to form a thick tube, the **urachus**. After birth, the urachus becomes a fibrous cord, the **median umbilical ligament**, which extends from the apex of the urinary bladder to the umbilicus (see Fig. 7.23D).

Allantoic Cysts

A cystic mass in the umbilical cord may represent the remains of the extraembryonic part of the allantois (Fig. 7.24). These cysts usually resolve, but they may be associated with an **omphalocele**, the congenital herniation of viscera into the proximal part of the umbilical cord (see Fig. 11.23).

MULTIPLE PREGNANCIES

The risks of chromosomal anomalies and fetal morbidity and mortality are higher in multiple gestations. As the number of fetuses increases, the risks are progressively greater. In most countries, multiple births are more common now because of greater access to fertility therapies, including induction of ovulation and assisted reproductive technology. In North America, twins naturally occur approximately once in every 85 pregnancies, triplets approximately once in 90^2 pregnancies, quadruplets once in 90^3 pregnancies, and quintuplets approximately once in every 90^4 pregnancies. It has also been observed that if the firstborns are twins, a repetition of twinning or some other form of multiple births is approximately five times more likely to occur with the next pregnancy than in the general population.

TWINS AND FETAL MEMBRANES

Twins that originate from two zygotes are **dizygotic** (DZ) (or fraternal) twins (Fig. 7.25), whereas twins that originate from one zygote are **monozygotic** (MZ) twins, or identical twins (Fig. 7.26). The fetal membranes and placentas vary according to the origin of the twins (Table 7.1). In the case of MZ twins, the type of placenta and membranes formed depend on when the twinning process occurs. Approximately two-thirds of twins are DZ.

The study of twins is important in human genetics because it is useful for comparing the effects of genes and the environment on development. If an abnormal condition does not show a simple genetic pattern, a comparison of its incidence in MZ and DZ twins may reveal that heredity is involved.

DIZYGOTIC TWINS

Because they result from the fertilization of two oocytes, DZ twins may be of the same sex or different sexes (see Fig. 7.25).

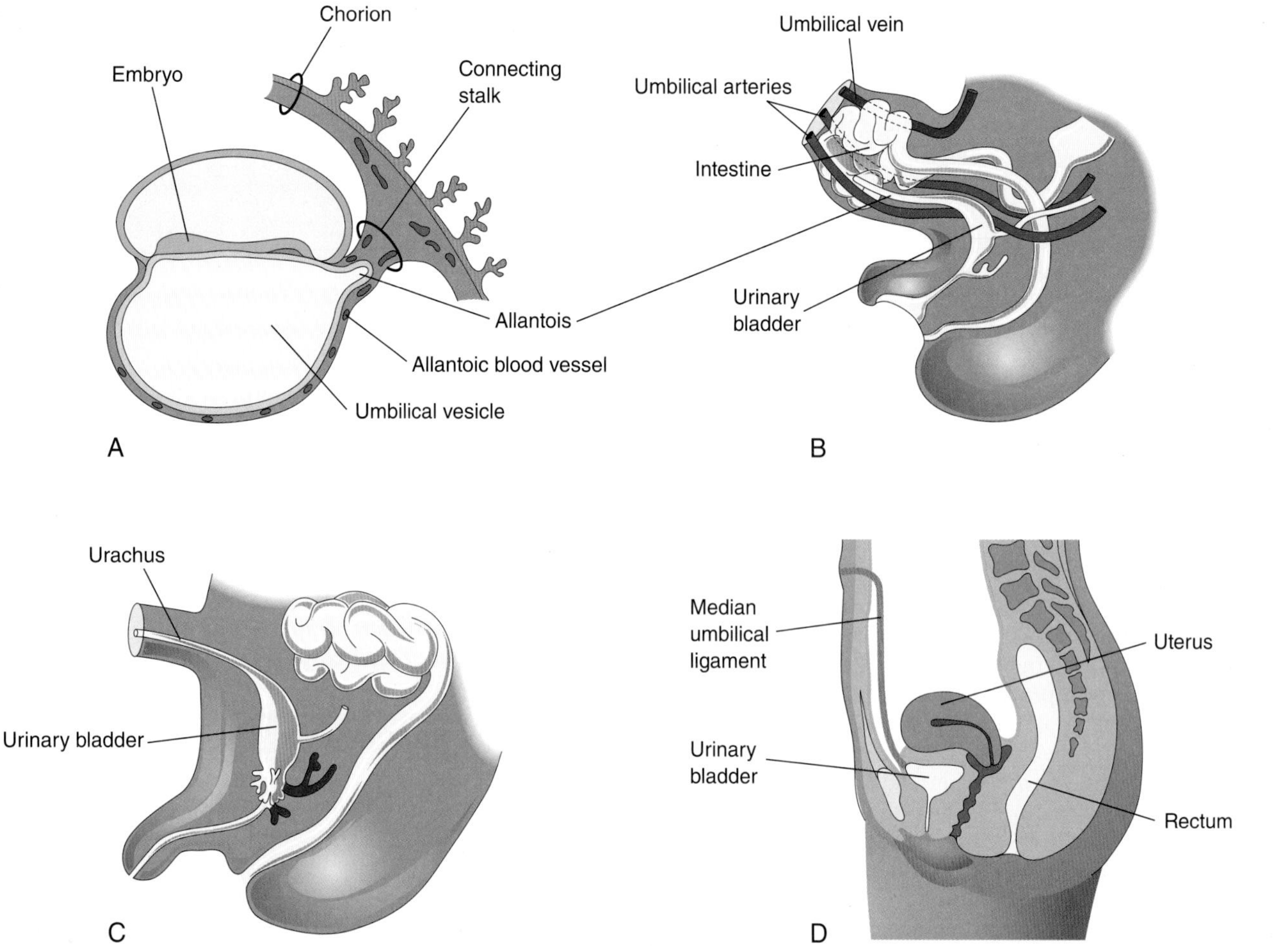

Fig. 7.23 Illustrations of the development and usual fate of the allantois. (A) A 3-week embryo. (B) A 9-week fetus. (C) A 3-month male fetus. (D) Adult female. The nonfunctional allantois form the urachus in the fetus and the median umbilical ligament in the adult.

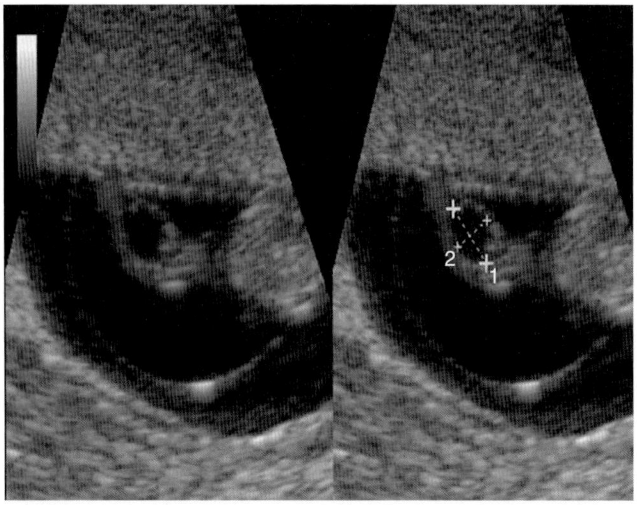

Fig. 7.24 Sonogram of the umbilical cord of a 7-week embryo exhibiting an allantoic cyst *(at calipers)*. (Courtesy Dr. E. A. Lyons, Professor of Radiology, Obstetrics and Gynecology and of Anatomy, Health Sciences Centre and University of Manitoba, Winnipeg, Manitoba, Canada.)

Anastomosis of Placental Blood Vessels

Anastomoses between blood vessels of fused placentas of DZ twins may result in erythrocyte **mosaicism**. The members of these DZ twins have red blood cells of two different blood groups because red cells were exchanged between the circulations of the twins. In cases in which one fetus is a male and the other is a female, masculinization of the female fetus does not occur.

For the same reason, they are no more alike genetically than brothers or sisters born at different times. The only thing they have in common is that they were in their mother's uterus at the same time. DZ twins always have two amnions and two chorions, but the chorions and placentas may be fused. DZ twinning shows a hereditary tendency. Recurrence in families is approximately three times that of the general population. The incidence of DZ twinning shows considerable racial variation, being approximately 1 in 500 Asians, 1 in 125 Whites, and as high as 1 in 20 in some African populations. The incidence of MZ twinning is approximately the same in all populations. In addition, the rate of MZ twinning shows little variation with the mother's age, whereas the rate of DZ twinning increases with maternal age.

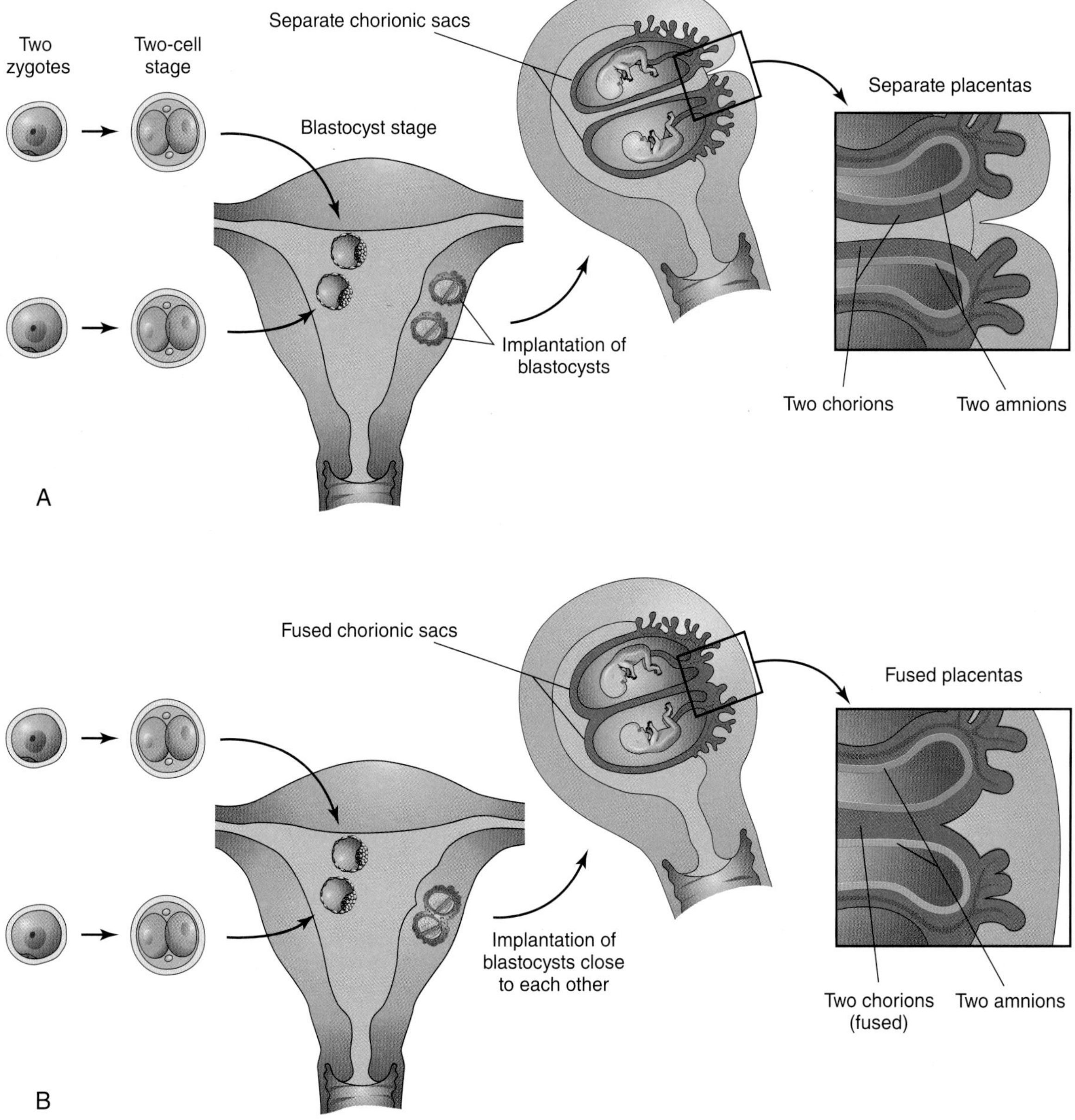

Fig. 7.25 Diagrams illustrating how dizygotic twins develop from two zygotes. The relationships of the fetal membranes and placentas are shown for instances in which the blastocysts implant separately (A) and the blastocysts implant close together (B). In both cases, there are two amnions and two chorions. The placentas are usually fused when they implant close together.

MONOZYGOTIC TWINS

Because they result from the fertilization of one oocyte and develop from one zygote (see Fig. 7.26), MZ twins are of the same sex, genetically identical, and very similar in physical appearance. Physical differences between MZ twins are caused by many factors (Fig. 7.27; also see the box titled "Establishing the Zygosity of Twins"). MZ twinning usually begins in the blastocyst stage, approximately at the end of the first week, and results from the division of the embryoblast into two embryonic primordia. Subsequently, two embryos, each in its own amniotic sac, develop within the same chorionic sac and share a common placenta, that is, a monochorionic-diamniotic twin placenta.

Uncommonly, early separation of embryonic blastomeres (e.g., during the two-cell to eight-cell stages) results in MZ twins with two amnions, two chorions, and two placentas that may or may not be fused (Fig. 7.28). In such cases, it is impossible to determine from the membranes alone whether the twins are MZ or DZ.

OTHER TYPES OF MULTIPLE BIRTHS

Triplets may be derived from:

- One zygote and be identical
- Two zygotes and consist of identical twins and a single
- Three zygotes and be of the same sex or different sexes

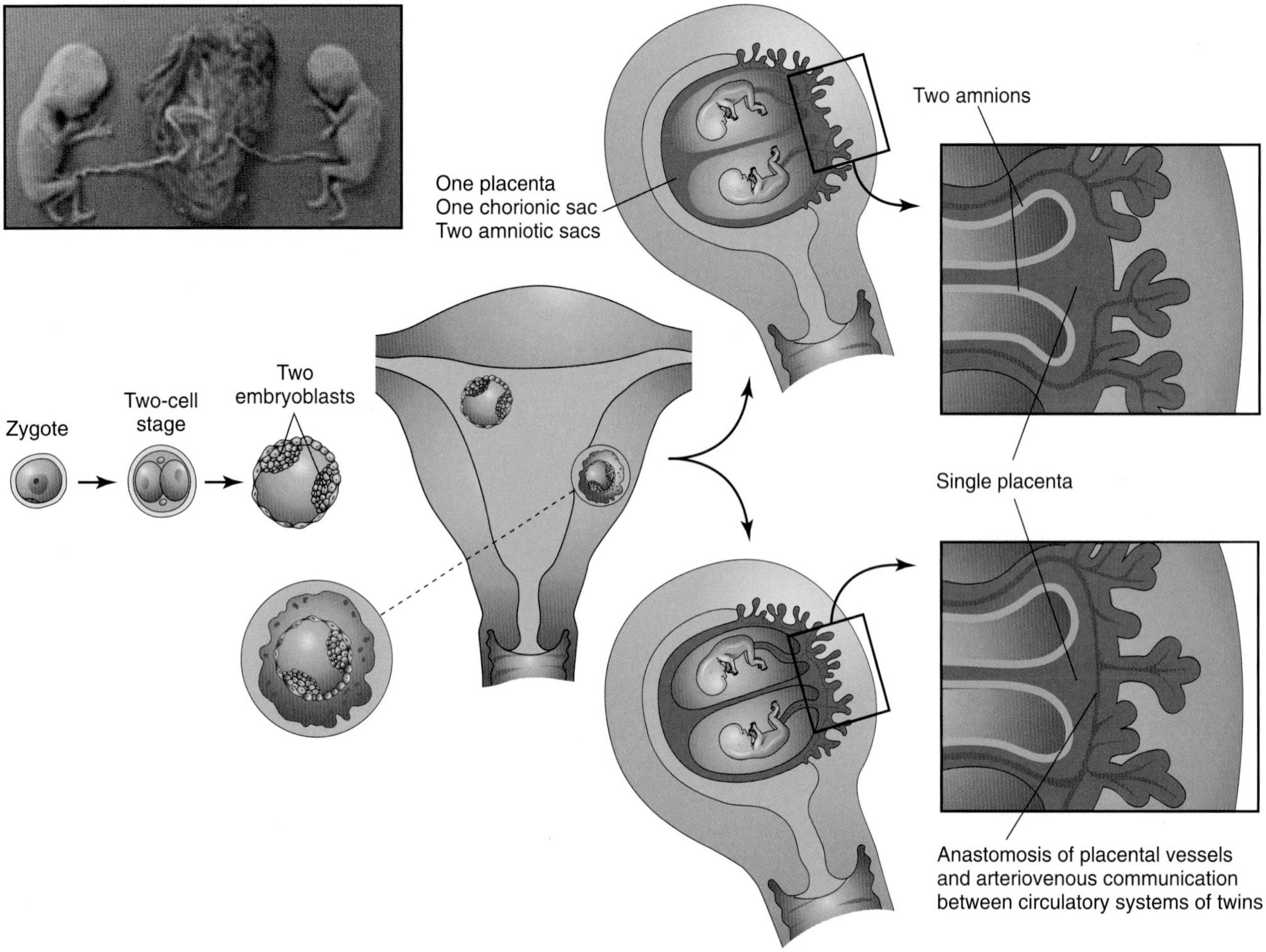

Fig. 7.26 Diagrams illustrating how approximately 65% of monozygotic twins develop from one zygote by division of the embryoblast of the blastocyst. These twins always have separate amnions, a single chorionic sac, and a common placenta. If there is anastomosis of the placental vessels, one twin may receive most of the nutrition from the placenta. *Inset*, Monozygotic twins, 17 weeks' gestation. (Courtesy Dr. Robert Jordan, St. George's University Medical School, Grenada.)

Table 7.1 Frequency of Types of Placentas and Fetal Membranes in Monozygotic (MZ) and Dizygotic (DZ) Twins

	Single Chorion (%)		Two Chorions (%)	
Zygosity	**Single Amnion**	**Two Amnions**	**Fused Placentas[a]**	**Two Placentas**
MZ	1	64	25	10
DZ	–	–	40	60

Adapted from Thompson MW, McInnes RR, Willard HF: *Thompson and Thompson genetics in medicine*, ed 5, Philadelphia, 1991, Saunders.
[a]Results from secondary fusion after implantation.

Twin Transfusion Syndrome

Twin transfusion syndrome occurs in 10% to 15% of monochorionic–diamniotic MZ twins. It usually appears in the second trimester of pregnancy. There is shunting of arterial blood from one twin through unidirectional umbilical-placental **arteriovenous anastomoses** into the venous circulation of the other twin. The donor twin is small, pale, and anemic (see Fig. 7.27), whereas the recipient twin is large and has **polycythemia** (an increase above the normal in the number of red blood cells). The placenta shows similar abnormalities; the part of the placenta supplying the anemic twin is pale, whereas the part supplying the polycythemic twin is dark red. In lethal cases, death results from anemia in the donor twin and congestive heart failure in the recipient twin. Fetoscopic laser coagulation of placental vascular anastomoses is the established method of treatment of severe twin transfusion syndrome. Survival of the fetuses after the procedure ranges from 65% for both fetuses to 88% for one fetus. However, preterm birth may follow the procedure. Follow-up studies of the children reveal significant cognitive and neurodevelopment problems in about 11% of the children.

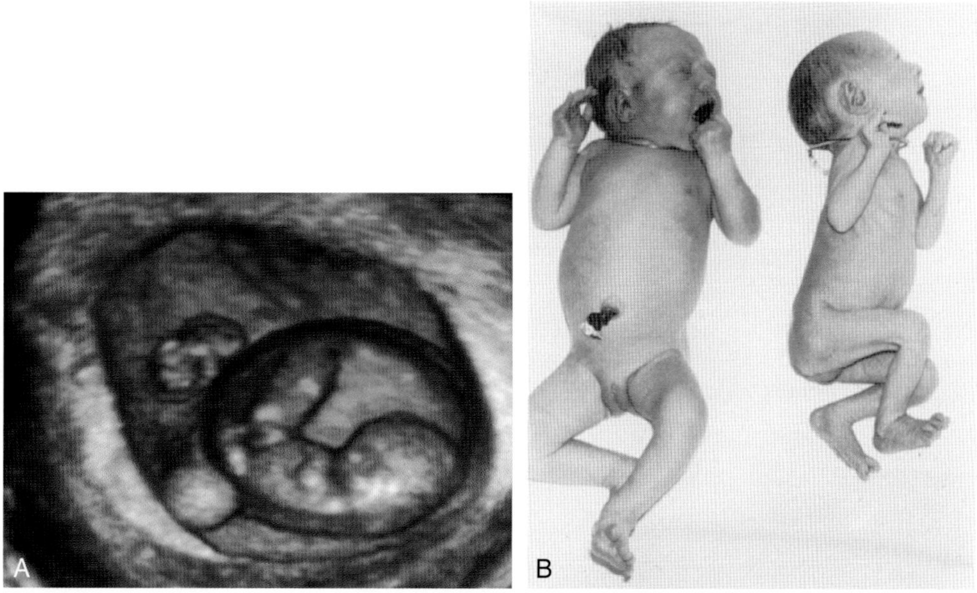

Fig. 7.27 (A) Three-dimensional ultrasound scan of 6-week monochorionic–diamniotic discordant twins. The normal twin *(right)* is seen surrounded by the amniotic membrane and adjacent to the umbilical vesicle. The arms and legs can also be seen. The smaller fetus is also visible *(above left)*. (B) Monozygotic-monochorionic-diamniotic twins showing a wide discrepancy in size resulting from an uncompensated arteriovenous anastomosis of placental vessels. Blood was shunted from the smaller twin to the larger one, producing the twin transfusion syndrome. (Courtesy Dr. E. A. Lyons, Professor of Radiology, Obstetrics and Gynecology and of Anatomy, Health Sciences Centre and University of Manitoba, Winnipeg, Manitoba, Canada.)

Establishing the Zygosity of Twins

Establishing the zygosity of twins is important for clinical care as well as in tissue and organ transplantation (e.g., bone marrow transplantations). The determination of twin zygosity is now done by molecular methods because any two people who are not MZ twins are virtually certain to show differences in some of the large number of DNA markers that can be studied.

Late division of early embryonic cells, such as the division of the embryonic disc during the second week, results in MZ twins that are in one amniotic sac and one chorionic sac (Fig. 7.29A). A monochorionic-monoamniotic twin placenta is associated with fetal mortality rates that are higher by up to 10%, with the cause being cord entanglement. This compromises the circulation of blood through the umbilical vessels, leading to the death of one or both fetuses. Sonography plays an important role in the diagnosis and management of twin pregnancies (Fig. 7.30; see also Fig. 7.27A). Ultrasound evaluation is necessary to identify various conditions that may complicate MZ twinning, such as IUGR, fetal distress, and premature labor.

MZ twins may be discordant for a variety of birth defects and genetic disorders, despite their origin from the same zygote. In addition to environmental differences and chance variation, the following have been implicated:

- Mechanisms of embryologic development, such as vascular abnormalities
- Postzygotic changes, such as somatic mutation, leading to discordance for cancer, or somatic rearrangement of immunoglobulin or T-cell–receptor genes
- Chromosome aberrations originating in one blastocyst after the twinning event
- Uneven X-chromosome inactivation between female MZ twins, with the result that one twin preferentially expresses the paternal X and the other the maternal X

Early Death of a Twin

Because ultrasonographic studies are a common part of prenatal care, it is known that early death and resorption of one member of a twin pair are common. Awareness of this possibility must be considered when discrepancies occur between prenatal cytogenetic findings and the karyotype of an infant. Errors in prenatal cytogenetic diagnosis may arise if extraembryonic tissues (e.g., part of a chorionic villus) from the resorbed twin are examined.

Conjoined Monozygotic Twins

If the embryonic disc does not divide completely or adjacent embryonic discs fuse, various types of conjoined MZ twins may form (Fig. 7.31; see also Fig. 7.29B). The twin phenotype is named according to the regions that are attached; for instance, the **thoracopagus** indicates that there is an anterior union of the thoracic regions. It has been estimated that the incidence of conjoined twins is 1 in 50,000 to 100,000 births. In some cases, the twins are connected to each other by skin only or by cutaneous and other tissues. Some conjoined twins can be successfully separated by surgical procedures (see Fig. 7.31B); however, the anatomic relations in many conjoined twins do not permit surgical separation with sustained viability. In rare circumstances (1:1,000,000), one of the conjoined twins is severely defective and becomes dependent on the cardiovascular system of the intact twin. These twins are called heteropagus or parasitic twins (see Figs. 7.31 and 7.29C).

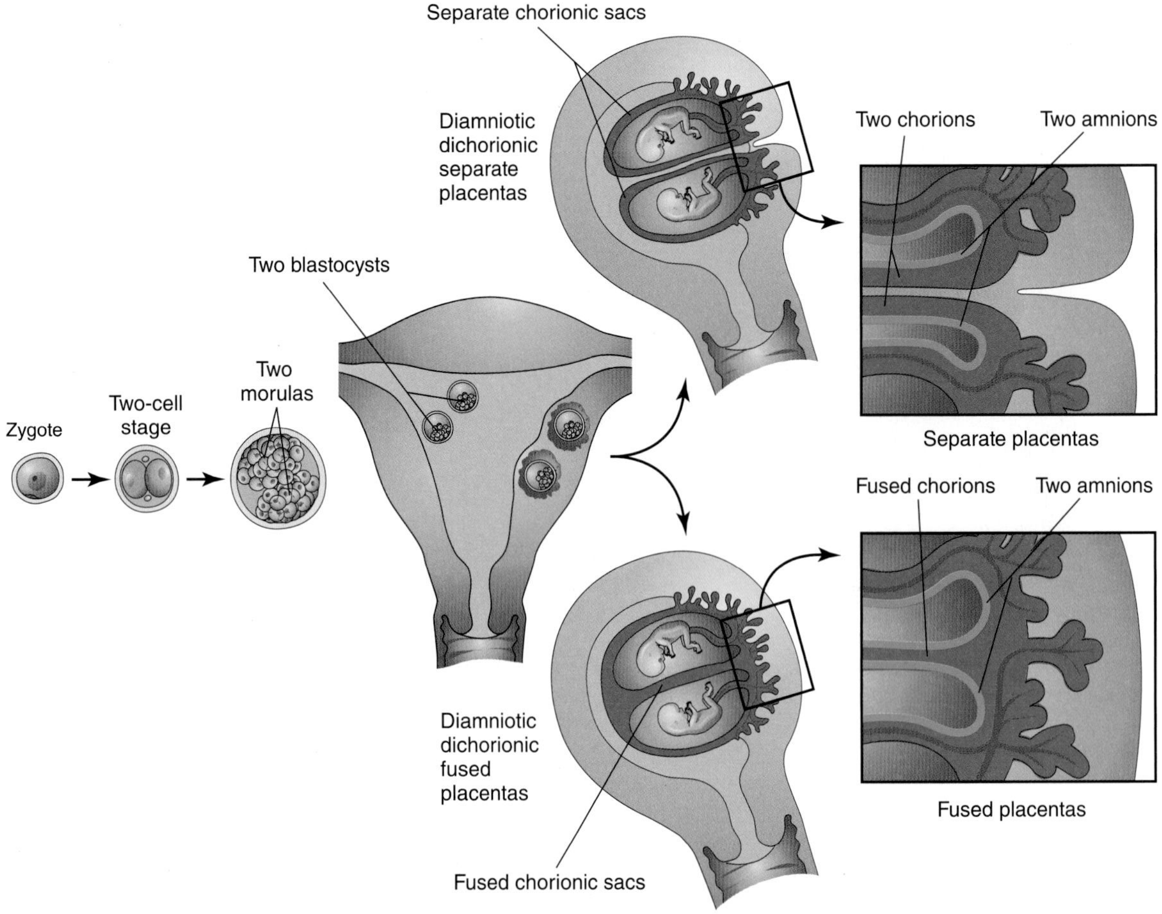

Fig. 7.28 Diagrams illustrating how approximately 35% of monozygotic twins develop from one zygote. Separation of the blastomeres may occur anywhere from the two-cell stage to the morula stage, producing two identical blastocysts. Each embryo subsequently develops its own amniotic and chorionic sacs. The placentas may be separate or fused. In 25% of cases, there is a single placenta resulting from secondary fusion, and in 10% of cases, there are two placentas. In the latter cases, examination of the placenta would suggest that the twins were dizygotic twins. This explains why some monozygotic twins are wrongly stated to be dizygotic twins at birth.

In the last case, the three infants are no more similar than infants from three separate pregnancies. Similar combinations occur in quadruplets, quintuplets, sextuplets, and septuplets.

SUMMARY OF PLACENTA AND FETAL MEMBRANES

- The **placenta** consists of two parts: a larger fetal part derived from the villous chorion and a smaller maternal part developed from the **decidua basalis**. The two parts are held together by stem **chorionic villi** that attach to the cytotrophoblastic shell surrounding the chorionic sac, which attaches the sac to the decidua basalis.
- The principal activities of the placenta are metabolism (synthesis of glycogen, cholesterol, and fatty acids), respiratory gas exchange (oxygen, carbon dioxide, and carbon monoxide), transfer of nutrients (vitamins, hormones, and antibodies), elimination of waste products, and endocrine secretion (e.g., of hCG) for the maintenance of pregnancy.
- The fetal circulation is separated from the maternal circulation by a thin layer of extrafetal tissues, the **placental membrane**. This permeable membrane allows water, oxygen, nutritive substances, hormones, and noxious agents to pass from the mother to the embryo/fetus. Excretory products pass through the placental membrane from the fetus to the mother.
- The fetal membranes and placentas in multiple pregnancies vary considerably, depending on the derivation of the embryos and the time when the division of embryonic cells occurs. The common type of twins is **dizygotic** twins, with two amnions, two chorions, and two placentas that may or may not be fused.
- **Monozygotic** twins, the less common type, represent approximately one-third of all twins; they are derived from one zygote. MZ twins commonly have one chorion, two amnions, and one placenta. Twins with one amnion, one chorion, and one placenta are always monozygotic, and their umbilical cords are often entangled. Other types of multiple births may be derived from one or more zygotes.
- The **umbilical vesicle** and **allantois** are vestigial structures; however, their presence is essential to normal embryonic development. Both are early sites of blood formation, and both are partly incorporated into the embryo. Primordial germ cells also originate in the wall of the umbilical vesicle.

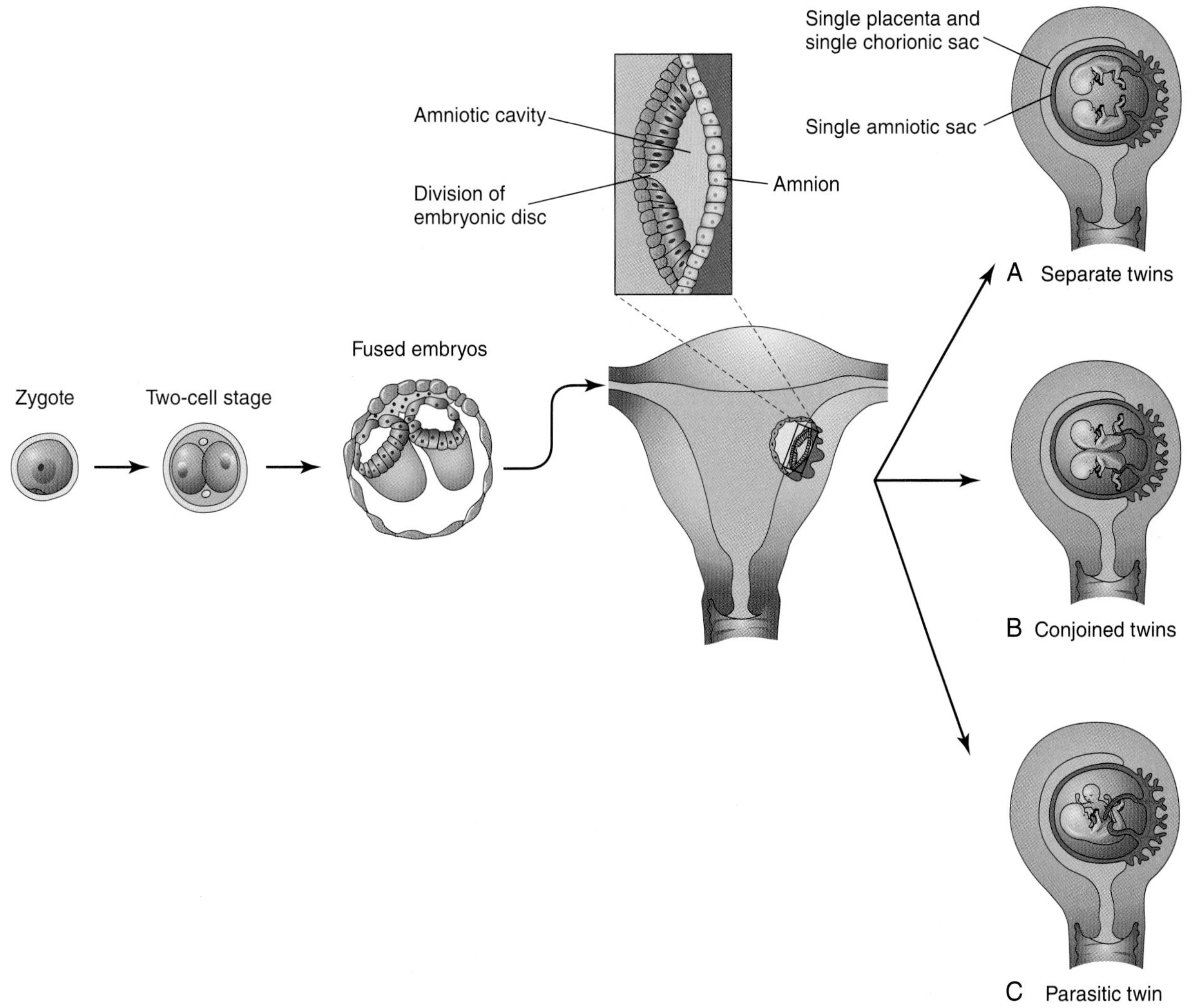

Fig. 7.29 Diagrams illustrating how some monozygotic twins develop. This method of development is very uncommon. Division of the embryonic disc results in two embryos within one amniotic sac. (A) Complete division of the embryonic disc gives rise to twins. Such twins rarely survive because their umbilical cords are often so entangled that interruption of the blood supply to the fetuses occurs. (B and C) Incomplete division of the embryonic disc results in various types of conjoined twins.

- The **amnion** forms an **amniotic sac** for amniotic fluid and provides a covering for the umbilical cord. The amniotic fluid has three main functions: to provide a protective buffer for the embryo/fetus, to allow room for fetal movements, and to assist in the regulation of fetal body temperature.

NEONATAL PERIOD

The neonatal period pertains to the first 4 weeks after birth. The **early neonatal period** is from birth to 7 days. The **neonate** is not a "miniature adult," and an extremely preterm infant is not the same as a full-term infant. The **late neonatal period** is from 7 to 28 days. The umbilical cord typically falls off 7 to 8 days after birth. The head of a neonate is large in proportion to the rest of its body, but, thereafter, the head grows more slowly than the trunk (torso). Usually, a neonate loses about 10% of its birth weight 3 to 4 days after birth, owing to the loss of excess extracellular fluid and the discharge of **meconium**, the first greenish intestinal discharge from the rectum.

When someone touches a neonate's hand, the baby will usually grasp a finger. If someone holds a baby close to his or her chest, the baby will search (root) for the breast to find the nipple. Similarly, a gentle stroke on the baby's cheek makes the baby turn toward the touch with its mouth open. Neonates quickly develop basic visual capacity, but this improves dramatically over the next 12 months as they prefer to look at faces. In some cases, the eyes of a neonate are crossed (**strabismus**) because the eye muscles are not yet fully developed, but this typically corrects itself within a few months.

CLINICALLY ORIENTED PROBLEMS

CASE 7-1

A physician told a pregnant female that she had polyhydramnios.

- If you were asked to explain the meaning of this clinical condition, what would be your answer?
- What conditions are often associated with polyhydramnios?
- Explain why polyhydramnios occurs and how it is identified.

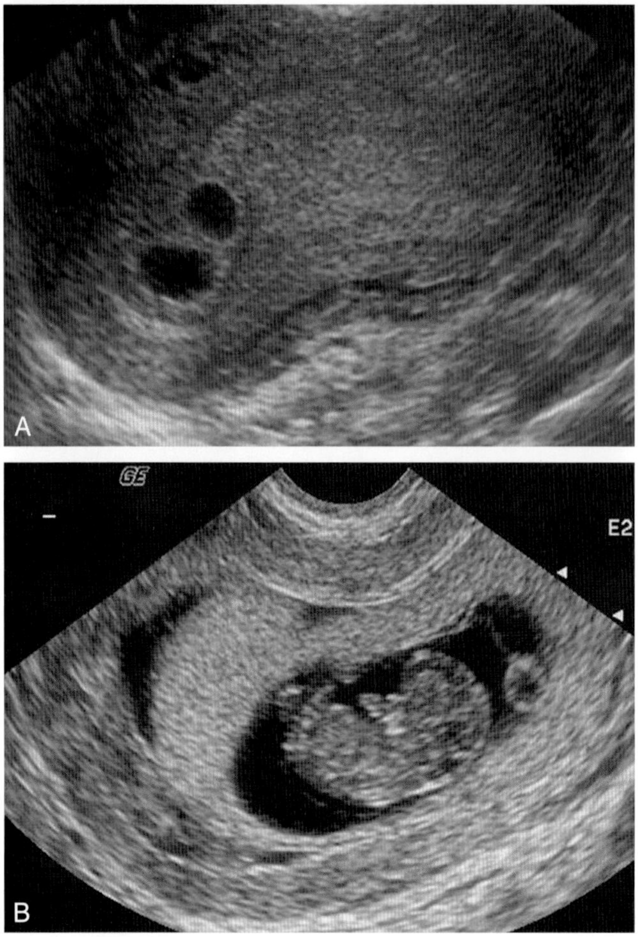

Fig. 7.30 Serial ultrasound scans of a dichorionic pregnancy: (A) at 3 weeks' gestation and (B) at 7 weeks' gestation. (Courtesy Dr. E. A. Lyons, Professor of Radiology, Obstetrics and Gynecology and of Anatomy, Health Sciences Centre and University of Manitoba, Winnipeg, Manitoba, Canada.)

CASE 7-2

A patient with a twin (dizygotic) sister asked her physician whether twinning runs in families.

- Is maternal age a factor?
- Is there a difference in the incidence of monozygotic and dizygotic twinning?

CASE 7-3

A pathologist noted that an umbilical cord had only one umbilical artery.

- How often does this anomaly occur?
- What kind of birth defects might be associated with this condition?

CASE 7-4

An ultrasound examination revealed a twin pregnancy with a single placenta. Chorionic villus sampling and chromosome analysis revealed that the twins were likely female. At birth, the twins were of different sexes.

- How could this error have occurred?

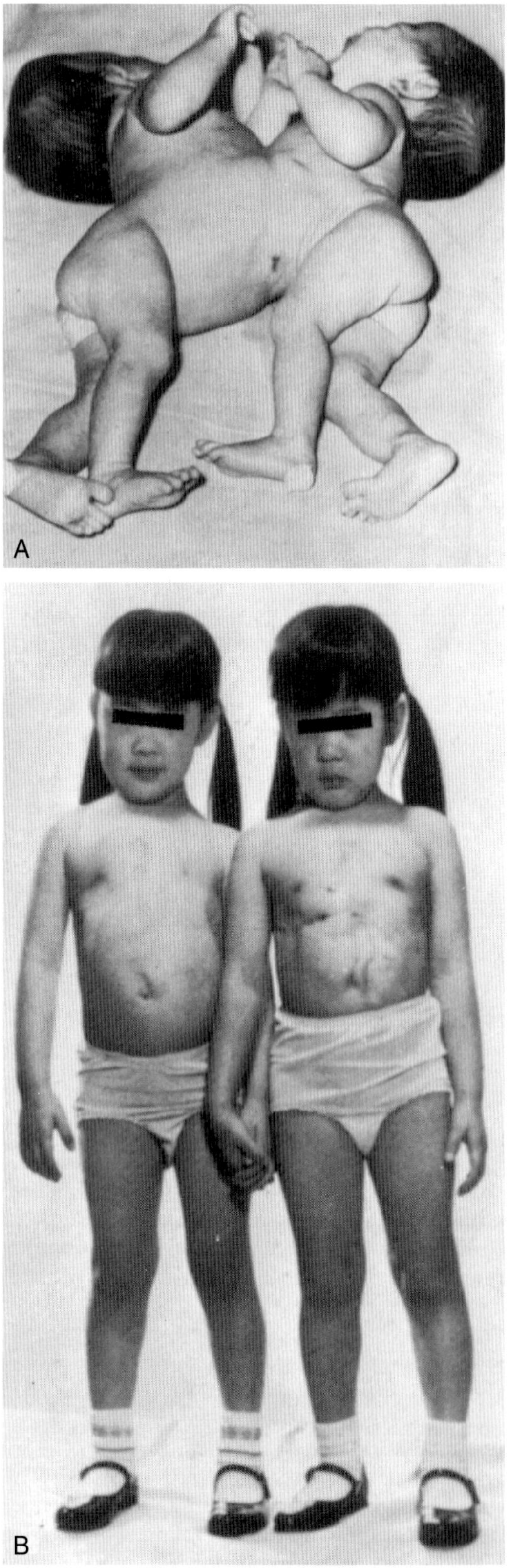

Fig. 7.31 (A) Newborn monozygotic conjoined twins showing union in the thoracic regions (thoracopagus). (B) The twins are approximately 4 years after separation. (From deVries PA: Case history: the San Francisco twins. In Bergsma D, editor: *Birth defects original article series: conjoined twins*, New York, 1967, Alan R. Liss for the National Foundation–March of Dimes, pp. 141–142.)

CASE 7-5

An ultrasound examination of a pregnant female during the second trimester revealed multiple amniotic bands associated with the fetus.

- What produces these bands?
- What birth defects may result from them?
- What is the syndrome called?

Discussion of these problems appears in the Appendix at the back of the book.

ACKNOWELDGEMENT

The authors are grateful to Dr. Peeyush Lala, Professor Emeritus, Department of Anatomy and Cell Biology, Schulich School of Medicine and Dentistry, Western University, London, Ontario, Canada, for preparing these sections: "Trophoblast stem cells and their differentiation," "The Placenta as an Allograft," "The Placenta as an Invasive Tumor-like Structure," and "Preeclampsia".

BIBLIOGRAPHY AND SUGGESTED READING

Alecsandru D, Garcia-Velasco JA: Immunology and human reproduction, *Curr Opin Obstet Gynecol* 27:231, 2015.

Alexander GR, Wingate MS, Salihu H, et al: Fetal and neonatal mortality risks of multiple births, *Obstet Gynecol Clin North Am* 32:1, 2005.

Amack JD: Structures and functions of cilia during vertebrate embryo development, *Mol Repro Dev* 1, 2022.

Bakhsh H, Alenizy H, Alenazi S, et al: Amniotic fluid disorders and the effects on prenatal outcome: a retrospective cohort study, *BMC Pregnancy Childbirth* 21:75, 2021. https://doi.org/10.1186/s12884-021-03549-3.

Brodowski L, Schröder-Heurich B, von Hardenberg S, et al: MicroRNA profiles of maternal and neonatal endothelial progenitor cells in preeclampsia, *Int J Mol Sci* 22(10):5320, 2021. https://doi.org/10.3390/ijms22105320.

Chen Y, Siriwardena D, Penfold C, et al: An integrated atlas of human placental development delineates essential regulators of trophoblast stem cells, *Development* 149(13):dev 200171, 2022. https://doi.org/10.1242/dev.200171.

Cindrova-Davies T, Sferruzzi-Perri AH. Human placental development and function, *Semin Cell Dev Biol*, 131:66–77, 2022. https://doi.org/10.1016/j.semcdb.2022.03.039.

Coorena THM, Oliver TRW, Sanghvi R, Sovio U, Cook E, Vento-Tormo R: Inherent mocaicism and extensive mutation of human plcentas, *Nature* 592:80, 2021.

D'Antonio F, Bhide A: Ultrasound in placental disorders, *Best Pract Res Clin Obstet Gynaecol* 28(3):429–442, 2014.

Dashe JS, Hoffman BL: Ultrasound evaluation of the placenta, membranes and umbilical cord. Ultrasound evaluation of normal fetal anatomy. In Norton ME, editor: *Callen's ultrasonography in obstetrics and gynecology*, ed 6, Philadelphia, 2017, Elsevier.

Egan JFX, Borgida AF: Ultrasound evaluation of multiple pregnancies. In Callen PW, editor: *Ultrasonography in obstetrics and gynecology*, ed 5, Philadelphia, 2008, Saunders.

Forbes K: IFPA Gabor Than Award lecture: molecular control of placental growth: the emerging role of microRNAs, *Placenta* 34(Suppl):S27–S33, 2013.

Gauster M, Moser G, Wernitznig S, Kupper N, Huppertz: Early human trophoblast development: from morphology to function, *Cell Mol Life Sci* 79:345, 2022.

Gibson J: Multiple pregnancy. In Magowan BA, Owen P, Thomson A, editors: *Clinical obstetrics and gynaecology*, ed 3, Philadelphia, 2014, Saunders.

Hubinont C, Lewi L, Bernard P, et al: Anomalies of the placenta and umbilical cord in twin gestations, *Am J Obstet Gynecol*:S91, 2015.

Jabrane-Ferrat N, Siewiera J: The up side of decidual natural killer cells: new developments in immunology of pregnancy, *Immunology* 141:490, 2014.

James JL, Whitley GS, Cartwright JE: Pre-eclampsia: fitting together the placental, immune and cardiovascular pieces, *J Pathol* 221:363, 2010.

Jeyarajah MJ, Bhattad J, Kelly RD, Bines KJ, Jarenem A, Yang FP: The multifaceted role of GCM1 during trophoblast differentiation in the human placenta, *Proc Natl Acad Sci* 119(49), 2020, e2203071119.

Khorami-Sarvestani S, Vanaki N, Shojaeian S, et al: Placenta: an old organ with new functions, *Front Immunol*, 15, 2024, 1385762. https://doi.org/ 10.3389/fimmu.2024.1385762.

Kosinska-Kaczynska K: Placental syndromes—a new paradigm in perinatology, *Int J Environ Res Public Health* 19, 2022. https://doi.org/10.3390/ijerph19127392t.

Knofler M, Haider S, Saleh L, et al: Human placenta and trophoblast development: key molecular mechanisms and model systems, *Cell Mol Life Sci* 76:3479, 2019.

Laing FC, Frates MC, Benson CB: Ultrasound evaluation during the first trimester. In Callen PW, editor: *Ultrasonography in obstetrics and gynecology*, ed 5, Philadelphia, 2008, Saunders.

Lala N, Girish GV, Cloutier-Bosworth A, et al: Mechanisms in decorin regulation of vascular endothelial growth factor-induced human trophoblast migration and acquisition of endothelial phenotype, *Biol Reprod* 87:59, 2012.

Lala PK, Chatterjee-Hasrouni S, Kearns M, et al: Immunobiology of the feto-maternal interface, *Immunol Rev* 75:87, 1983.

Lala PK, Nandi P: Mechanisms of trophoblast migrations, endometrial angiogenesis in preeclampsia: the role of decorin, *Cell Adh Migr* 10(1–2):111–125, 2016.

Lala PK, Nandi P, Hadi A, Halari C: A crossroad between placental and tumor biology: what have we learnt? *Placenta* 116:12–30, 2021. Epub 2021 Mar 12. PMID: 33958236 https://doi.org/10.1016/j.placenta.2021.03.003.

Linde LE, Rasmussen S, Kessler J, et al: Extreme umbilical cord lengths, cord knot and entanglement Risk factors and risk of adverse outcomes, a population-based study, *PLoS One* 13(3):e0194814, 2018. https://doi.org/10.1371/journal.pone.0194814.

Lo S, Kondon E, Chigusa Y, et al: New era of trophoblast research: intergrating morphological and molecular approaches, *Hum Reprod Update* 26:611, 2020.

Lurain JR: Gestational trophoblastic disease I: epidemiology, pathology, clinical presentation and diagnosis of gestational trophoblastic disease, and management of hydatidiform mole, *Am J Obstet Gynecol* 203:531, 2010.

Magann EF, Sandin AI: Amniotic fluid volume in fetal health and disease. In Norton ME, editor: *Callen's ultrasonography in obstetrics and gynecology*, ed 6, Philadelphia, 2017, Elsevier.

Manaster I, Mandelbolm O: The unique properties of uterine NK cells, *Am J Reprod Immunol* 63:434, 2010.

Masselli G, Gualdi G: MRI imaging of the placenta: what a radiologist should know, *Abdom Imaging* 38:573, 2013.

Mian A, Gabra NI, Sharma T, Topale N, Gielecki J, Tubbs RS, Loukas M: Conjoined twins: from conception to separation, a review, *Clin Anat* 30:385, 2017.

Miller JL: Twin to twin transfusion syndrome, *Transl Pediatr* 10:1518, 2021. https://doi.org/10.21037/tp-20-264.

Moffett A, Chazara O, Colucci F, et al: Variation of maternal KIR and fetal HLA-C genes in reproductive failure: too early for clinical intervention, *Reprod Biomed Online* 33:763, 2016.

Okae H, Toh H, Sato T, Hiura H, Takahashi S, Shirane K, Kabayama Y, Suyama M, Sasaki H, Arima T: Derivation of Human Trophoblast Stem Cells, *Cell Stem Cell* 22(1):50–63.e6, 2018. https://doi.org/10.1016/j.stem.2017.12.004. Epub 2017 Dec 14. PMID: 29249463.

Papúchová H, Meissner TB, Li Q, Strominger JL, Tilburgs T: The dual role of HLA-C in tolerance and immunity at the maternal-fetal interface, *Front Immunol* 10:2730, 2019. PMID: 31921098; PMCID: PMC6913657. https://doi.org/10.3389/fimmu.2019.02730.

Schust DJ, Bonney EA, Sugimoto J, Ezashi T, Roberts RM, Choi S, Zhou J: The immunology of syncytialized trophoblast, *Int J Mol Sci* 22:1767, 2021. https://doi.org/10.3390/ijms22041767.

Sherer DM, Al-Haddad S, Cheng R, Dalloul M: Current perspectives of prenatal sonography of umbilical cord morphology, *Int J Women's Health* 13:939, 2021.

Siddiqui MF, Nandi P, Girish GV, Nygard K, Eastabrook G, de Vrijer B, Han VKM, Lala PK: Decorin over-expression by decidual cells in preeclampsia: a potential blood biomarker, *Am J Obstet Gynecol* 2016; 215(3):361.e1–361.e15, 2016. Epub 2016 Mar 19.PMID: 27001218. https://doi.org/10.1016/j.ajog.2016.03.020.

Silasi M, Cohen B, Karumanchi SA, et al: Abnormal placentation, angiogenic factors, and the pathogenesis of preeclampsia, *Obstet Gynecol Clin North Am* 37:239, 2010.

Simpson LL: Ultrasound evaluation in multiple gestations. In Norton ME, editor: *Callen's ultrasonography in obstetrics and gynecology*, ed 6, Philadelphia, 2017, Elsevier.

Terzieva A, Dimitrova V, Djerov L, et al: Early pregnancy human decidua is enriched with activated, fully differentiated and pro-inflammatory gamma/delta T cells with diverse TCR repertoires, *Int J Mol Sci* 20(3):687, 2019. https://doi.org/10.1016/j.ajog.2016.03.020.

Turco MY, Moffett A: Development of the human placenta, *Development* 146:dev.163428, 2019. https://doi.org/10.3390/ijms20030687.

van der Schot AM, Sikkel E, Spaanderman MEA, Vandenbussche FPHA: Computer-assisted fetal laser surgery in the treatment of twin-to-twin transfusion syndrome: recent trends and prospects, *Prenat Diagn* 42(10):1225–1234, 2022. https://doi.org/10.1002/pd.6225.

Visentin S, Londero AP, Santoro L, et al: Abnormal umbilical cord insertions in singleton deliveries: placental histology and neonatal outcomes, *J Clin Path* 75:751, 2022.

Yang Y, Wang W, Weng J, Li H, Ma Y, Liu L, Ma W: Advances in the study of HLA class Ib in maternal-fetral immune tolerance, *Front. Immunol.*, 2022, Sec. Immunological Tolerance and Regulation. https://doi.org/10.3389/fimmu.2022.976289.

Zou L, Yang J, Min A, Yin Y, Li M: Clinical value and treatment progress of prenatal ultrasonography in twin pregnancy: a systematic review, *Contrast Media Mol Imaging* 2022:6748487, 2022. https://doi.org/10.1155/2022/6748487.

Zou Z, Forbes K, Harris LK, Heazell AEP: The potential role of the ESRRG pathway in placental dysfunction, *Reproduction* 161:R45–R60, 2021.

Zhang X, Wei H: Role of decidual natural killer cells in human pregnancy and related pregnancy complications, *Front Immunol* 12:728291, 2021. https://doi.org/10.3389/fimmu.2021.728291.

Body Cavities, Mesenteries, and Diaphragm

8

CHAPTER OUTLINE

Early in the fourth week, the **intraembryonic coelom** appears as a horseshoe-shaped cavity (Fig. 8.1A). The bend in the cavity at the cranial end of the embryo represents the future **pericardial cavity**, and its lateral extensions (limbs) indicate the future **pleural** and **peritoneal cavities**. The distal part of each limb of the intraembryonic coelom is continuous with the **extraembryonic coelom** at the lateral edges of the embryonic disc (see Fig. 8.1B). The intraembryonic coelom provides room for the organs to develop and move. For instance, it allows the normal herniation of the midgut into the umbilical cord (Fig. 8.2E; see Fig. 11.14). During embryonic folding in the horizontal plane, the limbs of the coelom are brought together on the ventral aspect of the embryo (see Fig. 8.2C). The ventral mesentery degenerates in the region of the future **peritoneal cavity** (see Fig. 8.2F), resulting in a large embryonic peritoneal cavity extending from the heart to the pelvic region.

EMBRYONIC BODY CAVITY

6

The intraembryonic coelom becomes the embryonic body cavity, which is divided into three well-defined cavities during the fourth week (Fig. 8.3; see Figs. 8.1A and 8.2):

- A pericardial cavity
- Two pericardioperitoneal canals
- A peritoneal cavity

These cavities have a **parietal** wall, lined by mesothelium (future parietal layer of the peritoneum), that is derived from the somatic lateral layer of mesoderm, and a **visceral** wall, also covered by mesothelium (future visceral layer of the peritoneum), that is derived from splanchnic mesoderm (see Fig. 8.3E). The peritoneal cavity is connected with the extraembryonic coelom at the umbilicus (Fig. 8.4A and D).

The peritoneal cavity loses its connection with the extraembryonic coelom during the 11th week of gestation as the intestines return to the abdomen from the umbilical cord (see Fig. 11.13C). Genetic lineage tracing studies suggest that the intraembryonic coelomic epithelium is a unique and highly active layer of mesenchymal cells that contribute to the development of major organs and systems, including the heart, lungs, and gastrointestinal tract.

During the formation of the head fold, the primordial heart and pericardial cavity are relocated ventrally, anterior to the foregut (see Fig. 8.2B). As a result, the pericardial cavity opens into pericardioperitoneal canals, which pass dorsal to the foregut (see Fig. 8.4B and D).

MESENTERIES

After embryonic folding, the caudal part of the foregut, midgut, and hindgut are suspended in the peritoneal cavity from the dorsal abdominal wall by the **dorsal mesentery** (see Figs. 8.2F and 8.3B, D, and E) A **mesentery** is a double layer of the peritoneum that begins as an extension of the visceral peritoneum covering an organ. The mesentery connects the organ to the body wall and conveys vessels and nerves to it. Transiently, the **dorsal and ventral mesenteries** divide the peritoneal cavity into right and left halves (see Fig. 8.3C). The ventral mesentery soon disappears (see Fig. 8.3E), except where it is attached to the caudal part of the foregut (primordium of stomach and proximal part of duodenum). The peritoneal cavity then becomes a continuous space (see Fig. 8.4D). The arteries supplying the primordial gut—celiac arterial trunk (foregut), superior mesenteric artery (midgut), and inferior mesenteric artery (hindgut)—pass between the layers of the dorsal mesentery (see Fig. 8.3C).

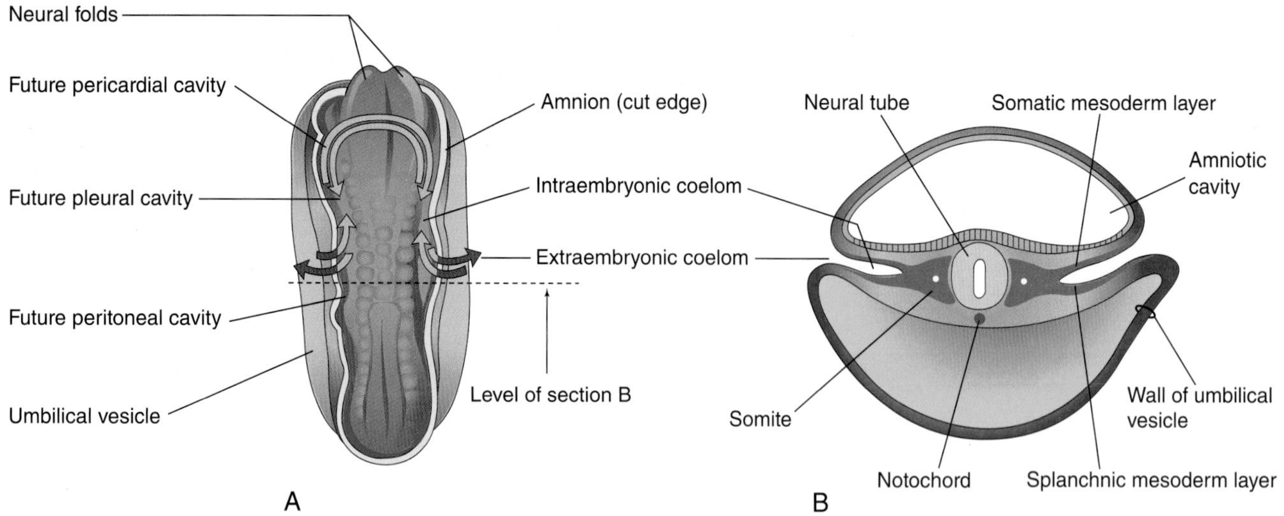

Fig. 8.1 (A) Drawing of a dorsal view of a 22-day embryo shows the outline of the horseshoe-shaped intraembryonic coelom. The amnion has been removed, and the coelom is shown as if the embryo were translucent. The continuity of the coelom and the communication of its right and left limbs with the extraembryonic coelom are indicated by arrows. (B) Transverse section through the embryo at the level shown in (A).

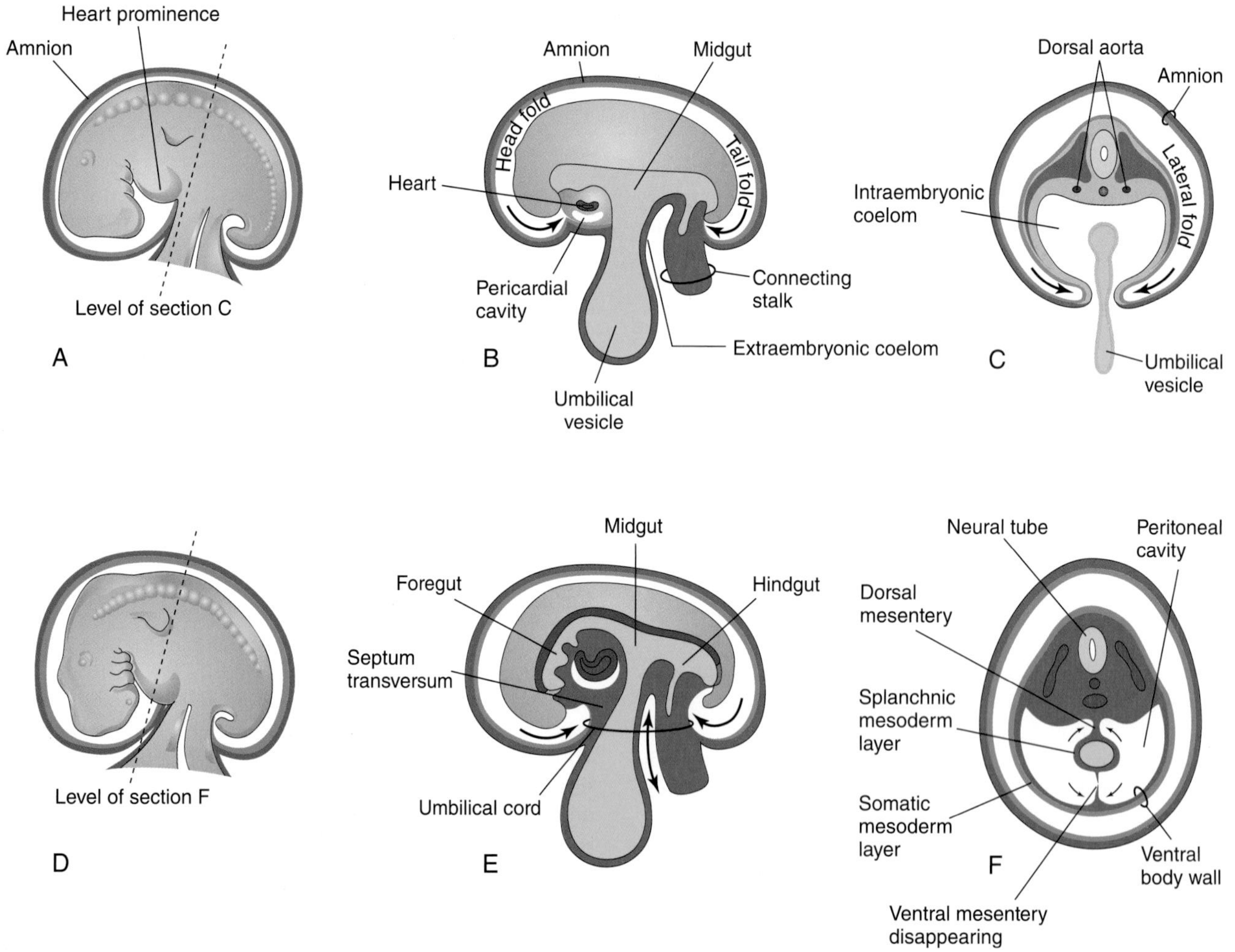

Fig. 8.2 Illustrations of embryonic folding and its effects on the intraembryonic coelom and other structures. (A) Lateral view of an embryo (approximately 26 days). (B) Schematic sagittal section of the same embryo shows the head and tail folds. (C) Transverse section at the level shown in (A) indicates how the fusion of the lateral folds gives the embryo a cylindrical form. (D) Lateral view of an embryo (at approximately 28 days). (E) Schematic sagittal section of the same embryo shows the reduced communication between the intraembryonic and extraembryonic coeloms *(double-headed arrow)*. (F) Transverse section at the level shown in (D) illustrates the formation of the ventral body wall and the disappearance of the ventral mesentery. The *arrows* indicate the junction of the somatic and splanchnic layers of the mesoderm. The somatic mesoderm will form the parietal peritoneum lining the abdominal wall, and the splanchnic mesoderm will form the visceral peritoneum covering the organs (e.g., the stomach).

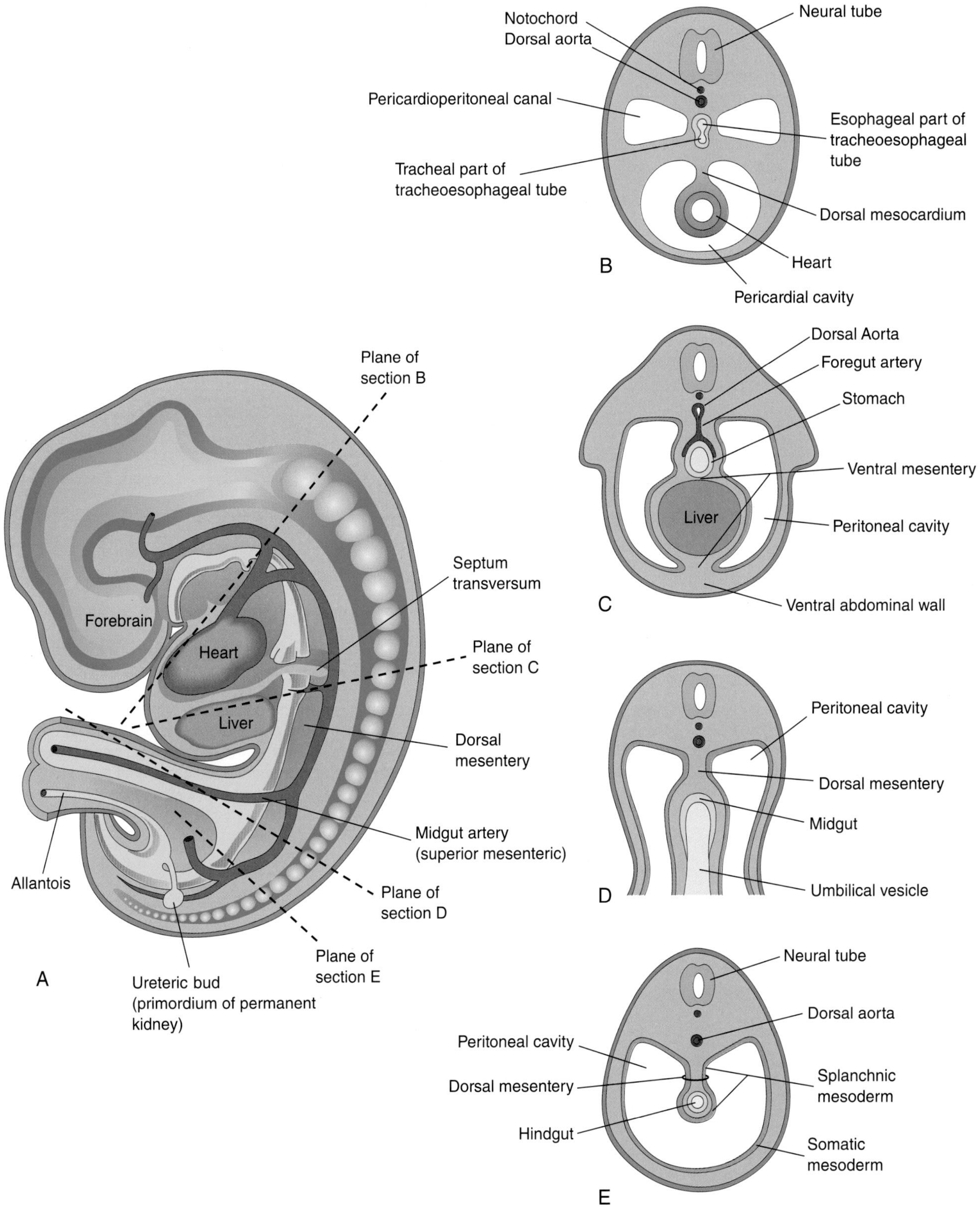

Fig. 8.3 Illustrations of the mesenteries and body cavities at the beginning of the fifth week of development. (A) Schematic sagittal section. Notice that the dorsal mesentery serves as a pathway for the arteries supplying the developing midgut. Nerves and lymphatics also pass between the layers of this mesentery. (B–E) Transverse sections through the embryo at the levels indicated in (A). The ventral mesentery disappears, except in the region of the terminal esophagus, stomach, and first part of the duodenum. Notice that the right and left parts of the peritoneal cavity separate in (C) but are continuous in (E).

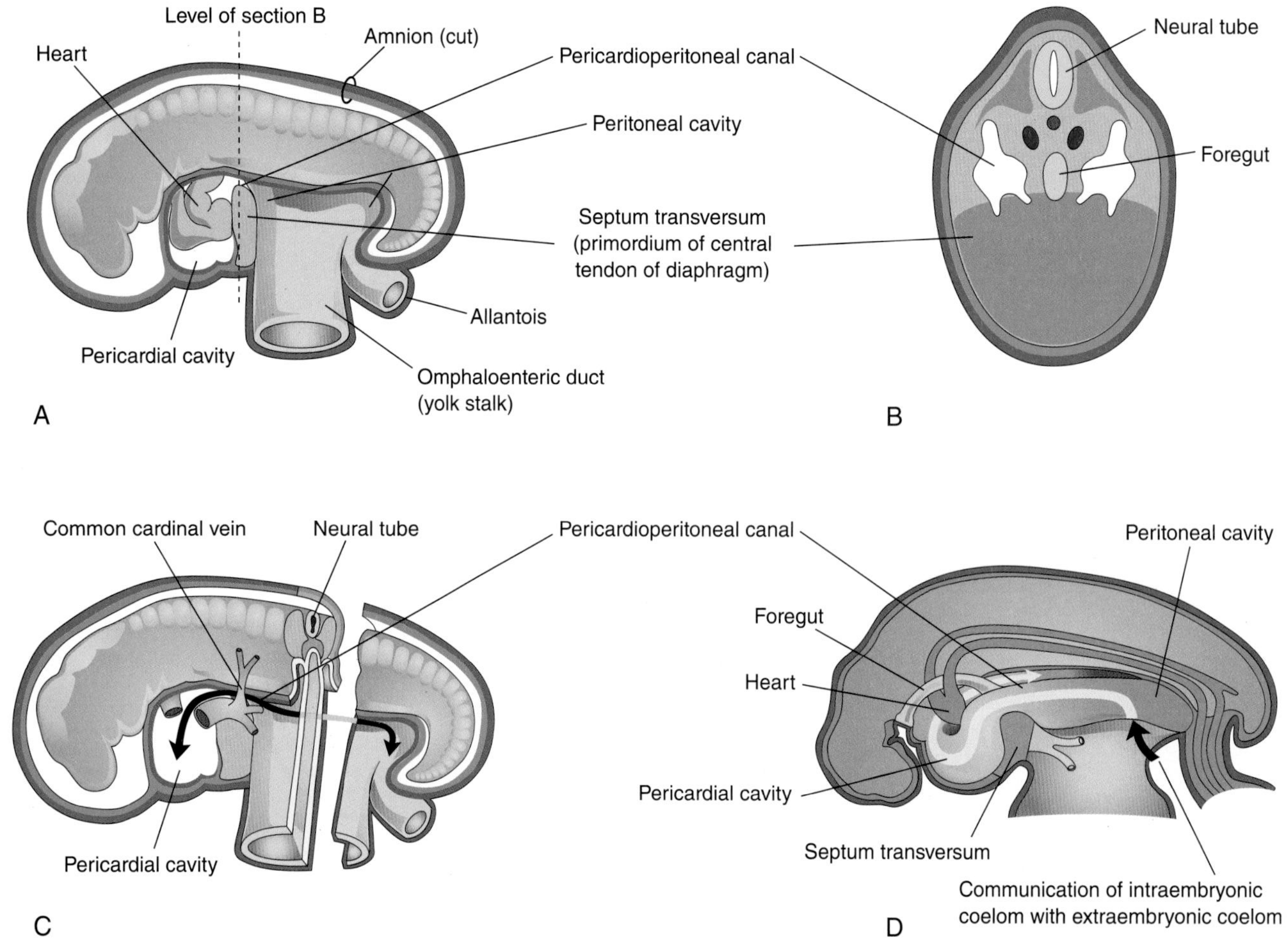

Fig. 8.4 Schematic drawings of an embryo (at approximately 24 days). (A) The lateral wall of the pericardial cavity has been removed to show the primordial heart. (B) Transverse section of the embryo illustrates the relationship of the pericardioperitoneal canals to the septum transversum (primordium of the central tendon of the diaphragm) and the foregut. (C) Lateral view of the embryo with heart removed. The embryo has also been sectioned transversely to show the continuity of the intraembryonic and extraembryonic coeloms *(arrow)*. (D) Sketch shows the pericardioperitoneal canals arising from the dorsal wall of the pericardial cavity and passing on each side of the foregut to join the peritoneal cavity. The *arrow* shows the communication of the extraembryonic coelom with the intraembryonic coelom and the continuity of the intraembryonic coelom at this stage.

DIVISION OF EMBRYONIC BODY CAVITY

Each pericardioperitoneal canal lies lateral to the proximal part of the foregut (future esophagus) and dorsal to the **septum transversum**—a plate of mesodermal (mesenchymal) tissue that occupies the space between the thoracic cavity and the omphaloenteric duct (see Fig. 8.4A and B).

The septum transversum is the primordium of the central tendon of the diaphragm. Partitions form in each pericardioperitoneal canal separating the pericardial cavity from the pleural cavities and the pleural cavities from the peritoneal cavity. Because of the growth of the **bronchial buds** (primordia of bronchi and lungs) into the pericardioperitoneal canals, a pair of membranous ridges is produced in the lateral wall of each canal (Fig. 8.5A and B):

- The cranial ridges—**pleuropericardial folds**—are located superior to the developing lungs.
- The caudal ridges—**pleuroperitoneal folds**—are located inferior to the lungs.

Congenital Pericardial Defect

Defective formation and/or fusion of the pleuropericardial membranes separating the pericardial and pleural cavities is uncommon. This rare anomaly results in a congenital defect of the pericardium, usually asymptomatic and more often on the left side. Consequently, the pericardial cavity communicates with the pleural cavity. In very unusual cases, a part of the left atrium of the heart herniates into the pleural cavity at each heartbeat.

PLEUROPERICARDIAL MEMBRANES

As the pleuropericardial folds enlarge, they form partitions that separate the pericardial cavity from the pleural cavities. These partitions—the **pleuropericardial membranes**—contain the common cardinal veins (see Figs. 8.4C and 8.5A), which drain the venous system into the sinus venosus of the heart. Initially, the bronchial buds are small relative to the heart and pericardial cavity (see Fig. 8.5A). They soon

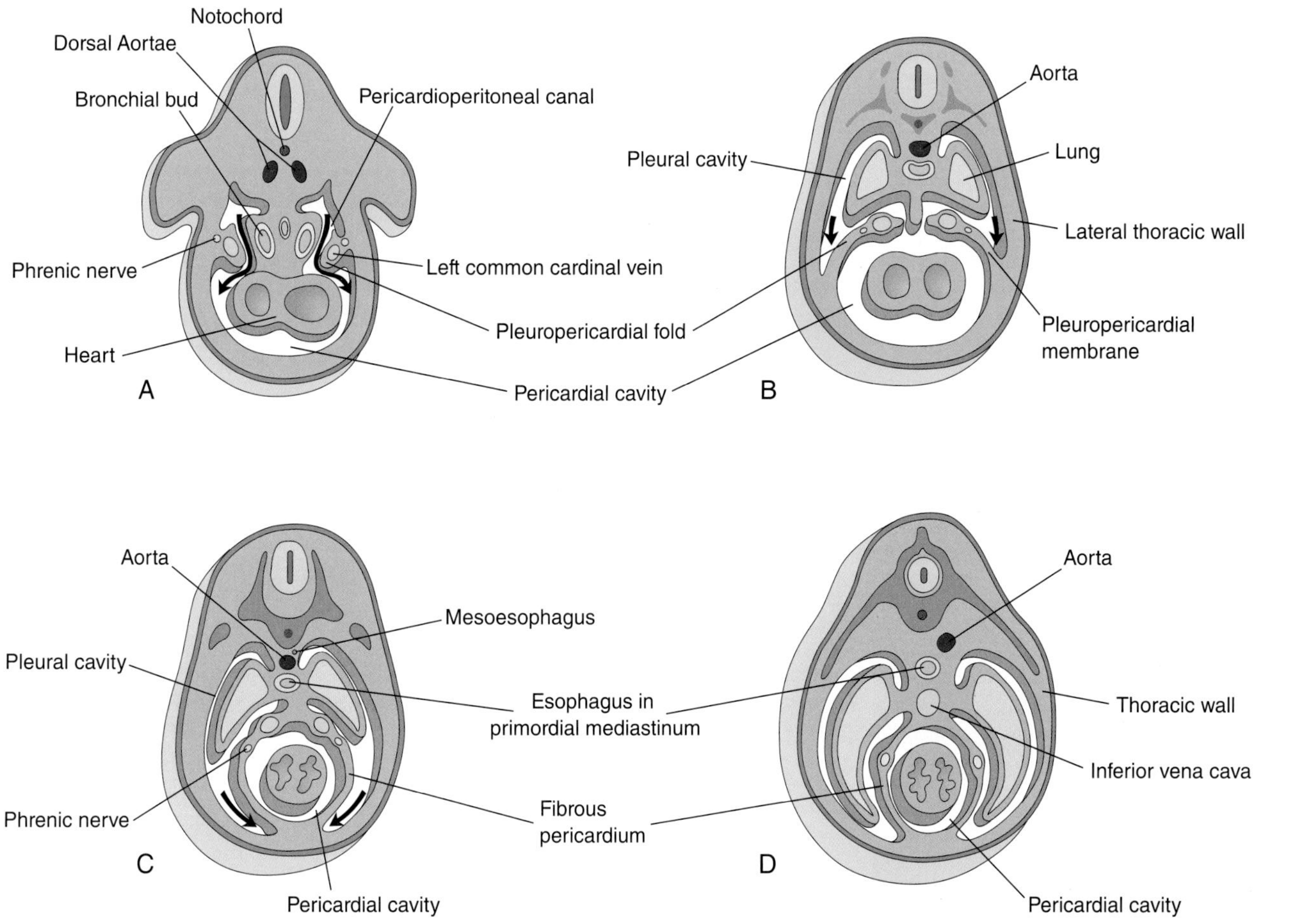

Fig. 8.5 Drawings of transverse sections through embryo cranial to the septum transversum illustrate successive stages in the separation of the pleural cavities from the pericardial cavity. Growth and development of the lungs, expansion of the pleural cavities, and formation of fibrous pericardium are also shown. (A) At 5 weeks. The arrows indicate the communications between the pericardioperitoneal canals and the pericardial cavity. (B) At 6 weeks. The *arrows* indicate the development of the pleural cavities as they expand into the body wall. (C) At 7 weeks. Expansion of the pleural cavities ventrally around the heart is shown. The pleuropericardial membranes are now fused in the median plane and with the mesoderm ventral to the esophagus. (D) At 8 weeks. Continued expansion of the lungs and pleural cavities and formation of the fibrous pericardium and thoracic wall are illustrated.

grow laterally from the caudal end of the trachea into the pericardioperitoneal canals (future pleural canals). As the primordial pleural cavities expand ventrally around the heart, they extend into the body wall, splitting the mesenchyme into:

- An outer layer that becomes the thoracic wall
- An inner layer that becomes the fibrous pericardium, the outer layer of the pericardial sac enclosing the heart (see Fig. 8.5C and D)

The pleuropericardial membranes project into the cranial ends of the pericardioperitoneal canals (see Fig. 8.5B). With subsequent growth of the **common cardinal veins,** positional displacement of the heart, and expansion of the pleural cavities, the membranes become mesentery-like folds extending from the lateral thoracic wall. By the seventh week, the membranes fuse with the mesenchyme ventral to the esophagus, separating the pericardial cavity from the pleural cavities (see Fig. 8.5C). This primordial mediastinum consists of a mass of mesenchyme that extends from the sternum to the vertebral column, separating the developing lungs (see Fig. 8.5D). The right pleuropericardial opening closes slightly earlier than the left one and produces a larger pleuropericardial membrane.

PLEUROPERITONEAL MEMBRANES

As the pleuroperitoneal folds enlarge, they project into the pericardioperitoneal canals. Gradually the folds become membranous, forming the pleuroperitoneal membranes (Figs 8.6 and 8.7). Eventually, these membranes separate the pleural cavities from the peritoneal cavity. The pleuroperitoneal membranes are produced as the developing lungs and pleural cavities expand and invade the body wall. They are attached dorsolaterally to the abdominal wall, and initially, their crescentic free edges project into the caudal ends of the pericardioperitoneal canals.

During the sixth week of gestation, the pleuroperitoneal membranes extend ventromedially until their free edges fuse with the dorsal mesentery of the esophagus and septum transversum (see Fig. 8.7C). This separates the pleural cavities from the peritoneal cavity. Closure of the pleuroperitoneal openings is completed by the migration of **myoblasts** (primordial muscle cells) from cervical somites into the pleuroperitoneal membranes (see Fig. 8.7E). The

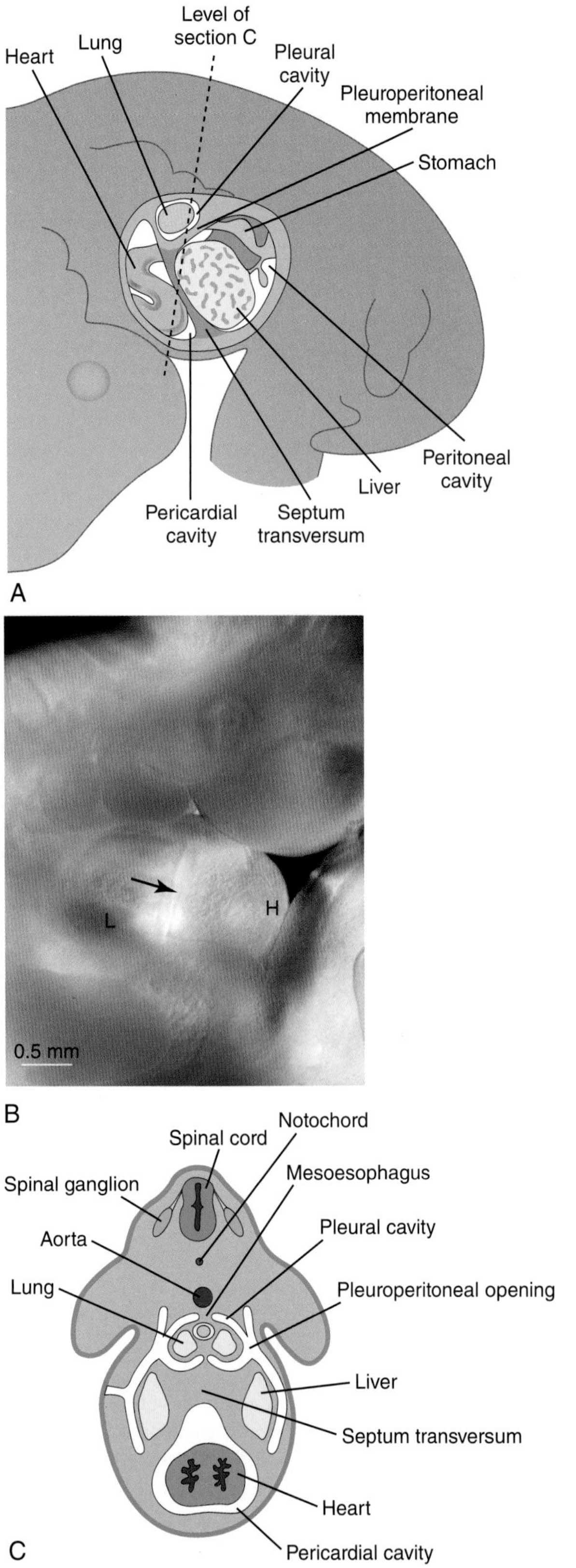

Fig. 8.6 (A) The primordial body cavities are viewed from the left side after removal of the lateral body wall. (B) Photograph of a 5-week-old embryo shows the developing septum transversum *(arrow)*, heart tube *(H)*, and liver *(L)*. (C) Transverse section through an embryo at the level shown in (A). ((B) Courtesy Dr. Bradley R. Smith, University of Michigan, Ann Arbor, Michigan.)

pleuroperitoneal opening on the right side closes slightly before the left one. The reason for this is uncertain, but it may be related to the relatively large size of the right lobe of the liver at this stage of development.

DEVELOPMENT OF DIAPHRAGM

6

The diaphragm is a dome-shaped, musculotendinous partition that separates the thoracic and abdominal cavities. It is a composite structure that develops from four embryonic components (see Fig. 8.7):

- Septum transversum
- Pleuroperitoneal membranes
- Dorsal mesentery of the esophagus
- Muscular ingrowth from lateral body walls

Several candidate genes on the long arm of chromosome 15 (15q) play a critical role in the development of the diaphragm.

SEPTUM TRANSVERSUM

The transverse septum grows dorsally from the ventrolateral body wall and forms a semicircular shelf that separates the heart from the liver (see Fig. 8.6A). This septum, which is composed of mesodermal tissue, forms the **central tendon of the diaphragm** (see Fig. 8.7D and E). After the head folds ventrally during the fourth week, the septum forms a thick, incomplete connective tissue partition between the pericardial and abdominal cavities (see Fig. 8.4). The septum does not completely separate the thoracic and abdominal cavities.

During early development, a large part of the liver is embedded in the septum transversum. There are large openings, the pericardioperitoneal canals, along the sides of the esophagus (see Fig. 8.7B). The septum expands and fuses with the dorsal mesentery of the esophagus and pleuroperitoneal membranes (see Fig. 8.7C).

PLEUROPERITONEAL MEMBRANES

The pleuroperitoneal membranes fuse with the dorsal mesentery of the esophagus and the septum transversum (see Fig. 8.7C). This completes the partition between the thoracic and abdominal cavities and forms the **primordial diaphragm**. Although the pleuroperitoneal membranes form large portions of the early fetal diaphragm, they represent relatively small portions of the neonate's diaphragm (see Fig. 8.7E).

DORSAL MESENTERY OF ESOPHAGUS

The septum transversum and pleuroperitoneal membranes fuse with the dorsal mesentery of the esophagus. This mesentery constitutes the median portion of the diaphragm. The **crura of the diaphragm**, a leg-like pair of diverging muscle bundles that cross in the median plane anterior to the aorta (see Fig. 8.7E), develop from myoblasts that grow into the dorsal mesentery of the esophagus.

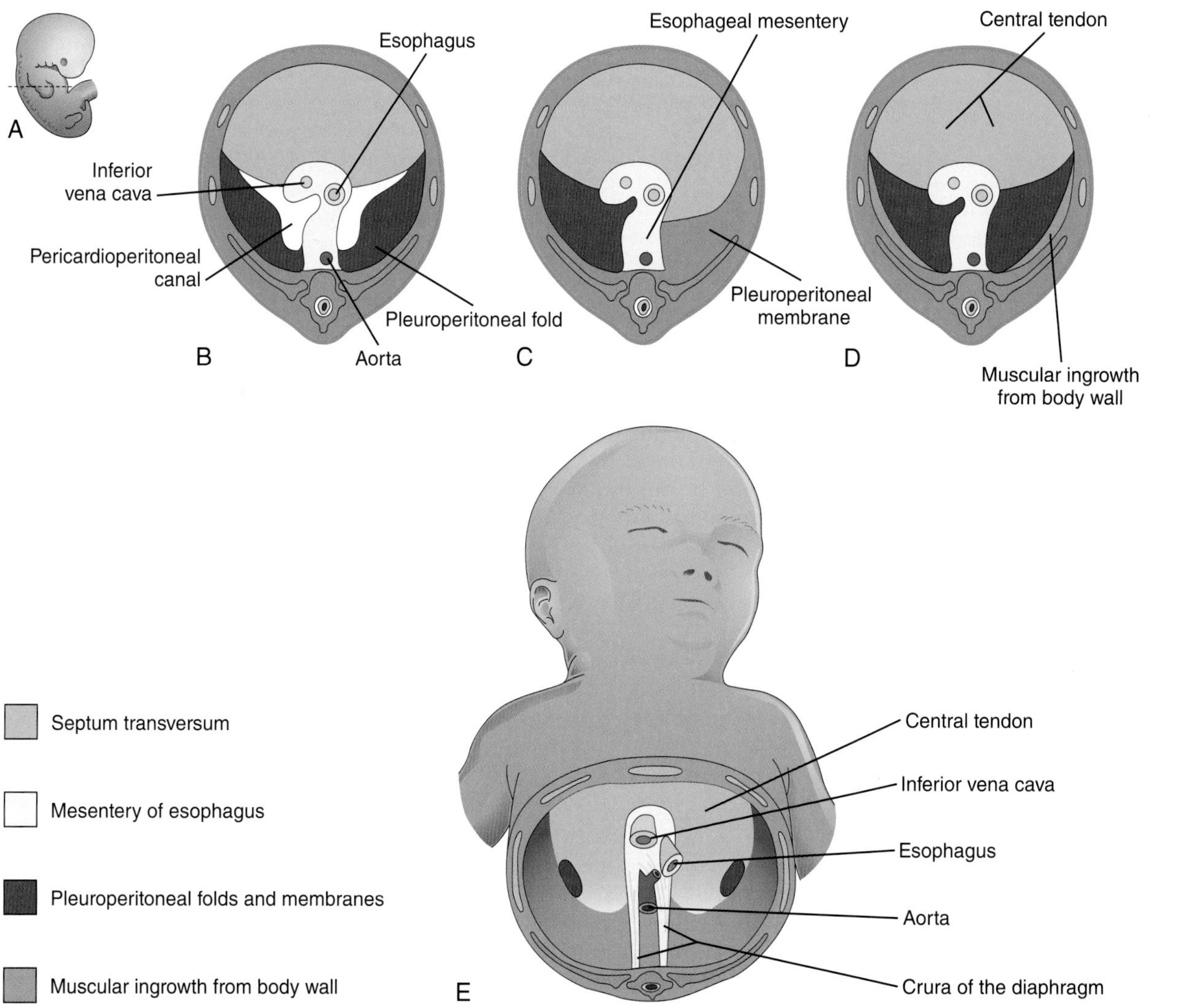

Fig. 8.7 Development of the diaphragm. (A) Lateral view of an embryo at the end of the fifth week (actual size) indicates the level of sections (B–D). (B) Transverse section shows the unfused pleuroperitoneal membranes. (C) Similar section at the end of the sixth week after fusion of the pleuroperitoneal membranes with the other two diaphragmatic components. (D) Transverse section of a 12-week fetus after ingrowth of the fourth diaphragmatic component from the body wall. (E) Inferior view of the diaphragm of a neonate indicates the embryologic origin of its components.

MUSCULAR INGROWTH FROM LATERAL BODY WALLS

During the ninth to 12th weeks, the lungs and pleural cavities enlarge, burrowing into the lateral body walls (see Fig. 8.5). During this process, the body-wall tissue is split into two layers:

- An external layer that becomes part of the definitive abdominal wall
- An internal layer that contributes to peripheral parts of the diaphragm, external to the parts derived from the pleuroperitoneal membranes (see Fig. 8.7D and E)

Further extension of the developing **pleural cavities** into the lateral body walls forms the **costodiaphragmatic recesses** (Fig. 8.8A and B), establishing the characteristic dome-shaped configuration of the diaphragm. After birth, the costodiaphragmatic recesses become alternately smaller and larger as the lungs move in and out during inspiration and expiration.

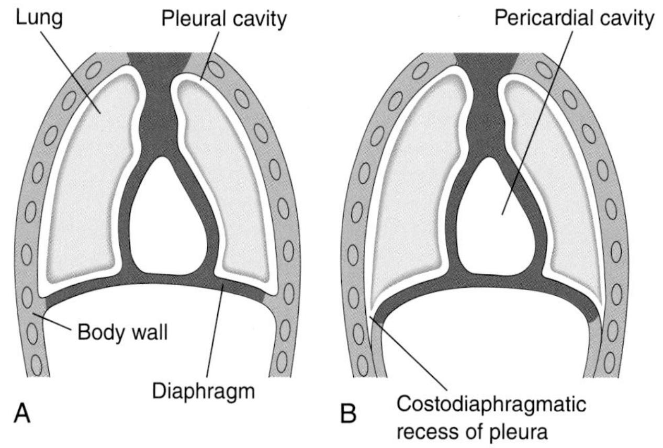

Fig. 8.8 (A and B) Extensions of the pleural cavities into the body walls form peripheral parts of the diaphragm and costodiaphragmatic recesses and establish the characteristic dome-shaped configuration of the diaphragm. Notice that body-wall tissue is added peripherally to the diaphragm as the lungs and pleural cavities enlarge.

POSITIONAL CHANGES AND INNERVATION OF DIAPHRAGM

During the fourth week of gestation, the septum transversum, before relocation of the heart, lies opposite the third to fifth cervical somites. During the fifth week, myoblasts from the third to the fifth cervical somites migrate into the developing diaphragm, bringing their nerve fibers with them. Consequently, the **phrenic nerves** that supply motor innervation to the diaphragm arise from the ventral primary rami of the third, fourth, and fifth cervical spinal nerves (see Fig. 8.5A and C). The three twigs on each side join to form a phrenic nerve. The phrenic nerves also supply sensory fibers to the superior and inferior surfaces of the right and left domes of the diaphragm.

The rapid growth of the dorsal part of the embryo's body results in an apparent descent of the diaphragm. By the sixth week, the diaphragm is at the level of the thoracic somites. The phrenic nerves now have a descending course. As the diaphragm appears relatively farther caudally in the body, the nerves are correspondingly lengthened. By the beginning of the eighth week, the dorsal part of the diaphragm lies at the level of the first lumbar vertebra. Because of the cervical origin of the phrenic nerves, they are approximately 30 cm long in adults.

The phrenic nerves in the embryo enter the diaphragm by passing through the pleuropericardial membranes. This explains why the phrenic nerves subsequently lie on the fibrous pericardium, the adult derivative of the pleuropericardial membranes (see Fig. 8.5C and D).

As the four parts of the diaphragm fuse (see Fig. 8.7), mesenchyme in the septum transversum extends into the other three parts. It forms myoblasts that differentiate into the skeletal muscle of the diaphragm. The costal border receives sensory fibers from the lower intercostal nerves because of the origin of the peripheral part of the diaphragm from the lateral body walls (see Fig. 8.7D and E).

Posterolateral Defect of Diaphragm

Congenital diaphragmatic hernia (CDH) is a defect in the diaphragm that may lead to herniation of abdominal contents (stomach and/or liver and/or intestine) into the thorax. CDH is classified according to its location in the diaphragm. The most common developmental defect of the diaphragm is a posterolateral defect (Figs. 8.9A and B and 8.10), which occurs in about 1 in 2200 neonates.

Life-threatening breathing difficulties may be associated with CDH because of inhibition of development and inflation of the lungs (Fig. 8.11). Moreover, fetal lung maturation may be delayed. **Polyhydramnios** (excess amniotic fluid) may also be present. The etiology and molecular pathways are not known but likely involve both environmental and multiple genetic factors (pathogenic variants in genes [mutations]). CDH is the most common cause of severe respiratory diseases, including pulmonary hypoplasia and pulmonary hypertension. *The candidate gene reported for CDH is a chromosome 15q26 gene pathogenic variant (mutation) that includes zinc finger formation (GATA6) and also transcription factors GATA4, ZFPM2, NR2F2, and WT1. Deletions in gene regions 8p23.1 and 4p16.3 have also been reported*. CDH, usually unilateral, results from defective formation and/or fusion of the pleuroperitoneal membranes with the other three parts of the diaphragm (see Fig. 8.7). This results in a large opening in the posterolateral region of the diaphragm. As a result, the peritoneal and pleural cavities are continuous with one another along the lumbocostal triangle at the posterior body wall. This birth defect (sometimes referred to as the *foramen of Bochdalek*) occurs on the left side in 85% to 90% of cases. The preponderance of left-sided defects may be related to the earlier closure of the right pleuroperitoneal opening. Prenatal diagnosis of CDH depends on ultrasound examination and MR imaging of abdominal organs in the thorax.

The pleuroperitoneal membranes normally fuse with the other three diaphragmatic components by the end of the sixth week of gestation (see Fig. 8.7C). If a pleuroperitoneal canal is still open when the intestines return to the abdomen from the physiological hernia of the umbilical cord in the 10th week, some of the intestines and other viscera may pass into the thorax. The presence of abdominal viscera in the thorax pushes the lungs and heart anteriorly and compresses the lungs. Often, the stomach, spleen, and most of the intestines herniate (see Fig. 8.11). Mortality in cases of CDH results not because there is a defect in the diaphragm or because the abdominal viscera are in the chest but because the lungs are hypoplastic due to compression during development.

The severity of pulmonary developmental abnormalities depends on when and to what extent the abdominal viscera herniate into the thorax (i.e., the timing and degree of compression of the fetal lungs). The effect on the ipsilateral lung is greater, but the contralateral lung also shows morphologic changes. If the abdominal viscera are in the thoracic cavity at birth, the initiation of respiration is likely to be impaired. The intestines dilate, and this compromises the functioning of the heart and lungs. Because the abdominal organs are most often on the left side of the thorax, the heart and mediastinum are usually displaced to the right.

The lungs in infants with CDH are often hypoplastic. The growth retardation of the lungs results from the lack of room for them to develop normally. Further complicating the neonatal course is the associated pulmonary hypertension resulting from decreased vascular cross-sectional area. Hypoxia may also trigger pulmonary vasoconstriction, which in some cases may be reversible with inhaled nitric oxide, a potent pulmonary vasodilator. The lungs often become aerated and achieve their normal size after the reduction (repositioning) of the herniated viscera and repair of the defect in the diaphragm. Prenatal detection of CDH occurs in about 50% of cases. Most infants with CDH now survive because of improvements in ventilator care.

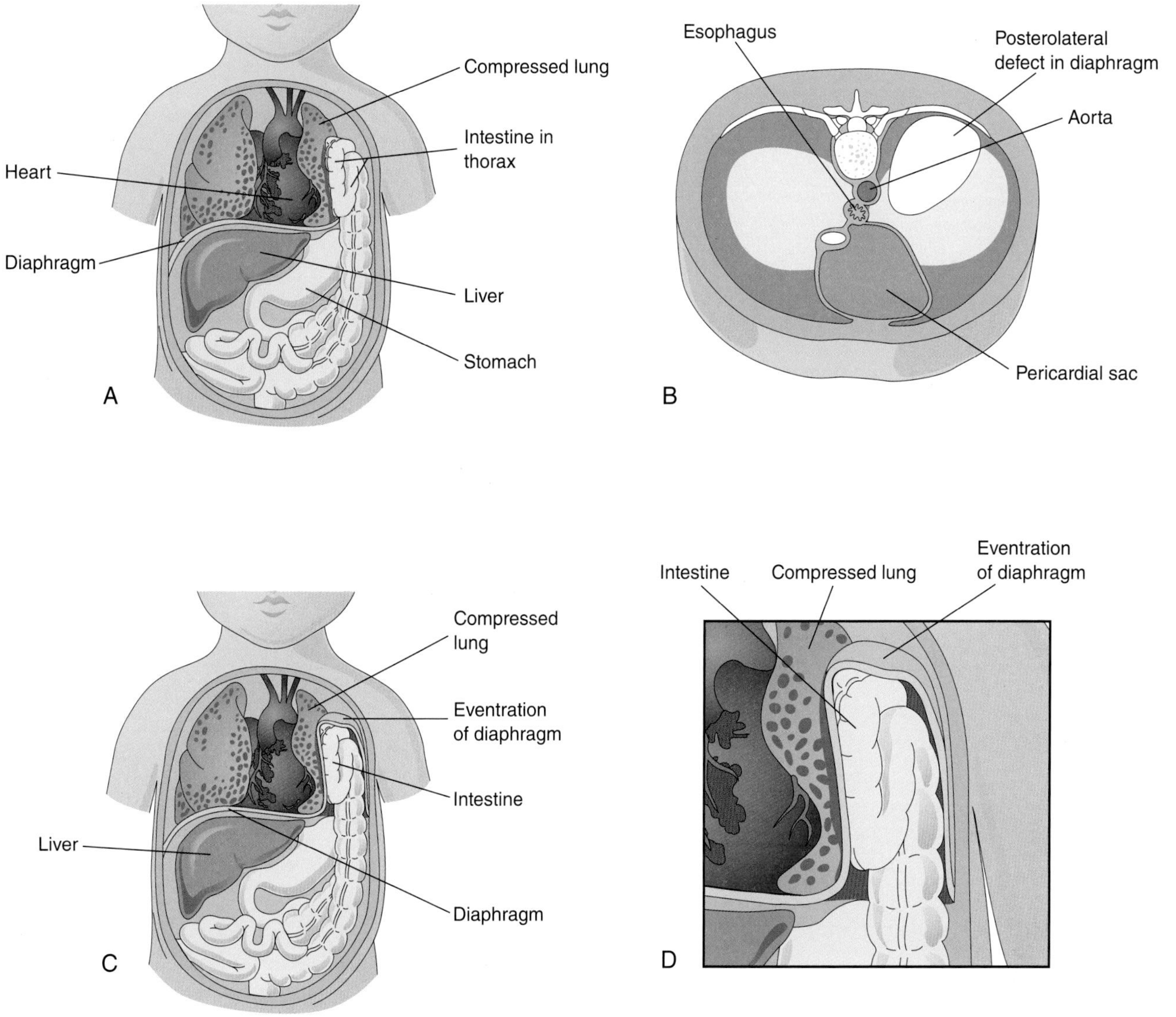

Fig. 8.9 (A) Diagram shows herniation of the intestine into the thorax through a posterolateral defect in the left side of the diaphragm. Notice that the left lung is compressed and hypoplastic. (B) Drawing of a diaphragm with a large posterolateral defect on the left side due to abnormal formation and/or abnormal fusion of the pleuroperitoneal membrane on the left side with the mesoesophagus and septum transversum. (C and D) Eventration of the diaphragm resulting from defective muscular development of the diaphragm. The abdominal viscera are displaced in the thorax within a pouch of diaphragmatic tissue.

Eventration of Diaphragm

In congenital eventration of the diaphragm, an uncommon condition, usually in the anteromedial region of the diaphragm, has defective musculature and balloons into the thoracic cavity as an aponeurotic (membranous) sheet, forming a **diaphragmatic pouch** (see Fig. 8.9C and D). The abdominal viscera are displaced superiorly into the pocket-like outpouching of the diaphragm. This defect results mainly from the failure of myoblasts (muscular tissue) from the body wall to extend into the pleuroperitoneal membrane on the affected side. Some cases of eventration of the diaphragm may be acquired as a result of phrenic nerve damage.

Eventration of the diaphragm is not a true diaphragmatic herniation; it is a superior displacement of viscera into a sac-like part of the diaphragm. However, the clinical manifestations of diaphragmatic eventration may simulate CDH.

Congenital Hiatal Hernia

Herniation of part of the fetal stomach may occur through an excessively large **esophageal hiatus**—the opening in the diaphragm through which the esophagus and the vagus nerves pass. A **hiatal hernia** is usually acquired during adult life; a congenitally enlarged esophageal hiatus may be the predisposing factor in some cases.

Retrosternal (Parasternal) Hernia

Herniations may occur through the **sternocostal hiatus** (also called the foramen of Morgagni)—the opening for the superior epigastric vessels in the retrosternal area. However, they are uncommon. This hiatus is located between the sternal and costal parts of the diaphragm. Herniation of the intestine into the pericardial sac may occur, or, conversely, part of the heart may descend into the peritoneal cavity in the epigastric region. Large defects are commonly associated with body-wall defects in the umbilical region. Radiologists and pathologists often observe fatty herniations through the sternocostal hiatus; however, they are usually of no clinical significance.

Accessory Diaphragm

More than 30 cases of the rare anomaly known as accessory diaphragm have been reported. It is a thin fibromuscular membrane, attached to the diaphragm anteriorly and extends posteriorly to the ribs. The accessory diaphragm is often on the right side and associated with lung hypoplasia and other respiratory complications. An accessory diaphragm can be diagnosed by magnetic resonance imaging or computed tomography. It is treated by surgical excision.

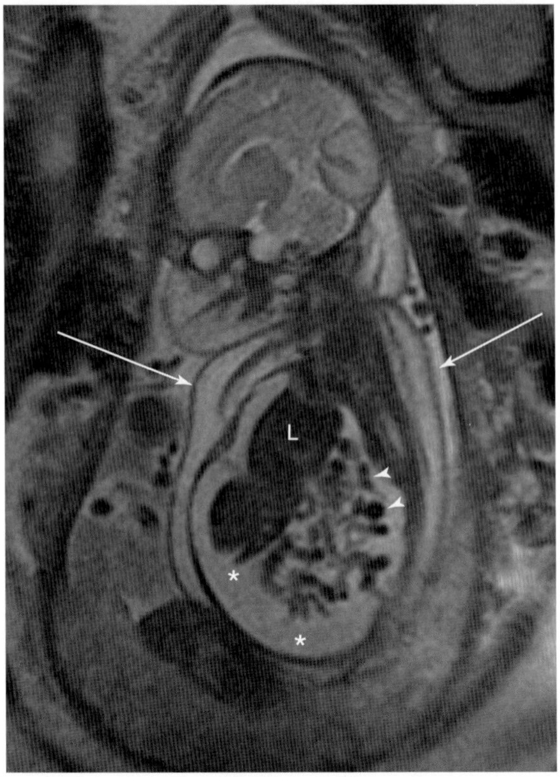

Fig. 8.10 Coronal magnetic resonance image of a fetus with right-sided congenital diaphragmatic hernia. Notice the liver *(L)* and loops of small intestine *(arrowheads)* in the thoracic cavity. Ascites are present *(asterisks)*, with the accumulation of serous fluid in the peritoneal cavity and extending into the thoracic cavity. *Arrows* indicate abnormal skin thickening. (Courtesy Deborah Levine, MD, Director of Obstetric and Gynecologic Ultrasound, Beth Israel Deaconess Medical Center, Boston, Massachusetts.)

SUMMARY OF DEVELOPMENT OF BODY CAVITIES, MESENTERIES, AND DIAPHRAGM

- The **intraembryonic coelom** begins to develop near the end of the third week. By the fourth week, it is a horseshoe-shaped cavity in the cardiogenic and lateral mesoderm. The bend in the cavity represents the future pericardial cavity, and its lateral extensions represent the future **pleural and peritoneal cavities**.
- During the folding of the embryonic disc in the fourth week (see Fig. 5.1B), lateral parts of the intraembryonic coelom move together on the ventral aspect of the embryo. When the caudal part of the ventral mesentery disappears, the right and left parts of the intraembryonic coelom merge to form the **peritoneal cavity**.
- As the peritoneal parts of the intraembryonic coelom come together, the splanchnic layer of mesoderm encloses the primordial gut and suspends it from the dorsal body wall by a double-layered peritoneal membrane, the **dorsal mesentery**.
- The parts of the parietal layer of mesoderm lining the peritoneal, pleural, and pericardial cavities become the parietal peritoneum, parietal pleura, and serous pericardium, respectively.
- By the seventh week, the embryonic pericardial cavity communicates with the peritoneal cavity through paired **pericardioperitoneal canals**. During the fifth and sixth weeks, folds (later to become membranes) form near the cranial and caudal ends of the canals.
- Fusion of the cranial pleuropericardial membranes with mesoderm ventral to the esophagus separates the **pericardial cavity** from the **pleural cavities**. Fusion of the caudal pleuroperitoneal membranes during the formation of the diaphragm separates the pleural cavities from the peritoneal cavity.
- The diaphragm develops from the septum transversum, mesentery of the esophagus, pleuroperitoneal folds and membranes, and muscular outgrowth from the body wall.
- The **diaphragm** divides the body cavity into thoracic and peritoneal cavities.
- **Congenital diaphragmatic hernia** (CDH) is a developmental defect in the diaphragm. It is classified according to its location. A defect (opening) in the pleuroperitoneal membrane on the left side may cause herniation of abdominal contents (stomach and intestine) into the thorax.

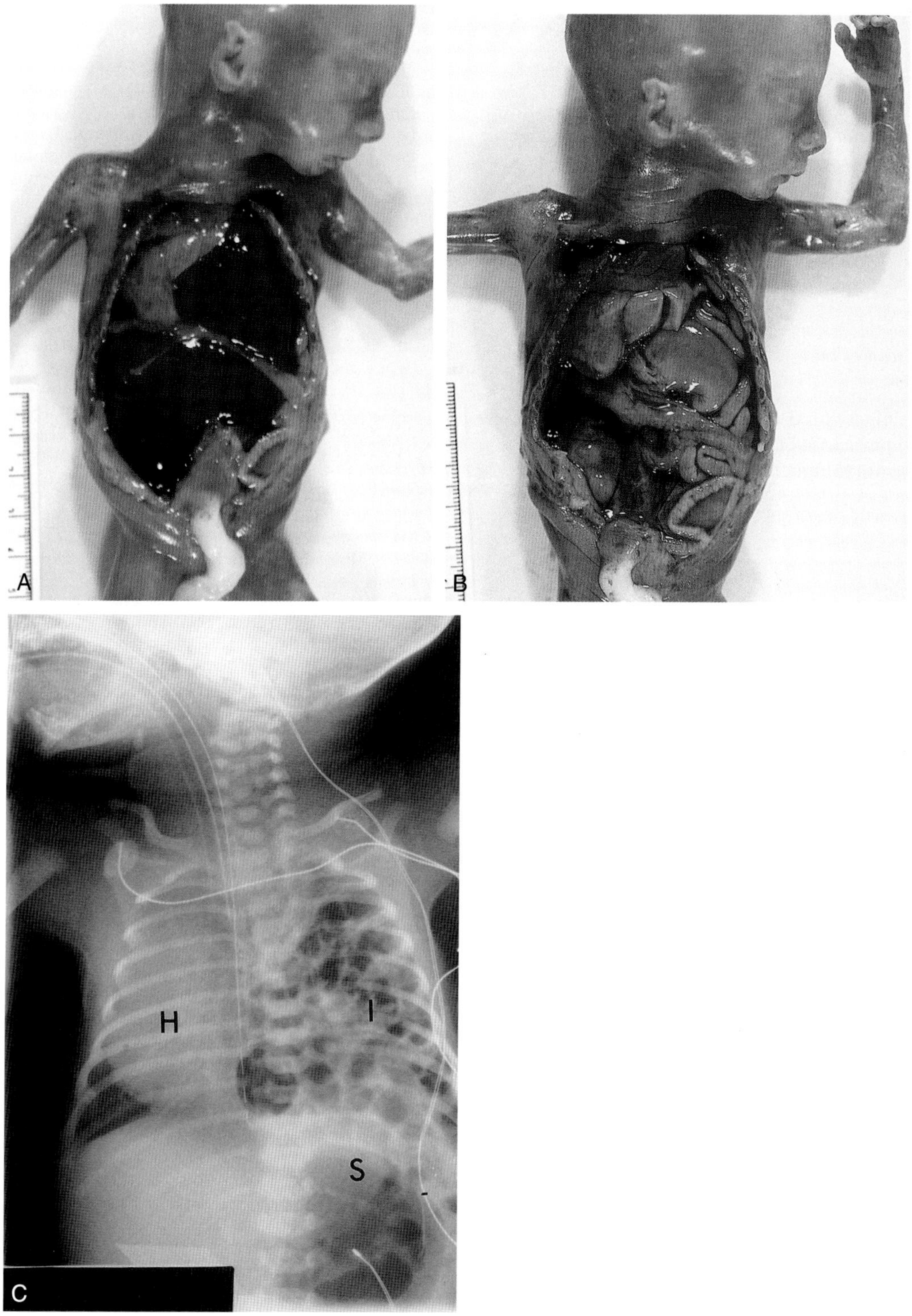

Fig. 8.11 Diaphragmatic hernia on the left side of a female fetus (19–20 weeks) with herniation of liver (A), stomach, and bowel (B) underneath the liver into left thoracic cavity. Notice the pulmonary hypoplasia visible after liver removal. (C) Diaphragmatic hernia (posterolateral defect). Chest radiograph of a neonate shows herniation of intestinal loops *(I)* into the left side of the thorax. Notice that the heart *(H)* is displaced to the right side and that the stomach *(S)* is on the left side of the upper abdominal cavity. ((A and B) Courtesy Dr. D.K. Kalousek, Department of Pathology, University of British Columbia, Children's Hospital, Vancouver, British Columbia, Canada. (C) Courtesy Dr. Prem S. Sahni, formerly of the Department of Radiology, Children's Hospital, Winnipeg, Manitoba, Canada.)

CLINICALLY ORIENTED PROBLEMS

CASE 8-1

A neonate had severe respiratory distress. The abdomen was unusually flat, and intestinal peristaltic movements were heard over the left side of the thorax.

- What birth defect do you think this is?
- Explain the basis of the signs described.
- How would the diagnosis likely be established?

CASE 8-2

An ultrasound scan of an infant's thorax revealed an intestine in the pericardial sac.

- What birth defect could result in herniation of the intestine into the pericardial cavity?
- What is the embryologic basis of this defect?

CASE 8-3

CDH was diagnosed prenatally during an ultrasound examination.

- How common is a posterolateral defect of the diaphragm?
- How do you think a neonate in whom this diagnosis is suspected should be positioned?
- Why would this positional treatment be given?
- Briefly describe the surgical repair of a CDH.

CASE 8-4

A baby was born with a hernia in the median plane, between the xiphoid process and the umbilicus.

- What is this type of hernia called?
- Is it common?
- What is the embryologic basis of this birth defect?

Discussion of these problems appears in the Appendix at the back of the book.

BIBLIOGRAPHY AND SUGGESTED READING

Ariza L, Carmona R, Cañete A, Cano E, Muñoz-Chápuli R: Coelomic epithelium-derived cells in visceral morphogenesis, *Dev Dyn* 245:307, 2016.

Badillo A, Gingalewski C: Congenital diaphragmatic hernia: treatment and outcome, *Semin Perinatol* 38:92, 2014.

Brosens E, Peters NCJ, van Weelden KS, et al: Unraveling the genetics of congenital diaphragmatic hernia: an ongoing challenge, *Front Pediatr* 9:800915, 2022. https://doi.org/10.3389/fped.2021.800915

Cannata G, Caporilli C, Grassi F, Perrone S, Esposito S: Management of congenital diaphragmatic hernia (CDH): role of molecular genetics, *Int J Mol Sci* 22(12):6353, 2021. https://doi.org/10.3390/ijms22126353. Published 2021 Jun 14.

Donahoe PK, Longoni M, High FA: Polygenic causes of congenital diaphragmatic hernia produce common lung pathologies, *Am J Pathol* 186:2532, 2016.

Groth SS, Andrade RS: Diaphragmatic eventration, *Thorac Surg Clin* 19:511, 2009.

Hedrick HL: Management of prenatally diagnosed congenital diaphragmatic hernia, *Semin Pediatr Surg* 22:37, 2013.

Kim W, Courtier J, Morin C, et al: Postnatal MRI for CDH: a pictorial review of late-presenting and recurrent diaphragmatic defects, *Clin Imaging* 43:1582017, 2017.

Koo CW, Johnson TF, Gierada DS, et al: The breadth of the diaphragm: updates in embryogenesis and role of imaging, *Br J Radiol* 91(1088):20170600, 2018. https://doi.org/10.1259/bjr.20170600

Mayer S, Metzger R, Kluth D: The embryology of the diaphragm, *Semin Pediatr Surg* 20:161, 2011.

Moore KL, Dalley AF, Agur AMR: *Clinically oriented anatomy,* ed 8 Baltimore, 2018, Williams & Wilkins.

Oh T, Chan S, Kieffer S: Fetal outcomes of prenatally diagnosed congenital diaphragmatic hernia: nine years of clinical experience in a Canadian tertiary hospital, *J Obstet Gynaecol Can* 38:17, 2016.

Pechriggl E, Blumer M, Tubbs RS, Olewnik Ł, Konschake M, Fortélny R, et al: Embryology of the abdominal wall and associated malformations-a review, *Front Surg* 9:891–896, 2022. https://doi.org/10.3389/fsurg.2022.891896. Published 07 July 2022

Wells LJ: Development of the human diaphragm and pleural sacs, *Contrib Embryol* 35:107, 1954.

Yu L, Hernan RR, Wynn J, Chung WK: The influence of genetics in congenital diaphragmatic hernia, *Semin Perinatol* 44(1):151169, 2020. https://doi.org/10.1053/j.semperi.2019.07.008

Pharyngeal Apparatus, Face, and Neck

9

CHAPTER OUTLINE

The **pharyngeal apparatus** consists of pharyngeal arches, pouches, grooves, and membranes (Fig. 9.1). These early embryonic structures contribute to the formation of the face, neck, and associated organs.

PHARYNGEAL ARCHES

7

The **pharyngeal arches** begin to develop early in the fourth week as **neural crest cells** migrate into the future head and neck regions (see Fig. 5.5). The first pair of arches, the primordial jaws, appears as surface elevations lateral to the developing pharynx (see Fig. 9.1A and B). Other arches soon appear as ridges on each side of the future head and neck regions (see Fig. 9.1C and D). By the end of the fourth week, four pairs of arches are visible externally (see Fig. 9.1D). The fifth and sixth arches are rudimentary and are not visible on the surface of the embryo. *The identity and fate of individual arches are determined by the migrating neural crest cells and the expression of Hox genes. Sonic hedgehog (Shh) and homeobox gene* Dlx2 *signaling play an important role in the formation and patterning (anterior-posterior and dorsoventral axes) of the pharyngeal arches.*

The pharyngeal arches are separated by **pharyngeal grooves** (clefts). Like the arches, the grooves are numbered in a craniocaudal sequence (see Fig. 9.1D). The **first arch** separates into the maxillary and mandibular prominences (Fig. 9.2; see Fig. 9.1E). The **maxillary prominence** forms the maxilla, zygomatic bone, and a portion of the vomer bone. The **mandibular prominence** forms the mandible and squamous temporal bone. Along with the third arch, the **second arch** contributes to the formation of the hyoid bone.

The arches support the lateral walls of the **primordial pharynx**, which is derived from the cranial part of the foregut. The **stomodeum** (primordial mouth) initially appears as a slight depression of the surface ectoderm (see Fig. 9.1D and G). It is separated from the cavity of the primordial pharynx by a bilaminar membrane, the **oropharyngeal membrane**, which is composed of ectoderm externally and endoderm internally (see Fig. 9.1E and F). This membrane ruptures at approximately 26 days, bringing the primordial pharynx and foregut into communication with the amniotic cavity. Persistence of the oropharyngeal membrane may result in orofacial defects. The ectodermal lining of the first arch forms the oral epithelium.

PHARYNGEAL ARCH COMPONENTS

Each arch consists of a core of **mesenchyme** (embryonic connective tissue) and is covered externally by ectoderm and internally by endoderm (see Fig. 9.1H and I). Originally, the mesenchyme is derived during the third week from mesoderm. During the fourth week, most of the mesenchyme is derived from **neural crest cells** that migrate into the arches. Migration of the multipotent neural crest stem cells into the arches is determined by the expression of paralogue groups of *Hox* genes (*Hox1-Hox4*) in the hindbrain. Their differentiation into mesenchyme produces the **maxillary** and **mandibular prominences** (see Fig. 9.2) in addition to all connective tissue, including the dermis and smooth muscle.

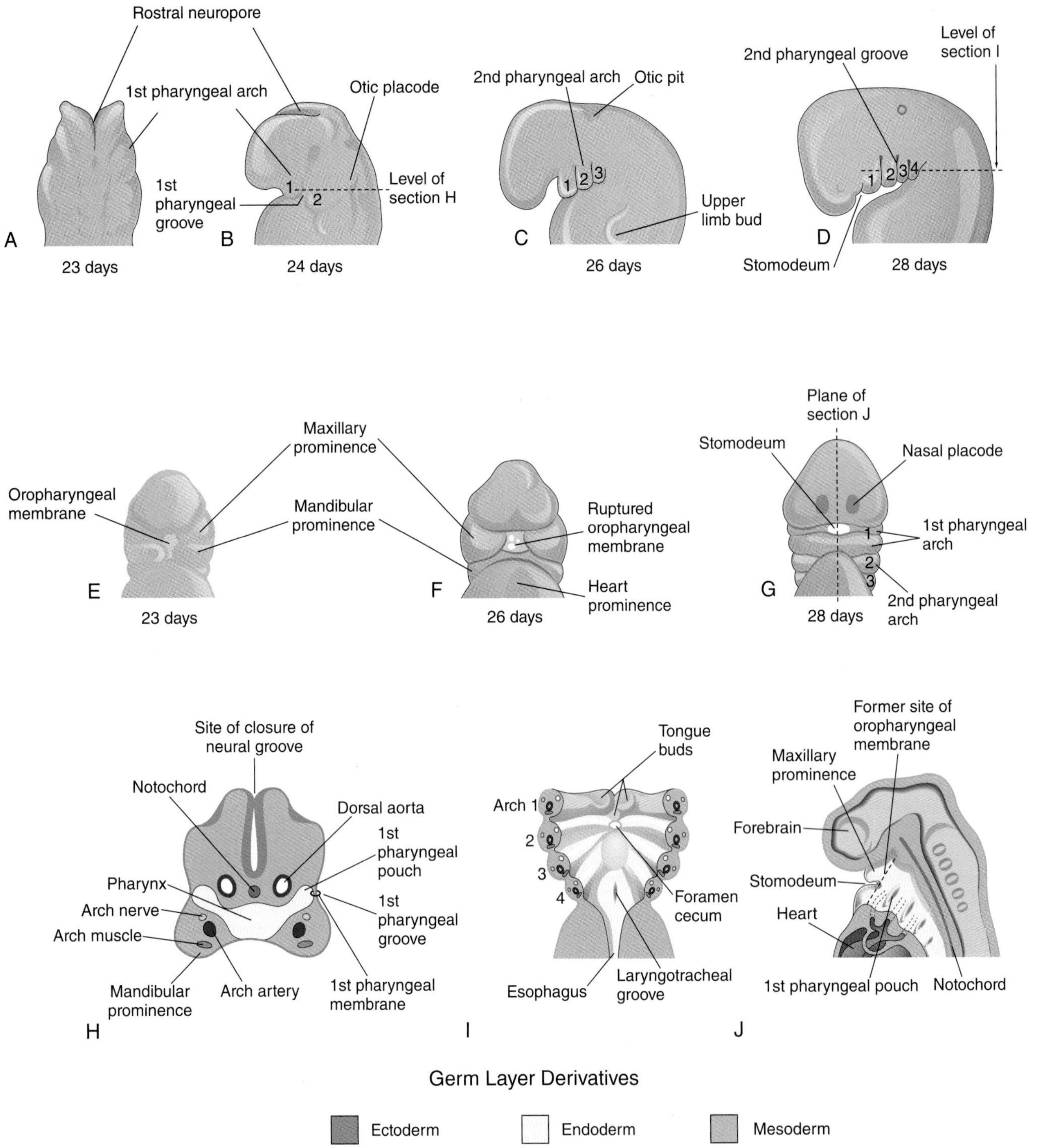

Fig. 9.1 Pharyngeal apparatus. (A) Dorsal view of the upper part of a 23-day embryo. (B–D) Lateral views show later development of the pharyngeal arches. (E–G) Ventral or facial views show the relationship of the first arch to the stomodeum. (H) Horizontal section through the cranial region of an embryo. (I) Similar section shows the arch components and floor of the primordial pharynx. (J) Sagittal section of the cranial region of an embryo shows the openings of the pouches in the lateral wall of the primordial pharynx.

Coincident with the immigration of neural crest cells, **myogenic mesoderm** from paraxial regions moves into each arch, forming a central core of **muscle primordium**. Endothelial cells in the arches are derived from the lateral mesoderm and invasive **angioblasts** (cells that differentiate into blood vessel endothelium) that move into the arches. The endothelium of the pharyngeal arches 3 to 6 is derived from endothelial progenitors of the second heart field. The **pharyngeal endoderm** plays an essential role in regulating the development of the arches.

A typical pharyngeal arch contains several structures:

- An **artery** arises from the **truncus arteriosus** of the primordial heart (Fig. 9.3B) and passes around the primordial pharynx to enter the dorsal aorta.

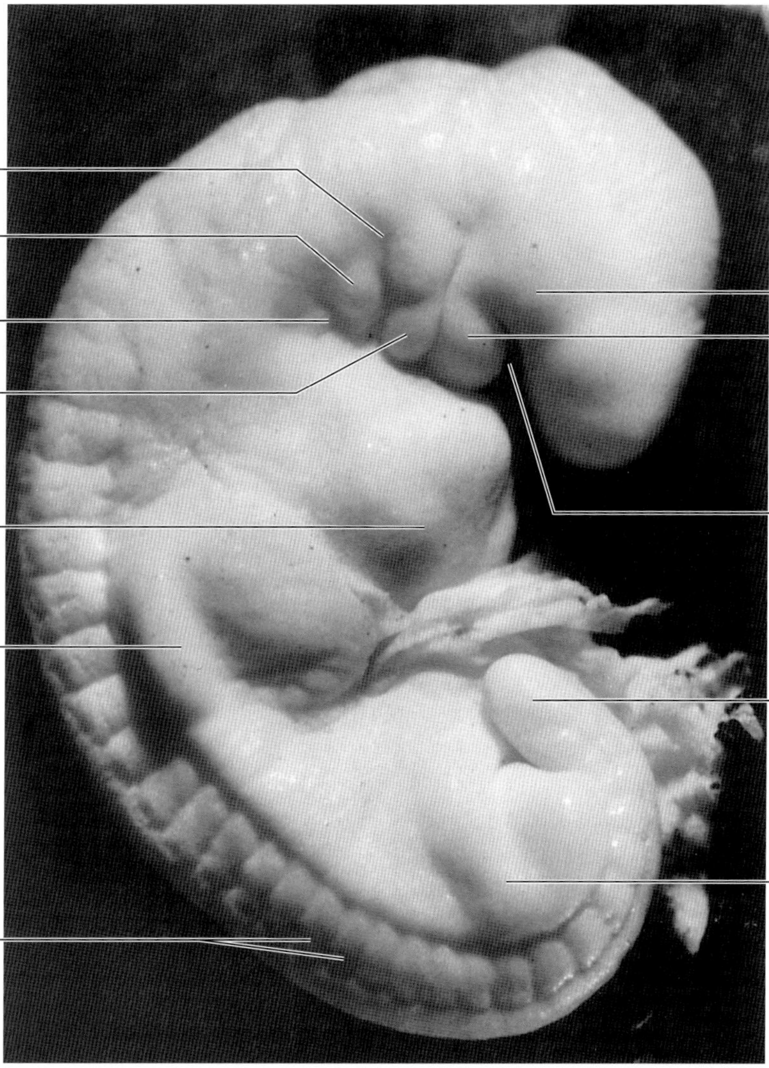

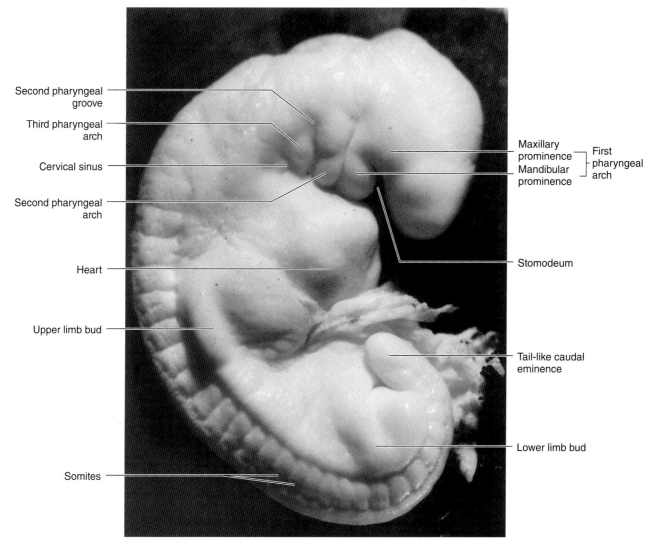

Fig. 9.2 Photograph of a stage 13, 4.5-week human embryo. (Courtesy the late Professor Emeritus Dr. K.V. Hinrichsen, Medizinische Fakultät, Institut für Anatomie, Ruhr-Universität Bochum, Bochum, Germany.)

- A **cartilaginous rod** forms the skeleton of the arch.
- A **muscular component** differentiates into muscles in the head and neck.
- **Sensory and motor nerves** supply the mucosa (tissue lining) and muscles derived from each arch. The nerves that grow into the arches are derived from the neuroectoderm of the primordial brain.

FATE OF PHARYNGEAL ARCHES

The arches contribute extensively to the formation of the face, nasal cavities, mouth, larynx, pharynx, and neck (see Figs. 9.3 and 9.25). During the fifth week, the second arch enlarges and overgrows the third and fourth arches, forming an ectodermal depression, the **cervical sinus** (see Figs. 9.2 and 9.7). By the end of the seventh week, the second to fourth grooves and cervical sinus have disappeared, giving the neck a smooth contour.

DERIVATIVES OF PHARYNGEAL ARCH CARTILAGES

The dorsal end of the **first arch cartilage** (Meckel cartilage) is closely related to the developing ear. Early in development, small nodules break away from the proximal part of the cartilage and form two of the middle ear bones, the **malleus** and **incus** (Fig. 9.4 and Table 9.1). The middle part of the cartilage regresses, but its **perichondrium** (connective tissue membrane around cartilage) forms the **anterior ligament of the malleus** and **sphenomandibular ligament**.

Ventral parts of the first arch cartilages form the horseshoe-shaped primordium of the mandible, and by keeping pace with its growth, they guide its early morphogenesis. Each half of the mandible forms lateral to and in close association with its cartilage. The first arch cartilage disappears as the mandible develops around it by **intramembranous ossification** (see Fig. 9.4B). TGF-β *signaling, homeobox genes (*BMP, PRRX1, *and* PRRX2*), and fibroblast growth factors regulate the morphogenesis of the mandible.*

An independent cartilage, the **anlage** (primordium) near the dorsal end of the **second arch cartilage** (Reichert cartilage), participates in ear development. It contributes to the formation of the **stapes** of the middle ear and the **styloid process of the temporal bone** (see Fig. 9.4B). The cartilage between the styloid process and hyoid bone regresses; its perichondrium forms the **stylohyoid ligament**. The ventral

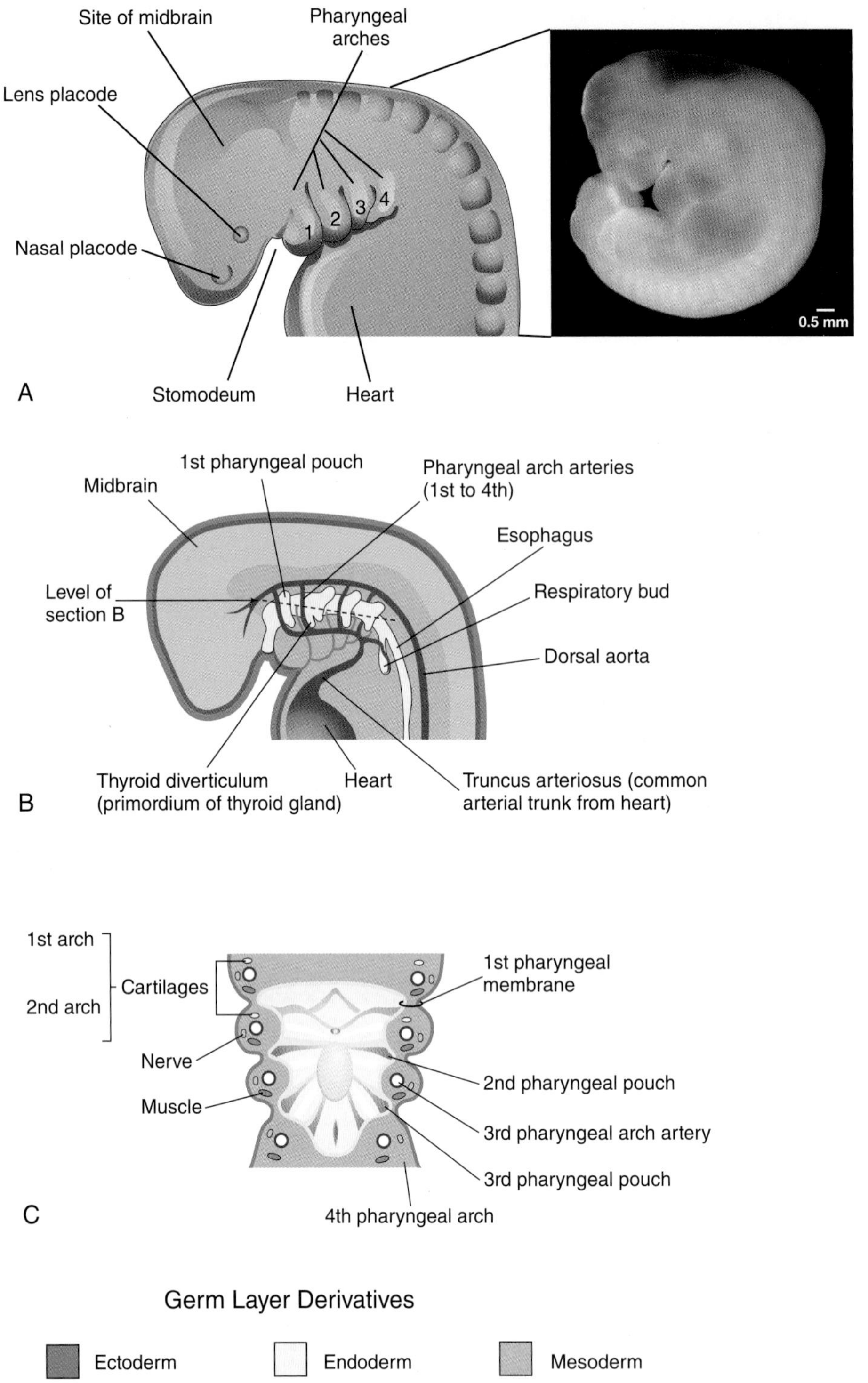

Fig. 9.3 (A) Drawing of the head, neck, and thoracic regions of an embryo at approximately 28 days' gestation shows the pharyngeal apparatus. *Inset*, Photograph of an embryo of approximately the same age as shown in (A). (B) Schematic drawing shows the pouches and arch arteries. (C) Horizontal section through the embryo shows the floor of the primordial pharynx and the germ layer of origin of the arch components. (*Inset*, Courtesy Dr. Bradley R. Smith, University of Michigan, Ann Arbor, Michigan.)

end of the second arch cartilage ossifies to form the hyoid **lesser cornu** (lesser horn; see Fig. 9.4B).

The **third arch cartilage**, located in the ventral part of the arch, ossifies to form the **greater cornu** of the hyoid bone and the superior cornu of the thyroid cartilage. The **body of the hyoid bone** is formed by the hypobranchial eminence (see Fig. 9.23).

The **fourth and sixth arch cartilages** fuse to form the **laryngeal cartilages** (see Fig. 9.4B and Table 9.1), except for the epiglottis. The cartilage of the epiglottis develops from mesenchyme in the **hypopharyngeal eminence** (see Fig. 9.23A), a prominence in the floor of the embryonic pharynx that is derived from the third and fourth arches. The **fifth arch**, if present, is rudimentary and has no derivatives.

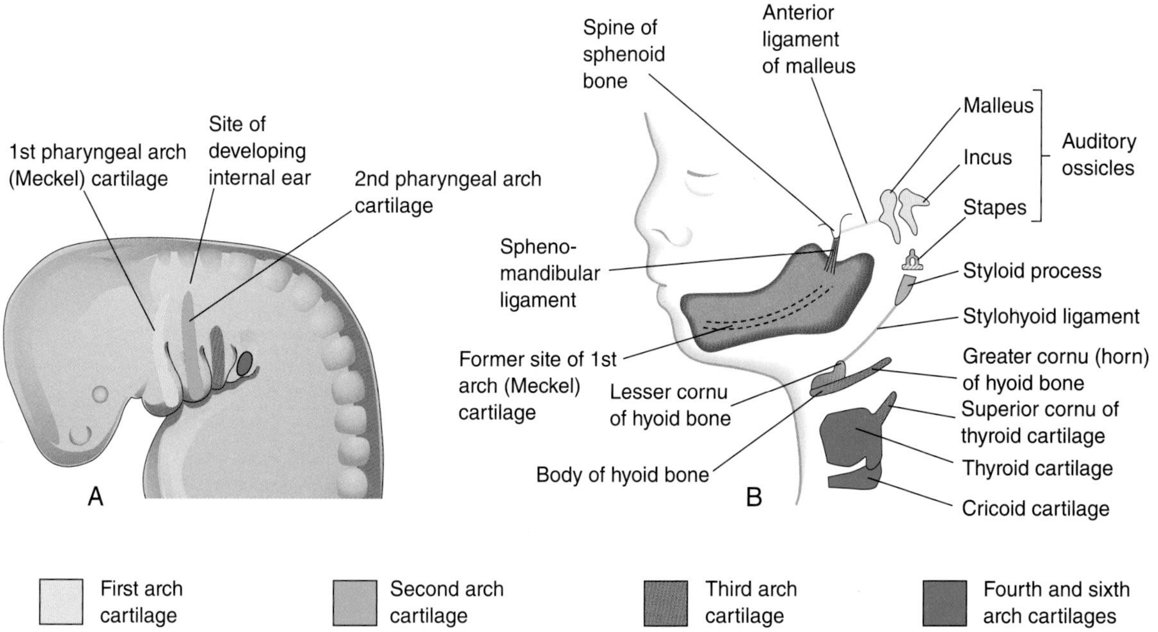

Fig. 9.4 (A) Schematic lateral view of the head, neck, and thoracic regions of a 4-week embryo shows the location of the cartilages in the pharyngeal arches. (B) Similar view of a 24-week fetus shows the derivatives of the arch cartilages. The mandible is formed by intramembranous ossification of mesenchymal tissue surrounding the first arch cartilage. The cartilage acts as a template for the development of the mandible but does not contribute directly to its formation. Occasionally, ossification of the second arch cartilage may extend from the styloid process along the stylohyoid ligament. When this occurs, it may cause pain in the region of the palatine tonsil.

Table 9.1 Structures Derived From Pharyngeal Arch Components

Arches[a]	Cranial Nerves	Muscles	Skeletal Structures	Ligaments
First (mandibular)	Trigeminal (CN V)[b]	Muscles of mastication[c] Mylohyoid and anterior belly of digastric Tensor tympani Tensor veli palatini	Malleus Incus	Anterior ligament of malleus Sphenomandibular ligament
Second (hyoid)	Facial (CN VII)	Muscles of facial expression[d] Stapedius Stylohyoid Posterior belly of digastric	Stapes Styloid process Upper part of the body and lesser cornu of the hyoid bone	Stylohyoid ligament
Third	Glossopharyngeal (CN IX)	Stylopharyngeus	Lower part of the body and greater cornu of the hyoid bone Superior cornu of the thyroid cartilage	
Fourth and sixth[e]	Superior laryngeal branch of vagus (CN X) Recurrent laryngeal branch of vagus (CN X)	Cricothyroid Levator veli palatini Constrictors of pharynx Intrinsic muscles of the larynx Striated muscles of the esophagus	Thyroid cartilage Cricoid cartilage Arytenoid cartilage Corniculate cartilage Cuneiform cartilage Body of hyoid bone	

[a]The derivatives of the pharyngeal arch arteries are described in Fig. 13.38.
[b]The ophthalmic division of the fifth cranial nerve (CN V) does not supply any pharyngeal arch components.
[c]Temporalis, masseter, medial, and lateral pterygoids.
[d]Buccinator, auricularis, frontalis, platysma, orbicularis oris, and orbicularis oculi.
[e]The fifth pharyngeal arch is often absent. When present, it is rudimentary and usually has no recognizable cartilage bar. The cartilaginous components of the fourth and sixth arches fuse to form the cartilages of the larynx.

DERIVATIVES OF PHARYNGEAL ARCH MUSCLES

The muscular components of the arches derived from unsegmented paraxial mesoderm and **prechordal plate** form various muscles in the head and neck. The musculature of the first arch forms the **muscles of mastication** and other muscles (Fig. 9.5; see Table 9.1). The musculature of the second arch forms the **stapedius**, stylohyoid, posterior belly of digastric, auricular, and **muscles of facial expression**. The musculature of the third arch forms the **stylopharyngeus**. The musculature of the fourth arch forms the **cricothyroid**, **levator veli palatini**, and **constrictors of the pharynx**. The musculature of the sixth arch forms the intrinsic muscles of the larynx.

DERIVATIVES OF PHARYNGEAL ARCH NERVES

Each arch is supplied by its **cranial nerve** (CN). The special visceral efferent (branchial) components of these nerves supply muscles derived from the arches (Fig. 9.6; see Table 9.1). Because mesenchyme from the arches contributes to the dermis and mucous membranes of the head and neck, these areas are supplied with special visceral afferent nerves.

The facial skin is supplied by the **trigeminal nerve** (CN V); however, only its caudal two branches (maxillary and mandibular) supply derivatives of the first arch (see Fig. 9.6B). CN V is the principal sensory nerve of the head and neck and is the motor nerve for the muscles of mastication (see Table 9.1). Its sensory branches innervate the face, teeth, and mucous membranes of nasal cavities, palate, mouth, and tongue (see Fig. 9.6C).

The **facial nerve** (CN VII), **glossopharyngeal nerve** (CN IX), and **vagus nerve** (CN X) supply the second, third, and fourth to sixth (caudal) arches, respectively. The fourth arch is supplied by the superior laryngeal branch of CN X and by its recurrent laryngeal branch. The nerves of the second to sixth arches have little cutaneous distribution (see Fig. 9.6C), but they innervate the mucous membranes of the tongue, pharynx, and larynx.

PHARYNGEAL POUCHES

The **primordial pharynx**, which is derived from the foregut, widens cranially as it joins the **stomodeum** (see Figs. 9.3A and B and 9.4B) and narrows as it joins the esophagus. The endoderm of the pharynx lines the internal aspects of the arches and the **pharyngeal pouches** (see Figs. 9.1H–J and 9.3B and C). The pouches develop as outpocketing of the endoderm in a craniocaudal sequence between the arches. The first pair of pouches, for example, lies between the first and second arches. Four pairs of pouches are well defined; the fifth pair (if present) is rudimentary. The endoderm of the pouches contacts the ectoderm of the pharyngeal grooves, and they form the double-layered **pharyngeal membranes** that separate the pouches from the grooves (see Figs. 9.1H and 9.3C). *Retinoic acid, Wnt, and fibroblast growth factor (Fgf) signaling play an essential role in the formation and differentiation of the pharyngeal pouches.*

DERIVATIVES OF PHARYNGEAL POUCHES

7

The endodermal epithelial lining of the pouches forms important organs in the head and neck.

FIRST PHARYNGEAL POUCH

The first pouch expands into an elongated **tubotympanic recess** (Fig. 9.7B). The expanded distal part of this recess contacts the first groove, where it later contributes to the

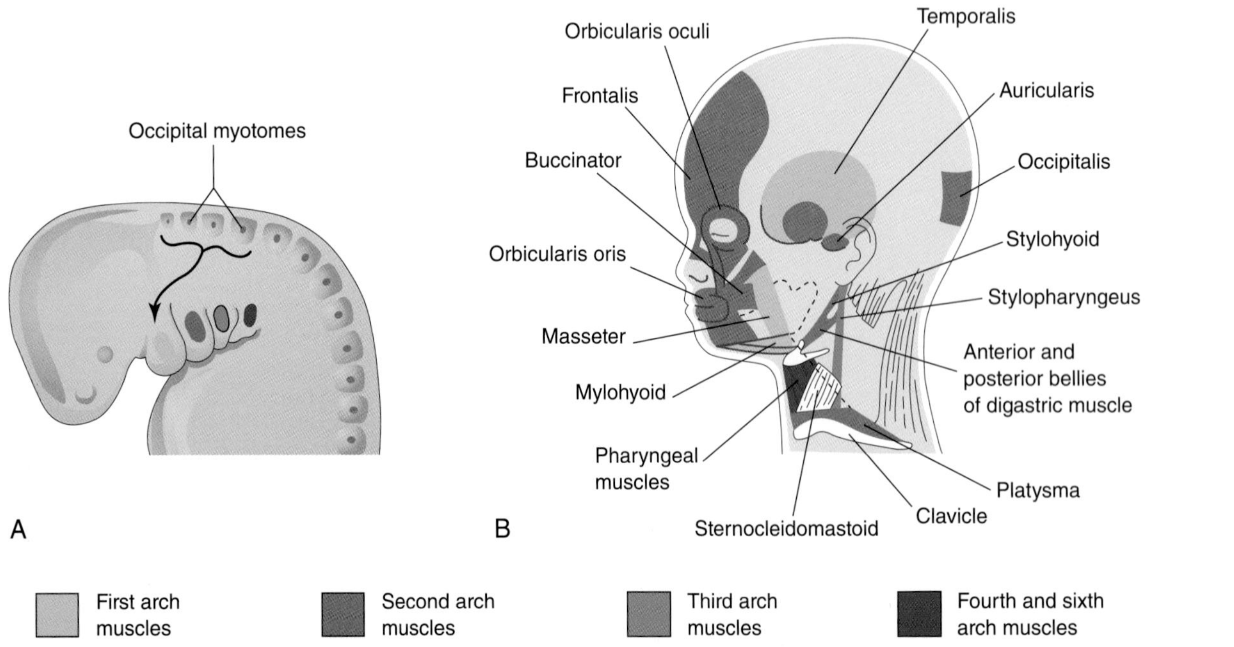

Fig. 9.5 (A) Lateral view of the head, neck, and thoracic regions of a 4-week embryo shows the muscles derived from the pharyngeal arches. The *arrow* shows the pathway taken by myoblasts from the occipital myotomes to form the tongue musculature. (B) Sketch of the dissected head and neck regions of a 20-week fetus shows the muscles derived from the arches. Parts of the platysma and sternocleidomastoid muscles have been removed to show the deeper muscles. The myoblasts from the second arch migrate from the neck to the head, where they give rise to the muscles of facial expression. These muscles are supplied by the facial nerve (cranial nerve VII), which is the nerve of the second arch.

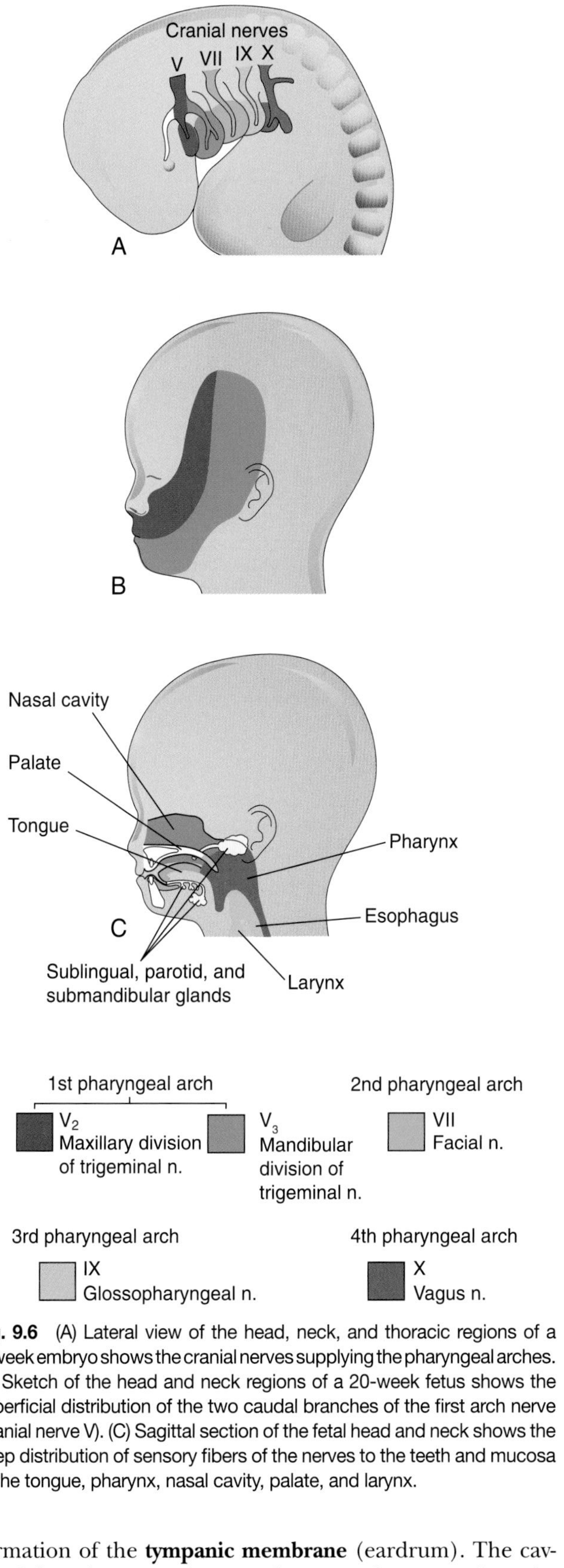

Fig. 9.6 (A) Lateral view of the head, neck, and thoracic regions of a 4-week embryo shows the cranial nerves supplying the pharyngeal arches. (B) Sketch of the head and neck regions of a 20-week fetus shows the superficial distribution of the two caudal branches of the first arch nerve (cranial nerve V). (C) Sagittal section of the fetal head and neck shows the deep distribution of sensory fibers of the nerves to the teeth and mucosa of the tongue, pharynx, nasal cavity, palate, and larynx.

formation of the **tympanic membrane** (eardrum). The cavity of the tubotympanic recess becomes the **tympanic cavity** and **mastoid antrum**. The connection of the tubotympanic recess with the pharynx gradually elongates to form the **pharyngotympanic tube** (auditory tube).

SECOND PHARYNGEAL POUCH

Although the second pouch is largely obliterated as the palatine tonsil develops, part of the cavity of this pouch remains as the **tonsillar sinus** (fossa), the depression between the **palatoglossal** and **palatopharyngeal arches** (Fig. 9.8; see Fig. 9.7C). The endoderm of the second pouch proliferates and grows into the underlying mesenchyme. The central parts of these buds break down, forming **tonsillar crypts**. The pouch endoderm forms the surface epithelium and lining of the tonsillar crypts. At approximately 20 weeks, the mesenchyme around the crypts differentiates into **lymphoid tissue**, which soon organizes into the **lymphatic nodules** of the palatine tonsil (see Fig. 9.7C). Initial lymphoid cell infiltration occurs at approximately the seventh month, with germinal centers forming in the neonatal period and active germinal centers within the first year of life.

THIRD PHARYNGEAL POUCH

The third pouch expands and forms a solid, dorsal, bulbar part and a hollow, elongated, ventral part (see Fig. 9.7B). Its connection with the pharynx is reduced to a narrow duct that soon degenerates. By the sixth week, the epithelium of each ***dorsal bulbar part*** of the pouch begins to differentiate into an **inferior parathyroid gland**. The epithelium of the elongated ***ventral parts*** of the pouch proliferates, obliterating their cavities. These parts come together in the median plane to form the **thymus**, which is a primary lymphoid organ (see Fig. 9.7C). The bilobed structure of this lymphatic organ remains throughout life, discretely encapsulated.

Each lobe has its own blood supply, lymphatic drainage, and nerve supply. The developing **thymus** and **inferior parathyroid glands** lose their connections with the pharynx when the brain and associated structures expand rostrally, and the pharynx and cardiac structures expand caudally. The derivatives of pouches two to four become displaced caudally. Later, the **parathyroid glands** separate from the thymus and lie on the dorsal surface of the thyroid gland (see Figs. 9.7C and 9.8). *The parathormone, GATA3, Gcm2, Sox3, fibroblast growth factor–signaling pathways, acting through fibroblast growth factor receptor substrate 2 (FRS2), are involved in the development of the thymus and parathyroid glands. Pathogenic variants (mutation) of the parathormone gene may lead to primary hypoparathyroidism.*

HISTOGENESIS OF THYMUS

The thymus is a primary lymphoid organ that develops from epithelial cells derived from the endoderm of the third pair of pouches and from mesenchyme into which epithelial tubes grow. The tubes soon become solid cords that proliferate and form side branches. Each side branch becomes the core of a lobule of the thymus. Some cells of the epithelial cords become arranged around a central point, forming small groups of degenerated reticular cells called **thymic corpuscles** (Hassall corpuscles). Other cells of the epithelial cords spread apart, but they retain connections with each other to form an epithelial reticulum. The mesenchyme between the epithelial cords forms thin, incomplete septa between the lobules.

Lymphocytes soon appear and fill the interstices between the epithelial cells. The lymphocytes are derived from **hematopoietic stem cells**. The thymic primordium is surrounded by a thin layer of mesenchyme that is essential for its development. Neural crest cells also contribute to thymic

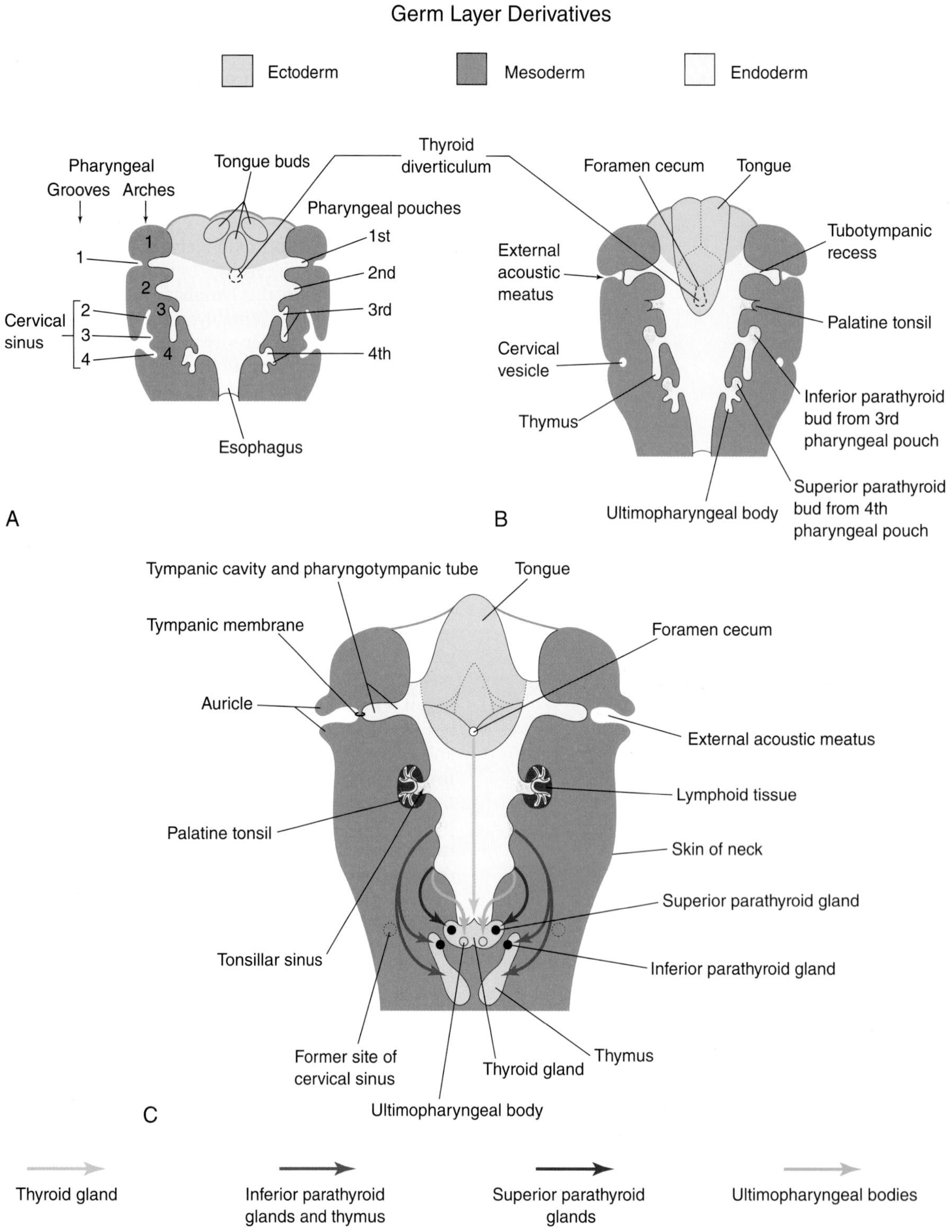

Fig. 9.7 Schematic horizontal sections at the level shown in Fig. 9.5A illustrate the adult derivatives of the pharyngeal pouches. (A) At 5 weeks, the second arch grows over the third and fourth arches, burying the second to fourth grooves in the cervical sinus. (B) Development at 6 weeks. (C) At 7 weeks, the developing thymus, parathyroid, and thyroid glands migrate into the neck *(arrows)*.

organogenesis. *The appearance and involvement of type 2 innate lymphoid cells (ILC2) and thymocytes (T-cell precursors) are important for the maintenance of immune homeostasis, resistance against infections, tissue reparation, and in general for the maintenance of health.*

Growth and development of the thymus are not complete at birth. It is a relatively large organ during the perinatal period and may extend through the superior thoracic aperture at the root of the neck. At puberty, the thymus undergoes involution. By adulthood, it is often scarcely recognizable because of fat infiltrating the cortex of the gland; however, the remnant of thymic tissue is still functional. In addition to secreting thymic hormones, the thymus primes **thymocytes** before releasing them to the periphery.

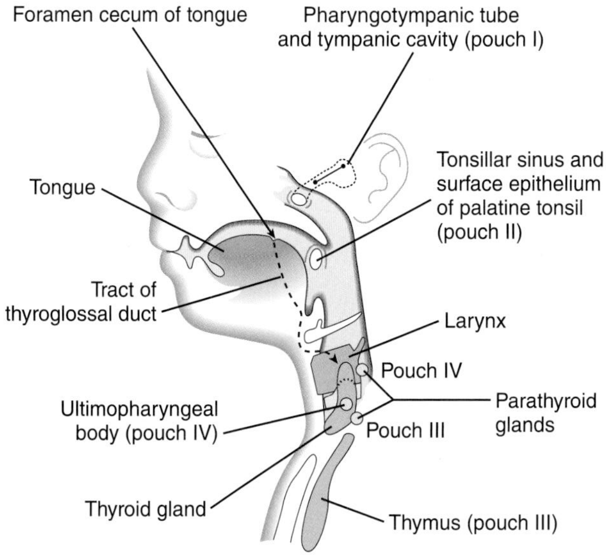

Fig. 9.8 Schematic sagittal section of the head, neck, and upper thoracic regions of a 20-week fetus shows the adult derivatives of the pharyngeal pouches and the descent of the thyroid gland into the neck *(broken line)*.

FOURTH PHARYNGEAL POUCH

The fourth pouch expands into a dorsal bulbar and elongated ventral parts (see Figs. 9.7 and 9.8). Its connection with the pharynx is reduced to a narrow duct that soon degenerates. By the sixth week, each dorsal part develops into a **superior parathyroid gland**, which lies on the dorsal surface of the thyroid gland. Because the parathyroid glands derived from the third pouches accompany the thymus, they are in a more inferior position than the parathyroid glands derived from the fourth pouches (see Fig. 9.8).

HISTOGENESIS OF PARATHYROID AND THYROID GLANDS

The epithelium of the dorsal parts of the third and fourth pouches proliferates during the fifth week and forms small nodules on the dorsal aspect of each pouch. Vascular mesenchyme soon grows into these nodules, forming a capillary network. The **chief** or **principal cells** differentiate during the embryonic period and are thought to become functionally active in regulating fetal calcium metabolism. The **oxyphil cells** of the parathyroid gland differentiate 5 to 7 years after birth.

The elongated ventral endodermal part of each fourth pouch develops into an **ultimopharyngeal body**, which fuses with the thyroid gland (see Fig. 9.8). Its cells disseminate within the thyroid and form **parafollicular cells**. These cells are also called C cells, indicating that they produce **calcitonin**, a hormone that lowers blood calcium levels. **C cells** differentiate from cephalic neural crest cells that migrate from the arches into the fourth pair of pouches. *The basic helix-loop-helix (bHLH) transcription factor MASH1 regulates C-cell differentiation.*

7

PHARYNGEAL GROOVES

The head and neck regions of the embryo exhibit four grooves (branchial clefts) on each side during the fourth and fifth weeks (see Figs. 9.1B–D and 9.2). These grooves separate the arches externally. Only one pair of grooves contributes to postnatal structures; the first pair persists as the **external acoustic meatus** (ear canals; see Fig. 9.7C). The other grooves lie in a slit-like depression **(cervical sinus)** and are normally obliterated along with the sinus as the neck develops (see Fig. 9.4A, D, and F). Birth defects of the second groove are relatively common.

PHARYNGEAL MEMBRANES

7

The pharyngeal membranes appear on the floors of the pharyngeal grooves (see Figs. 9.1H and 9.3C). These membranes form where the epithelia of the grooves and pouches approach each other. The endoderm of the pouches and ectoderm of the grooves are soon infiltrated and separated by both neural crest cells and mesenchyme. Only one pair of membranes contributes to the formation of adult structures; the first membrane becomes the **tympanic membrane** (see Fig. 9.7C).

Cervical (Branchial/Lateral) Sinuses

External cervical sinuses are uncommon, and most result from failure of the second groove and cervical sinus to obliterate (Figs. 9.9D and 9.10A and B). The sinus typically opens along the anterior border of the sternocleidomastoid muscle in the inferior third of the neck. Anomalies of the other pharyngeal grooves occur in approximately 5% of neonates. External sinuses are commonly detected during infancy because of the discharge of mucus from them (see Fig. 9.10A). The external cervical sinuses are bilateral in approximately 10% of affected neonates and are commonly associated with auricular sinuses.

Internal cervical sinuses open into the tonsillar sinus or near the palatopharyngeal arch (see Fig. 9.9D and F). These sinuses are rare. Most result from the persistence of the proximal part of the second pouch. This pouch usually disappears as the palatine tonsil develops; its normal remnant is the tonsillar sinus.

Cervical (Branchial/Lateral) Fistula

A cervical fistula is an abnormal canal that typically opens internally into the **tonsillar sinus** and externally in the side of the neck. The canal results from the persistence of parts of the second groove and second pouch (see Figs. 9.9E and F and 9.10B). The fistula ascends from its opening in the neck through the subcutaneous tissue and platysma muscle to reach the **carotid sheath**. The fistula then passes between the internal and external carotid arteries and opens into the tonsillar sinus.

Piriform Sinus Fistula

The piriform sinus fistula is thought to result from the persistence of remnants of the ultimopharyngeal body along its path to the thyroid gland (see Figs. 9.7C and 9.8).

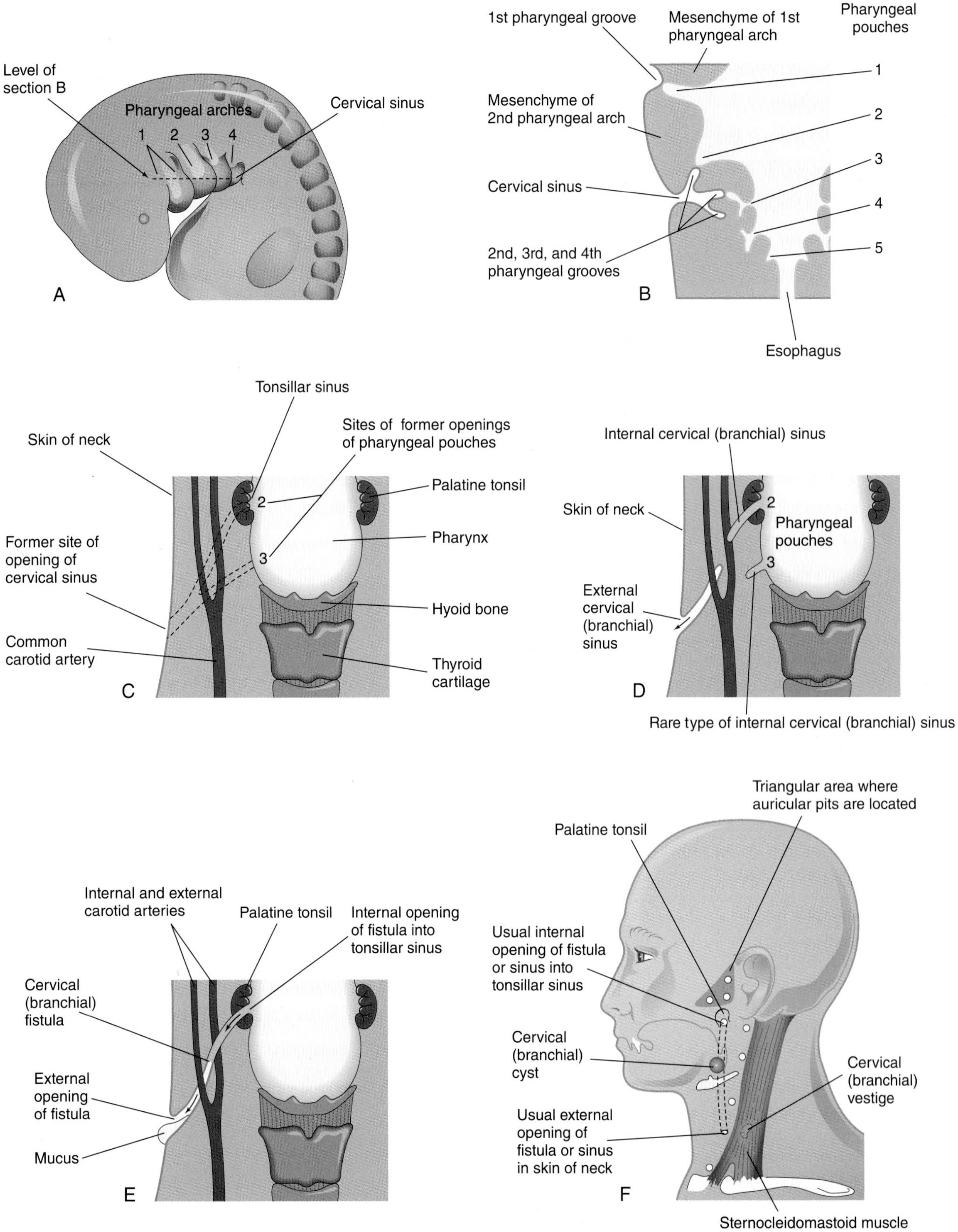

Fig. 9.9 (A) Lateral view of the head, neck, and thoracic regions of a 5-week embryo shows the cervical sinus that is normally present at this stage. (B) Horizontal section of the embryo at the level shown in (A) illustrates the relationship between the cervical sinus and the pharyngeal arches and pouches. (C) Diagrammatic sketch of the adult pharyngeal and neck regions shows the former sites of openings of the cervical sinus and pharyngeal pouches. The *broken lines* indicate possible tracts of cervical fistulas. (D) Similar sketch shows the embryologic basis of various cervical sinus types. (E) Drawing shows a cervical fistula that resulted from the persistence of parts of the second groove and second pouch. (F) Sketch shows possible sites of cervical cysts, the openings of cervical sinuses and fistulas, and a branchial vestige (see Fig. 9.13).

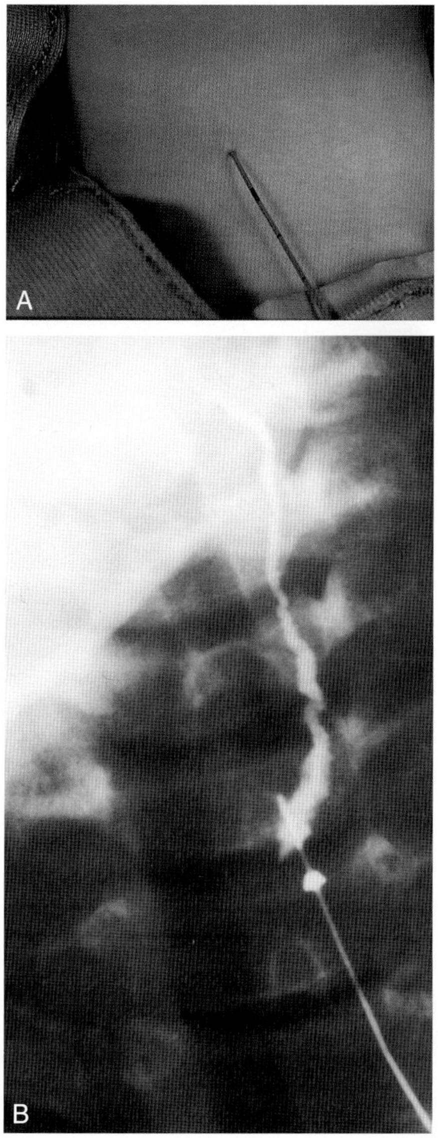

Fig. 9.10 (A) A catheter is inserted into the external opening of a cervical sinus in a child's neck. The catheter allows the definition of the length of the tract, which facilitates surgical excision. (B) After injection of contrast material, the fistulogram shows the course of a complete cervical fistula through the neck. (Courtesy Dr. Pierre Soucy, Division of Paediatric Surgery, Children's Hospital of Eastern Ontario, Ottawa, Ontario, Canada.)

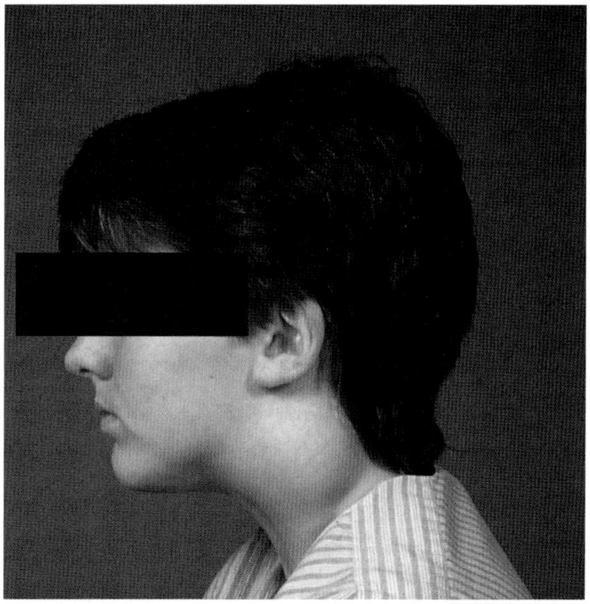

Fig. 9.11 The swelling in a boy's neck was produced by a cervical cyst. These large cysts often lie free in the neck just inferior to the angle of the mandible, but they may develop anywhere along the anterior border of the sternocleidomastoid muscle, as in this case. (Courtesy Dr. Pierre Soucy, Division of Paediatric Surgery, Children's Hospital of Eastern Ontario, Ottawa, Ontario, Canada.)

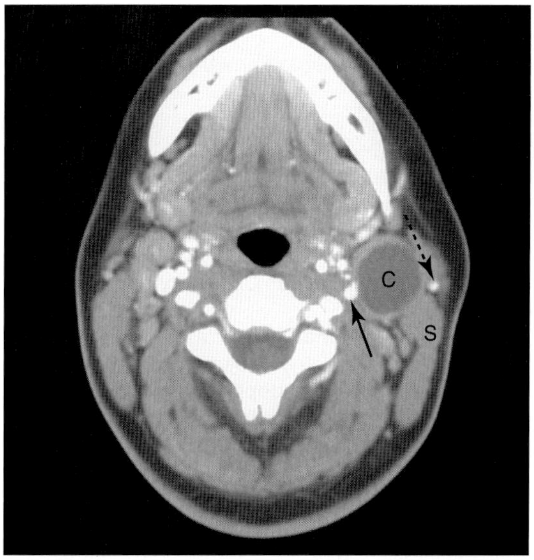

Fig. 9.12 Computed tomography of the neck region of a 24-year-old female with a 2-month history of a lump in the neck shows a low-density cervical cyst *(C)* that is anterior to the sternocleidomastoid muscle *(S)*. Notice the external carotid artery *(solid arrow)* and external jugular vein *(dotted arrow)*. (Courtesy Dr. Gerald S. Smyser, Altru Health System, Grand Forks, North Dakota.)

Cervical (Branchial/Lateral) Cysts

Remnants of the cervical sinus and/or the second groove may persist and form a spherical or elongated cyst (see Fig. 9.9F). Although they may be associated with cervical sinuses and drain through them, the cysts often lie free in the neck, just inferior to the angle of the mandible. However, they can develop anywhere along the anterior border of the sternocleidomastoid muscle or periauricular region. **Cervical cysts** usually become apparent between 30 and 50 years of age. These cysts produce a painless swelling in the neck (Fig. 9.11), which is easily diagnosed by ultrasonography. Cervical cyst enlarges because of the accumulation of fluid and cellular debris derived from the desquamation of their epithelial linings (Fig. 9.12).

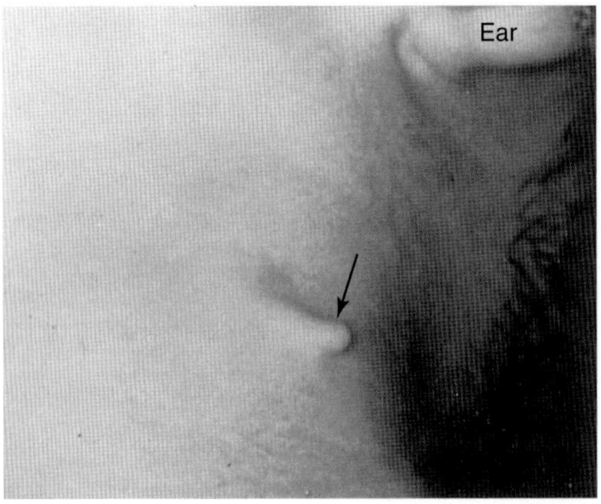

Fig. 9.13 A cartilaginous branchial vestige *(arrow)* in a child's neck (see Fig. 9.9F). (From Raffensperger JG: *Swenson's pediatric surgery*, ed 5, New York, 1990, Appleton-Century-Crofts.)

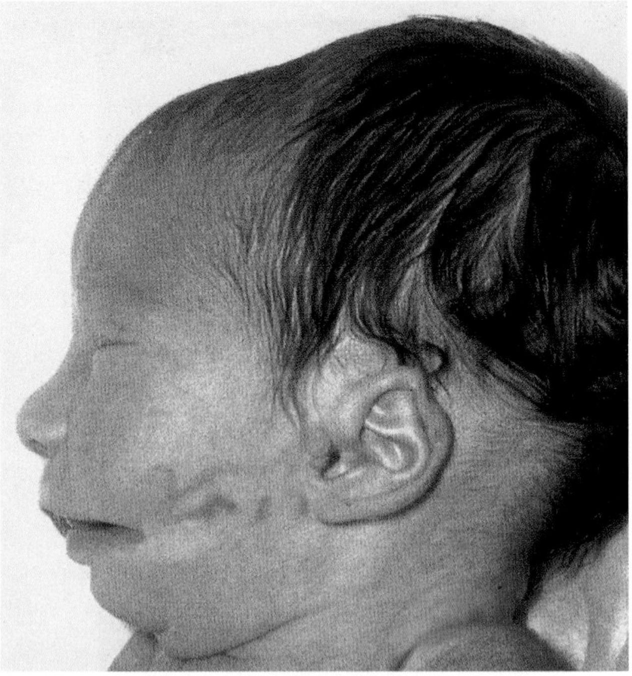

Fig. 9.14 This infant has the first arch syndrome, a pattern of birth defects that results from insufficient migration of neural crest cells into the first pharyngeal arch. Notice the deformed auricle of the external ear, preauricular appendage, defect in the cheek between the auricle and mouth, micrognathia (hypoplasia of the mandible), and macrostomia (large mouth).

Cervical (Branchial) Vestiges

The pharyngeal cartilages normally disappear, except for parts that form ligaments or bones. However, in unusual cases, cartilaginous or bony remnants of pharyngeal arch cartilages appear under the skin on the side of the neck (Fig. 9.13). They are usually found anterior to the inferior third of the sternocleidomastoid muscle (see Fig. 9.9F).

First Pharyngeal Arch Syndrome

Abnormal development of the components of the first arch results in various developmental birth defects of the eyes, ears, mandible, and palate, which together constitute the first arch syndrome (Fig. 9.14). This birth defect is thought to result from insufficient migration of neural crest cells into the first arch during the fourth week. There are two main manifestations of the first arch syndrome: **Treacher Collins syndrome** and **Pierre Robin sequence**.

Treacher Collins syndrome (1:50,000 incidence) (mandibulofacial dysostosis) is an autosomal dominant disorder characterized by **malar hypoplasia** (underdevelopment of zygomatic bones of the face) with down-slanting **palpebral fissures**, defects of the lower eyelids, deformed external ears, and sometimes defects of the middle and internal ears.

The Treacher Collins-Franceschetti syndrome 1 gene (TCOF1) *is responsible for the production of a protein called treacle. Treacle is involved in the biogenesis of ribosomal RNA that contributes to the development of bones and cartilage of the face. Pathogenic variants (mutation) in the* TCOF1 *gene are associated with Treacher Collins syndrome.*

Pierre Robin sequence (1:15,000 incidence) typically occurs de novo in most patients and is associated with **hypoplasia** (underdevelopment) of the mandible, cleft palate, and defects of the eyes and ears. Rarely, it is inherited in an autosomal dominant pattern. In the Robin morphogenetic complex, the initiating defect is a small mandible **(micrognathia)**, which results in posterior displacement of the tongue and obstruction to a full closure of the palatal processes, resulting in a **bilateral cleft palate** (see Figs. 9.40 and 9.41).

DiGeorge Syndrome

Infants with DiGeorge syndrome (1:5000 incidence) (also known as 22q11.2 deletion syndrome) are born without a thymus and parathyroid glands and have defects in the cardiac outflow tracts. In some cases, ectopic glandular tissue has been found (Fig. 9.15). The disease is characterized by **congenital hypoparathyroidism**, increased susceptibility to infections (from immune deficiency, specifically defective T-cell function), birth defects of the mouth (shortened philtrum of the upper lip), low-set and notched ears, nasal clefts, thyroid hypoplasia, and cardiac abnormalities (defects of the aortic arch and heart). Features of this syndrome vary widely, but most infants have some of the classic characteristics previously described. Only 1.5% of infants have the complete form of T-cell deficiency, and approximately 30% have only a partial T-cell deficiency.

DiGeorge syndrome occurs because the third and fourth pharyngeal pouches fail to differentiate into the thymus and parathyroid glands. This is the result of a breakdown in signaling between pharyngeal endoderm and adjacent neural crest cells. The facial abnormalities result primarily from abnormal development of the first arch components because neural crest cells are disrupted, and cardiac anomalies arise in the sites normally occupied by neural crest cells. *The microdeletion in the q11.2 region of chromosome 22 inactivates the* TBX1, HIRA, *and* UFDIL *genes. Disruption of CXCR4 signaling also affects neural crest cells and leads to similar anomalies.*

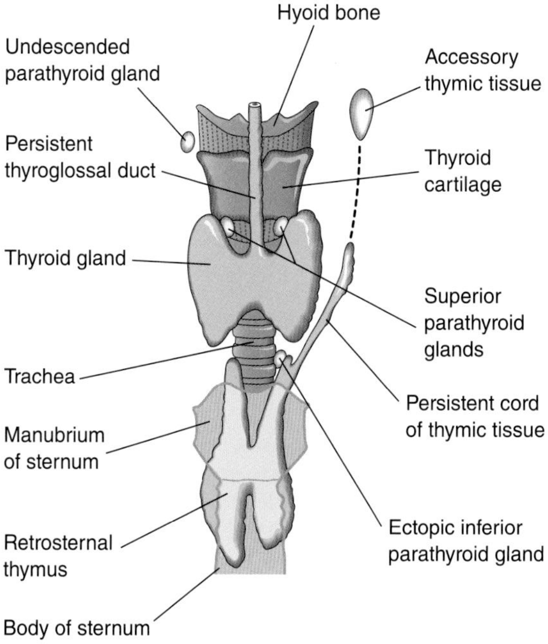

Fig. 9.15 Anterior view of the thyroid gland, thymus, and parathyroid glands illustrates various birth defects that may occur.

Accessory Thymic Tissue

An isolated mass of thymic tissue may persist in the neck and often lies close to an inferior parathyroid gland (see Fig. 9.15). This tissue breaks free from the developing thymus as it shifts caudally in the neck.

Ectopic Parathyroid Glands

Ectopic parathyroid glands may be found anywhere near or within the thyroid gland or thymus. The superior glands are more constant in position than the inferior ones. Occasionally, an inferior parathyroid gland remains near the bifurcation of the common carotid artery. In other cases, it may be in the thorax.

Abnormal Number of Parathyroid Glands

Uncommonly, there are more than four parathyroid glands. **Supernumerary parathyroid glands** probably result from the division of the primordia of the original glands. The absence of a gland results from the failure of one of the primordia to differentiate or from atrophy of a gland early in development. Nuclear diagnostic procedures are invaluable for the localization of hyperactive parathyroid glands.

DEVELOPMENT OF THYROID GLAND

7

The thyroid gland is the first endocrine gland to develop in the embryo. *Under the influence of Notch and Hedgehog signaling pathways,* it begins to form approximately 24 days after fertilization from a median endodermal thickening in the floor of the primordial pharynx. This thickening soon forms a small outpouching, the **thyroid primordium** (Fig. 9.16A).

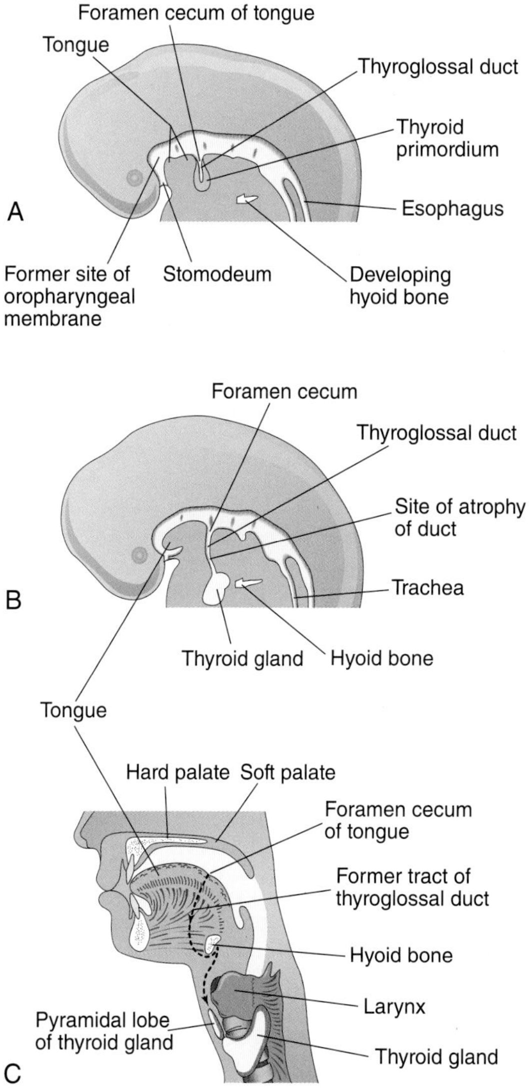

Fig. 9.16 Development of the thyroid gland. (A and B) Schematic sagittal sections of the head and neck regions of embryos at 5 and 6 weeks, respectively, illustrate successive stages in the development of the gland. (C) Similar section of an adult head and neck shows the path taken by the gland during its embryonic descent (indicated by the former tract of the thyroglossal duct).

Two lateral primordia form from the fourth pouch (ultimopharyngeal body) and fuse with the midline primordium. The lateral components primarily provide the parafollicular cell population while the midline component provides the majority of the follicular cells.

As the embryo and tongue grow, the developing thyroid gland changes position in the neck, passing ventral to the developing hyoid bone and laryngeal cartilages. For a short time, the gland is connected to the tongue by a narrow tube, the **thyroglossal duct** (see Fig. 9.16A and B). At first, the thyroid primordium is hollow, but it soon becomes a solid mass of cells. It divides into right and left lobes that are connected by the **isthmus of the thyroid gland** (Fig. 9.17), which lies anterior to the developing second and third tracheal rings.

At 7 weeks, the thyroid gland has assumed its definitive shape and is usually located in its final position in

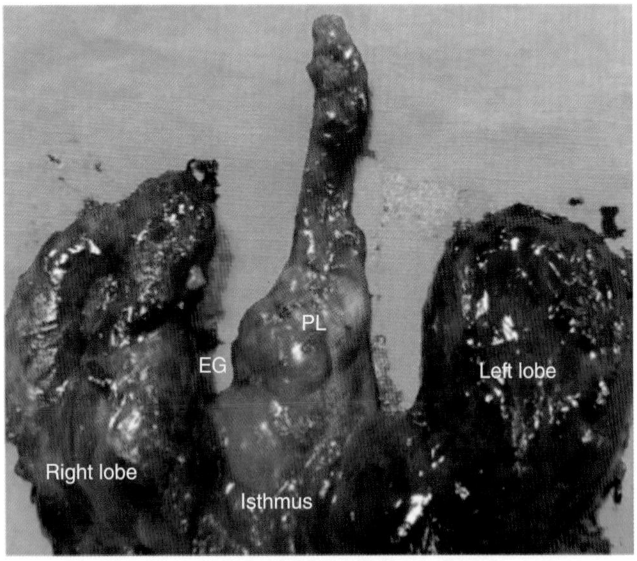

Fig. 9.17 The anterior surface of a dissected adult thyroid gland with euthyroid goiter (EG). Notice the pyramidal lobe (PL) ascending from the superior border of the isthmus of the gland. It represents a persistent portion of the inferior end of the thyroglossal duct that has formed thyroid tissue. (From Gurleyik E, Gurleyik G, Dogan S, Cobek U, Cetin F, Onsal U: Pyramidal lobe of the thyroid gland: surgical anatomy in patients undergoing total thyroidectomy, *Anat Res Int*, 384148, 2015.)

the neck (see Fig. 9.16C). By this time, the **thyroglossal duct** has normally degenerated and disappeared. The proximal opening of the duct persists as a small pit in the dorsum (posterosuperior surface) of the tongue, the **foramen cecum** (see Fig. 9.16D). A **pyramidal lobe** of the thyroid gland extends superiorly from the isthmus in approximately 50% of people (see Fig. 9.17). This lobe may be attached to the hyoid bone by fibrous tissue, smooth muscle, or both.

HISTOGENESIS OF THYROID GLAND

The thyroid primordium consists of a solid mass of endodermal cells. This cellular aggregation later breaks up into a network of epithelial cords as it is invaded by the surrounding vascular mesenchyme. By the 10th week, the cords have divided into small cellular groups. A lumen soon forms in each cell cluster, and the cells become arranged in a single layer around **thyroid follicles**. During the 11th week, follicular colloid begins to appear; thereafter, iodine concentration and synthesis of thyroid hormones can be demonstrated. Thyroid hormone is required by the fetal brain as early as the first trimester before the fetal thyroid gland is functioning; thyroid hormone is provided by the mother. By 20 weeks, the levels of fetal **thyroid-stimulating hormone** (TSH) and **thyroxine** begin to increase, reaching adult levels at 35 weeks. The placenta and fetal pancreas produce TSH before production by the hypothalamus. *Genes identified in the development of the thyroid include FGF 2, 8, 10, FGFR 2b, TPO, TITF1, FOXE1 and FOXE4, PAX 2, 5, 8, TSHR, and DUOX2. It also appears that NIS, a sodium/iodine symporter, plays a key role in the onset of thyroid functioning.*

Congenital Hypothyroidism

Congenital hypothyroidism is *the most common metabolic disorder in neonates* with an incidence of 2 to 4:1000 (females being affected two to four times as often as males). It is a **heterogeneous disorder** of the hypothalamic-pituitary-thyroid axis for which several candidate genes have been identified, including *IGSFI, FOXE1, NKX2-1, TBLIX, IRS4,* and those for the TSH receptor and thyroid transcription factors *(TTF1, TTF2,* and *PAX8)*. Congenital hypothyroidism may result in neurodevelopmental disorders and infertility if not treated early. An increased incidence of renal and urinary tract defects has been reported in infants with congenital hypothyroidism.

Thyroglossal Duct Cysts and Sinuses

Cysts may form anywhere along the course of the **thyroglossal duct** (Fig. 9.18). The duct typically atrophies and disappears, but a remnant of it may persist and form a cyst in the tongue or the anterior part of the neck, usually just inferior to the hyoid bone (Fig. 9.19). Most cysts are observed by the age of 5 years. Unless the lesions become infected, most of them are asymptomatic. The swelling produced by a **thyroglossal duct cyst** usually develops as a painless, progressively enlarging, movable mass (Fig. 9.20; see Figs. 9.18 and 9.19A and B). The cyst may contain some thyroid tissue. If infection of a cyst occurs, perforation of the skin may develop, forming a **thyroglossal duct sinus** that usually opens in the median plane of the neck anterior to the laryngeal cartilages.

Ectopic Thyroid Gland

An **ectopic thyroid gland** is an uncommon birth defect, and it is usually located along the course of the thyroglossal duct (see Fig. 9.16C). **Lingual thyroid glandular tissue** is the most common of ectopic thyroid tissues (90% of cases) and it is more prevalent in females. **Intralingual thyroid masses** are found in up to 10% of autopsies, although they are clinically relevant in only 1 of 4000 persons with thyroid disease.

Incomplete movement of the thyroid gland results in a **sublingual thyroid gland** that appears high in the neck at or just inferior to the hyoid bone (Figs. 9.21 and 9.22). In 70% of cases, an ectopic sublingual thyroid gland is the only thyroid tissue present. It is *clinically important* to differentiate an ectopic thyroid gland from a thyroglossal duct cyst or accessory thyroid tissue to prevent inadvertent surgical removal of the thyroid gland. Failure to do so may leave the person permanently dependent on thyroid medication. Ultrasound is commonly used to investigate an ectopic sublingual thyroid gland.

Agenesis of Thyroid Gland

The absence of a thyroid gland or one of its lobes is a rare anomaly. In **thyroid hemiagenesis** (unilateral failure of formation), the left lobe is more commonly absent. Pathogenic variants (mutations) in the receptor for TSH are probably involved in some cases.

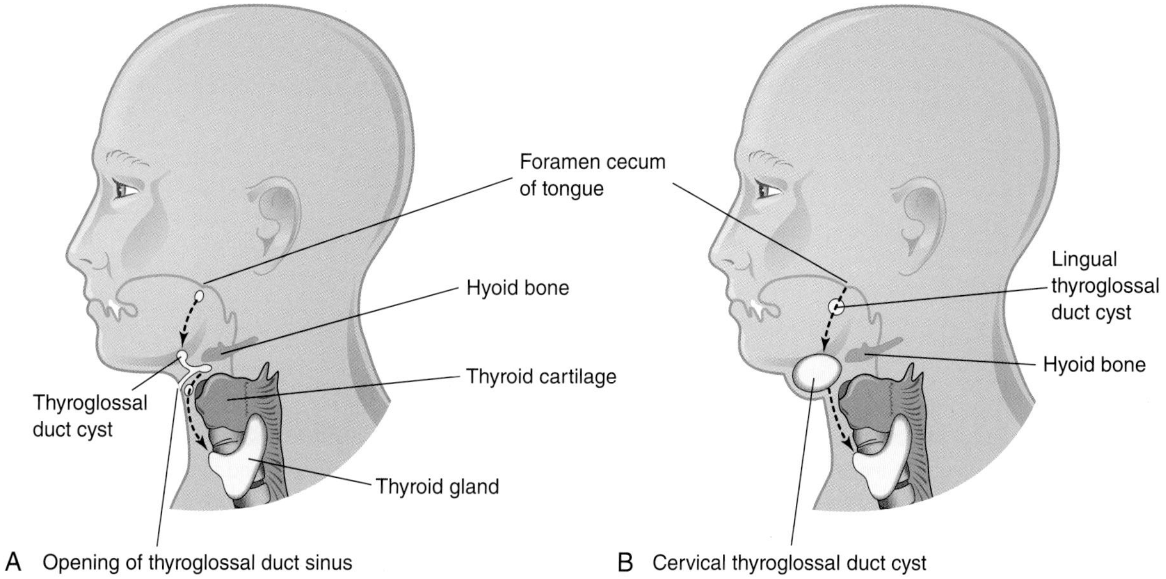

Fig. 9.18 (A) Sketch of the head and neck shows possible locations of thyroglossal duct cysts and a duct sinus. The *broken line* indicates the course taken by the duct during the descent of the developing thyroid gland from the foramen cecum to its final position in the anterior part of the neck. (B) Similar sketch illustrates lingual and cervical thyroglossal duct cysts. Most cysts are located inferior to the hyoid bone.

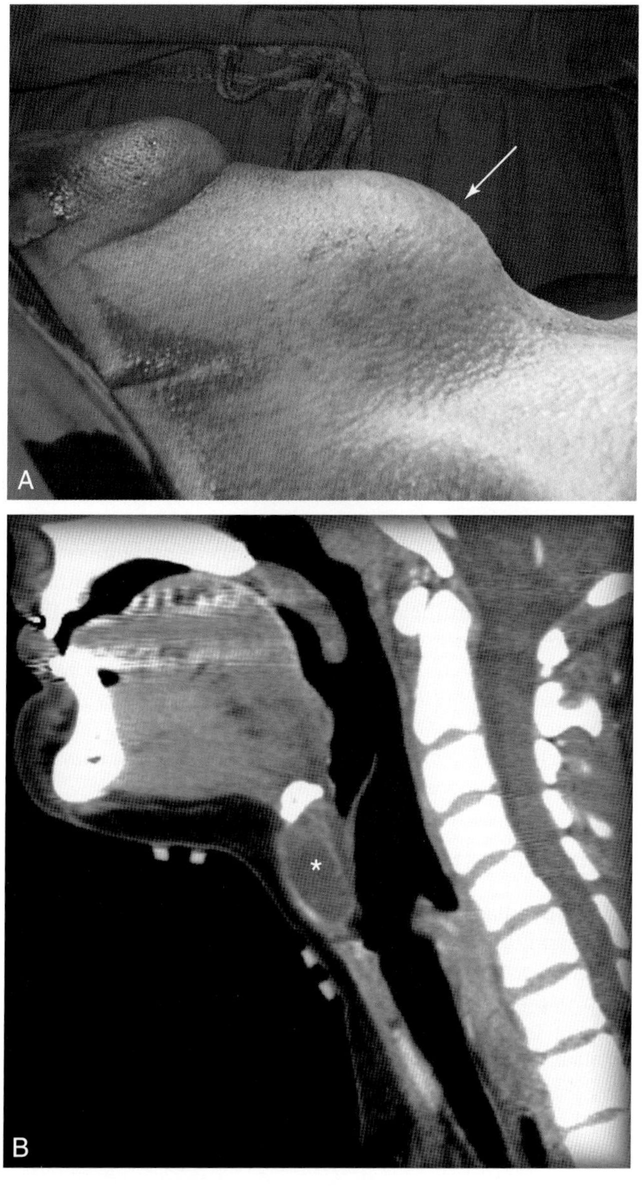

Fig. 9.19 (A) Large thyroglossal duct cyst *(arrow)* in a male patient. (B) Computed tomogram of a thyroglossal duct cyst (*) in a child shows that it is located in the neck anterior to the thyroid cartilage. ((A) Courtesy Dr. Srinivasa Ramachandra. (B) Courtesy Dr. Frank Gaillard, Radiopaedia.)

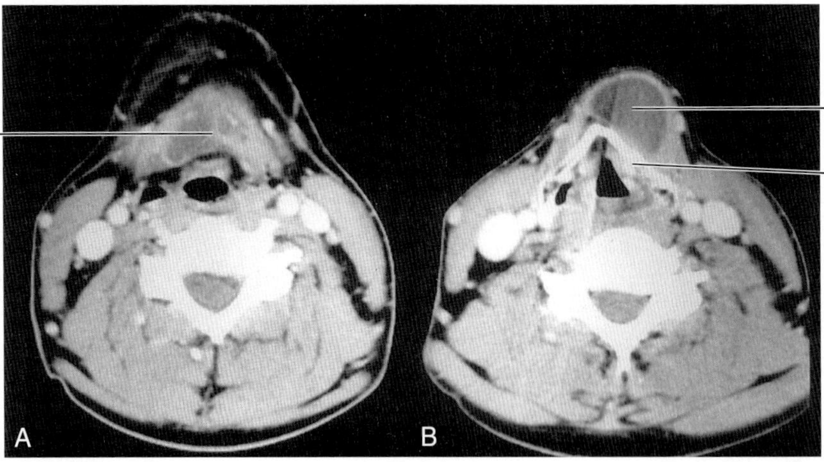

Fig. 9.20 Computed tomography at the level of the thyrohyoid membrane and base of the epiglottis (A) and the level of the calcified thyroid cartilage (B). The thyroglossal duct cyst extends cranially to the margin of the hyoid bone. (Courtesy Dr. Gerald S. Smyser, Altru Health System, Grand Forks, North Dakota.)

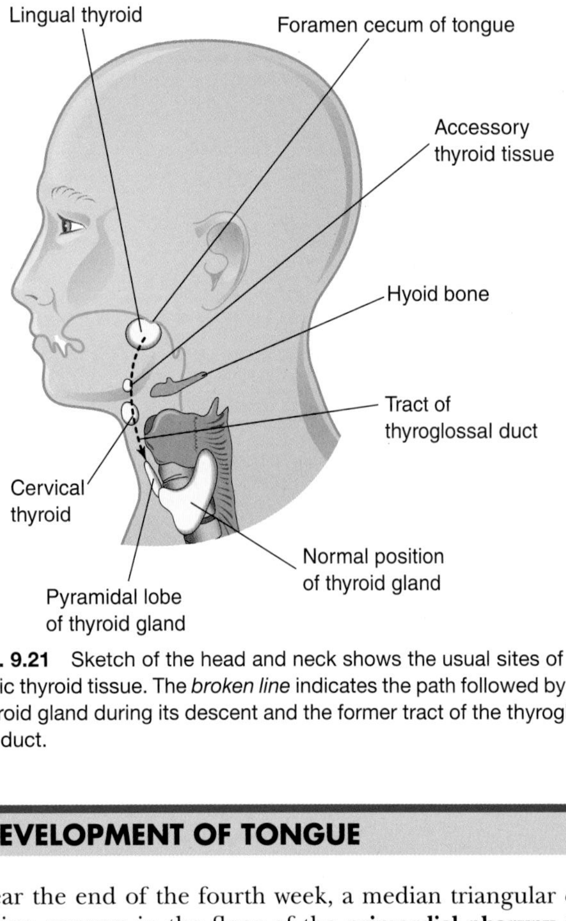

Fig. 9.21 Sketch of the head and neck shows the usual sites of ectopic thyroid tissue. The *broken line* indicates the path followed by the thyroid gland during its descent and the former tract of the thyroglossal duct.

DEVELOPMENT OF TONGUE

8

Near the end of the fourth week, a median triangular elevation appears in the floor of the **primordial pharynx** just rostral to the foramen cecum (Fig. 9.23A). This **median lingual swelling** (tongue bud) is the first indication of tongue development. Soon, two oval, **lateral lingual swellings** (distal tongue buds) develop on each side of the median lingual swelling. The three swellings result from the proliferation of mesenchyme in ventromedial parts of the first pair of pharyngeal arches. The lateral lingual swellings rapidly increase in size, merge, and overgrow the median lingual swelling.

The merged lateral lingual swellings form the anterior two-thirds of the tongue **(oral part)** (see Fig. 9.23C). The fusion site of the swellings is indicated by the **midline groove** and internally by the fibrous **lingual septum**. The median lingual swelling does not form a recognizable part of the adult tongue. Formation of the posterior third of the tongue (**pharyngeal part**) is indicated in the fetus by two elevations that develop caudal to the **foramen cecum** (see Fig. 9.23A). The **copula** forms by fusion of the ventromedial parts of the second pair of pharyngeal arches. The **hypopharyngeal eminence** develops caudal to the copula from a cluster of mesenchymal cells in the ventromedial parts of the third and fourth pairs of pharyngeal arches.

As the tongue develops, the copula is gradually overgrown by the hypopharyngeal eminence and disappears (see Fig. 9.23B and C). As a result, the posterior third of the tongue develops from the rostral part of the hypopharyngeal eminence. The line of fusion of the anterior and posterior parts of the tongue is roughly indicated by a V-shaped groove, the **terminal sulcus** (see Fig. 9.23C). Cranial neural crest cells migrate into the developing tongue and give rise to its connective tissue and vasculature.

Most of the tongue muscles are derived from **myoblasts** (primordial muscle cells) that migrate from the second to fifth occipital myotomes (see Fig. 9.5A). The **hypoglossal nerve** (CN XII) accompanies the myoblasts (myogenic precursors) during their migration and innervates the tongue muscles as they develop. The anterior and posterior parts of the tongue are located within the oral cavity at birth; the posterior third of the tongue descends into the **oropharynx** (oral part of the pharynx) by 4 years of age. *The molecular mechanisms regulating the morphogenesis of the tongue involve the expression of MRFs (myogenic regulatory factors), Sonic hedgehog (Shh), Dlx (distal-less homeobox) gene, TGFβ (transforming growth factor β), the Wnt/Notch pathway, and the paired box genes PAX3 and PAX7.*

LINGUAL PAPILLAE AND TASTE BUDS

Lingual papillae appear toward the end of the eighth week. The **vallate and foliate papillae** appear first and lie close to terminal branches of the glossopharyngeal nerve (CN IX). The **fungiform papillae** appear later near terminations of the chorda tympani branch of the facial nerve (CN VII). The **filiform papillae** develop during the early fetal period (10–11 weeks) and contain afferent nerve endings that are sensitive to touch.

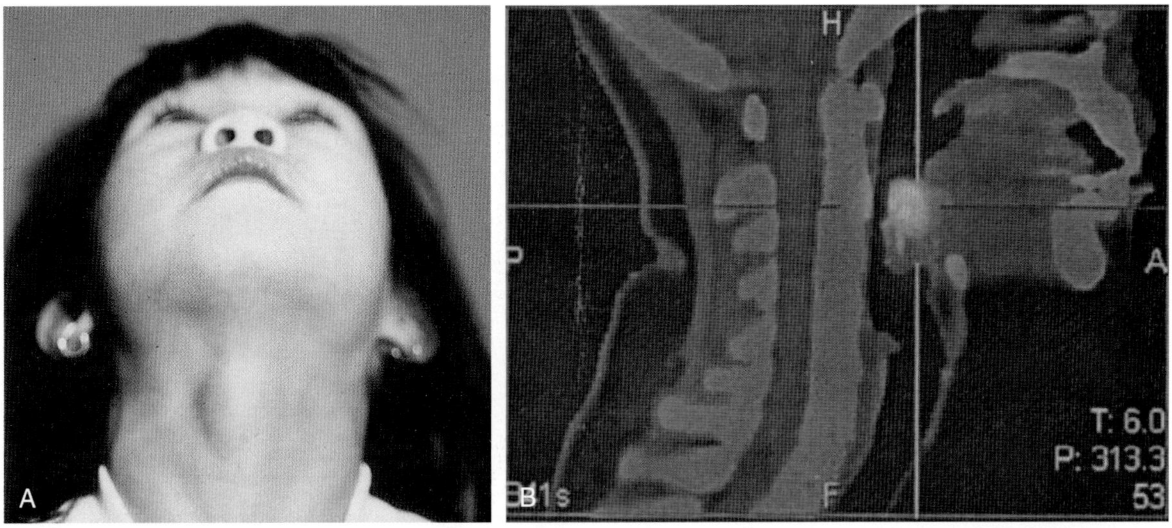

Fig. 9.22 (A) Sublingual thyroid mass in a 5-year-old girl. (B) Thyroid scintigraphy (of another patient) with technetium (99mTc) showed uptake of the radiotracer at the base of the tongue. Lingual thyroid was detected. No uptake was seen in the normal thyroid gland location. ((A) From Leung AK, Wong AL, Robson WL: Ectopic thyroid gland simulating a thyroglossal duct cyst, *Can J Surg* 38:87, 1995. (B) From Huang H, Lin Y-H: Lingual thyroid with severe hypothyroidism. A case report, *Medicine* 100:43, 2021.)

Taste buds (cell nests in the vallate, foliate, and fungiform papillae) develop during weeks 11 to 13 by inductive interaction between the epithelial cells of the tongue and invading gustatory (taste) nerve cells from the chorda tympani, glossopharyngeal, and vagus nerves. Most taste buds form on the dorsal surface of the tongue, and some develop on the palatoglossal (palate and tongue) arches, palate, posterior surface of the epiglottis, and posterior wall of the oropharynx. **Fetal facial responses** can be induced by bitter-tasting substances at 26 to 28 weeks, indicating that reflex pathways between taste buds and facial muscles are established.

NERVE SUPPLY OF THE TONGUE

The development of the tongue explains its nerve supply (see Fig. 9.23). The sensory supply to the mucosa of almost two-thirds of the tongue is from the lingual branch of the mandibular division of the **trigeminal nerve** (CN V), the nerve of the first pharyngeal arch. This arch forms the median and lateral lingual swellings. Although the **facial nerve** (CN VII) is the nerve of the second pharyngeal arch, its **chorda tympani branch** supplies the taste buds in the anterior two-thirds of the tongue except for the vallate papillae. Because the second arch component, the copula, is overgrown by the third arch, CN VII does not supply the tongue mucosa, except for the taste buds in the anterior part of the tongue. The vallate papillae in the anterior part of the tongue are innervated by the **glossopharyngeal nerve** (CN IX) of the third arch (see Fig. 9.23C). The usual explanation is that the mucosa of the posterior third of the tongue is pulled slightly anteriorly as the tongue develops.

The posterior third of the tongue is innervated mainly by the glossopharyngeal nerve (CN IX) of the third arch. The superior laryngeal branch of the **vagus nerve** (CN X) of the fourth arch supplies a small area of the tongue anterior to the epiglottis (see Fig. 9.23C). All muscles of the tongue are supplied by the hypoglossal nerve (CN XII), except for the palatoglossus, which is supplied from the pharyngeal plexus by fibers arising from the vagus nerve (CN X).

Congenital Anomalies of Tongue

Abnormalities of the tongue are uncommon, except for fissuring of the tongue and **hypertrophy** of the lingual papillae, which are characteristics of infants with Down syndrome (see Fig. 20.6D).

Congenital Lingual Cysts and Fistulas

Cysts in the tongue may be derived from remnants of the thyroglossal duct (see Fig. 9.16). They may enlarge and produce symptoms of pharyngeal discomfort, **dysphagia** (difficulty in swallowing), or both. Fistulas are also derived from persistent lingual parts of the thyroglossal duct. They open through the **foramen cecum** into the oral cavity.

Ankyloglossia

The **lingual frenulum** normally connects the inferior surface of the tongue to the floor of the mouth. In **ankyloglossia**, the frenulum is short and extends to the tip of the tongue (Fig. 9.24). This interferes with the tongue's free protrusion and may make breast-feeding difficult. Ankyloglossia (tongue-tie) occurs in approximately 1 of 300 North American neonates, but it usually has no permanent functional significance. A short frenulum usually stretches with time, making surgical correction of the defect unnecessary.

Macroglossia

An excessively large tongue is uncommon. It is caused by generalized hypertrophy of the developing tongue, usually resulting from **lymphangioma** (lymph tumor) or muscular hypertrophy. Macroglossia is often seen in infants with Down or Beckwith-Wiedemann syndrome.

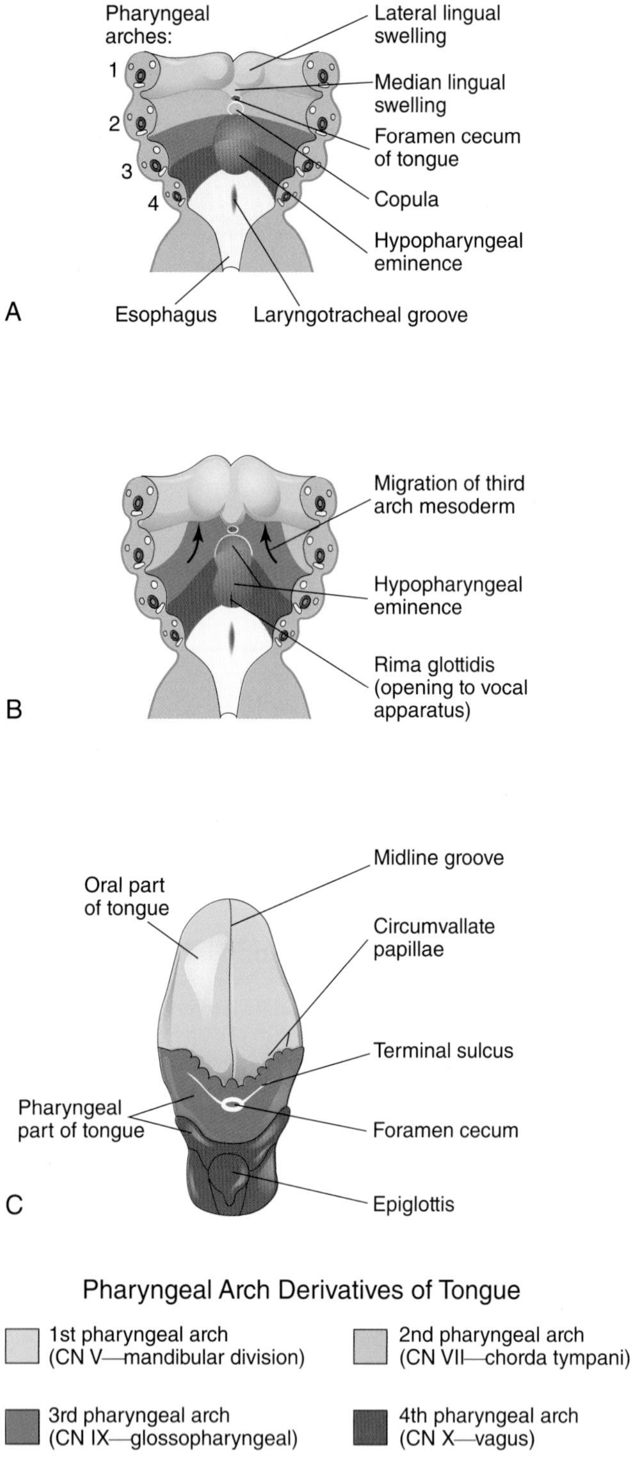

Fig. 9.23 (A and B) Schematic horizontal sections through the pharynx at the level shown in Fig. 9.5A illustrate successive stages in the development of the tongue during the fourth and fifth weeks. (C) Drawing of the adult tongue shows the pharyngeal arch derivation of the nerve supply of its mucosa. *CN*, Cranial nerve.

Microglossia

An abnormally small tongue is rare. It is usually associated with **micrognathia** (underdeveloped mandible and chin recession) and limb defects **(Hanhart syndrome)**.

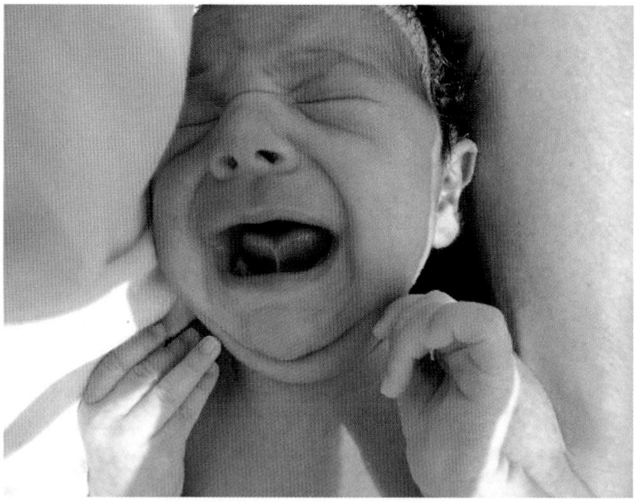

Fig. 9.24 Infant with ankyloglossia. Notice the short frenulum of the tongue, a fold of mucous membrane extending from the floor of the mouth to the midline of the undersurface of the tongue. (Courtesy Dr. Evelyn Jain, Lakeview Breastfeeding Clinic, Calgary, Alberta, Canada.)

Bifid or Cleft Tongue (Glossoschisis)

Incomplete fusion of the **lateral lingual swellings** (see Fig. 9.23A) results in a deep **midline groove** in the tongue (see Fig. 9.23A and C). This groove usually does not extend to the tip of the tongue. Occasionally the tongue is split at the tip, producing a bifid tongue.

DEVELOPMENT OF SALIVARY GLANDS

During the sixth and seventh weeks, the salivary glands, under the influence of the *Notch signaling pathway*, develop by branching morphogenesis from solid epithelial buds of the primordial oral cavity (see Fig. 9.6C). The club-shaped ends of these buds grow into the underlying mesenchyme. The connective tissue in the glands is derived from neural crest cells. All parenchymal (secretory) tissue arises from the proliferation of the oral epithelium. *Expression of the Fgf10 and Sox9 genes appears to be essential for the early development of the salivary glands by activating the Erk (extracellular signal–regulated) pathway through the FgfR2 gene.*

The **parotid glands** are the largest and first to develop and appear early in the sixth week (see Fig. 9.6C). They develop from buds that arise from the oral ectodermal lining near the angles of the stomodeum. Elongation of the jaws causes lengthening of the **parotid duct**, with the gland remaining close to its site of origin. Later the buds canalize (develop lumina) and become ducts by approximately 10 weeks. The rounded ends of the cords differentiate into serous **acini** (grape-shaped structures). The secretory activity begins at 18 weeks. The capsule and connective tissue of the glands develop from the surrounding mesenchyme.

The **submandibular glands** appear late in the sixth week. They develop from endodermal buds in the floor of the stomodeum. Solid cellular processes grow posteriorly, lateral to the developing tongue. Later, they branch and differentiate. Acini (mucous and serous) begin to form at

12 weeks, and secretory activity begins at 16 weeks. The growth of the glands continues after birth with the formation of mucous acini. Lateral to the developing tongue, a linear groove forms that soon closes to form the **submandibular duct**.

The **sublingual glands** are the smallest and appear during the eighth week, approximately 2 weeks later than the other glands (see Fig. 9.6C). They develop from multiple endodermal epithelial buds that branch and canalize to form 10 to 12 ducts that open independently into the floor of the mouth.

DEVELOPMENT OF FACE

8

The **facial primordia** appears early in the fourth week around the stomodeum (primordium of the mouth; Fig. 9.25A and B). Facial development depends on the inductive influence of the forebrain (through sonic hedgehog morphogenic gradients), frontonasal ectodermal zone, and developing eye. **Five facial primordia** appear as prominences around the stomodeum (see Fig. 9.25A):

- A frontonasal prominence
- Paired maxillary prominences
- Paired mandibular prominences

The maxillary and mandibular prominences are derivatives of the first pair of pharyngeal arches. The prominences are produced mainly by the expansion of *Hox*-negative **neural crest populations** that originate from the mesencephalic and rostral rhombencephalic neural folds during the fourth week. These cells are the major source of connective tissue components, including cartilage, bone, and ligaments in the facial and oral regions. *Neural crest cells migrate into the frontonasal process as a result of BMP signaling and undergo an epithelial-mesenchymal transformation from the expression of WNT. Formation of the frontonasal process is complex and controlled by highly integrated molecular signaling mechanisms involving at different stages expression of sonic hedgehog (SHH), fibroblast growth factors (FGF), transforming growth factor β (TGFβ), wingless (WNT) proteins, and bone morphogenetic protein (BMP).*

The **frontonasal prominence** surrounds the ventrolateral part of the forebrain, which gives rise to the **optic vesicles** that form the eyes (see Fig. 9.25C). The frontal part of the frontonasal prominence forms the forehead; the nasal part forms the rostral boundary of the stomodeum and nose. The **maxillary prominences** form the lateral boundaries of the stomodeum, and **mandibular prominences** constitute the caudal boundary of the stomodeum (Fig. 9.26). The facial prominences are **active centers of growth** in the underlying mesenchyme. This embryonic connective tissue is continuous from one prominence to the other.

Facial development occurs mainly between the fourth and eighth weeks (see Fig. 9.25A–G). By the end of the embryonic period, the face has an unquestionably human appearance. Facial proportions develop during the fetal period (see Fig. 9.25H and I). The lower jaw and lower lip are the first parts of the face to form. They result from the merging of the medial ends of the mandibular prominences in the median plane. The common chin dimple results from incomplete fusion of the prominences.

By the end of the fourth week, bilateral oval thickenings of the surface ectoderm (**nasal placodes**, the primordia of the **nasal epithelium**) have developed on the inferolateral parts of the frontonasal prominence (Figs. 9.27 and 9.28A and B). These placodes are initially convex, but they are later stretched to produce a flat depression in each **placode**. Mesenchyme in the margins of the placodes proliferates, producing horseshoe-shaped elevations, the **medial and lateral nasal prominences**. As a result, the nasal placodes lie in depressions, the **nasal pits** (see Fig. 9.28C and D). These pits are the primordia of the anterior **nares** (nostrils) and **nasal cavities** (see Fig. 9.28E), and the lateral nasal prominences form the alae (sides) of the nose.

The proliferation of mesenchyme in the maxillary prominences makes them enlarge and grow medially toward each other and the nasal prominences (see Figs. 9.25D–G, 9.26, and 9.27). This proliferation-driven expansion results in the movement of the medial nasal prominences toward the median plane and each other, a process regulated by *platelet-derived growth factor receptor α-polypeptide (PDGFRA) signaling.* Each lateral nasal prominence is separated from the maxillary prominence by a cleft, the **nasolacrimal groove** (see Figs. 9.25C and D).

By the end of the fifth week, the **primordia of the auricles** (the external part of ears) have begun to develop (Fig. 9.29; see Fig. 9.25E). **Six auricular hillocks** (three mesenchymal swellings on each side) form around the first pharyngeal groove, the primordia of the auricle, and the **external acoustic meatus**, respectively. Initially, the external ears are located in the neck region (Fig. 9.30); however, as the mandible develops, they become located on the side of the head at the level of the eyes (see Fig. 9.25H).

By the end of the sixth week, each maxillary prominence has begun to merge with the lateral nasal prominence along the line of the nasolacrimal groove (Figs. 9.31 and 9.32). This establishes continuity between the side of the nose, which is formed by the lateral nasal prominence, and the cheek region formed by the maxillary prominence.

The **nasolacrimal duct** develops from a rod-like thickening of ectoderm in the floor of the **nasolacrimal groove**. This thickening forms a solid epithelial cord that separates from the ectoderm and sinks into the mesenchyme. Later, as a result of apoptosis (programmed cell death), the epithelial cord canalizes to form a duct. The superior end of the duct expands to form the **lacrimal sac**. By the late fetal period, the nasolacrimal duct drains into the inferior meatus in the lateral wall of the nasal cavity. The duct becomes completely patent after birth.

Between the 7th and 10th weeks, the medial nasal prominences merge with the maxillary and lateral nasal prominences (see Fig. 9.25G and H). Fusion of the prominences requires the disintegration of their contacting surface epithelia, which results in the intermingling of the underlying mesenchymal cells. Merging the medial nasal and maxillary prominences results in the continuity of the upper jaw and lip and the separation of the nasal pits from the stomodeum.

As the medial nasal prominences merge, they form an **intermaxillary segment** (see Figs. 9.25H and 9.32E and F). This segment forms the middle part (philtrum) of the upper lip, the premaxillary part of the maxilla and its associated gingiva (gum), and the primary palate.

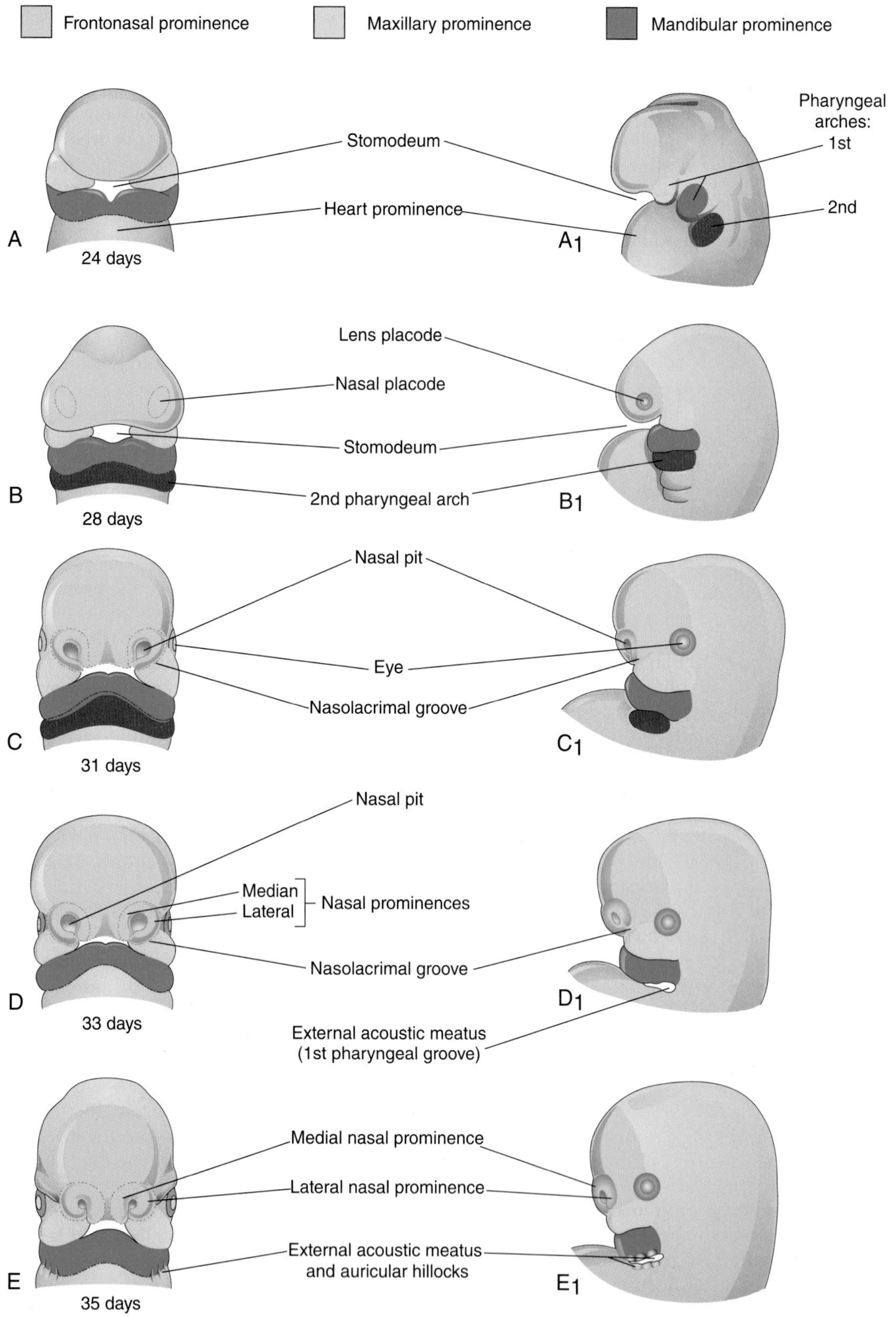

Fig. 9.25 (A–I) Diagrams show frontal and lateral views illustrating progressive stages in the development of the face.

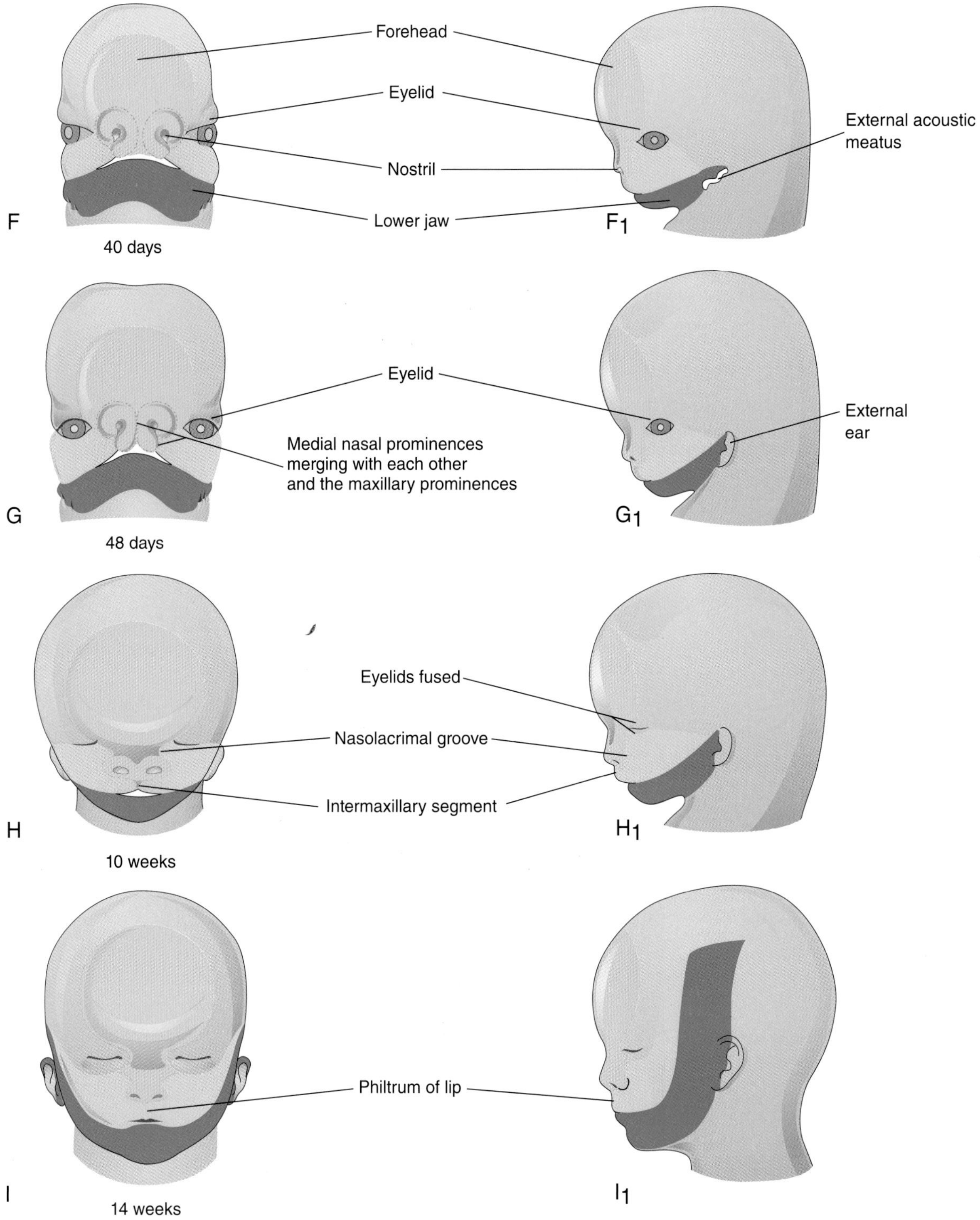
Forehead
Eyelid
Nostril
Lower jaw
External acoustic meatus
F
F1
40 days
Eyelid
Medial nasal prominences merging with each other and the maxillary prominences
External ear
G
G1
48 days
Eyelids fused
Nasolacrimal groove
Intermaxillary segment
H
H1
10 weeks
Philtrum of lip
I
I1
14 weeks

Fig. 9.25, Cont'd

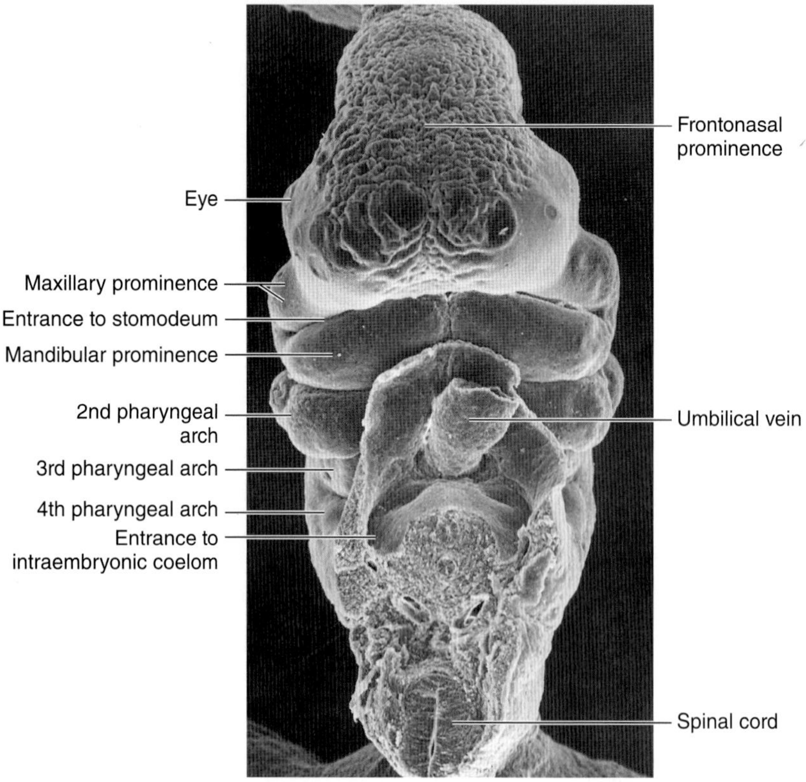

Fig. 9.26 Scanning electron micrograph shows the ventral view of a Carnegie stage 14 embryo (30–32 days). (Courtesy the late Professor Emeritus Dr. K.V. Hinrichsen, Medizinische Fakultät, Institut für Anatomie, Ruhr-Universität Bochum, Bochum, Germany.)

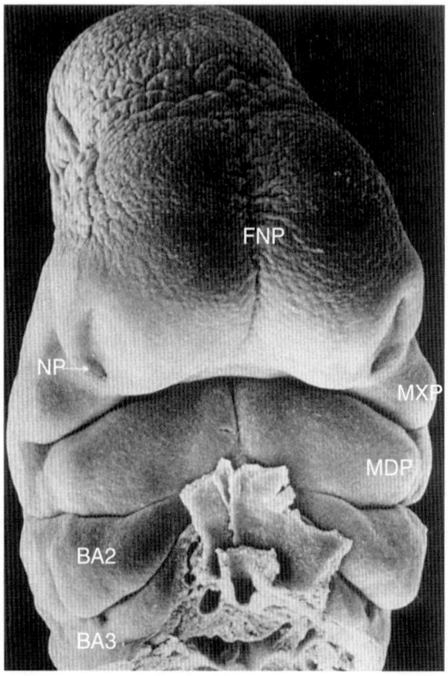

Fig. 9.27 Scanning electron micrograph shows the ventral view of a Carnegie stage 15 embryo of approximately 33 days with a crown-rump length of 8 mm. Notice the prominent frontonasal process *(FNP)* surrounding the telencephalon (forebrain) and the nasal pits *(NP)* located in the ventrolateral regions of the FNP. Medial and lateral nasal prominences surround these pits. The maxillary prominences *(MXP)* form the lateral boundaries of the stomodeum. The fusing mandibular prominences *(MDP)* are located just caudal to the stomodeum. The second pharyngeal arch *(BA2)* shows overhanging margins (opercula), and the third arch *(BA3)* is also clearly visible. (From Hinrichsen K: The early development of morphology and patterns of the face in the human embryo, *Adv Anat Embryol Cell Biol* 98:1, 1985.)

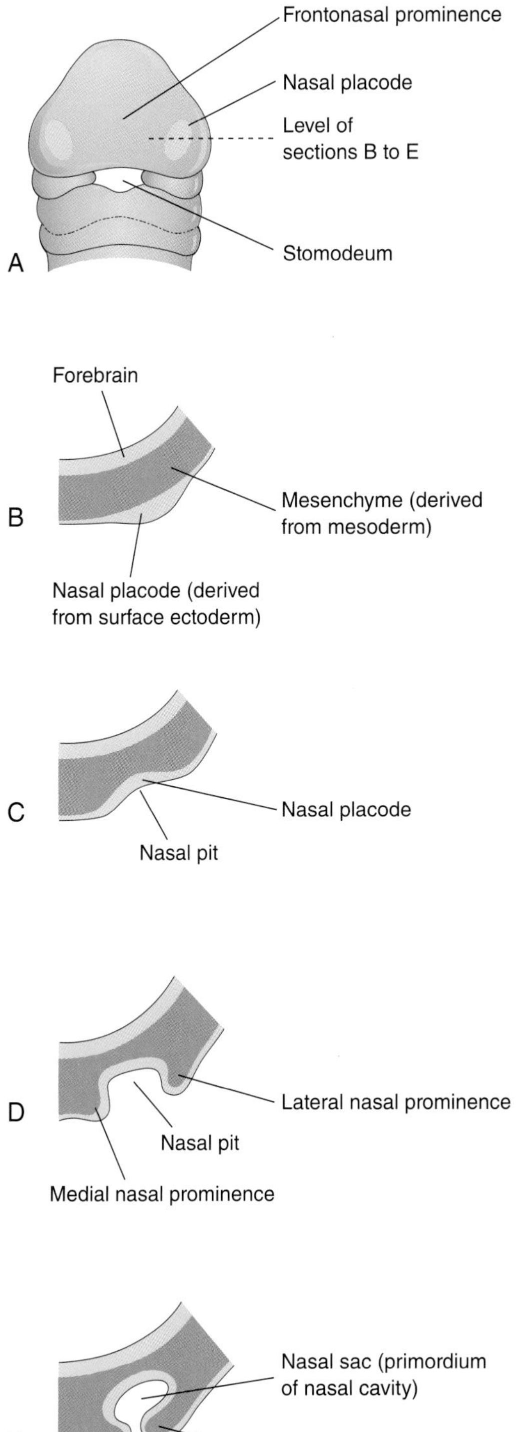

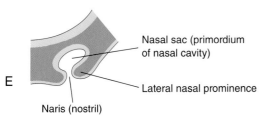

Fig. 9.28 Progressive stages in the development of a nasal sac (primordial nasal cavity). (A) Ventral view of an embryo of approximately 28 days. (B–E) Transverse sections through the left side of the developing nasal sac.

Clinical and embryologic studies indicate that the upper lip is formed entirely from the maxillary prominences. The lower parts of the medial nasal prominences appear to have become deeply positioned and covered by medial extensions of the maxillary prominences to form the **philtrum**

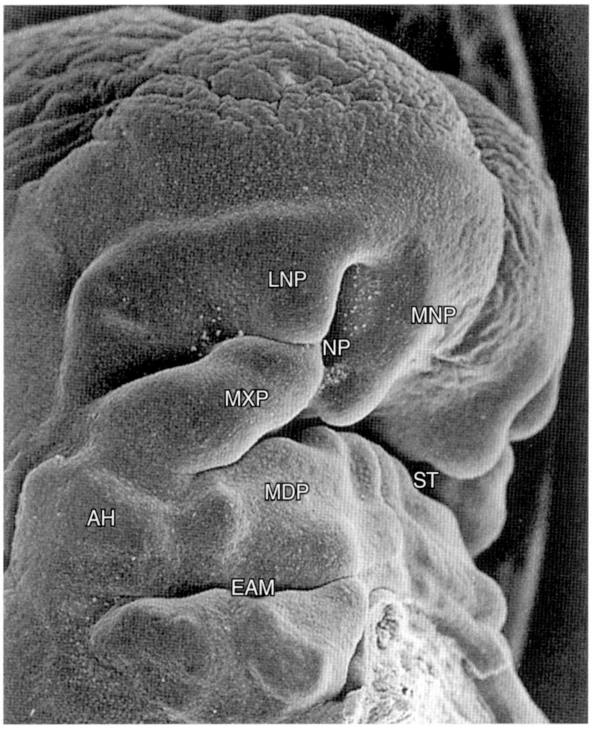

Fig. 9.29 Scanning electron micrograph shows the oblique view of the craniofacial region of a stage 16 embryo of approximately 41 days with a crown-rump length of 10.8 mm. The maxillary prominence *(MXP)* appears puffed up laterally and wedged between the lateral *(LNP)* and medial *(MNP)* nasal prominences surrounding the nasal pit *(NP)*. The auricular hillocks *(AH)* are present on both sides of the pharyngeal groove between the first and second arches, which will form the external acoustic meatus *(EAM)*. *MDP*, Mandibular prominence; *ST*, stomodeum. (From Hinrichsen K: The early development of morphology and patterns of the face in the human embryo, *Adv Anat Embryol Cell Biol* 98:1, 1985.)

(see Fig. 9.25H and I). In addition to connective tissue and muscular derivatives, various bones are derived from mesenchyme in the facial prominences.

Until the end of the sixth week, the primordial jaws are composed of masses of mesenchymal tissue. The lips and gingivae begin to develop when a linear thickening of the ectoderm, the **labiogingival lamina**, grows into the underlying mesenchyme (see Fig. 9.36B). Gradually, most of the lamina degenerates, leaving a **labiogingival groove** between the lips and gingivae (see Fig. 9.36H). A small area of the labiogingival lamina persists in the median plane to form the frenulum of the upper lip, which attaches the lip to the gum.

Further development of the face occurs slowly during the fetal period and results mainly from changes in the proportion and relative positions of the facial components. During the early fetal period, the nose is flat, and the mandible is underdeveloped (see Fig. 9.25H). At 14 weeks, the nose and mandible have their characteristic form as facial development is completed (see Fig. 9.25I).

As the brain enlarges, the **cranial cavity** (space occupied by the brain) expands bilaterally. This causes the orbits (bony cavities containing the eyeballs), which were oriented laterally, to assume a forward-facing orientation. The opening of the **external acoustic meatus** (**auditory canal**) appears to elevate, but it remains stationary; elongation of the lower

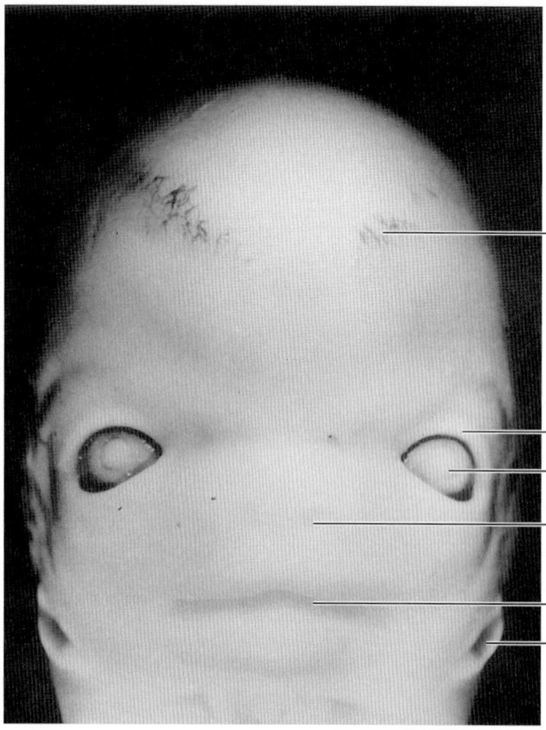

Fig. 9.30 Ventral view of the face of a stage 22 embryo at approximately 54 days. The eyes are widely separated at this stage, and the ears are low set. (From Nishimura H, Semba R, Tanimura T, Tanaka O: *Prenatal development of the human with special reference to craniofacial structures: an atlas*, Bethesda, Maryland, 1977, U.S. Department of Health, Education, and Welfare, National Institutes of Health.)

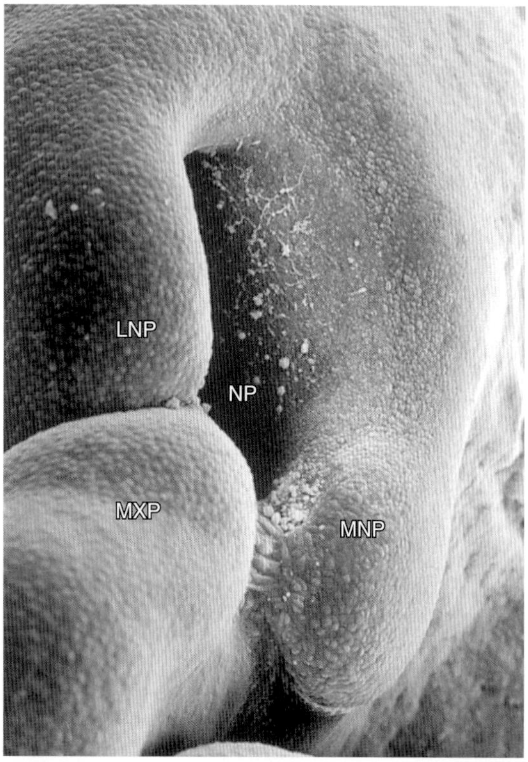

Fig. 9.31 Scanning electron micrograph of the right nasal region of a stage 17 embryo of approximately 41 days with a crown-rump length of 10.8 mm shows the maxillary prominence *(MXP)* fusing with the medial nasal prominence *(MNP)*. Epithelial bridges can be seen between these prominences. The furrow representing the nasolacrimal groove lies between the MXP and the lateral nasal prominence *(LNP)*. Notice the large nasal pit *(NP)*. (From Hinrichsen K: The early development of morphology and patterns of the face in the human embryo, *Adv Anat Embryol Cell Biol* 98:1, 1985.)

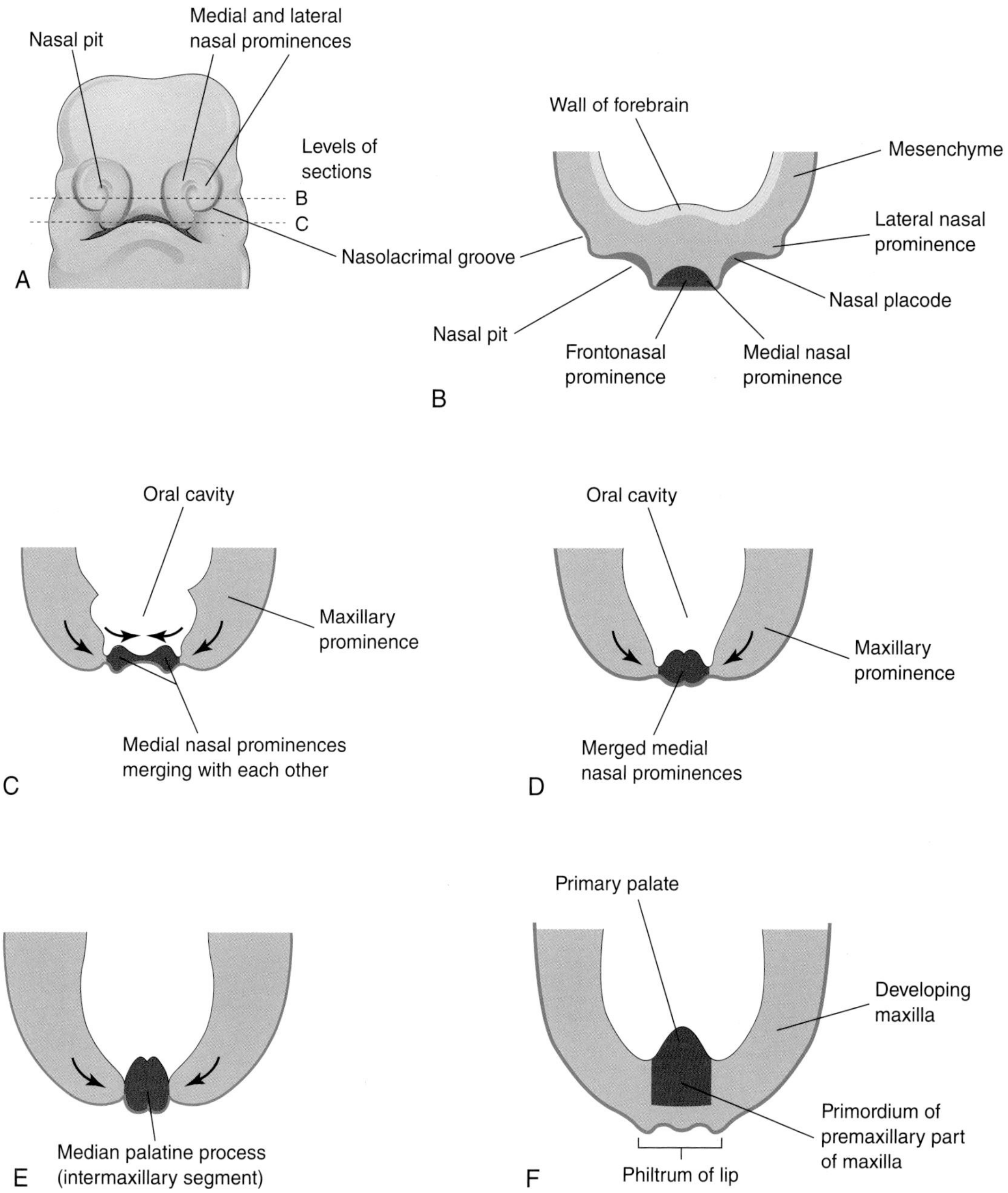

Fig. 9.32 Early development of the maxilla, palate, and upper lip. (A) Diagram of a facial view of a 5-week embryo. (B and C) Sketches of horizontal sections at the levels shown in (A). The *arrows* indicate subsequent growth of the maxillary and medial nasal prominences toward the median plane and merging of the prominences with each other. (D–F) Similar sections of older embryos illustrate the merging of the medial nasal prominences with each other and the maxillary prominences to form the upper lip. Studies suggest that the upper lip is formed entirely from the maxillary prominences.

jaw creates a false impression. The small appearance of the face prenatally results from the rudimentary upper and lower jaws, unerupted deciduous teeth (primary dentition), small nasal cavities, and maxillary sinuses.

Facial development requires all of the following components (see Fig. 9.25):

- The **frontal nasal prominence** forms the forehead and dorsum and apex of the nose.
- The **lateral nasal prominences** form the alae (sides) of the nose.
- The **medial nasal prominences** form the nasal septum, ethmoid bone, and **cribriform plate** (openings for passage of olfactory nerves).
- The **maxillary prominences** form the upper cheek regions and lip.
- The **mandibular prominences** form the chin, lower lip, and cheek regions.

Atresia of the Nasolacrimal Duct

Part of the nasolacrimal duct occasionally fails to canalize, resulting in **congenital atresia** (lack of an opening) of the nasolacrimal duct. Obstruction of this duct with clinical symptoms occurs in approximately 6% of neonates.

Congenital Auricular Sinuses and Cysts

Small auricular sinuses and cysts are usually located in a triangular area of skin anterior to the auricle of the external ear (see Fig. 9.9F); however, they may occur in other sites around the auricle or the lobule (earlobe). Although some sinuses and cysts are remnants of the first pharyngeal groove, others represent ectodermal folds sequestered during the formation of the auricle from six **auricular hillocks** (nodular masses of mesenchyme from the first and second arches that coalesce to form the auricle). The sinuses and cysts are classified as minor defects that have no serious medical consequences.

DEVELOPMENT OF NASAL CAVITIES

As the face develops, the **nasal placodes** become depressed, forming **nasal pits** (see Figs. 9.27, 9.28, and 9.31). The proliferation of the surrounding mesenchyme forms the medial and lateral **nasal prominences**, which results in the deepening of the nasal pits and the formation of **primordial nasal sacs**. Each sac grows dorsally and ventral to the developing forebrain. At first, the sacs are separated from the oral cavity by the **oronasal membrane** (Fig. 9.33A). This membrane ruptures by the end of the sixth week, bringing the nasal and oral cavities into communication (see Fig. 9.33B and C). Temporary epithelial plugs are formed in the nasal cavities from the proliferation of the cells lining them. By the middle of the 16th week, the nasal plugs disappear.

The regions of continuity between the nasal and oral cavities are the **primordial choanae** (openings from the nasal cavity into the nasal pharynx). After the **secondary palate** develops, the choanae are located at the junction of the nasal cavity and pharynx (see Figs. 9.33D and 9.36). While these changes are occurring, the superior, middle, and inferior **nasal conchae** develop as elevations of the lateral walls of the nasal cavities (see Fig. 9.33D). Concurrently, the ectodermal epithelium in the roof of each nasal cavity becomes specialized to form the **olfactory epithelium** (see Fig. 9.33C). Some epithelial cells differentiate into **olfactory receptor cells** (neurons). The neuronal axons constitute the **olfactory nerves**, which grow into the **olfactory bulbs** of the brain (see Fig. 9.33C and D).

Most of the upper lip, maxilla, and secondary palate forms from the maxillary prominences (see Fig. 9.25H). These prominences merge laterally with the mandibular prominences. The primordial lips and cheeks are invaded by mesenchyme from the second pair of pharyngeal arches, which differentiates into the facial muscles (see Fig. 9.5 and Table 9.1). The muscles of facial expression are supplied by

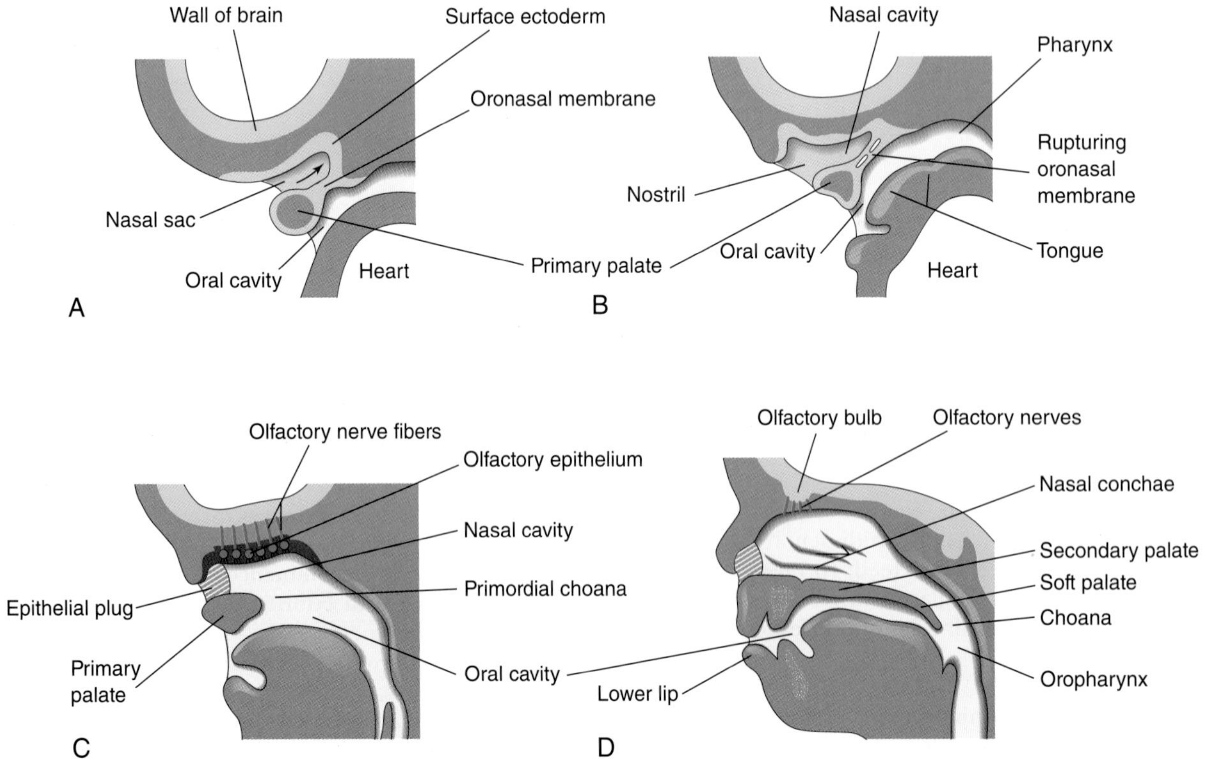

Fig. 9.33 Sagittal sections of the head show the development of the nasal cavities. The nasal septum has been removed. (A) Development at 5 weeks. (B) At 6 weeks, the oronasal membrane breaks down. (C) At 7 weeks, the nasal cavity communicates with the oral cavity, and the olfactory epithelium develops. (D) At 12 weeks, the palate and lateral wall of the nasal cavity develop.

the facial nerve (CN VII), the nerve of the second arch. The mesenchyme in the first pair of arches differentiates into the muscles of mastication and a few others, all of which are innervated by the trigeminal nerves (CN V), which supply the first pair of arches.

PARANASAL SINUSES

The ethmoid sinuses begin to develop during late fetal life; the remaining sinuses develop after birth (see Fig. 9.34). They form from diverticula of the walls of the nasal cavities and become pneumatic (air-filled) extensions of the nasal cavities in the adjacent bones, such as the **maxillary sinuses** in the maxillae, and the **frontal sinuses** in the frontal bones. The original openings of the diverticula persist as the orifices of the adult sinuses.

VOMERONASAL ORGAN

The first appearance of the **vomeronasal primordia** is in the form of bilateral epithelial thickenings on the nasal septum. Further invagination of the primordia and breaking away from the nasal septal epithelium forms a tubular **vomeronasal organ** (VNO) between days 37 and 43. This chemosensory structure, which ends blindly posteriorly, reaches its greatest development between 12 and 14 weeks. Later, the receptor population is gradually replaced with patchy ciliated cells. The VNO is consistently present in the form of a bilateral duct-like structure on the nasal septum, superior to the paraseptal cartilage. The tubular human VNO with its minute anterior opening is a true homolog of the VNO in other mammals, reptiles, and amphibians used as an auxiliary olfactory sense organ, typically to detect pheromones.

Postnatal Development of Paranasal Sinuses

The **maxillary sinuses** are small at birth but rapidly pneumatize from age 1 to 4 years and then slowly continue to pneumatize until early adulthood - they are not fully developed until all the permanent teeth have erupted.

No **frontal or sphenoidal sinuses** are present at birth. The **ethmoidal cells (sinuses)** are small before the age of 2 years, and they do not begin to grow rapidly until 6 to 8 years of age. At approximately 2 years of age, the two most anterior ethmoidal cells grow into the frontal bone, forming a **frontal sinus** on each side which slowly pneumatize. Usually, the frontal sinuses are visible in radiographs by the seventh year and have their adult appearance by age 12.

The two most posterior ethmoidal cells grow into the sphenoid bone at approximately 2 years of age, forming two **sphenoidal sinuses**. Growth of the paranasal sinuses is important in altering the size and shape of the face during infancy and childhood and in adding resonance to the voice during adolescence.

DEVELOPMENT OF PALATE

8

The palate develops from two primordia, the primary and secondary palates. **Palatogenesis** (regulated morphogenetic process) begins in the sixth week, but it is not completed until the 12th week. *Molecular interacting pathways, including WNT and PRICKLE1, Fgf18 gene, and the homeobox transcription factor Six2, PAX7, PAX9 RYK (receptor-like tyrosinase kinase) are involved in this process.* The critical period of palatogenesis is from the end of the sixth week until the beginning of the ninth week. The palate develops in two stages: primary and secondary.

PRIMARY PALATE

Early in the sixth week, the primary palate **(median process)** begins to develop (see Figs. 9.32F and 9.33). Formed by merging the medial nasal prominences, this segment is initially a wedge-shaped mass of mesenchyme between the internal surfaces of the maxillary prominences of the developing maxillae. The primary palate forms the anterior and midline aspect of the maxilla, the **premaxillary part of the maxilla** (Fig. 9.35B). It represents only a small part of the adult **hard palate** (anterior to the incisive fossa).

SECONDARY PALATE

The secondary palate (definitive palate) is the primordium of the hard and soft parts of the palate (see Figs. 9.33D and 9.35). The palate begins to develop early in the sixth week from two mesenchymal projections that extend from the internal aspects of the maxillary prominences. These **lateral**

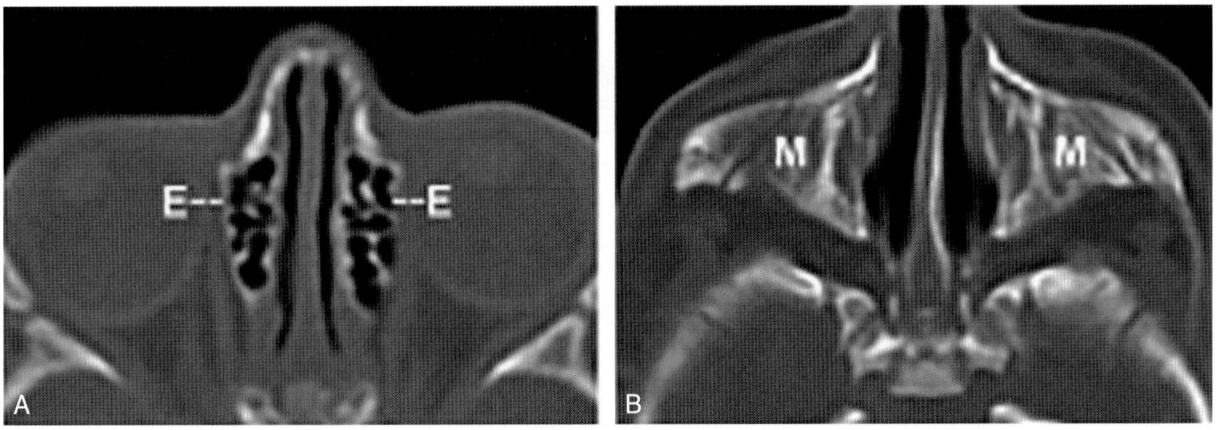

Fig. 9.34 Paranasal sinus development. CT images at birth, (A) pneumatized ethmoidal (*E*) labyrinth, and (B) none pneumatized maxillary (M) sinuses. (From Vaid S, Vaid, N: Sinonasal anatomy. *Neuroimag Clin N Am* 32:713, 2022.)

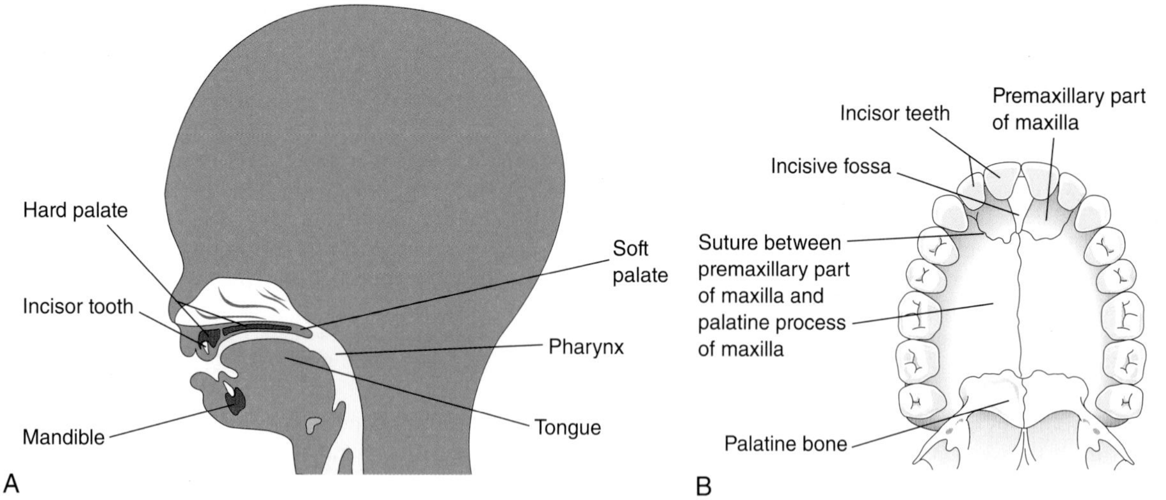

Fig. 9.35 (A) Sagittal section of the head of a 20-week fetus shows the location of the palate. (B) Bony palate and alveolar arch of a young adult. The suture between the premaxillary part of the maxilla and the fused palatine processes of the maxillae is usually visible in the cranium (skulls) of a young adult. Most dried crania are from older adults, and the suture is not visible.

palatine processes (palatal shelves) initially project inferomedially on each side of the tongue (Figs. 9.36B and 9.37A and B). As the jaws elongate, they pull the tongue away from its root, and it is brought lower in the mouth.

During the seventh and eighth weeks, the **lateral palatine processes** assume a horizontal position above the tongue (see Figs. 9.36E–H and 9.37C). This change in orientation occurs by a flowing process facilitated in part by the release of hyaluronic acid by the mesenchyme of the palatine processes.

Bone gradually develops in the primary palate, forming the **premaxillary part of the maxilla**, which lodges the incisor teeth (see Fig. 9.35B). Concurrently, bone extends from the maxillae and palatine bones into the lateral palatine processes to form the **hard palate** (see Fig. 9.36E and G). The posterior parts of these processes do not ossify. They extend posteriorly beyond the nasal septum and fuse to form the **soft palate**, including its soft conical projection, the **uvula** (see Fig. 9.36D, F, and H). The palatine raphe indicates the line of fusion of the palatine processes (see Fig. 9.36H). *It has been reported that expression of TBX15 and ADAMTS2 genes in the posterior palatal mesenchymal cells and their associated signaling pathway regulate the fusion of the soft palate.*

A small **nasopalatine canal** persists in the median plane of the palate between the anterior part of the maxilla and the palatine processes of the maxillae. This canal is represented in the adult hard palate by the **incisive fossa** (see Fig. 9.35B), which is the common opening for the small right and left incisive canals. An irregular suture runs on each side from the fossa to the alveolar process of the maxilla between the lateral incisor and canine teeth on each side (see Fig. 9.35B). It is visible in the anterior region of the palates of young persons. This suture indicates where the embryonic primary and secondary palates are fused.

The **nasal septum** develops as a down growth from internal parts of the merged medial nasal prominences (see Figs. 9.36 and 9.37). The fusion between the nasal septum and palatine processes begins anteriorly during the ninth week, and it is completed posteriorly by the 12th week superior to the primordium of the hard palate (see Fig. 9.36D–H).

Cleft Lip and Cleft Palate

Clefts of the upper lip and palate are common craniofacial birth defects. A 2014 report from the US Department of Health and Human Services indicated that approximately 7000 neonates have orofacial clefts each year in the United States. At the beginning of the second trimester (see Fig. 9.25), features of the fetal face can be identified using sonography. This imaging technique (Fig. 9.38) allows for the detection of facial defects such as a cleft lip.

The defects are usually classified according to developmental criteria, with the incisive fossa used as a reference landmark (see Fig. 9.35B). These clefts are especially conspicuous because they result in an abnormal facial appearance and defective speech. There are **two major groups of cleft lip and cleft palate** (Figs. 9.39, 9.40, and 9.41):

- **Anterior cleft defects** include cleft lip with or without a cleft of the alveolar part of the maxilla. In a complete anterior cleft defect, the cleft extends through the upper lip and alveolar part of the maxilla to the incisive fossa, separating the anterior and posterior parts of the palate (see Fig. 9.40E and F). Anterior cleft defects result from a deficiency of mesenchyme in the maxillary prominences and the median palatine process (see Fig. 9.32E).
- **Posterior cleft defects** include clefts of the secondary palate that extend through the soft and hard regions of the palate to the incisive fossa, separating the anterior and posterior parts of the palate (see Fig. 9.40G and H). Posterior cleft defects result from defective development of the secondary palate and growth distortions of the lateral palatine processes that prevent their fusion. Other factors such as the width of the stomodeum,

Cleft Lip and Cleft Palate—cont'd

mobility of the lateral **palatine processes** (palatal shelves), and altered focal degeneration sites of the palatal epithelium may contribute to these birth defects.

A cleft lip with or without a cleft palate occurs approximately once in 1000 births, but the frequency varies widely among ethnic groups. Between 60% and 80% of affected neonates are male. The clefts vary from incomplete cleft lip to those that extend into the nose and through the alveolar part of the maxilla (see Figs. 9.39 and 9.41A and B). Cleft lip may be unilateral or bilateral.

A **unilateral cleft lip** (see Figs. 9.39, 9.40E and F, and 9.41A) results from failure of the maxillary prominence on the affected side to unite with the merged medial nasal prominences. Failure of the mesenchymal masses to merge and mesenchyme to proliferate and smooth the overlying epithelium results in **a persistent labial groove** (Fig. 9.42D). The epithelium in the labial groove becomes stretched, and the tissue in the floor of the groove breaks down, resulting in a lip that is divided into medial and lateral parts (see Fig. 9.42G and H). A bridge of tissue, called the *Simonart band*, sometimes joins the parts of the incomplete unilateral cleft lip.

A **bilateral cleft lip** results from the failure of the mesenchymal masses in both maxillary prominences to meet and unite with the merged medial nasal prominences (Fig. 9.43C and D; see Fig. 9.41B). The epithelium in both labial grooves becomes stretched and breaks down (see Fig. 9.42H). In bilateral cases, the defects may be dissimilar, with various degrees of defect on each side. When there is a complete **bilateral cleft of the lip and alveolar part of the maxilla**, the median palatal process hangs free and projects anteriorly (see Fig. 9.41B). These defects are especially deforming because of the loss of continuity of the **orbicularis oris muscle** (see Fig. 9.5B), which closes the mouth and purses the lips.

A **median cleft lip** is a rare defect that results from a mesenchymal deficiency. This defect causes partial or complete failure of the medial nasal prominences to merge and form the median palatal process. A median cleft lip is a characteristic feature of the **Mohr syndrome**, which is transmitted as an autosomal recessive trait. A median cleft of the lower lip is also rare and results from the failure of the mesenchymal masses in the mandibular prominences to merge completely and smooth the embryonic cleft between them (see Fig. 9.25A).

A **cleft palate** with or without a cleft lip occurs approximately once in 2500 births, and it is more common in females than in males. It is thought that in isolated cleft palate only, the discrepancy of incidence is related to one one-week delay in palate shelf fusion in females compared to males. The cleft may involve only the uvula (a **cleft uvula** has a fishtail appearance; see Fig. 9.40B), or the cleft may extend through the soft and hard regions of the palate (see Figs. 9.40C and D and 9.43). In severe cases associated with a cleft lip, the cleft in the palate extends through the alveolar part of the maxilla and lips on both sides (see Figs. 9.40G and H and 9.41B).

A **complete cleft palate** is the maximum degree of clefting of any particular type. For example, a complete cleft of the posterior palate is a defect in which the cleft extends through the soft palate and anteriorly to the incisive fossa. The landmark for distinguishing anterior from posterior cleft defects is the incisive fossa. Unilateral and bilateral clefts of the palate are classified into three groups:

- *Clefts of the anterior palate* (clefts anterior to the incisive fossa) result from failure of mesenchymal masses in the lateral palatal processes to meet and fuse with the mesenchyme in the primary palate (see Fig. 9.40E and F).
- *Clefts of the posterior palate* (clefts posterior to the incisive fossa) result from the failure of mesenchymal masses in the lateral palatine processes to meet and fuse with each other and the nasal septum (see Fig. 9.40C and D).
- *Clefts of the secondary parts of the palate* (clefts of the anterior and posterior palates) result from failure of the mesenchymal masses in the lateral palatine processes to meet and fuse with mesenchyme in the primary palate, with each other, and the nasal septum (see Fig. 9.40G and H).

Most clefts of the upper lip and palate result from multiple genetic and nongenetic factors (**multifactorial inheritance**; see Fig. 20.1), with each causing a minor developmental disturbance. *Several studies show that the interferon regulatory factor 6 gene (IRF6), RYK, PAX7, and PAK9 expression are involved in the formation of isolated clefts*.

Some clefts of the lip and/or palate appear as part of syndromes determined by single mutant genes. Other clefts are parts of chromosomal syndromes, especially **trisomy 13** (see Fig. 20.8). A few cases of cleft lip and/or palate appear to have been caused by **teratogenic agents** (e.g., anticonvulsant drugs). Studies of twins indicate that genetic factors are more important in cases of cleft lip with or without a cleft palate than in cleft palate alone.

A sibling of a child with a cleft palate has an elevated risk of cleft palate but has no increased risk of cleft lip. A cleft of the lip and alveolar process of the maxilla that continues through the palate is usually transmitted through a male sex-linked gene. When neither parent is affected, the recurrence risk in subsequent siblings is approximately 4%.

Other Facial Defects

Congenital microstomia (small mouth) results from excessive merging of the mesenchymal masses in the maxillary and mandibular prominences of the first pharyngeal arch. In severe cases, the defect may be associated with underdevelopment (hypoplasia) of the mandible. A **single nostril** results when only one nasal placode forms. A **bifid nose** results when the medial nasal prominences do not merge completely; the nostrils are widely separated, and the nasal bridge is bifid. In mild forms, there is a groove in the tip of the nose.

Facial Clefts

Various types of facial clefts occur, but all are rare. Severe clefts are usually associated with gross defects of the head. **Oblique facial clefts** are often bilateral and extend from the upper lip to the medial margin of the **orbit** (bony cavity containing the eyeball). When this occurs, the nasolacrimal ducts are open grooves (persistent nasolacrimal grooves; Fig. 9.44). Oblique facial clefts associated with cleft lip result from failure of the mesenchymal masses in the maxillary prominences to merge with the lateral and medial nasal prominences. **Lateral or transverse facial clefts** run from the mouth toward the ear. **Bilateral clefts** result in a very large mouth **(macrostomia)**. In severe cases, the clefts in the cheeks extend almost to the ears.

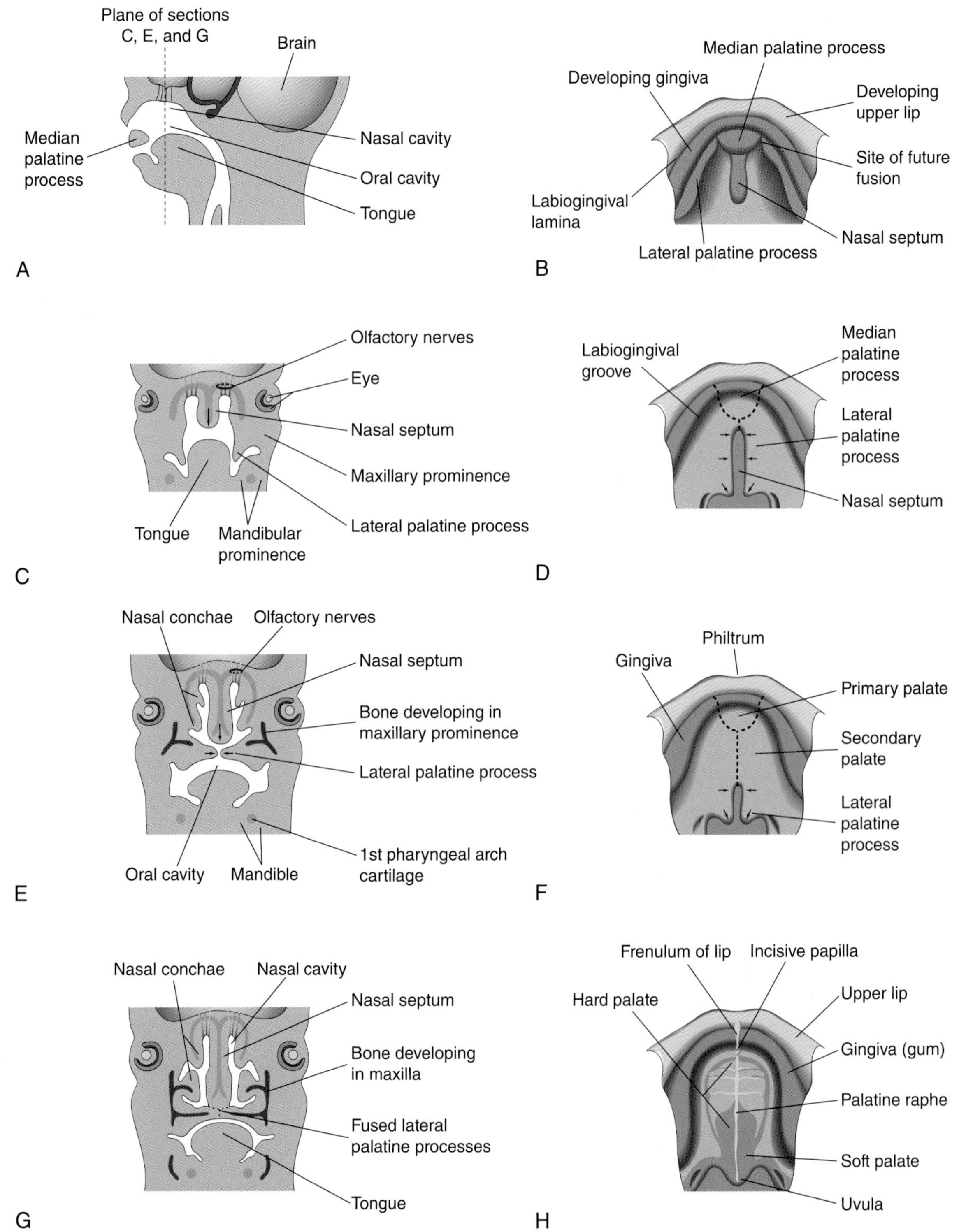

Fig. 9.36 (A) Drawings of the sagittal section of the embryonic head at the end of the sixth week show the median palatal process. (B, D, F, and H) Sections of the roof of the mouth from the 6th to 12th week show development of the palate. The *broken lines* in (D and F) indicate sites of fusion of the palatine processes. The *arrows* indicate medial and posterior growth of the lateral palatine processes. (C, E, and G) Frontal sections of the head show fusion of the lateral palatine processes with each other, the nasal septum, and separation of the nasal and oral cavities.

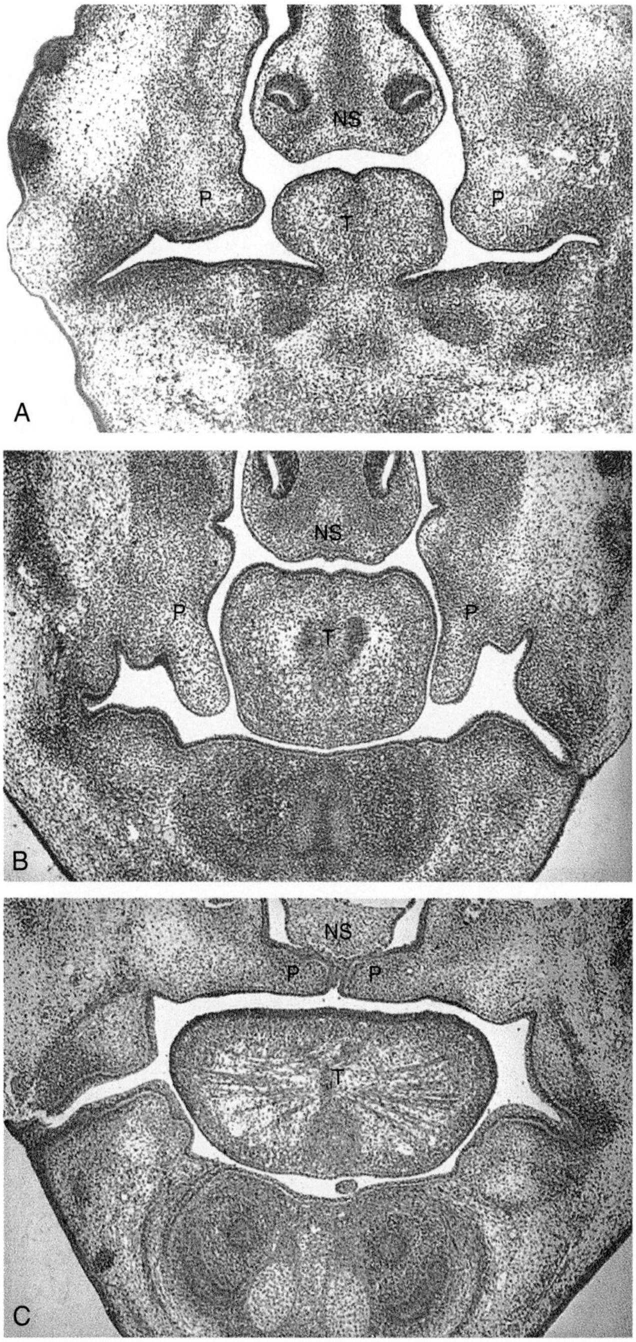

Fig. 9.37 Frontal sections of embryonic heads show the development of the lateral palatal processes *(P)*, nasal septum *(NS)*, and tongue *(T)* during the eighth week. (A) Section of an embryo with a crown-rump length (CRL) of 24 mm shows early development of the palatine processes. (B) Section of an embryo with a CRL of 27 mm shows the palate just before palatine process elevation. (C) In an embryo with a CRL of 29 mm (near the end of the eighth week), the palatine processes are elevated and fused. (From Sandham A: Embryonic facial vertical dimension and its relationship to palatal shelf elevation, *Early Hum Dev* 12:241, 1985.)

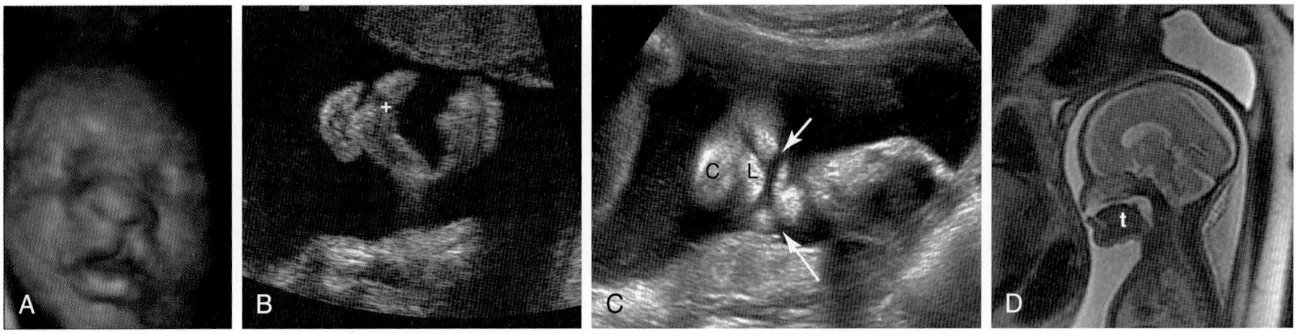

Fig. 9.38 (A) Three-dimensional ultrasound surface rendering of a fetus with a unilateral cleft lip. (B) Coronal sonogram shows a fetal mouth with a cleft lip extending into the left nostril *(+)*. (C) Coronal sonogram shows a fetus with a bilateral cleft lip *(arrows)*, lower lip *(L)*, and chin *(C)*. (D) Sagittal magnetic resonance image of a fetus shows the absence of the middle part of the hard palate. Notice the fluid above the tongue *(t)* without intervening palate. ((A and B) Courtesy Dr. G.J. Reid, Department of Obstetrics, Gynecology and Reproductive Sciences, University of Manitoba, Women's Hospital, Winnipeg, Manitoba, Canada. (C and D) Courtesy Deborah Levine, MD, Director of Obstetric and Gynecologic Ultrasound, Beth Israel Deaconess Medical Center, Boston, Massachusetts.)

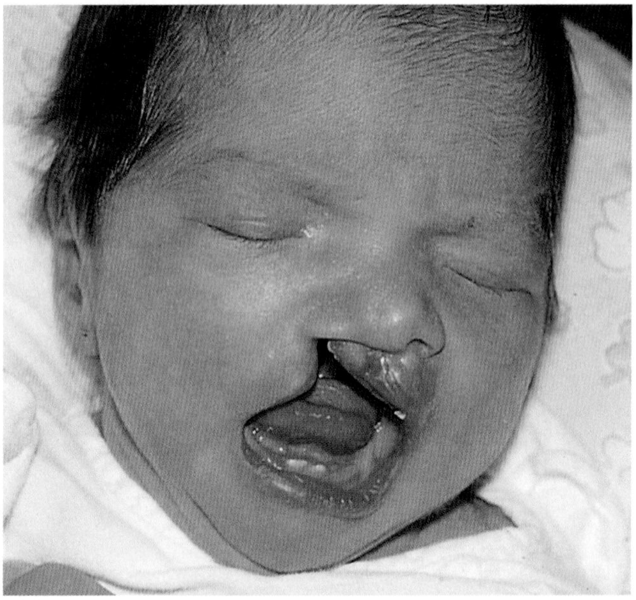

Fig. 9.39 An infant with a unilateral cleft lip and cleft palate. Clefts of the lip, with or without a cleft palate, occur in approximately 1 in 1000 births, and most affected infants are male. (Courtesy Dr. A.E. Chudley, Section of Genetics and Metabolism, Department of Pediatrics and Child Health, Children's Hospital, Winnipeg, Manitoba, Canada.)

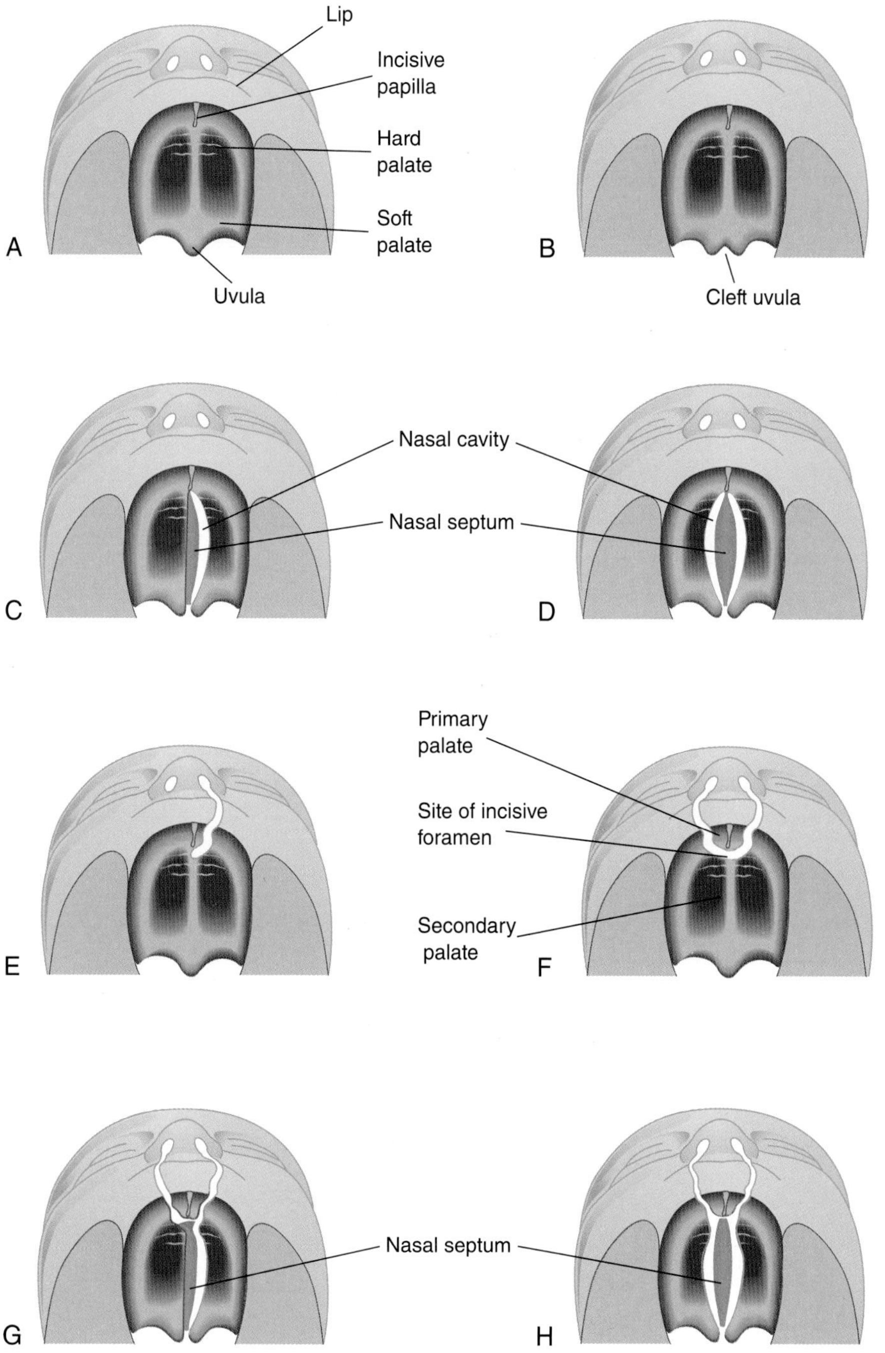

Fig. 9.40 Types of cleft lip and palate. (A) Normal lip and palate. (B) Cleft uvula. (C) Unilateral cleft of the secondary (posterior) palate. (D) Bilateral cleft of the posterior part of the palate. (E) Complete unilateral cleft of the lip and alveolar process of the maxilla with a unilateral cleft of the primary (anterior) palate. (F) Complete bilateral cleft of the lip and alveolar processes of the maxillae with bilateral cleft of the anterior part of the palate. (G) Complete bilateral cleft of the lip and alveolar processes of the maxillae with bilateral cleft of the anterior part of the palate and unilateral cleft of the posterior part of the palate. (H) Complete bilateral cleft of the lip and alveolar processes of the maxillae with complete bilateral cleft of the anterior and posterior palate.

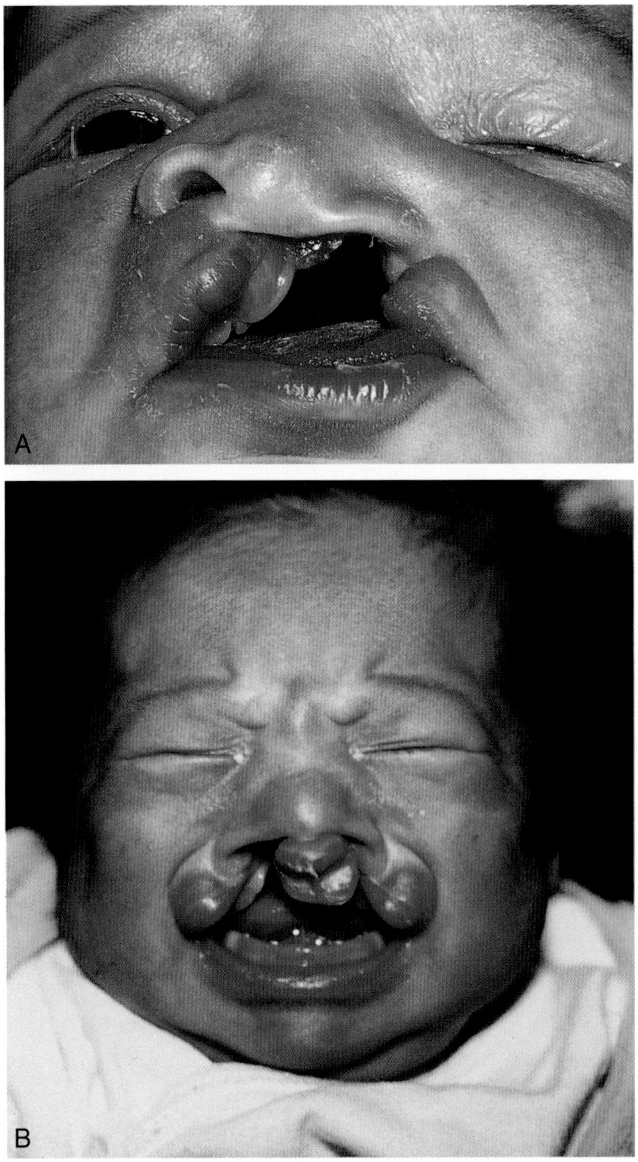

Fig. 9.41 Birth defects of the lip and palate. (A) Infant with a left unilateral cleft lip and cleft palate. (B) Infant with a bilateral cleft lip and cleft palate. (Courtesy Dr. Barry H. Grayson and Dr. Bruno L. Vendittelli, New York University Medical Center, Institute of Reconstructive Plastic Surgery, New York, New York.)

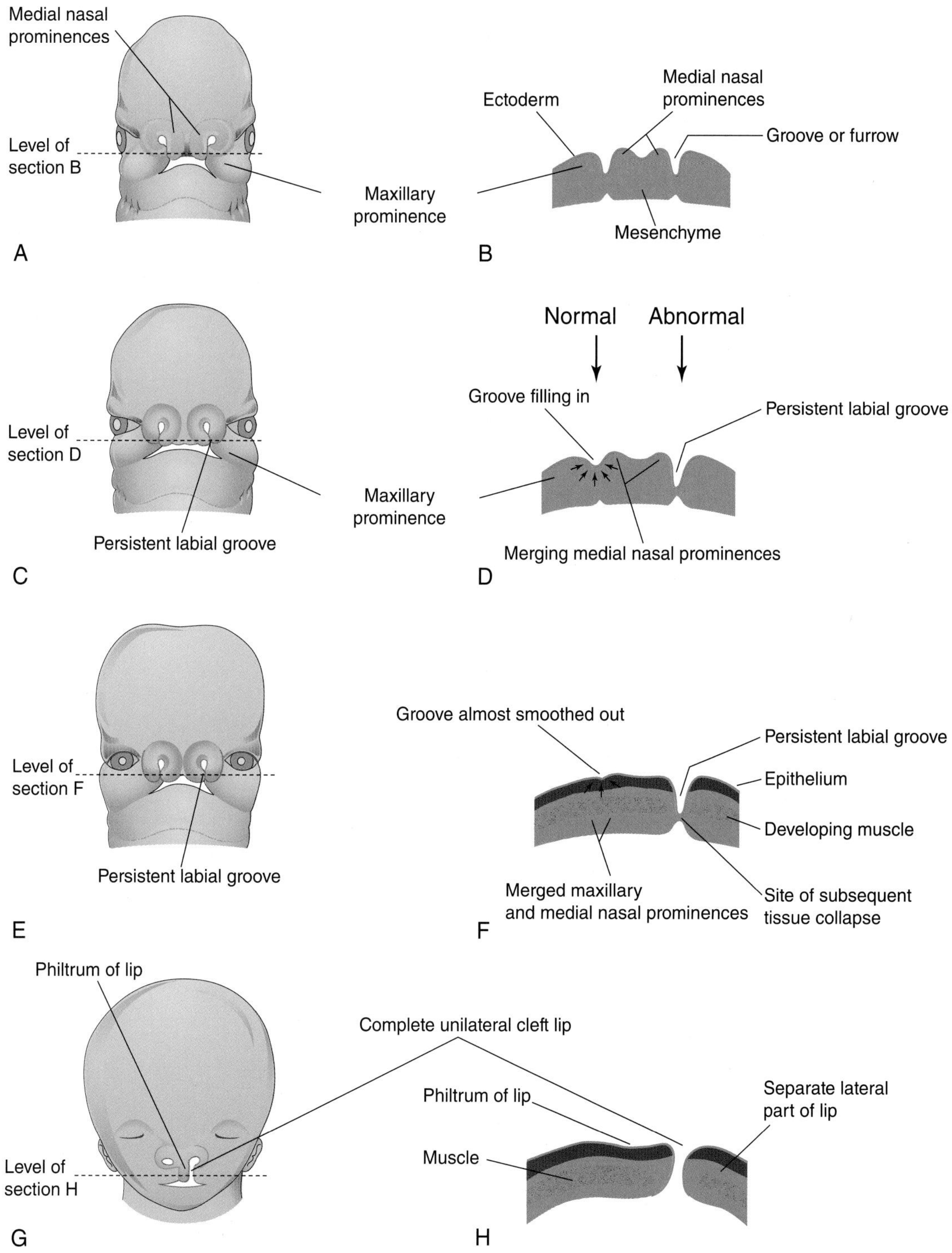

Fig. 9.42 Embryologic basis of complete unilateral cleft lip. (A) Drawing of a 5-week embryo. (B) Horizontal section through the head shows the grooves between the maxillary prominences and merging medial nasal prominences. (C) Drawing of a 6-week embryo shows a persistent labial groove on the left side. (D) Horizontal section through the head shows the groove gradually filling in on the right side after the proliferation of mesenchyme *(arrows)*. (E) Drawing of a 7-week embryo. (F) Horizontal section through the head shows that the epithelium on the right has almost been pushed out of the groove between the maxillary and medial nasal prominences. (G) Drawing of a 10-week fetus with a complete unilateral cleft lip. (H) Horizontal section through the head after stretching of the epithelium and breakdown of the tissues in the floor of the persistent labial groove on the left side shows the formation of a complete unilateral cleft lip.

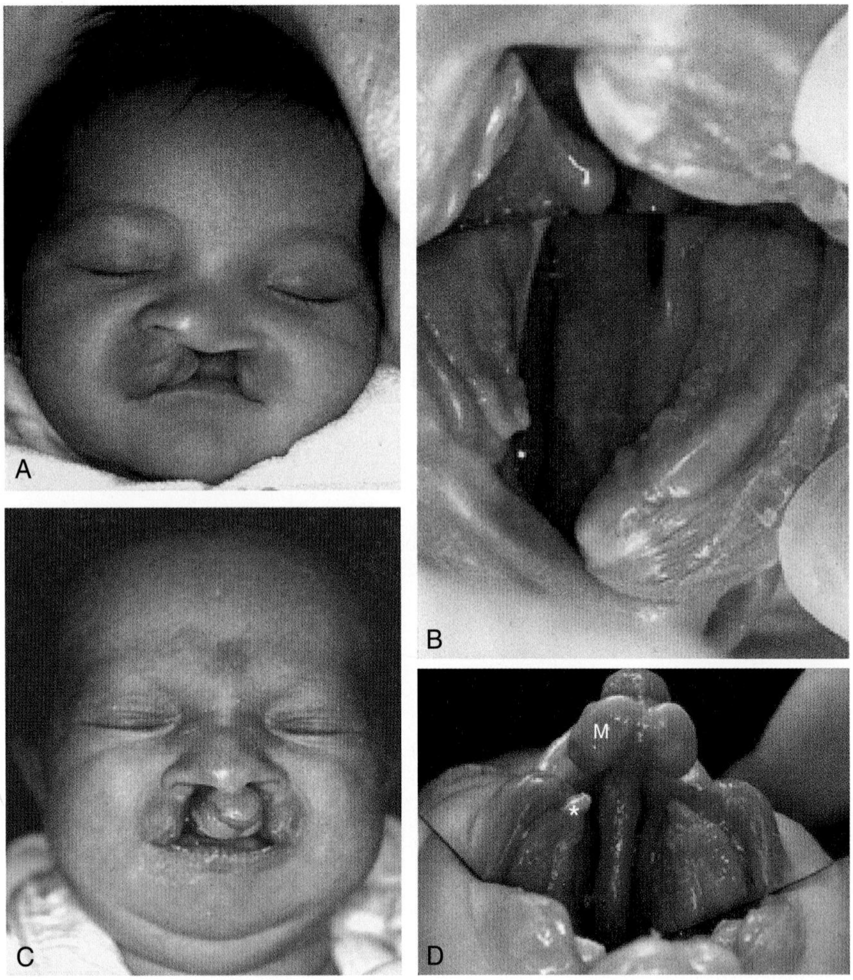

Fig. 9.43 Birth defects of the lip and palate. (A) Male neonate with a unilateral complete cleft lip and cleft palate. (B) Intraoral photograph (taken with a mirror) shows a left unilateral complete cleft of the primary and secondary parts of the palate. (C) Female neonate with a bilateral complete cleft lip and cleft palate. (D) Intraoral mirror photograph shows a bilateral complete cleft palate. Notice the maxillary protrusion *(M)* and natal tooth *(*)* (present at birth) in the gingival apex in each lesser segment. (Courtesy Dr. John B. Mulliken, Children's Hospital Boston, Harvard Medical School, Boston, Massachusetts.)

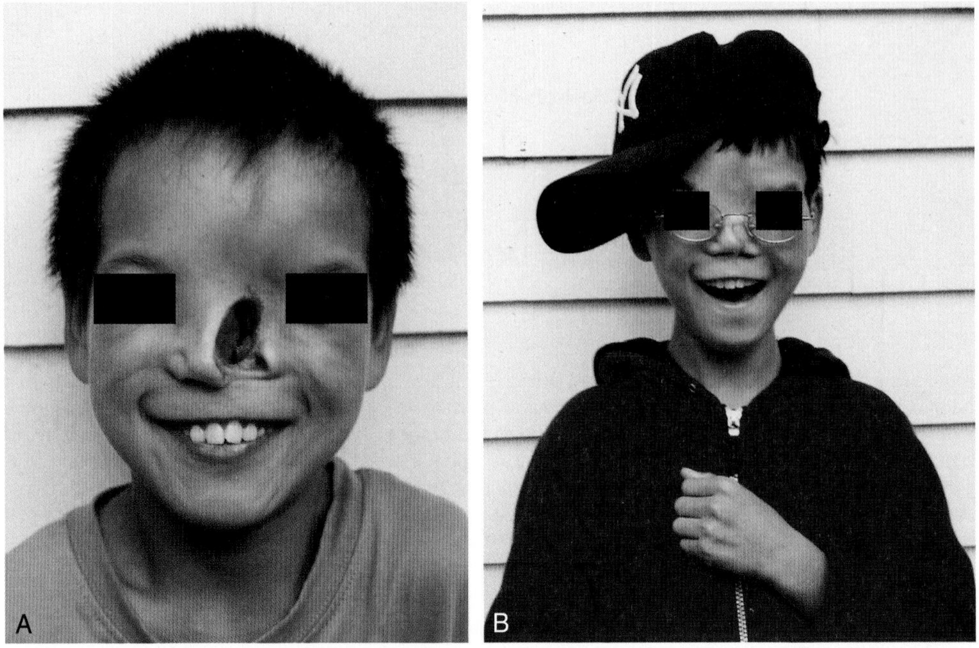

Fig. 9.44 Photographs of a child with an oblique facial cleft. Notice the persistent nasolacrimal cleft. (A) Before surgical correction. (B) After surgical correction. (Courtesy Dr. J.A. Ascherman, Department of Surgery, Division of Plastic Surgery, Columbia University Medical Center, New York, New York.)

SUMMARY OF PHARYNGEAL APPARATUS, FACE, AND NECK

- The **primordial pharynx** is bounded laterally by **pharyngeal arches**. Each arch consists of a core of mesenchyme covered externally by ectoderm and internally by endoderm. The original mesenchyme of each arch is derived from mesoderm. Later, **neural crest cells** migrate into the arches and are the major source of the connective tissue components, including cartilage, bone, and ligaments in the oral and facial regions. Each arch contains an artery, cartilage rod, nerve, and a muscular component.
- Externally, **the pharyngeal arches** are separated by pharyngeal grooves. Internally, the arches are separated by evaginations (outpocketings) of the pharynx **(pharyngeal pouches)**. Where the ectoderm of a groove contacts the endoderm of a pouch, **pharyngeal membranes** are formed. The adult derivatives of the various pharyngeal arch components are summarized in Table 9.1, and the derivatives of the pouches are illustrated in Fig. 9.7.
- The **pharyngeal grooves** disappear except for the first pair, which persists as the external acoustic meatus. The pharyngeal membranes also disappear, except for the first pair, which becomes the tympanic membranes. The **first pharyngeal pouch** forms the tympanic cavity, mastoid antrum, and pharyngotympanic tube. The **second pharyngeal pouch** is associated with the development of the palatine tonsil.
- The **thymus** is derived from the **third pair of pharyngeal pouches**, and the **parathyroid glands** are formed from the **third and fourth pairs of pouches**.
- The **thyroid gland** develops from a down growth from the floor of the primordial pharynx in the region where the tongue develops. The parafollicular cells (C cells) in the thyroid gland are derived from the **ultimopharyngeal bodies**, which are derived mainly from the fourth pair of pharyngeal pouches.
- Cervical cysts, sinuses, and fistulas may develop from parts of the second pharyngeal groove, the **cervical sinus**, or the second pharyngeal pouch that fail to obliterate.
- An **ectopic thyroid gland** results when the gland fails to descend completely from its site of origin in the tongue. The **thyroglossal duct** may persist, or remnants of it may form **thyroglossal duct cysts** and ectopic thyroid tissue masses. Infected cysts may perforate the skin and form thyroglossal duct sinuses that open anteriorly in the median plane of the neck.
- **Cleft of the upper lip** is a common birth defect. Although frequently associated with cleft palate, cleft lip, and cleft palate are etiologically distinct defects that involve different developmental processes occurring at different times. A cleft of the upper lip results from the failure of mesenchymal masses in the medial nasal and maxillary prominences to merge, whereas a cleft palate results from the failure of mesenchymal masses in the palatal processes to meet and fuse. Most cases of cleft lip, with or without cleft palate, are caused by a combination of genetic and environmental factors (**multifactorial inheritance**; see Chapter 20).

CLINICALLY ORIENTED PROBLEMS

CASE 9-1

The mother of a 2-year-old boy consulted her pediatrician about an intermittent discharge of mucoid material from a small opening in the side of the boy's neck. There was also extensive redness and swelling in the inferior third of his neck just anterior to the sternocleidomastoid muscle.

- What is the most likely diagnosis?
- What is the probable embryologic basis of this intermittent mucoid discharge?
- Discuss the cause of this birth defect.

CASE 9-2

During a subtotal thyroidectomy, the surgeon located only one inferior parathyroid gland.

- Where might the other one be located?
- What is the embryologic basis for the ectopic location of this gland?

CASE 9-3

A young female consulted her physician about a swelling in the anterior part of her neck, just inferior to the hyoid bone.

- What kind of a cyst is this?
- Are these cysts always in the median plane?
- Discuss the embryologic basis of these cysts.
- What other condition may be confused with the swelling?

CASE 9-4

A male neonate has a unilateral cleft lip extending into his nose and through the alveolar process of his maxilla.

- Are the terms *harelip* and *cleft lip* synonymous?
- What is the embryologic basis of this birth defect?
- Neither parent had a cleft lip or cleft palate. Are genetic factors likely involved?
- Are these defects more common in males?
- What is the chance that the next child will have a cleft lip?

CASE 9-5

A mother with epilepsy who was treated with an anticonvulsant drug during pregnancy gave birth to a child with a cleft lip and palate.

- Is there evidence indicating that these drugs increase the incidence of these birth defects?
- Discuss the causes of these two birth defects.

Discussion of these problems appears in the Appendix at the back of the book.

BIBLIOGRAPHY AND SUGGESTED READING

Bajaj Y, Ifeacho S, Tweedie D, Jephson CG, Albert DM, Cochrane LA: Branchial anomalies in children, *Int J Pediatr Otorhinolaryngol* 75:1020, 2011.

Berkovitz BKB, Holland GR, Moxham B: *Oral anatomy, histology, and embryology*, ed 5, Edinburgh, 2018, Elsevier.

Bothe I, Tenin G, Oseni A, Dietrich S: Dynamic control of head mesoderm patterning, *Development* 138:2807, 2011.

Burford CM, Mason MJ: Early development of the malleus and incus in humans, *J Anat* 229:857, 2016.

Cordes M, Coerper S, Kuwert T, Schmidkonz C: Ultrasound imaging of cervical anatomic variants, *Curr Med Imaging* 17:966, 2021.

Danescu A, Mattson M, Dool C, Diewert VM, Richman JM: Analysis of human soft palate morphogenesis supports regional regulation of palatal fusion, *J. Anat* 227:474, 2015.

Danescu A, Rens EG, Rehki J, et al: Symmetry and fluctuation of cell movements in neural crest-derived facial mesenchyme, *Development* 148(9):dev193755, 2021. https://doi.org/10.1242/dev.193755.

de Paula F, Teshima THN, Hsieh R, Souza MM, Nico MMS, Lourenco SV: Overview of human salivary glands: highlights of morphology and developing processes, *Anat Rec* 300:1180, 2017.

Fabik J, Psutkova V, Machon O: The mandibular and hyoid arches-from molecular patterning to shaping bone and cartilage, *Int J Mol Sci* 22(14):7529, 2021. https://doi.org/10.3390/ijms22147529.

Ferreira ACF, Szeto ACH, Heycock MWD, Clark PA, Walker JA, Crisp A: RORα is a critical checkpoint for T cell and ILC2 commitment in the embryonic thymus, *Nat Immunol* 22(2):166–178, 2021. https://doi.org/10.1038/s41590-020-00833-w.

Frisdal A, Trainor PA: Development and evolution of the pharyngeal apparatus, *Wiley Interdiscip Rev Dev Biol* 6:403, 2014.

Gitton Y, Heude E, Vieux-Rochas M, et al: Evolving maps in craniofacial development, *Semin Cell Develop Biol* 21:301, 2010.

Gross E, Sichel JY: Congenital neck lesions, *Surg Clin North Am* 86:383, 2006.

Gupta P, Tripathi T, Singh N, et al: A review of genetics of nasal development and morphological variation, *J Family Med Prim Care* 9(4): 1825–1833, 2020. https://doi.org/10.4103/jfmpc.jfmpc_126519.

Hennekam R, Allanson J, Krantz I: *Gorlin's syndromes of the head and neck,* ed 5, New York, 2010, Oxford University Press.

Hinrichsen K: The early development of morphology and patterns of the face in the human embryo, *Adv Anat Embryol Cell Biol* 98:1, 1985.

Honkura Y, Yamamoto M, Yoshimoto T, et al: Is the ultimobranchial body a reality or myth: a study using serial sections of human embryos, *Okajimas Folia Anat Jpn* 93:29, 2016.

Houssin NS, Bharathan NK, Turner SD, Dickinson AJ: Role of JNK during buccopharyngeal membrane perforation, the last step of embryonic mouth formation, *Dev Dyn* 246(2):100–115, 2016.

Jirasek JE: *An atlas of human prenatal developmental mechanics.* In *Anatomy and staging,* London, 2004, Taylor & Francis.

Jones KL, Jones MC, Campo MD: *Smith's recognizable patterns of human malformation,* ed 8, Philadelphia, 2021, Elsevier.

Khan MI, Cs P, Srinath NM: Genetic factors in non-syndromic orofacial clefts, *Glob Med Genet* 7(4):101–108, 2020. https://doi.org/10.1055/s-0041-1722951.

Kostopoulou E, Miliordos K, Spiliotis B: Genetics of primary congenital hypothyroidism – a review, *Hormones* 20:225, 2021.

Lale SM, Lele MS, Anderson VM: The thymus in infancy and childhood, *Chest Surg Clin North Am* 11:233, 2001.

Lauffer P, Zwaveling-Soonawala N, Naafs JC, Boelen A, van Trotsenburg ASP: Diagnosis and management of central congenital hypothyroidism, *Front Endocrinol* 2:686317, 2021. https://doi.org/10.3389/fendo.2021.686317.

Leitch VD, Basssett JHD, Williams GR: Role of thyroid hormones in craniofacial development, *Nat Rev Endocrinol* 16:147, 2020.

Mai CT, Isenburg JL, Canfield MA, et al: National population-based estimates for major birth defects, 2010–2014, *Birth Defect Res* 111(18): 1420–1435, 2019.

Martinelli M, Palmieri A, Carinci F, Scapoli L: Non-syndromic cleft palate: an overview on human genetic and environmental risk factors, *Front Cell Dev Biol* 8:592271, 2020.

Minoux M, Rijii FM: Molecular mechanisms of cranial neural crest cell migration and patterning in craniofacial development, *Development* 137:2605, 2010.

Mueller DT, Callanan VP: Congenital malformations of the oral cavity, *Otolaryngol Clin North Am* 40:141, 2007.

Nanci O: *Ten Cate's oral histology,* ed 9, Philadelphia, 2018, Elsevier.

Naqvi S, Hoskens H, Wilke F, Weinberg SM, Shaffer JR, Walsh S: Decoding the human face: progress and challenges in understanding the genetics of craniofacial morphology, *Annu Rev Genom Hum Genet* 23:383, 2022.

Nishimura Y: Embryological study of nasal cavity development in human embryos with reference to congenital nostril atresia, *Acta Anat* 147:140, 1993.

Noden DM, Francis-West P: The differentiation and morphogenesis of craniofacial muscles, *Dev Dyn* 235:1194, 2006.

Noden DM, Trainor PA: Relations and interactions between cranial mesoderm and neural crest populations, *J Anat* 207:575, 2005.

Passos-Bueno MR, Ornelas CC, Fanganiello RD: Syndromes of the first and second pharyngeal arches: a review, *Am J Med Genet A* 149A:1853, 2009.

Pechriggl E., Blumer M., Tubbs R.S., Olewnik Ł, Konschake M., Fortélny R., et al: Embryology of the abdominal wall and associated malformations-a review. Front Surg, published 07 July 2022; 9:891896. https://doi.org/10.3389/fsurg.2022.891896.

Petit KE, Tran NV, Pretorius DH: Ultrasound evaluation of the fetal face and neck. In Norton ME, editor: *Callen's ultrasonography in obstetrics and gynecology,* ed 6, Philadelphia, 2017, Elsevier.

Rodriguez-Vázquez JF: Development of the stapes and associated structures in human embryos, *J Anat* 207:165, 2005.

Sarnat HB, Flores-Sarnat L: Olfactory development, part 2: neuroanatomic maturation and dysgeneses, *J Child Neurol* 32:579, 2017.

Som PM, Grapin-Botton A: The current embryology of the foregut and its derivatives, *Neurographics* 6:43, 2016.

Sweat YY, Sweat M, Mansaray M, Cao H, Eliason S, Adeyemo WL: Six2 regulates PAX9 expression, palatogenesis and craniofacial bone formation, *Dev Biol* 458:246, 2020.

Takanashi Y, Honkura Y, Rodriguez-Vazquez JF, Murakami G, Kawase T, Katori Y: Pyramidal lobe of the thyroid gland and the thyroglossal duct remnant: a study using human fetal sections, *Ann Anat* 197:29, 2015.

Thi Thu HN, Haw Tien SF, Loh SL: Tbx2a is required for specification of endodermal pouches during development of the pharyngeal arches, *PLoS One* 10:e77171, 2013.

Thompson H, Ohazama A, Sharpe PT, Tucker AS: The origin of the stapes and relationship to the otic capsule and oval window, *Dev Dyn* 241:1396, 2012.

Vid S, Vaid N: Sinonasla anatomy, *Neuroimag Clin N Am* 32:713, 2022.

van Trotsenburg P, Stoupa A, Léger J, Rohrer T, Peters C, Fugazzola L: Congenital hypothyroidism: a 2020-2021 consensus guidelines update-an ENDO-European Reference Network Initiative Endorsed by the European Society for Pediatric Endocrinology and the European Society for Endocrinology, *Thyroid* 31(3):387–419, 2021. https://doi.org/10.1089/thy.2020.0333.

Wang X, Chen D, Chen K, Jubran A, Ramirez A, Astrof S: Endothelium in the pharyngeal arches 3, 4 and 6 is derived from the second heart field, *Dev Biol* 421:108, 2017.

Wang X, Li C, Zhu Z, Yuan L, Chan WY, Sha O: Extracellular matrix remodeling during palate development, *Organogenesis* 16(2):43–60, 2020. https://doi.org/10.1080/15476278.2020.1735239.

Yatzey KE: DiGeorge syndrome, Tbx1, and retinoic acid signaling come full circle, *Circ Res* 106:630, 2010.

Zhang Y, Li J, Ji Y, Cheng Y, Fu X: Mutations in the TBX15-ADAMTS2 pathway associate with a novel soft palate dysplasia, *Hum Mutat,* 2022. https://doi.org/10.1002/humu.24473.

Respiratory System 10

CHAPTER OUTLINE

The lower respiratory organs (larynx, trachea, bronchi, and lungs) begin to form during the fourth week of development.

9

RESPIRATORY PRIMORDIUM

The respiratory system starts as a median outgrowth, the **laryngotracheal groove**, which appears in the floor of the caudal end of the anterior foregut (primordial pharynx) (Fig. 10.1B and C; see also Fig. 10.4A). This primordium of the **tracheobronchial tree** develops caudal to the fourth pair of pharyngeal pouches. The endodermal lining of the laryngotracheal groove forms the pulmonary epithelium and glands of the larynx, trachea, and bronchi. The connective tissue, cartilage, and smooth muscle in these structures develop from the splanchnic mesoderm surrounding the foregut (see Fig. 10.5A).

By the end of the fourth week, the laryngotracheal groove has evaginated (protruded) to form a pouch-like **laryngotracheal diverticulum**, located ventral to the caudal part of the foregut (Fig. 10.2A, and see also Fig. 10.1B). As this diverticulum elongates, it is invested with **splanchnic mesenchyme**. Its distal end enlarges to form a globular **respiratory bud** (lung bud) that denotes the single bud from which the tracheobronchial (respiratory) tree originates (see Fig. 10.2B).

The laryngotracheal diverticulum soon separates from the primordial pharynx; however, they maintain communication through the **primordial laryngeal inlet** (see Fig. 10.2C). Longitudinal **tracheoesophageal folds** develop in the diverticulum, approach each other, and fuse to form a partition, the **tracheoesophageal septum**, at the end of the fifth week (see Fig. 10.2D and E). This septum divides the cranial portion of the foregut into a ventral part, the **laryngotracheal tube** (the primordium of the larynx, trachea, bronchi, and lungs), and a dorsal part (the primordium of the oropharynx and esophagus; see Fig. 10.2F). The opening of the laryngotracheal tube into the pharynx becomes the **primordial laryngeal inlet** (see Figs. 10.2C and 10.4B–D). *The separation of the single foregut tube into the trachea and esophagus results from a complex and coordinated process of multiple signaling pathways and transcription factors* (Fig. 10.3).

9

DEVELOPMENT OF LARYNX

The epithelial lining of the larynx develops from the endoderm of the cranial end of the **laryngotracheal tube** (see Fig. 10.2C). The **laryngeal cartilages** may develop from the fourth and sixth pairs of pharyngeal arches (see Fig. 10.1A and C) from mesenchyme that is derived from **neural crest cells**. The mesenchyme at the cranial end of the laryngotracheal tube proliferates rapidly, producing paired **arytenoid swellings** (Fig. 10.4B). The swellings grow toward the tongue, converting the slit-like aperture, the **primordial glottis**, into a T-shaped **laryngeal inlet** (see Fig. 10.4C). *Osteochondroblastic differentiation of the mesenchyme and maturation is controlled by Wnt signaling and expression of Sox9, RUN2, and SP9 transcription factors.*

The laryngeal epithelium proliferates rapidly, resulting in temporary occlusion of the laryngeal lumen. Recanalization normally occurs by the 10th week (see Fig. 10.4D); **laryngeal ventricles** form during this recanalization process. These recesses are bounded by folds of mucous membranes that become the **vocal folds** (cords) and **vestibular folds**.

The **epiglottis** develops from the caudal part of the hypopharyngeal eminence, a prominence produced by the proliferation of mesenchyme in the ventral ends of the third and fourth pharyngeal arches (see Fig. 10.4B–D). The rostral part of this eminence forms the posterior third or pharyngeal part of the tongue (see Fig. 10.4C and D).

Because the **laryngeal muscles** develop from myoblasts in the fourth and sixth pairs of pharyngeal arches, they are innervated by the laryngeal branches of the **vagus nerves** (cranial nerve X) that supply these arches (see Table 9.1). The larynx is found in a high position in the neck of the neonate; this positioning allows the epiglottis to come into

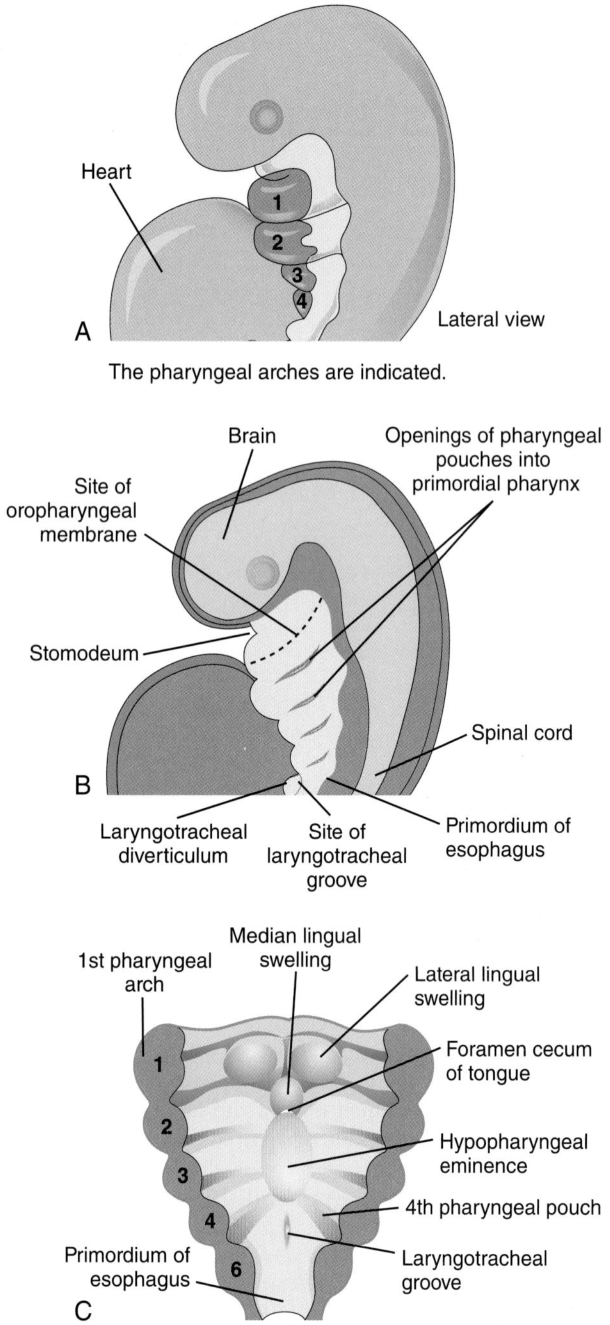

Fig. 10.1 (A) Lateral view of a 4-week embryo illustrating the relationship of the pharyngeal apparatus to the developing respiratory system. (B) Sagittal section of the cranial half of the embryo. (C) Horizontal section of the embryo illustrating the floor of the primordial pharynx and the location of the laryngotracheal groove.

Laryngeal Atresia

Laryngeal atresia (obstruction), an extremely rare birth defect (1:50,000 incidence), results from failure of recanalization of the larynx, which produces obstruction of the upper fetal airway, or **congenital high airway obstruction syndrome (CHAOS syndrome)**. Distal to the region of atresia or stenosis (narrowing), the fetal airways become dilated, and the lungs are enlarged and filled with fluid. CHAOS syndrome is often fatal due to fetal heart failure. In some cases, postpartum airway intervention (tracheostomy) may lead to survival.

Incomplete atresia, or laryngeal web, is a defect in which the connective tissue between the vocal folds is covered with a mucous membrane; this causes airway obstruction and a hoarse cry in the neonate. This defect results from incomplete recanalization of the larynx during the 10th week. Treatment is by endoscopic dilation of the laryngeal web.

Tracheoesophageal Fistula

A **fistula** (abnormal passage) between the trachea and esophagus occurs once in 3000 to 4500 infants (Figs. 10.6 and 10.7); most affected infants are males (male:female relative incidence 3:2). In more than 85% of cases, the **tracheoesophageal fistula** (TEF) is associated with esophageal **atresia**. A TEF results from the incomplete division of the cranial part of the foregut into respiratory and esophageal parts during the fourth week. Incomplete fusion of the tracheoesophageal folds results in a defective tracheoesophageal septum and a TEF between the trachea and esophagus.

TEF is the most common birth defect of the lower respiratory tract. Four main varieties of TEF may develop (see Fig. 10.6). The usual defect is for the superior part of the esophagus to end blindly **(esophageal atresia)** and for the inferior part to join the trachea near its bifurcation (see Figs. 10.6A and 10.7). Other varieties of this defect are illustrated in Fig. 10.6B–D.

Infants with the common type of TEF and esophageal atresia cannot swallow, so they frequently drool saliva and immediately regurgitate milk when fed. Gastric and intestinal contents may also reflux from the stomach through the fistula into the trachea and lungs. This refluxed acid, and in some cases bile, can cause **pneumonitis** (inflammation of the lungs), leading to respiratory compromise. **Polyhydramnios** is often associated with esophageal atresia. The excess amniotic fluid develops because fluid cannot enter the stomach and intestines for absorption and subsequent transfer through the placenta to the mother's blood for disposal.

contact with the soft palate. This provides an almost separate respiratory and digestive tract, facilitating breast-feeding, but also means that neonates almost obligatorily breathe through their noses. Structural descent of the larynx occurs over the first 2 years of life.

9

DEVELOPMENT OF TRACHEA

During its separation from the foregut, the laryngotracheal diverticulum forms the primordium of the trachea and two lateral outpouchings, the **primary bronchial buds** (see Figs. 10.2C, 10.8A, and 10.9). The endodermal lining of the laryngotracheal tube distal to the larynx differentiates into the epithelium and glands of the trachea and the pulmonary epithelium. The cartilage, connective tissue, and muscles of the trachea are derived from the splanchnic mesenchyme surrounding the laryngotracheal tube (Fig. 10.5). *The cargo receptor Evi/Wis is involved in the dorsal-ventral patterning of the endodermal lining of the laryngotracheal tube. The proliferation of the surrounding mesenchyme and formation of cartilage and smooth muscle differentiation and tracheal development are regulated by Wnt/β–catenin, Bmp, Shh, fgf, and retinoic acid signaling pathways.*

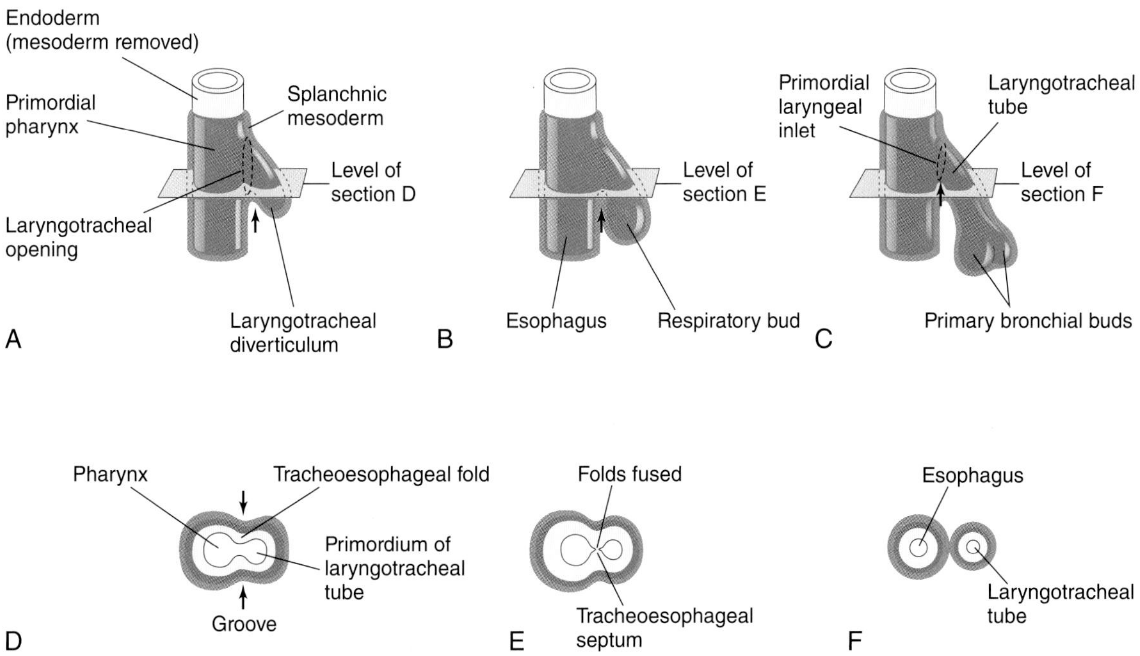

Fig. 10.2 Successive stages in the development of the tracheoesophageal septum during the fourth and fifth weeks. (A–C) Lateral views of the caudal part of the primordial pharynx showing the laryngotracheal diverticulum and partitioning of the foregut into the esophagus and laryngotracheal tube. (D–F) Transverse sections illustrating the formation of the tracheoesophageal septum and showing how it separates the foregut into the laryngotracheal tube and esophagus. The *arrows* indicate cellular changes resulting from growth.

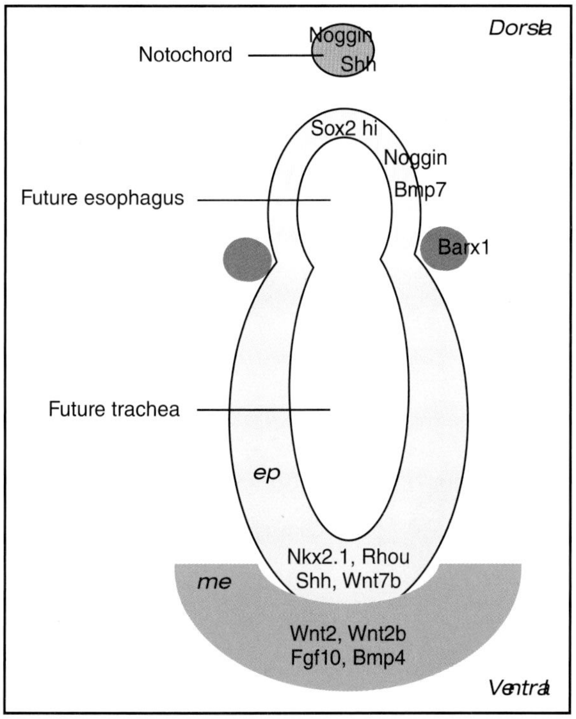

Fig. 10.3 Schematic section showing dorsal-ventral patterning of the anterior foregut (mouse). The unseparated anterior foregut tube shows high levels of Sox2, Noggin, and Bmp7 in the dorsal epithelium that will give rise to the esophagus. The ventral epithelium, which will contribute to the trachea, highly expresses transcription factor Nkx2.1 and signaling molecules Shh and Wnt7b, along with Rhou. Homeobox gene *Barx1* is expressed at the demarcation between the dorsal and ventral foregut separation. The ventral mesenchyme factors Wnt2, Wnt2b, Fgf10, and Bmp4 support gene expression in the epithelium. Defects in the Shh, Wnt, or Bmp pathway or mutations of Sox2, Nkx2.1, or Rhou can result in abnormal foregut development, leading to esophageal atresia with or without tracheoesophageal fistula. (From Jacobs IJ, Ku WY, Que J: Genetic and cellular mechanisms regulating anterior foregut and esophageal development, *Dev Biol* 369(1):54–64, 2012.)

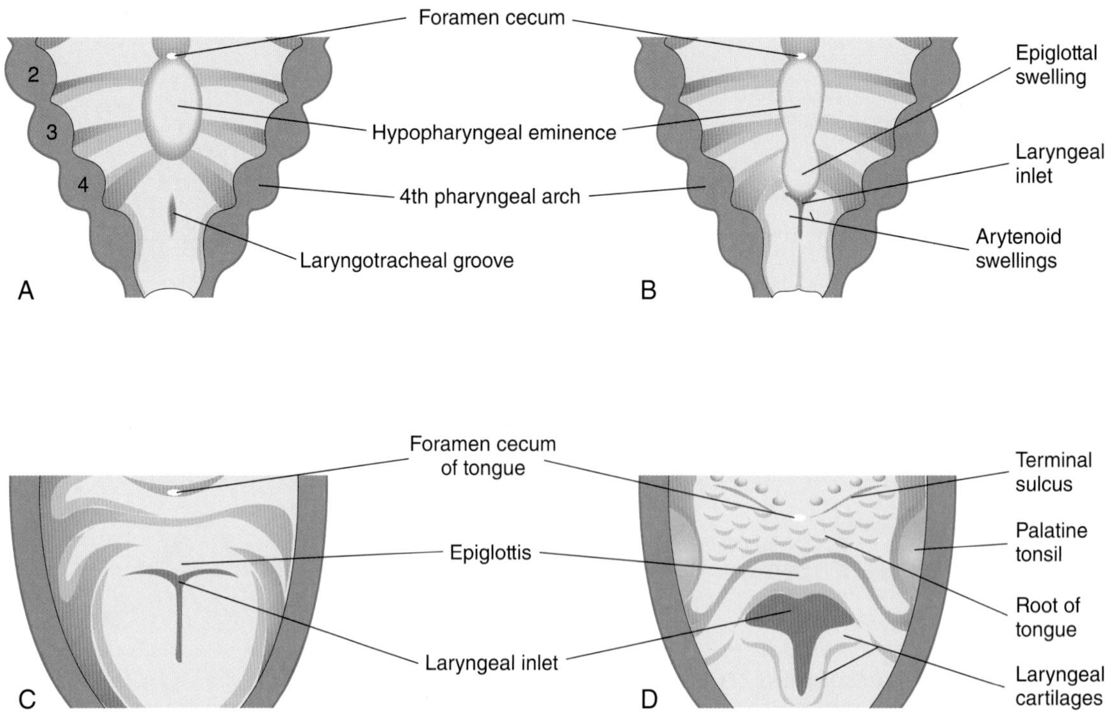

Fig. 10.4 Successive stages in the development of the larynx: (A) 4 weeks, (B) 5 weeks, (C) 6 weeks, (D) 10 weeks. The epithelium lining the larynx is of endodermal origin. The cartilages and muscles of the larynx arise from mesenchyme in the fourth and sixth pairs of pharyngeal arches. Note that the laryngeal inlet changes in shape from a slit-like opening to a T-shaped inlet as the mesenchyme surrounding the developing larynx proliferates.

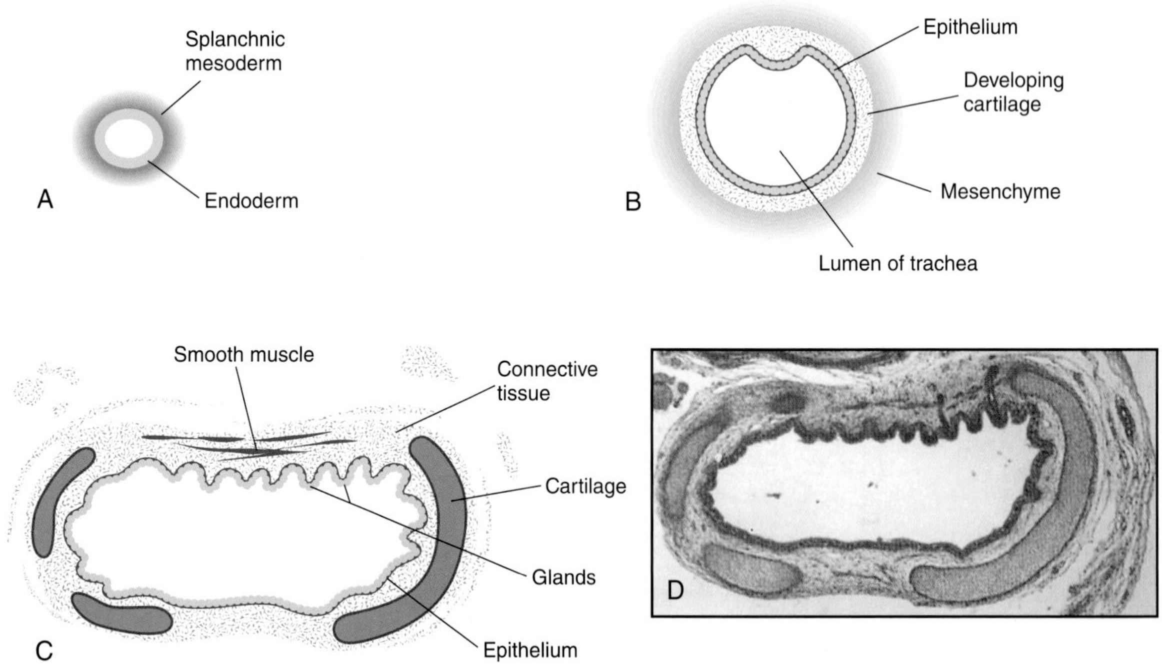

Fig. 10.5 Transverse sections through the laryngotracheal tube illustrating progressive stages in the development of the trachea: (A) 4 weeks, (B) 10 weeks, (C) 12 weeks (drawing of micrograph in (D)). Note that the endoderm of the tube gives rise to the epithelium and glands of the trachea and that mesenchyme surrounding the tube forms the connective tissue, muscle, and cartilage. (D) Photomicrograph of a transverse section of the developing trachea at 12 weeks. ((D) From Moore KL, Persaud TVN, Shiota K: *Color atlas of clinical embryology*, ed 2, Philadelphia, 2000, Saunders.)

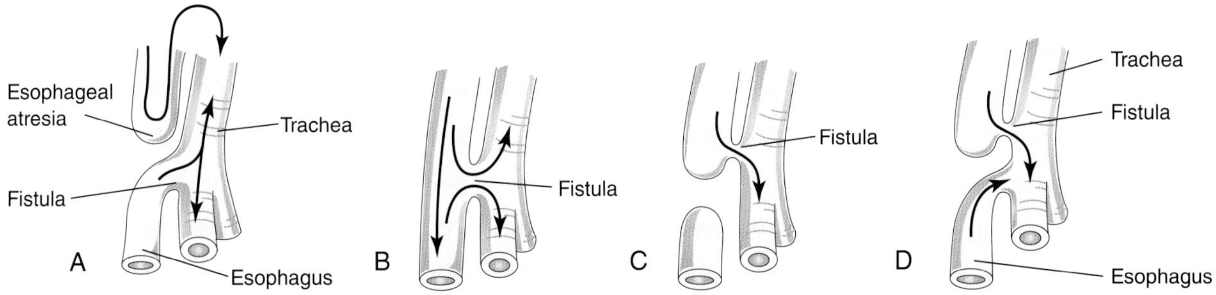

Fig. 10.6 The four main varieties of tracheoesophageal fistula (TEF) are shown in order of frequency. Possible directions of the flow of the contents are indicated by *arrows*. Esophageal atresia, as illustrated in (A) is associated with TEF in more than 85% of cases. (B) Fistula between the trachea and esophagus. (C) Air cannot enter the distal esophagus and stomach. (D) Air can enter the distal esophagus and stomach, and the esophageal and gastric contents may enter the trachea and lungs.

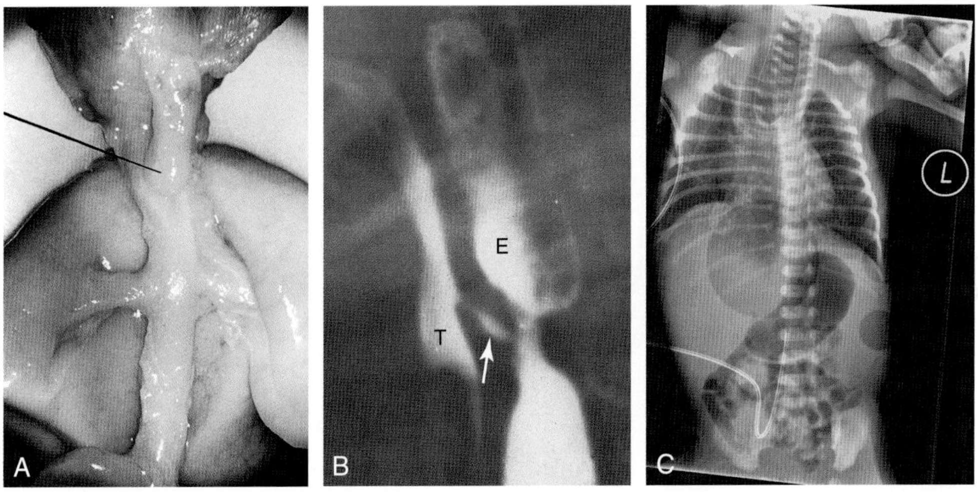

Fig. 10.7 (A) Tracheoesophageal fistula (TEF) in a 17-week male fetus. The upper esophageal segment ends blindly *(pointer)*. (B) Contrast radiograph of a neonate with TEF. Note the communication *(arrow)* between the esophagus *(E)* and trachea *(T)*. (C) Radiograph of esophageal atresia and tracheoesophageal fistula. The blind proximal esophageal sac is visible. Note the air present in the distal gastrointestinal tract, indicating the presence of the tracheoesophageal fistula. An umbilical venous catheter can also be seen. (A, From Kalousek DK, Fitch N, Paradice B: *Pathology of the human embryo and previable fetus*, New York, 1990, Springer-Verlag. B, Courtesy Dr. Prem S. Sahni, formerly of the Department of Radiology, Children's Hospital, Winnipeg, Manitoba, Canada. C, Courtesy Dr. J. V. Been and Dr. M. J. Schuurman, Department of Pediatrics, and Dr. S. G. Robben, Department of Radiology, Maastricht University Medical Centre, Maastricht, the Netherlands.)

Laryngotracheoesophageal Cleft

Uncommonly, the larynx and upper trachea may fail to separate completely from the esophagus. This results in a persistent connection of variable lengths between these normally separated structures, or **laryngotracheoesophageal cleft**. Symptoms of this birth defect are similar to those of TEF because of aspiration of fluid and/or food into the lungs. **Aphonia** (inability to speak) is a distinguishing feature. Laryngotracheoesophageal clefts occur sporadically but hereditary factors (familial) may be involved.

Tracheal Stenosis and Atresia

Stenosis (narrowing) and atresia of the trachea are uncommon birth defects, which are usually associated with one of the varieties of TEF. Stenoses and atresias probably result from unequal partitioning of the foregut into the esophagus and trachea (see Fig. 10.6). Sometimes there is a web of tissue obstructing airflow **(incomplete tracheal atresia)**. Atresia or **agenesis** (absence) of the trachea is uniformly fatal.

Tracheal Diverticulum (Tracheal Bronchus)

Tracheal diverticulum, or **bronchus**, consists of a blind, bronchus-like projection from the trachea. The outgrowth may terminate in normal-appearing lung tissue, forming a tracheal lobe of the lung. This diverticulum may cause recurrent infection and respiratory distress in infants.

DEVELOPMENT OF BRONCHI AND LUNGS

9

The respiratory bud (lung bud) develops at the caudal end of the laryngotracheal diverticulum during the fourth week (see Fig. 10.2A and B). The bud soon divides into right and left outpouchings, the **primary bronchial buds** (Figs. 10.8A, 10.9, and 10.2C). These buds grow laterally into the **pericardioperitoneal canals**, the primordia of the pleural cavities (see Fig. 10.8B). **Secondary** and **tertiary bronchial buds** soon develop.

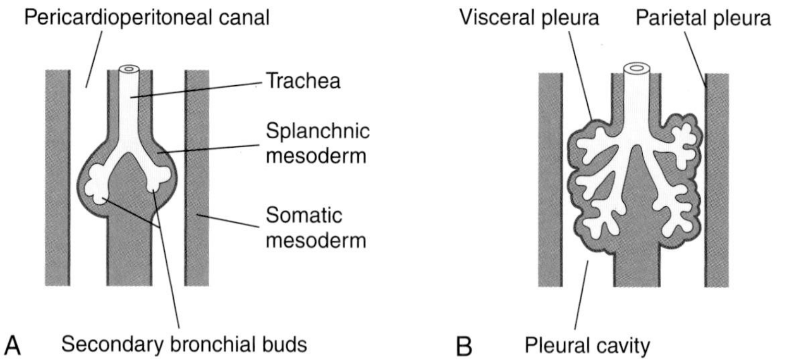

Fig. 10.8 Illustrations of the growth of the developing lungs into the splanchnic mesenchyme adjacent to the medial walls of the pericardioperitoneal canals (primordial pleural cavities). Development of the layers of the pleura is also shown: (A) 5 weeks and (B) 6 weeks.

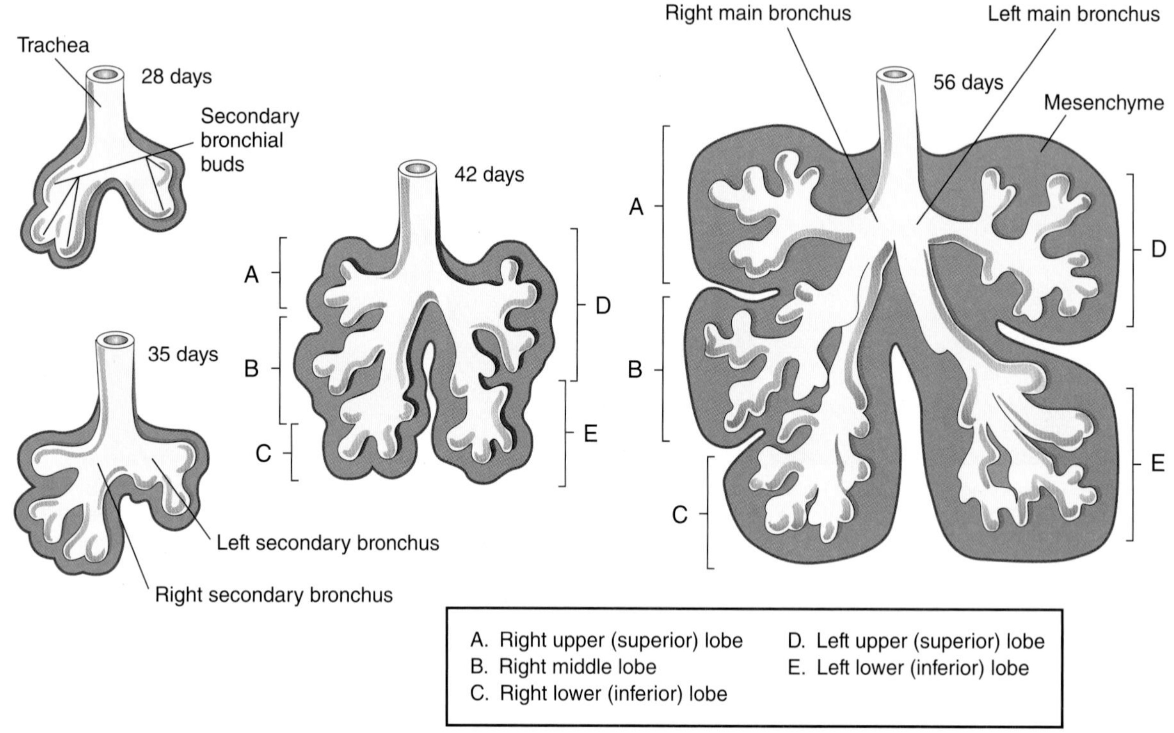

Fig. 10.9 Successive stages in the development of the bronchial buds, bronchi, and lungs.

Together with the surrounding splanchnic mesenchyme, the bronchial buds differentiate into bronchi and their branches in the lungs. Early in the fifth week, the connection of each bronchial bud with the trachea enlarges to form the primordia of the **main bronchi** (see Fig. 10.9).

The embryonic right main bronchus is slightly larger than the left one and is oriented more vertically. This relationship persists in the adult; consequently, a foreign body is more likely to enter the right main bronchus than the left one.

The main bronchi subdivide into **secondary bronchi** that form **lobar**, **segmental**, and **intrasegmental** branches (see Fig. 10.9). On the right, the superior lobar bronchus will supply the upper (superior) lobe of the lung, whereas the inferior bronchus subdivides into two bronchi, one to the middle lobe of the right lung and the other to the lower (inferior) lobe. On the left, the two secondary bronchi supply the upper and lower lobes of the lung. Each **lobar bronchus** undergoes progressive branching.

The **segmental bronchi**, 10 in the right lung and 8 or 9 in the left lung, begin to form by the seventh week. As this occurs, the surrounding mesenchyme also divides. The segmental bronchi, with the surrounding mass of mesenchyme, form the primordia of the **bronchopulmonary segments**. By 24 weeks, approximately 17 orders of branches have formed, and **respiratory bronchioles** have developed (Fig. 10.10B). An additional seven orders of airways develop after birth.

As the bronchi develop, cartilaginous plates develop from the surrounding splanchnic mesenchyme. The bronchial smooth muscle and connective tissue and the pulmonary connective tissue and capillaries are also derived from this mesenchyme. As the lungs develop, they acquire a layer of **visceral pleura** from the splanchnic mesenchyme (see Fig. 10.8). With expansion, the lungs and pleural cavities grow caudally into the mesenchyme of the body wall and soon lie close to the heart. The thoracic body wall becomes lined by a layer of **parietal pleura** derived from

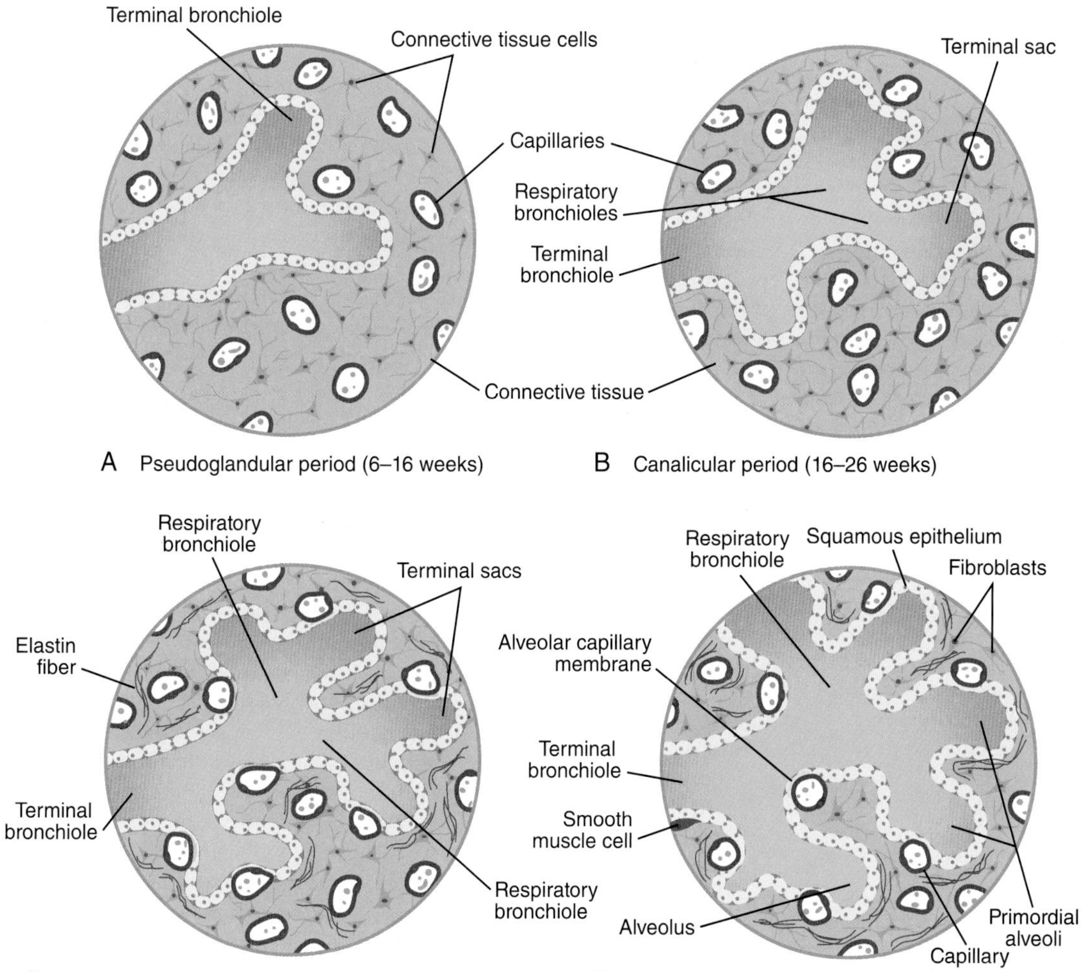

Fig. 10.10 Diagrammatic sketches of histologic sections illustrating the stages of lung development. (A and B) Early stages of lung development. (C and D) Note that the alveolocapillary membrane is thin and that some capillaries bulge into the terminal sacs and alveoli.

the somatic mesoderm (see Fig. 10.8B). The space between the parietal and visceral pleura is the **pleural cavity**.

MATURATION OF LUNGS

The maturation of the lungs is classified into four overlapping microscopic stages: the **pseudoglandular**, **canalicular**, **terminal sac (saccular)**, and **alveolar stages**.

PSEUDOGLANDULAR STAGE (5–17 WEEKS)

From a histologic standpoint, the developing lungs somewhat resemble exocrine glands during the **pseudoglandular stage** (Fig. 10.11A, and see Fig. 10.10A). By 16 weeks, all major elements of the lung have formed, except those involved with gas exchange. Respiration is not possible; therefore, *fetuses born during this period are unable to survive.*

CANALICULAR STAGE (16–25 WEEKS)

The **canalicular stage** overlaps the pseudoglandular stage because cranial segments of the lungs mature faster than caudal ones. During the canalicular stage, the lumina of the bronchi and **terminal bronchioles** become larger, and the lung tissue becomes highly vascular (see Figs. 10.10B and 10.11B). By 24 weeks, each terminal bronchiole has formed two or more **respiratory bronchioles**, each of which divides into three to six passages, the **primordial alveolar ducts**.

Respiration is possible at the end of the canalicular stage (26 weeks) because some thin-walled **terminal sacs** (primordial alveoli) have developed at the ends of the respiratory bronchioles, and lung tissue is well vascularized. Although a fetus born toward the end of this period may survive if given intensive care, this premature neonate may die because its respiratory and other systems are still relatively immature.

TERMINAL SAC STAGE (SACCULAR) (24 WEEKS TO LATE FETAL PERIOD)

During the **terminal sac stage**, many more terminal sacs (primordial alveoli) develop (see Figs. 10.10C and 10.11D), and their epithelium becomes very thin. Capillaries begin to bulge into these sacs. The intimate contact between epithelial and endothelial cells establishes a **blood-air barrier**, which permits adequate gas exchange for the survival of the fetus if it is born prematurely.

At 26 weeks, the terminal sacs are lined mainly by squamous epithelial cells of endodermal origin, **type I pneumocytes**, across which gas exchange occurs. The capillary network proliferates rapidly in the mesenchyme around the developing alveoli, and there is concurrent active development of lymphatic capillaries. Scattered among the squamous epithelial cells are rounded secretory epithelial cells (from the same endodermal origin), **type II pneumocytes**, which secrete **pulmonary surfactant**, a complex mixture of phospholipids and proteins.

Surfactant forms as a monomolecular film over the internal walls of the **alveolar sacs**, and the functional units of the lung, and counteracts surface tension forces at the air-alveolar interface. This facilitates the expansion of the terminal sacs by preventing **atelectasis** (collapse of sacs during exhalation). The maturation of type II pneumocytes and surfactant production varies widely in fetuses of different gestational ages. The production of surfactant increases during the terminal stages of pregnancy, particularly during the last 2 weeks.

Surfactant production begins at 20 to 22 weeks, but surfactant is present in only small amounts in premature infants; it does not reach adequate levels until the late fetal period. By 26 to 28 weeks, the fetus usually weighs approximately 1000 g, and sufficient alveolar sacs and surfactant are present to permit the survival of a prematurely born infant. Before this, the lungs are usually incapable of providing adequate gas exchange, partly because the alveolar surface area is insufficient, and the vascularity is underdeveloped.

It is not the presence of thin terminal sacs or a primordial alveolar epithelium so much as the development of an adequate pulmonary vasculature and surfactant that is critical to the survival and neurodevelopmental outcome of premature infants.

Fetuses born at 24 to 26 weeks after fertilization may survive if given intensive care; however, they may suffer from **respiratory distress** because of surfactant deficiency. Survival of these infants has improved with the use of antenatal corticosteroids, which induce surfactant production, and also with postnatal surfactant replacement therapy.

ALVEOLAR STAGE (LATE FETAL PERIOD TO 8 YEARS)

Exactly when the terminal sac stage ends and the **alveolar stage** begins depends on the definition of the term ***alveolus***. Terminal sacs analogous to alveoli are present at 32 weeks. The epithelial lining of the sacs attenuates to a thin squamous epithelial layer. The type I pneumocytes become so thin that the adjacent capillaries bulge into the alveolar sacs (see Figs. 10.10D and 10.11D). By the late fetal period (38 weeks), the lungs are capable of respiration because the **alveolocapillary membrane** (pulmonary diffusion barrier or respiratory membrane) is sufficiently thin to allow gas exchange. Although the lungs do not begin to perform this vital function until birth, they are well developed so that they are capable of functioning as soon as the baby is born.

At the beginning of the alveolar stage (34 weeks), each respiratory bronchiole terminates in a cluster of thin-walled **alveolar sacs**, separated from one another by loose connective tissue. These sacs represent future **alveolar ducts** (see Figs. 10.10D and 10.11D). The transition from dependence on the placenta for gas exchange to autonomous gas exchange requires the following adaptive changes in the lungs:

- Production of surfactant in the alveolar sacs
- Transformation of the lungs from secretory organs into organs capable of gas exchange
- Establishment of parallel pulmonary and systemic circulations

Approximately 95% of mature alveoli develop postnatally. Before birth, the primordial alveoli appear as small bulges on the walls of respiratory bronchioles and alveolar sacs, and terminal dilations of alveolar ducts (see Fig. 10.10D). After birth, the primordial alveoli enlarge as the lungs expand, but the greatest increase in the size of the lungs results from an increase in the number of respiratory bronchioles and primordial alveoli rather than from an increase in the size of the alveoli (see Fig. 10.11B and D).

Alveolar development is largely completed by 3 years of age, but new alveoli are added until approximately 8 years of age. Unlike mature alveoli, immature alveoli have the potential for forming additional primordial alveoli. As these alveoli increase in size, they become mature alveoli. However, the major mechanism for increasing the number of alveoli is the formation of secondary connective tissue septa that subdivide existing primordial alveoli. Initially, the septa are relatively thick, but they are soon transformed into mature thin septa that are capable of gas exchange.

Lung development during the first few months after birth is characterized by an exponential increase in the surface area of the air-blood barrier through the multiplication of alveoli and capillaries. Approximately 150 million primordial alveoli, one-half of the adult number, are present in the lungs of a full-term neonate. On chest radiographs, therefore, the lungs of neonates are denser than adult lungs. Between the third and eighth years, the adult complement of 300 million alveoli is achieved.

Molecular studies *(Fig. 10.12) indicate that lung development is controlled by a cascade of signaling pathways that are regulated by the temporal and sequential expression of highly conserved genes. The commitment and differentiation of endodermal foregut cells to form respiratory-type epithelial cells are associated with the expression of several transcription factors, including thyroid transcription factor 1, hepatocyte nuclear factor 3β, and GATA-6, as well as other zinc-finger family members, retinoic acid receptors, and homeobox (Hox) domain-containing genes. Hox genes specify the anteroposterior axis in the embryo. Fibroblast growth factor 10 and other signals from splanchnic mesenchyme probably induce the formation of the respiratory buds.*

Branching of the buds (branching morphogenesis) and its proliferation depend on epithelial (endodermal foregut)-mesenchymal (mesoderm) interactions. Regulated expression of the Hedgehog (HH) and Wnt signaling pathways play an essential role in the inductive interactions between epithelium and mesenchyme. The transcription factor SOX17 and Wnt7b signaling from the epithelium regulate mesenchymal proliferation and blood vessel formation in the lung. The patterning morphogen sonic hedgehog (Shh-Gli) modulates Fgf10 expression, which is a critical regulator of smooth muscle differentiation and controls the branching of the bronchial buds. Also, the morphogen retinoic acid regulates Hox a5, b5, and c4, which are expressed in the developing lung.

It appears that an autonomic nerve-myofibroblast circuit may regulate the formation of alveoli through neurotransmitters under control of VANGL planar cell polarity protein 2.

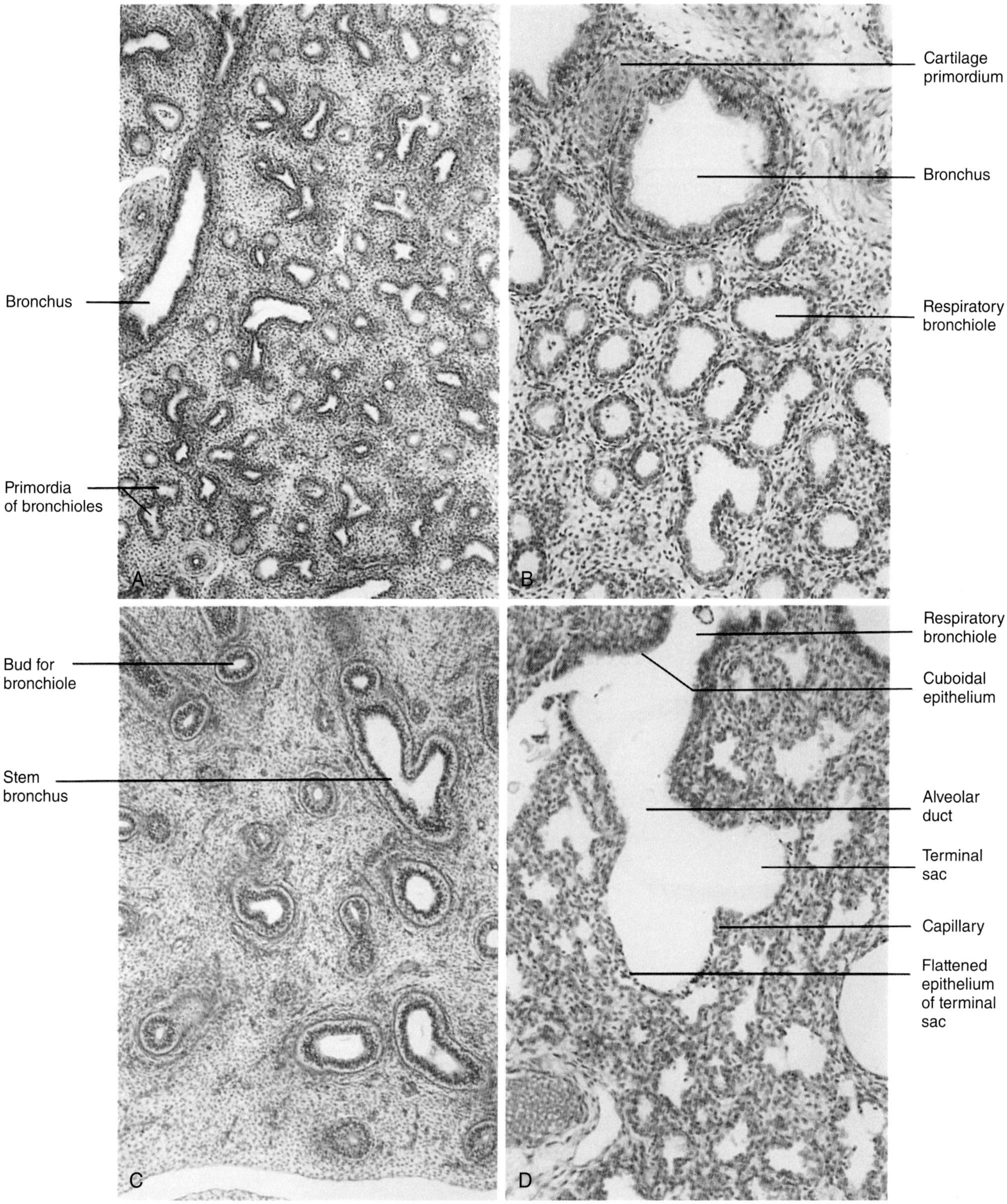

Fig. 10.11 Photomicrographs of sections of developing embryonic and fetal lungs. (A) Pseudoglandular stage, 8 weeks. Note the "glandular" appearance of the lung. (B) Canalicular stage, 16 weeks. The lumina of the bronchi and terminal bronchioles are enlarging. (C) Canalicular stage, 18 weeks. (D) Terminal sac stage, 24 weeks. Observe the thin-walled terminal sacs (primordial alveoli) that have developed at the ends of the respiratory bronchioles. Also, observe that the numbers of capillaries have increased and that some of them are closely associated with the developing alveoli. (From Moore KL, Persaud TVN, Shiota K: *Color atlas of clinical embryology*, ed 2, Philadelphia, 2000, Saunders.)

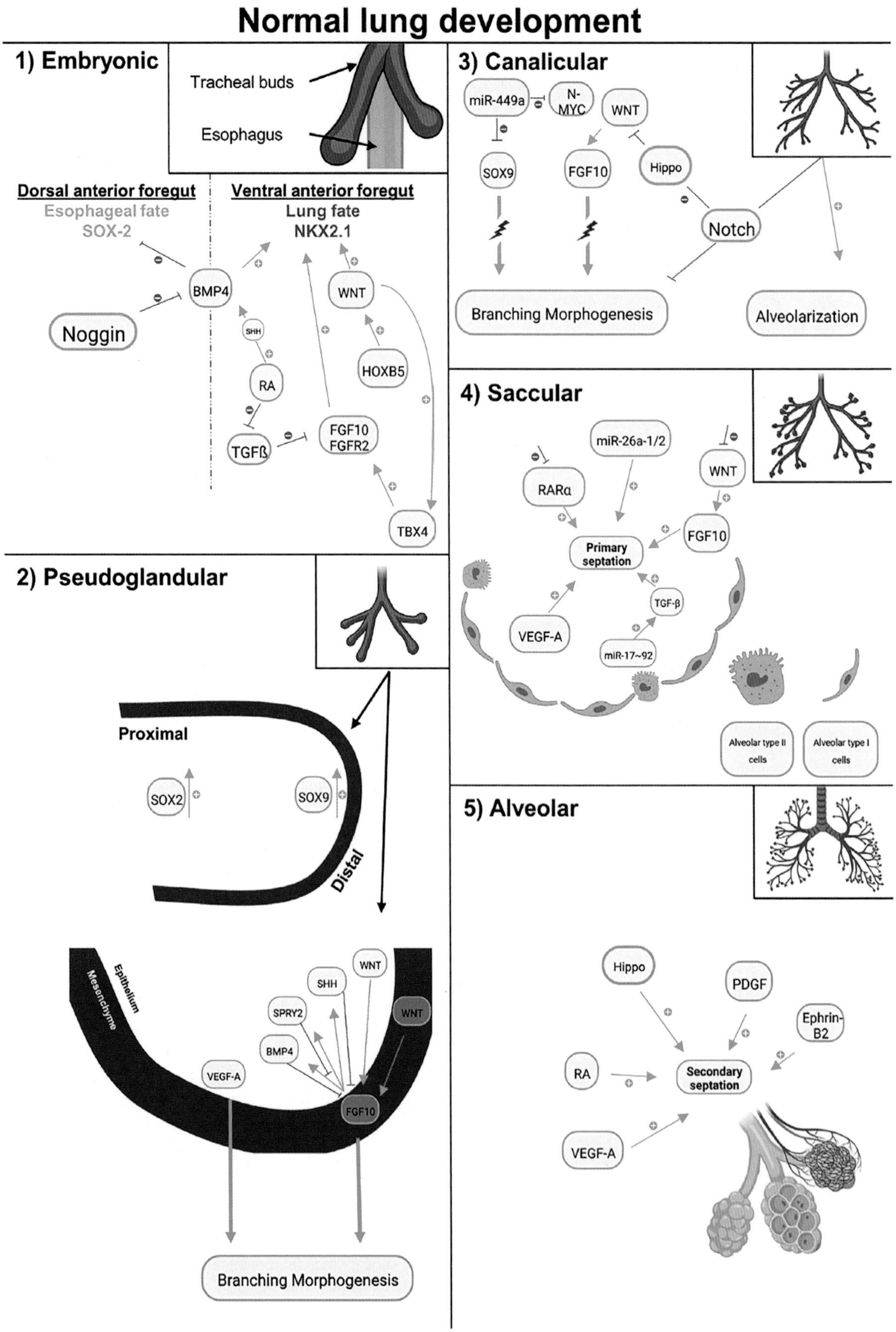

Fig. 10.12 Processes and pathways involved in the five stages of lung development. (From Doktor F, Antounians L, Lacher M, Zani A: Congenital lung malformations: dysregulated lung developmental processes and altered signaling pathways. *Semin Pediatr Surg* 31(6):151228, 2022.)

Fetal breathing movements (FBMs), which can be detected by real-time ultrasonography, occur before birth and exert sufficient force to cause aspiration of some amniotic fluid into the lungs. FBMs occur intermittently (approximately 30% of them during rapid eye movement [REM] sleep) and are essential for normal lung development (Fig. 10.13). The pattern of FBMs is widely used in the monitoring of labor and as a predictor of fetal outcome in preterm delivery. By birth, the fetus has had the advantage of several months of breathing exercises. FBMs, which increase as the time of delivery approaches, probably condition the respiratory muscles. In addition, these movements stimulate lung development, possibly by creating a pressure gradient between the lungs and the amniotic fluid.

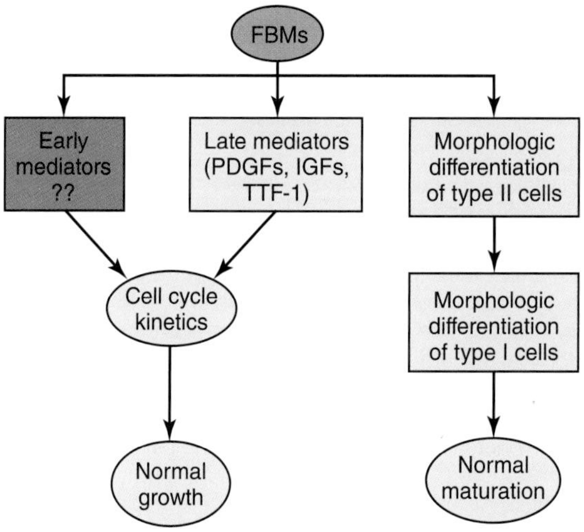

Fig. 10.13 Fetal breathing movements (*FBMs*) seem to play a role in lung growth through their effects on lung cell cycle kinetics by regulating the expression of growth factors, such as platelet-derived growth factors (*PDGFs*) and insulin-like growth factors (*IGFs*) and establishing the gradient of thyroid transcription factor 1 (*TTF-1*) expression at the last stage of lung organogenesis (i.e., late mediators). It is also suggested that FBMs influence the expression of other unknown growth factors (i.e., early mediators) that are responsible for changes in cell cycle kinetics at earlier stages of lung development. FBMs appear to also be required for the accomplishment of the morphologic differentiation of type I and II pneumocytes. (From Inanlou MR, Baguma-Nibasheka M, Kablar B: The role of fetal breathing–like movements in lung organogenesis, *Histol Histopathol* 20:1261, 2005.)

Three factors are important for normal lung development: adequate thoracic space for lung growth, FBMs, and adequate amniotic fluid volume (Fig. 10.14).

At birth, the lungs are approximately half-filled with fluid derived from the amniotic cavity, lungs, and tracheal glands. Aeration of the lungs at birth is not so much the inflation of empty, collapsed organs but rather the rapid replacement of intra-alveolar fluid by air.

The fluid in the lungs is cleared at birth by three routes:

- Through the mouth and nose by pressure on the fetal thorax during vaginal delivery
- Into the pulmonary capillaries, arteries, and veins
- Into the lymphatics

In the near-term fetus, the pulmonary lymphatic vessels are relatively larger and more numerous than in the adult. Lymph flow is rapid during the first few hours after birth and then diminishes.

Oligohydramnios and Lung Development

When **oligohydramnios** (insufficient amount of amniotic fluid) is severe and chronic, because of amniotic fluid leakage or decreased production, lung development is retarded, and severe **pulmonary hypoplasia** may result from restriction of the fetal thorax and breathing movements. The risk of pulmonary hypoplasia increases significantly with oligohydramnios before 26 weeks. It has also been shown that oligohydramnios results in decreased hydraulic pressure on the lungs, which affects stretch receptors, which in turn affect Ca^+ regulation and lung growth.

Lungs of Neonates

Healthy lungs of neonates always contain some air; consequently, pulmonary tissue removed from them will float in water. A diseased lung, partly filled with fluid, may not float. Of medicolegal significance is the fact that the lungs of a stillborn infant are firm and sink when placed in water because they contain fluid, not air.

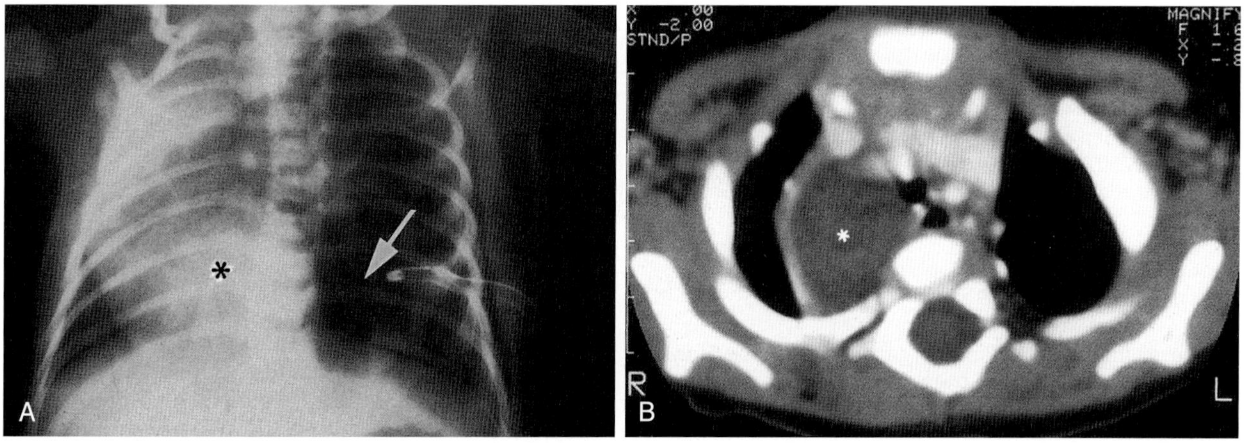

Fig. 10.14 Congenital lung cysts. (A) Chest radiograph (posteroanterior) of an infant showing a large left-sided congenital cystic adenomatoid malformation (*arrow*). The heart (*asterisk*) has shifted to the right. Note the chest tube on the left side, which was placed on the initial diagnosis of a pneumothorax (air in the pleural cavity). (B) Axial computed tomography image of the thorax in an infant with a large right-sided congenital bronchogenic cyst (*asterisk*). (Courtesy Dr. Prem S. Sahni, formerly of the Department of Radiology. Children's Hospital, Winnipeg, Manitoba, Canada.)

Respiratory Distress Syndrome

Respiratory distress syndrome (RDS) affects approximately 2% of neonates; those born prematurely are most susceptible. These infants develop rapid, labored breathing shortly after birth. RDS is also known as **hyaline membrane** disease. An estimated 30% of all neonatal diseases result from RDS or its complications.

Deficiency of surfactant produces RDS. The lungs are underinflated, and the alveoli contain a fluid with a high protein content that resembles a glassy, or hyaline, membrane. This membrane is thought to be derived from a combination of substances in the circulation and the injured pulmonary epithelium. It has been suggested that prolonged intrauterine **asphyxia** may produce irreversible changes in the **type II alveolar cells**, making them incapable of producing surfactant. Other factors such as sepsis, aspiration, and pneumonia may inactivate surfactant, leading to an absence or deficiency of surfactant in premature and full-term infants.

All growth factors and hormones controlling surfactant production have not been identified, but corticosteroids and thyroxine, which are involved in fetal lung maturation, are potent stimulators of surfactant production. Maternal glucocorticoid treatment during pregnancy accelerates fetal lung development and surfactant production. This finding has led to the routine antenatal use of corticosteroids for the prevention of RDS in preterm labor. In addition, administration of exogenous (animal-derived or synthetic) surfactant **(surfactant replacement therapy)** reduces the severity of RDS and the chance of neonatal mortality.

Lobe of Azygos Vein

A **lobe of the azygos vein** appears in the right lung in approximately 1% of people. It develops when the apical bronchus grows superiorly, medial to the arch of the azygos vein, instead of lateral to it. As a result, the vein lies at the bottom of a fissure in the superior (upper) lobe, which produces a linear marking on a radiograph of the lungs.

Congenital Lung Malformation (CLM)

CLMs are uncommon with an incidence of 1:6000–24,000. The most common CLM is congenital pulmonary adenomatoid malformation, where a multicystic mass replaces some alveoli. CPAM is thought to result from abnormal bronchiole branching. Other CLMs include congenital lobar emphysema and bronchogenic cysts (see Fig. 10.14).

Agenesis of Lungs

Absence of the lungs results from failure of the respiratory bud to develop. **Agenesis** of one lung is more common than bilateral agenesis, but both conditions are rare. Unilateral pulmonary agenesis is compatible with life. The heart and other mediastinal structures are shifted to the affected side, and the existing lung is hyperexpanded.

Primary Ciliary Dyskinesia

Primary ciliary dyskinesia (PCD) is a disease caused by motile cilia dysfunction and has an incidence of 1:10–20,000 births. The most common feature of PCD in neonates is respiratory distress. PCD is genetically heterogeneous, with over 45 genes currently identified. Individuals with PCD have poor mucociliary clearance, productive cough, lower respiratory infections, progressive COPD, and chronic rhinosinusitis. In addition, other abnormalities resulting from motile ciliary dysfunction in PCD include situs abnormalities (50%; see Chapter 13, discussion of situs inversus—dextrocardia), including a smaller percentage with situs ambiguous (heterotaxy syndrome; disturbance in the right-left distribution of thoracic and abdominal organs); male and female reduced fertility due to dysmobility of sperm and cilia dysfunction in the uterine tube, respectively; pectus excavatum; and scoliosis.

Lung Hypoplasia

In infants with **congenital diaphragmatic hernia** see Figs. 8.9A and B and 8.10), the lung is unable to develop normally because it is compressed by the abnormally positioned abdominal viscera. **Lung hypoplasia** is characterized by a markedly reduced lung volume and hypertrophy of smooth muscle in the pulmonary arteries. Pulmonary hypertension leads to decreased blood flow through the pulmonary vascular system as the blood continues to shunt through the ductus arteriosus.

Approximately 25% of infants with congenital diaphragmatic hernia die of pulmonary insufficiency and respiratory failure, despite optimal postnatal care, because their lungs are too hypoplastic for air exchange and there is too much resistance for pulmonary blood flow to support extrauterine life.

Accessory Lung

A small **accessory mass of lung tissue (pulmonary sequestration)** is uncommon. It may be intralobar or extralobar and is usually located at the base of the left lung and is nonfunctional. Pulmonary sequestration does not communicate with the tracheobronchial tree, and its blood supply is usually from one or more systemic arteries. Larger masses should be removed because they tend to circulate from their systemic arterial blood supply. Computed tomography (CT) scanning is invaluable for the diagnosis of pulmonary sequestration.

SUMMARY OF RESPIRATORY SYSTEM

- By the fourth week, a **laryngotracheal diverticulum** develops from the floor of the primordial pharynx.
- The laryngotracheal diverticulum becomes separated from the foregut by **tracheoesophageal folds** that fuse to form a tracheoesophageal septum. This septum results in the formation of the esophagus and laryngotracheal tube (see Fig. 10.2C and E).
- The endoderm of the laryngotracheal tube gives rise to the epithelium of the lower respiratory organs and

tracheobronchial glands. The splanchnic mesenchyme surrounding the laryngotracheal tube forms the connective tissue, cartilage, muscle, and blood and lymphatic vessels of these organs.

- Pharyngeal arch mesenchyme contributes to the formation of the epiglottis and connective tissue of the larynx. The laryngeal muscles are derived from mesenchyme in the caudal pharyngeal arches. The laryngeal cartilages are derived from neural crest cells.
- The distal end of the laryngotracheal diverticulum forms a **respiratory bud** that divides into two **bronchial buds**. Each bronchial bud soon enlarges to form a **main bronchus**, and then the main bronchus subdivides to form lobar, segmental, and subsegmental branches (see Figs. 10.2C and 10.9).
- **Each tertiary bronchial bud** (segmental bronchial bud), with its surrounding mesenchyme, is the primordium of a **bronchopulmonary segment**. Branching continues until *approximately* 17 orders of branches have formed. Additional airways are formed after birth until *approximately* 24 orders of branches are present.
- Lung development is divided into four stages: the **pseudoglandular** (6–16 weeks), **canalicular** (16–26 weeks), **terminal sac** (26 weeks to birth), and **alveolar** (32 weeks to approximately 8 years of age) **stages**.
- By 20 to 22 weeks, **type II pneumocytes** begin to secrete pulmonary **surfactant**. The deficiency of surfactant results in **RDS** or **hyaline membrane disease**.
- A **tracheoesophageal fistula**, which results from faulty partitioning of the foregut into the esophagus and trachea, is usually associated with esophageal atresia.

CLINICALLY ORIENTED PROBLEMS

CASE 10-1

Choking and continuous coughing were observed in a male neonate. There was an excessive amount of secreted mucus and saliva in his mouth. He also experienced considerable difficulty in breathing. The pediatrician was unable to pass a catheter through the esophagus into the stomach.

- What birth defect would be suspected?
- Discuss the embryologic basis of these defects.
- What kind of examination or testing do you think would be used to confirm the tentative diagnosis?

CASE 10-2

A premature infant develops rapid, shallow respiration shortly after birth. A diagnosis of RDS was made.

- How do you think the infant might attempt to overcome his or her inadequate exchange of oxygen and carbon dioxide?
- What usually causes RDS?
- What treatment is currently used clinically to prevent RDS?
- A deficiency of what substance is associated with RDS?

CASE 10-3

The parents of a neonate were told that their son had a fistula between his trachea and esophagus.

- What is the most common type of TEF?
- What is its embryologic basis?
- What defect of the alimentary (digestive) tract is frequently associated with this abnormality?

CASE 10-4

A neonate with esophageal atresia experienced respiratory distress with cyanosis shortly after birth. Radiographs demonstrated air in the infant's stomach.

- How did the air enter the stomach?
- What other problem might result in an infant with this fairly common type of birth defect?

Discussion of these problems appears in the Appendix at the back of the book.

BIBLIOGRAPHY AND SUGGESTED READING

Belgacemi R, Danopoulos S, Deutsch G, et al: Hedgehog signaling pathway orchestrates human lung branching morphogenesis, *Int J Mol Sci* 23(9):5265, 2022. https://doi.org/10.3390/ijms23095265.

Berman DR, Treadwell MC: Ultrasound evaluation of fetal thorax. In Norton ME, editor: *Callen's ultrasonography in obstetrics and gynecology*, ed 6, Philadelphia, 2017, Elsevier.

Caldeira I, Fernandes-Silva H, Machado-Costa D, Correia-Pinto J, Moura RS: Developmental pathways underlying lung development and congenital lung disorders, *Cells* 10(11):2987, 2021. https://doi.org/10.3390/cells10112987.

Coshal H, Mukerji A, Lemyre B, Ng EH, Alvaro R, Ethier G: Characteristics and outcomes of preterm neonates according to number of doses of surfactant received, *J Perinatol* 41(1):39–46, 2021. https://doi.org/10.1038/s41372-020-00779-9.

Edwards NA, Shacham-Silverberg V, Weitz L, Kingma PS, Shen Y, Wells JM: Developmental basis of trachea-esophageal birth defects, *Dev Biol* 477:85, 2021.

Fabik J, Psutkova V, Machon O: The Mandibular and hyoid arches from molecular patterning to shaping bone and cartilage, *Int J Mol Sci.* 22(14):7529, 2021. https://doi.org/10.3390/ijms22147529.

Hentschel R, Bohlin K, van Kaam A, Fuchs H, Danhaive O: Surfactant replacement therapy: from biological basis to current clinical practice, *Pediatric Research* 88:176, 2020.

Herriges M, Morrisey EE: Lung development: orchestrating the generation and regeneration of a complex organ, *Development* 141:502, 2014.

Kallapur SG, Jobe AH: Lung development and maturation. In Martin RJ, Fanaroff AA, Walsh MC, editors: *Fanaroff and Martin's neonatal-perinatal medicine: diseases of the fetus and infant*, ed 10, Philadelphia, 2014, Mosby.

Kardon G, Ackerman KG, McCulley DJ, Shen Y, Wynn J, Shang L: Congenital diaphragmatic hernias: from genes to mechanisms to therapies, *Dis Model Mech* 10:955, 2017.

Kina YP, Khadim A, Seeger W: The lung vasculature: a driver or passenger in lung branching morphogenesis? *Front Cell Dev Biol* 8:623868, 2021. https://doi.org/10.3389/fcell.2020.623868.

Lange AW, Haitchi HM, LeCras TD, Sridharan A, Xu Y, Wert SE: Sox17 is required for normal pulmonary vascular morphogenesis, *Dev Biol* 387:109, 2014.

Mariani TJ: Update on molecular biology of lung development—transcriptomics, *Clin Perinatol* 42:685, 2015.

Morrisey EE, Cardoso WV, Lane RH, Rabinovitch M, Abman SH, Ai X: Molecular determinants of lung development, *Ann Am Thorac Soc* 10:S12–S16, 2013.

O'Rahilly R, Boyden E: The timing and sequence of events in the development of the human respiratory system during the embryonic period proper, *Z Anat Entwicklungsgesch* 141:237, 1973.

Palla J, Sockrider MM: Congenital lung malformations, *Ped Ann* 48(4):e169, 2019.

Perin S, McCann CJ, Borrelli O, De Coppi P, Thapar N: Update on foregut molecular embryology and role of regenerative medicine therapies, *Front Pediatr* 5:91, 2017. https://doi.org/10.3389/fped.2017.00091.

Sardesai S, Biniwale M, Wertheimer F, Garingo A, Ramanathan R: Evolution of surfactant therapy for respiratory distress syndrome: past, present, and future, *Pediatr Res* 81(1-2):240–248, 2017. https://doi.org/10.1038/pr.2016.203.

Schittny JC: Development of the lung, *Cell Tissue Res* 367:427, 2017.

Shoemark A, Harman K: Primary ciliary dyskinesia, *Semin Respir Crit Care Med* 42:537, 2021.

Snowball J, Ambalavanan M, Whitsett J, Sinner D: Endodermal Wnt signaling is required for tracheal cartilage formation, *Dev Biol* 405:56, 2015.

Som PM, Grapin-Botton A: The current embryology of the foregut and its derivatives, *Neurographics* 6:43, 2016.

Sun D, Batlle OL, van den Ameele J, Thomas JC, He P, Lim K: SOX9 maintains human foetal lung tip progenitor state by enhancing WNT and RTK signalling, *EMBO J* 41:e111338, 2022.

Warburton D: Overview of lung development in the newborn human, *Neonatology* 111:398, 2017.

Wells LJ, Boyden EA: The development of the bronchopulmonary segments in human embryos of horizons XVII and XIX, *Am J Anat* 95:163, 1954.

Whitsett JA: The molecular era of surfactant biology, *Neonatology* 105:337, 2014.

Yamazake Y, Kanahashi T, Yamada S, Männer J, Takakuwa T: Three-dimensional analysis of human laryngeal and tracheobronchial cartilages during the late embryonic and early fetal period, *Cells Tissues Organs* 211(1):1, 2022.

Zhang K, Yao E, Wang S-A, Chuang E, Wong J, Minichiello L: A functional circuit formed by the autonomic nerves and myofibrils controls mammalian alveolar formation for gas exchange, *Dev Cell* 57:1566, 2022.

Zepp JA, Morrisey EE: Cellular crosstalk in the development and regeneration of the respiratory system, *Nat Rev Mol Cell Biol* 20:551, 2019. https://doi.org/10.1038/s41580-019-0141-3.

Alimentary System

11

CHAPTER OUTLINE

The **alimentary system** (digestive system) is the digestive tract from the mouth to the anus, with all its associated glands and organs. The **primordial gut** forms during the fourth week as the head, caudal eminence (tail), and lateral folds incorporate the dorsal part of the umbilical vesicle (see Fig. 5.1). The primordial gut is initially closed at its cranial end by the **oropharyngeal membrane** (see Fig. 9.1E) and at its caudal end by the **cloacal membrane** (Fig. 11.1B). The endoderm of the primordial gut and the surrounding splanchnic mesoderm form most of the gut, epithelium, and glands. The endoderm specifies temporal and positional information, which is essential for the development of the gut. The muscular, connective tissue and other layers of the wall of the alimentary tract are derived from the splanchnic mesenchyme surrounding the primordial gut. Mesenchymal cells derived from the coelomic epithelium, through epithelial-mesenchymal transformation, contribute to the mesoderm already surrounding the primordial gut and are also involved in the formation of connective tissue and blood vessels in the gut. *Mesenchymal factors, FoxF proteins, control the proliferation of the endodermal epithelium that secretes sonic hedgehog (Shh).* The epithelium of the cranial and caudal ends of the alimentary tract is derived from the ectoderm of the **stomodeum and anal pit (proctodeum)**, respectively (see Fig. 11.1A and B).

Fibroblast growth factors (FGFs) play an important role in early anteroposterior axial patterning. The WNT and Nodal signaling pathways are essential for the formation of the endoderm. and it appears that FOXA2, SOX17, GAT 4-6, and FGF-4 signals from the adjacent ectoderm and mesoderm induce the endoderm. Other secreted factors, such as activins, members of the transforming growth factor-β superfamily, contribute to the formation of the endoderm.

For descriptive purposes, the primordial gut is divided into three parts: foregut, midgut, and hindgut. *Molecular studies indicate that Nodal signals,* expression of *Hox and ParaHox genes, as well as Shh, BMP, and Wnt regulate the regional differentiation of the primordial gut to form its three parts.*

FOREGUT

The derivatives of the foregut are as follows:

- Primordial pharynx and its derivatives
- Lower respiratory system
- Esophagus and stomach
- Duodenum, including the opening of the bile duct
- Liver, biliary apparatus (hepatic ducts, gallbladder, and bile duct), and pancreas

These foregut derivatives, other than the pharynx, lower respiratory tract, and most of the esophagus, are supplied by the **celiac trunk**, the artery of the foregut (see Fig. 11.1B).

DEVELOPMENT OF ESOPHAGUS

10

The **esophagus** develops from the foregut immediately caudal to the pharynx (see Fig. 11.1B). The partitioning of the trachea from the esophagus by the **tracheoesophageal**

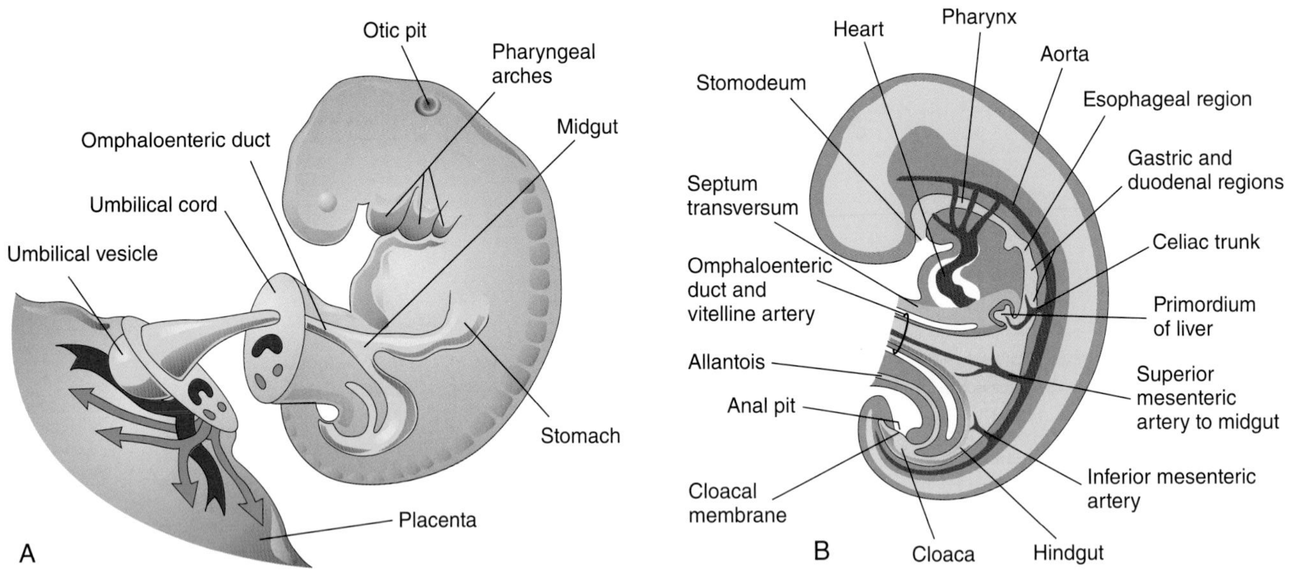

Fig. 11.1 (A) Lateral view of a 4-week embryo showing the relationship of the primordial gut to the omphaloenteric duct. (B) Drawing of the median section of the embryo showing the early alimentary system and its blood supply.

Esophageal Atresia

Atresia (blockage) of the esophageal lumen occurs with an incidence of 1 in 3000 to 4500 neonates. Approximately one-third of affected infants are born prematurely. This defect is associated with **tracheoesophageal fistula** and other anomalies in more than 90% of cases (see Fig. 10.6). Esophageal atresia results from deviation of the tracheoesophageal septum in a posterior direction (see Fig. 10.7) and incomplete separation of the esophagus from the laryngotracheal tube. Isolated atresia (5%–7% of cases) appears to result from insufficient vascular perfusion. *BMP and TGFβ signaling, and other pathways, such as SHH, Wnt7b, SOX2, and NXX2-1, play an important role in foregut development. Incomplete separation which causes tracheoesophageal fistula or esophageal atresia is likely caused by both genetic and environmental factors.*

A fetus with esophageal atresia is unable to swallow amniotic fluid; consequently, the fluid cannot pass to the intestine for absorption and transfer through the placenta to the maternal blood for disposal resulting in **polyhydramnios**. Neonates with esophageal atresia usually appear healthy initially. Excessive drooling may be noted soon after birth, and the diagnosis of esophageal atresia should be considered if the baby rejects oral feeding with immediate regurgitation and coughing.

The inability to pass a catheter through the esophagus into the stomach strongly suggests esophageal atresia. A radiographic examination shows the nasogastric tube arrested in the proximal esophageal pouch. In neonates weighing more than 2 kg and without associated cardiac anomalies, the survival rate now approaches 100% with surgical repair. As the birth weight decreases and cardiovascular anomalies become more severe; the survival rate decreases to as low as 1%.

Esophageal Stenosis

Stenosis of the lumen of the esophagus can occur anywhere along the esophagus, but it usually occurs in its distal third, either as a web or a long segment with a thread-like lumen. Stenosis likely results from a failure of esophageal blood vessels to develop in the affected area.

septum is described in Fig. 10.2E. Initially, the esophagus is short, but it elongates rapidly, mainly because of the growth and relocation of the heart and lungs.

The esophagus reaches its final relative length by the seventh week. Its epithelium and glands are derived from endoderm and mesenchymal. The **striated muscle** forming the muscularis externa (external muscle) of the superior third of the esophagus is derived from mesenchyme in the fourth and sixth pharyngeal arches. The **smooth muscle**, mainly in the inferior third of the esophagus, develops from the surrounding splanchnic mesenchyme. *The regional segmentation and the concentric layering of the endodermal-lined foregut (muscles, connective tissue, nerves, and blood vessels) are regulated by the Notch, SHH, and BMP signaling pathways. Molecular studies reported the expression of multiple genes in esophageal development, including SOX2, JNK 1 and 2, FOXC, FOX 2, and NKX 2-1.*

Recent studies indicate transdifferentiation of smooth muscle cells in the superior part of the esophagus to striated muscle is dependent on myogenic regulatory factors. Both types of muscle are innervated by branches of the vagus nerves (cranial nerve X), which supply the caudal pharyngeal arches (see Table 9.1).

DEVELOPMENT OF STOMACH

10

Initially, the distal part of the foregut is a tubular structure (see Fig. 11.1B). During the fourth week, a slight dilation indicates the site of the primordial stomach. The dilation first appears as a fusiform enlargement of the caudal (distal) part of the foregut and is initially oriented in the median plane (see Figs. 11.1 and 11.2B). The left wall of the primordial stomach soon enlarges and broadens ventrodorsally. During the next 2 weeks, on account of the polarization and radial rearrangement of the epithelium, the dorsal border of the right wall of the stomach grows faster than its ventral

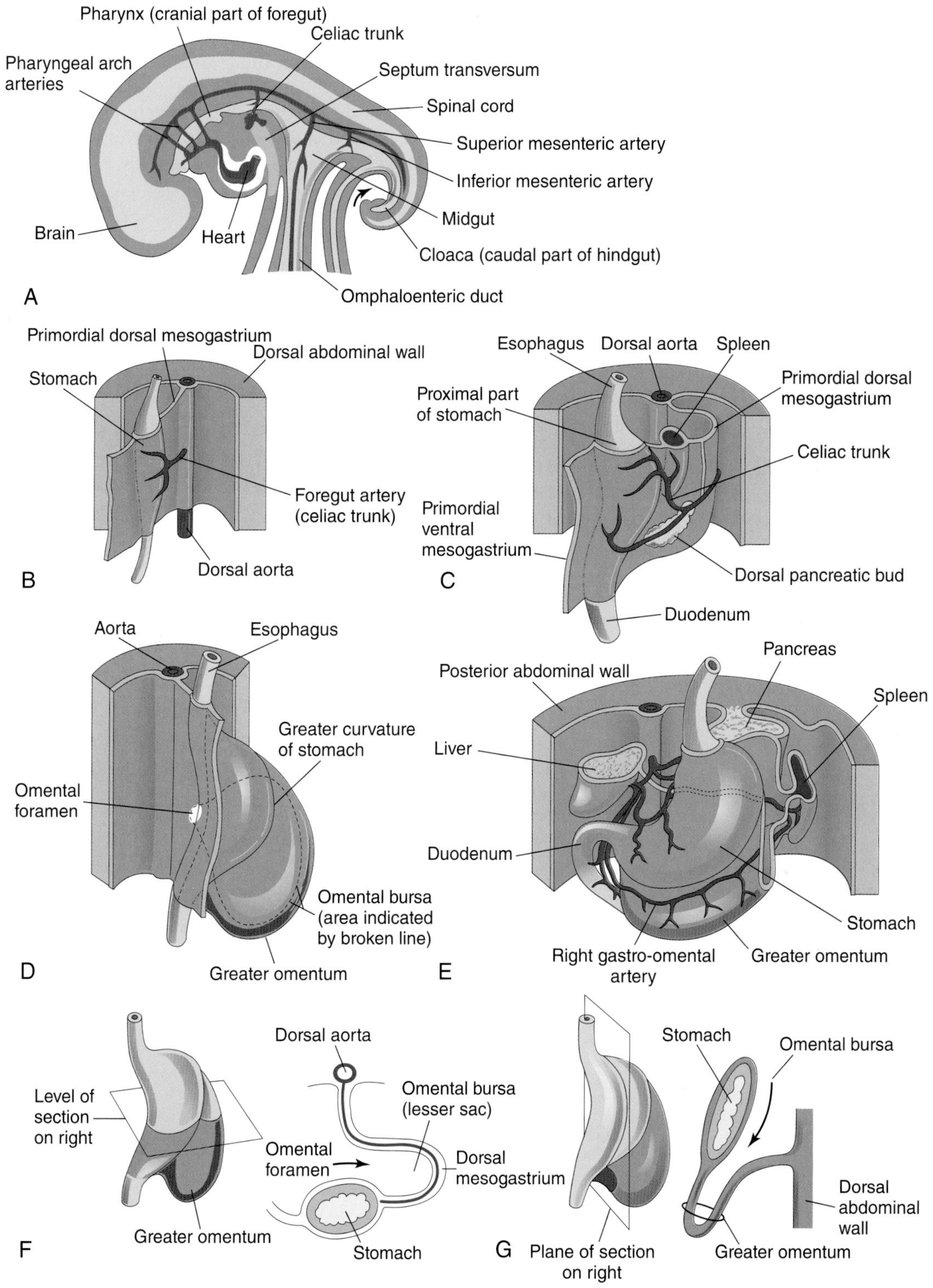

Fig. 11.2 Development of the stomach and formation of the omental bursa and greater omentum. (A) Median section of the abdomen of a 28-day embryo. (B) Anterolateral view of the embryo shown in (A). (C) Embryo of approximately 35 days. (D) Embryo of approximately 40 days. (E) Embryo of approximately 48 days. (F) Lateral view of the stomach and greater omentum of an embryo of approximately 52 days. (G) Sagittal section showing the omental bursa and greater omentum. The *arrow* in (F) and (G) indicates the site of the omental foramen.

border; this demarcates the developing **greater curvature of the stomach** (see Fig. 11.2D). *Such left-right asymmetry and rotation of the gut are regulated by extrinsic forces and the expression of left-right patterning genes Pitx2, JNK family, Foxj1, FoxC1, Nodal, and Sim2 (Single-minded 2) transcription factor.*

ROTATION OF STOMACH

Changes in the position and relocation of the stomach and intestine are described as a passive rotation. Enlargement of the mesentery and adjacent organs, as well as the growth of the stomach walls, contributes to the rotation of the stomach.

As the stomach enlarges and acquires its final shape, it slowly rotates 90 degrees in a clockwise direction (viewed from the cranial end) around its longitudinal axis. The effects of rotation on the stomach are as follows (Figs. 11.2 and 11.3):

- The ventral border (lesser curvature) moves to the right, and the dorsal border (greater curvature) moves to the left (see Fig. 11.2C and F).
- The original left side becomes the ventral surface, and the original right side becomes the dorsal surface.
- Before rotation, the cranial and caudal ends of the stomach are in the median plane (see Fig. 11.2B). During rotation and growth of the stomach, its cranial region moves to the left and slightly inferiorly, and its caudal region moves to the right and superiorly.

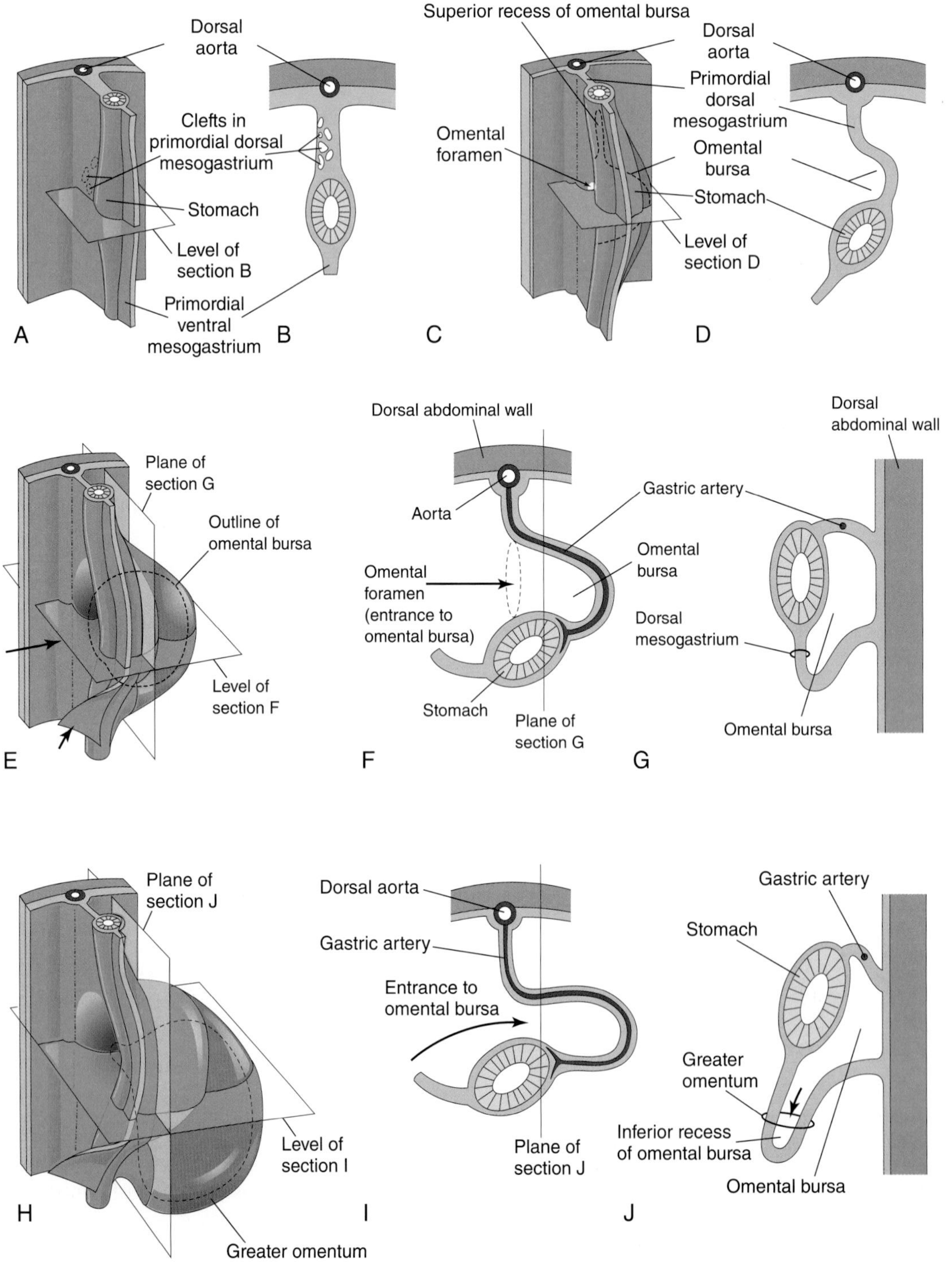

Fig. 11.3 Development of stomach and mesenteries and formation of omental bursa. (A) Embryo of 5 weeks. (B) Transverse section showing clefts in the dorsal mesogastrium. (C) Later stage after coalescence of the clefts to form the omental bursa. (D) Transverse section showing the initial appearance of the omental bursa. (E) The dorsal mesentery has elongated, and the omental bursa has enlarged. (F and G) Transverse and sagittal sections, respectively, show elongation of the dorsal mesogastrium and expansion of the omental bursa. (H) Embryo of 6 weeks showing the greater omentum and expansion of the omental bursa. (I and J) Transverse and sagittal sections, respectively, show the inferior recess of the omental bursa and the omental foramen. The *arrows* in (E, F, and I) indicate the site of the omental foramen. In (J) the *arrow* indicates the inferior recess of the omental bursa.

- After rotation, the stomach assumes its final position, with its long axis almost transverse to the long axis of the body (see Fig. 11.2E).

The rotation and growth of the stomach explain why the **left vagus nerve** supplies the anterior wall of the adult stomach and the **right vagus nerve** innervates its posterior wall.

MESENTERIES OF STOMACH

The stomach is suspended from the dorsal wall of the abdominal cavity by a dorsal mesentery, the **primordial dorsal mesogastrium** (see Figs. 11.2B and C and 11.3A). This mesentery, originally in the median plane, is carried to the left during rotation of the stomach and formation of the **omental bursa** or lesser sac of the peritoneum (see Fig. 11.3A–E). The mesentery also contains the spleen and celiac artery. The **primordial ventral mesogastrium** attaches to the stomach; it also attaches the duodenum to the liver and ventral abdominal wall (see Figs. 11.2C and 11.3A and B).

10 OMENTAL BURSA

Isolated clefts develop in the mesenchyme, forming the thick **dorsal mesogastrium** (see Fig. 11.3A and B). The clefts soon coalesce to form a single cavity, the **omental bursa** or lesser peritoneal sac (see Fig. 11.3C and D). Rotation of the stomach pulls the mesogastrium to the left, thereby enlarging the bursa, a large recess in the peritoneal cavity. The bursa expands transversely and cranially and soon lies between the stomach and posterior abdominal wall. The pouch-like bursa facilitates movements of the stomach (see Fig. 11.3H).

The superior part of the omental bursa is cut off as the diaphragm develops, forming a closed space, the **infracardiac bursa**. If the space persists, it usually lies medial to the base of the right lung. The inferior region of the superior part of the bursa persists as the **superior recess of the omental bursa** (see Fig. 11.3C).

As the stomach enlarges, the omental bursa expands and acquires an **inferior recess of the omental bursa** between the layers of the elongated dorsal mesogastrium, the **greater omentum** (see Fig. 11.3J). This membrane overhangs the developing intestines. The inferior recess disappears as the layers of the greater omentum fuse (see Fig. 11.15F). The omental bursa communicates with the peritoneal cavity through an opening, the **omental foramen** (see Figs. 11.2D and F and 11.3C and F).

Hypertrophic Pyloric Stenosis

Anomalies of the stomach are uncommon, except for **hypertrophic pyloric stenosis**. This defect affects one in every 150 males and one in every 750 females. In affected infants there is a marked **muscular thickening of the pylorus**, the distal sphincteric region of the stomach (Fig. 11.4A and B). The circular muscles and, to a lesser degree, the longitudinal muscles in the pyloric region are hypertrophied. This results in severe stenosis of the pyloric canal and obstruction of the passage of food. As a result, the stomach becomes markedly distended (see Fig. 11.4C), and the infant expels the stomach's contents with considerable force (projectile vomiting).

Surgical relief of the pyloric obstruction by **pyloromyotomy**, in which a longitudinal incision is made through the anterior wall of the pyloric canal, is the usual treatment. The cause of congenital pyloric stenosis is unknown, but the high rate of concordance in monozygotic twins suggests genetic factors may be involved.

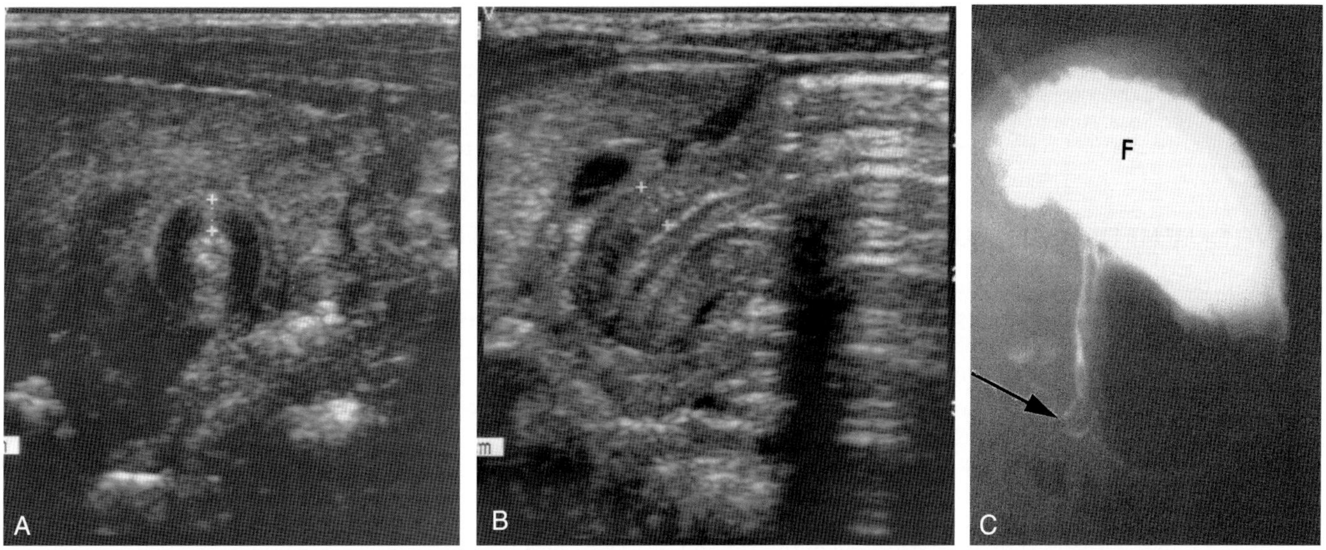

Fig. 11.4 (A) Transverse abdominal sonogram demonstrating a pyloric muscle wall thickness of greater than 4 mm *(distance between crosses)* and the "target sign". (B) Horizontal image demonstrating the wall thickness of greater than 4 mm (crosses) and a pyloric channel length greater than 14 mm (asterisks) in an infant with hypertrophic pyloric stenosis. (C) Contrast radiograph of the stomach in a 1-month-old male infant with pyloric stenosis. Note the narrowed pyloric end *(arrow)* and the distended fundus *(F)* of the stomach, filled with contrast material. (A and B, From Wyllie R: Pyloric stenosis and other congenital anomalies of the stomach. In Behrman RE, Kliegman RM, Arvin AM, editors: *Nelson textbook of pediatrics*, ed 6, Philadelphia, 2000, Saunders. C, Courtesy Dr. Prem S. Sahni, formerly of the Department of Radiology, Children's Hospital, Winnipeg, Manitoba, Canada.)

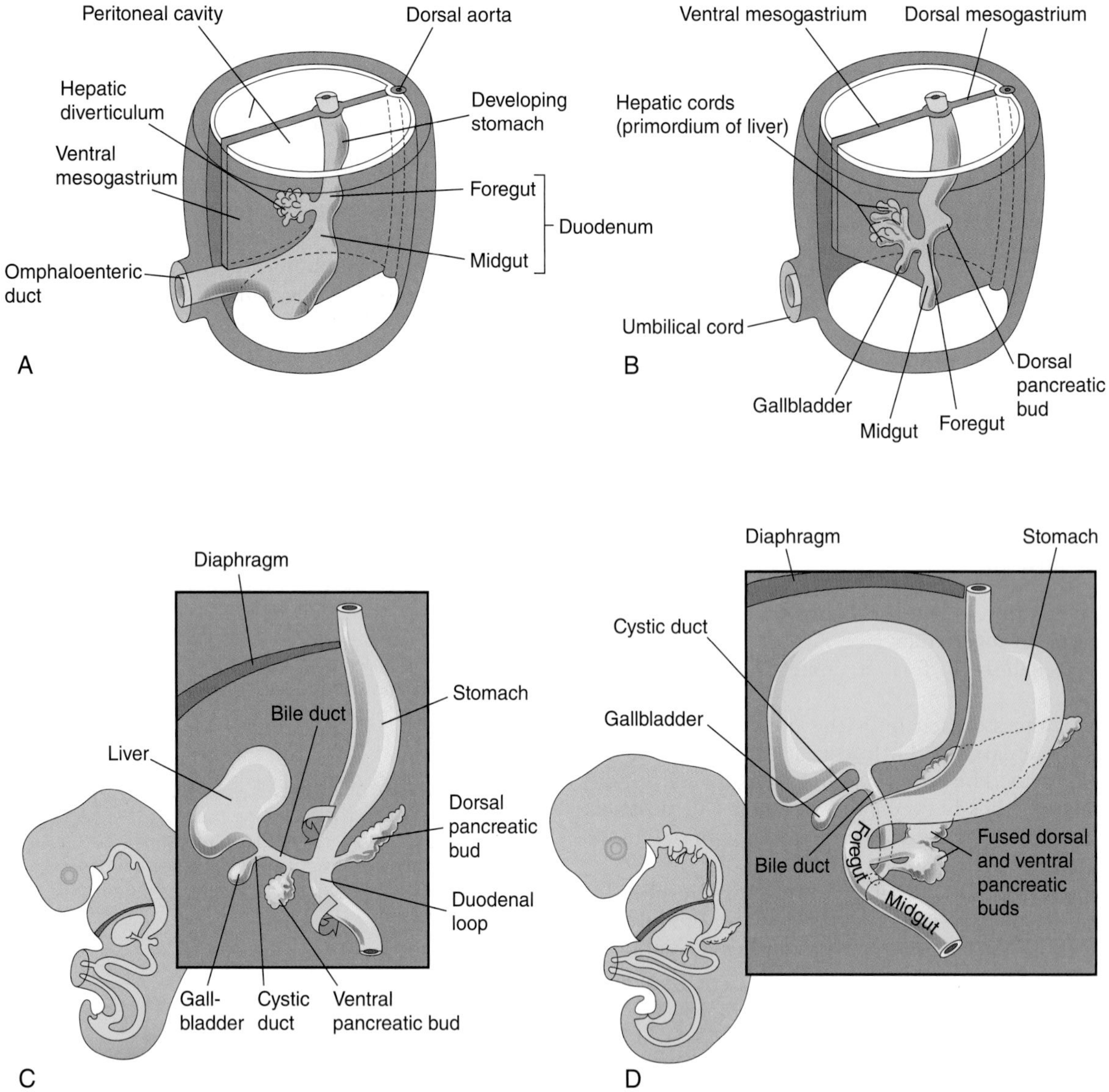

Fig. 11.5 Progressive stages in the development of the duodenum, liver, pancreas, and extrahepatic biliary apparatus. (A) Embryo of 4 weeks. (B and C) Embryo of 5 weeks. (D) Embryo of 6 weeks. During embryologic development, the dorsal and ventral pancreatic buds eventually fuse, forming the pancreas. Note that the entrance of the bile duct into the duodenum gradually shifts from its initial position to a posterior one. This explains why the bile duct in adults passes posterior to the duodenum and the head of the pancreas.

DEVELOPMENT OF DUODENUM

10

Early in the fourth week, the duodenum begins to develop from the caudal part of the foregut, cranial part of the midgut, and splanchnic mesenchyme associated with these parts of the primordial gut (Fig. 11.5A). The junction of the two parts of the duodenum is just distal to the origin of the bile duct (see Fig. 11.5D). The developing duodenum grows rapidly, forming a C-shaped loop that projects ventrally (see Fig. 11.5B–D).

As the stomach rotates, the duodenal loop rotates to the right and is pressed against the posterior wall of the abdominal cavity, or in a retroperitoneal position (external to the peritoneum). Because of its derivation from the foregut and midgut, the duodenum is supplied by branches of the celiac trunk and superior mesenteric arteries that supply these parts of the primordial gut (see Fig. 11.1).

During the fifth and sixth weeks, the lumen of the duodenum becomes progressively smaller and is temporarily obliterated because of the proliferation of its epithelial cells. By this time, most of the ventral mesentery of the duodenum has disappeared.

DEVELOPMENT OF LIVER AND BILIARY APPARATUS

10

The liver, gallbladder, and biliary duct system arise as a ventral endodermal outgrowth, the **hepatic diverticulum**, from the distal part of the foregut early in the fourth week (Fig. 11.8A, and see also Fig. 11.5A). *The Wnt/β-catenin signaling pathway plays a key role in this process, which includes the proliferation and differentiation of the hepatic progenitor cells (hepatoblasts) to form hepatocytes and cholangiocytes (epithelial cells of the intrahepatic bile ducts). Both the hepatic diverticulum and the ventral bud of the pancreas develop from two cell populations in*

Duodenal Stenosis and Atresia

Duodenal stenosis and atresia appear to result from reduced vascular perfusion, leading to duodenal narrowing or complete obliteration of the lumen (Fig. 11.6). Most stenoses involve the horizontal (third) and/or ascending (fourth) parts of the duodenum. Because of the stenosis, the stomach's contents (usually containing bile) are often vomited. **Duodenal atresia**, is not common. The blockage usually occurs at the junction of the bile duct and pancreatic duct, or **hepatopancreatic ampulla**, a dilated area within the major duodenal papilla that receives the bile duct and main pancreatic duct; occasionally, the blockage involves the horizontal (third) part of the duodenum. Investigation of families with **familial duodenal atresia** suggests an autosomal recessive inheritance pattern.

In neonates with duodenal atresia, vomiting begins a few hours after birth. The vomitus almost always contains bile; often there is distention of the epigastrium, the upper central area of the abdomen, resulting from an overfilled stomach and superior part of the duodenum. The atresia is associated with bilious emesis (vomiting of bile) because the blockage occurs distal to the opening of the bile duct. The atresia may occur as an isolated birth defect, but other defects are often associated with it, such as the annular pancreas (see Fig. 11.11C), cardiovascular defects, anorectal defects, and malrotation of the gut (see Fig. 11.20). The presence of nonbilious emesis does not exclude duodenal atresia as a diagnosis because some infants will have obstruction proximal to the ampulla. Importantly, approximately one-third of affected infants have 21 trisomy (Down syndrome), and an additional 20% are premature.

Polyhydramnios also occurs because duodenal atresia prevents normal intestinal absorption of swallowed amniotic fluid. The diagnosis of duodenal atresia is suggested by the presence of a "double-bubble" sign on plain radiographs and ultrasound scans (Fig. 11.7). This appearance is caused by a distended, gas-filled stomach and the proximal duodenum.

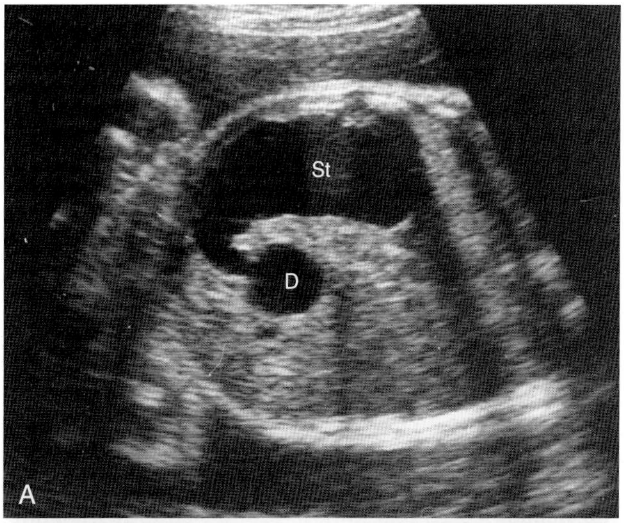

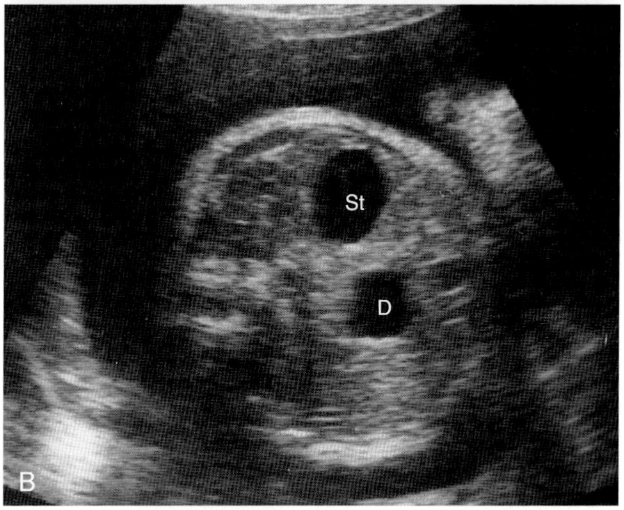

Fig. 11.7 Ultrasound scans of a fetus of 33 weeks showing duodenal atresia. (A) An oblique scan showing the dilated, fluid-filled stomach (*St*) entering the proximal duodenum (*D*), which is also enlarged because of atresia (blockage) distal to it. (B) Transverse scan illustrating the characteristic "double-bubble" appearance of the stomach and duodenum when there is duodenal atresia. (Courtesy Dr. Lyndon M. Hill, Magee-Women's Hospital, Pittsburgh, PA.)

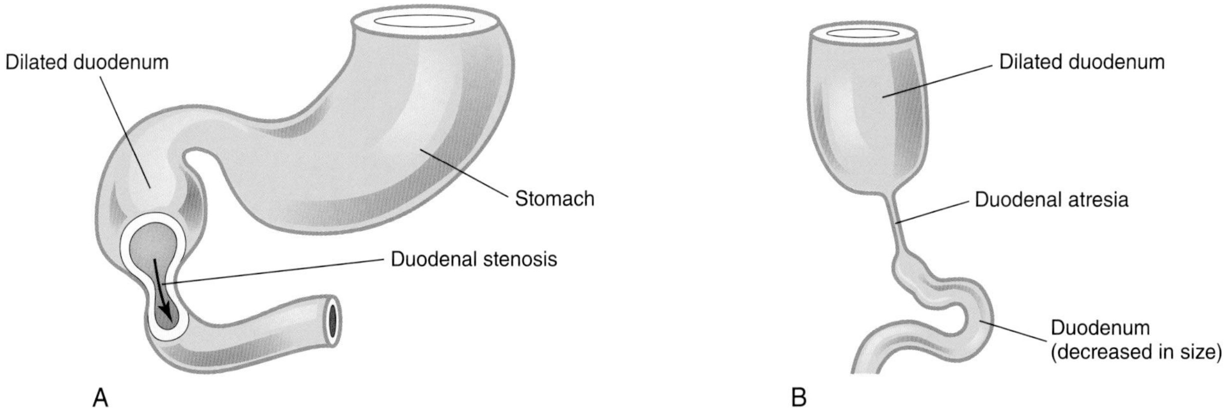

Fig. 11.6 Drawings showing the embryologic basis of common types of congenital intestinal obstruction: (A) duodenal stenosis and (B) duodenal atresia.

the embryonic endoderm. At sufficient levels, FGFs secreted by the developing heart interact with the bipotential cells and induce the formation of the hepatic diverticulum.

The diverticulum invades into the **septum transversum**, a mass of splanchnic mesoderm, separating the pericardial and peritoneal cavities. The septum forms the ventral mesogastrium in this region. The hepatic diverticulum enlarges rapidly and divides into two parts as it grows between the layers of the **ventral mesogastrium**, or mesentery of the dilated portion of the foregut and the future stomach (see Fig. 11.5A).

The larger cranial part of the **hepatic diverticulum** is the primordium of the liver (see Figs. 11.8A and C and 11.10A and B); the smaller caudal part becomes the primordium of the **gallbladder**. The proliferating endodermal cells form interlacing cords of hepatocytes and give rise to the epithelial lining of the intrahepatic part of the biliary apparatus. The **hepatic cords** anastomose around endothelium-lined spaces, the primordia of the **hepatic sinusoids**. *Vascular endothelial growth factor Flk-1 signaling appears to be important for the early morphogenesis of the hepatic sinusoids (primitive vascular system).* The fibrous and hematopoietic tissues are derived from mesenchyme in the septum transversum, whereas Kupffer cells of the liver originate from precursors from the umbilical vesicle. *Development of the intrahepatic biliary system depends on Notch signaling.*

The liver grows rapidly from the 5th to 10th weeks and fills a large part of the upper abdominal cavity (see Fig. 11.8C and D). The quantity of oxygenated blood flowing from the umbilical vein into the liver determines the development and functional segmentation of the liver. Initially, the right and left lobes are approximately the same size, but the right lobe soon becomes larger.

Hematopoiesis begins in the liver during the sixth week, with hematopoietic stem cells migrating from the dorsal aorta to the liver. The formation of blood gives the liver a bright reddish appearance. By the ninth week, the liver accounts for approximately 10% of the total weight of the fetus. Bile formation by hepatic cells begins during the 12th week.

The small caudal part of the hepatic diverticulum becomes the **gallbladder**, and the stalk of the diverticulum forms the **cystic duct** (see Fig. 11.5C). Initially, the **extrahepatic biliary**

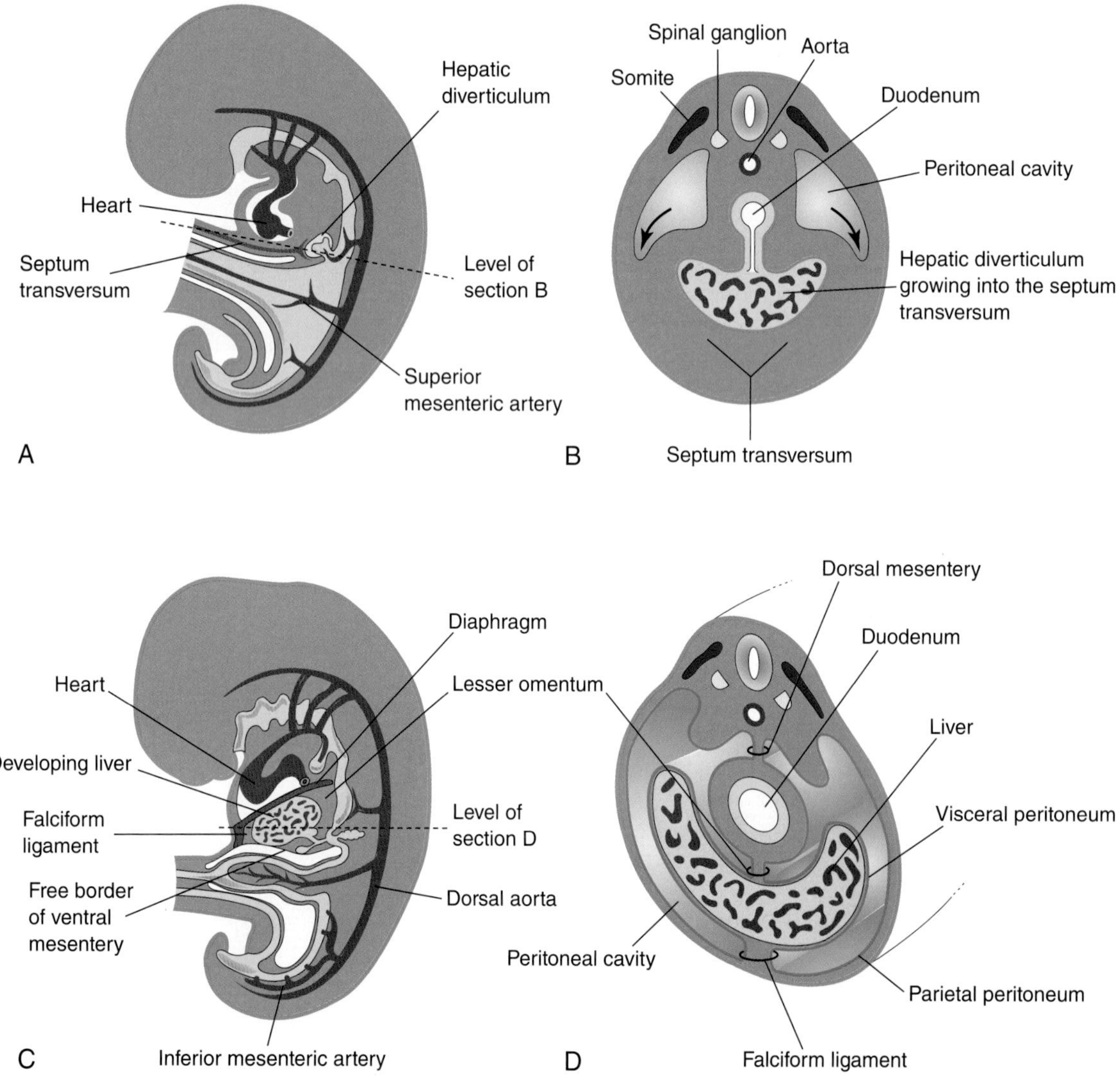

Fig. 11.8 (A) Median section of a 4-week embryo. (B) Transverse section of the embryo showing expansion of the peritoneal cavity (*arrows*). (C) Sagittal section of a 5-week embryo. (D) Transverse section of the embryo after formation of the dorsal and ventral mesenteries.

apparatus is occluded with epithelial cells, but it is later canalized because of vacuolation resulting from degeneration of these cells. The cholangiocytes (epithelial cells) of the extrahepatic ducts are derived from the endoderm. *The YAP 1 gene (Yes1 Associated Transcriptional Regulator) plays a critical role in the development of the gall bladder bile ducts.*

The stalk of the diverticulum connecting the hepatic and cystic ducts to the duodenum becomes the **bile duct**. Initially, this duct attaches to the ventral aspect of the duodenal loop; however, as the duodenum grows and rotates, the entrance of the bile duct is carried to the dorsal aspect of the duodenum (see Fig. 11.5C and D). The bile entering the duodenum through the bile duct after the 13th week, combined with intestinal gland secretions, produces **meconium**, the dark green intestinal discharge of the fetus. By 25 weeks, almost all fetuses have meconium throughout the colon.

VENTRAL MESENTERY

The **ventral mesentery**, a thin, double-layered membrane (see Fig. 11.8C and D), gives rise to:

- The **lesser omentum**, passing from the liver to the lesser curvature of the stomach **(hepatogastric ligament)** and from the liver to the duodenum **(hepatoduodenal ligament)**
- The **falciform ligament**, extending from the liver to the ventral abdominal wall

The **umbilical vein** passes through the free border of the **falciform ligament** on its way from the umbilical cord to the liver. The ventral mesentery, derived from the mesogastrium, also forms the visceral peritoneum of the liver. The liver is covered by the peritoneum, except for the **bare area**, which is in direct contact with the diaphragm (Fig. 11.9).

Anomalies of Liver

Minor variations of liver lobulation are common; however, birth defects of the liver are rare. Variations of the hepatic ducts, bile ducts, and cystic ducts are common and clinically significant. **Accessory hepatic ducts** are present in approximately 5% of the population, and awareness of their possible presence is of importance in surgery (e.g., liver transplantation). The accessory ducts are narrow channels running from the right lobe of the liver into the anterior surface of the body of the gallbladder. In some cases, the **cystic duct** opens into an accessory hepatic duct rather than into the common hepatic duct.

Extrahepatic Biliary Atresia

Extrahepatic biliary atresia is the most serious defect of the extrahepatic biliary system, and it occurs in 1 in 5000 to 20,000 live births. The most common form of extrahepatic biliary atresia (present in 85% of cases) is the **obliteration of the bile ducts** at or superior to the **porta hepatis**, a deep transverse fissure on the visceral surface of the liver.

Previous speculations that there is a failure of the bile ducts to canalize may not be true. Biliary atresia (absence of a normal opening) of the major bile ducts could result from a failure of the remodeling process at the hepatic hilum from viral infections, immunologic reactions, or defects of circulation during late fetal development.

Jaundice occurs soon after birth, the stools are acholic (clay colored), and the urine appears dark-colored. Biliary atresia can be palliated surgically in most patients, but in more than 70% of those treated, the disease continues to progress.

Agenesis of the gallbladder occurs rarely and is usually associated with the absence of the cystic duct.

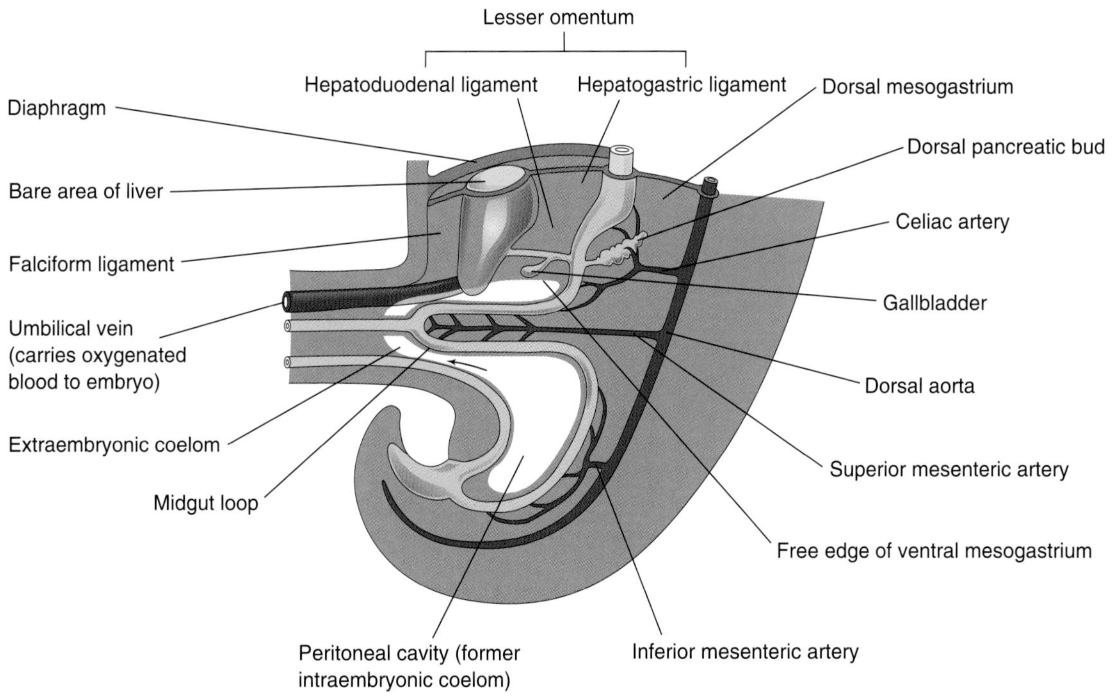

Fig. 11.9 Median section of the caudal half of an embryo at the end of the fifth week, showing the liver and associated ligaments. The *arrow* indicates the communication of the peritoneal cavity with the extraembryonic coelom.

DEVELOPMENT OF PANCREAS

10

The pancreas develops between the layers of the mesentery from dorsal and ventral **pancreatic buds** of endodermal cells, which arise from the caudal part of the foregut (Fig. 11.10A and B, and see also Fig. 11.9). Most of the pancreas is derived from the larger **dorsal pancreatic bud**, which appears first and develops at a slight distance cranial to the ventral bud.

The smaller **ventral pancreatic bud** develops near the entry of the bile duct into the duodenum and grows between the layers of the ventral mesentery. As the duodenum rotates to the right and becomes C-shaped, the bud is carried dorsally with the bile duct (see Fig. 11.10C–G). It soon lies posterior to the dorsal pancreatic bud and later fuses with it. The ventral pancreatic bud forms the **uncinate process** and part of the **head of the pancreas**.

As the stomach, duodenum, and ventral mesentery rotate, the pancreas comes to lie along the dorsal abdominal wall (in a retroperitoneal position). As the pancreatic buds fuse, their ducts anastomose, or open into one

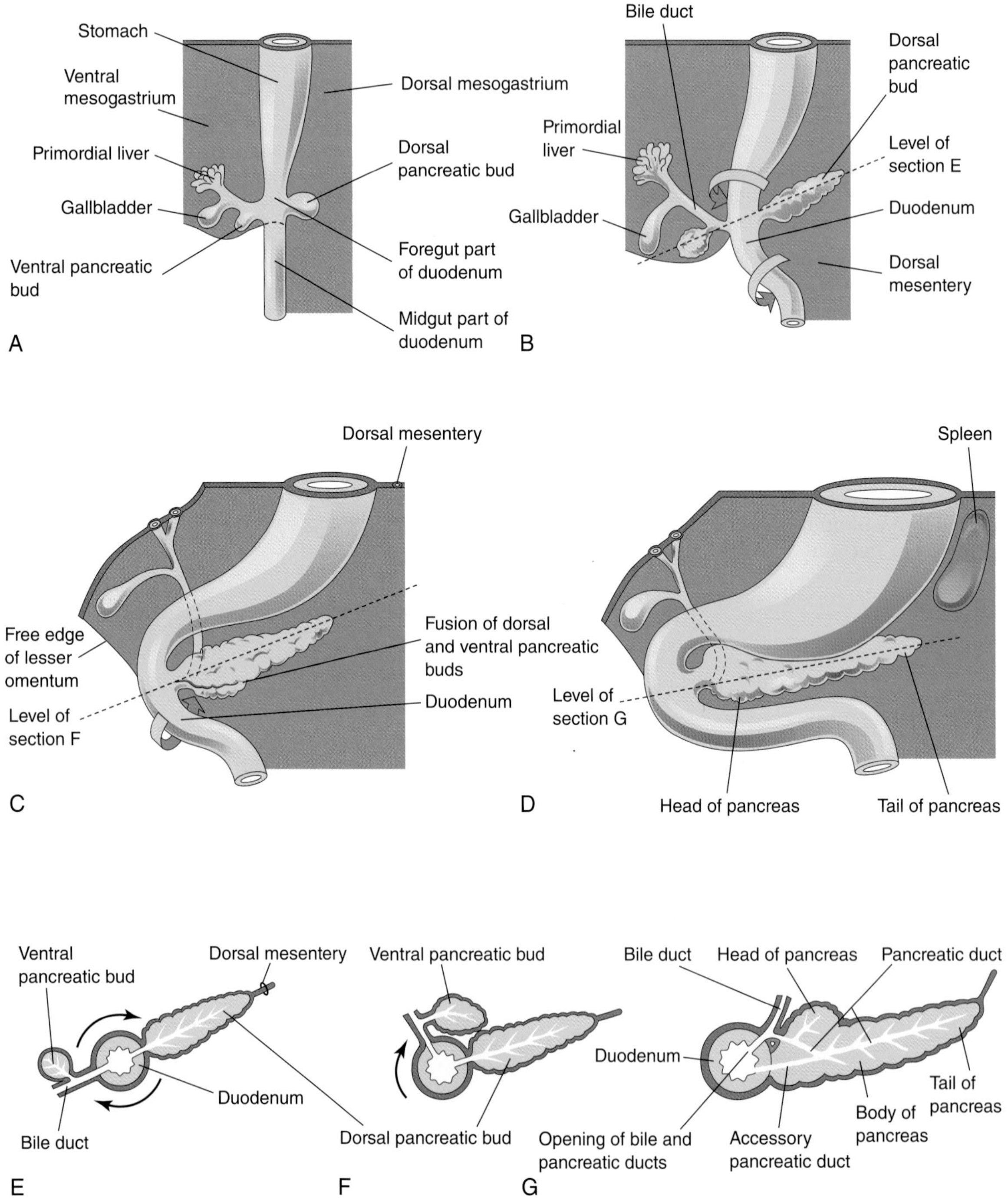

Fig. 11.10 (A–D) Successive stages in the development of the pancreas from the fifth to eighth weeks. (E–G) Diagrammatic transverse sections through the duodenum and developing pancreas. Growth and rotation (*arrows*) of the duodenum bring the ventral pancreatic bud toward the dorsal bud, and the two buds subsequently fuse.

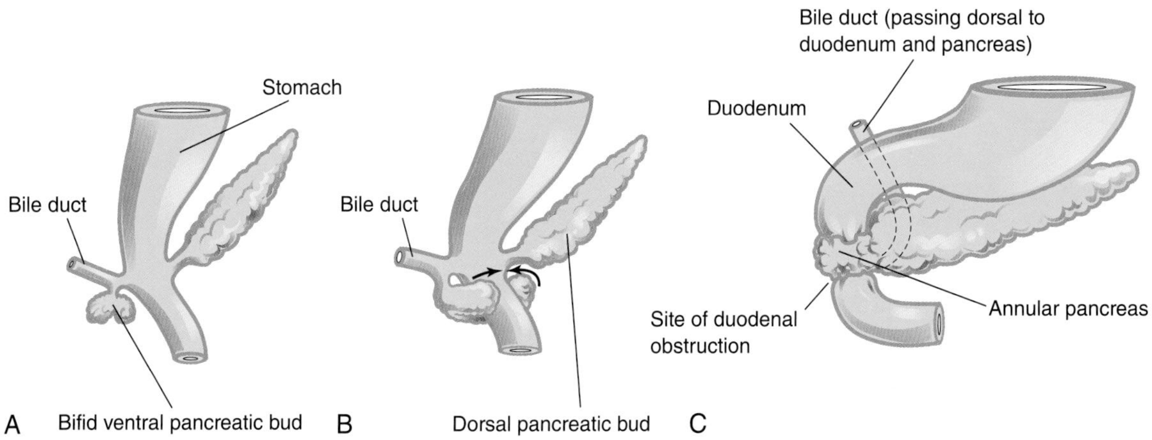

Fig. 11.11 (A and B) show the probable basis of an annular pancreas. (C) An annular pancreas encircling the duodenum. This birth defect produces complete obstruction (atresia) or partial obstruction (stenosis) of the duodenum.

another (see Fig. 11.10C). The **pancreatic duct** forms from the duct of the ventral bud and the distal part of the duct of the dorsal bud (see Fig. 11.10G). The proximal part of the duct of the dorsal bud often persists as an **accessory pancreatic duct** that opens into the **minor duodenal papilla**, located approximately 2 cm cranial to the main duct (see Fig. 11.10G). The two ducts often communicate with each other. In approximately 9% of people, the pancreatic ducts fail to fuse, resulting in two ducts.

Molecular studies show that the ventral pancreas develops from a bipotential cell population in the ventral region of the duodenum where the transcription factor PDX1 is expressed. A default mechanism involving FGF-2, which is secreted by the developing heart, plays a role. Formation of the dorsal pancreatic bud depends on the notochord secreting activin and FGF-2, which block the expression of Shh in the associated endoderm, and the transcription factor Myte, which is expressed in the endocrine progenitor cells of the pancreas. FGF and other signaling pathways control the branching of the pancreatic ducts.

HISTOGENESIS OF PANCREAS

The **parenchyma** of the pancreas is derived from the endoderm of the pancreatic buds, which forms a network of tubules **(primordial pancreatic ducts)**. Early in the fetal period, **pancreatic acini** (secretory portions of an acinous gland) begin to develop from cell clusters around the ends of these tubules. The **pancreatic islets** develop from groups of cells that separate from the tubules and lie between the acini.

Recent studies show that the chemokine stromal-cell derived factor 1 (SDF-1), expressed in the mesenchyme, controls the formation and branching of the tubules. Expression of transcription factor neurogenin-3 is required for the differentiation of pancreatic islet endocrine cells.

Insulin secretion begins during the early fetal period (at 10 weeks). The cells containing glucagon and somatostatin develop before the differentiation of the **beta cells that secrete insulin**. Glucagon has been detected in fetal plasma at 15 weeks.

The connective tissue sheath and interlobular septa of the pancreas develop from the surrounding splanchnic mesenchyme. When there is **maternal diabetes mellitus**, the beta cells that secrete insulin in the fetal pancreas are chronically exposed to high levels of glucose. As a result, these cells undergo hypertrophy to increase the rate of insulin secretion.

Ectopic Pancreas

Ectopic pancreatic tissue is located separately from the pancreas. Locations for the tissue are the mucosa of the stomach, the proximal duodenum, the jejunum, the pyloric antrum, and an ileal diverticulum (of Meckel). This defect is usually asymptomatic and is discovered incidentally (e.g., by computed tomography scanning); however, it may present with gastrointestinal symptoms, obstruction, bleeding, or even cancer.

Annular Pancreas

Although an **annular pancreas** is rare, the defect warrants description because it may cause duodenal obstruction (Fig. 11.11C). The ring-like, annular part of the pancreas consists of a thin, flat band of pancreatic tissue surrounding the descending or second part of the duodenum which may cause obstruction. Infants present with symptoms of complete or partial bowel obstruction.

Blockage of the duodenum develops if inflammation **(pancreatitis)** develops in the annular pancreas. The defect may be associated with trisomy 21 (Down syndrome), intestinal malrotation, and cardiac defects. Females are affected more frequently than males. An annular pancreas probably results from the growth of a bifid ventral pancreatic bud around the duodenum (see Fig. 11.11A–C). The parts of the bifid ventral bud then fuse with the dorsal bud, forming a pancreatic ring. Surgical intervention may be required for the management of this condition.

DEVELOPMENT OF SPLEEN

The **spleen** is derived from a mass of mesenchymal cells located between the layers of the **dorsal mesogastrium** (Fig. 11.12A and B). The spleen, a vascular lymphatic organ, begins to develop during the fifth week, but it does not acquire its characteristic shape until early in the fetal period. 10

Gene-targeting experiments show that capsulin, a basic helix-oop transcription factor, and homeobox genes NKx2-5, Hox11, and Bapx1 regulate the development of the spleen.

The fetal spleen is lobulated, but the lobules normally disappear before birth. The notches in the superior border

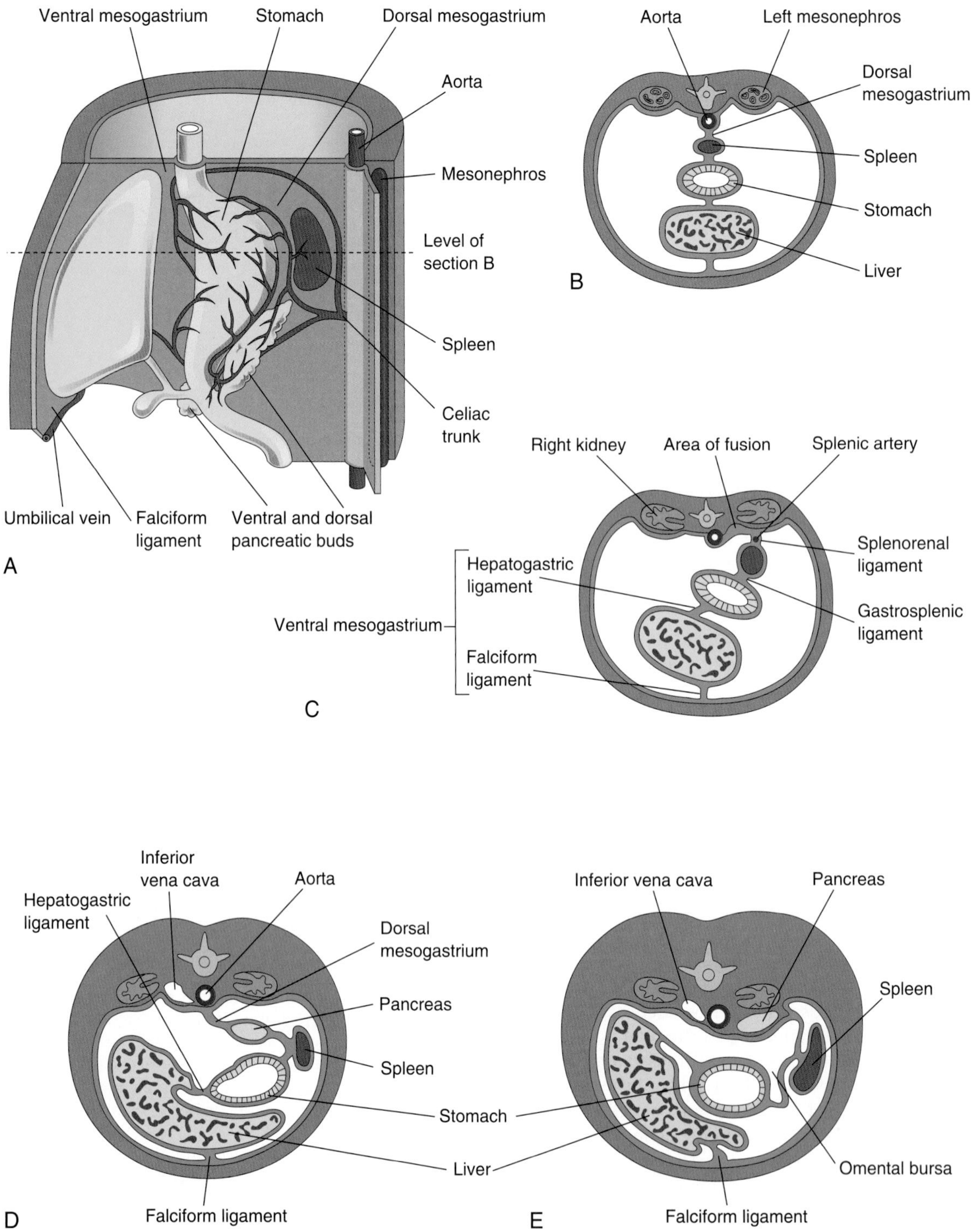

Fig. 11.12 (A) Left side of the stomach and associated structures at the end of the fifth week. Note that the pancreas, spleen, and celiac trunk are between the layers of the dorsal mesogastrium. (B) Transverse section of the liver, stomach, and spleen at the level shown in (A) illustrating the relationship of these structures to the dorsal and ventral mesenteries. (C) Transverse section of a fetus showing fusion of the dorsal mesogastrium with the peritoneum on the posterior abdominal wall. (D and E) Similar sections showing the movement of the liver to the right and rotation of the stomach. Observe the fusion of the dorsal mesogastrium with the dorsal abdominal wall. As a result, the pancreas becomes situated in a retroperitoneal position.

of the adult spleen are remnants of the grooves that separate the fetal lobules. As the stomach rotates, the left surface of the mesogastrium fuses with the peritoneum over the left kidney. This fusion explains why the **splenorenal ligament** has a dorsal attachment and why the adult **splenic artery**, the largest branch of the **celiac trunk**, follows a tortuous course posterior to the omental bursa and anterior to the left kidney (see Fig. 11.12C).

The mesenchymal cells in the splenic primordium differentiate to form the capsule, connective tissue framework,

Accessory Spleens

One or more small splenic masses (~1 cm in diameter) of fully functional splenic tissue may exist in addition to the main body of the spleen. Accessory spleens are commonly found in one of the peritoneal folds near the hilum of the spleen, in the tail of the pancreas, or within the gastrosplenic ligament (see Fig. 11.10D). An accessory spleen occurs in approximately 10% of people. In **polysplenia**, multiple small accessory spleens are present in an infant without a main body of the spleen. Although the multiple spleens are functional tissue, the infant's immune function may still be compromised, resulting in an increased susceptibility to infection (functional asplenia).

and parenchyma of the spleen. The spleen functions as a **hematopoietic center** until late fetal life; however, it retains its potential for blood cell formation even in adult life.

MIDGUT

The derivatives of the midgut are as follows:

- Small intestine, including the duodenum distal to the opening of the bile duct
- Cecum, appendix, ascending colon, and right one-half to two-thirds of the transverse colon

These derivatives are supplied by the **superior mesenteric artery** (see Figs. 11.1 and 11.9).

HERNIATION OF MIDGUT LOOP

As the midgut elongates, it forms a ventral U-shaped **midgut loop**, that projects into the remains of the **extraembryonic coelom** in the proximal part of the umbilical cord (Fig. 11.13A). The loop is a **physiological umbilical herniation**, which occurs at the beginning of the sixth week (Fig. 11.14A, and see also Fig. 11.13A and B). The loop communicates with the **umbilical vesicle** through the narrow **omphaloenteric duct** until the 10th week.

The herniation occurs because there is not enough room in the abdominal cavity for the rapidly growing midgut. The shortage of space is caused mainly by the relatively massive liver and kidneys. The midgut loop has a cranial (proximal) limb and a caudal (distal) limb and is suspended from the dorsal abdominal wall by an elongated mesentery, the **dorsal mesogastrium** (see Fig. 11.13A).

The **omphaloenteric duct** is attached to the apex of the midgut loop where the two limbs join (see Fig. 11.13A). The cranial limb grows rapidly and forms **small intestinal loops** (see Fig. 11.13B), but the caudal limb undergoes very little change except for the development of the **cecal swelling** (diverticulum), the primordium of the cecum and appendix (see Fig. 11.13C).

ROTATION OF MIDGUT LOOP

While the midgut loop is in the umbilical cord, components of the loop rotate 90 degrees counterclockwise around the axis of the **superior mesenteric artery** (see Fig. 11.13B and C). This brings the **cranial limb** (small intestine) of the loop to the right and the **caudal limb** (large intestine) to the left. During rotation, the cranial limb elongates and forms **intestinal loops** (e.g., the primordia of the jejunum and ileum). The rotation of the midgut loop results from the differential growth of the various components; the rotation is a passive process.

RETRACTION OF INTESTINAL LOOPS

10

During the 10th week, the intestines return to the abdomen; this is the **reduction of the midgut hernia** (see Fig. 11.13C and D). It is not known what causes the intestine to return; however, the enlargement of the abdominal cavity and the relative decrease in the size of the liver and kidneys are important factors. The small intestine (formed from the cranial limb) returns first, passing posterior to the superior mesenteric artery, and occupies the central part of the abdomen.

As the large intestine returns, it undergoes a further 180-degree counterclockwise rotation (see Fig. $11.13C_1$ and D_1). The descending colon and sigmoid colon move to the right side of the abdomen. The ascending colon becomes recognizable with the elongation of the posterior abdominal wall (see Fig. 11.13E).

FIXATION OF INTESTINES

Rotation of the stomach and duodenum causes the duodenum and pancreas to fall to the right. The enlarged colon presses the duodenum and pancreas against the posterior abdominal wall. As a result, most of the **duodenal mesentery** is absorbed (Fig. 11.15C, D, and F). Consequently, the duodenum, except for the first part (derived from the foregut), has no mesentery and lies retroperitoneally. Similarly, the head of the pancreas becomes retroperitoneal.

The attachment of the dorsal mesentery to the posterior abdominal wall is greatly modified after the intestines return to the abdominal cavity. At first, the dorsal mesentery is in the median plane. As the intestines enlarge, lengthen, and assume their final positions, their mesenteries are pressed against the posterior abdominal wall. The mesentery of the ascending colon fuses with the parietal peritoneum on this wall and disappears; consequently, the ascending colon also becomes retroperitoneal (see Fig. 11.15B and E).

Other derivatives of the midgut loop (e.g., jejunum and ileum) retain their mesenteries. The mesentery is at first attached to the median plane of the posterior abdominal wall (see Fig. 11.13B and C). After the mesentery of the ascending colon disappears, the fan-shaped mesentery of the small intestine acquires a new line of attachment that passes from the duodenojejunal junction inferolaterally to the ileocecal junction.

CECUM AND APPENDIX

10

The primordium of the cecum and appendix, the **cecal swelling**, appears in the sixth week as an elevation on the antimesenteric border of the caudal limb of the midgut loop (Fig. 11.16A–C, and see also Fig. 11.13C and E). The apex of the cecal swelling does not grow as rapidly as the rest of it; therefore, the **appendix** is initially a small pouch or sac

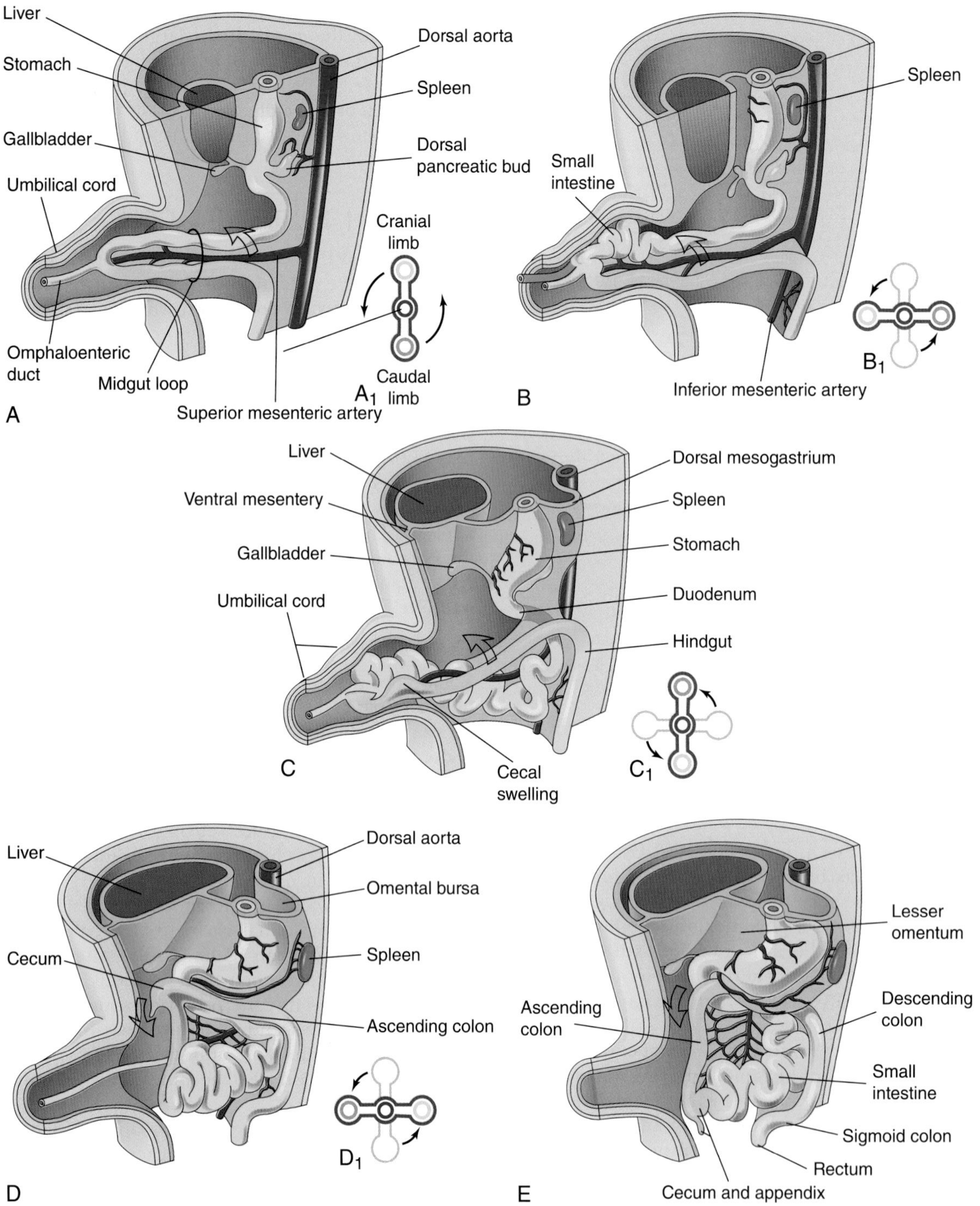

Fig. 11.13 Drawings illustrating herniation and rotation of the midgut loop. (A) At the beginning of the sixth week. (A_1) Transverse section through the midgut loop, illustrating the initial relationship of the limbs of the loop to the superior mesenteric artery. Note that the midgut loop is in the proximal part of the umbilical cord. (B) Later stage showing the beginning of midgut rotation. (B_1) Illustration of the 90-degree counterclockwise rotation that carries the cranial limb of the midgut to the right. (C) At approximately 10 weeks, the intestine returning to the abdomen. (C_1) Illustration of a further rotation of 90 degrees. (D) At approximately 11 weeks, showing the location of the viscera after retraction of the intestine. (D_1) Illustration of a further 90-degree rotation of the viscera, for a total of 270 degrees. (E) Later in the fetal period, the cecum rotating to its normal position in the lower right quadrant of the abdomen.

opening from the cecum (see Fig. 11.16B). The appendix increases rapidly in length, so at birth, it is a relatively long tube arising from the distal end of the cecum (see Fig. 11.16D and E). After birth, the wall of the cecum grows unequally, with the result that the appendix comes to enter its medial side.

There are variations in the position of the appendix. As the ascending colon elongates, the appendix may pass posterior to the cecum **(retrocecal appendix)** or colon **(retrocolic appendix)**. It may also descend over the brim of the pelvis **(pelvic appendix)**. In approximately 64% of people, the appendix is located **retrocecally** (see Fig. 11.16E).

Congenital Omphalocele

Congenital omphalocele is a birth defect of persistent herniation of abdominal contents into the proximal part of the umbilical cord. (Figs. 11.17 and 11.18). Herniation of the intestine into the cord occurs in approximately 1 in 5000 births, and herniation of the liver and intestine occurs in approximately 1 in 10,000 births. Up to 50% of cases are associated with chromosomal abnormalities. The abdominal cavity is proportionately small when there is an omphalocele because the impetus for it to grow is absent.

Surgical repair of omphaloceles is required. Minor omphaloceles may be treated with primary closure. A staged reduction is often planned if the visceral-abdominal disproportion is large. Infants with very large omphaloceles can also suffer from pulmonary and thoracic hypoplasia (underdevelopment).

The covering of the hernia sac is the peritoneum and the amnion. Omphalocele results from impaired growth of mesodermal (muscle) and ectodermal (skin) components of the abdominal wall. Because the formation of the abdominal compartment occurs during gastrulation, a critical failure of growth at this time is often associated with other birth defects of the cardiovascular and urogenital systems.

Umbilical Hernia

When the intestines return to the abdominal cavity during the 10th week and later herniate again through an imperfectly closed umbilicus, an **umbilical hernia** forms. This common type of hernia is different from an omphalocele. In an umbilical hernia, the protruding mass (usually the greater omentum and part of the small intestine) is covered by subcutaneous tissue and skin.

Usually, the hernia does not reach its maximum size until the end of the neonatal period (28 days). It usually ranges in diameter from 1 to 5cm. The defect through which the hernia occurs is in the linea alba (fibrous band in the median line of the anterior abdominal wall between the rectus muscles). The hernia protrudes during crying, straining, or coughing and can be easily reduced through the fibrous ring at the umbilicus. Surgery is not usually performed unless the hernia persists to the age of 3 to 5 years.

Gastroschisis

Gastroschisis, a birth defect of the abdominal wall (prevalence 1 in 2000; Fig. 11.19), results from a defect lateral to the median plane of the anterior abdominal wall. The linear defect permits the extrusion of the abdominal viscera without involving the umbilical cord. The viscera protrude into the amniotic cavity and are bathed by amniotic fluid. The term *gastroschisis*, which literally means a "split or open stomach," is a misnomer because it is the anterior abdominal wall that is split, not the stomach.

This defect usually occurs on the right side lateral to the umbilicus; it is more common in males than females. The exact cause of gastroschisis is uncertain, but various suggestions have been proposed, such as genetic factors, ischemic injury to the anterior abdominal wall, absence of the right omphalomesenteric artery, rupture of the abdominal wall, weakness of the wall caused by abnormal involution of the right umbilical vein, and perhaps rupture of an omphalocele (herniation of viscera into the base of the umbilical cord) before the sides of the anterior abdominal wall have closed.

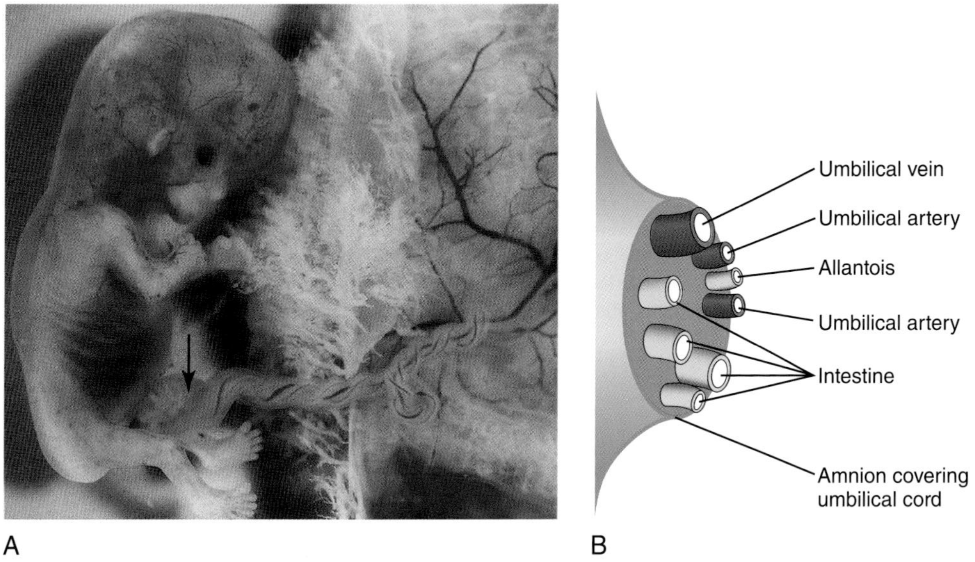

Fig. 11.14 (A) Physiological hernia in a fetus of approximately 58 days (attached to its placenta). Note the herniated intestine (*arrow*) in the proximal part of the umbilical cord. (B) Schematic drawing showing the structures in the distal part of the umbilical cord. (A, Courtesy Dr. D. K. Kalousek, Department of Pathology, University of British Columbia, Children's Hospital, Vancouver, British Columbia, Canada.)

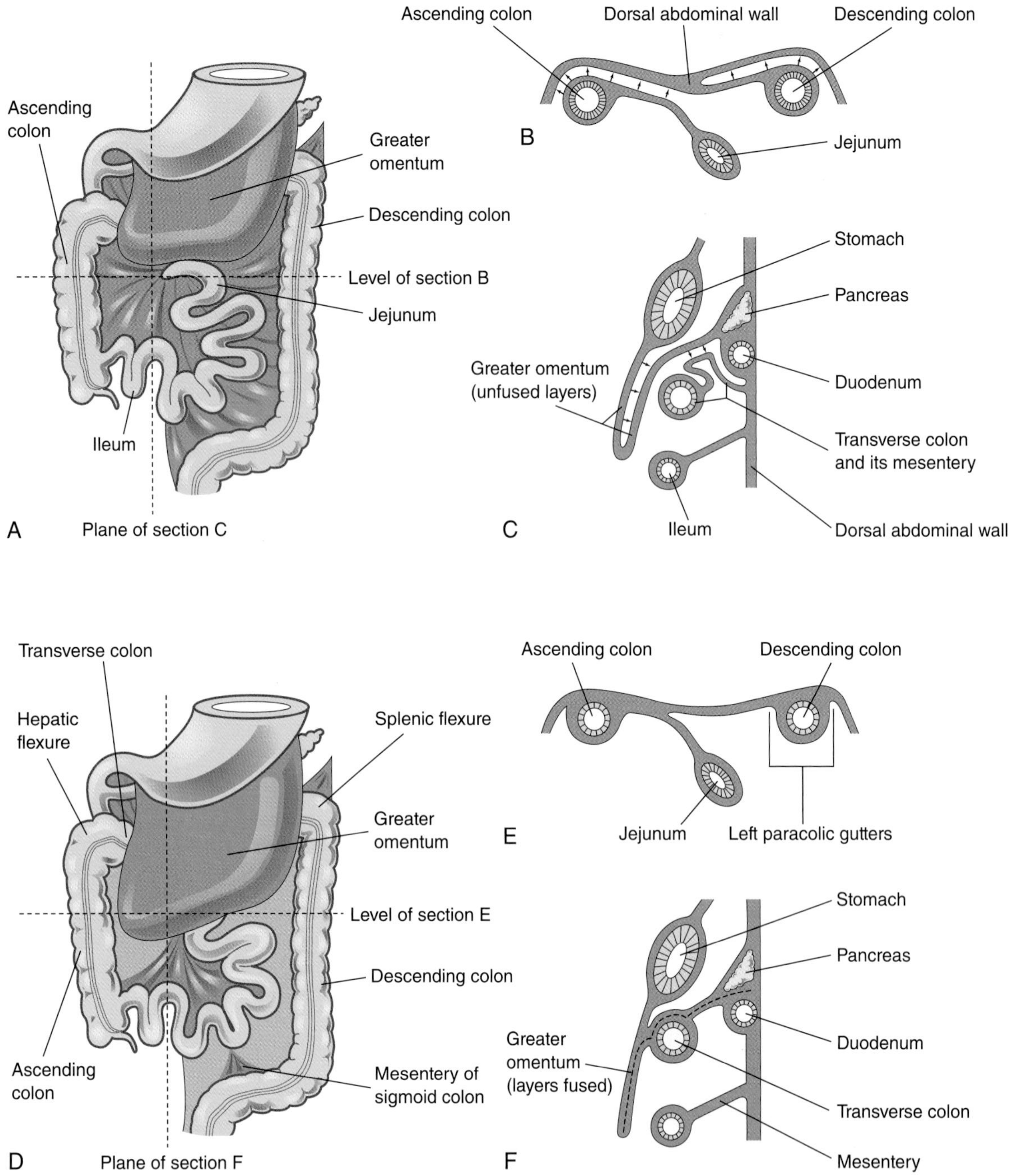

Fig. 11.15 Illustrations showing the mesenteries and fixation of the intestine. (A) Ventral view of the intestines before fixation. (B) Transverse section at the level shown in (A). The *arrows* indicate areas of subsequent fusion. (C) Sagittal section at the plane shown in (A) illustrating the greater omentum overhanging the transverse colon. The *arrows* indicate areas of subsequent fusion. (D) Ventral view of the intestine after fixation. (E) Transverse section at the level shown in (D) after the disappearance of the mesentery of the ascending colon and descending colon. (F) Sagittal section at the plane shown in (D) illustrating the fusion of the greater omentum with the mesentery of the transverse colon and fusion of the layers of the greater omentum.

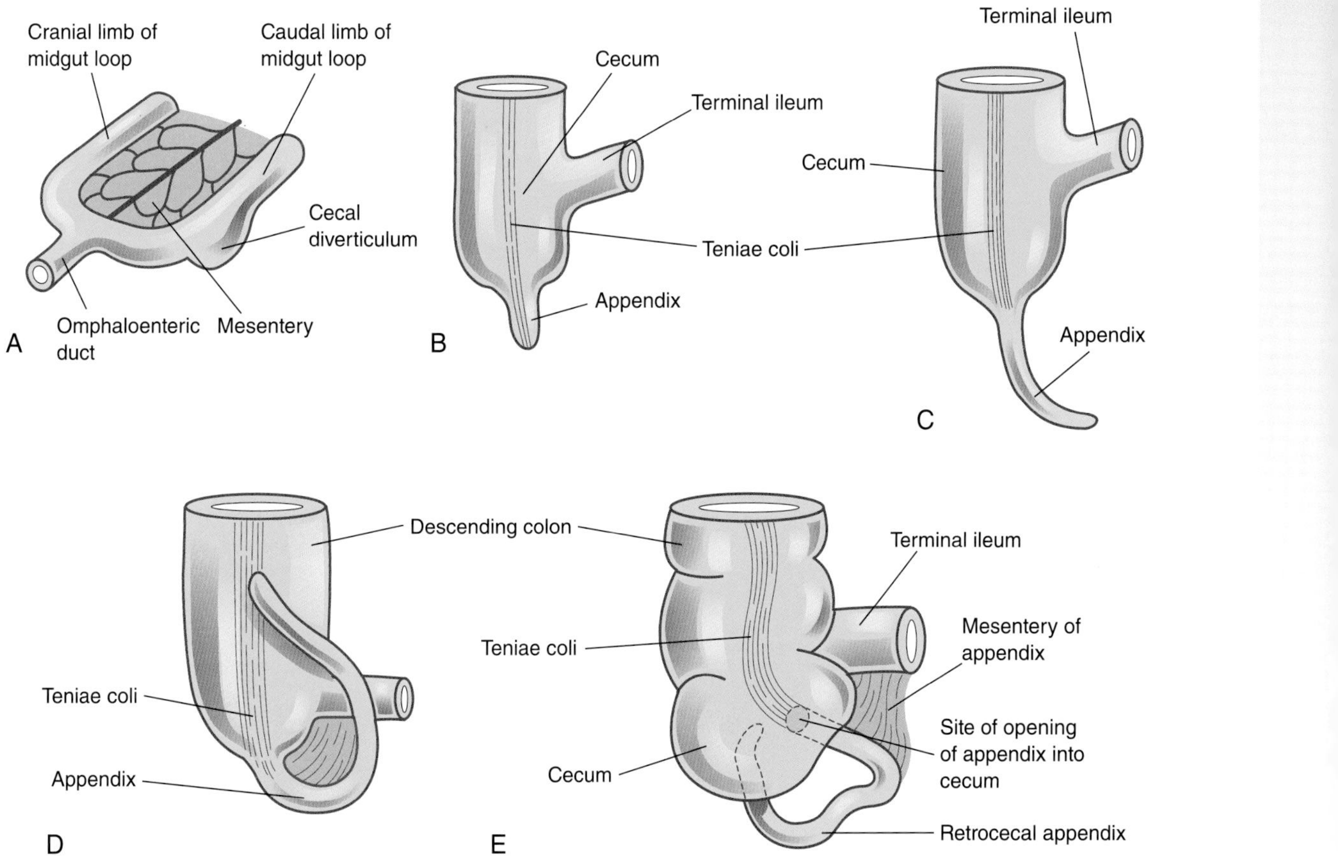

Fig. 11.16 Successive stages in the development of the cecum and appendix. (A) Embryo of 6 weeks. (B) Embryo of 8 weeks. (C) Fetus of 12 weeks. (D) Fetus at birth. Note that the appendix is relatively long and is continuous with the apex of the cecum. (E) Child. Note that the opening of the appendix lies on the medial side of the cecum. In approximately 64% of people, the appendix is located posterior to the cecum (retrocecal). The teniae coli is a thickened band of longitudinal muscle in the wall of the colon.

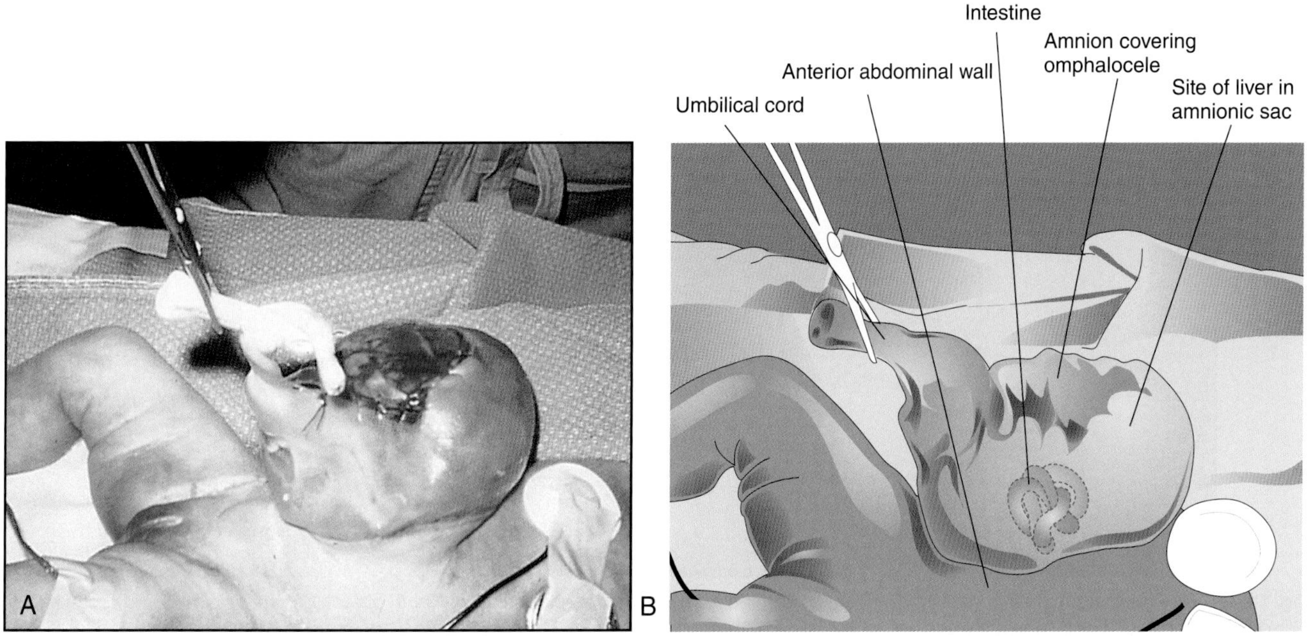

Fig. 11.17 (A) A neonate with a large omphalocele. (B) Drawing of the neonate with an omphalocele resulting from a median defect of the abdominal muscles, fascia, and skin near the umbilicus. This defect resulted in the herniation of intra-abdominal structures (liver and intestine) into the proximal end of the umbilical cord. The omphalocele is covered by a membrane composed of peritoneum and amnion. (A, Courtesy Dr. N. E. Wiseman, pediatric surgeon, Children's Hospital, Winnipeg, Manitoba, Canada.)

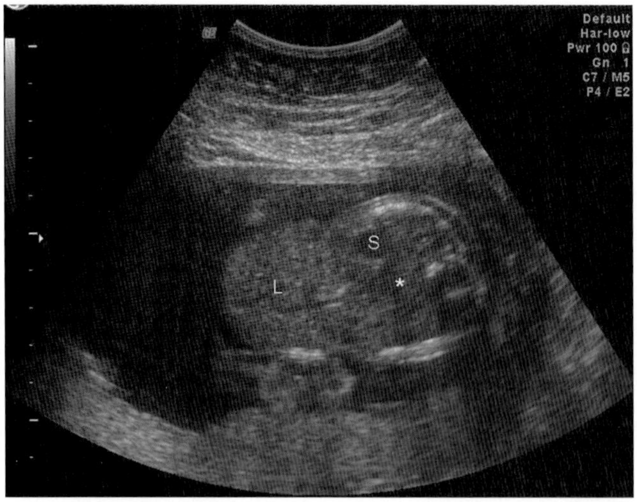

Fig. 11.18 Sonogram of the abdomen of a fetus showing a large omphalocele. Note that the liver (*L*) is protruding (herniating) from the abdomen (*asterisk*). Also, observe the stomach (*S*). (Courtesy Dr. G. J. Reid, Department of Obstetrics, Gynecology and Reproductive Sciences, University of Manitoba, Women's Hospital, Winnipeg, Manitoba, Canada.)

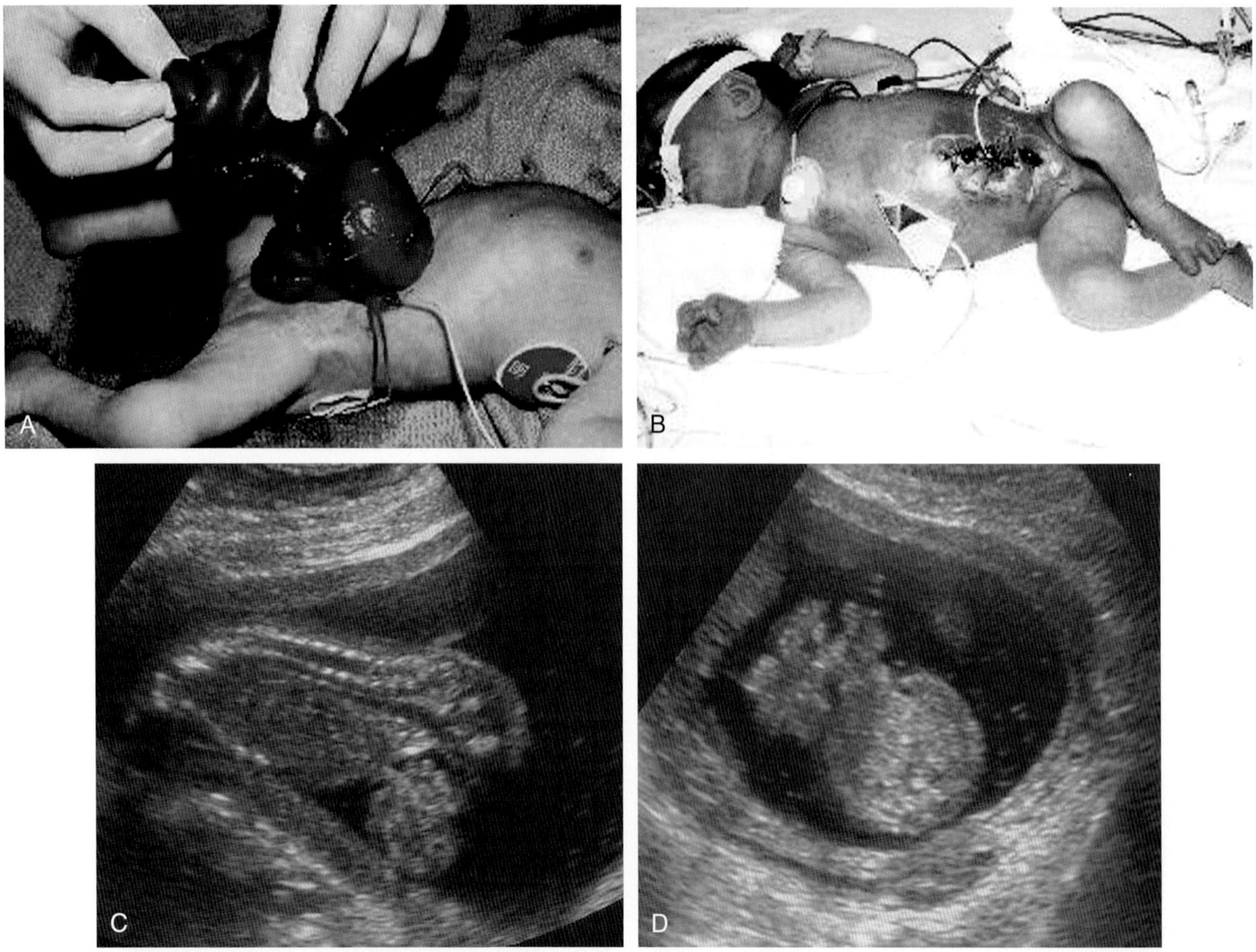

Fig. 11.19 (A) Photograph of a neonate with viscera protruding from an anterior abdominal wall birth defect (gastroschisis). The defect was 2 to 4 cm long and involved all layers of the abdominal wall. (B) Photograph of the infant after the viscera were returned to the abdomen and the defect was surgically closed. (C) (sagittal) and (D) (axial) sonograms of a fetus at 18 weeks with gastroschisis. Loops of the intestine can be seen in the amniotic fluid anterior to the fetus *(F)*. (A and B, Courtesy A. E. Chudley, MD, Section of Genetics and Metabolism, Department of Pediatrics and Child Health, Children's Hospital, Winnipeg, Manitoba, Canada. C and D, Courtesy Dr. E. A. Lyons, Departments of Radiology, Obstetrics and Gynecology, and Anatomy, Health Sciences Centre and University of Manitoba, Winnipeg, Manitoba, Canada.)

Anomalies of Midgut

Birth defects of the intestine are common; most of them are **malrotation of the gut**, which results from incomplete rotation and/or fixation of the intestine. **Nonrotation of the midgut** occurs when the intestine does not rotate as it reenters the abdomen. As a result, the caudal limb of the midgut loop returns to the abdomen first, the small intestine lies on the right side of the abdomen, and the entire large intestine is on the left side (Fig. 11.20A). The usual 270-degree counterclockwise rotation is not completed, and the cecum and appendix lie just inferior to the pylorus of the stomach, a condition known as **subhepatic cecum and appendix** (see Fig. 11.20D). The cecum is fixed to the posterolateral abdominal wall by peritoneal bands that pass over the duodenum (see Fig. 11.20B). The peritoneal bands and the volvulus (twisting) of the intestine cause **intestinal atresia** (duodenal obstruction). This type of malrotation results from the failure of the midgut loop to complete the final 90 degrees of rotation (see Fig. 11.13D). Only two parts of the intestine are attached to the posterior abdominal wall, the duodenum and the proximal colon. This improperly positioned and incompletely fixed intestine may lead to a twisting of the midgut, or **midgut volvulus** (see Fig. 11.20F). The small intestine hangs by a narrow stalk that contains the superior mesenteric artery and vein.

When midgut volvulus occurs, the superior mesenteric artery may be obstructed, resulting in **infarction** and **gangrene** of the intestine supplied by it (see Fig. 11.20A and B). Infants with intestinal malrotation are prone to volvulus and present with **bilious emesis** (vomiting bile). A contrast X-ray study can determine the presence of rotational abnormalities.

Reversed Rotation

In rare cases, the midgut loop rotates in a clockwise rather than a counterclockwise direction (see Fig. 11.20C). As a result, the duodenum lies anterior to the superior mesenteric artery rather than posterior to it, and the transverse colon lies posterior instead of anterior to it. In these infants, the transverse colon may be obstructed by pressure from the superior mesenteric artery. In more unusual cases, the small intestine lies on the left side of the abdomen, and the large intestine lies on the right side, with the cecum in the center. This unusual situation results from malrotation of the midgut followed by failure of fixation of the intestines.

Subhepatic Cecum and Appendix

If the cecum adheres to the inferior surface of the liver when it returns to the abdomen, it will be drawn superiorly as the liver diminishes in size; as a result, the cecum and appendix remain in their fetal positions (see Fig. 11.20D). **Subhepatic cecum and appendix** are more common in males and occur in approximately 6% of fetuses. A subhepatic cecum and "high-riding" appendix may be seen in adults. When this situation occurs, it may create a problem in the diagnosis of appendicitis and during surgical removal of the appendix **(appendectomy)**.

Mobile Cecum

In approximately 10% of people, the cecum has an abnormal amount of freedom. In very unusual cases, it may herniate into the right inguinal canal. A **mobile cecum** results from incomplete fixation of the ascending colon (see Fig. 11.20F). This condition is clinically significant because of the possible variations in the position of the appendix and because twisting, or **volvulus**, of the cecum, may occur (see Fig. 11.20B).

Internal Hernia

In **internal hernia**, a rare birth defect, the small intestine passes into the mesentery of the midgut loop during the return of the intestine to the abdomen (see Fig. 11.20E). As a result, a hernia-like sac forms. This usually does not produce symptoms and is often detected only on postmortem examination.

Stenosis and Atresia of Intestine

Partial occlusion and complete occlusion **(atresia)** of the intestinal lumen account for approximately one-third of cases of **intestinal obstruction** (see Fig. 11.6A and B). The obstructive lesion occurs most often in the duodenum (25%) and ileum (50%). The length of the area affected varies. These birth defects result from the failure of an adequate number of vacuoles to form during recanalization **(restoration of the lumen)** of the intestine. In some cases, a transverse septum or web forms, producing the blockage.

Another possible cause of stenoses and atresias is an interruption of the blood supply to a loop of the fetal intestine resulting from a **fetal vascular accident** caused by impaired microcirculation associated with *fetal distress*, *drug exposure*, or a *volvulus*. The loss of blood supply leads to **necrosis** of the intestine and the development of a fibrous cord connecting the proximal and distal ends of the normal intestine. Malfixation of the gut most likely occurs during the 10th week; it predisposes the gut to volvulus, strangulation, and impairment of its blood supply.

Ileal Diverticulum and Omphaloenteric Remnants

Outpouching of part of the ileum is a common defect of the alimentary tract (Figs. 11.21 and 11.22A). A **congenital ileal diverticulum (Meckel diverticulum)** occurs in about 2% of people, and it is three to five times more prevalent (2:1) in males than females. *An ileal diverticulum is of clinical significance* because it may become inflamed and cause symptoms that mimic appendicitis. Meckel diverticulum is the most common anomaly of the gastrointestinal tract in children. The leading symptoms are abdominal pain, bleeding, and bowel obstruction. Management of this condition is by surgical intervention.

The wall of the diverticulum contains all layers of the ileum and may contain small patches of gastric and pancreatic tissues. This ectopic gastric mucosa often secretes acid, producing ulceration (ulcer) and bleeding (see Fig. 11.22A). An ileal diverticulum is the remnant of the proximal part of the omphaloenteric duct. It typically appears as a blind-ending finger-like pouch approximately 3 to 6 cm long that arises from the antimesenteric border of the ileum (see Fig. 11.21), 40 to 50 cm from the ileocecal junction. An ileal diverticulum may be connected to the umbilicus by a fibrous cord. This may predispose the person to intestinal obstruction because the intestine may wrap around this cord or may form an **omphaloenteric fistula** (Fig. 11.23; also see Fig. 11.22B and C). Similarly, cysts may form within a remnant of the duct and can be found within the abdominal cavity or the anterior abdominal wall (see Figs. 11.22D and 11.23); other possible remnants of the omphaloenteric duct are illustrated in Fig. 11.22E and F.

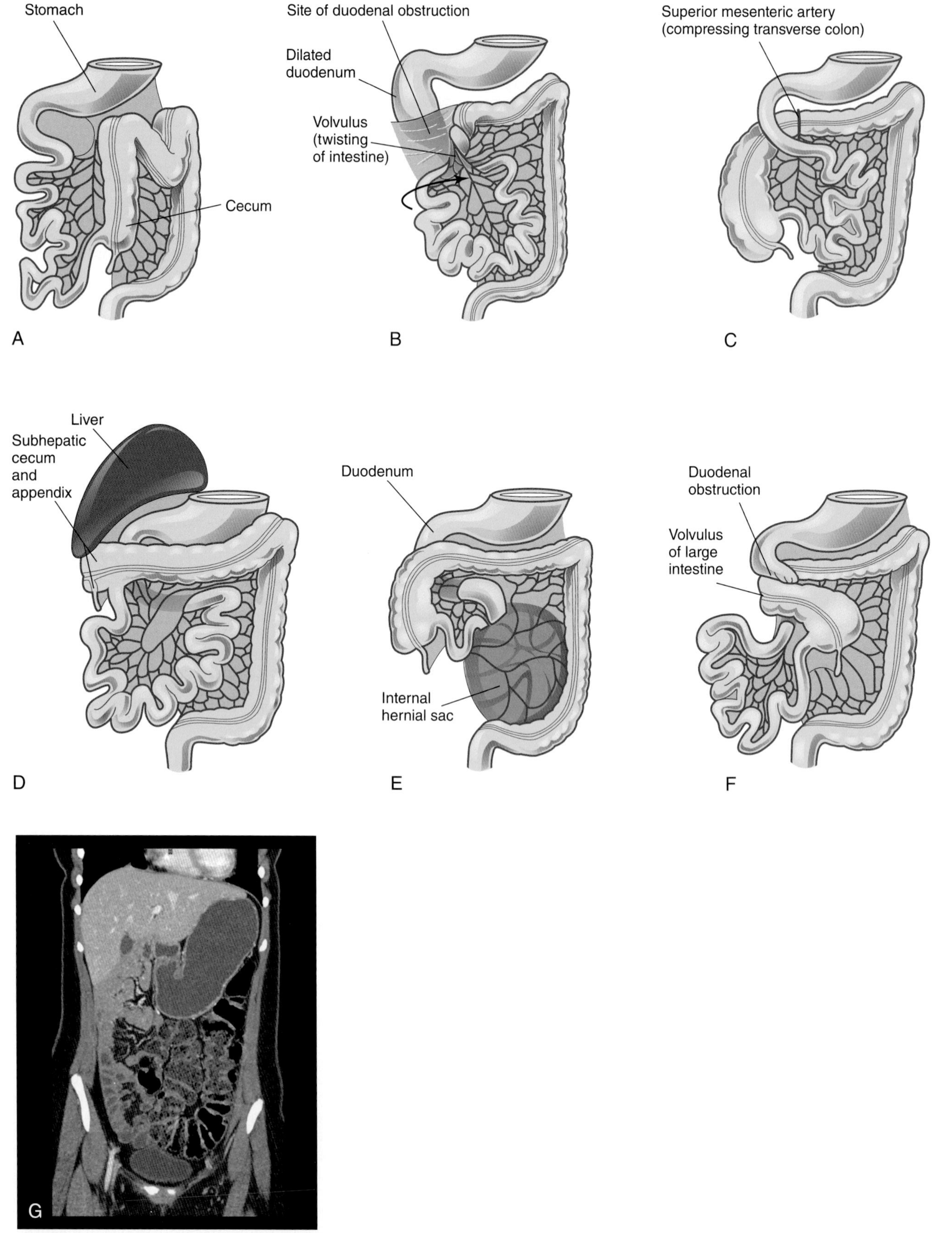

Fig. 11.20 Birth defects of midgut rotation. (A) Nonrotation. (B) Mixed rotation and volvulus (twisting); the *arrow* indicates the twisting of the intestine. (C) Reversed rotation. (D) Subhepatic (below liver) cecum and appendix. (E) Internal hernia. (F) Midgut volvulus. (G) Computed tomography enterographic image of nonrotation in an adolescent patient with chronic abdominal pain. The large intestine is completely on the left side of the abdomen (stool-filled). The small intestine (fluid-filled) is seen on the right. (G, Courtesy Dr. S. Morrison, Children's Hospital, the Cleveland Clinic, Cleveland, OH.)

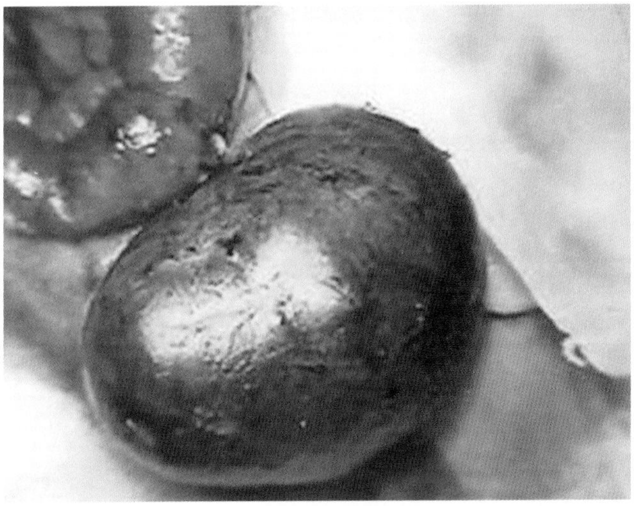

Fig. 11.21 Photograph of a large ileal diverticulum (Meckel diverticulum). Only a small percentage of these diverticula produce symptoms. Ileal diverticula are some of the most common birth defects of the alimentary tract. (Courtesy Dr. M. N. Golarz De Bourne, St. George's University Medical School, Grenada.)

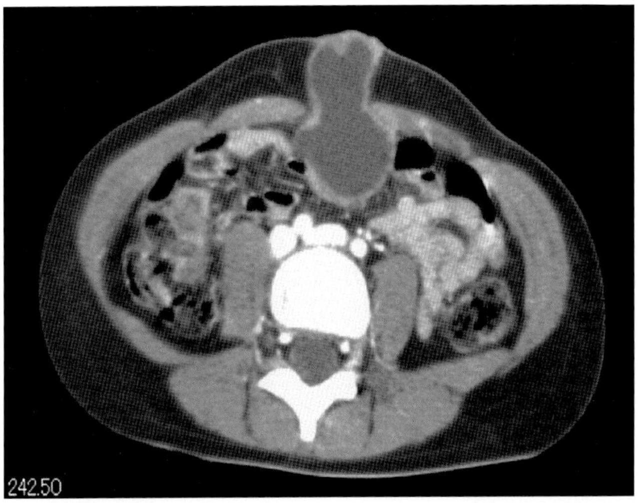

Fig. 11.23 A contrast-enhanced computed tomogram of the abdomen of a 6-year-old girl demonstrating a cyst within an omphaloenteric duct remnant, located just below the level of the umbilicus. A portion of the cyst wall contained ectopic gastric tissue with obvious glandular components. (From Iwasaki M, Taira K, Kobayashi H, et al: Umbilical cyst containing ectopic gastric mucosa originating from an omphalomesenteric duct remnant, *J Pediatr Surg* 44:2399, 2009.)

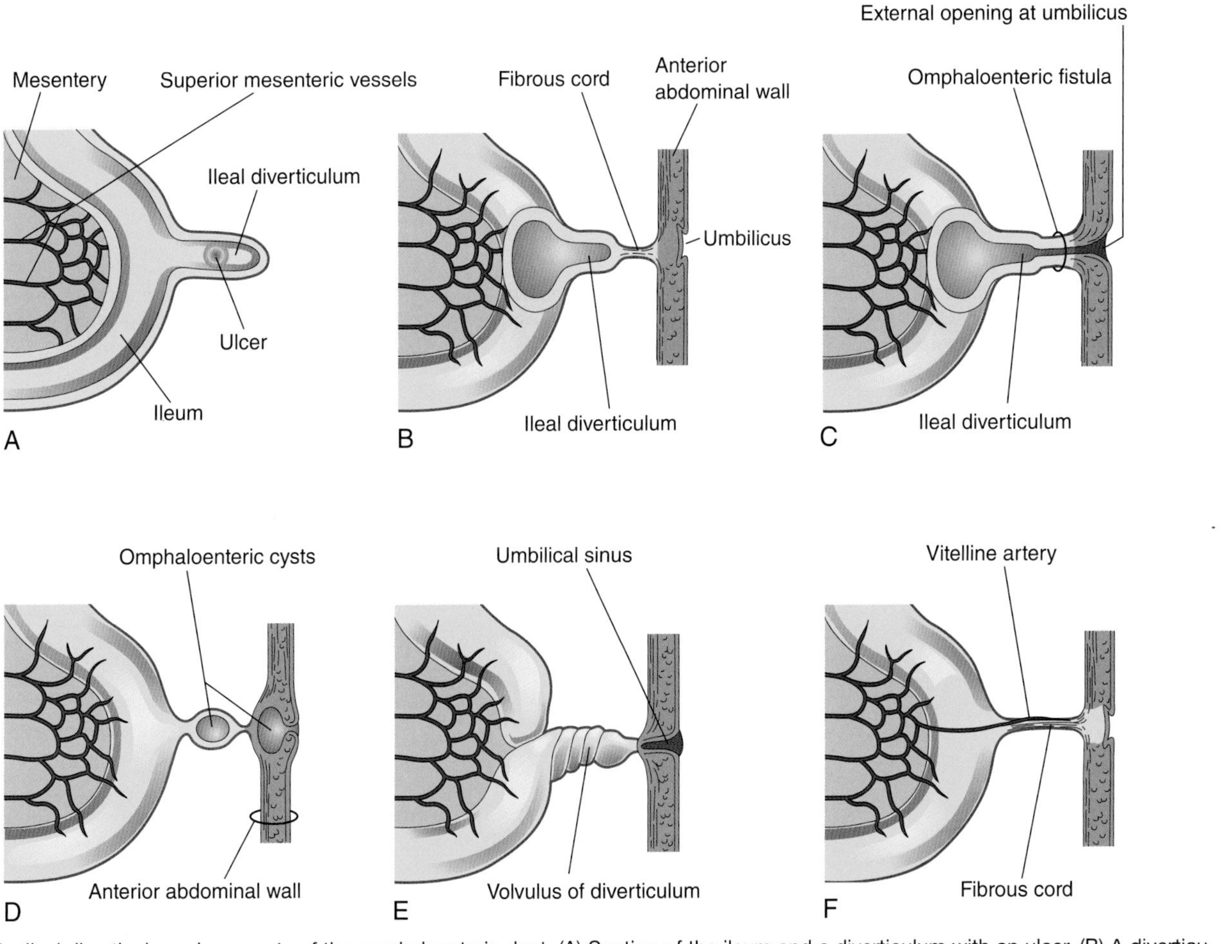

Fig. 11.22 Ileal diverticula and remnants of the omphaloenteric duct. (A) Section of the ileum and a diverticulum with an ulcer. (B) A diverticulum connected to the umbilicus by a fibrous remnant of the omphaloenteric duct. (C) Omphaloenteric fistula resulting from persistence of the intra-abdominal part of the omphaloenteric duct. (D) Omphaloenteric cysts at the umbilicus and in the fibrous remnant of the omphaloenteric duct. (E) Volvulus (twisted) ileal diverticulum and an umbilical sinus resulting from the persistence of the omphaloenteric duct in the umbilicus. (F) The omphaloenteric duct has persisted as a fibrous cord connecting the ileum with the umbilicus. A persistent vitelline artery extends along the fibrous cord to the umbilicus. This artery carries blood to the umbilical vesicle from the anterior wall of the embryo.

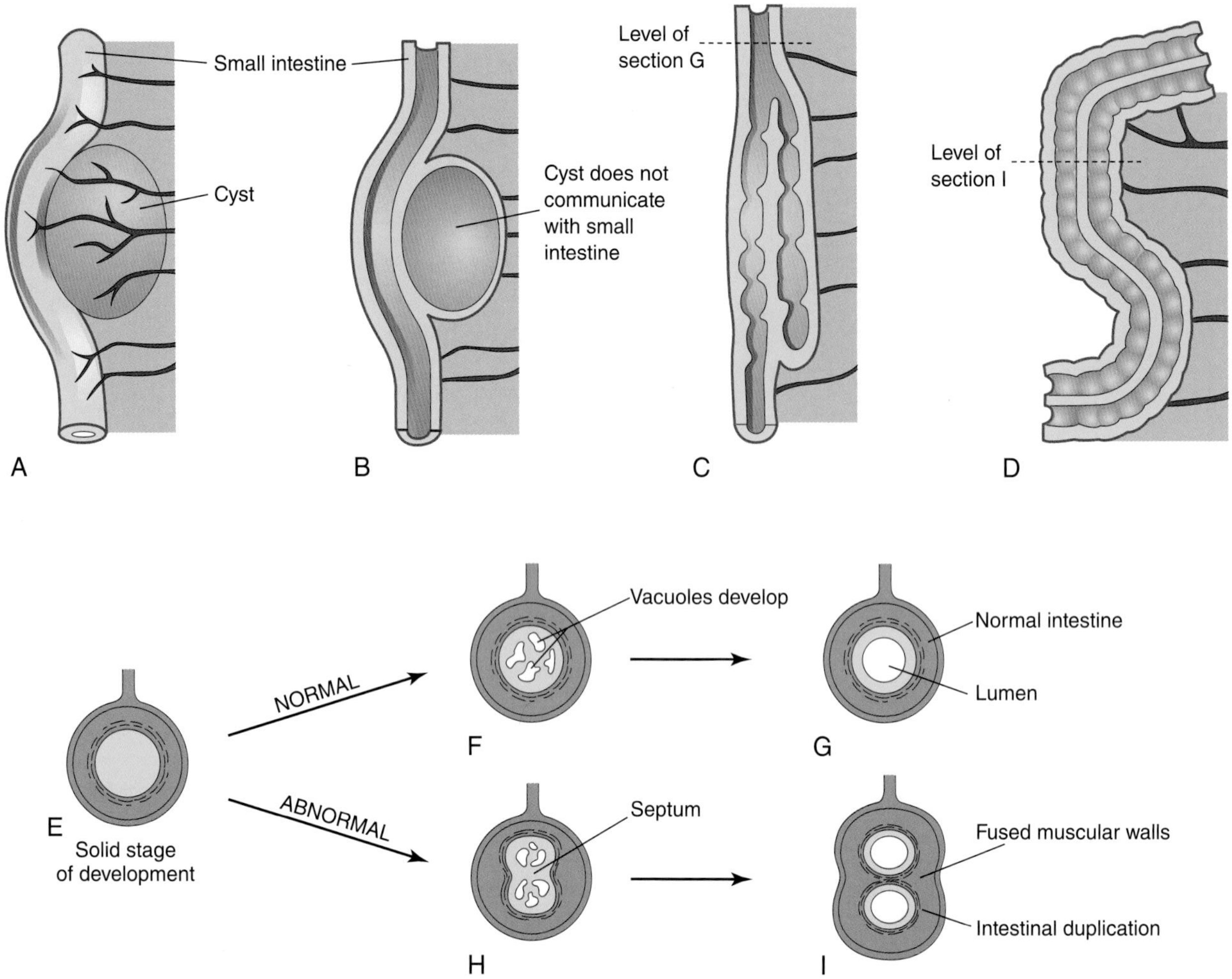

Fig. 11.24 (A) Cystic duplication of the small intestine on the mesenteric side of the intestine; it receives branches from the arteries supplying the intestine. (B) Longitudinal section of the duplication shown in (A); its musculature is continuous with the intestinal wall. (C) A short tubular duplication. (D) A long duplication showing a partition consisting of the fused muscular walls. (E) Transverse section of the intestine during the solid stage. (F) Normal vacuole formation. (G) Coalescence of the vacuoles and reformation of the lumen. (H) Two groups of vacuoles have formed. (I) Coalescence of vacuoles illustrated in (H) results in intestinal duplication.

Duplication of Intestine

Cystic duplications are more common than **tubular duplications** (Fig. 11.24A–D). Tubular duplications usually communicate with the intestinal lumen (see Fig. 11.24C). Almost all duplications are caused by the failure of normal recanalization of the small intestine; as a result, two lumina form (see Fig. 11.24H and I). The duplicated segment lies on the mesenteric side of the intestine. The duplication often contains **ectopic gastric mucosa**, which may result in local peptic ulceration and gastrointestinal bleeding. The incidence of intestinal duplication is approximately 1:5000.

HINDGUT

The derivatives of the hindgut are as follows:

- Left one-third to one-half of the transverse colon, the descending colon, the sigmoid colon, the rectum, and the superior part of the anal canal
- Epithelium of the urinary bladder and most of the urethra

All hindgut derivatives are supplied by the **inferior mesenteric artery**. The junction between the segment of the transverse colon derived from the midgut and that originating from the hindgut is indicated by the change in blood supply from a branch of the superior mesenteric artery to a branch of the inferior mesenteric artery. *The colon is formed as an extension of the hindgut and is regulated by Wnt3a-β-catenin-Sp5 signaling pathway along the dorsal and ventral hindgut endoderm.*

The descending colon becomes retroperitoneal as its mesentery fuses with the parietal peritoneum on the left posterior abdominal wall and then disappears (see Fig. 11.15B and E). The mesentery of the fetal sigmoid colon is retained, but it is smaller than in the embryo (see Fig. 11.15D).

CLOACA

In early embryos, the **cloaca** is a chamber into which the hindgut and allantois empty. The expanded terminal part of the hindgut, the cloaca, is an endoderm-lined chamber that is in contact with the surface ectoderm at the **cloacal membrane** (Fig. 11.25A and B). This membrane is composed of

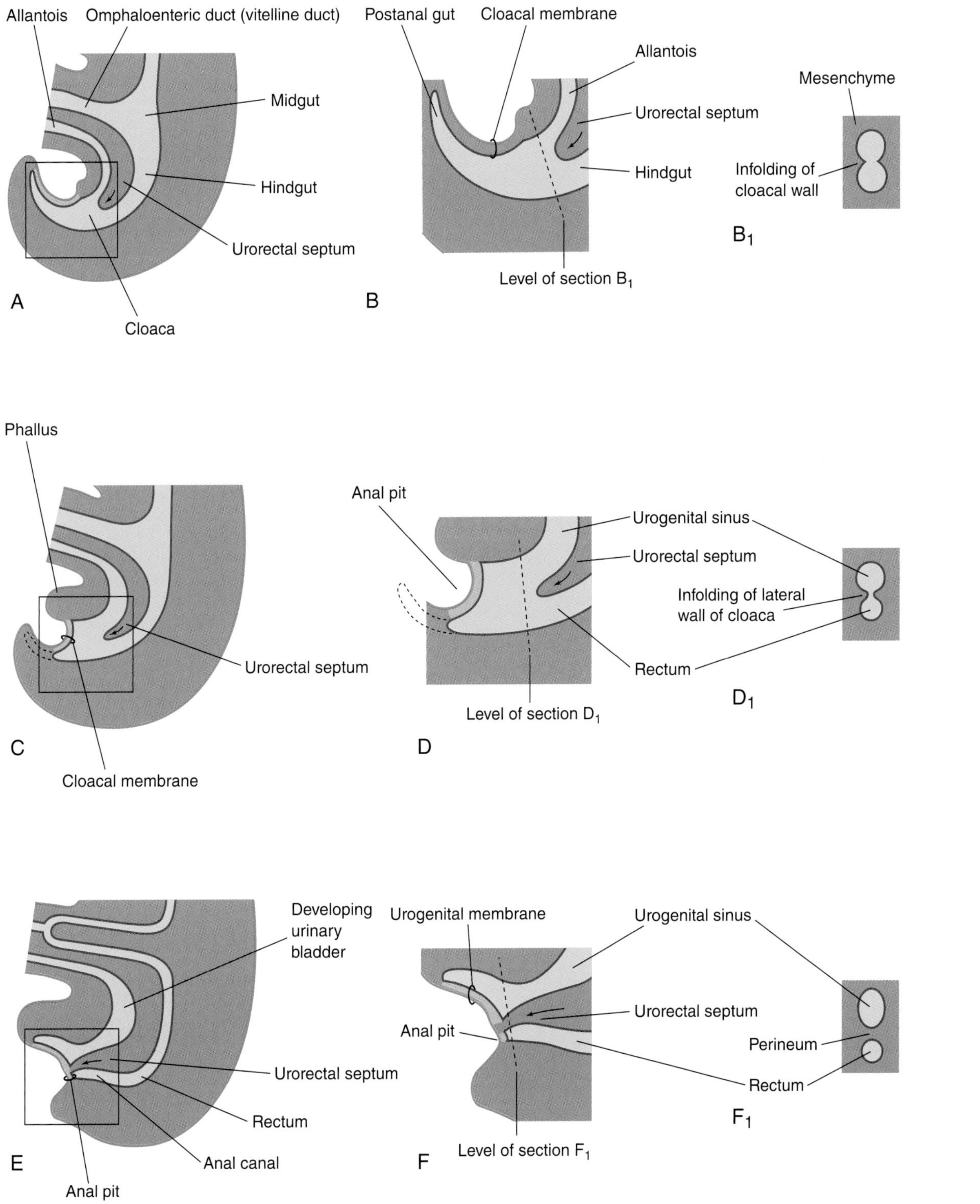

Fig. 11.25 Successive stages in the partitioning of the cloaca into the rectum and urogenital sinus by the urorectal septum. (A, C, and E) Views from the left side at 4, 6, and 7 weeks, respectively. (B, D, and F) Enlargements of the cloacal region. (B_1 and D_1) Transverse sections of the cloaca at the levels shown in (B and D). Note that the postanal portion (shown in B) degenerates and disappears as the rectum forms.

the endoderm of the cloaca and the ectoderm of the anal pit (see Fig. 11.25D). The cloaca receives the **allantois** ventrally, which is a finger-like diverticulum (see Fig. 11.25A).

PARTITIONING OF THE CLOACA

The cloaca is divided into dorsal and ventral parts by a wedge of mesenchyme, the **urorectal septum**, that develops in the angle between the allantois and hindgut. *Endodermal Shh-Wifi and β-catenin signaling pathways are required for mesenchymal proliferation and formation of the urorectal septum.* As the septum grows toward the cloacal membrane, it develops fork-like extensions that produce infoldings of the lateral walls of the cloaca (see Fig. 11.25B). These folds grow toward each other and fuse, forming a partition that divides the cloaca into three parts: the **rectum**, the cranial part of the anal canal, and the **urogenital sinus** (see Fig. 11.25D and E).

The cloaca plays a crucial role in anorectal development. New information indicates that the urorectal septum does not fuse with the cloacal membrane; therefore, an anal membrane does not exist. After the cloacal membrane ruptures by **apoptosis** (programmed cell death), the **anorectal lumen** is temporarily closed by an **epithelial plug** (which may have been misinterpreted as the anal membrane). Mesenchymal proliferations produce elevations of the surface ectoderm around the epithelial anal plug. Recanalization of the anorectal canal occurs by apoptotic cell death of the epithelial anal plug, which forms the **anal pit** (proctodeum; see Fig. 11.25E).

ANAL CANAL

10 The superior two-thirds of the adult anal canal is derived from the **hindgut**; the inferior one-third develops from the **anal pit** (Fig. 11.26). The junction of the epithelium derived from the ectoderm of the anal pit and endoderm of the hindgut is roughly indicated by the irregular **pectinate line**, located at the inferior limit of the anal valves. Approximately 2 cm superior to the anus is the **anocutaneous line** (white line). This is approximately where the composition of the anal epithelium changes from columnar to stratified squamous cells. At the anus, the epithelium is **keratinized** (made keratinous) and continuous with the skin around the anus. The other layers of the wall of the anal canal are derived from splanchnic mesenchyme. *The formation of the anal sphincter appears to be under* Hox D *genetic control.*

Because of its hindgut origin, the superior two-thirds of the anal canal is mainly supplied by the **superior rectal artery**, the continuation of the inferior mesenteric artery (hindgut artery). The venous drainage of this superior part is mainly via the **superior rectal vein**, a tributary of the inferior mesenteric vein. The lymphatic drainage of the superior part is eventually to the **inferior mesenteric lymph nodes**. Its nerves are from the **autonomic nervous system**.

Because of its origin in the anal pit, the inferior one-third of the anal canal is supplied mainly by the **inferior rectal arteries**, branches of the internal pudendal artery. The venous drainage is through the **inferior rectal vein**, a tributary of the internal pudendal vein that drains into the internal iliac vein. The lymphatic drainage of the inferior part of the anal canal is to the **superficial inguinal lymph nodes**. Its nerve supply is from the **inferior rectal nerve**; hence, it is sensitive to pain, temperature, touch, and pressure.

The differences in blood supply, nerve supply, and venous and lymphatic drainage of the anal canal are important clinically, as when one may be considering the **metastasis**

Congenital Megacolon

Congenital aganglionic megacolon (Hirschsprung disease, HSCR) is a dominantly inherited multigenic neurocristopathy with incomplete penetrance and variable expressivity. Of the genes so far identified, the RET proto-oncogene is the major susceptibility gene and accounts for most cases. This disorder affects 1 in 5000 newborns and is defined as an absence of ganglion cells **(aganglionosis)** in a variable length of distal bowel, although more proximal and longer segments can also be involved.

Infants with HSCR lack autonomic ganglion cells in the myenteric plexus distal to the dilated segment of the colon (Fig. 11.27). The enlarged colon, or megacolon, has the normal number of ganglion cells. The dilation results from failure of relaxation of the aganglionic segment, which prevents movement of the intestinal contents, resulting in dilation. In most cases, only the rectum and sigmoid colon are involved; occasionally, ganglia are also absent from more proximal parts of the colon.

HSCR is the most common cause of neonatal obstruction of the colon and accounts for 33% of all neonatal obstructions; males are affected more often than females (4:1). HSCR results from the failure of neural crest cells to migrate into the wall of the colon during the fifth to seventh weeks. This results in the failure of parasympathetic ganglion cells to develop in the myenteric and submucosal plexuses.

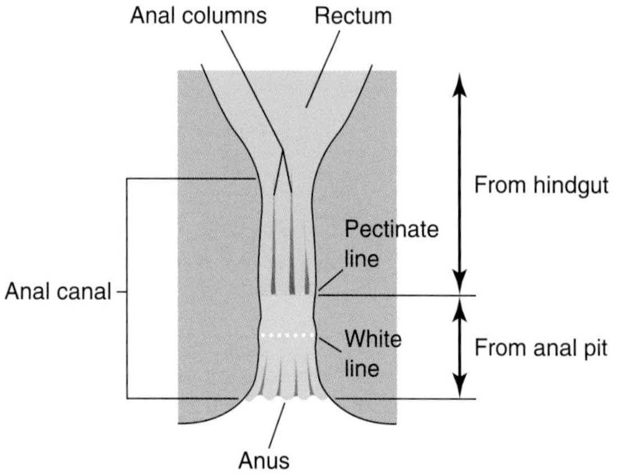

Fig. 11.26 Sketch of the rectum and anal canal showing their developmental origins. Note that the superior two-thirds of the anal canal is derived from the hindgut, whereas the inferior one-third of the canal is derived from the anal pit. Because of their different embryologic origins, the superior and inferior parts of the anal canal are supplied by different arteries and nerves and have different venous and lymphatic drainages.

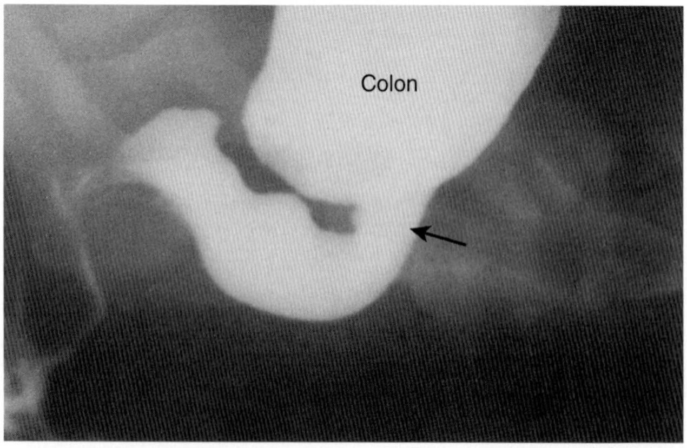

Fig. 11.27 Radiograph of the colon after a barium enema in a 1-month-old infant with congenital megacolon (Hirschsprung disease). The aganglionic distal segment (rectum and distal sigmoid colon) is narrow, with a distended normal ganglionic bowel, full of fecal material, proximal to it. Note the transition zone *(arrow)*. (Courtesy Dr. Martin H. Reed, Department of Radiology, University of Manitoba and Children's Hospital, Winnipeg, Manitoba, Canada.)

Anorectal Anomalies

Most anorectal anomalies result from abnormal development of the urorectal septum, resulting in incomplete separation of the cloaca into urogenital and anorectal parts (see Fig. 11.29A). *The pathogenesis of hindgut anomalies possibly involves the disruption of several genes, including DKK4, Wnt, Hox, Gli2, and CDX1. Shh and FGF-10, and the β-catenin signaling pathways have also been implicated*. There is normally a temporary communication between the rectum and anal canal dorsally from the bladder and urethra ventrally (see Fig. 11.25C). Lesions are classified as low or high depending on whether the rectum ends superior or inferior to the puborectalis muscle, which maintains fecal continence and relaxes to allow defecation. Other anomalies (genitourinary, cardiovascular, spinal, vertebral) are present in 50% to 60% of infants born with anorectal malformation.

BIRTH DEFECTS OF LOW ANORECTAL REGION

- **Imperforate anus** occurs in 1 in 5000 neonates and is more common in males than females (Figs. 11.28 and 11.29C). The anal canal may end blindly, or there may be an ectopic anus or an **anoperineal fistula (abnormal passage)** that opens into the perineum (see Fig. 11.29D and E). However, the abnormal canal may open into the vagina in females or urethra in males (see Fig. 11.29F and G).
- In **anal stenosis**, the anus is in the normal position, but the anus and anal canal are narrow (see Fig. 11.29B). This defect is probably caused by a slight dorsal deviation of the urorectal septum as it grows caudally.
- In **membranous atresia**, the anus is in the normal position, but a thin layer of tissue separates the anal canal from the exterior (see Figs. 11.28 and 11.29C). The remnant of the epithelial anal plug is thin enough to bulge on straining and appears blue from the presence of **meconium** (feces of neonate) superior to it. This defect results from the failure of the epithelial plug to perforate at the end of the eighth week.

BIRTH DEFECTS OF HIGH ANORECTAL REGION

In **anorectal agenesis**, an anomaly of the high anorectal region, the rectum ends superior to the puborectalis muscle. *This is the most common type of anorectal birth defect*. Although the rectum ends blindly, there is usually a **fistula (abnormal passage)** to the bladder **(rectovesical fistula)** or urethra **(rectourethral fistula)** in males, or to the vagina **(rectovaginal fistula)** or the vestibule of the vagina **(rectovestibular fistula)** in females (see Fig. 11.29F and G).

Anorectal agenesis with a fistula is the result of incomplete separation of the cloaca from the urogenital sinus by the urorectal septum (see Fig. 11.25C–E). In newborn males with this condition, meconium may be observed in the urine, whereas fistulas in females result in the presence of meconium in the vestibule of the vagina. More than 90% of high anorectal defects are associated with a **fistula**.

In **rectal atresia**, the anal canal and rectum are present but separated (see Fig. 11.29H and I). Sometimes the two segments of the intestine are connected by a fibrous cord, the remnant of an atretic portion of the rectum. The cause of rectal atresia may be abnormal recanalization of the colon or, more likely, a defective blood supply.

of cancer cells. Tumors inferior to the pectinate line metastasize to the femoral and inguinal nodes, whereas tumors superior to the pectinate lines metastasize to the internal iliac, retroperitoneal, and perirectal nodes.

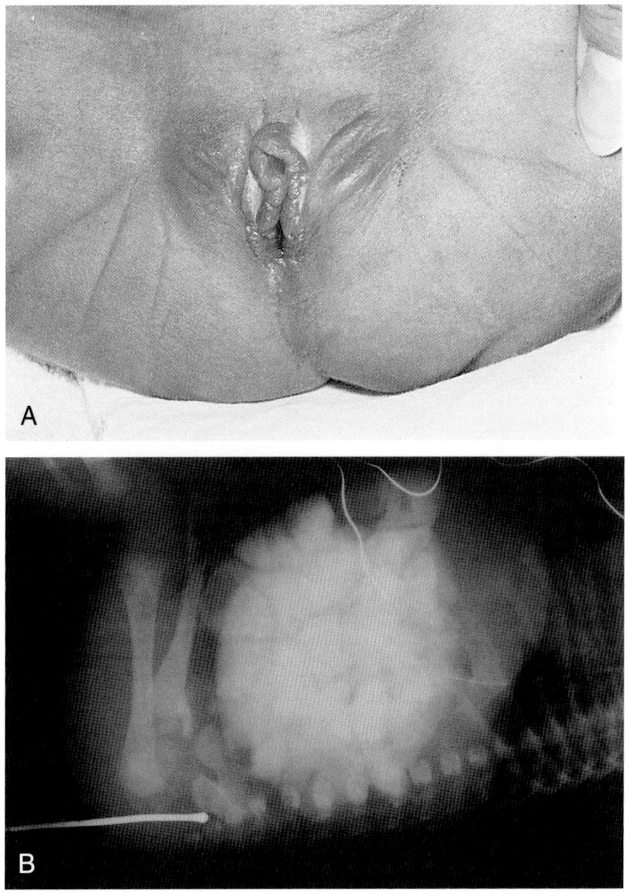

Fig. 11.28 Imperforate anus. (A) Female neonate with anal atresia (imperforate anus). In most cases, a thin layer of tissue separates the anal canal from the exterior. Some form of imperforate anus occurs approximately once in every 5000 neonates; it is more common in males. (B) Radiograph of an infant with an imperforate anus. The dilated end of the radiopaque probe is at the bottom of the blindly ending anal pit. The large intestine is distended with feces and contrast material. (A, Courtesy A. E. Chudley, MD, Section of Genetics and Metabolism, Department of Pediatrics and Child Health, Children's Hospital, Winnipeg, Manitoba, Canada. B, Courtesy Dr. Prem S. Sahni, formerly of the Department of Radiology, Children's Hospital, Winnipeg, Manitoba, Canada.)

MORPHOGENESIS OF GUT CELLS AND MICROSTRUCTURE

Intestinal villi appear approximately at the end of week 8. The villi extend in length by the proliferation of underlying mesenchyme cells, which also create the villi core. Gut epithelium continues to proliferate beyond the time of the muscular layer formation. This results in the development of luminal furrows or wrinkles. The intestinal crypts appear around week 9 with crypt stem cells (related to enterocyte formation) appearing by approximately week 11. Panteth cells, goblet cells, and Brunner's glands also appear in week 11. The development of early follicles within Peyer's patches occurs during weeks 16–20, but full maturations only occur postpartum by stimulation from luminal antigens.

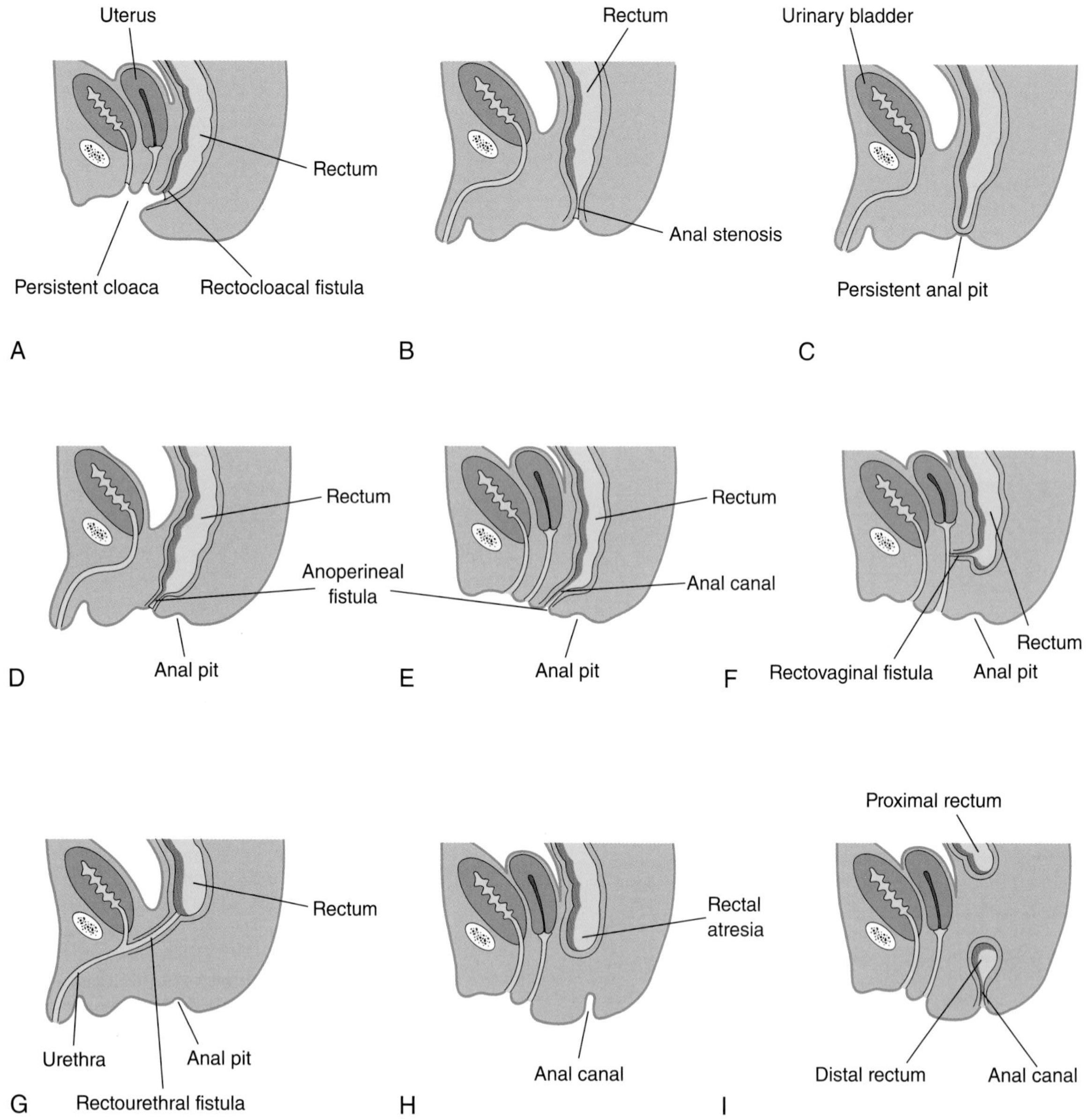

Fig. 11.29 Various types of anorectal birth defects. (A) Persistent cloaca. Note the common outlet for the intestinal, urinary, and reproductive tracts. (B) Anal stenosis. (C) Anal atresia. (D and E) Anal agenesis with a perineal fistula. (F) Anorectal agenesis with a rectovaginal fistula. (G) Anorectal agenesis with a rectourethral fistula. (H and I) Rectal atresia.

ENTERIC NERVOUS SYSTEM

The gastrointestinal system has numerous functions, including transportation, secretion, digestion, and protection. All of these are controlled by the enteric nervous system (ENS), comprised of both extrinsic and intrinsic components. The ENS can maintain functions autonomously, without input from the brain or spinal cord. The extrinsic ENS is mainly comprised of nerve fibers along the arterial supply of the gut. The intrinsic ENS is comprised of ganglionic plexuses and enteric neurons and is highly complex, with more than 200 million neurons and more than 20 different neuron subtypes. Neural crest cells migrate to the foregut during its development, and once reaching this location, they travel along the length of the developing gut, populating and differentiating into neurons, glial cells, and other cell types. The foregut is populated by neural crest cells by week 3, and the most distal portion of the gut receives neural crest cells by week 7. *Studies have reported that several interacting genes, including RET, EDNRB, GDNF, SOX10, PHOX2B, EDN3, and other signaling pathways are associated with the development of the ENS.* Defects in the migration, proliferation, and differentiation of neural crest cells with failure in the formation of associated ganglia can lead to Hirschsprung disease (see Fig. 11.27).

SUMMARY OF ALIMENTARY SYSTEM

- The **primordial gut** forms from the dorsal part of the umbilical vesicle, which is incorporated into the embryo. The endoderm of the primordial gut gives rise to the epithelial lining of the alimentary tract, except for the cranial and caudal parts, which are derived from the ectoderm of the stomodeum and cloacal membrane, respectively. The muscular and connective tissue components of the alimentary tract are derived from splanchnic mesenchyme surrounding the primordial gut.

- The **foregut** gives rise to the pharynx, lower respiratory system, esophagus, stomach, proximal part of the duodenum, liver, pancreas, and biliary apparatus. Because the trachea and esophagus have a common origin from the foregut, incomplete partitioning by the tracheoesophageal septum results in stenoses or atresias, with or without fistulas between them.
- The **hepatic diverticulum**, the primordium of the liver, gallbladder, and biliary duct system, is an outgrowth of the endodermal epithelial lining of the foregut. Epithelial liver cords develop from the hepatic diverticulum and grow into the **septum transversum**. Between the layers of the ventral mesentery, derived from the septum transversum, primordial cells differentiate into hepatic tissues and linings of the ducts of the biliary system.
- **Congenital duodenal atresia** results from failure of the vacuolization and recanalization process to occur after the normal solid developmental stage of the duodenum. Usually, the epithelial cells degenerate, and the lumen of the duodenum is restored. Obstruction of the duodenum can also be caused by an **annular pancreas** or pyloric stenosis.
- The **pancreas** develops from two pancreatic buds that form from the endodermal lining of the foregut. When the duodenum rotates to the right, the **ventral pancreatic bud** moves dorsally and fuses with the dorsal pancreatic bud. The ventral pancreatic bud forms most of the head of the pancreas, including the uncinate process. The **dorsal pancreatic bud** forms the remainder of the pancreas. In some fetuses, the duct systems of the two buds fail to fuse, and an accessory pancreatic duct forms.
- The **midgut** gives rise to the duodenum (the part distal to the entrance of the bile duct), jejunum, ileum, cecum, appendix, ascending colon, and right one-half to two-thirds of the transverse colon. The midgut forms a U-shaped **umbilical loop of the intestine** that herniates into the umbilical cord during the sixth week because there is no room for it in the abdomen. While in the umbilical cord, the midgut loop rotates counterclockwise 90 degrees. During the 10th week, the intestine returns to the abdomen, rotating a further 180 degrees.
- **Omphaloceles**, **malrotations**, and **abnormal fixation of the gut** result from failure of return or abnormal rotation of the intestine. Because the gut is normally occluded during the fifth and sixth weeks, stenosis (partial obstruction), atresia (complete obstruction), and duplications result if recanalization fails to occur or occurs abnormally. Remnants of the omphaloenteric duct may persist. **Ileal diverticula** are common; however, very few of them become inflamed and produce pain.
- The **hindgut** gives rise to the left one-third to one-half of the transverse colon, the descending colon and sigmoid colon, the rectum, and the superior part of the anal canal. The inferior part of the anal canal develops from the anal pit. The caudal part of the hindgut divides the **cloaca** into the urogenital sinus and rectum. The urogenital sinus gives rise to the urinary bladder and urethra. The rectum and superior part of the anal canal are separated from the exterior by the epithelial plug. This mass of epithelial cells breaks down by the end of the eighth week.
- Most **anorectal defects** result from abnormal partitioning of the cloaca into the rectum and anal canal posteriorly and urinary bladder and urethra anteriorly. Arrested growth and/or deviation of the urorectal septum cause most anorectal defects, such as rectal atresia and fistulas between the rectum and urethra, urinary bladder, or vagina.

CLINICALLY ORIENTED PROBLEMS

CASE 11-1

A female infant was born prematurely at 32 weeks' gestation to a 39-year-old woman whose pregnancy was complicated by polyhydramnios. Amniocentesis at 16 weeks showed that the fetus had trisomy 21. The baby began to vomit within a few hours after birth. Marked dilation of the epigastrium was noted. Radiographs of the abdomen showed gas in the stomach and superior part of the duodenum, but no other intestinal gas was observed. A diagnosis of duodenal atresia was made.

- Where does obstruction of the duodenum usually occur?
- What is the embryologic basis of this congenital defect?
- What caused distention of the infant's epigastrium?
- Is duodenal atresia commonly associated with other defects such as trisomy 21 (Down syndrome)?
- What is the embryologic basis of the polyhydramnios in this case?

CASE 11-2

The umbilicus of a neonate failed to heal normally. It was swollen, and there was a persistent discharge from the umbilical stump. A sinus tract was outlined with contrast media during fluoroscopy. The tract was resected on the ninth day after birth, and its distal end was found to terminate in a diverticulum of the ileum.

- What is the embryologic basis of the sinus tract?
- What is the usual clinical name given to this type of ileal diverticulum?
- Is this birth defect common?

CASE 11-3

A female infant was born with a small dimple where the anus should have been. Examination of her vagina revealed meconium and an opening of a sinus tract in the posterior wall of the vagina. Radiographic examination using a contrast medium injected through a tiny catheter inserted into the opening revealed a fistulous connection.

- With which part of the lower bowel would the fistula probably be connected?
- Name this birth defect.
- What is the embryologic basis of this condition?

CASE 11-4

A newborn infant was born with a light gray, shiny mass measuring the size of an orange that protruded from the umbilical region. The mass was covered by a thin transparent membrane.

- What is this birth defect called?
- What is the origin of the membrane covering the mass?
- What would be the composition of the mass?
- What is the embryologic basis of this protrusion?

CASE 11-5

A newborn infant appeared normal at birth; however, excessive vomiting and abdominal distention developed after a few hours. The vomitus contained bile, and a little meconium was passed. A radiographic examination showed a gas-filled stomach and dilated, gas-filled loops of small bowel, but no air was present in the large intestine. This indicated a congenital obstruction of the small bowel.

- What part of the small bowel was probably obstructed?
- What would this condition be called?
- Why was only a little meconium passed?
- What would likely be observed at operation?
- What was the probable embryologic basis of the condition?

Discussion of these problems appears in the Appendix at the back of the book.

BIBLIOGRAPHY AND SUGGESTED READING

Ambartsumyan L, Smith C, Kapur RP: Diagnosis of Hirschung disease, *Pediatr Dev Pathol* 23:8, 2020.

Bastidas-Ponce A, Scheibner K, Lickert L: Cellular and molecular mechanisms coordinating pancreas development, *Development* 144:2873, 2017.

Belo J1, Krishnamurthy M, Oakie A, Wang R: The role of SOX9 transcription factor in pancreatic and duodenal development, *Stem Cells Dev* 22:2935, 2013.

Bishop WP, Ebach DR: The digestive system. In Marcdante KJ, Kliegman KJ, editors: *Nelson essentials of pediatrics,* ed 7, Philadelphia, 2015, Saunders.

Choi SY, Hong SS, Park H, Lee HK, Shin HC, Choi GC: The many faces of Meckel's diverticulum and its complications, *J Med Imaging Radiat Oncol* 61:225, 2017.

De Bakker BS, Babar A, Tol KCN: Reconsidering the 'non-recanalization theory" of the gut, *J Dev Orig Health Dis,* 2021. https://doi.org/10.1017/S2040174421000490.

DeLaForest A, Di Furio F, Jing R. et al.: HNF4A regulates the formation of hepatic progenitor cells from human iPSC-derived endoderm by facilitating efficient recruitment of RNA Pol II, *Genes* 10(1):21, 2018. https://doi.org/10.3390/genes10010021.

DeSesso JM: Comparative anatomy, pre- and postnatal changes during the development and maturation of the small intestine: life-stage influences on exposure, *Birth Defects Res* 114:449, 2022.

Diposarosa R, Bustam NA, Sahiratmadja E, Susanto PS, Sribudiani Y: Literature review: enteric nervous system development, genetic and epigenetic regulation in the etiology of Hirschsprung's disease, *Heliyon.* 7(6):e07308, 2021. https://doi.org/10.1016/j.heliyon.2021.e0730.

Đuknić M, Puškaš N, Labudović-Borović M, Janković R: Signaling pathways in the control of embryonic development of the enteric nervous system, Zdravstvena zaštita 51(3):18–31, 2022. https://doi.org/10.5937/zdravzast51-39735Heliyon 2021 Jun 15;7(6):e07308. doi: 10.1016/j.heliyon.2021.e07308.

Garriock RJ, Chalamalasetty RB, Zhu J, et al: A dorsal-ventral gradient of Wnt3a/β-catenin signals controls mouse hindgut extension and colon formation, *Development* 147(8):dev185108, 2020. https://doi.org/10.1242/dev.185108.

Gordillo M, Evans T, Gouon-Evans V: Orchestrating liver development, *Development* 142:2094, 2015.

Keplinger KM, Bloomston M: Anatomy and embryology of the biliary tract, *Surg Clin North Am* 94:203, 2014.

Khanna K, Sharma S, Pabalan N, Singh N, Gupta DK: A review of genetic factors contributing to the etiopathogenesis of anorectal malformations, *Pediatr Surg Int* 34:9, 2018.

Klein M, Varga I: Hirschsprung's Disease-recent understanding of embryonic aspects, etiopathogenesis and future treatment avenues, *Medicina (Kaunas)* 56(11):611, 2020. https://doi.org/10.3390/medicina56110611

Kluth D, Fiegel HC, Metzger R: Embryology of the hindgut, *Semin Pediatr Surg* 20:152, 2011.

Kostouros A, Koliarakis I, Natsis K, Spandidos DA, Tsatsakis A, Tsiaoussis J: Large intestine embryogenesis: molecular pathways and related disorders (Review), *Int J Mol Med* 46:27, 2020.

Kruepunga N, Hikspoors JPJM, Hülsman CJM, Mommen GMC, Köhler SE, Lamers WH: Development of extrinsic innervation in the abdominal intestines of human embryos, *J Anat* 237:655, 2020.

Kuwahara A, Lewis AE, Coombes C, Leung FS, Percharde M, Bush JO: Delineating the early transcriptional specification of the mammalian trachea and esophagus, *Elife* 9:e55526, 2020. https://doi.org/10.7554/eLife.55526

Ledbetter DJ: Gastroschisis and omphalocele, *Surg Clin North Am* 86:249, 2006.

Levitt MA, Pena A: Cloacal malformations: lessons learned from 490 cases, *Semin Pediatr Surg* 9:118, 2010.

Marine MB, Forbes-Amrhein MM: Magnetic resonance imaging of the fetal gastrointestinal system, *Pediatr Radiol* 50:1895, 2020.

Metzger R, Metzger U, Fiegel HC, Kluth D: Embryology of the midgut, *Semin Pediatr Surg* 20:145, 2011.

Metzger R, Wachowiak R, Kluth DL: Embryology of the early foregut, *Semin Pediatr Surg* 20:136, 2011.

Mueller JL, Goldstein AM: The science of Hirschsprung disease: what we know and where we are headed, *Sem Ped Surg* 31:151157, 2022.

Muniz T.D, Rolo L.C, Araujo Júnior E.: Gastroschisis: embriology, pathogenesis, risk factors, prognosis, and ultrasonographic markers for adverse neonatal outcomes, *J Ultrasound* 2024. https://doi.org/10.1007/s40477-024-00887-8.

Miyagawa S, Harada M, Matsumaru D: Disruption of the temporally regulated cloaca endodermal β-catenin signaling causes anorectal malformations, *Cell Death Differ,* 2014.

Molina LM, Zhu J, Li Q, Pradhan-Sundd T, Krutsenko Y, Sayed K: Compensatory hepatic adaptation accompanies permanent absence of intrahepatic biliary network due to YAP1 loss in liver progenitors, *Cell Rep* 36(1):109310, 2021. https://doi.org/10.1016/j.celrep.2021.109310.

Nadel A: The fetal gastrointestinal tract and abdominal wall. In Norton ME, Scoutt LM, Feldstein VA, editors: *Callen's ultrasonography in obstetrics and gynecology,* ed 6, Philadelphia, 2017, Elsevier.

Nagy N, Goldstein AM: Enteric nervous system development: a crest cell's journey from neural tube to colon, *Semin Cell Dev Biol* 66:94, 2017.

Naik-Mathuria B, Olutoye OO: Foregut abnormalities, *Surg Clin North Am* 86:261, 2006.

Nakamura T, Yamada S, Funatomi T, Takakuwa T, Shinohara H, Sakai Y: Three-dimensional morphogenesis of the omental bursa from four recesses in staged human embryos, *J Anat* 237(1):166–175, 2020. https://doi.org/10.1111/joa.13174.

Chuaire Noack L: New clues to understand gastroschisis. Embryology, pathogenesis and epidemiology, *Colomb Med (Cali)* 30;52(3):e4004227, 2021. https://doi.org/10.25100/cm.v52i3.4227.

Oh C, Youn JK, Han JW, Yang HB, Kim HY, Jung SE: Analysis of associated anomalies in anorectal malformation: major and minor anomalies, *J Korean Med Sci* 35(14):e98, 2020. https://doi.org/10.3346/jkms.2020.35.

Schierz IAM, Piro E, Giuffrè M, et al: Clinical and genetic approach in the characterization of newborns with anorectal malformation, *J Matern Fetal Neonatal Med* 35:4513, 2022.

Som PM, Grapin-Botton A: The current embryology of the foregut and its derivatives, *Neurographics* 6:43, 2016.

Thomas DFM: The embryology of persistent cloaca and urogenital sinus malformations, *Asian J Androl* 22:124, 2020.

Van der Putte SCJ: The development of the human anorectum, *Anat Rec* 292:952, 2009.

Wyatt BH, Amin NM, Bagley K, et al: Single-minded 2 is required for left-right asymmetric stomach morphogenesis, *Development* 148(17):dev199265, 2021. https://doi.org/10.1242/dev.199265.

Zangen D, Kaufman Y, Banne E, Weinberg-Shukron A, Abulibdeh A, Garfinkel BP: Testicular differentiation factor SF-1 is required for human spleen development, *J Clin Invest* 124:2071, 2014.

Zhang Y, Yang Y, Jiang M, Huang SX, Zhang W, Al Alam D: 3D modeling of esophageal development using human PSC-derived basal progenitors reveals a critical role for notch signaling, *Cell Stem Cell* 23(4):516–529.e5, 2018. https://doi.org/10.1016/j.stem.2018.08.009.

Urogenital System 12

CHAPTER OUTLINE

The **urogenital system** is divided functionally into two different embryological parts: the **urinary system** and the **genital system**. The urogenital system includes all the organs involved in reproduction and forming and voiding urine. Embryologically, the systems are closely associated, especially during their early stages of development. The kidneys and internal genitalia and their ducts develop from the **intermediate mesenchyme** derived from the dorsal body wall of the embryo (Fig. 12.1A and B).

During the folding of the embryo in the horizontal plane, the mesenchyme is carried ventrally and loses its connection with the **somites** (Fig. 12.1B–D). A longitudinal elevation of mesoderm, the **urogenital ridge**, forms on each side of the **dorsal aorta** (Fig. 12.1D and F). The part of the ridge giving rise to the urinary system is the **nephrogenic cord** (see Fig. 12.1D–F); the part of the ridge giving rise to the genital system is the **gonadal ridge** (see Fig. 12.29C).

Expression of the following genes is needed for the formation and anterior-posterior patterning (regionalization) of the urogenital ridge: HOX, GATA 4, Wilms tumor suppressor 1 (WT1), steroidogenic factor 1, and DAX1.

DEVELOPMENT OF THE URINARY SYSTEM

11

The urinary system (kidneys, ureters, urinary bladder, and urethra) begins to develop before the genital system.

DEVELOPMENT OF KIDNEYS AND URETERS

Three sets of successive kidneys develop in the embryos. The first set, the **pronephroi**, is rudimentary. The second set, the **mesonephroi**, functions briefly during the early fetal period. The third set, the **metanephroi**, forms the permanent kidneys.

PRONEPHROI

Pronephroi are bilateral transitory structures that appear early in the fourth week. They are represented by a few cell clusters and tubular structures in the developing neck region (Fig. 12.2A). The pronephric ducts run caudally and open into the **cloaca**, the chamber into which the hindgut and allantois emptied (Fig. 12.2B). The pronephroi soon degenerate; however, most parts of the ducts persist and are used by the second set of kidneys.

MESONEPHROI

Mesonephroi, which are large, elongated excretory organs, appear late in the fourth week (see Fig. 12.2). The mesonephroi function as interim kidneys for approximately 4 weeks, until the permanent kidneys develop and function (Fig. 12.3). The **mesonephric kidneys** consist of **glomeruli** (10–50 per kidney) and **mesonephric tubules** (Figs. 12.4 and 12.5; see also Fig. 12.3). The tubules open into bilateral **mesonephric ducts** and, in turn, open into the **cloaca** (see Fig. 12.2B and Fig. 11.25A). The mesonephroi degenerate

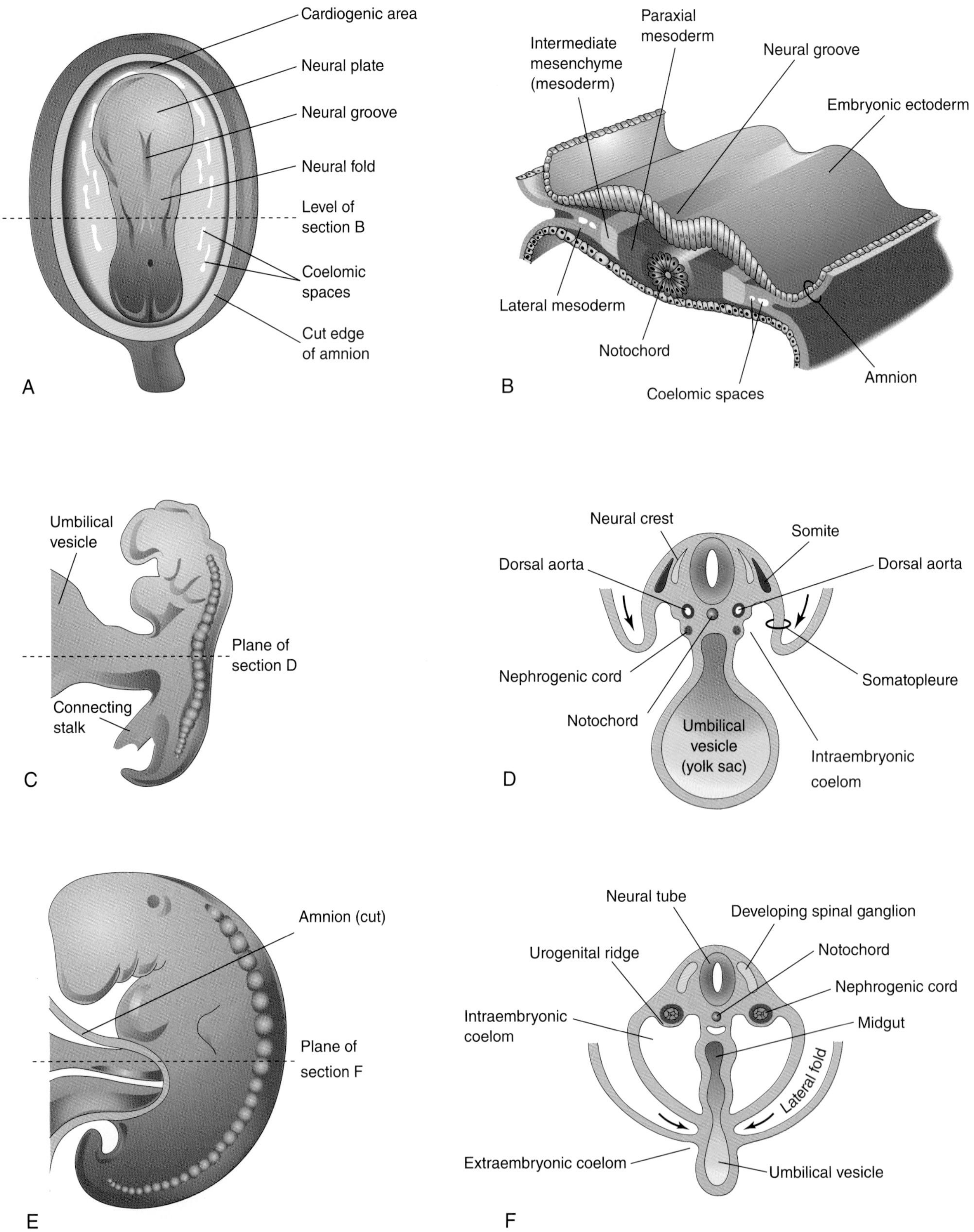

Fig. 12.1 (A) Dorsal view of an embryo during the third week (approximately 18 days). (B) Transverse section of the embryo, showing the position of the intermediate mesenchyme before lateral folding occurs. (C) Lateral view of an embryo during the fourth week (approximately 24 days). (D) Transverse section of the embryo after the commencement of folding, showing the nephrogenic cords. (E) Lateral view of an embryo later in the fourth week (approximately 26 days). (F) Transverse section of the embryo, showing the lateral folds meeting each other ventrally.

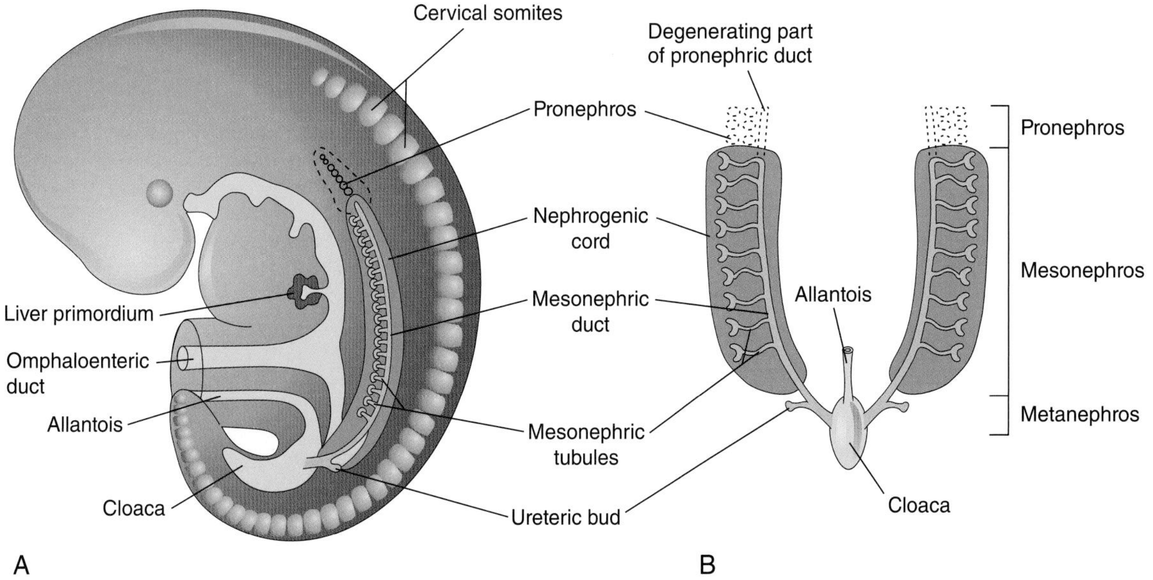

Fig. 12.2 Illustrations of the three sets of nephric systems in an embryo during the fifth week. (A) Lateral view. (B) Ventral view. The mesonephric tubules are pulled laterally; their normal position is shown in (A).

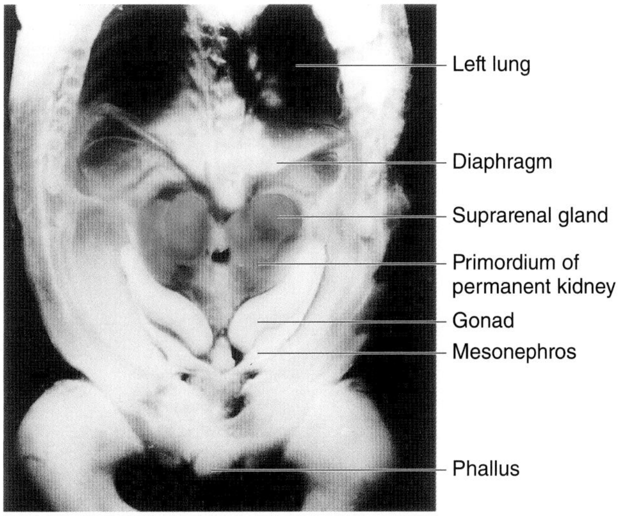

Fig. 12.3 Dissection of thorax, abdomen, and pelvis of an embryo at approximately 54 days, during the indifferent stage of development. Observe the large suprarenal glands and elongated mesonephroi (interim kidneys). Also, observe the gonads (testes or ovaries) and the phallus, the primordium of the penis or clitoris, which develops from the genital tubercle (see Fig. 12.37A and B). (From Nishimura H, editor: *Atlas of human prenatal histology*, Tokyo, 1983, Igaku-Shoin.)

toward the end of week 12; however, the metanephric tubules become the efferent ductules of the **testes**. The mesonephric ducts have several adult derivatives in males (Table 12.1).

METANEPHROI

Metanephroi, or the **primordia of the permanent kidneys**, begin to develop in the fifth week (Fig. 12.6) and become functional approximately 4 weeks later. Urine formation continues throughout fetal life; the urine is excreted through the urethra into the amniotic cavity and forms a component of the amniotic fluid. The kidneys develop from two sources (see Fig. 12.6):

- The **ureteric bud** (metanephric diverticulum)
- The **metanephrogenic blastema** (metanephric mass of mesenchyme)

The ureteric bud is a diverticulum from the mesonephric duct near its entrance into the cloaca (see Fig. 12.6A and B). The metanephrogenic blastema is derived from the caudal part of the nephrogenic cord. As the ureteric bud elongates, it penetrates the blastema.

The stalk of the ureteric bud becomes the **ureter** (see Fig. 12.6B). The cranial part of the bud undergoes repetitive branching, resulting in the bud differentiating into the **collecting tubules** (Fig. 12.7A and B; see also Fig. 12.6E). The first four generations of tubules enlarge and become confluent to form the **major calices** (see Fig. 12.6C and D). The second four generations coalesce to form the **minor calices**. The end of each arched collecting tubule induces clusters of mesenchymal cells in the metanephrogenic blastema to form small **metanephric vesicles** (see Fig. 12.7A and B).

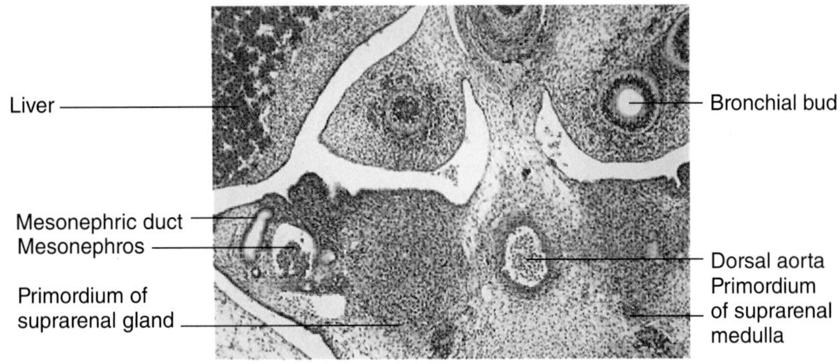

Fig. 12.4 Photomicrograph of a transverse section of an embryo at approximately 42 days, showing the mesonephros and developing suprarenal glands. (From Moore KL, Persaud TVN, Shiota K: *Color atlas of clinical embryology*, ed 2, Philadelphia, 2000, Saunders.)

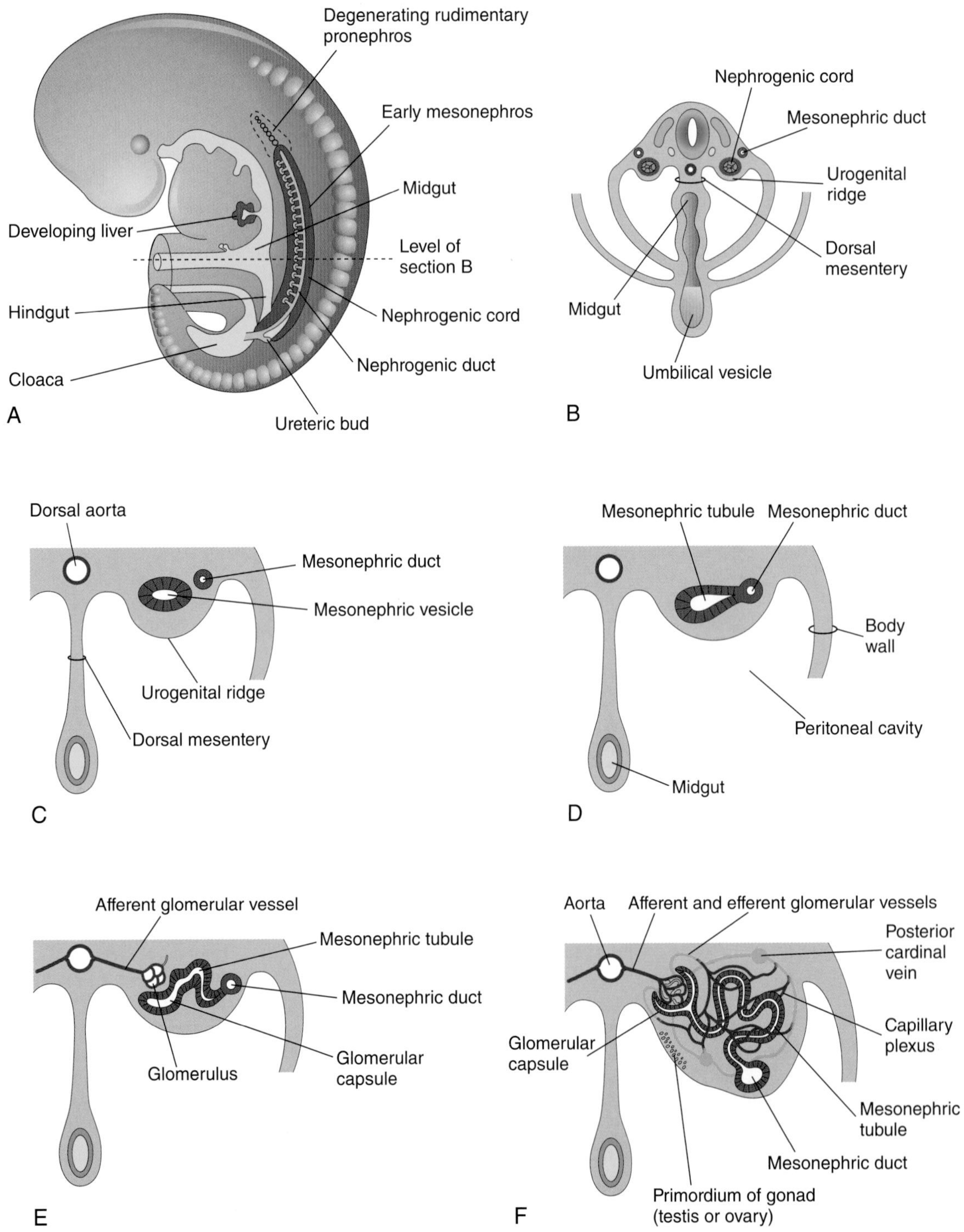

Fig. 12.5 Schematic drawings illustrating the development of kidneys. (A) Lateral view of a 5-week embryo, showing the extent of the early mesonephros and ureteric bud, the primordium of the metanephros (primordium of permanent kidney). (B) Transverse section of the embryo, showing the nephrogenic cords from which the mesonephric tubules develop. (C–F) Successive stages in the development of mesonephric tubules between the 5th and 11th weeks. The expanded medial end of the mesonephric tubule is invaginated by blood vessels to form a glomerular capsule.

Table 12.1 Derivatives and Vestigial Remnants of Embryonic Urogenital Structures[a]

Embryonic Structure	Female	Male
Indifferent gonad	*Ovary*	*Testis*
Cortex	*Ovarian follicles*	*Seminiferous tubules*
Medulla	*Rete ovarii*	*Rete testis*
Gubernaculum	*Ovarian ligament* *Round ligament of uterus*	Gubernaculum testis
Mesonephric tubules	Epoophoron	*Efferent ductules of testis*
	Paroophoron	Paradidymis
Mesonephric duct	Appendix vesiculosa	Appendix of epididymis
	Duct of epoophoron	*Duct of epididymis*
	Longitudinal duct (Gartner duct)	*Ductus deferens*
		Ejaculatory duct and seminal gland
Stalk of ureteric bud	*Ureter, pelvis, calices, and collecting tubules*	*Ureter, pelvis, calices, and collecting tubules*
Paramesonephric duct	Paraovarian or paratubular cyst	Appendix of testis
	Uterine tube	
	Uterus, Cervix	
Urogenital sinus	*Urinary bladder*	*Urinary bladder*
	Urethra	*Urethra (except navicular fossa)*
	Vagina	Prostatic utricle
	Urethral and paraurethral glands	*Prostate*
	Greater vestibular glands	*Bulbourethral glands*
Sinus tubercle	Hymen	Seminal colliculus
Primordial phallus	*Clitoris*	*Penis*
	Glans clitoris	*Glans penis*
	Corpora cavernosa of clitoris	*Corpora cavernosa of penis*
	Bulb of vestibule	*Corpus spongiosum of penis*
Urogenital folds	*Labia minora*	*Ventral aspect of penis*
Labioscrotal swellings	*Labia majora*	*Scrotum*

[a]Functional derivatives are in italics.

These vesicles elongate and become **metanephric tubules** (see Fig. 12.7B and C).

As branching occurs, some of the metanephric mesenchyme cells condense and form **cap mesenchyme cells**; these undergo mesenchymal-to-epithelial transition and further develop into the majority of the nephron's epithelium. The proximal ends of the tubules are invaginated by **glomeruli**. The tubules differentiate into proximal and distal convoluted tubules; the **nephron loop (Henle loop)**, together with the **glomerulus** and the **glomerular capsule**, constitute a **nephron** (see Fig. 12.7D).

Transgenic knockout mouse studies show that proliferation of the nephron progenitor cells and formation of the nephrons are dependent on GLDC (glycine decarboxylase), expression of irx3b and irx1a, PTEN, and BMP7- and Wnt-mediated signals ([Notch]/β-catenin signaling). Bone morphogenetic protein 7 (BMP7) expressed in the progenitor cells and the ureteric bud determine the number of nephrons formed. Each distal convoluted tubule contacts an arched collecting tubule, and the tubules become confluent. A **uriniferous tubule** consists of two embryologically different parts (see Figs. 12.6 and 12.7):

- A **nephron** derived from the metanephrogenic blastema
- A **collecting tubule** derived from the ureteric bud

Between the 10th and 18th weeks, the number of **glomeruli** increases gradually and then increases rapidly until the 36th week, when an upper limit is reached. Nephron formation is complete at birth, with each kidney containing between 200,000 and 2 million nephrons. No new nephrons are formed after this time, and limited numbers may result in significant consequences for health in the child and adult. In some particular population groups (e.g., Aboriginal Australians) with lower numbers of nephrons developed in utero, there is also a higher incidence of adult chronic renal failure.

The fetal kidneys are subdivided into lobes (Fig. 12.8). The lobulation usually disappears at the end of the first

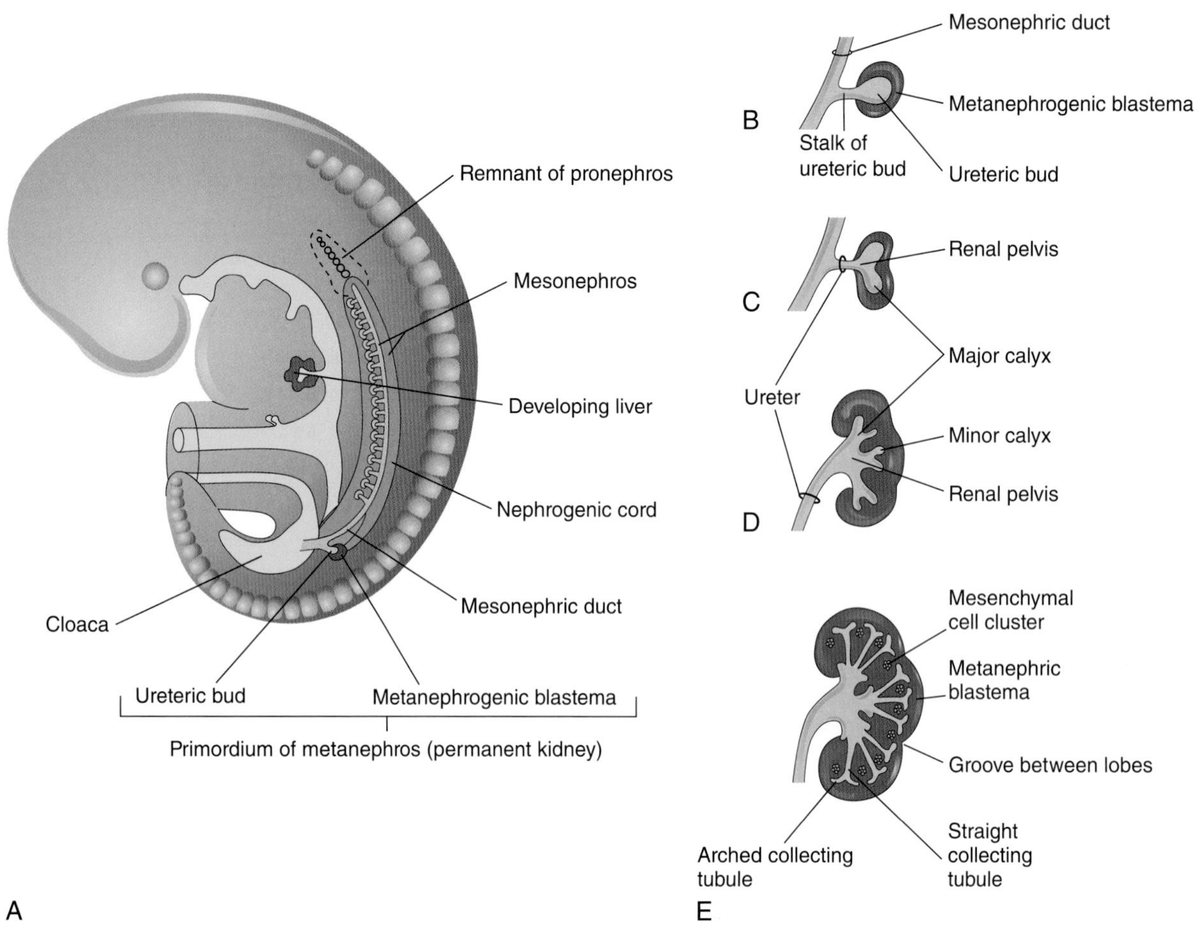

Fig. 12.6 Development of permanent kidney. (A) Lateral view of a 5-week embryo, showing the ureteric bud, the primordium of the metanephros. (B–E) Successive stages in the development of the ureteric bud (fifth to eighth weeks). Observe the development of the kidney: ureter, renal pelvis, calices, and collecting tubules.

year of infancy as the nephrons increase and grow. The increase in kidney size after birth results mainly from the elongation of the proximal convoluted tubules as well as an increase in interstitial tissue (see Fig. 12.7D). Glomerular filtration begins between the 9th and 10th fetal weeks, functional maturation of the kidneys occurs between 14 and 16 weeks, and increasing rates of filtration follow after birth.

Branching of the ureteric bud is dependent on induction by the metanephric mesenchyme. Differentiation of the nephrons depends on induction by the collecting tubules. The ureteric bud and the metanephrogenic blastema interact and induce each other, a process known as **reciprocal induction**, to form the permanent kidneys.

Laboratory studies, especially knockout and transgenic analyses in the mouse, show that this process involves two principal signaling systems that use conserved molecular pathways. Recent research has provided insight into the complex interrelated molecular events regulating the development of the kidneys (Fig. 12.9). *Before induction, a transcription factor, WT1, is expressed in the metanephrogenic blastema supporting the survival of the as-yet uninduced mesenchyme. Expression of Pax2, Eya1, and Sall1 is required for the expression of glial-derived neurotrophic factor (GDNF) in the metanephric mesenchyme. The transcription factors WIST1, POU3F4, vHNF1 (HNF1β), Wnt1b, CRKL, AIFM3, AIF (apoptosis-inducing factor), BCL2, UBASH3A, and GDNF are essential in the induction and lateral branching of the ureteric bud* ***(branching morphogenesis)****. The receptor for GDNF, c-ret, is first expressed in the mesonephric duct but later becomes localized on the tip of the ureteric bud. Subsequent branching is controlled by transcription factors, including Emx2 and Pax2, and growth factor signals of the Wnt, fibroblast growth factor (FGF), and BMP families. Transformation of the metanephric mesenchyme to the epithelial cells of the nephron, mesenchymal-epithelial transition, is regulated by diverse mesenchyme factors, including FGFR1, FGFR2, and Wnt4. Related studies reveal that RET tyrosinase signaling system, pathogenic variant (mutation) of the angiotensin-type 2 receptor gene, vitamin A, and retinoic acid are involved in kidney and urinary tract congenital anomalies.*

POSITIONAL CHANGES OF KIDNEYS

Initially, the primordial permanent kidneys lie close to each other in the pelvis, ventral to the sacrum (Fig. 12.10A). As the abdomen and pelvis grow, the kidneys gradually become repositioned to the abdomen and move farther apart (see Fig. 12.10B and C). The kidneys attain their adult position during the beginning of the fetal period (see Fig. 12.10D) from straightening of the vertebral curvature and growth of the embryo's thorax and abdomen so that they progressively occupy their normal position on either side of the vertebral column.

Initially, the **hilum** of each kidney, where the blood vessels, ureter, and nerves enter and leave, faces ventrally; however, as the kidneys relocate, the hilum rotates medially

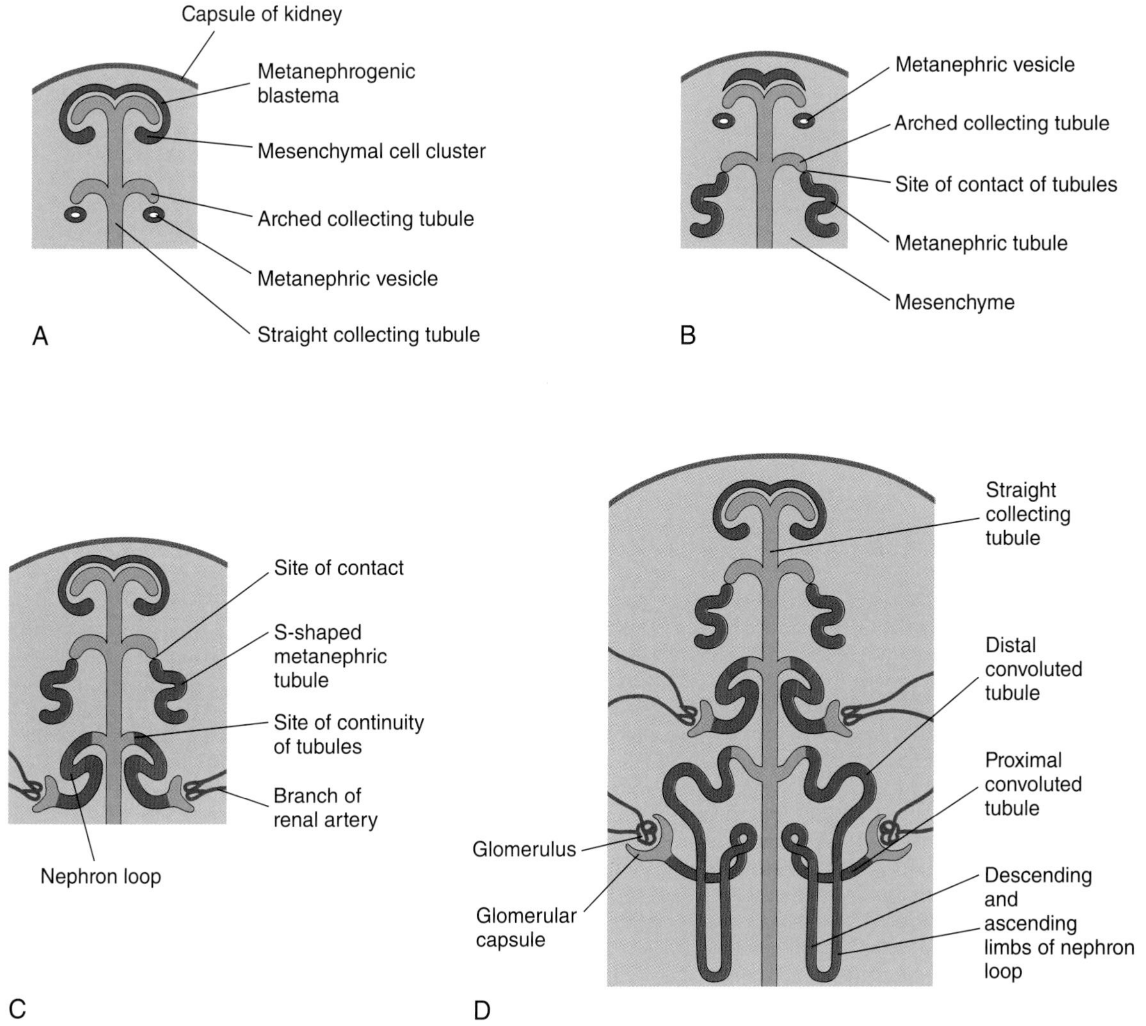

Fig. 12.7 Development of nephrons. (A) Nephrogenesis commences around the beginning of the eighth week. (B and C) Note that the metanephric tubules, the primordia of the nephrons, connect with the collecting tubules to form uriniferous tubules. (D) Observe that nephrons are derived from the metanephrogenic blastema, and the collecting tubules are derived from the ureteric bud.

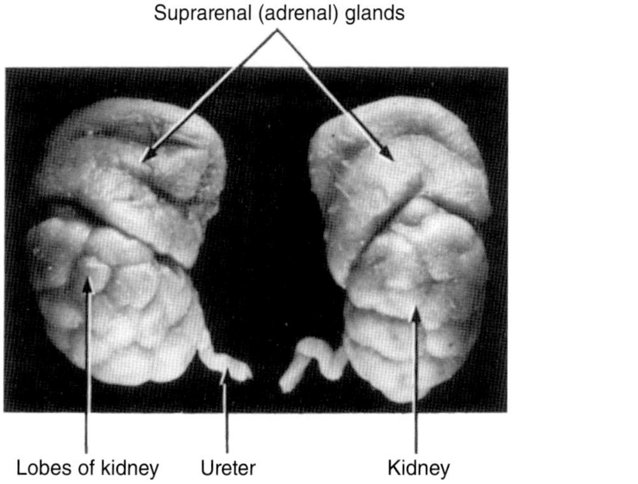

Fig. 12.8 Kidneys and suprarenal glands of a 28-week fetus (×2). The kidneys are subdivided into lobes; this lobulation usually disappears at the end of the first postnatal year. Note that the suprarenal glands are large compared with the kidneys; they will rapidly become smaller during the first year of infancy (see Fig. 12.27).

almost 90 degrees. By the ninth week, the hila are directed anteromedially (see Fig. 12.10C and D). Eventually, the kidneys become retroperitoneal structures on the posterior abdominal wall. By this time, the kidneys are in contact with the suprarenal glands (see Fig. 12.10D).

CHANGES IN THE BLOOD SUPPLY OF KIDNEYS

During the changes in the kidneys' positions, the kidneys receive their blood supply from vessels that are close to them. Initially, the **renal arteries** are branches of the **common iliac arteries** (see Fig. 12.10A and B). Later, the kidneys receive their blood supply from the distal end of the **abdominal aorta** (see Fig. 12.10B). When the kidneys are located at a higher level, they receive new branches from the aorta (see Fig. 12.10C and D). Normally, the caudal branches of the renal vessels undergo involution and disappear.

The positions of the kidneys become fixed once the kidneys come into contact with the suprarenal glands in the ninth week. The kidneys receive their most cranial arterial branches from the **abdominal aorta**; these branches become the permanent **renal arteries**. The right renal artery is longer and often in a more superior position than the left renal artery.

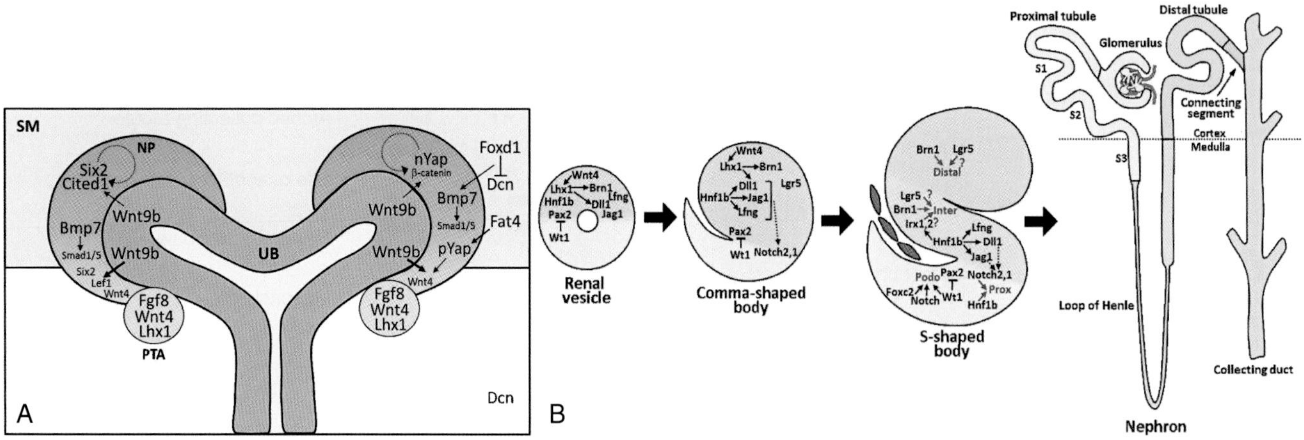

Fig. 12.9 Molecular control of kidney development. (A) Regulation of nephron progenitor induction. The self-renewing nephron progenitors are demarcated by the expression of Six2 and Cited1. Six2 promotes self-renewal, in addition to Wnt9b signals from the ureteric bud, which directly promote the expression of progenitor genes such as Cited1. nYap signaling may also cooperate with β-catenin induced by canonical Wnt9b signals to promote progenitor self-renewal. Bmp7-SMAD signaling promotes the conversion of nephron progenitors to a Six2+Cited1 state, where they can be induced by Wnt9b and turn on differentiation markers Lef1 and Wnt4. These cells form the pretubular aggregate highlighted by the expression of critical differentiation factors Fgf8, Wnt4, and Lhx1. Foxd1+ stromal cells promote Bmp7-SMAD signaling in the nephron progenitors by repressing Dcn, an antagonist of Bmp7 activity. Stromal Fat4 regulates the induction process by inducing nuclear export and phosphorylation of Yap, which allows Wnt9b inductive signals to promote differentiation of the nephron progenitors. *NP*, Nephron progenitors; *PTA*, pretubular aggregate; *SM*, stromal mesenchyme; *UB*, ureteric bud; *dotted arrow*, promotion of self-renewal. (B) Regulation of nephron patterning. Proximal/distal polarity is established in the renal vesicle and demarcated by the expression of several genes, including three Notch ligands: *Dll1, Lfng*, and *Jag1*. The Notch pathway establishes a proximal polarity that is carried through the comma- and S-shaped body stages and integral for proximal tubule and podocyte development. Wt1 also promotes proximal fate, specifically that of the podocyte, by antagonizing Pax2, and cooperating with Notch pathway components and Foxc2, to regulate genes necessary for podocyte development. Endothelial cells are recruited by signals from developing podocytes of the S-shaped body. Hnf1b promotes proximal and intermediate/medial fate through the regulation of Notch ligand expression and other factors such as Irx1/2, which may play a role in medial segment differentiation. Intermediate and distal fates are regulated by Brn1, which establishes distal polarity starting at the renal vesicle stage. Lgr5 is expressed in the distal segment of the comma-shaped body and the distal and intermediate segments of the S-shaped body; however, a direct role in establishing or maintaining these segments has not been shown. Proximal polarity establishes the glomerulus and S1 to S3 segments of the proximal tubule. Intermediate segments give rise to the loop of Henle. Distal segments establish the distal tubule, which hooks up to the collecting duct through a connecting segment. *Inter*, Intermediate; *Podo*, podocyte; *Prox*, proximal; *?*, direct role not established; *dashed arrow*, ligand-receptor engagement. (From O'Brien LL, McMahon AP: Induction and patterning of the metanephric nephron. *Semin Cell Devel Biol* 36:31–38, 2014.)

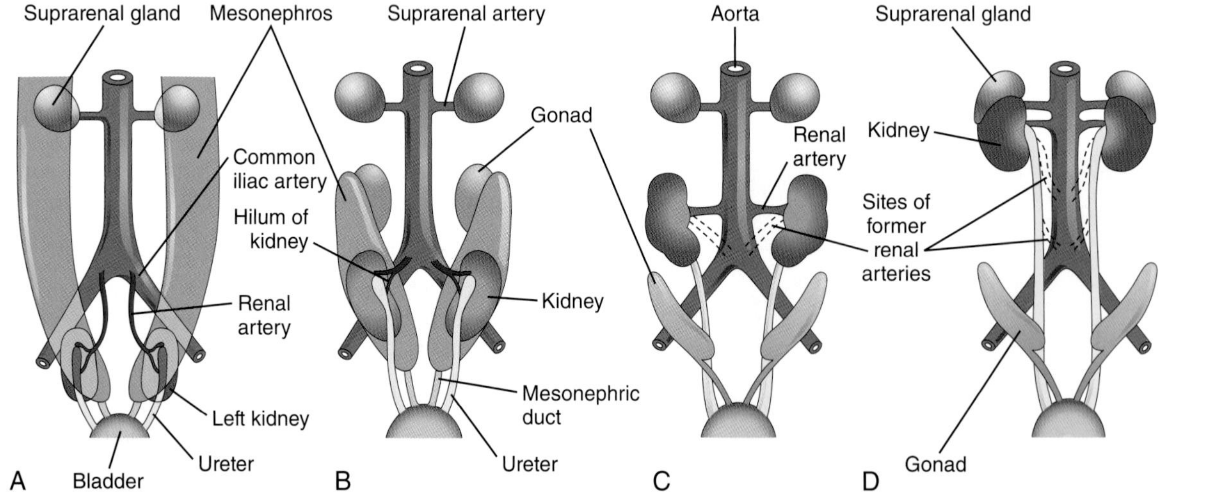

Fig. 12.10 (A–D) Diagrammatic ventral views of the abdominopelvic region of embryos and fetuses (sixth to ninth weeks), showing medial rotation and relocation of the kidneys from the pelvis to the abdomen. (C and D) Note that as the kidneys relocate (ascend), they are supplied by arteries at successively higher levels and that the hila of the kidneys, where the nerves and vessels enter are directed anteromedially.

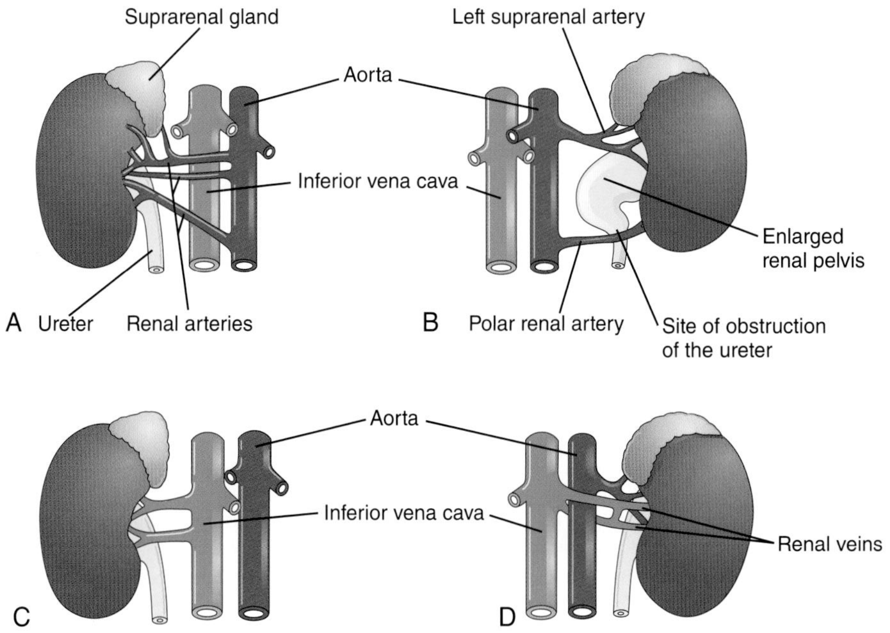

Fig. 12.11 Common variations of renal vessels. (A) Multiple renal arteries. (B) Note the accessory vessel entering the inferior pole of the kidney and that it is obstructing the ureter and producing an enlarged renal pelvis. (C and D) Supernumerary renal veins.

Accessory Renal Arteries

The common variations in the blood supply to the kidneys reflect how the blood supply continually changes during embryonic and early fetal life (see Fig. 12.10). Approximately 10% to 25% of kidneys in the general population have two to four renal arteries. **Accessory (supernumerary) renal arteries** usually arise from the aorta superior or inferior to the main renal artery and follow it to the hilum of the kidney (Fig. 12.11A, C, and D). Accessory arteries may also enter the kidneys directly, usually via the superior or inferior pole (see Fig. 12.11B). An accessory artery to the inferior pole (polar renal artery) may cross anterior to the ureter and obstruct it, causing **hydronephrosis**, or distention of the renal pelvis and calices with urine. If the artery enters the inferior pole of the right kidney, it usually crosses anterior to the inferior vena cava and ureter.

Accessory renal arteries are end arteries; consequently, if an accessory artery is damaged or ligated, the part of the kidney supplied by it will become ischemic. Accessory arteries are approximately twice as common as accessory veins. Diagnostic CT imaging and identification of accessory renal arteries are essential for surgical procedures to avoid significant morbidity.

Congenital Anomalies of Kidneys and Urinary Tract

Congenital anomalies of the kidneys and urinary tract occur frequently in newborns (3%–4%) and account for 20% to 30% of all major birth defects. Kidney and urinary tract anomalies are present in more than 200 clinical syndromes and can be detected prenatally by ultrasonography.

Renal Agenesis

Unilateral renal agenesis (absence) occurs approximately once in every 1000 neonates. Males are affected more often than females, and the left kidney is usually the absent one (Figs. 12.12A and B and 12.13A). Unilateral renal agenesis often causes no symptoms and is usually not discovered during infancy because the other kidney usually undergoes compensatory hypertrophy and performs the function of the missing kidney. Unilateral renal agenesis may be present in infants with a *single umbilical artery* (see Fig. 7.18).

Bilateral renal agenesis (see Fig. 12.12C) is associated with **oligohydramnios or anhydramnios**, a condition that develops because little or no urine is excreted into the amniotic cavity. This condition occurs approximately once in 3000 births and is incompatible with postnatal life. About 20% of cases of **Potter syndrome** are caused by bilateral renal agenesis. Infants with Potter syndrome have a characteristic facial appearance: the eyes are widely separated and have **palpebronasal folds** (epicanthic folds), the ears are low set, the nose is broad and flat, the chin is receding, and there are limb and respiratory anomalies. Infants with bilateral renal agenesis usually die shortly after birth from pulmonary hypoplasia, leading to respiratory insufficiency.

Renal agenesis results when the ureteric buds do not develop or the primordia (stalks of buds) of the ureters degenerate. Failure of the buds to penetrate the metanephrogenic blastema results in the failure of kidney development because no nephrons are induced by the collecting tubules to develop from the blastema. Renal agenesis probably has a multifactorial cause. There is clinical evidence that complete in utero involution of **polycystic kidneys** could lead to renal agenesis, with a blind ending ureter on the same side.

Malrotated Kidney

If a kidney fails to rotate, the hilum faces anteriorly; that is, the fetal kidney retains its embryonic position (see Figs. 12.10A and 12.13C). If the hilum faces posteriorly, rotation of the kidney proceeds too far; if it faces laterally, lateral instead of medial rotation occurs. **Malrotation** of the kidneys is often associated with ectopic kidneys.

Ectopic Kidneys

One or both kidneys may be in an abnormal position (see Fig. 12.13B, E, and F). Most **ectopic kidneys** are located in the pelvis (Fig. 12.14), but some lie in the inferior part of the abdomen. **Pelvic kidneys** and other forms of ectopia result from the failure of

Continued

Congenital Anomalies of Kidneys and Urinary Tract—cont'd

the kidneys to ascend. Pelvic kidneys are close to each other and usually fuse to form a discoid (pancake) kidney (see Fig. 12.13E). Ectopic kidneys receive their blood supply from blood vessels near them (internal or external iliac arteries and/or abdominal aorta). They are often supplied by several vessels. Sometimes a kidney crosses to the other side, resulting in **crossed renal ectopia**, and 90% of these kidneys are fused (Fig. 12.15). An unusual type of abnormal kidney is the **unilateral fused kidney**. In such cases, the developing kidneys fuse after they leave the pelvis, and one kidney attains its normal position, carrying the other kidney with it (see Fig. 12.13D).

Horseshoe Kidney

Horseshoe kidney is the most common renal fusion defect. In 0.2% of the population, the poles of the kidneys are fused; usually, it is the inferior poles that fuse. The large **U-shaped kidney** usually lies in the pubic region, anterior to the inferior lumbar vertebrae (Fig. 12.16A). In 60% of cases, the horseshoe kidney is found below the level of the inferior mesenteric artery or in the pelvis (see Fig. 12.16B).

A horseshoe kidney usually produces no symptoms because its collecting system develops normally, and the ureters enter the bladder. If urinary flow is impeded, signs and symptoms of obstruction (urinary stones, hydronephrosis) and/or infection may appear. Approximately 7% of persons with **Turner syndrome** have horseshoe kidneys (see Figs. 20.3 and 20.4).

Duplications of Urinary Tract

Duplications of the abdominal part of the ureter and renal pelvis are common (see Fig. 12.13F). These defects result from abnormal division of the ureteric bud. Incomplete division results in a divided kidney with a **bifid ureter** (see Fig. 12.13B). Complete division results in a double kidney with a bifid ureter (see Fig. 12.13C) or separate ureters (Fig. 12.17). A **supernumerary kidney** with its ureter, which is rare, probably results from the formation of two ureteric buds (see Fig. 12.13F).

Ectopic Ureter

An ectopic ureter results when the ureter is not incorporated into the **trigone** between the openings of the ureters in the posterior part of the urinary bladder. Instead, it is carried caudally with the mesonephric duct and is incorporated into the middle pelvic portion of the vesical part of the urogenital sinus. In males, the ectopic ureter will open into the neck of the bladder or the prostatic part of the urethra. The ureter may also enter the ductus deferens, prostatic utricle, or seminal gland. In females, the ectopic ureter may also open into the neck of the bladder or the urethra, vagina, or vestibule of the vagina (Fig. 12.18). Incontinence is the common complaint resulting from an ectopic ureter because urine flowing from the orifice of the ureter does not enter the bladder; instead, it continually dribbles from the urethra in males and the urethra and/or vagina in females.

When two ureters form on one side (see Fig. 12.17), they usually open into the urinary bladder (see Fig. 12.13F).

Cystic Kidney Diseases

Autosomal dominant polycystic kidney disease (ADPKD) is the most common of all heritable cystic kidney diseases (1:500). Mostly PKD-1 and PKD-2 pathogenic variants (mutations) are responsible; these encode for polycystin 1 and 2, respectively. These two molecules are mechanoreceptors localized to the primary cilia of the kidney—they detect urine flow in the tubules. The main clinical findings in ADPKD are cysts involving <5% of nephrons. These cysts can enlarge and reduce normal kidney function.

In **autosomal recessive polycystic kidney disease** (1 in 20,000 live births), diagnosed at birth or in utero by ultrasonography, both kidneys contain many small cysts (Fig. 12.19A), which results in **renal insufficiency**. Death of the infant may occur shortly after birth, with up to 50% of cases associated with pulmonary hypoplasia; however, more than 80% of these infants survive beyond 1 year because of postnatal dialysis and kidney transplantation. Most cases have a pathogenic variant (mutation) of the *PKHD1* gene and, less commonly, the DZIP1L gene, that results in polycystic kidney and congenital hepatic fibrosis.

Multicystic dysplastic kidney disease results from dysmorphology and abnormal development of the renal system (see Fig. 12.19B). The outcome for most children with this disease is generally good because the disease is unilateral in 75% of the cases. In this kidney disease, fewer cysts are seen than in autosomal recessive polycystic kidney disease, and they range in size from a few millimeters to many centimeters in the same kidney. It was thought that the cysts were the result of the failure of the ureteric bud derivatives to join the tubules derived from the metanephrogenic blastema. It is now believed that the cystic structures are wide dilations of parts of the otherwise continuous nephrons, particularly the **nephron loops** (of Henle).

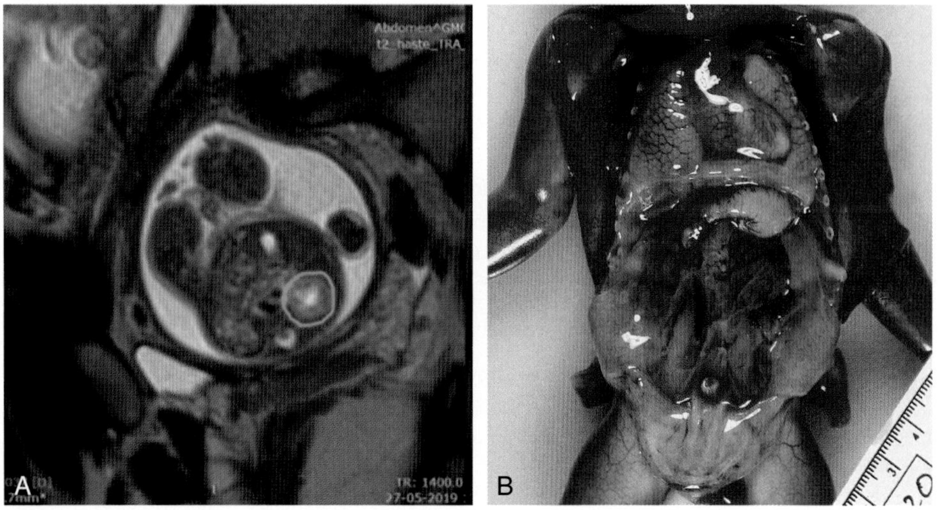

Fig. 12.12 Sonograms of a fetus with unilateral renal agenesis. (A) Magnetic resonance imaging (MRI) image of a fetus at just over 24 weeks showing one normal fetal kidney with a bright MRI signal (*green* tracing) while the on the contralateral side the renal fossa is empty, and bright signal is missing (*red* arc). (B) Dissection of a male fetus of 19.5 weeks with bilateral renal agenesis. ((A) Adapted from Gupta S, Mohi JK, Gambhir P, et al: Prenatal diagnosis of congenital anomalies of genito-urinary system on fetal magnetic resonance imaging. *Egypt J Radiol Nucl Med* 51:155, 2020. (B) Courtesy Dr. D.K. Kalousek, Department of Pathology, University of British Columbia, Children's Hospital, Vancouver, British Columbia, Canada.)

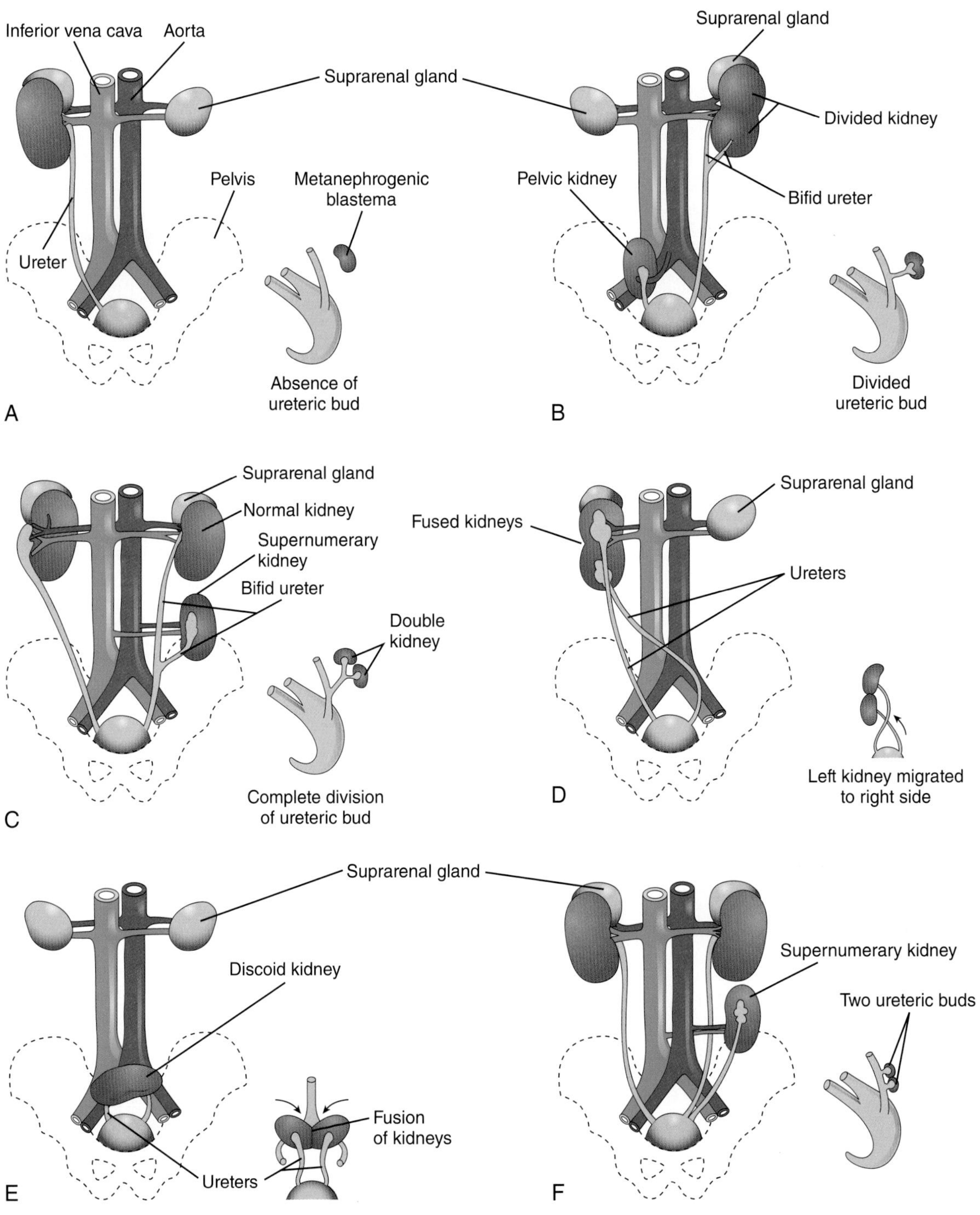

Fig. 12.13 Illustrations of various birth defects of the urinary system. The small sketch to the lower right of each drawing illustrates the probable embryologic basis of the defect. (A) Unilateral renal agenesis. (B) *Right side*, pelvic kidney; *left side*, divided kidney with a bifid ureter. (C) *Right side*, malrotation of the kidney; the hilum is facing laterally. *Left side*, bifid ureter and supernumerary kidney. (D) Crossed renal ectopia. The left kidney crossed to the right side and fused with the right kidney. (E) Pelvic kidney (discoid kidney), resulting from fusion of the kidneys while they were in the pelvis. (F) Supernumerary left kidney resulting from the development of two ureteric buds.

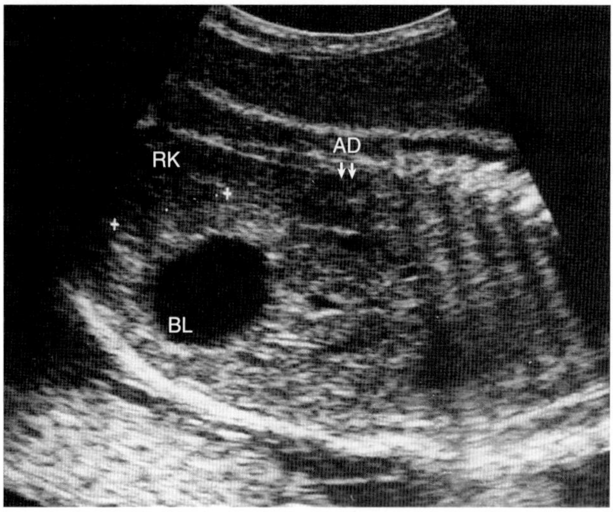

Fig. 12.14 Sonogram of the pelvis of a fetus at 29 weeks. Observe the low position of the right kidney *(RK)* near the urinary bladder *(BL)*. This pelvic kidney resulted from its failure to ascend during the sixth to ninth weeks. Observe the normal location of the right suprarenal gland *(AD)*, which develops separately from the kidney. (Courtesy Dr. Lyndon M. Hill, Director of Ultrasound, Magee-Women's Hospital, Pittsburgh, Pennsylvania.)

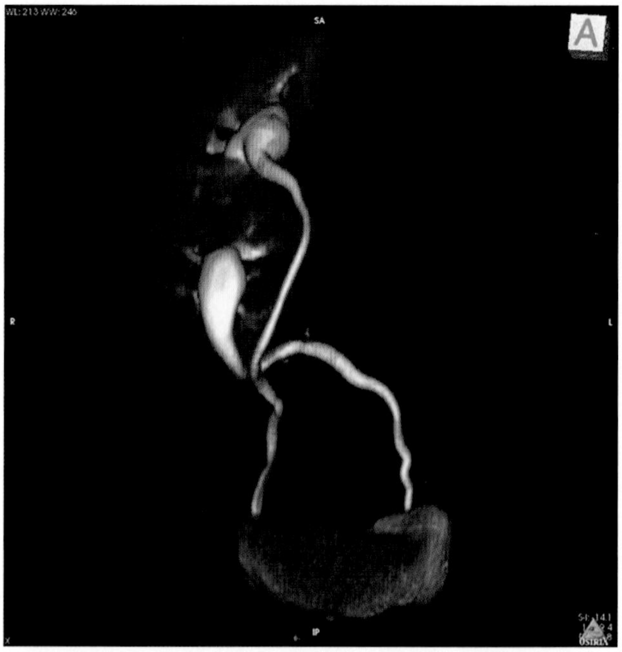

Fig. 12.15 Computed tomography scan showing congenital renal malformation in a 69-year-old female. Crossed fused renal ectopia is an anomaly in which the kidneys are fused and located on the same side of the midline. (From Di Muzzio B: Crossed fused renal ectopia. Radiopaedia.org.)

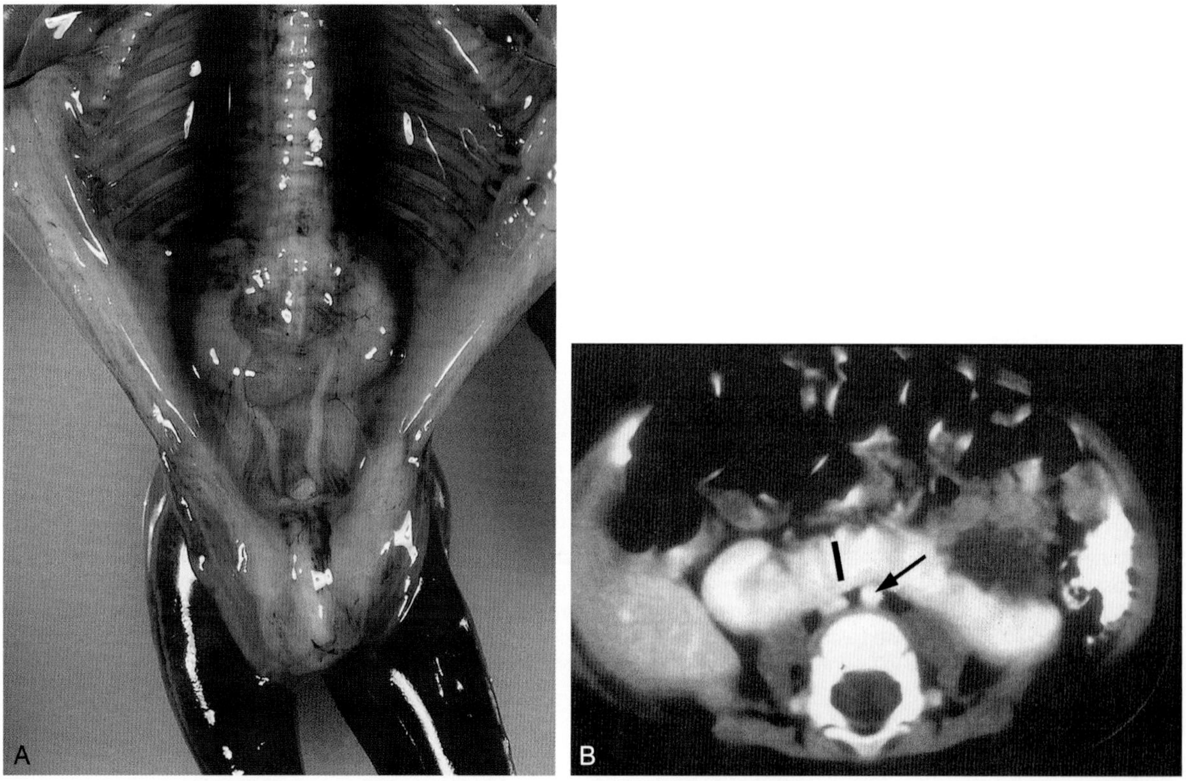

Fig. 12.16 (A) Horseshoe kidney in the lower abdomen of a 13-week female fetus. (B) Contrast-enhanced computed tomography scan of the abdomen of an infant with a horseshoe kidney. Note the isthmus (vascular) of renal tissue *(thick vertical line)* connecting the right and left kidneys just anterior to the aorta *(arrow)* and inferior vena cava. (A) Courtesy Dr. D.K. Kalousek, Department of Pathology, University of British Columbia, Children's Hospital, Vancouver, British Columbia, Canada. (B) Courtesy Dr. Prem S. Sahni, formerly of the Department of Radiology, Children's Hospital, Winnipeg, Manitoba, Canada.

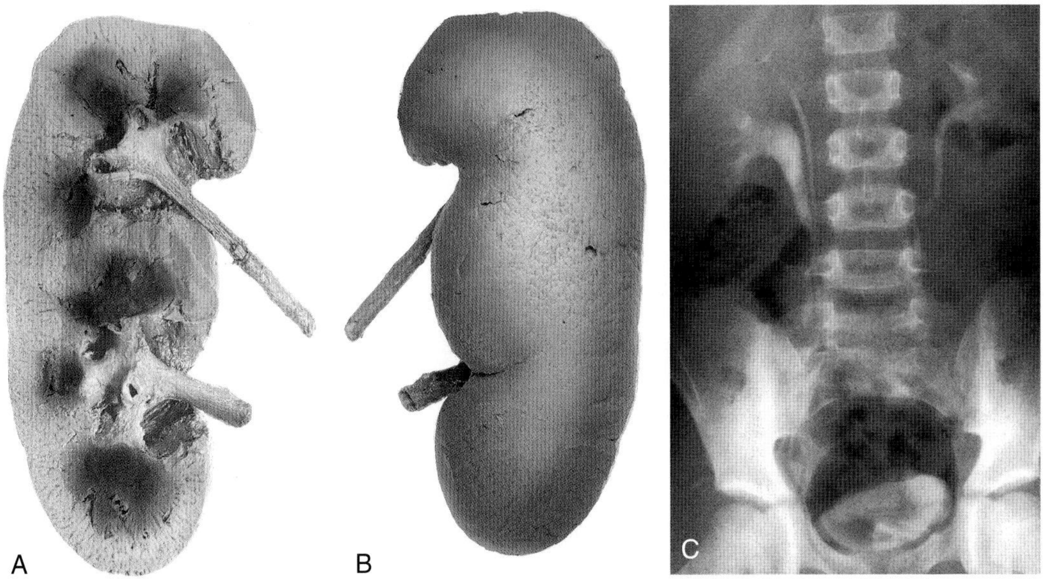

Fig. 12.17 A duplex kidney with two ureters and renal pelves. (A) Longitudinal section through the kidney showing two renal pelves and calices. (B) Anterior surface of the kidney. (C) Intravenous urography showing duplication of the right kidney and ureter in a 10-year-old male. The distal ends of the right ureter are fused at the level of the first sacral vertebra. (Courtesy Dr. Prem S. Sahni, formerly of the Department of Radiology, Children's Hospital, Winnipeg, Manitoba, Canada.)

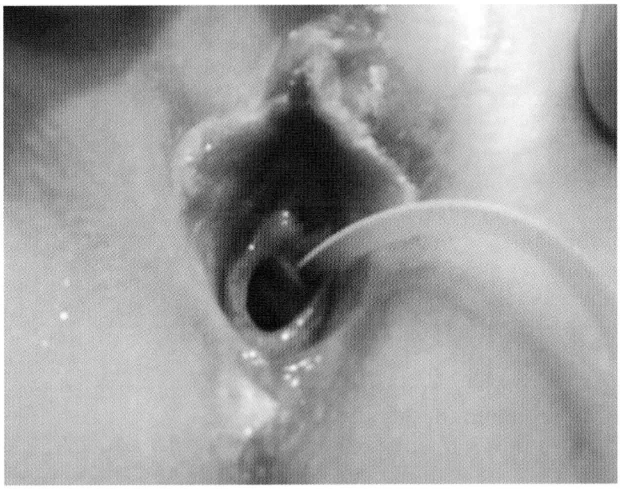

Fig. 12.18 Ureteral duplication with ectopic ureteral orifice. A catheter has been placed into the ureter via the ectopic orifice in the vagina. (From MacLennan GT: *Hinman's atlas of urosurgical anatomy*, 2012, Saunders.)

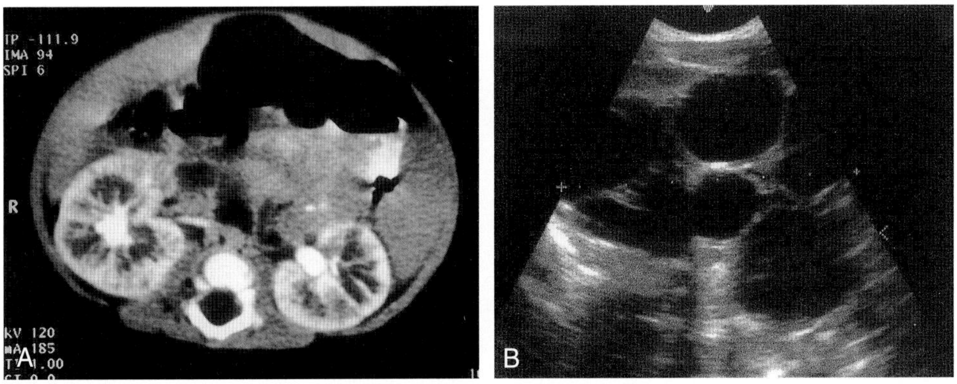

Fig. 12.19 Cystic kidney disease. (A) Computed tomography scan (with contrast enhancement) of the abdomen of a 5-month-old male infant with autosomal recessive polycystic kidney disease. Note the linear ectasia (cysts) of collecting tubules. (B) Ultrasound scan of the left kidney of a 15-day-old male infant showing multiple noncommunicating cysts with no renal tissue (unilateral multicystic dysplastic kidney). (Courtesy Dr. Prem S. Sahni, formerly of the Department of Radiology, Children's Hospital, Winnipeg, Manitoba, Canada.)

DEVELOPMENT OF URINARY BLADDER

For descriptive purposes, the **urogenital sinus** is divided into three parts (Fig. 12.20C):

- A **vesical part** that forms most of the urinary bladder and is continuous with the allantois
- A **pelvic part** that becomes the urethra in the neck of the bladder, the prostatic part of the urethra in males, and the entire urethra in females
- A **phallic part** that grows toward the genital tubercle (primordium of the penis or clitoris; see)

The bladder develops mainly from the vesical part of the **urogenital sinus** (see Fig. 12.20C). The entire epithelium of the bladder is derived from the endoderm of the vesical part of the urogenital sinus, or ventral part of the cloaca (see Fig. 12.20C). The other layers of its wall develop from the adjacent splanchnic mesenchyme.

Initially, the bladder is continuous with the **allantois** (see Fig. 12.20C and Chapter 4, p.56). The allantois soon constricts and becomes a thick fibrous cord, the **urachus**. It extends from the apex of the bladder to the **umbilicus** (Fig. 12.21; see also Fig. 12.20G and H). In adults, the urachus is represented by the **median umbilical ligament**.

As the bladder enlarges, distal parts of the **mesonephric ducts** are incorporated into its dorsal wall (see Fig. 12.20B–H). These ducts contribute to the formation of the connective tissue in the **trigone of the bladder**. As these ducts are absorbed, the ureters open separately into the urinary bladder (see Fig. 12.20C–H). Partly because of traction exerted by the kidneys as they ascend, the orifices of the ureters move superolaterally and enter obliquely through the base of the bladder (see Fig. 12.20F). In males, the orifices of the ducts move close together and enter the prostatic part of the urethra as the caudal ends of the ducts develop into the **ejaculatory ducts** (see Fig. 12.33A). In females, the distal ends of the mesonephric ducts degenerate (see Fig. 12.33B).

In infants and children, the urinary bladder, even when empty, is in the abdomen. It begins to enter the greater pelvis at approximately 6 years of age; however, the bladder does not enter the lesser pelvis and becomes a pelvic organ until after puberty. The **apex of the bladder** in adults is continuous with the **median umbilical ligament**, which extends posteriorly along the posterior surface of the anterior abdominal wall.

Urachal Birth Defects

In infants, a remnant of the urachal lumen may persist in the inferior part of the urachus. In approximately 50% of cases, the lumen is continuous with the cavity of the bladder. Remnants of the epithelial lining of the urachus may give rise to midline fluid-filled **urachal cysts** (Fig. 12.22A), which are not usually detected unless the cysts become infected and enlarged. The patent inferior end of the urachus may dilate to form a **urachal sinus** that opens into the bladder. The lumen in the superior part of the urachus may also remain patent and form a **urachal sinus** that opens at the umbilicus (see Fig. 12.22B). Very rarely, the entire urachus remains patent and forms a **urachal fistula** that allows urine to escape from its umbilical orifice (see Fig. 12.22C). Imaging (ultrasound, MRI) of the urachal anomalies provides a reliable diagnosis for surgical treatment of this condition.

Congenital Megacystis

A pathologically large urinary bladder, **megacystis (megalocystis)**, may result from a congenital disorder of the ureteric bud, which in turn can dilate the renal pelvis. The large bladder may also result from posterior urethral valves (Fig. 12.23). Many infants with megacystitis suffer from renal failure in early childhood.

Exstrophy of Bladder

Exstrophy of the bladder, a severe birth defect, occurs approximately once in every 30,000 to 50,000 births. **Exstrophy (eversion) of the bladder** usually occurs in males (Fig. 12.24). Exposure and protrusion of the mucosal surface of the posterior wall of the bladder characterize this defect. The trigone of the bladder and ureteric orifices are exposed, and urine dribbles intermittently from the everted bladder.

Exstrophy of the bladder, a deficiency of the anterior abdominal wall, is caused by incomplete median closure of the inferior part of the wall (Fig. 12.25). The defect involves both the abdominal wall and the anterior wall of the urinary bladder. The defect results from the failure of the mesoderm to migrate between the ectoderm and endoderm of the abdominal wall (see Fig. 12.25B and C). As a result, the inferior parts of the rectus muscles are absent, and the external and internal oblique and transversus abdominis muscles are deficient.

No muscle or connective tissue forms in the anterior abdominal wall over the urinary bladder. Rupture of the cloacal membrane results in wide communication between the exterior and the mucous membrane of the bladder. Rupture of the cloacal membrane before connection of the urogenital septum results in exstrophy of the cloaca, resulting in exposure of the posterior wall of the bladder (Fig. 12.25F) and hindgut.

DEVELOPMENT OF URETHRA

The epithelium of most of the male urethra and the entire female urethra is derived from the endoderm of the **urogenital sinus** (Fig. 12.26; see Figs. 12.20E and H). The distal part of the urethra in the **glans penis** is derived from a solid cord of ectodermal cells, which grows inward from the tip of the glans penis and joins the rest of the spongy urethra (Fig. 12.26A–C). Consequently, the epithelium of the terminal part of the urethra is derived from the surface ectoderm. The connective tissue and smooth muscle of the urethra in both sexes are derived from splanchnic mesenchyme.

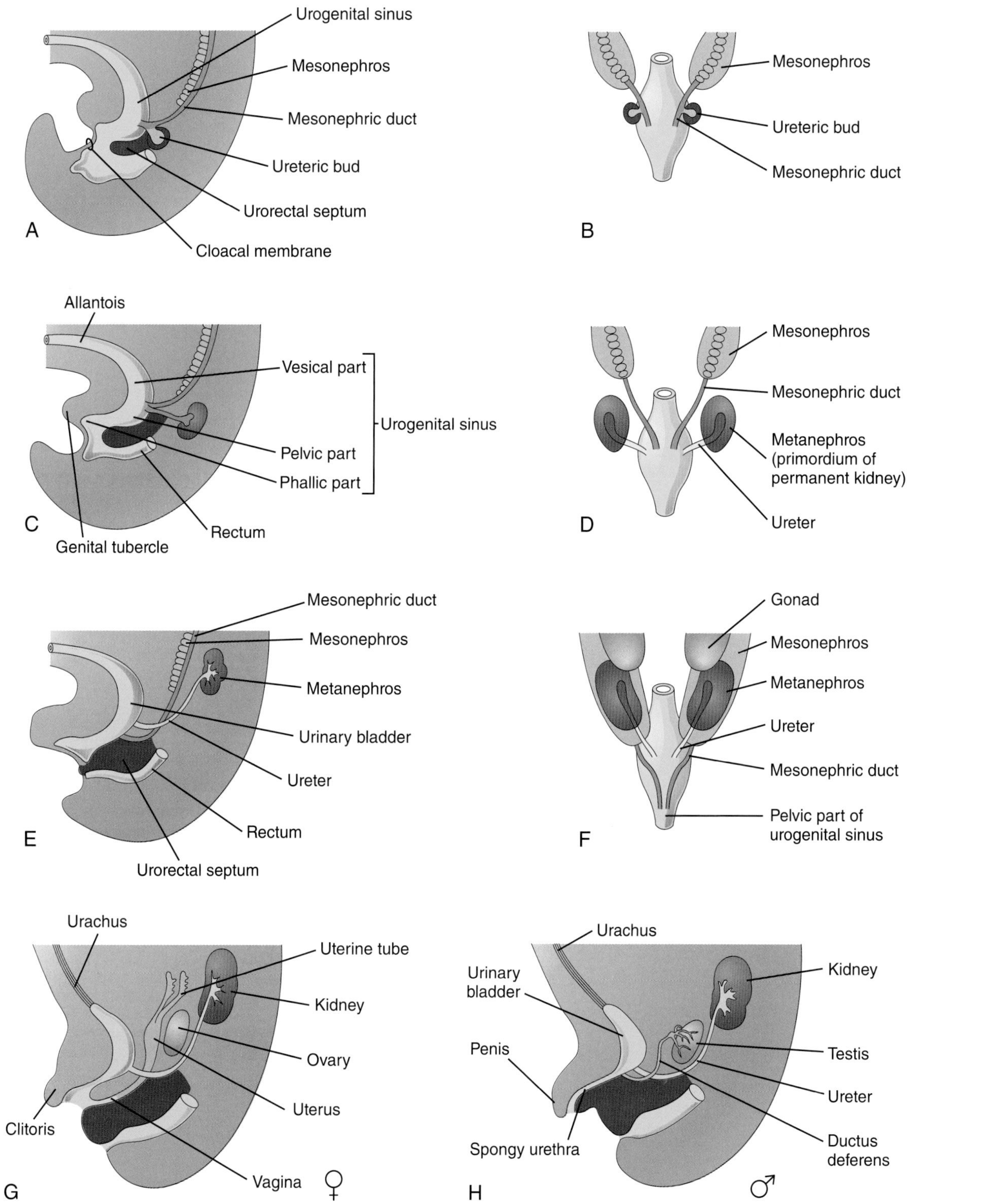

Fig. 12.20 (A) Lateral view of a 5-week embryo showing the division of the cloaca by the urorectal septum into the urogenital sinus and rectum. (B, D, and F) Dorsal views showing the development of the kidneys and bladder and changes in the location of the kidneys. (C, E, G, and H) Lateral views. The stages shown in (G and H) are reached by the 12th week.

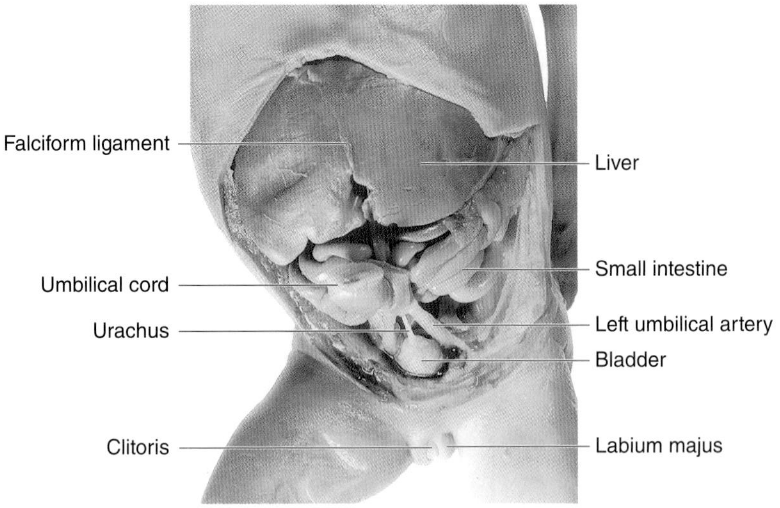

Fig. 12.21 Dissection of the abdomen and pelvis of an 18-week female fetus showing the relation of the urachus to the urinary bladder and umbilical arteries.

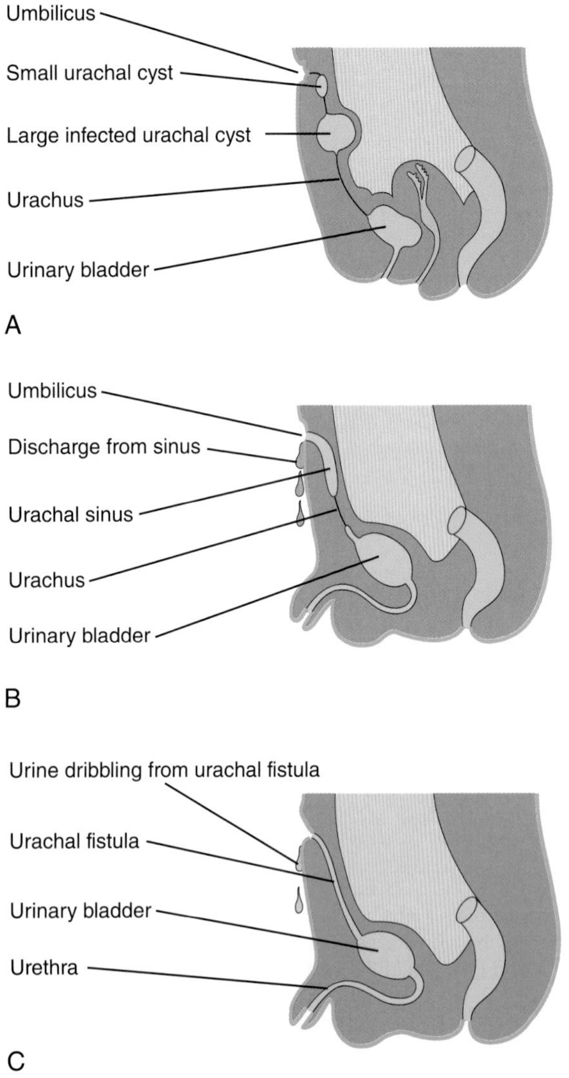

Fig. 12.22 Urachal anomalies. (A) Urachal cysts; the common site for them is in the superior end of the urachus, just inferior to the umbilicus. (B) Two types of urachal sinus are shown: one opens into the bladder, and the other opens at the umbilicus. (C) A urachal fistula connects the bladder and umbilicus.

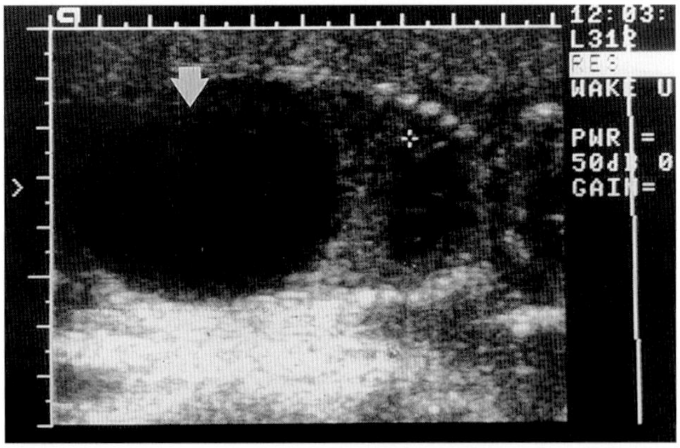

Fig. 12.23 Sonogram of an 18-week male fetus with megacystis (enlarged bladder) caused by posterior urethral valves. The *cross* is placed on the fourth intercostal space, the level to which the diaphragm has been elevated by this very large fetal bladder (*arrow*; *black* = urine). In this case, the fetus survived because of the in utero placement of a catheter within the fetal bladder, allowing the drainage of urine into the amniotic cavity. (Courtesy Dr. C.R. Harman, Department of Obstetrics and Gynecology and Reproductive Health, University of Maryland Medical Center, Baltimore, Maryland.)

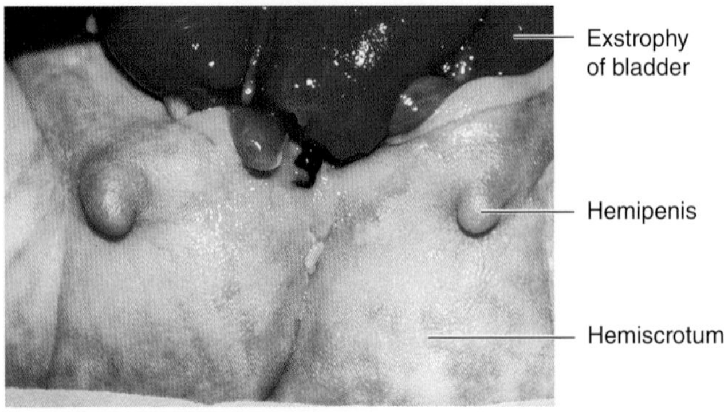

Fig. 12.24 Exstrophy (eversion) of bladder and bifid penis in a male neonate. The red bladder mucosa is visible, and the halves of the penis and scrotum are widely separated. (Courtesy A.E. Chudley, MD, Section of Genetics and Metabolism, Department of Pediatrics and Child Health, Children's Hospital and University of Manitoba, Winnipeg, Manitoba, Canada.)

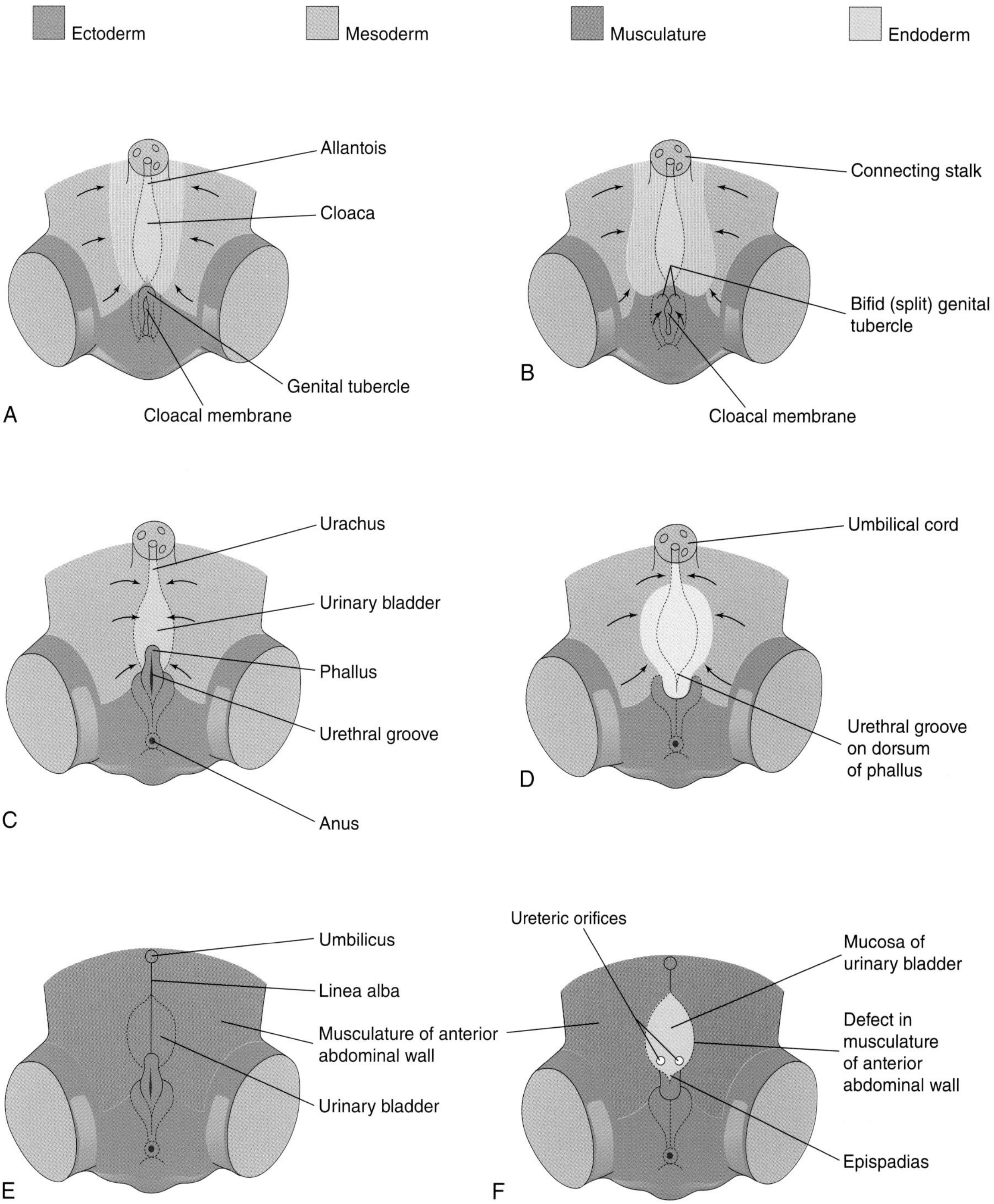

Fig. 12.25 (A, C, and E) Normal stages in the development of the infraumbilical abdominal wall and the penis during the fourth to eighth weeks. (B, D, and F) Probable stages in the development of epispadias and exstrophy of the bladder. (B and D) Note that the mesoderm fails to extend into the anterior abdominal wall anterior to the urinary bladder. Also note that the genital tubercle is located in a more caudal position than usual, and the urethral groove has formed on the dorsal surface of the penis. (F) The surface ectoderm and anterior wall of the bladder have ruptured, resulting in exposure of the posterior wall of the bladder. Note that the musculature of the anterior abdominal wall is present on each side of the defect. (Based on Patten BM, Barry A: The genesis of exstrophy of the bladder and epispadias. *Am J Anat* 90:35, 1952.)

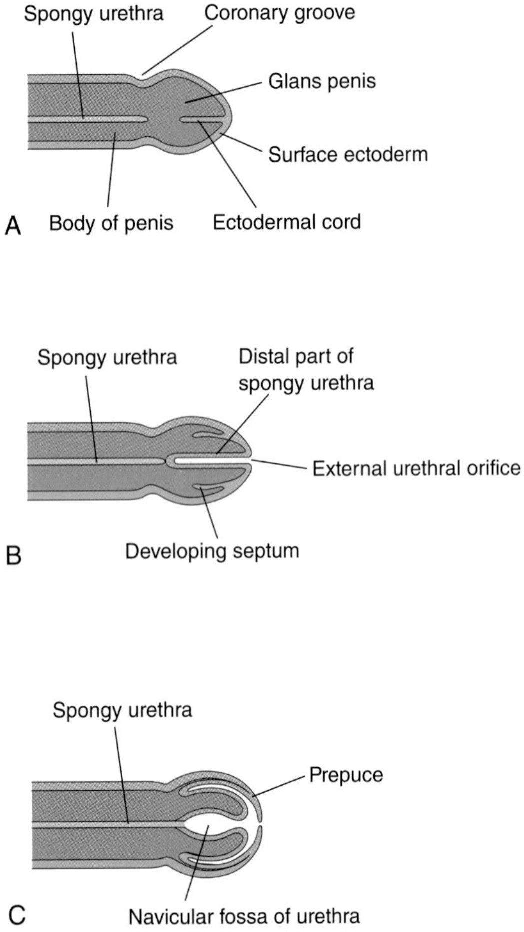

Fig. 12.26 Schematic longitudinal sections of the developing penis illustrating the development of the prepuce (foreskin) and the distal part of the spongy urethra. (A) At 11 weeks. (B) At 12 weeks. (C) At 14 weeks. The epithelium of the spongy urethra has a dual origin; most of it is derived from the endoderm of the phallic part of the urogenital sinus; the distal part of the urethra lining the navicular fossa is derived from the surface ectoderm.

DEVELOPMENT OF SUPRARENAL GLANDS

11

The cortex and medulla of the **suprarenal glands** (adrenal glands) have different origins (Fig. 12.27). The **cortex** develops from the mesenchyme of the urogenital ridge, and the **medulla** develops from neural crest cells. During the sixth week, the cortex begins as an aggregation of mesenchymal cells on each side of the embryo between the root of the dorsal mesentery and the developing gonad (see Fig. 12.28C). The cells that form the medulla are derived from an adjacent sympathetic ganglion, which is derived from neural crest cells.

Initially, the neural crest cells form a mass on the medial side of the embryonic cortex (see Fig. 12.27B). As they are surrounded by the cortex, the cells differentiate into the secretory cells of the suprarenal medulla. Later, more mesenchymal cells arise from the mesothelium (a single layer of flattened cells) and enclose the cortex. These cells give rise to the permanent cortex of the suprarenal gland (see Fig. 12.27C). *Factors Sf1, DAX1, and Pbx1 have important roles in the development of the adrenal cortex.*

Immunohistochemical studies identify a "transitional zone" that is located between the permanent cortex and fetal cortex. It has been suggested that the **zona fasciculata** is derived from this third layer. The **zona glomerulosa** and zona fasciculata are present at birth, but the **zona reticularis** is not recognizable until the end of the third year (see Fig. 12.27H).

Relative to body weight, the **suprarenal glands** of the fetus are 10 to 20 times larger than the adult glands and are large compared with the kidneys (see Figs. 12.3 and 12.8). These large glands result from the extensive size of the fetal cortex, which produces steroid precursors that are used by the placenta for the synthesis of estrogen. The suprarenal medulla remains relatively small until after birth.

The suprarenal glands rapidly become smaller as the fetal cortex regresses during the first year of infancy (see Fig. 12.27H). The glands lose approximately one-third of their

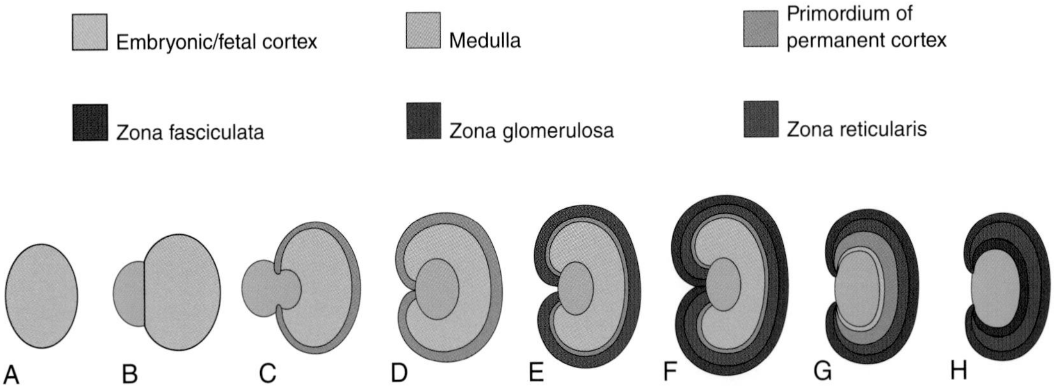

Fig. 12.27 Schematic drawings illustrating the development of the suprarenal glands. (A) At 6 weeks, showing the mesodermal primordium of the embryonic/fetal cortex. (B) At 7 weeks, showing the addition of neural crest cells (medulla). (C) At 8 weeks, showing the fetal cortex and early permanent cortex beginning to encapsulate the medulla. (D and E) Later stages of encapsulation of the medulla by the cortex. (F) Gland of a neonate showing the fetal cortex and two zones of the permanent cortex. (G) At 1 year, the fetal cortex has almost disappeared. (H) At 4 years, showing the adult pattern of cortical zones. Note that the fetal cortex has disappeared, and the gland is much smaller than it was at birth (F).

weight during the 2 to 3 weeks of the neonatal period, and they do not regain their original weight until the end of the second year.

DEVELOPMENT OF GENITAL SYSTEM

12

The chromosomal sex of an embryo is determined at fertilization by the chromosomal complement of sperm (X or Y) that fertilizes the oocyte. Male and female morphologic characteristics do not begin to develop until the seventh week. The early genital systems in the two sexes are similar; therefore the initial period of genital development is an *indifferent stage of sexual development.*

DEVELOPMENT OF GONADS

12

The **gonads (testes or ovaries)** produce sex cells (sperms or oocytes). The gonads are derived from three sources (Fig. 12.28):

- **Mesothelium** (mesodermal epithelium) lining the posterior abdominal wall
- **Underlying mesenchyme**
- **Primordial germ cells** (earliest undifferentiated sex cells)

INDIFFERENT (BIPOTENTIAL) GONADS

The initial stages of gonadal development occur during the fifth week, when a thickened area of mesothelium develops on the medial side of the mesonephros, the primordium of a permanent kidney (see Fig. 12.28A). The proliferation of this epithelium and underlying mesenchyme produces a bulge on the medial side of the mesonephros, the **gonadal ridge** (Fig. 12.29). Fingerlike epithelial cords, **gonadal cords**, soon grow into the underlying mesenchyme (see Fig. 12.28D). The **indifferent gonads** (primordial organs before differentiation) now consist of an external cortex and an internal medulla. *It appears that FOG2, WT1, and NR5A1 are required for bipotential gonad development.*

In embryos with an **XX sex chromosome complex**, the cortex of the indifferent gonad differentiates into an ovary, and the medulla regresses. In embryos with an **XY sex chromosome complex**, the medulla differentiates into a testis, and the cortex regresses.

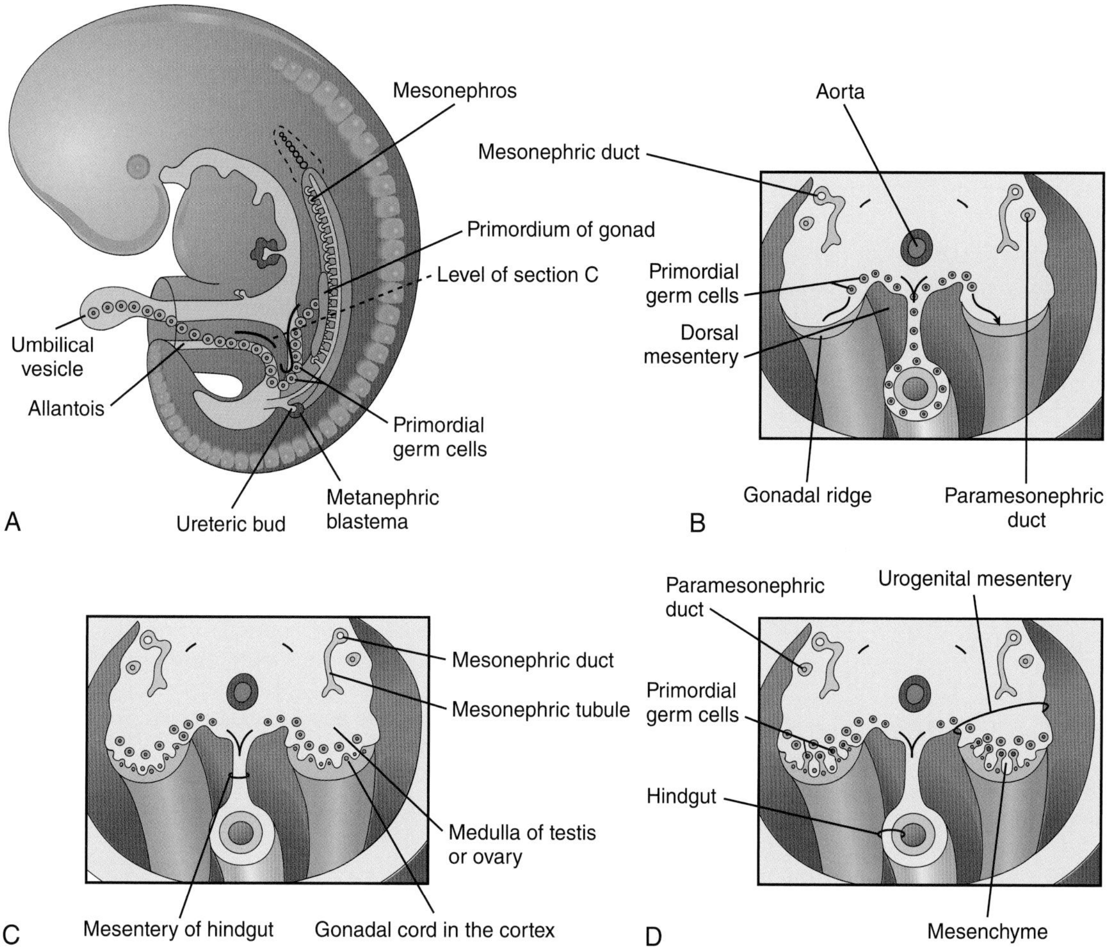

Fig. 12.28 (A) Sketch of a 5-week embryo illustrating the migration of primordial germ cells from the umbilical vesicle into the embryo. (B) Transverse section showing the primordium of the suprarenal glands, the gonadal ridges, and the migration of primordial germ cells into the developing gonads. (C) Transverse section of a 6-week embryo showing the gonadal cords. (D) Similar section at a later stage showing the indifferent gonads and paramesonephric ducts.

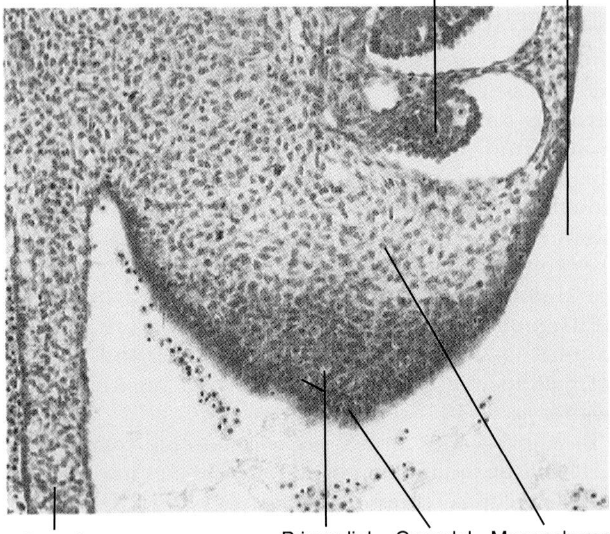

Fig. 12.29 Photomicrograph of a transverse section of the abdomen of an embryo at approximately 40 days, showing the gonadal ridge, which will develop into a testis or ovary depending on the chromosomal sex. Most of the developing gonad is composed of mesenchyme derived from the coelomic epithelium of the gonadal ridge. The large round cells in the gonad are primordial germ cells. (From Moore KL, Persaud TVN, Shiota K: *Color atlas of clinical embryology*, ed 2, Philadelphia, 2000, Saunders.)

PRIMORDIAL GERM CELLS

Primordial germ cells are large, spherical progenitors of sex cells that are first recognizable 24 days after fertilization among the endodermal cells of the umbilical vesicle near the origin of the allantois (see Figs. 12.28A and 12.29). During the folding of the embryo (see Fig. 5.1), the dorsal part of the umbilical vesicle is incorporated into the embryo. As this occurs, the primordial germ cells migrate along the dorsal mesentery of the hindgut to the gonadal ridges (see Fig. 12.28C). During the sixth week, the primordial germ cells enter the underlying mesenchyme and are incorporated in the **gonadal cords** (see Fig. 12.28C). *The migration of primordial germ cells is regulated by the genes* stella, fragilis, *and* BMP-4.

SEX DETERMINATION

Determination of chromosomal and genetic sex depends on whether an X-bearing sperm or a Y-bearing sperm fertilizes the X-bearing oocyte. Before the seventh week, the gonads of the two sexes are identical in appearance and are called **indifferent gonads** (see Fig. 12.28D). The indifferent gonad then determines the type of sexual differentiation that occurs in the genital ducts and external genitalia.

Development of a male phenotype (characteristics of an individual) requires a functional Y chromosome. The ***SRY* gene (sex-determining region on the Y chromosome)** for a testis-determining factor has been localized in the short-arm region of the Y chromosome. It is the testis-determining factor regulated by the Y chromosome that determines **testicular differentiation** (Fig. 12.30). Under the influence of this organizing factor, the **gonadal cords** differentiate into **seminiferous cords** (primordia of **seminiferous tubules**). *Sry activates testis-specific enhancers of Sox9. Two gene regulatory networks then prevent ovarian development (Wnt4, Foxl2, Fst, and Rspo1) while enhancing testicular development (Fgf9, Amh, and Dhh).* **Testosterone**, produced by the fetal testes, **dihydrotestosterone** (a metabolite of testosterone), and **antimüllerian hormone (AMH)** determine normal male sexual differentiation, which begins during the seventh week.

The absence of a Y chromosome results in the formation of an ovary. Development of the female phenotype requires two X chromosomes. Several genes and regions of the X chromosome have special roles in sex determination. Ovarian development begins about the 12th week and requires germ cell presence. *Ovary formation also requires DAX1, encoded by the X chromosome. Other factors thought to be important include FOXL2, WNT, and Iroquois-3.* Primary female sexual differentiation does not depend on hormones; it occurs even if the ovaries are absent.

DEVELOPMENT OF TESTES

Testis-determining factor induces the **seminiferous cords** to condense and extend into the medulla of the **indifferent gonad**, where they branch and anastomose to form the **rete testis**, a network of canals (see Fig. 12.30). The connection of the seminiferous cords with the surface epithelium is lost when a thick fibrous capsule, the **tunica albuginea**, develops. The development of the dense tunica albuginea is the characteristic feature of testicular development. Gradually, the enlarging testis separates from the degenerating mesonephros and is suspended by its own mesentery, the **mesorchium**.

The seminiferous cords develop into the seminiferous tubules, **tubuli recti**, and **rete testis** (see Fig. 12.30). The **seminiferous tubules** are separated by mesenchyme, which gives rise to the **interstitial cells** (Leydig cells). By the eighth week, these cells begin to secrete androgenic hormones, **testosterone**, and **androstenedione**, which induce masculine differentiation of the mesonephric ducts and external genitalia.

Testosterone production is stimulated by human chorionic gonadotropin, which reaches peak amounts during the 8th to 12th week period. In addition to testosterone, the fetal testes produce a glycoprotein, **AMH**, or müllerian-inhibiting substance (MIS) beginning in week 8. AMH is produced by the **sustentacular cells** (Sertoli cells); production continues until puberty, after which the levels of the hormone decrease. AMH suppresses the development of the paramesonephric ducts, which form the uterus and uterine tubes.

The seminiferous tubules have no lumina until puberty. The walls of the seminiferous tubules are composed of two types of cells (see Fig. 12.30):

- **Sertoli cells** support spermiogenesis; they are derived from the surface epithelium of the testis
- **Spermatogonia**, primordial sperm cells, are derived from primordial germ cells

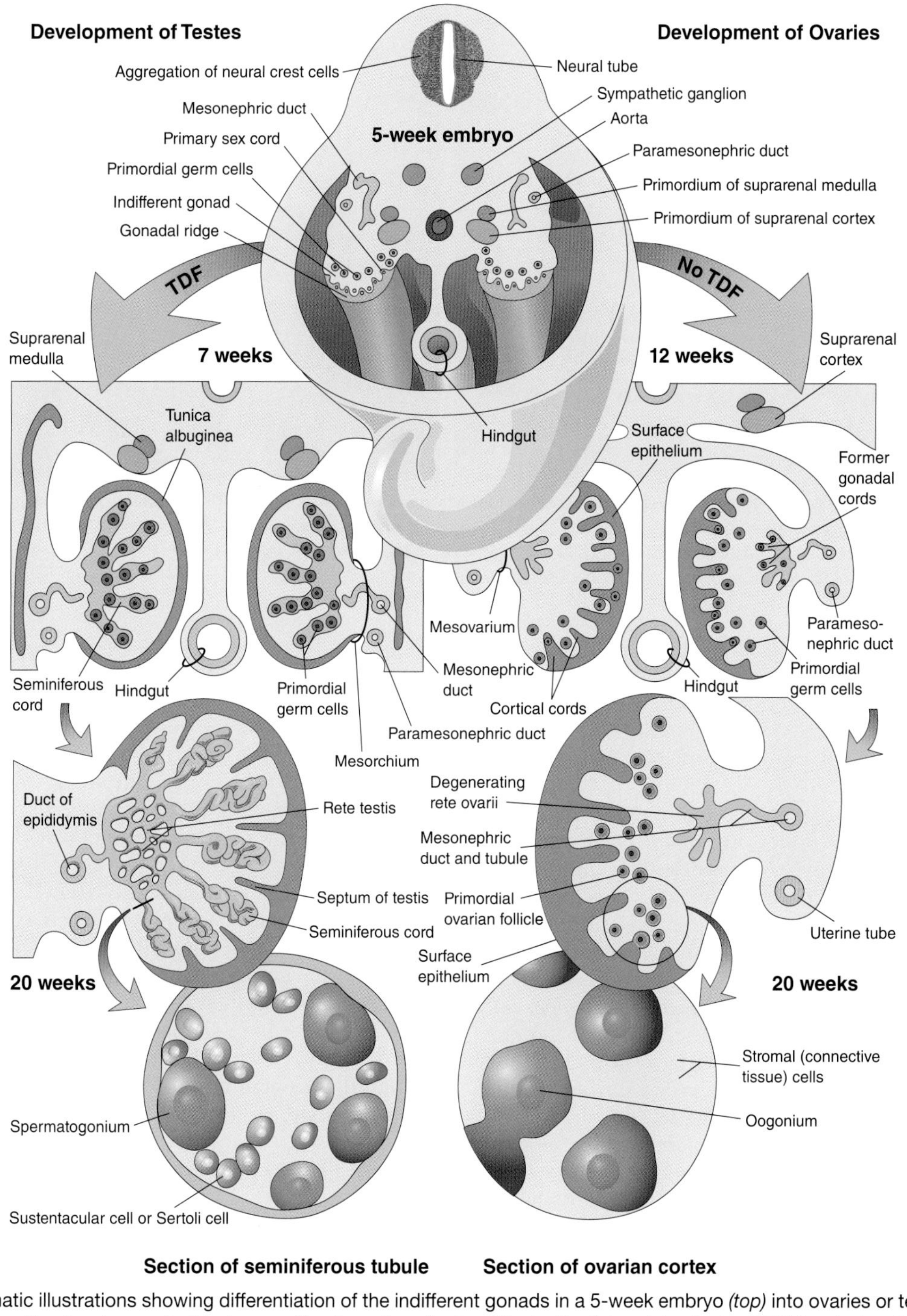

Fig. 12.30 Schematic illustrations showing differentiation of the indifferent gonads in a 5-week embryo *(top)* into ovaries or testes. The left side of the drawing shows the development of testes resulting from the effects of the testis-determining factor (TDF) located on the Y chromosome. Note that the gonadal cords become seminiferous cords, the primordia of the seminiferous tubules. The parts of the gonadal cords that enter the medulla of the testis form the rete testis. In the section of the testis at the bottom left, observe that there are two kinds of cells: spermatogonia, derived from the primordial germ cells, and sustentacular or Sertoli cells, derived from mesenchyme. The right side of the drawing shows the development of ovaries in the absence of TDF. Cortical cords have extended from the surface epithelium of the gonad, and primordial germ cells have entered them. They are the primordia of the oogonia. Follicular cells are derived from the surface epithelium of the ovary.

Sertoli cells constitute most of the seminiferous epithelium in the fetal testis (Fig. 12.31A; see also Fig. 12.30). During later fetal development, the surface epithelium of the testis flattens to form **mesothelium (a layer of cells)** on the external surface of the testis. The **rete testis** becomes continuous with 15 to 20 **mesonephric tubules** that become **efferent ductules**. These ductules are connected with the mesonephric duct, which becomes the **duct of the epididymis** (Fig. 12.32A; see also Fig. 12.30).

DEVELOPMENT OF OVARIES

Gonadal development occurs slowly in female embryos (see Fig. 12.31). The ovary is not identifiable histologically until approximately the 10th week. **Gonadal cords** are not

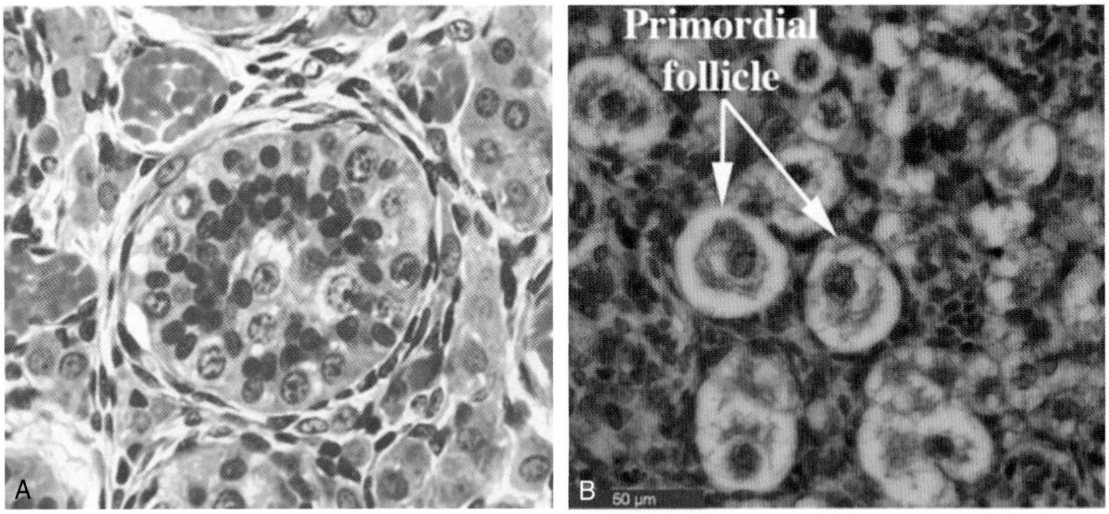

Fig. 12.31 Transverse sections of gonads of human fetuses. (A) Testis from a 24-week-old fetus. The seminiferous tubules contain Sertoli cells (small dark nuclei) (B) Ovarian primordial follicles. ((A) From Cheng L, MacLennan GT, Bostwick DG: *Urologic surgical pathology*, ed 4, 2020, Elsevier; (B) From Overland MR, Li Y, Derpinghaus A, Aksel S, Cao M, Ladwig N, Cunha GR, Himelreich-Perić M, Baskin LS: Development of the human ovary: fetal through pubertal ovarian morphology, folliculogenesis and expression of cellular differentiation markers. *Differentiation* 129:27–59, 2023.)

prominent in the developing ovary, but they extend into the medulla and form a rudimentary **rete ovarii** (see Fig. 12.30). This network of canals and the gonadal cords normally degenerate and disappear (see Fig. 12.30).

Cortical cords extend from the surface epithelium of the developing ovary into the underlying mesenchyme during the early fetal period. This epithelium is derived from the mesothelium of the peritoneum. As the cortical cords increase in size, **primordial germ cells** are incorporated into them (see Fig. 12.30). At approximately 16 weeks, these cords begin to break up into isolated cell clusters, or **primordial follicles**, each of which contains an **oogonium (primordial germ cell)**. The follicles are surrounded by a single layer of flattened **follicular cells** derived from the surface epithelium (see Fig. 12.30). Active mitosis of oogonia occurs during fetal life, producing primordial follicles (see Fig. 12.31B).

No oogonia form postnatally. Although many oogonia degenerate before birth, the 2 million or so that remain enlarge to become **primary oocytes**. After birth, the surface epithelium of the ovary flattens to a single layer of cells continuous with the mesothelium of the peritoneum at the **hilum of the ovary**, where vessels and nerves enter or leave. The surface epithelium becomes separated from the follicles in the cortex by a thin fibrous capsule, the **tunica albuginea**. As the ovary separates from the regressing mesonephros, it is suspended by a mesentery, the **mesovarium** (see Fig. 12.30).

DEVELOPMENT OF GENITAL DUCTS

During the fifth and sixth weeks, the genital system is in an indifferent state, and two pairs of genital ducts are present. The **mesonephric ducts** (wolffian ducts) play an important part in the development of the male reproductive system (see Fig. 12.32A). The **paramesonephric ducts** (müllerian ducts) have a leading role in the development of the female reproductive system.

The paramesonephric ducts develop lateral to the gonads and mesonephric ducts (see Fig. 12.30) on each side from longitudinal invaginations of the mesothelium on the lateral aspects of the mesonephroi (primordial kidneys). The edges of these grooves approach each other and fuse to form the paramesonephric ducts (Fig. 12.33A; see also Fig. 12.28C and E). The cranial ends of these ducts open into the peritoneal cavity (see Fig. 12.32B and C). Caudally, the paramesonephric ducts run parallel to the mesonephric ducts until they reach the future pelvic region of the embryo. Here they cross ventral to the mesonephric ducts, approach each other in the median plane, and fuse to form a Y-shaped **uterovaginal primordium** (see Fig. 12.33B). This tubular structure projects into the dorsal wall of the urogenital sinus and produces an elevation, the **sinus tubercle**.

DEVELOPMENT OF MALE GENITAL DUCTS AND GLANDS

The fetal testes produce masculinizing hormones (e.g., testosterone) and AMH. The Sertoli cells produce AMH at 6 to 7 weeks. The interstitial cells begin producing testosterone in the eighth week. Testosterone stimulates the mesonephric ducts to form male genital ducts, whereas AMH causes the paramesonephric ducts to regress. *It has been suggested that AMH-induced regression of the paramesonephric ducts in the male involves homeobox genes Dlx5 and Dlx6.* Under the influence of testosterone produced by the fetal testes in the eighth week, the proximal part of each mesonephric duct becomes highly convoluted to form the **epididymis** (see Fig. 12.32A). As the mesonephros degenerates, some mesonephric tubules persist and are transformed into **efferent ductules**. These ductules open into the **duct of the epididymis**. Distal to the epididymis, the mesonephric duct acquires a thick investment of smooth muscle and becomes the **ductus deferens** (see Fig. 12.32A).

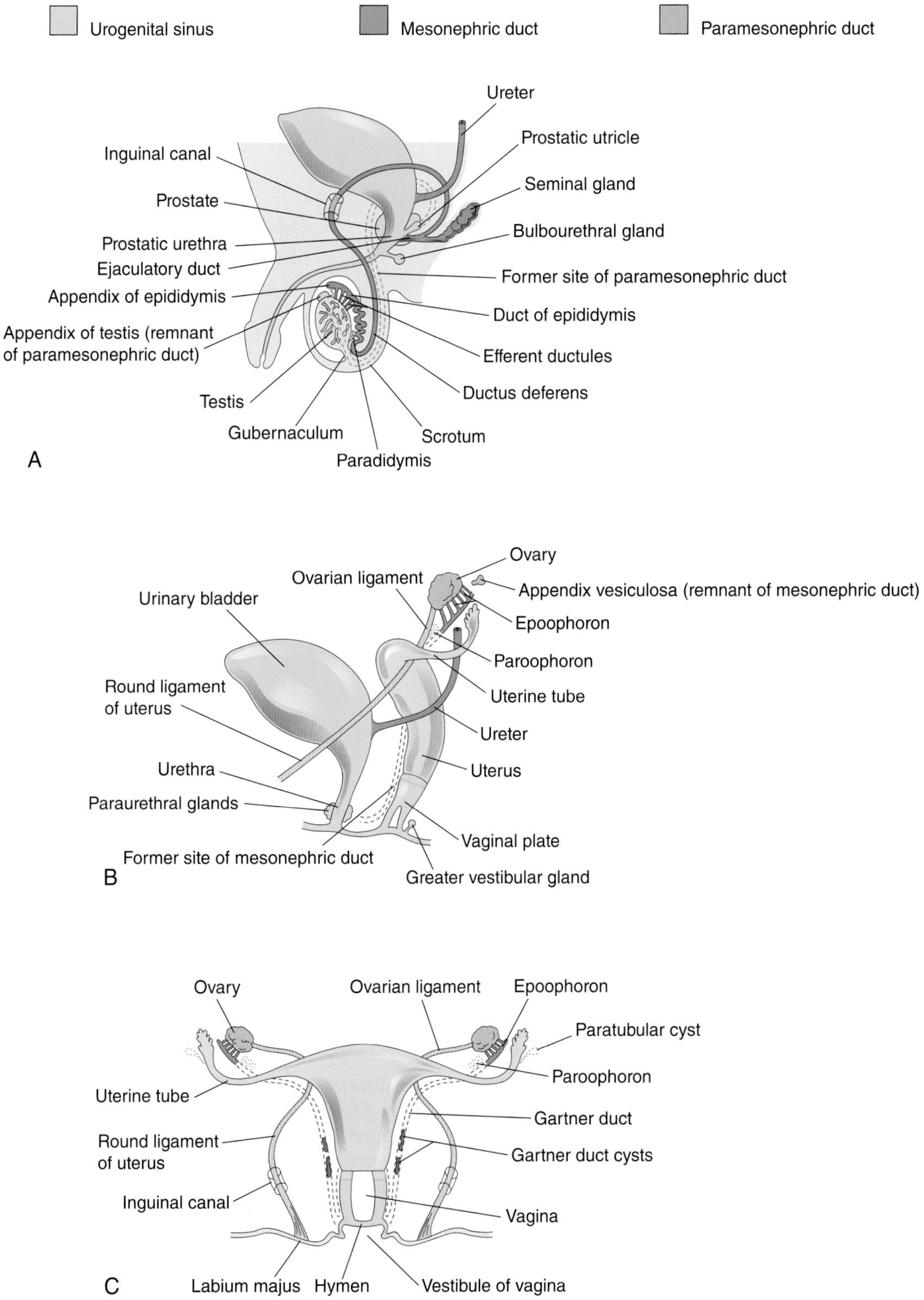

Fig. 12.32 Schematic drawings illustrating the development of the male and female reproductive systems from the genital ducts and urogenital sinus. Vestigial structures are also shown. (A) Reproductive system in a male neonate. (B) Female reproductive system in a 12-week fetus. (C) Reproductive system in a female neonate.

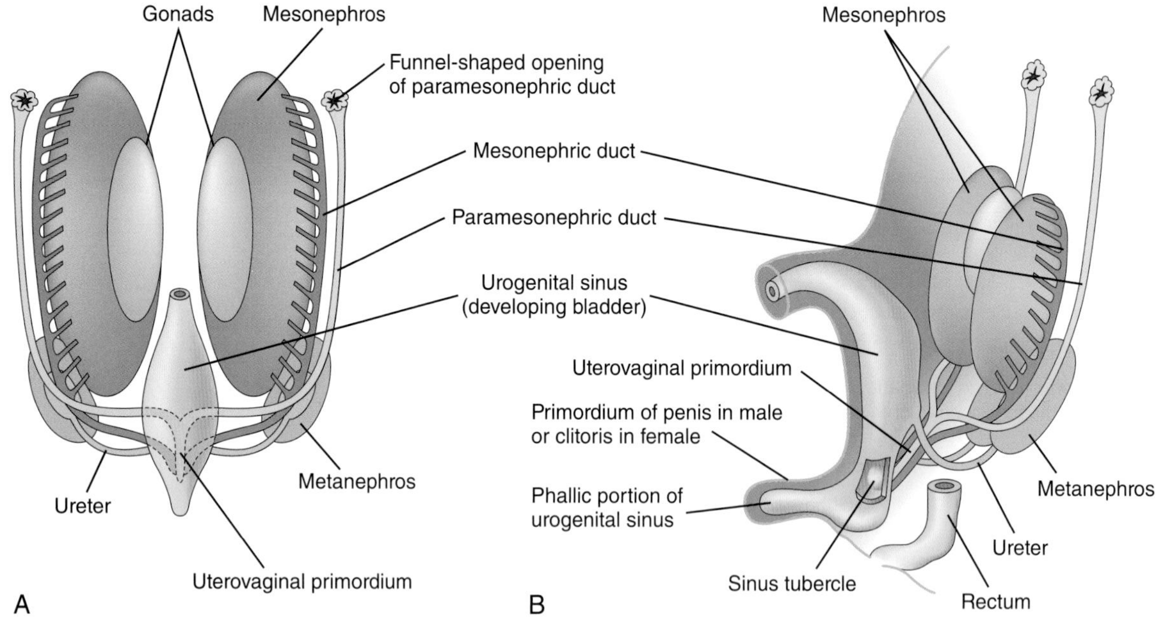

Fig. 12.33 (A) Sketch of a ventral view of the posterior abdominal wall of a 7-week embryo showing the two pairs of genital ducts present during the indifferent stage of sexual development. (B) Lateral view of a 9-week fetus showing the sinus tubercle on the posterior wall of the urogenital sinus. It becomes the hymen in females (see Fig. 12.33C) and the seminal colliculus in males. The colliculus is an elevated part of the urethral crest on the posterior wall of the prostatic urethra (see Fig. 12.33A).

SEMINAL GLANDS

Lateral outgrowths from the caudal end of each mesonephric duct become **seminal glands** (vesicles), which produce a secretion that makes up the majority of the fluid in **semen** and nourishes the sperms (see Fig. 12.32A). The part of the mesonephric duct between the duct of this gland and the urethra becomes the **ejaculatory duct**.

PROSTATE

Multiple endodermal outgrowths arise from the prostatic part of the urethra and grow into the surrounding urogenital sinus mesenchyme (Fig. 12.34A–C; see also Fig. 12.32A). The glandular epithelium of the prostate differentiates from these endodermal cells, and the associated mesenchyme differentiates into the dense **stroma** (framework of connective tissue) and smooth muscle of the prostate. *Hox genes control the development of the prostate gland as well as the seminal glands.* Secretions from the prostate contribute to the semen.

BULBOURETHRAL GLANDS

These pea-sized glands develop from paired outgrowths derived from the spongy part of the urethra (see Fig. 12.32A). The smooth muscle fibers and stroma differentiate from the adjacent mesenchyme. The secretions of these glands also contribute to the semen.

DEVELOPMENT OF FEMALE GENITAL DUCTS AND GLANDS

12

The **mesonephric ducts** of female embryos regress because of the absence of testosterone; only a few nonfunctional remnants persist (see Fig. 12.32B and C and Table 12.1). The **paramesonephric ducts** develop because of the absence of AMH. Later, **estrogens** produced by the maternal ovaries and the placenta stimulate the development of the uterine tube, uterus, and superior part of the vagina.

The paramesonephric ducts form most of the female genital tract. The uterine tubes develop from the unfused cranial parts of these ducts (see Figs. 12.32B and C and 12.33). The caudal fused portions of the paramesonephric ducts form the **uterovaginal primordium**, which gives rise to the **uterus** and the superior part of the **vagina** (see Fig. 12.33). The endometrial stroma and myometrium are derived from splanchnic mesenchyme. *Uterine development is regulated by the homeobox gene HOXA10.* Parts of the uterus remain underdeveloped until puberty (including the cervix, endometrium, and myometrium).

Fusion of the paramesonephric ducts also forms a peritoneal fold that becomes the **broad ligament** and forms two peritoneal compartments, the **rectouterine pouch** and **vesicouterine pouch** (Fig. 12.35A–D). Along the sides of the uterus, between the layers of the broad ligament, the mesenchyme proliferates and differentiates into cellular tissue, or **parametrium**, which is composed of loose connective tissue and smooth muscle.

FEMALE AUXILIARY GENITAL GLANDS

Outgrowths from the urethra into the surrounding mesenchyme form the bilateral mucus-secreting **urethral glands** and **paraurethral glands** (see Fig. 12.32B). Outgrowths from the **urogenital sinus** form the **greater vestibular glands** in the lower third of the labia majora (see Fig. 12.33B). These tubuloalveolar glands also secrete mucus and are homologous to the bulbourethral glands in males (see Table 12.1).

DEVELOPMENT OF VAGINA

12

The fibromuscular wall of the vagina develops from the surrounding mesenchyme. Contact of the **uterovaginal**

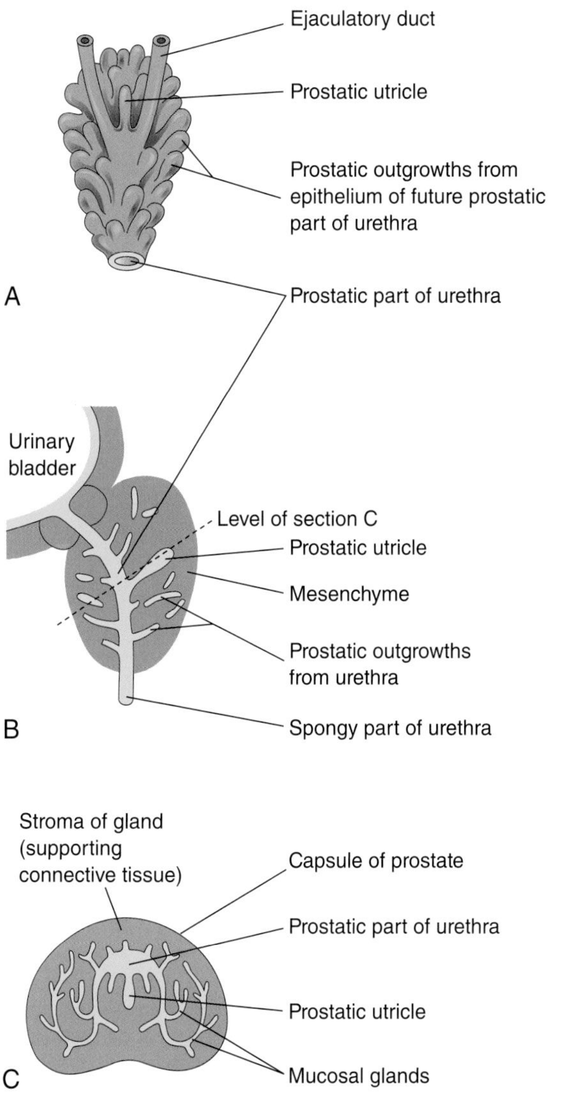

Fig. 12.34 (A) Dorsal view of the developing prostate in an 11-week fetus. (B) Sketch of a median section of the developing urethra and prostate showing numerous endodermal outgrowths from the prostatic urethra. The vestigial prostatic utricle is also shown. (C) Section of the prostate (16 weeks) at the level shown in (B).

primordium with the urogenital sinus, forming the **sinus tubercle** (see Fig. 12.33B), induces the formation of paired endodermal outgrowths, **sinovaginal bulbs** (see Fig. 12.35A). They extend from the urogenital sinus to the caudal end of the uterovaginal primordium. The sinovaginal bulbs fuse to form a **vaginal plate** (see Fig. 12.32B). Later the central cells of this plate break down, forming the **lumen of the vagina**. The epithelium of the vagina is derived from the peripheral cells of the vaginal plate (see Fig. 12.32C).

Until late fetal life, the lumen of the vagina is separated from the cavity of the urogenital sinus by a membrane, the **hymen** (Fig. 12.36H; see also Fig. 12.32C). The membrane is formed by invagination of the posterior wall of the urogenital sinus, resulting from expansion of the caudal end of the vagina. The hymen usually ruptures, leaving a small opening during the perinatal period and remains as a thin fold of mucous membrane just within the vaginal orifice (see Fig. 12.36H).

VESTIGIAL REMAINS OF EMBRYONIC GENITAL DUCTS

During the conversion of the mesonephric and paramesonephric ducts into adult structures, some parts of the ducts remain as **vestigial structures** (see Fig. 12.32 and Table 12.1). These vestiges are rarely seen unless pathologic changes develop in them (e.g., Gartner duct cysts arising from vestiges of mesonephric ducts; see Fig. 12.32C).

In males, the cranial end of the mesonephric duct may persist as an **appendix of the epididymis**, which is usually attached to the head of the epididymis (see Fig. 12.32A). Caudal to the efferent ductules, some mesonephric tubules may persist as a small body, the **paradidymis**. In females, the cranial end of the mesonephric duct may persist as an **appendix vesiculosa** (see Fig. 12.32B). A few blind tubules and a duct, or epoophoron, may persist in the mesovarium between the ovary and uterine tube (see Fig. 12.32B and C). Closer to the uterus, some rudimentary tubules may persist as the paroophoron (see Fig. 12.32B). Parts of the mesonephric duct, corresponding to the ductus deferens and ejaculatory duct in males, may persist as **Gartner duct cysts** between the layers of the broad ligament along the lateral wall of the uterus and in the wall of the vagina (see Fig. 12.32C).

In males, the cranial end of the paramesonephric duct may persist as a vesicular appendix of the testis, which is attached to the superior pole of the testis (see Fig. 12.32A). The prostatic utricle, a small sac-like structure arising from the paramesonephric duct, opens into the prostatic urethra. The lining of the prostatic utricle is derived from the epithelium of the urogenital sinus. Within its epithelium, endocrine cells containing neuron-specific enolase and serotonin have been detected. The seminal colliculus, a small elevation in the posterior wall of the prostatic urethra, is the adult derivative of the sinus tubercle (see Fig. 12.33B). In females, part of the cranial end of the paramesonephric duct that does not contribute to the infundibulum of the uterine tube may persist as a paraovarian or paratubular cyst (see Fig. 12.32C), called a hydatid.

DEVELOPMENT OF EXTERNAL GENITALIA

12

Up to the seventh week, the external genitalia are similar in both sexes (see Fig. 12.36A and B). Distinguishing sexual characteristics begin to appear during the 9th week, but the external genitalia are not fully differentiated until the 12th week. Early in the fourth week, proliferating mesenchyme produces a **genital tubercle** (primordium of the penis or clitoris) in both sexes at the cranial end of the **cloacal membrane** (see Fig. 12.36A). *The cloacal ectoderm is believed to be the source of the genital initiation signal that involves Fgf8 expression.*

Labioscrotal swellings and **urogenital folds** soon develop on each side of the cloacal membrane. The genital tubercle elongates to form a **primordial phallus** (penis or clitoris). In female fetuses, the urethra and vagina open into a common cavity, the **vestibule of the vagina** (see Fig. 12.36H).

DEVELOPMENT OF MALE EXTERNAL GENITALIA

Masculinization of the indifferent external genitalia is induced by testosterone produced by the interstitial cells of the fetal testes (see Fig. 12.36C, E, and G). The

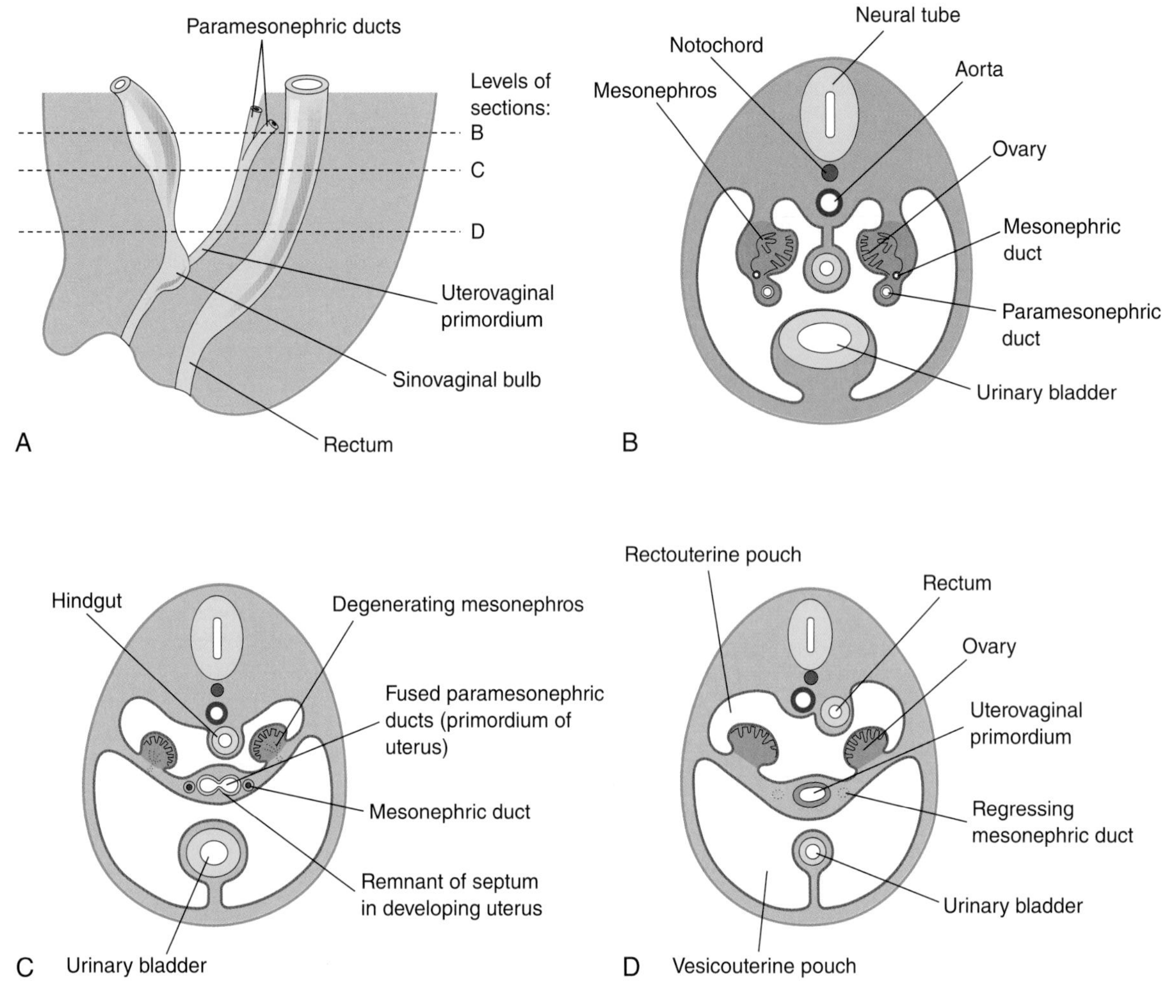

Fig. 12.35 Early development of ovaries and uterus. (A) Schematic drawing of a sagittal section of the caudal region of an 8-week female embryo. (B) Transverse section showing the paramesonephric ducts approaching each other. (C) Similar section at a more caudal level illustrating fusion of the paramesonephric ducts. A remnant of the septum in the developing uterus that separates the paramesonephric ducts is shown. (D) Similar section showing the uterovaginal primordium, broad ligament, and pouches in the pelvic cavity. Note that the mesonephric ducts have regressed.

primordial phallus enlarges and elongates to form the **penis**. A **urethral plate** forms on the ventral side of the primordial phallus. The urethral plate canalizes, in a proximal to distal direction, and opens to form the **urethral groove**. This groove is bounded by the **urethral folds**, which form the lateral walls (Fig. 12.37A and B; see also Fig. 12.36C). This groove is lined by a proliferation of endodermal cells from the urethral plate (see Fig. 12.36C), which extends from the phallic portion of the urogenital sinus. Under the influence of androgens, the **urethral folds** fuse with each other, in a proximal to distal direction, along the ventral surface of the penis to form the **spongy urethra** (see Figs. 12.36E and G and 12.37C_1 and C_3). This fusion occurs in three layers: the epithelium of the folds, forming the urethra; the stroma, forming a portion of the spongiosum; and the surface ectoderm, forming the **penile raphe** and enclosing the spongy urethra within the penis (see Fig. 12.36G).

At the tip of the **glans penis**, an ectodermal ingrowth forms a cellular **ectodermal cord**, which grows toward the root of the penis to meet the spongy urethra (see Figs. 12.6A and 12.37C). As this cord canalizes, its lumen joins the previously formed spongy urethra. This juncture completes the terminal part of the urethra and moves the **external urethral orifice** to the tip of the glans penis (see Figs. 12.26B and C and 12.36G). *HOX, FGF, SHH (sonic hedgehog) and IHH (Indian hedgehog) genes regulate the development of the penis from the primordial phallus* (see Fig.12.36A and B).

During the 12th week, a circular ingrowth of the ectoderm occurs at the periphery of the glans penis (see Fig. 12.26B). When this ingrowth breaks down, it forms the **prepuce** (foreskin), a covering fold of skin (see Fig. 12.26C). The **corpus cavernosum penis** (one of two columns of erectile tissue) and **corpus spongiosum penis** (median column of erectile tissue between the two corpora cavernosa) develop from mesenchyme in the phallus. The two **labioscrotal swellings** grow toward each other and fuse to form the **scrotum** (see Fig. 12.36A, E, and G). The line of fusion of these folds is clearly visible as the **scrotal raphe** (see Figs. 12.36G and 12.37C).

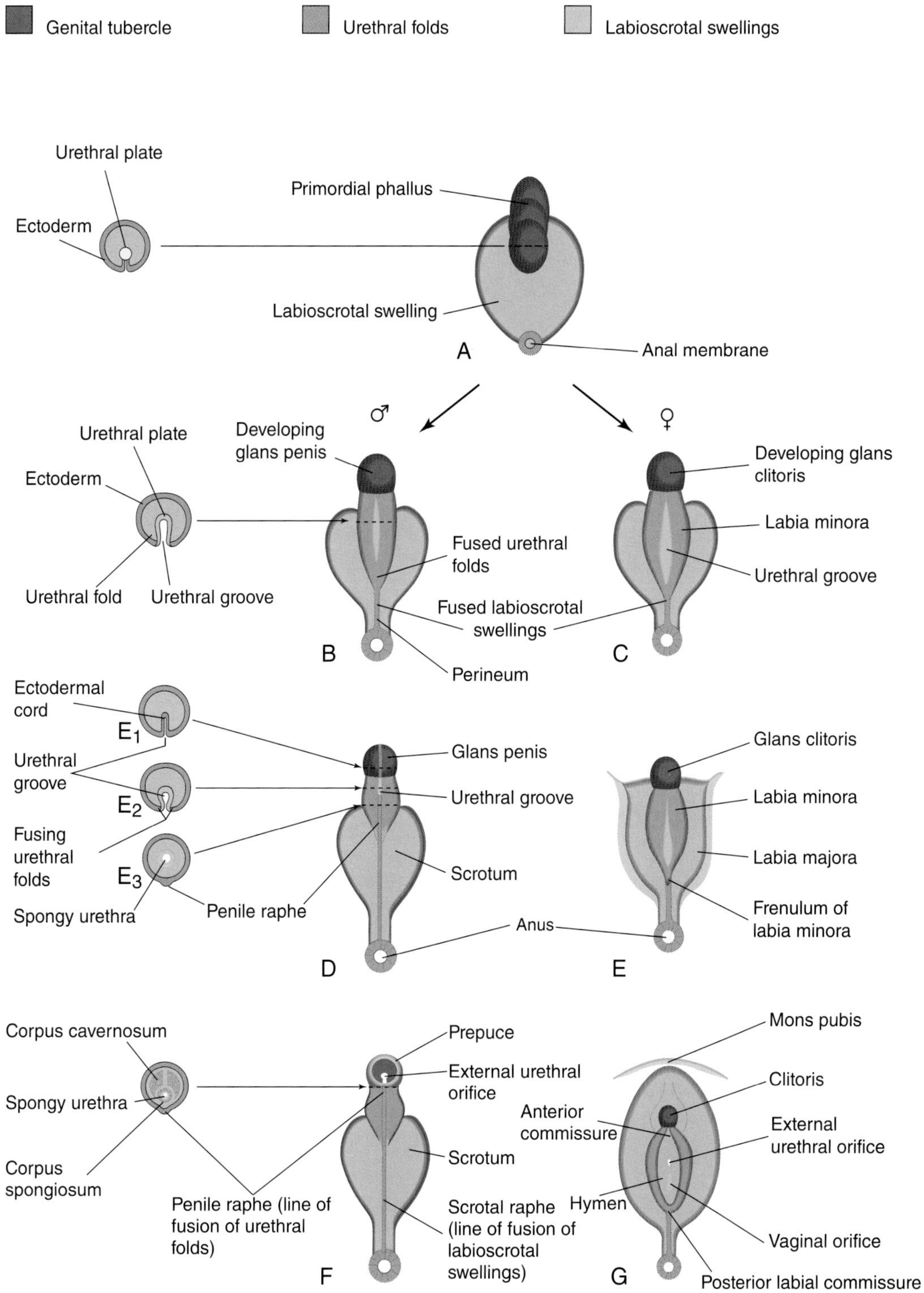

Fig. 12.36 Development of external genitalia. (A) Diagram illustrating the appearance of the genitalia during the indifferent (bipotential) stage (fourth to seventh weeks). (B, D, and F) Stages in the development of male external genitalia at 9, 11, and 12 weeks, respectively. To the left are schematic transverse sections of the developing penis illustrating the formation of the spongy urethra. (C, E, and G) Stages in the development of female external genitalia at 9, 11, and 12 weeks, respectively. The mons pubis is a pad of fatty tissue over the symphysis pubis.

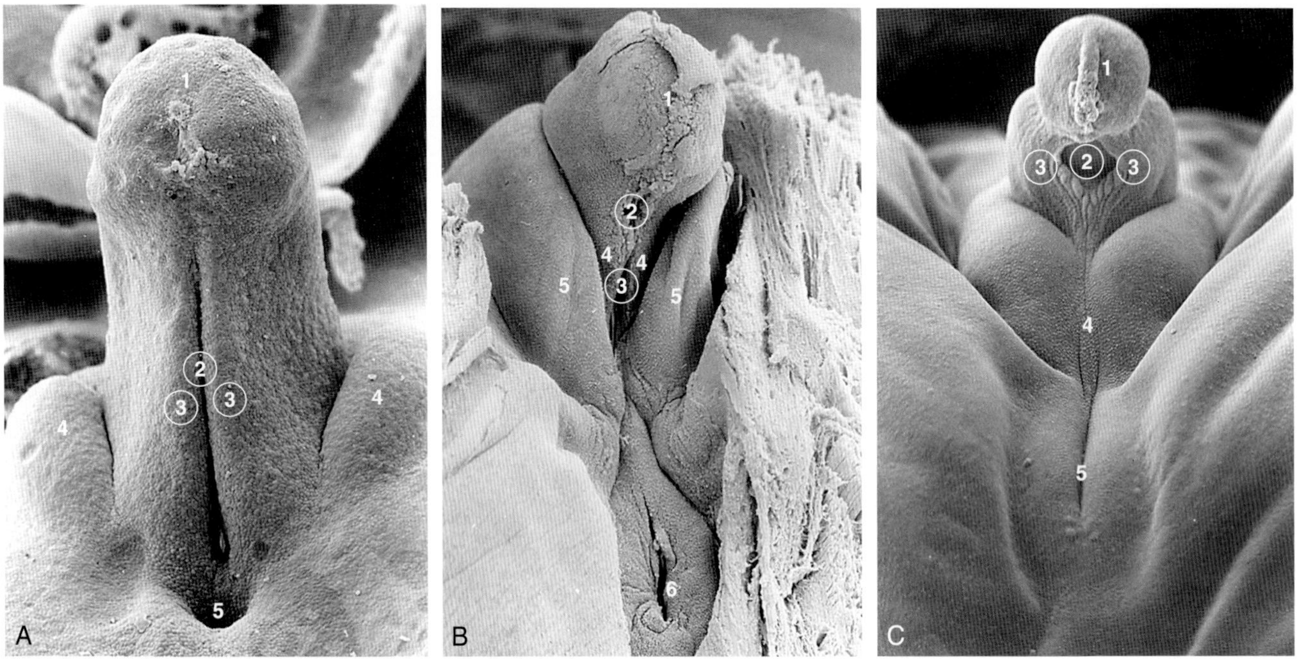

Fig. 12.37 Scanning electron micrographs of the developing external genitalia. (A) The perineum during the indifferent stage of a 17-mm, 7-week embryo (×100). *1*, Developing glans penis with the ectodermal cord; *2*, urethral groove continuous with the urogenital sinus; *3*, urethral folds; *4*, labioscrotal swellings; *5*, anus. (B) The external genitalia of a 7.2-cm, 10-week female fetus (×45). *1*, Glans clitoris; *2*, external urethral orifice; *3*, opening into urogenital sinus; *4*, urethral fold (primordium of labium minora); *5*, labioscrotal swelling (labium majora); *6*, anus. (C) The external genitalia of a 5.5-cm, 10-week male fetus (×40). *1*, Glans penis with ectodermal cord; *2*, remains of urethral groove; *3*, urethral folds in the process of closing; *4*, labioscrotal swellings fusing to form the scrotal raphe; *5*, anus. (From Hinrichsen KV: Embryologische Grundlagen. In Sohn C, Holzgreve W, editors: *Ultraschall in Gynäkologie und Geburtshilfe*, New York, 1995, Georg Thieme Verlag.)

DEVELOPMENT OF FEMALE EXTERNAL GENITALIA

The **primordial phallus** in the female fetus gradually becomes the **clitoris** (see Figs. 12.20G, 12.36B–D, F, and H, and 12.37B). The clitoris is still relatively large at 18 weeks (see Fig. 12.21). The **urethral folds** do not fuse, except posteriorly, where they join to form the **frenulum of the labia minora** (see Fig. 12.36F). The unfused parts of the urogenital folds form the **labia minora**. The labioscrotal folds fuse posteriorly to form the **posterior labial commissure** and anteriorly to form the **anterior labial commissure** and **mons pubis** (Fig. 12.36H). Most parts of the **labioscrotal folds** remain unfused but develop into two large folds of skin, the **labia majora**.

Sex Chromosome DSDs

In embryos with **abnormal sex chromosome complexes**, such as XXX or XXY (see Fig. 20.9), the number of X chromosomes appears to be unimportant in sex determination. If a normal Y chromosome is present, the embryo develops as a male. If no Y chromosome is present or the testis-determining region of the Y chromosome is absent, female development occurs. The loss of an X chromosome does not appear to interfere with the migration of primordial germ cells to the gonadal ridges because some germ cells have been observed in the fetal gonads of 45,XO females with **Turner syndrome** (see Figs. 20.3 and 20.4). Two X chromosomes are needed, however, to bring about normal ovarian development.

Determination of Fetal Sex

Visualization of external genitalia during ultrasonography is clinically important for several reasons, including the detection of fetuses at risk of severe X-linked disorders (Fig. 12.38). Careful examination of the perineum may detect **ambiguous genitalia** (Fig. 12.39B). Ultrasonographic confirmation of testes in the scrotum provides only 100% gender determination, which is not possible in utero until 22 to 36 weeks. In 30% of fetuses, the fetal position prevents good visualization of the **perineum** (area between the thighs).

When there is normal sexual differentiation, the appearance of the external and internal genitalia is consistent with the **sex chromosome complement**. Errors in sex determination and differentiation result in various degrees of intermediate sex. Advances in molecular genetics have led to a better understanding of abnormal sexual development and **ambiguous genitalia**.

The term **disorders of sex development (DSD)** implies a discrepancy between the morphology of the gonads (testes or ovaries) and the appearance of the external genitalia. DSDs can be classified as follows:

- **Sex-chromosome DSD**, including Turner syndrome and Klinefelter syndrome
- **Gonadal dysgenesis**, including ovotesticular DSD, XX testicular DSD, and XY gonadal dysgenesis
- **Virilizing congenital adrenal hyperplasia (CAH)**
- **Disorders of androgen action**

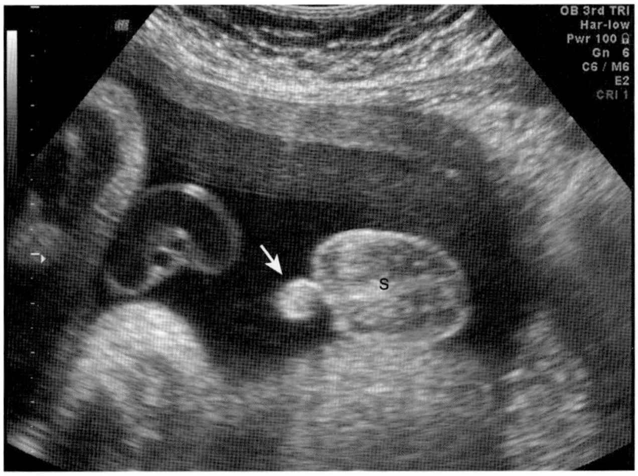

Fig. 12.38 Sonogram of a 33-week-old male fetus showing normal external genitalia. Observe the penis *(arrow)* and scrotum *(S)*. Also, note the testes in the scrotum. (Courtesy Dr. G.J. Reid, Department of Obstetrics, Gynecology and Reproductive Sciences, University of Manitoba, Women's Hospital, Winnipeg, Manitoba, Canada.)

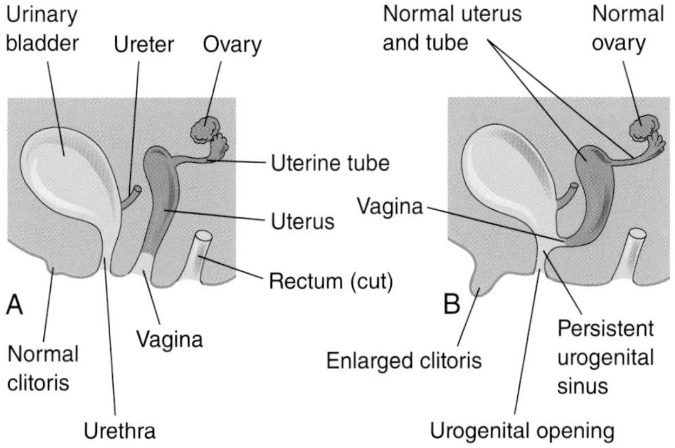

Fig. 12.39 Schematic lateral views of the female urogenital system. (A) Normal. (B) Female with 46,XX disorder of sex development caused by congenital adrenal hyperplasia. Note the enlarged clitoris and persistent urogenital sinus that were induced by androgens produced by the hyperplastic suprarenal glands.

Gonadal Dysgenesis

Ovotesticular DSD

Persons with **ovotesticular DSD**, a rare intersexual condition, usually have **chromatin-positive nuclei** (sex chromatin in cells observed in a buccal smear). Approximately 70% of these persons have a 46,XX chromosome constitution; approximately 20% have 46,XX/46,XY **mosaicism** (the presence of two or more cell lines); and approximately 10% have a 46,XY chromosome constitution. The causes of ovotesticular DSD are still poorly understood.

Persons with this condition can have both testicular and ovarian tissue within one gonad (an **ovotestis**) or on opposite sides. These tissues are not usually functional. An ovotestis forms if both the medulla and cortex of the indifferent gonads develop. Ovotesticular DSD results from an error in sex determination. The phenotype may be male or female, but the external genitalia are always ambiguous.

XX Testicular DSD

In 80% of persons with **XX testicular DSD**, the *SRY* gene is translocated to an X chromosome, resulting in a male appearance of the external genitalia, although some individuals may have ambiguous-appearing genitalia. The testes are often small and azoospermic and there are often increased gonadotropin levels. The individual may also have hypospadias (Figs. 12.40 and 12.42; see also Fig. 12.39B). In 20% of affected individuals, there is no translocation of the SRY gene, and the exact cause of the condition is unknown, although individuals with SRY-negative 46,XX testicular DSD more commonly have ambiguous genitalia.

XY Gonadal Dysgenesis

In complete XY gonadal dysgenesis, the individuals have internal and external structures that appear female and underdeveloped (streak) gonads, and they do not develop secondary sexual characteristics at puberty. This is due to a failure of testicular development with several genes being implicated (SRY deletion or loss of function, DHH, NR5A1, and MAP3K1). In partial XY gonadal dysgenesis, the Leydig and Sertoli cell functions are partially absent, and persons have external and internal genitalia that are developmentally variable. Pathogenic variants (mutations) in SF-1 and SRY are often detected. Overall, these anomalies are caused by inadequate production of testosterone and AMH by the fetal testes, and affected individuals are at higher risk of germ cell tumors.

Virilizing CAH

CAH refers to clinical conditions that result from autosomal defects in the synthesis of adrenal steroids. In more than 90% of cases, the defect is due to a deficiency 21-hydroxylase; approximately 5% of cases result from 11-β hydroxylase deficiency, with the remainder caused by other adrenal steroid dysfunctions. In cases of 21-hydroxylase deficiency, there is an overall reduced production of mineralocorticoid and glucocorticoid production (adrenal insufficiency). The pituitary reacts to this insufficiency by increasing the production of adrenocorticotropic hormone, causing the overproduction of androgens by the adrenal gland.

In females, this usually causes masculinization of the external genitalia (Fig. 12.40). Commonly, there is **clitoral hypertrophy**, partial fusion of the labia majora, and a persistent urogenital sinus (see Fig. 12.40).

In rare cases, the masculinization may be so intense that a complete clitoral urethra results. Affected male infants have normal external genitalia, and the syndrome may go undetected in early infancy. Later in childhood in both sexes, androgen excess leads to rapid growth and accelerated skeletal maturation.

The **adrenogenital syndrome**, associated with CAH, manifests itself in various forms that can be correlated with enzymatic deficiencies of **cortisol biosynthesis**. In some male infants, though, the first presentation may be related to insufficient production of aldosterone, leading to a salt-wasting state that clinically presents as shock from dehydration. *Pathogenic variants (mutations) of* DAX1 *result in X-linked adrenal hypoplasia congenita*.

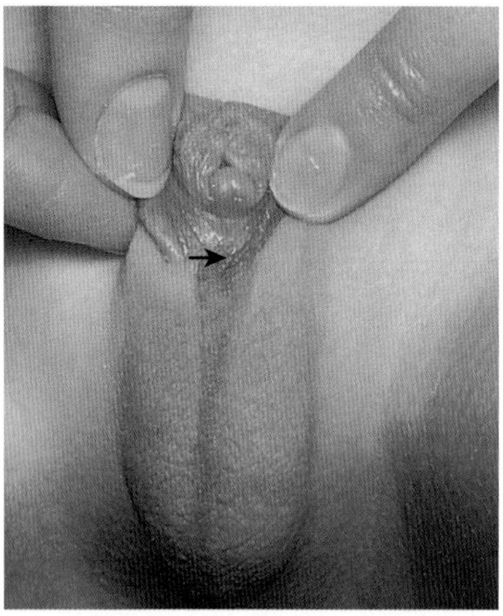

Fig. 12.40 External genitalia of a 6-year-old girl showing an enlarged clitoris and fused labia majora that have formed a scrotum-like structure. The *arrow* indicates the opening into the urogenital sinus. This extreme masculinization is the result of congenital adrenal hyperplasia. (Courtesy Dr. Heather Dean, Department of Pediatric and Child Health, University of Manitoba, Winnipeg, Manitoba, Canada.)

Disorders of Androgen Action

Androgen Insensitivity Syndrome

Persons with androgen insensitivity syndrome, which occurs in 1 in 20,000 live births, are **normal-appearing females**, despite the presence of testes and a 46,XY chromosome constitution (Fig. 12.41). **The external genitalia are female**; however, the vagina usually ends in a blind pouch, and the uterus and uterine tubes are absent or rudimentary. At puberty, there is normal development of breasts and female characteristics; however, menstruation does not occur.

The testes are usually in the abdomen or inguinal canals, but they may be within the labia majora. The failure of masculinization to occur in these persons results from a resistance to the action of testosterone at the cellular level in the genital tubercle and labioscrotal and urethral folds (see Fig. 12.36A, B, D, F, and H).

Persons with **partial androgen insensitivity syndrome** exhibit some masculinization at birth, such as ambiguous external genitalia, and they may have an enlarged clitoris. The vagina ends blindly, and the uterus is absent. Testes are in the inguinal canals or *labia majora*. There are usually point mutations in the sequence that codes for the **androgen receptor**. Hundreds of AG gene pathogenic variants (mutations) have been described. Usually, the testes of these persons are removed as soon as they are discovered because in approximately one-third of these individuals, malignant tumors develop by 50 years of age. Androgen insensitivity syndrome follows X-linked recessive inheritance, and the gene encoding the androgen receptor has been localized.

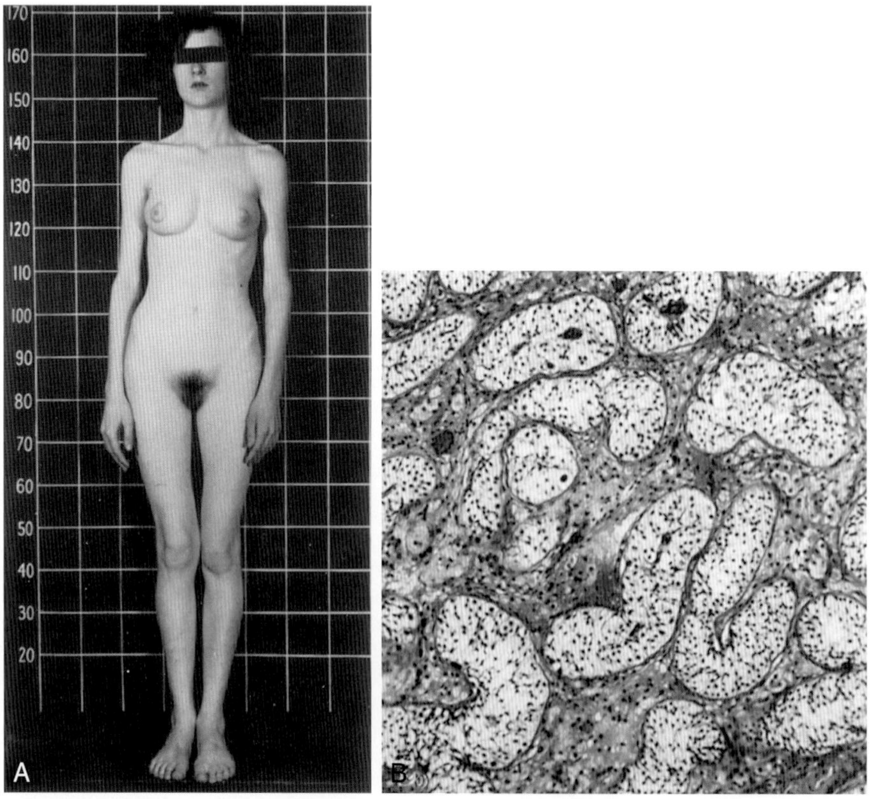

Fig. 12.41 (A) Photograph of a 17-year-old female with androgen insensitivity syndrome. The external genitalia are female; however, she has a 46,XY karyotype and testes in the inguinal region. (B) Photomicrograph of a section through a testis removed from the inguinal region of this female showing seminiferous tubules lined by Sertoli cells. There are no germ cells, and the interstitial cells are hypoplastic. (From Jones HW, Scott WW: *Hermaphroditism, genital anomalies and related endocrine disorders*, Baltimore, Maryland, 1958, Williams & Wilkins.)

Hypospadias

Hypospadias is the most common defect of the penis. There are four main types:

- Glanular hypospadias, the most common type
- Penile hypospadias
- Penoscrotal hypospadias
- Perineal hypospadias

In 1 of every 125 male neonates, the **external urethral orifice** is on the ventral surface of the glans penis **(glanular hypospadias)** or the ventral surface of the body of the penis **(penile hypospadias)**. Usually, the penis is underdeveloped and curved ventrally (**chordee**; Fig. 12.42).

Glanular hypospadias and penile hypospadias constitute approximately 80% of all cases of hypospadias. In **penoscrotal hypospadias**, the urethral orifice is at the junction of the penis and scrotum. In **perineal hypospadias**, the labioscrotal folds (swellings) fail to fuse (see Figs. 12.36 and 12.37) and the external urethral orifice is located between the unfused halves of the scrotum. Because the external genitalia in this severe type of hypospadias are ambiguous, persons with perineal hypospadias and cryptorchidism (undescended testes) are sometimes misdiagnosed as having XY gonadal dysgenesis.

Hypospadias results from inadequate production of androgens by the fetal testes and/or inadequate receptor sites for the hormones. Most likely, both genomic and environmental factors are involved. Hypospadias has been found to be associated with pathogenic variants (mutation) of several genes, including *AR*, *BNC2*, *CTNNB1*, *FGFR2*, *FGF10*, *HOXA13*, and *SHH*. It has been suggested that the expression of testosterone-related genes is affected. These defects result in failure of canalization of the ectodermal cord in the glans penis and/or failure of fusion of the urethral folds; as a consequence, there is an incomplete formation of the spongy urethra.

Epispadias

In one of every 30,000 male infants, the urethra opens on the dorsal surface of the penis; note that when the penis is flaccid, its dorsal surface is directed anteriorly. Although epispadias may occur as a separate entity, it is often associated with **exstrophy of the bladder** (see Figs. 12.24 and 12.25F). Epispadias may result from inadequate ectodermal-mesenchymal interactions during the development of the genital tubercle (see Fig. 12.36A). As a consequence, the genital tubercle develops more dorsally than in normal embryos. Consequently, when the **urogenital membrane** ruptures, the urogenital sinus opens on the dorsal surface of the penis (see Fig. 12.36B and C). Urine is expelled at the root of the malformed penis, which is located in the superficial perineal pouch.

Agenesis of External Genitalia

Congenital absence of the penis or clitoris is an extremely rare condition (Fig. 12.43) with about 100 cases reported worldwide. Often, rectovesical or urogenital anomalies were also present in these infants. Failure of the **genital tubercle** to develop (see Fig. 12.36A and B) may result from inadequate ectodermal-mesenchymal interactions during the seventh week. The urethra usually opens into the perineum near the anus. *Transcription factor SOX9 and Hedgehog genes—SHH and IHH—have been reported in association with the closure of the urethra and the formation of the penis.*

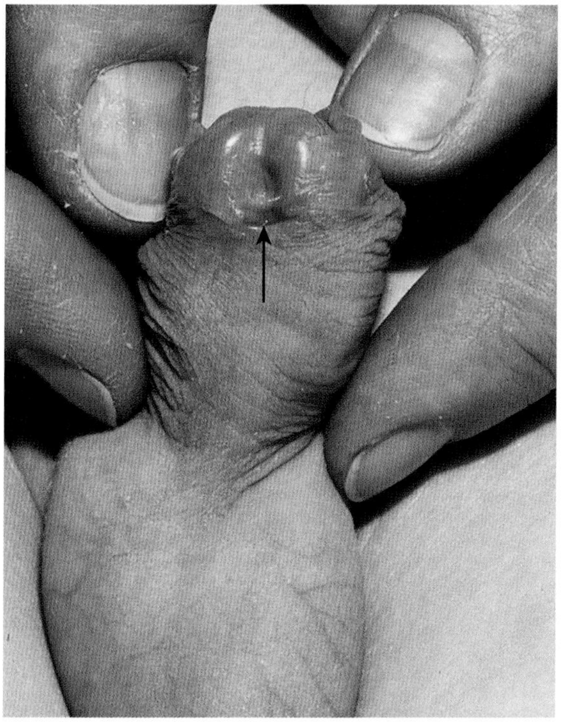

Fig. 12.42 Glanular hypospadias in an infant. The external urethral orifice is on the ventral surface of the glans penis *(arrow)*. (Courtesy A.E. Chudley, MD, Section of Genetics and Metabolism, Department of Pediatrics and Child Health, University of Manitoba, Children's Hospital, Winnipeg, Manitoba, Canada.)

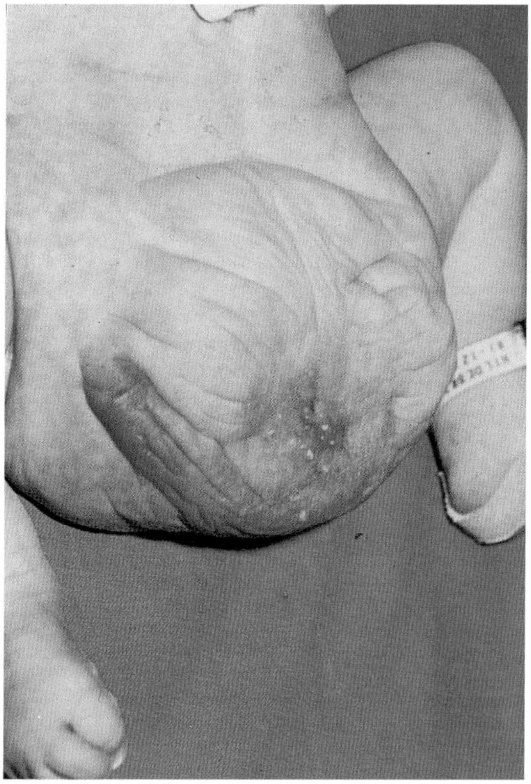

Fig. 12.43 Perineum of an infant with agenesis of the external genitalia. There are no external genitalia. (Courtesy A.E. Chudley, MD, Section of Genetics and Metabolism, Department of Pediatrics and Child Health, University of Manitoba, Children's Hospital, Winnipeg, Manitoba, Canada.)

Bifid Penis and Diphallia

These defects are very rare. **Bifid penis** is usually associated with **exstrophy of the bladder** (see Fig. 12.24). It may also be associated with urinary tract abnormalities and imperforate anus. **Diphallia** (double penis) results when two genital tubercles develop; fewer than 100 cases have been reported worldwide.

Micropenis

In this condition, the penis is so small that it is almost hidden by the suprapubic fat pad. **Micropenis** results from fetal testicular failure and is commonly associated with hypopituitarism (diminished activity of the anterior lobe of the hypophysis). *Epigenetic factors are likely involved. Molecular studies have shown decreased levels of nuclear androgen receptor and SOX expression in association with penile anomalies, including micropenis.*

Anomalies of Uterine Tubes, Uterus, and Vagina

Defects of the uterine tubes are rare; there are only a few irregularities, including hydatid cysts, accessory ostia (openings), complete and segmental absence of the tubes, duplication of a uterine tube, lack of the muscular layer, and failure of the tube to canalize. Various types of uterine duplications and vaginal anomalies result from arrests of development of the uterovaginal primordium during the eighth week (Fig. 12.44) by:

- Incomplete development of a paramesonephric duct
- Failure of parts of one or both paramesonephric ducts to develop
- Incomplete fusion of the paramesonephric ducts
- Incomplete canalization of the vaginal plate to form the vagina

Double uterus (uterus didelphys) results from failure of fusion of the inferior parts of the paramesonephric ducts. It may be associated with a double or a single vagina (see Fig. 12.44B–D). In some cases, the uterus appears normal externally but is divided internally by a thin septum (see Fig. 12.44F). If the duplication involves only the superior part of the body of the uterus, the condition is called **bicornuate uterus** (Fig. 12.45; see also Fig. 12.44D and E).

If the growth of one paramesonephric duct is retarded and the duct does not fuse with the second duct, a **bicornuate uterus with a rudimentary horn** (cornu) develops (see Fig. 12.44E). The rudimentary horn may not communicate with the cavity of the uterus. A **unicornuate uterus** develops when one paramesonephric duct fails to develop; this results in a uterus with one uterine tube (see Fig. 12.44G). In many cases, the individuals are fertile but may have an increased incidence of preterm delivery or recurrent pregnancy loss.

Absence of Vagina and Uterus

Once in approximately every 5000 births, absence of the vagina occurs. This results from the failure of the **sinovaginal bulbs** to develop and form the vaginal plate (see Figs. 12.32B and 12.35A). When the vagina is absent, the uterus is usually absent because the developing uterus (uterovaginal primordium) induces the formation of sinovaginal bulbs, which fuse to form the vaginal plate.

Other Vaginal Anomalies

Failure of canalization of the vaginal plate results in **atresia** (blockage) of the vagina. A transverse **vaginal septum** occurs in approximately one in 80,000 females. Usually, the septum is located at the junction of the middle and superior thirds of the vagina. Failure of the inferior end of the vaginal plate to perforate results in an **imperforate hymen**, the most common anomaly of the female reproductive tract that results in obstruction. Variations in the appearance of the hymen are common (Fig. 12.46). The vaginal orifice varies in diameter from very small to large, and there may be more than one orifice.

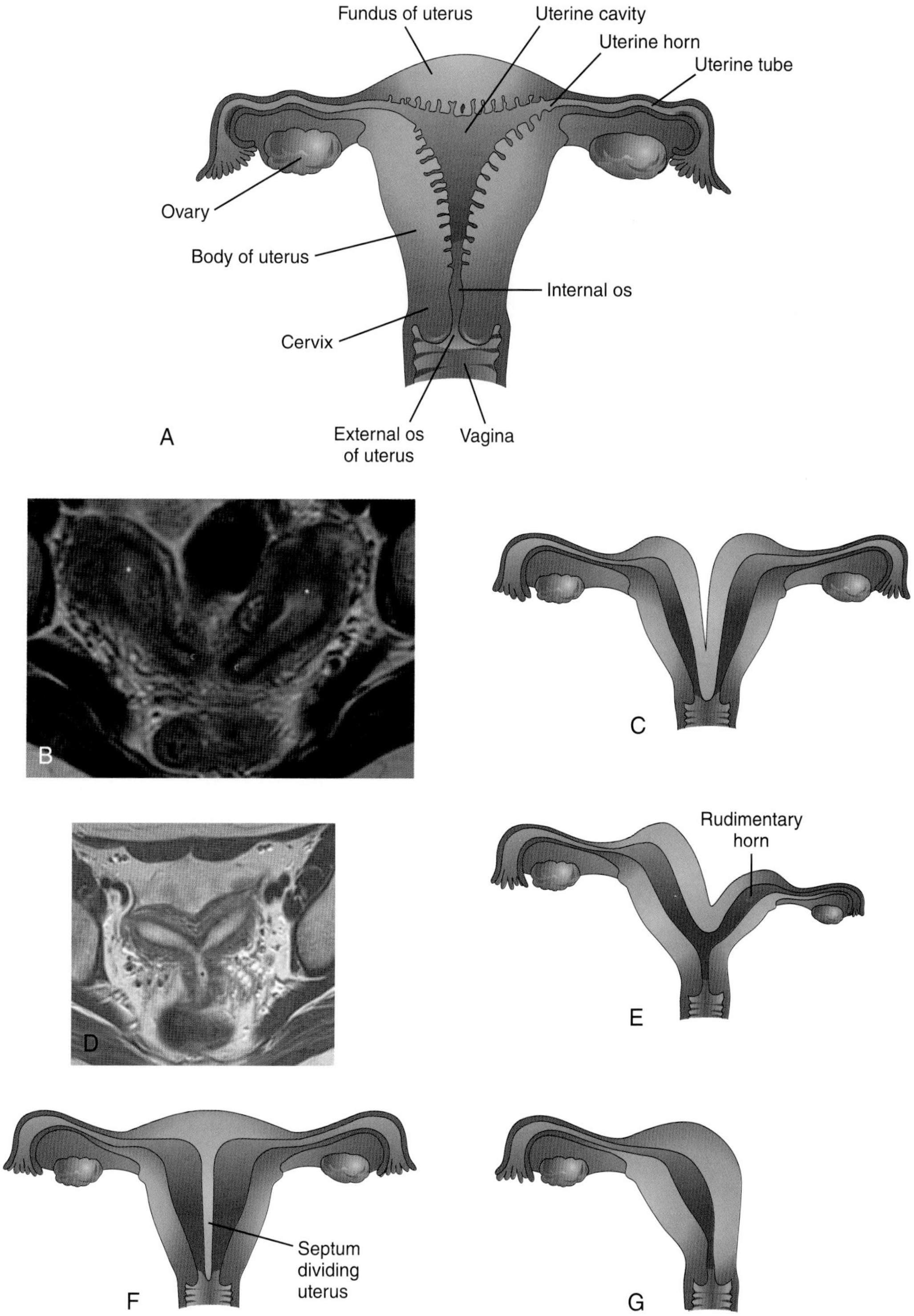

Fig. 12.44 Uterine birth defects. (A) Normal uterus and vagina. (B) Uterus didelphys (double uterus) Axial T2-weighted magnetic resonance (MR) image demonstrates two widely divergent uterine horns (*). Two separate cervices are (C) likewise visualized in the image. (C) Double uterus with single vagina. (D) Bicornuate uterus (two uterine horns). Axial T2-weighted MR image through the level of the proximal vagina in a patient with known bicornate uterus. A prominent vaginal septum (*) is noted. (E) Bicornuate uterus with a rudimentary left horn. (F) Septate uterus; the septum separates the body of the uterus. (G) Unicorn uterus; only one lateral horn exists. ((B, D) From Olpin JD, Moeni A, Willmore RJ, Heilbrun ME: MR imaging of Müllerian fusion anomalies, *Magn Reson Imaging Clin N Am* 25:563, 2017.)

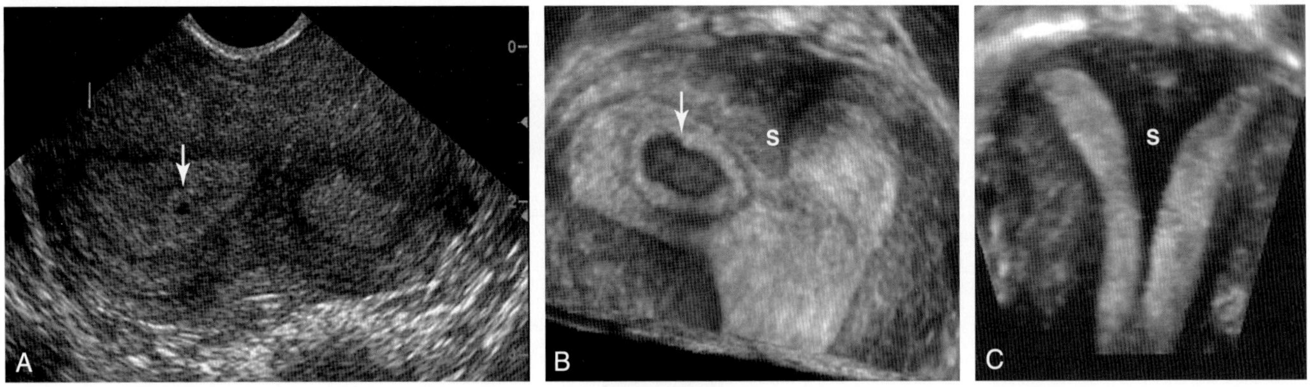

Fig. 12.45 Sonogram of bicornuate uterus. (A) Axial sonogram of the fundus of the uterus showing two separate endometrial canals with a 1-week chorionic (gestational) sac *(arrow)*. (B) A three-dimensional ultrasound scan of the same patient with a 4-week chorionic sac *(arrow)* on the right of a uterine septum *(S)*. (C) Coronal ultrasound scan of a uterus with a large septum *(S)* extending down to the cervix. (Courtesy Dr. E.A. Lyons, Department of Radiology, Health Sciences Centre and University of Manitoba, Winnipeg, Manitoba, Canada.)

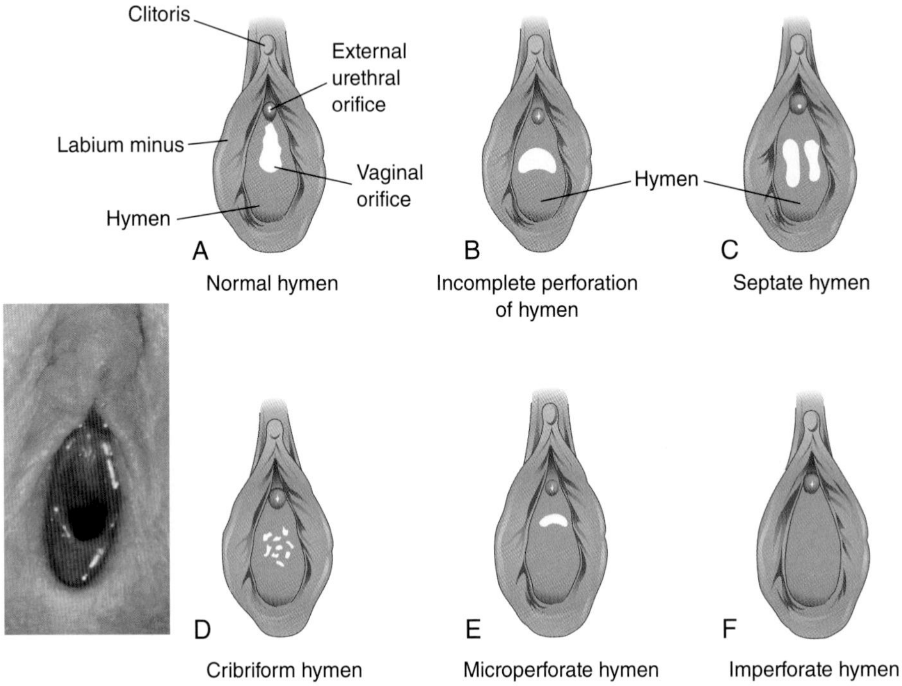

Fig. 12.46 (A–F) Congenital anomalies of the hymen. The normal appearance of the hymen is illustrated in (A) and in the black-and-white photograph *(left)*, which is a normal crescentic hymen in a prepubertal child. (Courtesy Dr. Margaret Morris, Professor of Obstetrics, Gynaecology and Reproductive Sciences, Women's Hospital and University of Manitoba, Winnipeg, Manitoba, Canada.)

12

DEVELOPMENT OF INGUINAL CANALS

The **inguinal canals** form pathways for the testes to descend from the dorsal abdominal wall through the anterior abdominal wall into the scrotum. Inguinal canals develop in both sexes because of the morphologically indifferent stage of sexual development. Through a series of condensations of mesenchyme, a connective tissue structure, the **gubernaculum**, develops on each side of the abdomen from the caudal pole of the gonad (Fig. 12.47A). The gubernaculum passes obliquely through the developing anterior abdominal wall at the site of the future inguinal canal (Fig. 12.47B–D) and is associated cranially with the mesenchyme of the mesonephros.

The **processus vaginalis**, an evagination of the peritoneum, develops ventral to the gubernaculum (a fibrous cord connecting two structures, e.g., the testis and scrotum) and herniates through the abdominal wall along the path formed by this cord (see Fig. 12.47B). The processus vaginalis carries extensions of the layers of the abdominal wall before it, which form the walls of the inguinal canal. These layers also form the coverings of the spermatic cord and testis (see Fig. 12.47D to F). The opening in the transversalis fascia produced by the processus vaginalis becomes the **deep inguinal ring**, and the opening created in the external oblique aponeurosis (broad, flat tendinous portion of the external abdominal oblique muscle) forms the **superficial inguinal ring**.

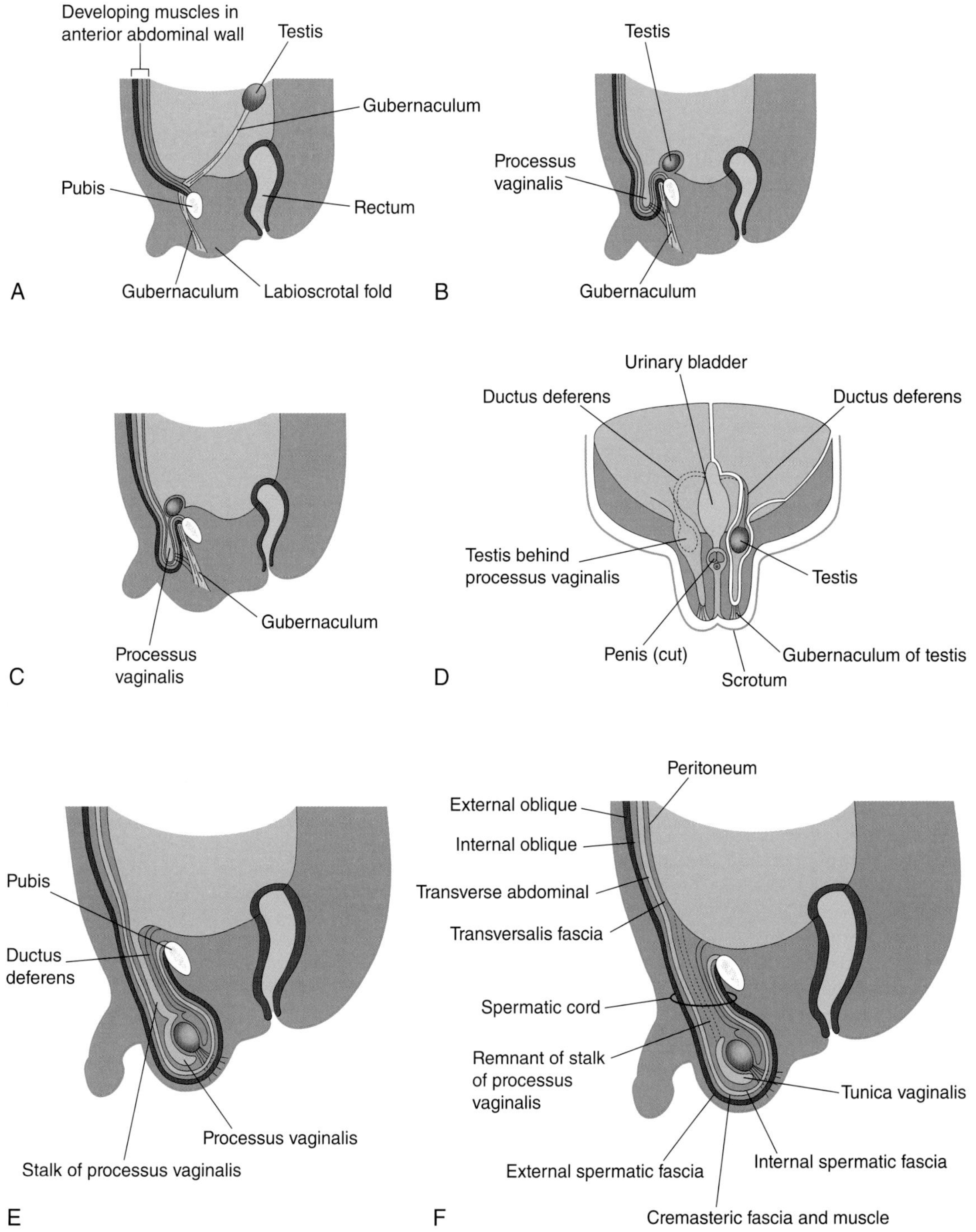

Fig. 12.47 Formation of the inguinal canals and descent of the testes. (A) Sagittal section of a 7-week embryo showing the testis before its descent from the dorsal abdominal wall. (B and C) Similar sections at approximately 28 weeks showing the processus vaginalis and testis beginning to pass through the inguinal canal. Note that the processus vaginalis carries fascial layers of the abdominal wall before it. (D) Frontal section of a fetus approximately 3 days later, illustrating descent of the testis posterior to the processus vaginalis. The processus has been cut away on the left side to show the testis and ductus deferens. (E) Sagittal section of a male neonate showing the processus vaginalis communicating with the peritoneal cavity by a narrow stalk. (F) Similar section of a 1-month-old male infant after obliteration of the stalk of the processus vaginalis. Note that the extended fascial layers of the abdominal wall now form the coverings of the spermatic cord.

12

RELOCATION OF TESTES AND OVARIES

TESTICULAR DESCENT

This descent is associated with:

- Enlargement of the testes and atrophy of the ***mesonephroi*** allowing movement of the testes caudally along the posterior abdominal wall
- Atrophy of the ***paramesonephric ducts*** induced by MIS, enabling the testes to move transabdominally to the deep inguinal rings
- Enlargement of the **processus vaginalis** guiding the testis through the inguinal canal into the scrotum
- Increasing in intraabdominal pressure

By 26 weeks, the testes have usually descended retroperitoneally from the superior lumbar region to the posterior abdominal wall to the deep inguinal rings (see Fig. 12.47B and C). This change in position occurs as the fetal pelvis enlarges and the body or trunk of the embryo elongates. **Transabdominal relocation of the testes** is largely a relative movement that results from the growth of the cranial part of the abdomen away from the future pelvic region. The descent of the testes through the inguinal canals into the scrotum is controlled by androgens (e.g., testosterone) produced by the fetal testes (see Fig. 12.32A). The **gubernaculum** forms a path through the anterior abdominal wall for the processus vaginalis to follow during the formation of the inguinal canal (see Fig. 12.47B–E). Passage of the testis through the inguinal canal may also be aided by the increase in intraabdominal pressure resulting from the growth of abdominal viscera.

Descent of the testes through the inguinal canals into the scrotum usually begins during the 26th week, and in some fetuses, it takes 2 or 3 days. By 32 weeks, both testes are present in the scrotum in most cases. The testes pass external to the peritoneum and processus vaginalis. After the testes enter the scrotum, the inguinal canal contracts around the spermatic cord. More than 97% of full-term neonates have both testes in the scrotum. During the first 3 months after birth, most undescended testes descend into the scrotum.

The mode of descent of the testis explains why the **ductus deferens** crosses anterior to the ureter (see Fig. 12.32A); it also explains the course of the **testicular vessels**. These vessels form when the testes are located high on the posterior abdominal wall. As the testes descend, they carry the ductus deferens and vessels with them, and they are sheathed by the fascial extensions of the abdominal wall (see Fig. 12.47F).

- The extension of the transversalis fascia becomes the **internal spermatic fascia**.
- The extensions of the internal oblique muscle and fascia become the **cremasteric muscle** and **fascia**.
- The extension of the external oblique muscle and aponeurosis become the **external spermatic fascia**.

Within the scrotum, the testis projects into the distal end of the **processus vaginalis**. During the perinatal period, the connecting stalk of the processus normally obliterates, forming a serous membrane, the **tunica vaginalis**, which covers the front and sides of the testis (see Fig. 12.47F).

OVARIAN DESCENT

The ovaries also descend from the lumbar region of the posterior abdominal wall and relocate to the lateral wall of the pelvis; however, they do not pass from the pelvis and enter the inguinal canals. The **gubernaculum** is attached to the uterus near the attachment of the uterine tube. The cranial part of the gubernaculum becomes the **ovarian ligament**, and the caudal part forms the **round ligament of the uterus** (see Fig. 12.32C). The round ligaments pass through the inguinal canals and terminate in the labia majora. The relatively small **processus vaginalis** in the female usually obliterates and disappears long before birth. A persistent processus in the fetus is known as the **processus vaginalis of the peritoneum** (canal of Nuck).

Cryptorchidism

Cryptorchidism (hidden testes) is the most common defect in neonates; it occurs in about 30% of premature males and 3% to 5% of full-term males. This reflects the fact that the testes begin to descend into the scrotum by the end of the second trimester. Cryptorchidism may be unilateral or bilateral. Cryptorchid testes may be in the abdominal cavity or anywhere along the usual path of descent of the testis, but they are usually in the inguinal canal (Fig. 12.48A). The cause of most cases of cryptorchidism is unknown. *Insulin-like peptide 3 (INSL3) is secreted by Leydig cells in the male fetus shortly after sex determination. This hormone controls the formation and shortening of the gubernaculum, which plays a crucial role in the descent of the testes. Disruption in the expression of INSL3 may lead to cryptorchidism.* A deficiency of androgen production by the fetal testes is also an important factor.

In most cases, undescended testes descend into the scrotum by the end of the first year. If both testes remain within or just outside the abdominal cavity, they fail to mature, and sterility is common. Surgical correction is usually carried out by 6 months of age or later when detected.

If cryptorchidism is uncorrected, these males have a significantly higher risk of developing **germ cell tumors**, especially in cases of abdominal cryptorchidism. Undescended testes are often histologically normal at birth, but failure of development and atrophy are detectable by the end of the first year.

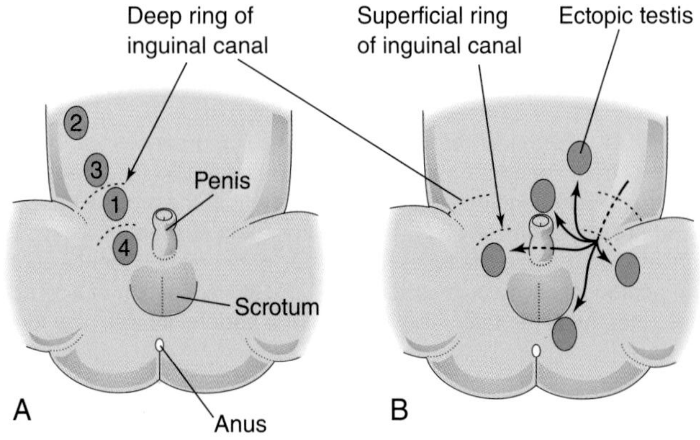

Fig. 12.48 Possible sites of cryptorchid and ectopic testes. (A) Positions of cryptorchid testes, numbered (*1–4*) in order of frequency. (B) Usual locations of ectopic testes.

Ectopic Testes

As the testes pass through the inguinal canal, they may deviate from their usual path of descent and arrive in various abnormal locations (see Fig. 12.48B):

- Interstitial (external to the aponeurosis of the external oblique muscle)
- In the proximal part of the medial thigh
- Dorsal to the penis
- On the opposite side (crossed ectopia)

All types of ectopic testes are rare, but **interstitial ectopia** occurs most frequently. An ectopic testis occurs when a part of the gubernaculum passes to an abnormal location and the testis follows it.

Congenital Inguinal Hernia

If the communication between the tunica vaginalis and the peritoneal cavity fails to close (Fig. 12.49A and B), a **persistent processus vaginalis** exists. A loop of the intestine may herniate through it into the scrotum or labium majora (see Fig. 12.49B).

Embryonic remnants resembling the ductus deferens or epididymis are often found in **inguinal hernial sacs**. Congenital inguinal hernia is much more common in males, especially when there are undescended testes. These hernias are also common with ectopic testes and **androgen insensitivity syndrome** (see Fig. 12.41).

Hydrocele

Occasionally, the abdominal end of the **processus vaginalis** remains open; however, it is too small to permit herniation of the intestine. Peritoneal fluid passes into the **patent processus vaginalis** and forms a **scrotal hydrocele** (see Fig. 12.49D). If only the middle part of the processus vaginalis remains open, fluid may accumulate and give rise to a **hydrocele of the spermatic cord** (see Fig. 12.49C).

SUMMARY OF UROGENITAL SYSTEM

- Development of the urinary and genital systems is intimately associated.
- The urinary system develops before the genital system.
- Three successive kidney systems develop **pronephroi** (nonfunctional), **mesonephroi** (temporary excretory organs), and **metanephroi** (primordia of permanent kidneys).
- The **metanephroi** develop from two sources: the **ureteric buds**, which give rise to the **ureter**, renal pelvis, calices, and collecting tubules, and the metanephrogenic blastema, which gives rise to the **nephrons**.
- At first, the **kidneys** are located in the pelvis; however, they gradually shift position to the abdomen. This apparent migration results from disproportionate growth of the fetal lumbar and sacral regions.

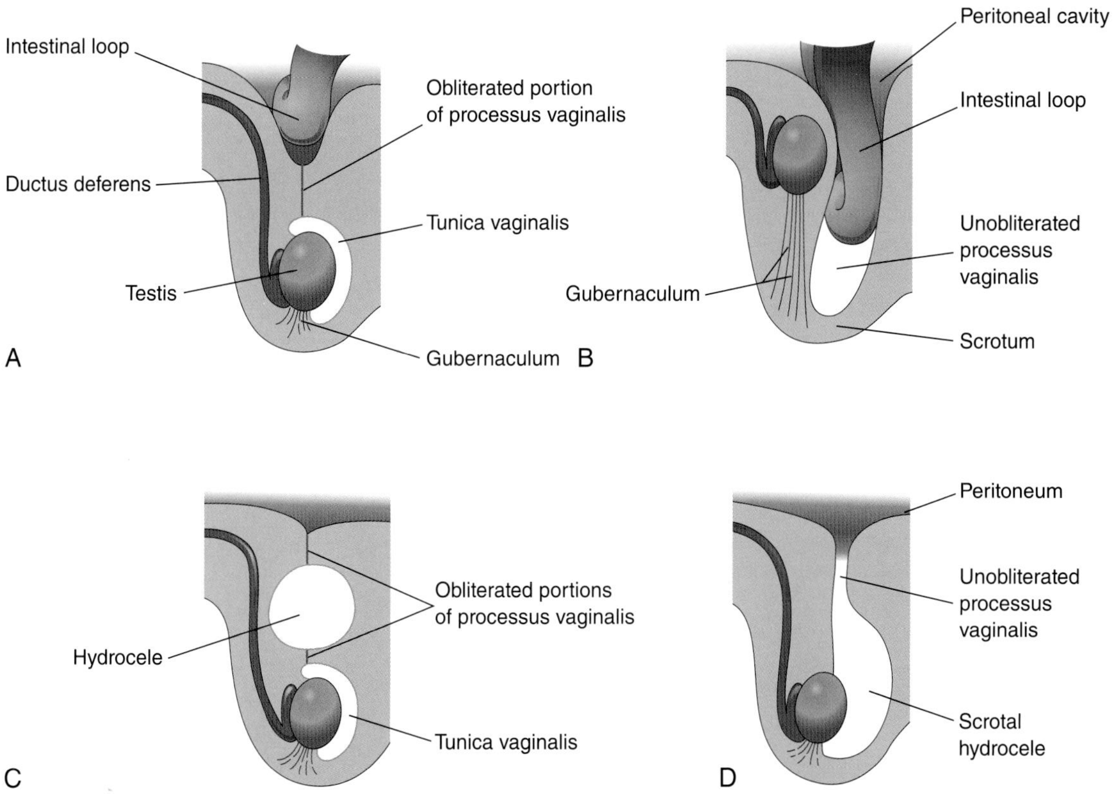

Fig. 12.49 Diagrams of sagittal sections illustrating conditions resulting from failure of closure of the processus vaginalis. (A) Incomplete congenital inguinal hernia resulting from the persistence of the proximal part of the processus vaginalis. (B) Complete congenital inguinal hernia into the scrotum resulting from persistence of the processus vaginalis. Cryptorchidism, a commonly associated defect, is also illustrated. (C) Large hydrocele that resulted from an unobliterated portion of the processus vaginalis. (D) Hydrocele of the testis and spermatic cord resulting from the peritoneal fluid passing into an unobliterated processus vaginalis.

- Birth defects of the kidneys and ureters are common. Incomplete division of the ureteric bud results in a **double ureter** and **supernumerary kidney**. An ectopic kidney that is abnormally rotated results if the developing kidney remains in its embryonic position in the pelvis.
- The **urinary bladder** develops from the **urogenital sinus** and the surrounding splanchnic mesenchyme. The female urethra and most of the male urethra have a similar origin.
- **Exstrophy of the bladder** results from a rare ventral body wall defect through which the posterior wall of the urinary bladder protrudes onto the abdominal wall. **Epispadias** is a commonly associated defect in males; the urethra opens on the dorsum of the penis.
- The **genital system** develops in close association with the urinary system. **Chromosomal sex** is established at fertilization; however, the gonads do not attain sexual characteristics until the seventh week.
- **Primordial germ cells** form in the wall of the **umbilical vesicle** during the fourth week and migrate into the developing gonads, where they differentiate into germ cells (oogonia/spermatogonia).
- The **external genitalia** do not acquire distinct masculine or feminine characteristics until the 12th week. The genitalia develop from primordia that are identical in both sexes.
- **Gonadal sex** is determined by a **testes-determining factor**, which is located on the Y chromosome. Testes-determining factor directs testicular differentiation. The **interstitial cells** (Leydig cells) produce **testosterone**, which stimulates the development of the **mesonephric ducts** into male genital ducts. Testosterone also stimulates the development of the indifferent external genitalia into the penis and scrotum. Anti-müllerian substance (**MIS**), produced by the **Sertoli cells**, inhibits the development of the **paramesonephric ducts** (primordia of the female genital ducts).
- In the absence of a Y chromosome and the presence of two X chromosomes, ovaries develop, the **mesonephric ducts** regress, and the **paramesonephric ducts** develop into the uterus and uterine tubes. The vagina develops from the **vaginal plate** derived from the **urogenital sinus**, and the indifferent external genitalia develops into the clitoris and labia majora and minora.
- Most defects of the female genital tract, such as **double uterus**, result from incomplete fusion of the paramesonephric ducts. **Cryptorchidism** and **ectopic testes** result from abnormalities of testicular descent.
- **Congenital inguinal hernia** and **hydrocele** result from the persistence of the **processus vaginalis**. Failure of the urethral folds to fuse in males results in various types of **hypospadias**.

CLINICALLY ORIENTED PROBLEMS

CASE 12-1

A 4-year-old girl was still in diapers because she was continually wet. The pediatrician saw urine coming from the infant's vagina. An intravenous urogram showed two renal pelves and two ureters on the right side. One ureter was clearly observed to enter the bladder, but the termination of the other one was not clearly seen. A pediatric urologist examined the child under general anesthesia and observed a small opening in the posterior wall of the vagina. The urologist passed a tiny catheter into it and injected contrast media. This procedure showed that the opening in the vagina was the orifice of the second ureter.

- What is the embryologic basis for the two renal pelves and ureters?
- Describe the embryologic basis of an ectopic ureteric orifice.
- What is the anatomic basis of the continual dribbling of urine into the vagina?

CASE 12-2

A radiologist carried out femoral artery catheterization and aortography (radiographic visualization of the aorta and its branches) on a patient who had no brain activity because of having been injured in a motor vehicle collision. The patient's family had agreed to organ donation. The examination showed a single large renal artery on the right but one normal and one small renal artery on the left. Only the right kidney was used for transplantation. Grafting of the small accessory renal artery into the aorta would be difficult because of its size, and part of the kidney would die if one of the arteries was not successfully grafted.

- Are accessory renal arteries common?
- What is the embryologic basis of the two left renal arteries?
- In what other circumstance might an accessory renal artery be of clinical significance?

CASE 12-3

A 32-year-old female with a short history of cramping, lower abdominal pain, and tenderness underwent a laparotomy because of a suspected ectopic pregnancy. The operation revealed a pregnancy in a rudimentary right uterine horn.

- Is this type of uterine birth defect common?
- What is the embryologic basis of the rudimentary uterine horn?

CASE 12-4

During the physical examination of a male neonate, it was observed that the urethra opened on the ventral surface of the penis at the junction of the glans penis and the body of the penis. The penis was curved toward the undersurface of the penis.

- Give the medical terms for the birth defects described.
- What is the embryologic basis of the abnormal urethral orifice?
- Is this anomaly common? Discuss its etiologic basis.

CASE 12-5

A female had previously been prevented from competing in the Olympics because genetic testing revealed an XY chromosome complement.

- Is she a male or a female?
- What is the probable basis for the results of this test?
- Is there an anatomic basis for not allowing her to compete in the Olympics?

CASE 12-6

A 10-year-old boy suffered pain in his left groin while attempting to lift a heavy box. Later he noticed a lump in his groin. When he told his mother about the lump, she arranged an appointment with the family physician. After a physical examination, a diagnosis of indirect inguinal hernia was made.

- Explain the embryologic basis of this type of inguinal hernia.
- Based on your embryologic knowledge, list the layers of the spermatic cord that would cover the hernial sac.

Discussion of problems appears in the Appendix at the back of the book.

BIBLIOGRAPHY AND SUGGESTED READING

Ali MAA, Maalman RS-U, Dankar YO: Ambiguous genitalia: clinical management of adult female with male assigned gender: case report, *J Med Case Rep* 15:362, 2021.

Amândio AR, Lopez-Delisle L, Bolt CC, Mascrez B, Duboule D: A complex regulatory landscape involved in the development of mammalian external genitals. *eLife* 9:e52962, 2020. https://doi.org/10.7554/eLife.5296.

Bakhsh H, Alenizy H, Alenazi S, Alnasser S, Alanazi N, Alsowinea M: Amniotic fluid disorders and the effects on prenatal outcome: a retrospective cohort study, *BMC Pregnancy Childbirth* 21(1):75, 2021. https://doi.org/10.1186/s12884-021-03549-3.

Billmire DF: Germ cell tumors, *Surg Clin North Am* 86:489, 2006.

Bunce C, McKey J, Capel B: Concerted morphogenesis of genital ridges and nephric ducts in the mouse captured through whole-embryo imaging, *Development* 148(18):dev199208, 2021. https://doi.org/10.1242/dev.199208.

Chang J, Wang S, Zheng Z: Etiology of Hypospadias: a comparative review of genetic factors and developmental processes between human and animal models, *Res Rep Urol* 12:673–686, 2020. https://doi.org/10.2147/RRU.S276141.

Cordido A, Vizoso-Gonzalez M, Garcia-Gonzalez MA: Molecular pathophysiology of autosomal recessive polycystic kidney disease, *Int J Mol Sci* 22:6523, 2021.

Cunha GR, Vezina CM, Isaacson D, Ircke WA, Timms BG, Cao M: Development of the human prostate, *Differenitation* 103:24, 2018.

Davies R, Davies L, Alleemudder D, et al: Differences of sexual development and their clinical implications, *TOG Obstetr Gynaecol* 22:257, 2020.

de Bakker BS, van den Hoff MJB, Vize PD, Oostra RJ: The Pronephros; a fresh perspective, *Integr Comp Biol* 59:29, 2019.

Diaz A, Lipman Diaz EG: Disorders of sex development, *Ped Rev* 42(8):414, 2021.

Faa G, Gerosa C, Fanni D, et al: Morphogenesis and molecular mechanisms involved in human kidney development, *J Cell Physiol* 227:1257, 2012.

Fiegel HC, Rolle U, Metzger R, Gfroerer S, Kluth D: Embryology of the testicular descent, *Semin Pediatr Surg* 20:161, 2011.

Fukuoka K, Wilting J, Rodríguez-Vázquez JF, Murakami G, Ishizawa A, Matsubara A: The Embryonic Ascent of the Kidney Revisited, *Anat Rec* 302:278, 2019.

Gates RL, Shelton J, Diefenbach KA, Arnold M, St Peter SD, Renaud EJ: Management of the undescended testis in children: An American Pediatric Surgical Association Outcomes and Evidence Based Practice Committee Systematic Review, *J Pediatr Surg* 57:1293, 2022.

Gulas E, Wysiadecki G, Szymański J, et al: Morphological and clinical aspects of the occurrence of accessory (multiple) renal arteries, *Arch Med Sci* 14(2):442–453, 2018. https://doi.org/10.5114/aoms.2015.55203.

Haller M, Ma L: Temporal, spatial, and genetic regulation of external genitalia development, *Diffrentiation* 110:1, 2019.

Herlin K, Petersen MB, Brannstrom M: Mayer-Rokitansky-Kuster-Hauser (MRKH) syndrome: a comprehensive update, *Orphanet J Rare Dis* 15(1):214, 2020. https://doi.org/10.1186/s13023-020-01491-9.

Hornig NC, Holterhus P-M: Molecular. Basis of androgen insensitivity syndromes, *Mol Cell Endocrin* 523:1, 2021.

Ivell R, Mamsen LS, Andersen CY, Anand-Ivell R: Expression and role of INSL3 in the fetal testis, *Front Endocrinol* 13:868313, 2022. 3389/fendo.2022.868313

Habiba M, Heyn R, Bianchi P, Brosens I, Benagiano G: The development of the human uterus: morphogenesis to menarche, *Hum Reprod Update* 27(1), 2021.

Haynes JH: Inguinal and scrotal disorders, *Surg Clin North Am* 86:371, 2006.

Khan N, Khaliq M, Azam MM, Raja R: Mayer-Rokitansky-Kuster-Hauser syndrome: MR manifestations of typical and atypical cases, *J Ayub Med Coll Abbottabad* 33(Suppl 1):711–716, 2021.

Kluth D, Fiegel HC, Geyer C: Embryology of the distal urethra and external genitals, *Semin Pediatr Surg* 20:176, 2011.

Kraft KH, Shukla AR, Canning DA: Hypospadia, *Urol Clin North Am* 37:167, 2010.

Kutney K, Konczal L, Kaminski B, Uli N: Review – challenges in the diagnosis and management of disorders of sex development, *Birth Defects Res C Embryo Today* 108:293, 2016.

Kuure S, Vuolteenaho R, Vainio S: Kidney morphogenesis: cellular and molecular regulation, *Mech Dev* 92:19, 2000.

Larney C, Bailey TYL, Koopman P: Switching on sex: transcriptional regulation of the testis-determining gene *Sry*, *Development* 141:2195, 2014.

Lindström NO, Lawrence ML, Burn SF, et al: Integrated β-catenin, BMP, PTEN, and Notch signaling patterns the nephron, *eLife* 3:e04000, 2015. https://doi.org/10.7554/eLife.04000.

Little M, Georgas K, Pennisi D, Wilkinson L: Kidney development: two tales of tubulogenesis, *Curr Top Dev Biol* 90:193, 2010.

Lozic M, Minarik L, Racetin A, et al: *AIF*, *BCL2*, and *UBASH3A* during human kidney development, *Int J Mol Sci* 22(17):9183, 2021. https://doi.org/10.3390/ijms22179183.

Meeks J, Schaeffer EM: Genetic regulation of prostate development, *J Androl* 32:210, 2011.

Mehmood KT, Rentea RM: *Ambiguous genitalia and disorders of sexual differentiation. [Updated 2022 May 8]*. In *StatPearls [Internet]*, Treasure Island, 2022, StatPearls Publishing. Available from: https://www.ncbi.nlm.nih.gov/books/NBK557435/.

Mullen RD, Bellessort B, Levi G, Behringer RR: *Distal-less* homeobox genes *Dlx5/6* regulate Müllerian duct regression, *Front Endocrinol (Lausanne)* 13:916173, 2022. https://doi.org/10.3389/fendo.2022.916173 PMID: 35909540; PMCID: PMC9334558.

Murugapoopathy V, Gupta IR: A primer on congenital anomalies of the kidneys and urinary tracts (CAKUT), *Clin J Am Soc Nephrol* 15(5):723–731, 2020. Epub 2020 Mar 18. PMID: 32188635; PMCID: PMC7269211. https://doi.org/10.2215/CJN.12581019.

Nebot-Cegarra J, Fàbregas PJ, Sánchez-Pérez I: Cellular proliferation in the urorectal septation complex of the human embryo at Carnegie stages 13–18: a nuclear area-based morphometric analysis, *J Anat* 207:353, 2005.

Nguyen V, Ngo L, Jaqua EE. Cryptorchidism (undescended testicle). *Am Fam Physician* 108(4):378–385, 2023.

Odiba AO, Dick JM: Fetal genitourinary tract. In Norton ME, editor: *Callen's ultrasonography in obstetrics and gynecology*, ed 6, Philadelphia, 2017, Elsevier.

Overland MR, Li Y, Derpinghaus A, et al: Development of the human ovary: fetal through pubertal ovarian morphology, folliculogenesis, and expression of cellular differentiation markers. *Differentiation* 129:37–59, 2023. Available from: https://doi.org/j.diff.2022.10.005.

Persaud TVN: Embryology of the female genital tract and gonads. In Copeland LJ, Jarrell J, editors: *Textbook of gynecology*, ed 2, Philadelphia, 2000, Saunders.

Poder L: Ultrasound evaluation of the uterus. In Norton ME, editor: *Callen's ultrasonography in obstetrics and gynecology*, ed 6, Philadelphia, 2017, Elsevier.

Profeta G, Micangeli G, Tarani F, Paparella R, Ferraguti G, Spaziani M: Sexual developmental disorder in pediatrics, *Clin Ter* 173:475, 2022.

Pradhay G, Gopidas GS, Karumathil Pullara S, Mathew G, Mathew AJ, Sukumaran TT: Prevalence and relevance of multiple renal arteries: a radioanatomical perspective, *Cureus* 13(10):e18957, 2021. https://doi.org/10.7759/cureus.18957.

Rieke JM, Zhang R, Braun D, Yilmaz Ö, Japp AS, Lopes FM: *SLC20A1* is involved in urinary tract and urorectal development, *Front Cell Dev Biol* 8:567, 2020. SLC20A1Is Involved in Urinary Tract and Urorectal Development. https://doi.org/10.3389/fcell.2020.00567

Rodprasert W, Virtanen HE, Mäkelä JA, Toppari J: Hypogonadism and Cryptorchidism, *Front Endocrinol (Lausanne)* 10:906, 2020. https://doi.org/10.3389/fendo.2019.00906.

Schuh MP, Alkhudairy L, Potter A, Potter SS, Chetal K, Thakkar K: The Rhesus Macaque serves as a model for human lateral branch nephrogenesis, *J Am Soc Nephrol* 32(5):1097–1112, 2021. https://doi.org/10.1681/ASN.2020101459.

Seth A, Rivera A, Chahdi A, Choi IS, Medina-Martinez O, Lewis S: Gene dosage changes in *KCTD13* result in penile and testicular anomalies via diminished androgen receptor function, *FASEB J*(11), 2022. https://doi.org/10.1096/fj.202200558R.

Smyth IM: Development of the metanephric kidney. (Chapter) *Curr Top Developmental Biol* 14(3):111–1150, 2020. https://www.doi.org.10.1016/bs.ctdb.2020.09.003.

Sreenivasan R, Gonen N, Sinclair A: SOX genes and their role in disorders of sex development, *Sex Dev* 16:80, 2022.

Stec AA: Embryology and bony and pelvic floor anatomy in the bladder and exstrophy-epispadias complex, *Semin Pediatr Surg* 20:66, 2011.

Stein D, McNamara E: Congenital anomalies of the kidneys and urinary tract, *Clin Perinatol* 49:791, 2022.

Taglienti M, Graf D, Schumacher V, Kreidberg JA: BMP7 drives proximal tubule expansion and determines nephron number in the developing kidney, *Development* 149, 2022. https://doi.org/10.1242/dev.200773.

van der Ven AT, Connaughton DM, Ityel H, Mann N, Nakayama M, Chen J: Whole-Exome sequencing identifies causative mutations in families with congenital anomalies of the kidney and urinary tract, *J Am Soc Nephrol* 29(9):2348–2361, 2018 Sep. https://doi.org/10.1681/ASN.2017121265.

Witschi E: Migration of the germ cells of human embryos from the yolk sac to the primitive gonadal folds, *Contr Embryol Carnegie Inst* 32:67, 1948.

Yatsenko SA, Witchel SF: Genetic approach to ambiguous genitalia and disorders of sex development: what clinicians need to know, *Semin Perinatol* 41(4):232–243, 2017.

Cardiovascular System

13

CHAPTER OUTLINE

The cardiovascular system is the first major system to function in the embryo. The primordial heart and vascular system appear in the middle of the third week (Fig. 13.1). This precocious cardiac development occurs because diffusion alone cannot supply the nutritional and oxygen requirements of the rapidly developing embryo. Consequently, there is a need for an efficient method of acquiring oxygen and nutrients from the maternal blood and disposing of carbon dioxide and waste products.

Multipotential cardiac progenitor cells from several sources contribute to the formation of the heart. Specified cardiac progenitor cells expressing *Nkx2-5* can already be identified during gastrulation. These include two distinct mesodermal populations of cardiac precursor cells, a primary (first) heart field, and a second heart field. Neural crest cells also contribute to the heart. Mesodermal cells from the primitive streak migrate to form bilaterally paired strands of the **primary heart field.** Cardiac progenitor cells from the pharyngeal mesoderm are constituted as the **second heart field**, which is located medial to the first heart field. The first heart field contributes to the formation of the left ventricle and part of the atrium; the right ventricle, the atria, and the sinus venosus are derived from cardiac progenitor cells of the second heart field.

Successive stages in the development of blood and blood vessels are described in Fig. 4.11. Primordial blood vessels cannot be distinguished structurally as arteries or veins; however, they are named according to their future fates and relationship to the heart.

EARLY DEVELOPMENT OF HEART AND BLOOD VESSELS

13

By day 18, the bilateral mesoderm has somatopleure and splanchnopleure components; the latter gives rise to almost

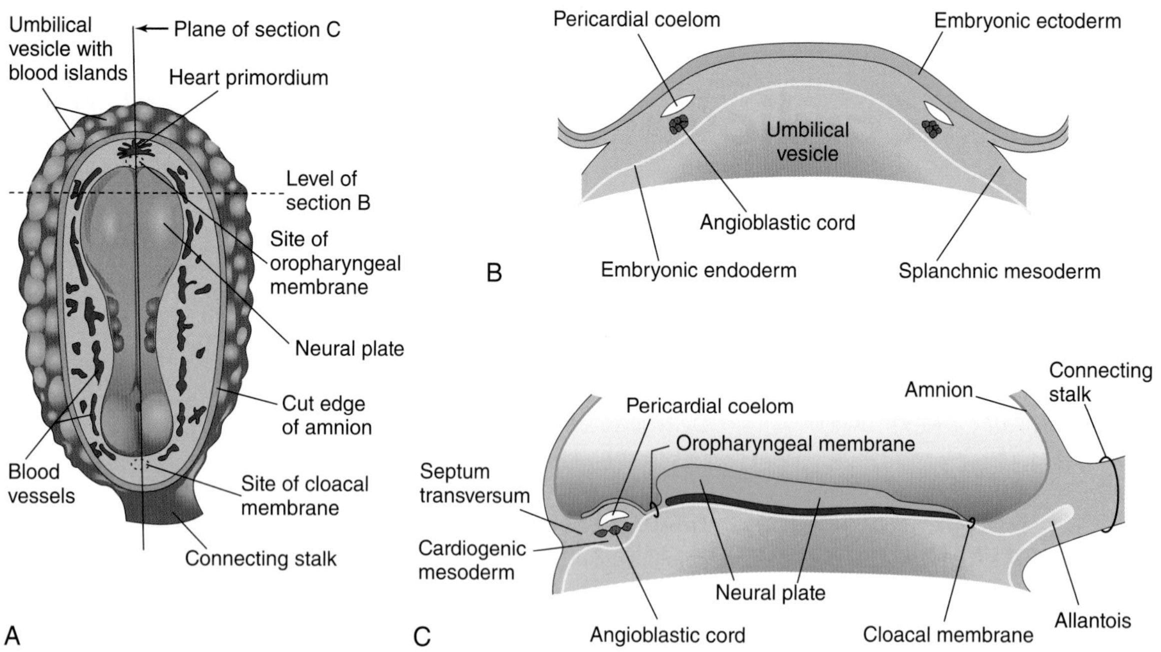

Fig. 13.1 Early development of the heart. (A) Drawing of a dorsal view of an embryo (approximately 18 days). (B) Transverse section of the embryo showing the angioblastic cords in the cardiogenic mesoderm and their relationship to the pericardial coelom. (C) Longitudinal section of the embryo illustrating the relationship of the angioblastic cords to the oropharyngeal membrane, pericardial coelom, and septum transversum.

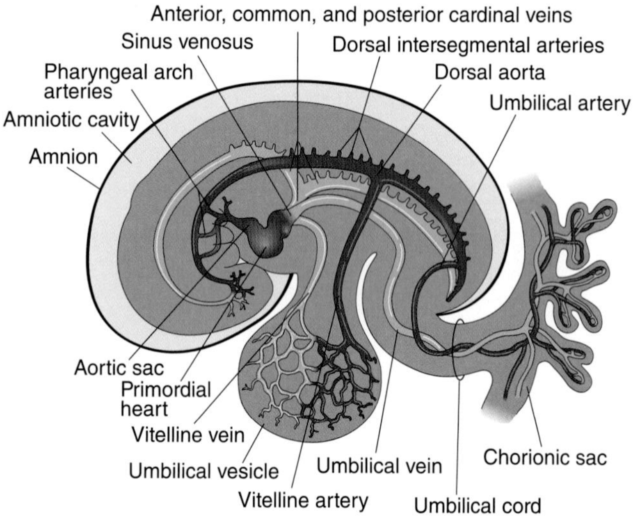

Fig. 13.2 Drawing of the embryonic cardiovascular system (approximately 26 days), showing vessels on the left side. The umbilical vein carries well-oxygenated blood and nutrients from the chorionic sac to the embryo. The umbilical arteries carry poorly oxygenated blood and waste products from the embryo to the chorionic sac (outermost embryonic membrane).

all of the heart components. These early endocardial progenitor cells separate from the mesoderm to create paired heart tubes. As lateral embryonic folding occurs, the **endocardial heart tubes** approach each other and fuse to form a single **heart tube** (see Figs. 13.7C and 13.9C). Shortening of the endoderm plays an important mechanical role in the formation of the tubular heart. Fusion of the heart tubes begins at the cranial end of the developing heart and extends caudally. *The embryonic heart begins to beat* at approximately days 22 and 23 (Fig. 13.2). Blood flow begins during the fourth week, and heartbeats can be visualized by Doppler ultrasonography (Fig. 13.3).

A multitude of genes and transcription factors (*Pax, NKX, Brachyury, Msp1and others*), are involved in the development of the mammalian heart, which includes lineage determination, specification of the cardiac chambers, valvuloseptal development, and formation of the conducting system.

Gene expression analysis and lineage tracing experiments suggest that progenitor cells from the pharyngeal mesoderm, located anterior to the early heart tube **(anterior heart field)**, give rise to ventricular myocardium and the myocardial wall of the outflow tract. *Expression of Smarcd3, Nkx2.5, Pax 3, Pax 9, and Id genes, an inhibitor of DNA binding 1, HLH protein, are important for the early specification of cardiogenic progenitors of the first heart field that will form the heart tubes.* Moreover, another wave of progenitor cells from the pharyngeal mesoderm **(second heart field)** also contributes to the rapid growth and elongation of the heart tube. The myocardium of the left ventricle and the anterior pole of the heart tube are derived mostly from the second field. *Pax genes and expression of transcription factors Nkx2.5 and Hes-1 in pharyngeal endoderm and mesoderm (second heart field) play an essential role in the development of the outflow tract.*

The basic helix-loop-helix genes, dHAND *and* eHAND, *are expressed in the paired primordial endocardial tubes and the later stages of cardiac morphogenesis. The* MEF2C *and* Pitx-2 *genes, which are expressed in cardiogenic precursor cells emerging from the primitive streak before the formation of the heart tubes (Wnt 3a mediated), are essential regulators in early cardiac development.*

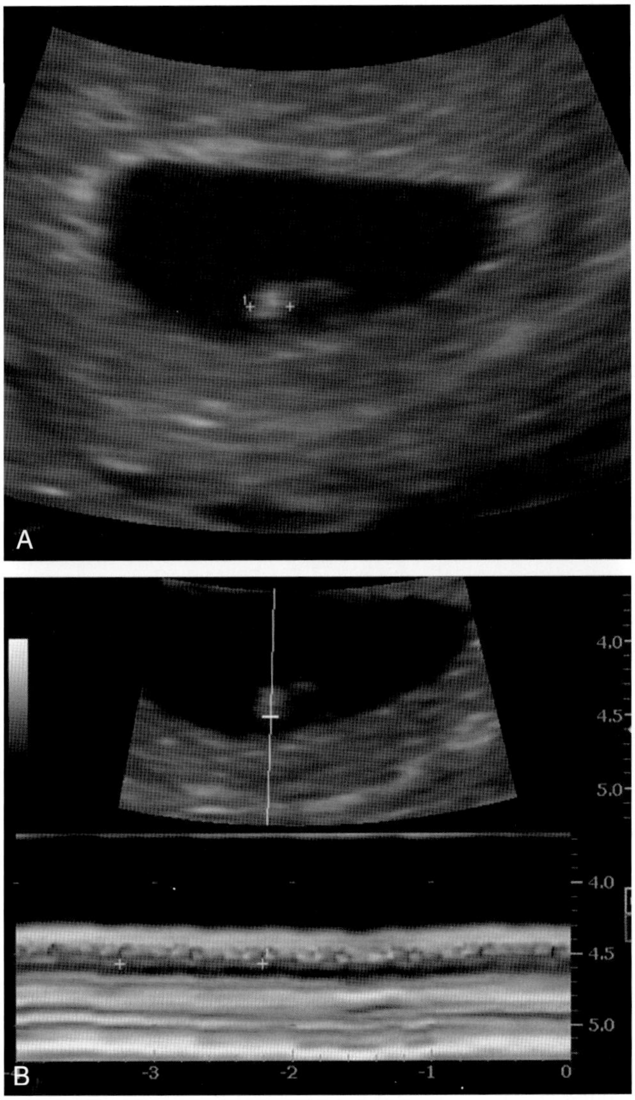

Fig. 13.3 Endovaginal scan of a 4-week embryo. (A) Bright (echogenic) 2.4-mm embryo *(calipers)*. (B) Cardiac activity of 116 beats/min demonstrated with motion mode. *Calipers* used to encompass two beats. (Courtesy Dr. E.A. Lyons, Professor of Radiology, Obstetrics and Gynecology, and Human Anatomy, University of Manitoba and Health Sciences Centre, Winnipeg, Manitoba, Canada.)

DEVELOPMENT OF VEINS ASSOCIATED WITH EMBRYONIC HEART

Three paired veins drain into the primordial heart of a 4-week embryo (see Fig. 13.2):

- **Vitelline veins** return poorly oxygenated blood from the umbilical vesicle.
- **Umbilical veins** carry well-oxygenated blood from the placenta.
- **Common cardinal veins** return poorly oxygenated blood from the body of the embryo to the heart.

The **vitelline veins** follow the omphaloenteric duct into the embryo. This duct is the narrow tube connecting the umbilical vesicle with the midgut (see Fig. 11.1). After passing through the septum transversum, which provides a pathway for blood vessels, the vitelline veins enter the venous end of the heart, the **sinus venosus** (Fig. 13.4A; see also Fig. 13.2). The left vitelline vein regresses, and the right vitelline vein forms most of the **hepatic portal system** (see Fig. 13.5B and C), as well as a portion of the **inferior vena cava (IVC)**. As the **liver primordium** grows into the septum transversum, the **hepatic cords** anastomose around preexisting endothelium-lined spaces. These spaces, the primordia of the **hepatic sinusoids**, later become linked to the vitelline veins.

The **umbilical veins** run on each side of the liver and carry well-oxygenated blood from the placenta to the sinus venosus (see Fig. 13.2). As the liver develops, the umbilical veins lose their connection with the heart and empty into the liver.

Transformation of the umbilical veins may be summarized as follows (Fig. 13.5):

- The right umbilical vein and the cranial part of the left umbilical vein between the liver and the sinus venosus degenerate.
- The persistent caudal part of the left umbilical vein becomes the **umbilical vein**, which carries all the blood from the placenta to the embryo.
- A large venous shunt, the **ductus venosus**, develops within the liver (see Fig. 13.5B) and connects the umbilical vein with the IVC. The ductus venosus forms a bypass through the liver, enabling most of the blood from the placenta to pass directly to the heart without passing through the developing capillary networks of the liver.

The **cardinal veins** constitute the main venous drainage system of the embryo (see Figs. 13.2 and 13.4A). The **anterior and posterior cardinal veins**, the earliest veins to develop, drain cranial and caudal parts of the embryo, respectively. They join the **common cardinal veins**, which enter the sinus venosus (see Fig. 13.2). During the eighth week, the **anterior cardinal veins** are connected by an **anastomosis** (see Fig. 13.5A and B), which shunts blood from the left to the right anterior cardinal vein. This anastomotic shunt becomes the **left brachiocephalic vein** when the caudal part of the left anterior cardinal vein degenerates (see Figs. 13.4D and 13.5C). The **superior vena cava (SVC)** forms from the right anterior cardinal vein and the right common cardinal vein.

The **posterior cardinal veins** develop primarily as the vessels of the **mesonephroi** and largely disappear with these transitory kidneys (see Fig. 12.5F). The only adult derivatives of these veins are the root of the azygos vein and common iliac veins (see Fig. 13.4D). The subcardinal and supracardinal veins gradually develop and replace and supplement the posterior cardinal veins (see Fig. 13.4A–D).

The **subcardinal veins** appear first (see Fig. 13.4A). They are connected through the **subcardinal anastomosis** and with the posterior cardinal veins through the mesonephric sinusoids. The subcardinal veins form the stem of the left renal vein, the suprarenal veins, the gonadal veins (testicular and ovarian), and a segment of the IVC (see Fig. 13.4D). The supracardinal veins become disrupted in the region of the kidneys (see Fig. 13.4C). Cranial to this region, they are united by an anastomosis that is represented in the adult by the **azygos** and **hemiazygos veins** (see Figs. 13.4D and 13.5C). Caudal to the kidneys, the left supracardinal vein degenerates; however, the right supracardinal vein becomes the inferior part of the IVC (see Fig. 13.4D).

DEVELOPMENT OF INFERIOR VENA CAVA

The IVC forms during a series of changes in the primordial veins of the trunk, which occur when blood, returning from the caudal part of the embryo, is shifted from the left to the right side of the body. The IVC is composed of four main segments (Fig. 13.4C):

- A **hepatic segment** derived from the hepatic vein (proximal part of the right vitelline vein) and hepatic sinusoids
- A **prerenal segment** derived from the right subcardinal vein
- A **renal segment** derived from the subcardinal-supracardinal anastomosis
- A **postrenal segment** derived from the right supracardinal vein

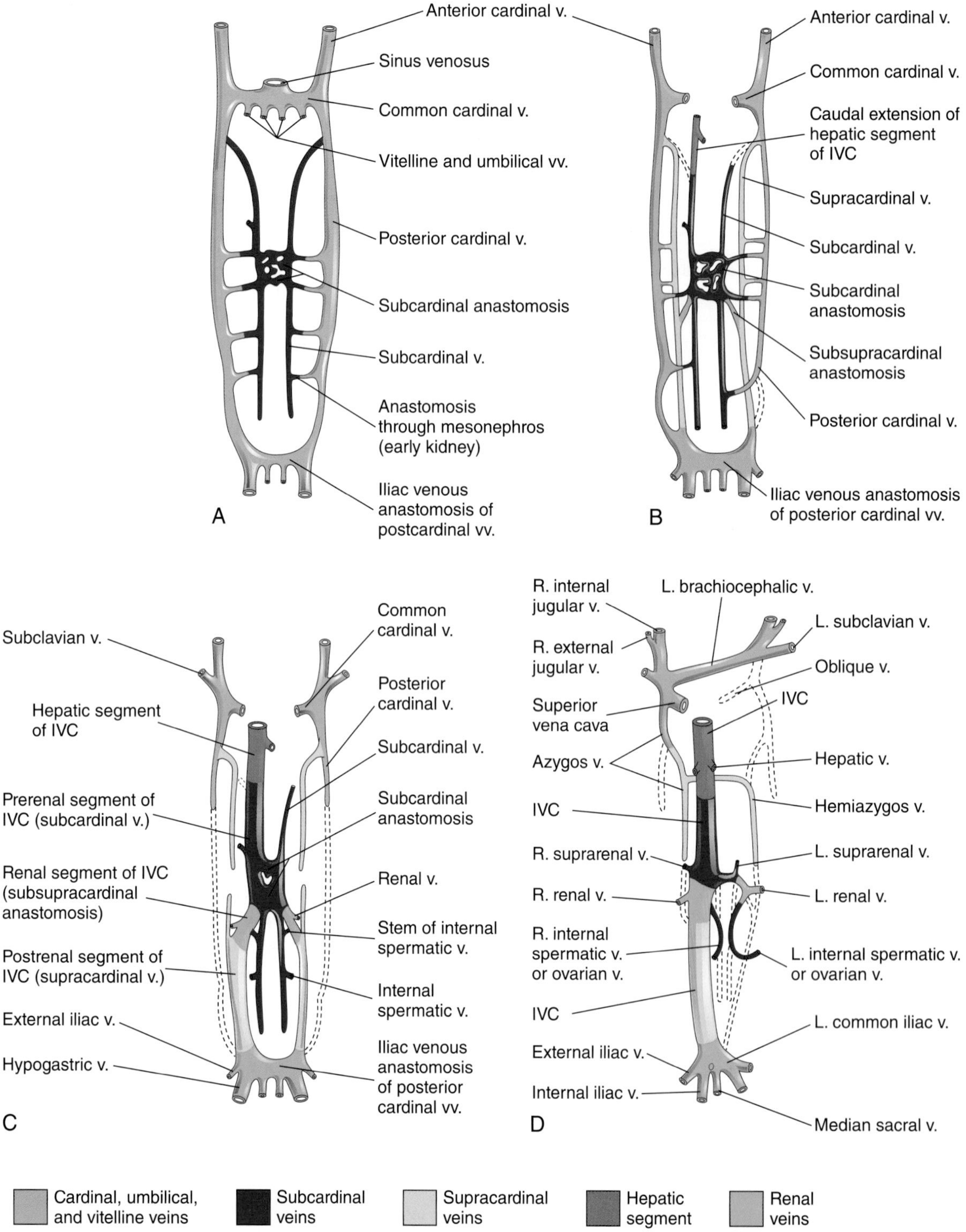

Fig. 13.4 (A) Illustrations of the primordial veins of bodies (trunks) of embryos (ventral views). Initially, three systems of veins are present: the umbilical veins from the chorion, vitelline veins from the umbilical vesicle, and cardinal veins from the body of the embryos. Next the subcardinal veins appear, and finally the supracardinal veins develop. (A) At 6 weeks. (B) At 7 weeks. (C) At 8 weeks. (D) Adult. This drawing illustrates the transformations that produce the adult venous pattern. *IVC,* Inferior vena cava; *L.,* left; *R.,* right; *v.,* vein; *vv.,* veins. Modified from Arey LB: *Developmental anatomy,* revised ed 7, Philadelphia, 1974, Saunders.)

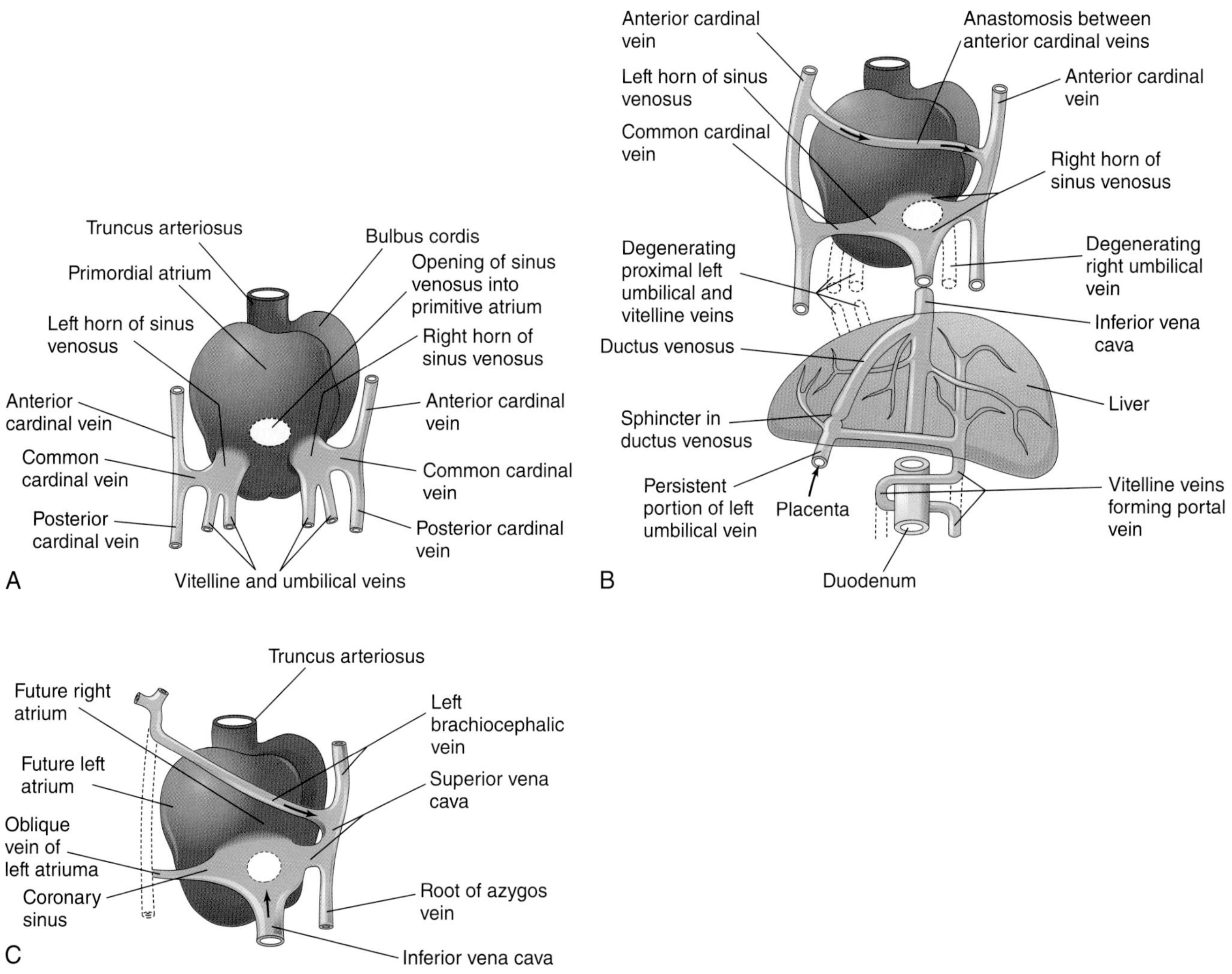

Fig. 13.5 Dorsal views of the developing heart. (A) During the fourth week (approximately 24 days), showing the primordial atrium and sinus venosus and the veins draining into them. (B) At 7 weeks, showing the enlarged right sinus horn and venous circulation through the liver. The organs are not drawn to scale. (C) At 8 weeks, indicating the adult derivatives of the cardinal veins shown in (A) and (B).

Anomalies of Venae Cavae

Because of the many transformations that occur during the formation of the SVC and IVC, variations in their adult forms may occur. The most common anomaly of the IVC is for its abdominal course to be interrupted; as a result, blood drains from the lower limbs, abdomen, and pelvis to the heart through the azygos system of veins.

Double Superior Venae Cavae

Persistence of the left anterior cardinal vein results in a **persistent left SVC** (~3:1000); hence, there are two superior venae cavae (Fig. 13.6). The anastomosis that usually forms the left brachiocephalic vein is small or absent. The abnormal left SVC, derived from the left anterior cardinal and common cardinal veins, opens into the right atrium through the coronary sinus. Almost all cases are asymptomatic.

Persistent Left Superior Vena Cava

The left anterior cardinal vein and common cardinal vein may form a left SVC, and the right anterior cardinal vein and common cardinal vein, which usually form the SVC, degenerate. As a result, blood from the right side is carried by the brachiocephalic vein to the unusual left SVC, which, in 80% to 90% of cases, empties into a dilated coronary sinus. The incidence is approximately 3–5:1000.

Interrupted IVC With Azygous Continuation

Occasionally, the hepatic segment of the IVC fails to form (6:1000). As a result, blood from inferior parts of the body drains into the right atrium through the azygos and hemiazygos veins. The hepatic veins open separately into the right atrium.

Double Inferior Venae Cavae

In these cases (2–30:1000), the IVC inferior to the renal veins is represented by two vessels; usually, the left one is much smaller. This condition probably results from the failure of an anastomosis to develop between the veins of the trunk (see Fig. 13.4B). As a result, the inferior part of the left supracardinal vein persists as a second IVC. Less frequent is the absence of the infrarenal IVC with an interrupted IVC and azygous involvement.

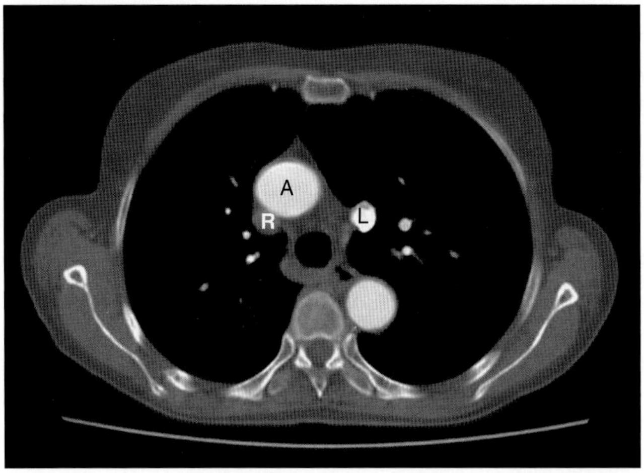

Fig. 13.6 Computed tomography scan showing a duplicated superior vena cava. Note the aorta *(A)*, the right superior vena cava (*R*, unopacified), and the left superior vena cava (*L*, with contrast from left arm injection). (Courtesy Dr. Blair Henderson, Department of Radiology, Health Sciences Centre, University of Manitoba, Winnipeg, Manitoba, Canada.)

PHARYNGEAL ARCH ARTERIES AND OTHER BRANCHES OF DORSAL AORTAE

As the pharyngeal arches form during the fourth and fifth weeks, they are supplied by arteries, the **pharyngeal arch arteries** that arise from the **aortic sac** and terminate in the **dorsal aortae** (see Fig. 13.2). Neural crest cells contribute to the formation of the outflow tract of the heart and the pharyngeal arch arteries. Initially, the paired dorsal aortae run through the entire length of the embryo. Later, the caudal portions of the aortae fuse to form a single lower thoracic/abdominal aorta. Of the remaining paired dorsal aortae, the right one regresses, and the left one becomes the primordial aorta.

INTERSEGMENTAL ARTERIES

Thirty or so branches of the dorsal aorta, the **intersegmental arteries**, pass between and carry blood to the somites and their derivatives (see Fig. 13.2). These arteries in the neck join to form a longitudinal artery on each side, the **vertebral artery**. Most of the original connections of the arteries to the dorsal aorta disappear. Rarely, the second cervical intersegmental artery may persist.

In the thorax, the intersegmental arteries persist as **intercostal arteries**. Most of the intersegmental arteries in the abdomen become **lumbar arteries**; however, the fifth pair of lumbar intersegmental arteries remains as the **common iliac arteries**. In the sacral region, the intersegmental arteries form the **lateral sacral arteries**.

FATE OF VITELLINE AND UMBILICAL ARTERIES

The unpaired ventral branches of the **dorsal aorta** supply the umbilical vesicle, allantois, and chorion (see Fig. 13.2). The **vitelline arteries** pass to the umbilical vesicle and later to the primordial gut, which forms from the incorporated part of the umbilical vesicle. Only three vitelline artery derivatives remain: the celiac arterial trunk to the foregut, the superior mesenteric artery to the midgut, and the inferior mesenteric artery to the hindgut.

The paired **umbilical arteries** pass through the connecting stalk (primordial umbilical cord) and become continuous with vessels in the **chorion**, the embryonic part of the placenta (see Fig. 7.5). The umbilical arteries carry poorly oxygenated blood to the placenta (see Fig. 13.2). The proximal parts of these arteries become **internal iliac arteries** and **superior vesical arteries**. The distal parts of the umbilical arteries become modified and form the **medial umbilical ligaments**.

LATER DEVELOPMENT OF HEART

The external layer of the embryonic heart tube, the primordial **myocardium**, is formed from splanchnic mesoderm surrounding the pericardial cavity (cardiac precursors of the anterior, or second, heart field; Figs. 13.7A and B and 13.8B). At this stage, the developing heart is composed of a thin endothelial tube, separated from a thick myocardium by a gelatinous extracellular matrix of connective tissue, cardiac jelly (see Fig. 13.8C and D). Cardiac jelly not only provides a form of skeletal framework for the development of the heart but also appears to assist in the pumping function of the early valveless heart.

The **endothelial tube** becomes the internal endothelial lining of the heart, or **endocardium**, and the primordial myocardium becomes the muscular wall of the heart, or **myocardium**. The visceral pericardium, or epicardium, is derived from mesothelial cells that arise from the external surface of the **sinus venosus** and spread over the myocardium (see Fig. 13.7D and F).

As folding of the head region occurs, the heart and pericardial cavity come to lie ventral to the foregut and caudal to the **oropharyngeal membrane** (Fig. 13.9A–C). Concurrently, the tubular heart elongates and develops alternate dilations and constrictions (see Fig. 13.7C–E): the **bulbus cordis** (composed of the **truncus arteriosus, conus arteriosus,** and **conus cordis**), ventricle, atrium, and **sinus venosus**. The growth of the heart tube results from the addition of cells, cardiomyocytes, differentiating from mesoderm at the dorsal wall of the pericardium. Progenitor cells added to the rostral and caudal poles of the heart tube form a proliferative pool of mesodermal cells located in the dorsal wall of the pericardial cavity and the pharyngeal arches.

The **truncus arteriosus** is continuous cranially with the aortic sac from which the pharyngeal arch arteries arise (Fig. 13.10A). Progenitor cells from the **second heart field** and cranial neural crest cells contribute to the formation of the arterial and venous ends of the developing heart. The **sinus venosus** receives the umbilical, vitelline, and common cardinal veins from the chorion, umbilical vesicle, and embryo, respectively (Fig. 13.10B). The arterial and venous ends of the heart are fixed by the pharyngeal arches and septum transversum, respectively. The tubular heart undergoes a dextral (right-handed) looping at approximately 23 to 28 days, forming a U-shaped D-loop **(bulboventricular loop)** that results in a heart with its apex pointing to the left (see Figs. 13.7D and E and 13.8E). *Before the formation of the heart tube, the homeobox transcription factor (Pitx2c) is expressed in the left heart-forming field and plays an important role in the left-right patterning of the heart tube during the formation of the cardiac loop.* As the primordial

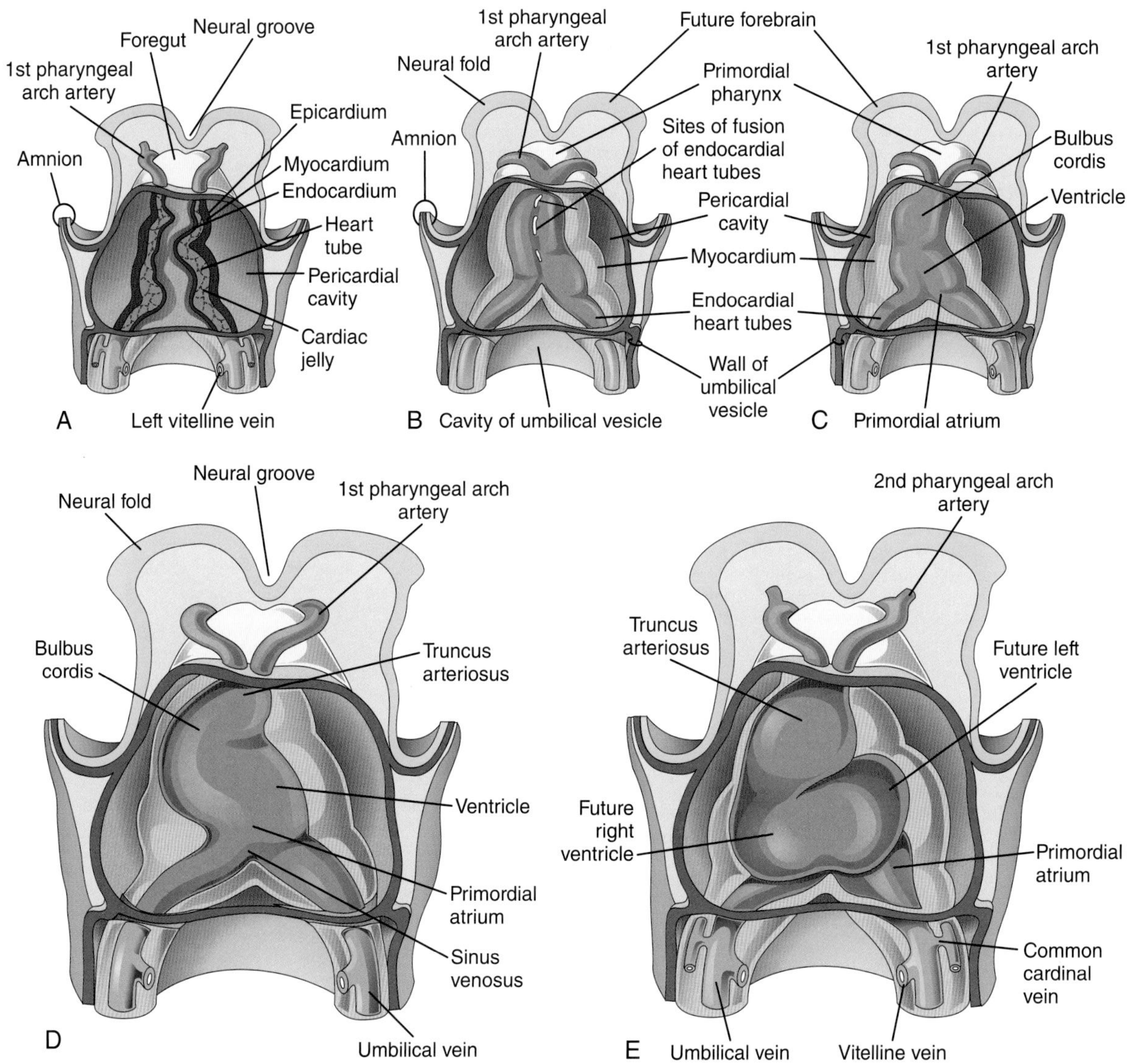

Fig. 13.7 Drawings showing fusion of the heart tubes and looping of the tubular heart. (A–C) Ventral views of the developing heart and pericardial region (22–35 days). The ventral pericardial wall has been removed to show the developing myocardium and fusion of the two heart tubes to form a tubular heart. The endothelium of the heart tube forms the endocardium of the heart. (D and E) As the straight tubular heart elongates, it bends and undergoes looping, which forms a D-loop (D, dextro; rightward) that produces an S-shaped heart.

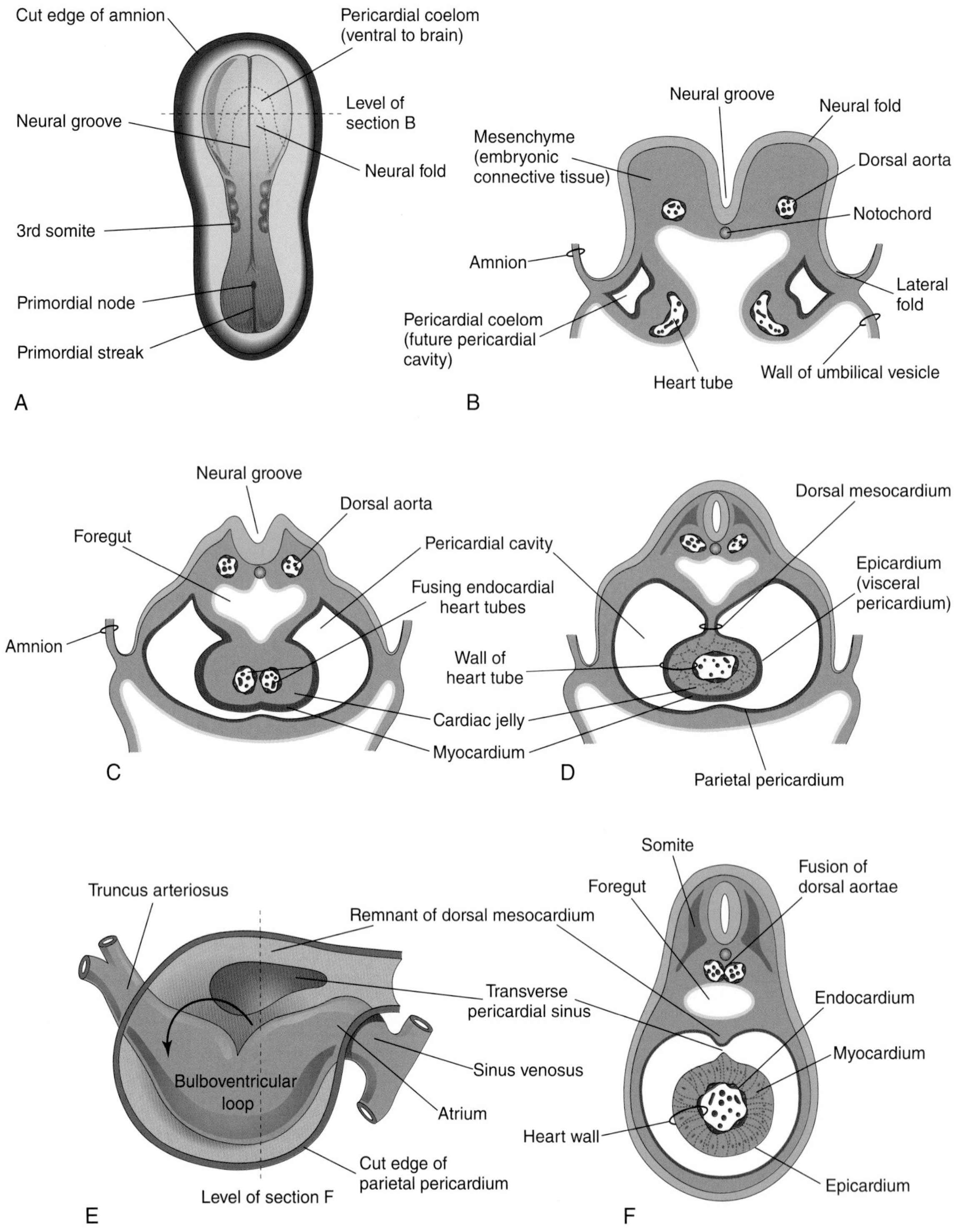

Fig. 13.8 (A) Dorsal view of an embryo (approximately 20 days). (B) Schematic transverse section of the heart region of the embryo illustrated in (A) showing the two heart tubes and lateral folds of the body. (C) Transverse section of a slightly older embryo showing the formation of the pericardial cavity and fusion of the heart tubes. (D) Similar section (approximately 22 days) showing the tubular heart suspended by the dorsal mesocardium. (E) Schematic drawing of the heart (approximately 28 days) showing degeneration of the central part of the dorsal mesocardium and formation of the transverse pericardial sinus. The *arrow* shows the bending of the primordial heart. The tubular heart now has a D-loop (D, dextro; rightward). (F) Transverse section of the embryo at the level seen in (E) showing the layers of the heart wall.

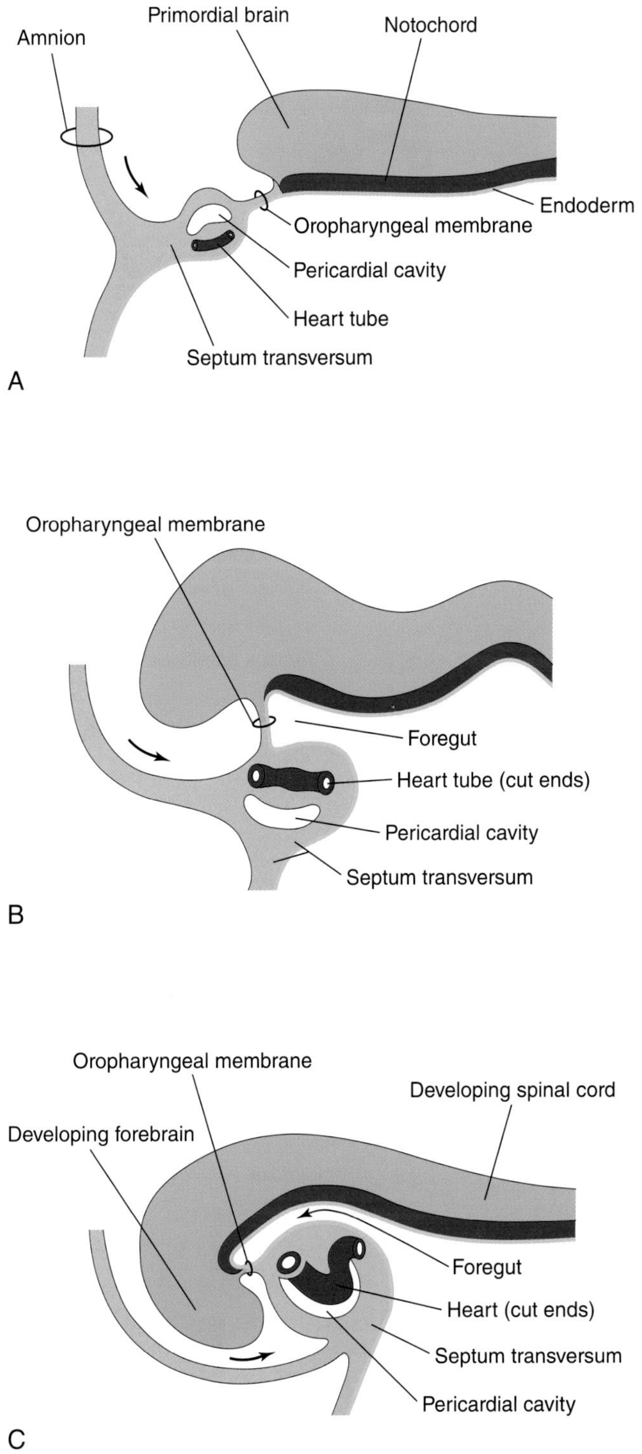

Fig. 13.9 Illustrations of longitudinal sections through the cranial half of embryos during the fourth week, showing the effect of the head fold *(arrows)* on the position of the heart and other structures. (A and B) As the head fold develops, the tubular heart and pericardial cavity move ventral to the foregut and caudal to the oropharyngeal membrane. (C) Note that the positions of the pericardial cavity and septum transversum have reversed with respect to each other. The septum transversum now lies posterior to the pericardial cavity, where it will form the central tendon of the diaphragm.

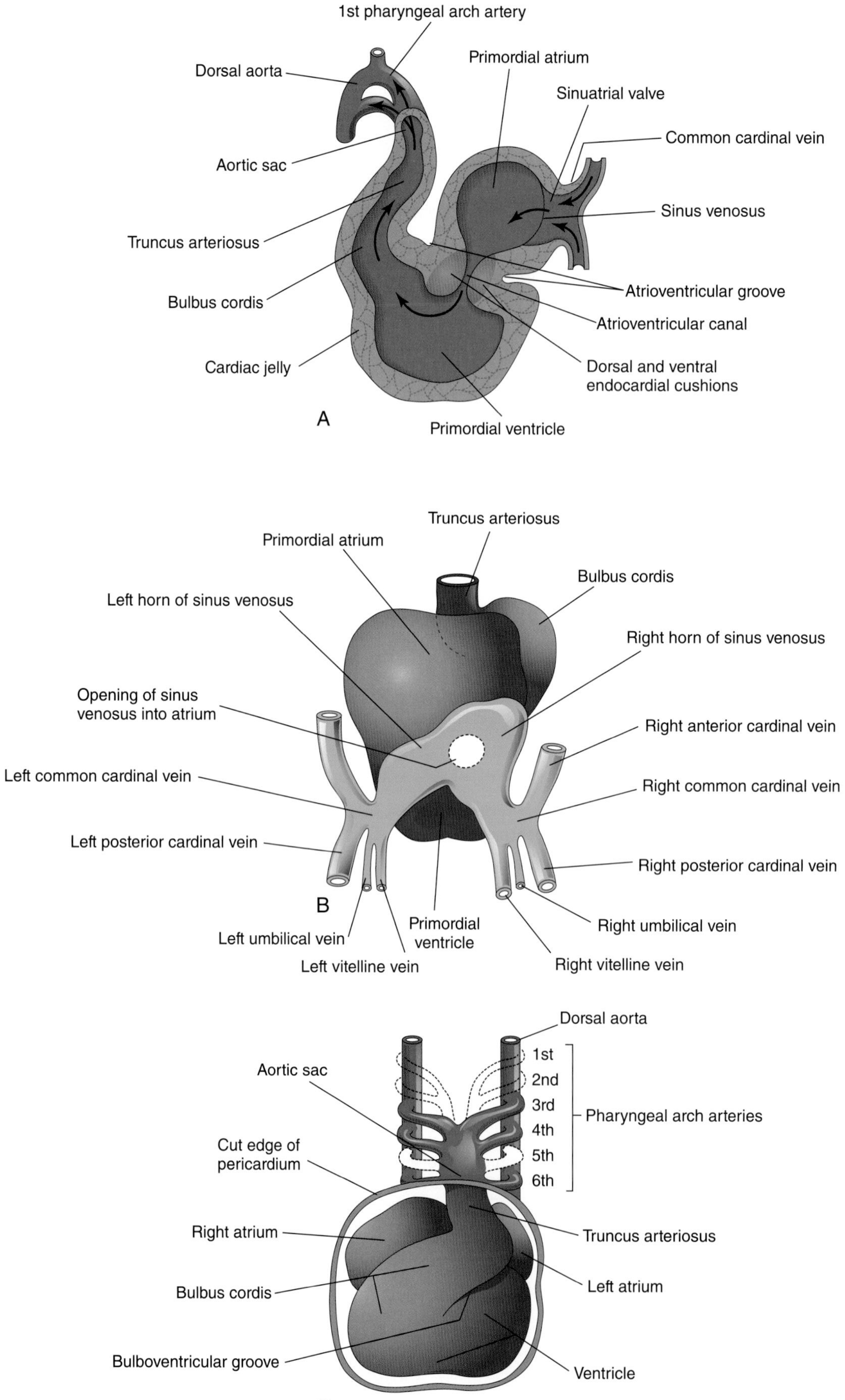

Fig. 13.10 (A) Sagittal section of the primordial heart at approximately 24 days, showing blood flow through it *(arrows)*. (B) Dorsal view of the heart at approximately 26 days showing the horns of the sinus venosus and the dorsal location of the primordial atrium. (C) Ventral view of the heart and pharyngeal arch arteries at approximately 35 days. The ventral wall of the pericardial sac has been removed to show the heart in the pericardial cavity.

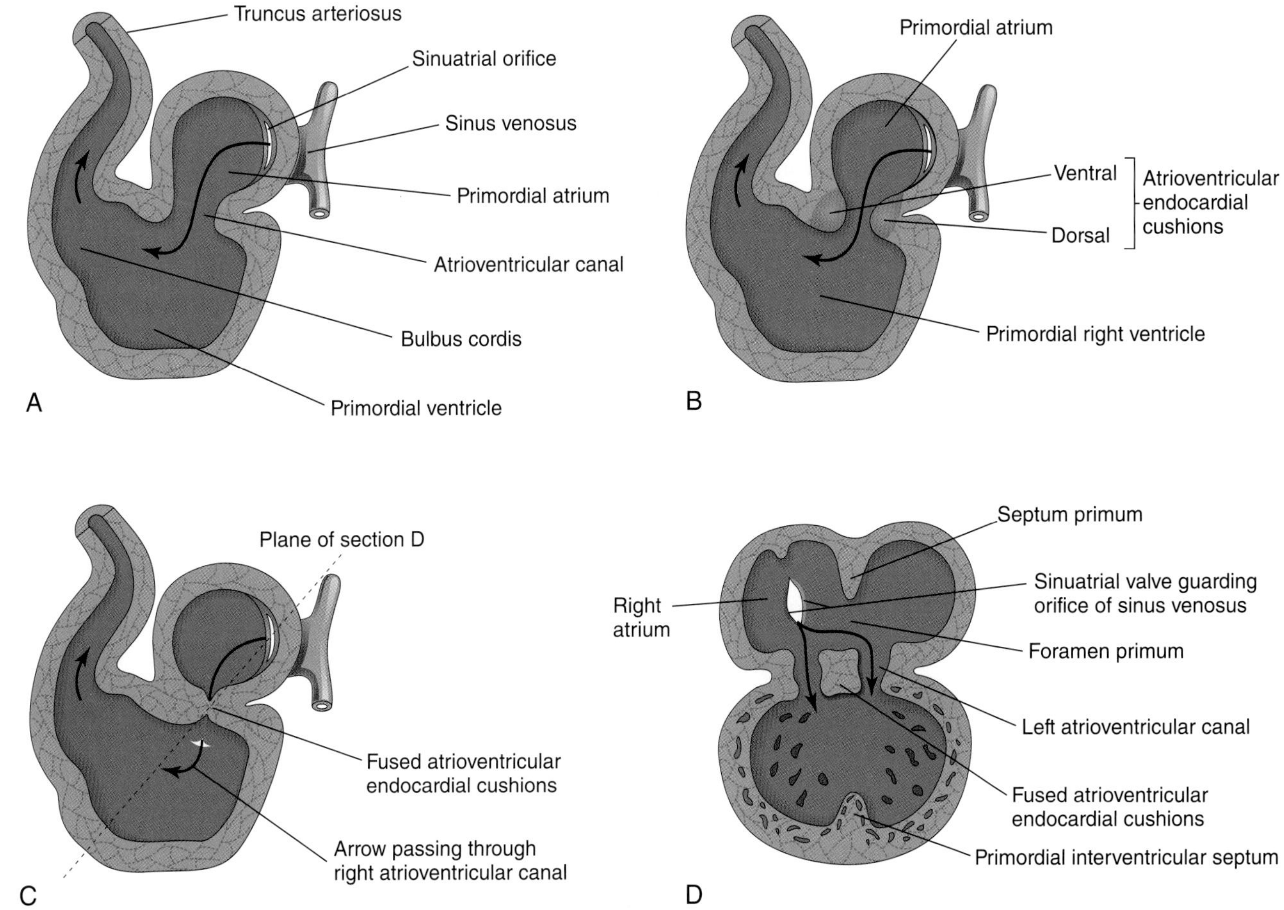

Fig. 13.11 (A and B) Sagittal sections of the heart during the fourth and fifth weeks, illustrating blood flow through the heart and division of the atrioventricular canal. The *arrows* are passing through the sinuatrial orifice. (C) Fusion of the atrioventricular endocardial cushions. (D) Coronal section of the heart at the plane shown in (C). Note that the septum primum and interventricular septa have started to develop.

heart bends, the atrium and sinus venosus come to lie dorsal to the truncus arteriosus, bulbus cordis, and ventricle (see Fig. 13.10B and C). By this stage, the sinus venosus has developed lateral expansions, the right and left **sinus horns** (see Fig. 13.5A). *The signaling molecule(s) and cellular mechanisms responsible for cardiac looping and remodeling are complex and involve the homeobox gene Nbx2-5, GATA, TBX5, HANDS, BMP, Notch, Wnt, and SHH pathways.*

As the primordial heart elongates and bends, it gradually invaginates into the pericardial cavity (see Figs. 13.7B–D and 13.8C and D). The primordial heart is initially suspended from the dorsal wall by a mesentery (double layer of peritoneum), the dorsal mesocardium. The central part of the mesentery soon degenerates, forming a communication, the **transverse pericardial sinus**, between the right and left sides of the pericardial cavity (see Fig. 13.8E and F). The primordial heart is now attached only at its cranial and caudal ends.

CIRCULATION THROUGH PRIMORDIAL HEART

The initial contractions of the heart are of myogenic origin. The muscle layers of the atrium and ventricle outflow tract are continuous, and contractions occur in peristalsis-like waves that begin in the sinus venosus. At first, circulation through the primordial heart is an ebb-and-flow type; however, by the end of the fourth week, coordinated contractions of the heart result in unidirectional flow. Blood enters the sinus venosus (see Fig. 13.10A and B) from the:

- Embryo through the common cardinal veins
- Developing placenta through the umbilical veins
- Umbilical vesicle through the vitelline veins

Blood from the sinus venosus enters the **primordial atrium**; flow from it is controlled by sinuatrial (SA) valves (Fig. 13.11A to D). The blood then passes through the **atrioventricular (AV) canal** into the primordial ventricle. When the ventricle contracts, blood is pumped through the bulbus cordis and truncus arteriosus into the aortic sac, from which it is distributed to the pharyngeal arch arteries in the pharyngeal arches (see Fig. 13.10C). The blood then passes into the **dorsal aortae** for distribution to the embryo, umbilical vesicle, and placenta (see Fig. 13.2).

PARTITIONING OF PRIMORDIAL HEART

Partitioning of the AV canal, primordial atrium, ventricle, and outflow tract begins during the middle of the fourth week. Partitioning is essentially completed by the end of the eighth week. Although described separately, these processes occur concurrently.

PARTITIONING OF ATRIOVENTRICULAR CANAL

Toward the end of the fourth week, **AV endocardial cushions** form on the dorsal and ventral walls of the AV canal (see Fig. 13.11A and B). The AV endocardial cushions develop initially from cardiac jelly, as well as neural crest cells (see Fig. 13.8C and D). After inductive signals emanate from the myocardium of the AV canal, a segment of the inner endocardial cells undergoes **epithelial-mesenchymal transformation**, and the resulting cells then invade the extracellular matrix. During the fifth week, the AV endocardial cushions approach each other and fuse, dividing the AV canal into **right and left canals** (see Fig. 13.11C and D). These canals partially separate the primordial atrium from the primordial ventricle, and the endocardial cushions function as **AV valves**. The septal valves are derived from the fused superior and inferior endocardial cushions. The mural leaflets are mesenchymal in origin.

Transforming growth factor-β (TGF-β_1 and TGF-β_2), bone morphogenetic proteins (BMP-2A and BMP-4) expression in the endocardial lineage, the zinc finger protein Slug, and an activin receptor–like kinase (ChALK2) have been reported to be involved in the epithelial-mesenchymal transformation and formation of the endocardial cushions.

PARTITIONING OF PRIMORDIAL ATRIUM

Beginning at the end of the fourth week, the primordial atrium is divided into right and left atria by the formation of, and subsequent modification and fusion of, two septa: the septum primum and septum secundum (Figs. 13.12 and 13.13).

The **septum primum**, a thin crescent-shaped membrane, grows toward the fusing endocardial cushions from the roof of the **primordial atrium**, partially dividing the common atrium into right and left halves. As the curtain-like muscular septum primum grows, a large opening, or **foramen primum**, remains between its crescentic-free edge and the endocardial cushions (see Figs. 13.12C and 13.13A–C). This foramen serves as a shunt, enabling oxygenated blood to pass from the right to the left atrium. The foramen becomes progressively smaller and disappears as the mesenchymal cap of the septum primum fuses with the fused AV endocardial cushions to form a **primordial AV septum** (see Fig. 13.13D and D_1). *Molecular studies have revealed that a distinct population of extracardiac progenitor cells from the second heart field migrates through the dorsal mesocardium to complete the lateral septum; Shh signaling plays a critical role in this process.*

Before the foramen primum disappears, perforations produced by **apoptosis** appear in the central part of the septum primum. These perforations coalesce to form another opening in the septum primum, the **foramen secundum**. The free edge of the septum primum fuses with the left side of the fused endocardial cushions, obliterating the foramen primum (see Figs. 13.12D and 13.13D). The foramen secundum ensures continued shunting of oxygenated blood from the right to the left atrium.

The **septum secundum**, a thick crescentic muscular fold, grows from the muscular ventrocranial wall of the right atrium, immediately adjacent to the septum primum (see Fig. 13.12D_1). As this thick septum grows during the fifth and sixth weeks, it gradually overlaps the foramen secundum in the septum primum (see Fig. 13.13E). The septum secundum forms an incomplete partition between the atria; consequently, a **foramen ovale** forms. The cranial part of the septum primum, initially attached to the roof of the left atrium, gradually disappears (see Fig. 13.13G_1 and H_1). The remaining part of the septum, attached to the fused endocardial cushions, forms the flap-like valve of the foramen ovale.

Before birth, the foramen ovale allows most of the oxygenated blood entering the right atrium from the IVC to pass into the left atrium (Fig. 13.14A; see also Fig. 13.13H). It also prevents the passage of blood in the opposite direction because the septum primum closes against the relatively rigid septum secundum (see Fig. 13.14B).

After birth, the foramen ovale functionally closes because the pressure in the left atrium is higher than that in the right atrium. At approximately 3 months, the valve of the foramen ovale fuses with the septum secundum, forming the **oval fossa** (fossa ovalis; see Fig. 13.14B). By the age of 2, the fossa ovalis is completely sealed in 75% of people. As a result, the interatrial septum becomes a complete partition between the atria.

CHANGES IN SINUS VENOSUS

Initially, the sinus venosus opens into the center of the dorsal wall of the **primordial atrium**, and its right and left horns are approximately the same size (see Fig. 13.5A). Progressive enlargement of the right horn results from two **left-to-right shunts of blood**:

- The first shunt results from the transformation of the vitelline and umbilical veins.
- The second shunt occurs when the anterior cardinal veins are connected by an anastomosis (see Fig. 13.5B and C). This communication shunts blood from the left to the right anterior cardinal vein; this shunt becomes the **left brachiocephalic vein**. The right anterior cardinal vein and right common cardinal vein become the **SVC** (Fig. 13.15C).

By the end of the fourth week, the right horn of the sinus venosus is noticeably larger than the left horn (Fig. 13.15A). As this occurs, the **SA orifice** moves to the right and opens in the part of the primordial atrium that will become the adult right atrium (see Figs. 13.11 and 13.15C). As the right horn of the sinus enlarges, it receives all the blood from the head and neck through the SVC and from the placenta and caudal regions of the body through the IVC. Initially, the **sinus venosus** is a separate chamber of the heart and opens into the dorsal wall of the right atrium (see Fig. 13.10A and B). The left horn becomes the **coronary sinus**, and the right horn is incorporated into the wall of the right atrium (see Fig. 13.15B and C).

Because it is derived from the sinus venosus, the smooth part of the wall of the right atrium is called the **sinus venarum of the right atrium** (see Fig. 13.15B and C). The remainder of the anterior internal surface of the atrial wall and the conical muscular pouch, the **right auricle**, has a rough trabeculated appearance. These two parts are derived from the primordial atrium. The smooth part and the rough part are demarcated internally in the right atrium by a vertical ridge, the **crista terminalis**, and externally by a shallow groove, the **sulcus terminalis** (see Fig. 13.15B). The crista terminalis represents the cranial part of the right SA valve (see Fig. 13.15C). The caudal part of the SA valve forms the valves of the IVC and coronary sinus. The left SA valve fuses with the septum secundum and is incorporated with it into the interatrial septum.

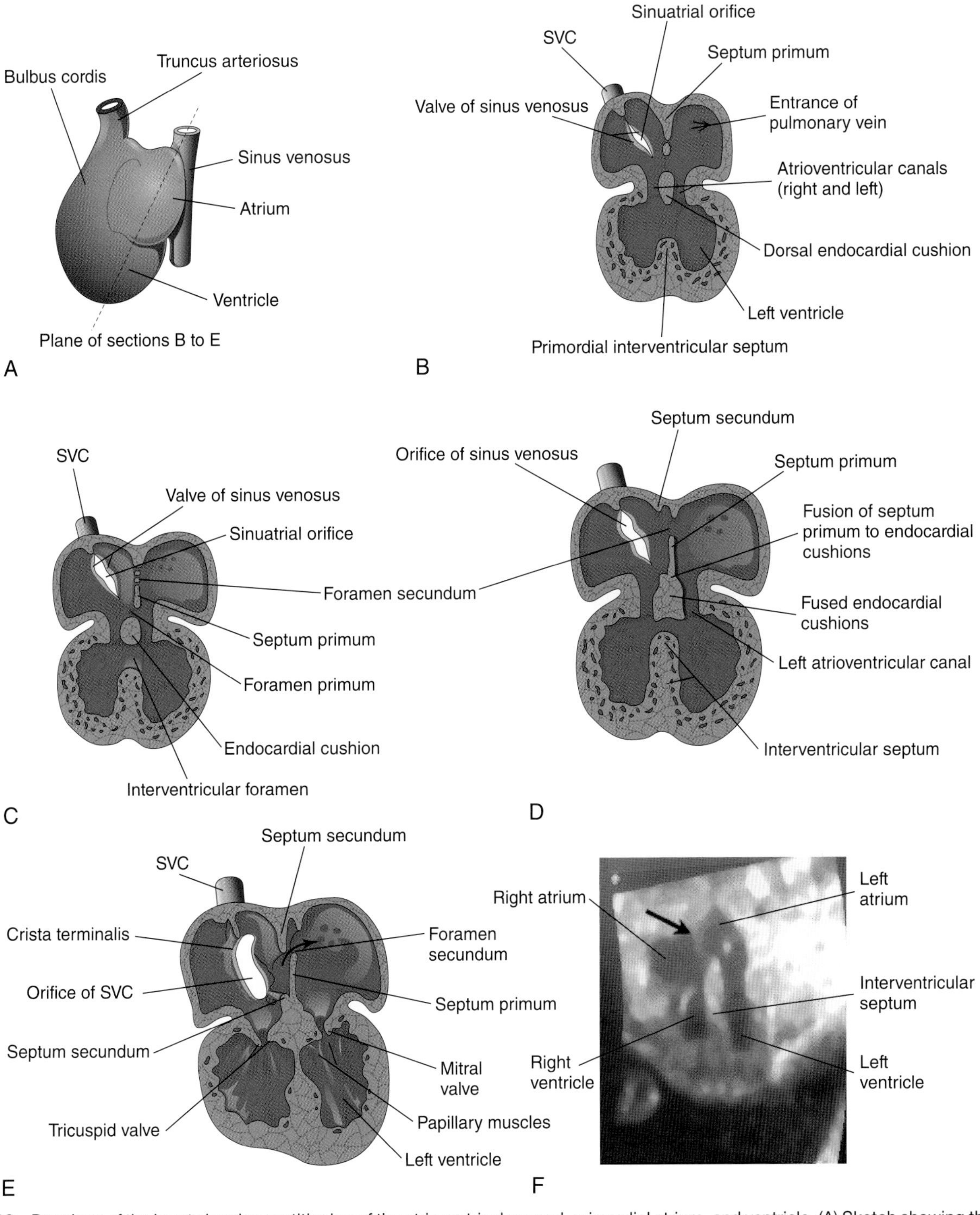

Fig. 13.12 Drawings of the heart showing partitioning of the atrioventricular canal, primordial atrium, and ventricle. (A) Sketch showing the plane of the sections (B–E). (B) Frontal section of the heart during the fourth week (approximately 28 days) showing the early appearance of the septum primum, interventricular septum, and dorsal atrioventricular endocardial cushion. (C) Frontal section of the heart (approximately 32 days) showing perforations in the dorsal part of the septum primum. (D) Section of the heart (approximately 35 days) showing the foramen secundum. (E) Section of the heart (at approximately 8 weeks) showing the heart after it is partitioned into four chambers. The *arrow* indicates the flow of well-oxygenated blood from the right into the left atrium. (F) Sonogram of a second-trimester fetus showing the four chambers of the heart. Note the septum secundum *(arrow)*. *SVC*, Superior vena cava. (Courtesy Dr. G.J. Reid, Department of Obstetrics, Gynecology and Reproductive Sciences, University of Manitoba, Women's Hospital, Winnipeg, Manitoba, Canada.)

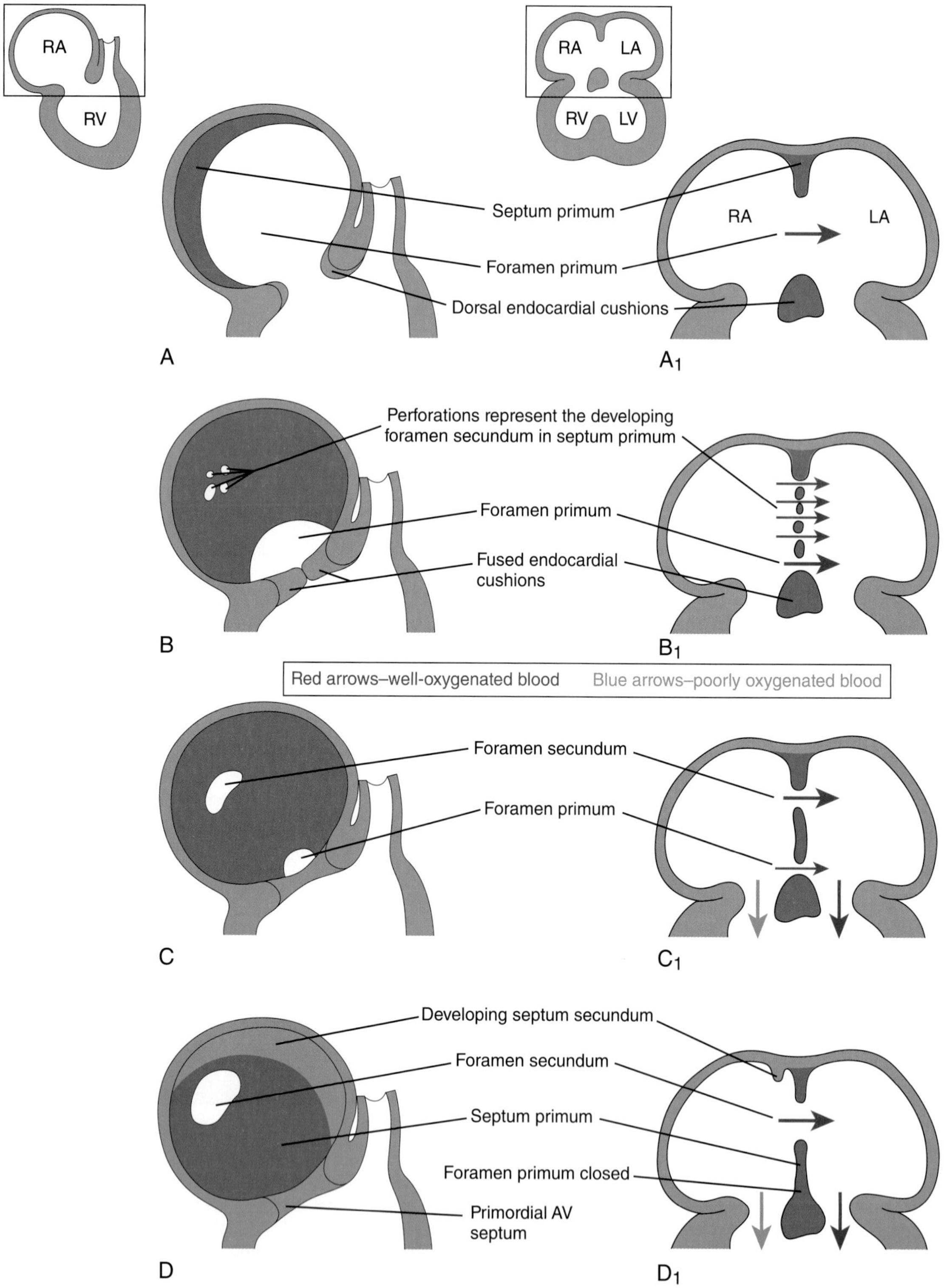

Fig. 13.13 Diagrammatic sketches illustrating progressive stages in the partitioning of the primordial atrium. (A–H) Sketches of the developing interatrial septum as viewed from the right side. (A_1–H_1) are coronal sections of the developing interatrial septum. Note that as the septum secundum grows, it overlaps the opening in the septum primum, the foramen secundum. Observe the valve of the foramen ovale in (G_1 and H_1). When the pressure in the right atrium *(RA)* exceeds that in the left atrium *(LA)*, blood passes from the right to the left side of the heart. When the pressures are equal or higher in the left atrium, the valve closes the foramen ovale (G_1). *AV*, Atrioventricular; *LV*, left ventricle; *RV*, right ventricle.

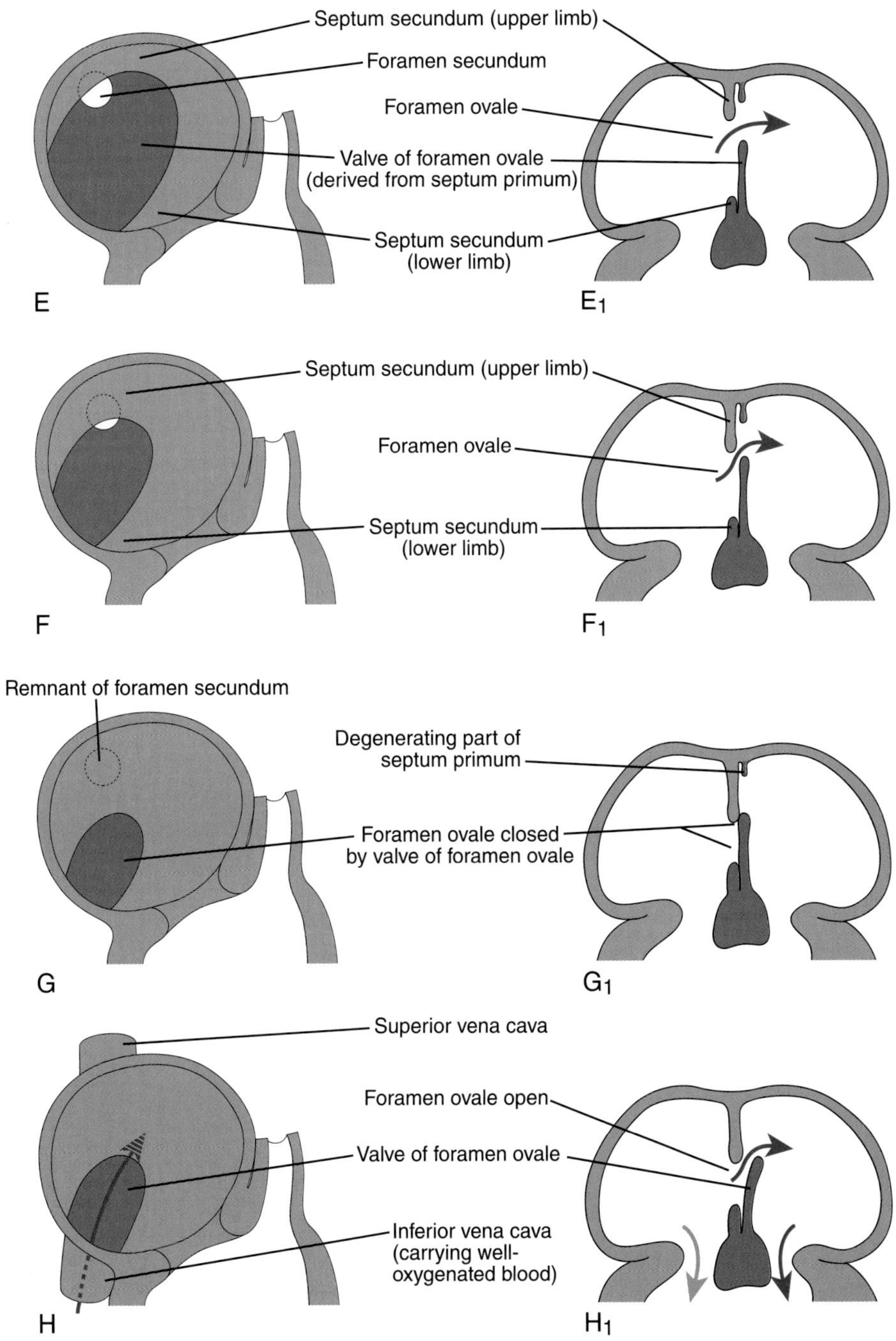
Septum secundum (upper limb)
Foramen secundum
Foramen ovale
Valve of foramen ovale (derived from septum primum)
Septum secundum (lower limb)
E
E1
Septum secundum (upper limb)
Foramen ovale
Septum secundum (lower limb)
F
F1
Remnant of foramen secundum
Degenerating part of septum primum
Foramen ovale closed by valve of foramen ovale
G
G1
Superior vena cava
Foramen ovale open
Valve of foramen ovale
Inferior vena cava (carrying well-oxygenated blood)
H
H1

Fig. 13.13, Cont'd

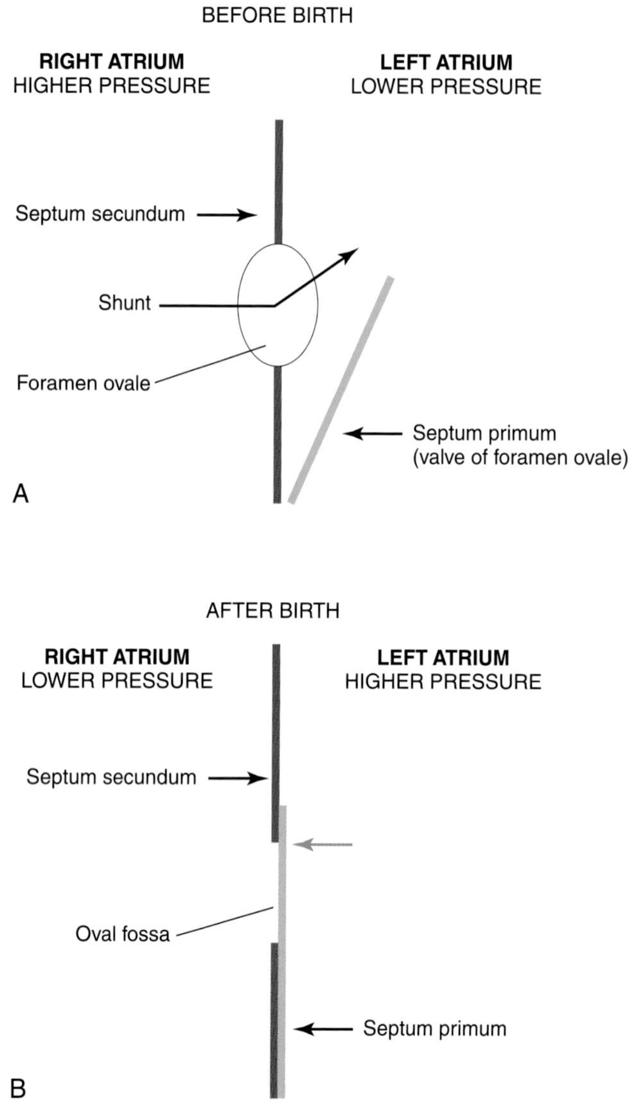

Fig. 13.14 Diagrams illustrating the relationship of the septum primum to the foramen ovale and septum secundum. (A) Before birth, well-oxygenated blood is shunted from the right atrium through the foramen ovale into the left atrium when the pressure increases. When the pressure decreases in the right atrium, the flap-like valve of the foramen ovale is pressed against the relatively rigid septum secundum. This closes the foramen ovale. (B) After birth, the pressure in the left atrium increases as the blood returns from the lungs. Eventually the septum primum is pressed against the septum secundum and adheres to it, permanently closing the foramen ovale and forming the oval fossa.

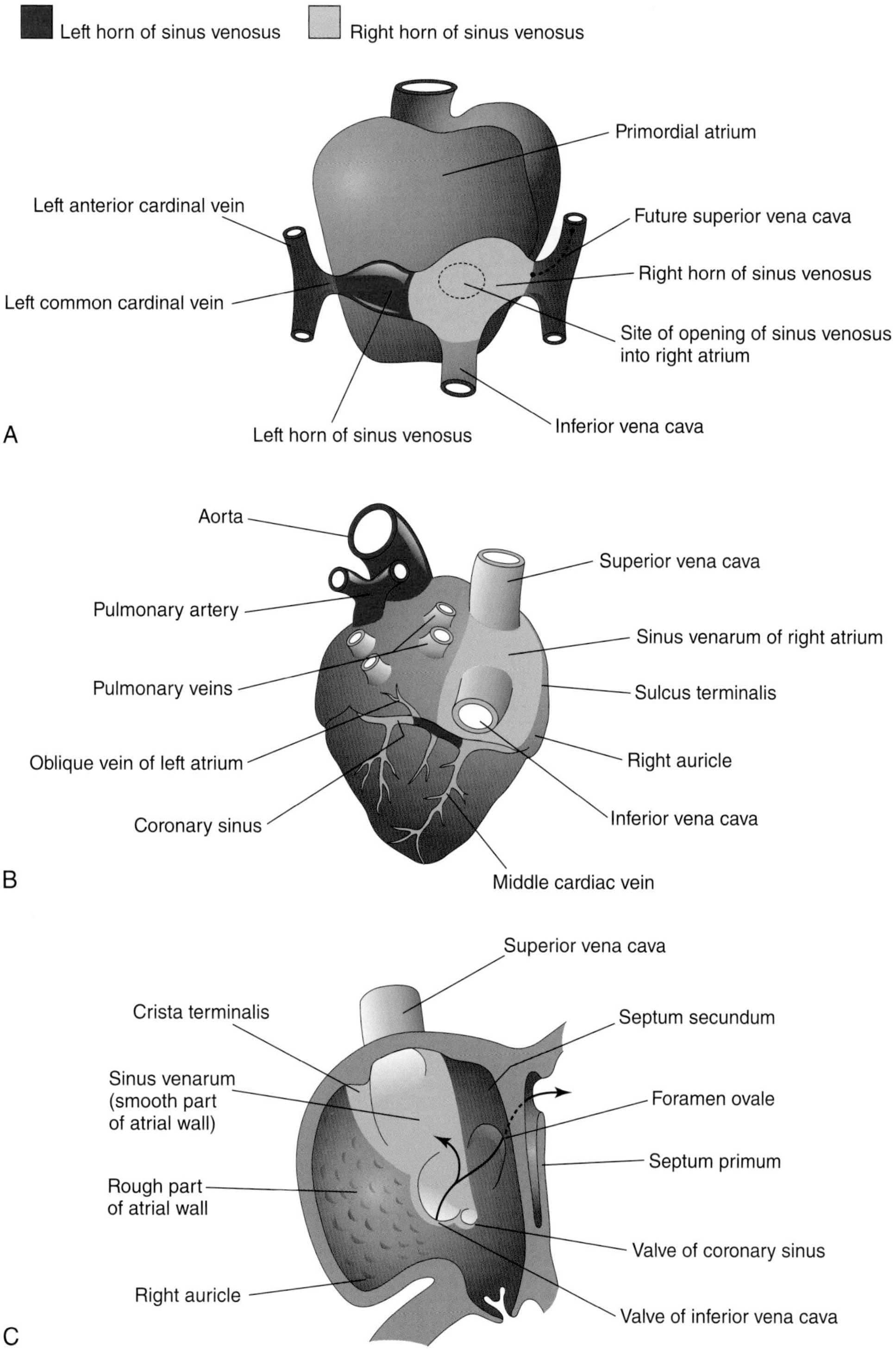

Fig. 13.15 Diagrams illustrating the fate of the sinus venosus. (A) Dorsal view of the heart (approximately 26 days) showing the primordial atrium and sinus venosus. (B) Dorsal view at 8 weeks after incorporation of the right horn of the sinus venosus into the right atrium. The left horn of the sinus horn becomes the coronary sinus. (C) Internal view of the fetal right atrium showing: (1) the smooth part of the wall of the right atrium (sinus venarum) derived from the right horn of the sinus venosus and (2) the crista terminalis and valves of the inferior vena cava and coronary sinus that are derived from the right sinuatrial valve. The primordial right atrium becomes the right auricle, a conical muscular pouch. The *arrows* indicate the flow of blood.

PRIMORDIAL PULMONARY VEIN AND FORMATION OF LEFT ATRIUM

Most of the wall of the left atrium is smooth because it is formed by the incorporation of the **primordial pulmonary vein** (Fig. 13.16A). This vein develops as an outgrowth of the dorsal atrial wall, just to the left of the septum primum. As the atrium expands, the primordial pulmonary vein and its main branches are incorporated into the wall of the left atrium. As a result, four pulmonary veins are formed (Fig. 13.16C and D).

Molecular studies have confirmed that atrial mesenchymal cells migrate into the walls of the pulmonary veins and differentiate into specific myocytes (NKX2-5, TH18 +ve cells). The functional significance of this **pulmonary cardiac muscle** (pulmonary myocardium) at the base of the pulmonary vein is uncertain. The small left auricle is derived from the primordial atrium; its internal surface has a rough trabeculated appearance.

Anomalous Pulmonary Venous Connections

In the disorder involving total anomalous pulmonary venous connections, none of the pulmonary veins connect with the left atrium. Most commonly, the veins coalesce into a confluence of one of the systemic veins posterior to the left atrium and then drain into this chamber of the heart. Less commonly the veins may descend below the diaphragm and empty into the hepatic venous system, where they commonly become obstructed and produce increased pressure, leading to significant congestive heart failure. In the disorder involving partial anomalous pulmonary venous connections, one or more pulmonary veins have similar anomalous connections, but the others have normal connections.

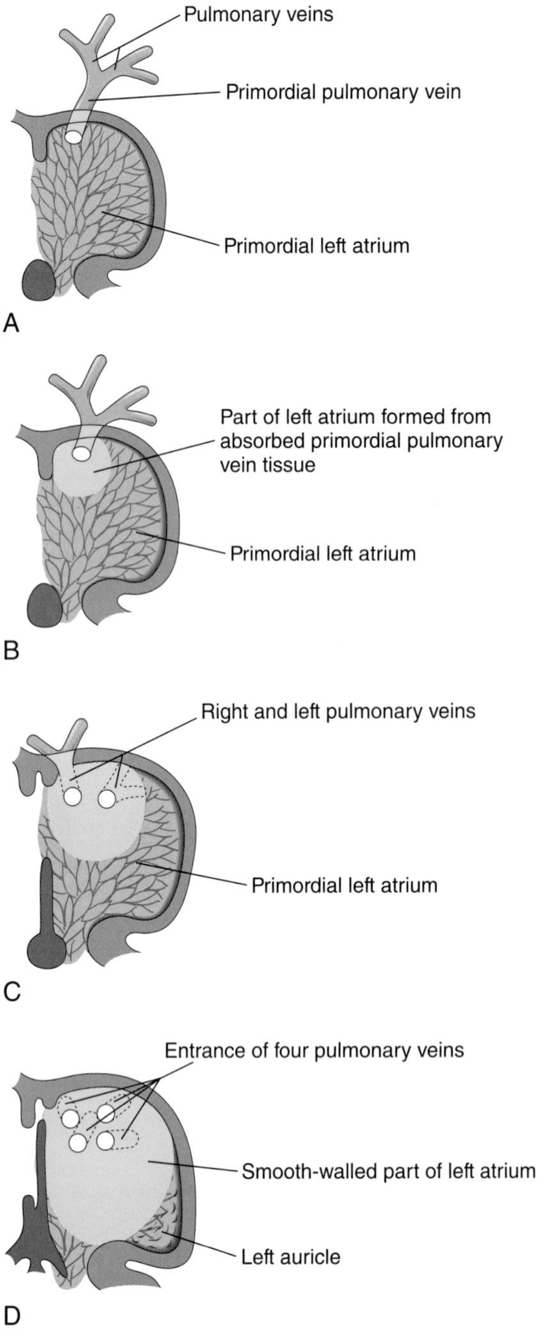

Fig. 13.16 Diagrammatic sketches illustrating absorption of the pulmonary vein into the left atrium. (A) At 5 weeks, showing the primordial pulmonary vein opening into the primordial left atrium. (B) Later stage showing partial absorption of the primordial pulmonary vein. (C) At 6 weeks, showing the openings of two pulmonary veins into the left atrium resulting from absorption of the primordial pulmonary vein. (D) At 8 weeks, showing four pulmonary veins with separate atrial orifices. The primordial left atrium becomes the left auricle, a tubular appendage of the atrium. Most of the left atrium is formed by absorption of the primordial pulmonary vein and its branches.

PARTITIONING OF PRIMORDIAL VENTRICLE

Division of the ventricle is indicated by a median ridge, the muscular **interventricular septum**, in the floor of the ventricle near its apex (see Fig. 13.12B). Myocytes (muscle cells) from both the left and right primordial ventricles contribute to the formation of the **muscular part of the interventricular septum**. The septum has a concave free edge (Fig. 13.17A). Initially, it attains most of its height from dilation of the ventricles on each side of the muscular interventricular septum (Fig. 13.17B). Later, there is active proliferation of myoblasts in the septum, which increases the size of the septum.

Until the seventh week, there is a crescent-shaped **interventricular foramen** between the free edge of the interventricular septum and the fused endocardial cushions. The foramen permits communication between the right and left ventricles (Fig. 13.18B; see also Fig. 13.17). The foramen usually closes by the end of the seventh week as the **bulbar ridges** fuse with the endocardial cushion (Fig. 13.18C–E).

Closure of the interventricular foramen and formation of the membranous part of the interventricular septum results from the fusion of tissues from three sources: the right bulbar ridge, the left bulbar ridge, and the endocardial cushion. The **membranous part of the interventricular septum** is derived from an extension of tissue from the right side of the endocardial cushion to the muscular part of the septum as well as neural crest cells. This tissue merges with the **aorticopulmonary septum** and the thick muscular part of the interventricular septum (Fig. 13.19C; see also Fig. 13.18E). After the closure of the interventricular foramen and formation of the membranous part of the interventricular septum, the pulmonary trunk is in communication with the right ventricle, and the aorta communicates with the left ventricle (see Fig. 13.18E).

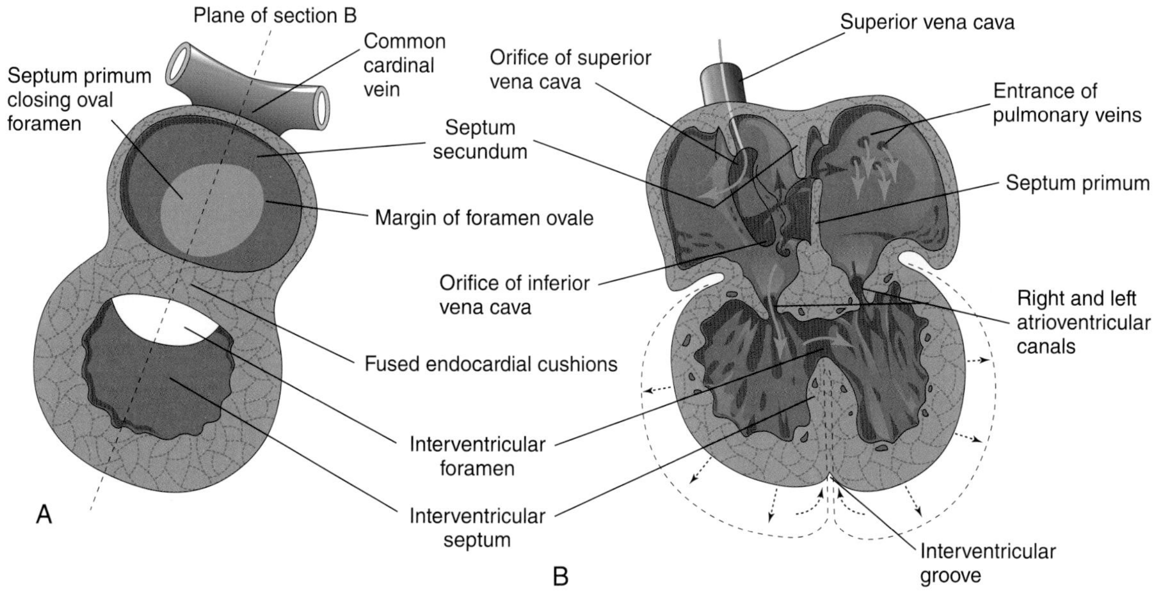

Fig. 13.17 Schematic diagrams illustrating partitioning of the primordial heart. (A) Sagittal section late in the fifth week showing the cardiac septa and foramina. (B) Coronal section at a slightly later stage illustrating the directions of blood flow through the heart *(blue arrows)* and expansion of the ventricles *(black arrows)*.

Cavitation of the ventricular walls forms a spongy mass of muscular bundles, **trabeculae carneae**. Some of these bundles become **papillary muscles** and **tendinous cords (chordae tendineae)**. The cords run from the papillary muscles to the AV valves (see Fig. 13.19C and D).

Fetal Cardiac Ultrasonography

Cardiac screening using high-resolution real-time ultrasonography is usually first performed between 18 and 22 weeks of gestation (Fig. 13.20) when the heart is large enough to examine. Based on international convention, a four-chamber view of the heart is obtained (see Fig. 13.20) and the great vessels are also examined for anomalies.

PARTITIONING OF BULBUS CORDIS AND TRUNCUS ARTERIOSUS

During the fifth week, the active proliferation of mesenchymal cells in the walls of the bulbus cordis results in the formation of **bulbar ridges** (Fig. 13.21B and C; see also Fig. 13.18C and D). Similar ridges that are continuous with the bulbar ridges form in the **truncus arteriosus**. The **bulbar** and **truncal ridges** are derived largely from neural crest mesenchyme (see Fig. 13.21B and C).

Neural crest cells migrate through the primordial pharynx and pharyngeal arches to reach the ridges. As this occurs, the bulbar and truncal ridges undergo a 180-degree spiraling. The spiral orientation of the ridges, caused in part by the streaming of blood from the ventricles, results in the formation of a spiral **aorticopulmonary septum** when the ridges fuse (see Fig. 13.21D–G). This septum divides the bulbus cordis and truncus arteriosus into two arterial channels, the ascending aorta and pulmonary trunk. Because of the spiraling of the aorticopulmonary septum, the **pulmonary trunk** twists around the **ascending aorta** (see Fig. 13.21H).

The **bulbus cordis** is incorporated into the walls of the definitive ventricles (see Fig. 13.18A and B):

- In the right ventricle, the bulbus cordis is represented by the **conus arteriosus** (infundibulum), which is the origin of the pulmonary trunk.
- In the left ventricle, the bulbus cordis forms the walls of the **aortic vestibule**, the part of the ventricular cavity just inferior to the aortic valve.

DEVELOPMENT OF CARDIAC VALVES

When partitioning of the truncus arteriosus is nearly completed (see Fig. 13.21A–C), the **semilunar valves** begin to develop from three swellings of subendocardial tissue around the orifices of the aorta and pulmonary trunk. Cardiac precursor neural crest cells also contribute to this tissue. These swellings are hollowed out and reshaped to form three thin-walled cusps (Fig. 13.22; see also Fig. 13.19C and D). The **AV valves** (tricuspid and mitral valves) develop similarly from localized proliferations of tissue around the AV canals.

CONDUCTING SYSTEM OF HEART

Initially, the muscle in the primordial atrium and ventricle is continuous. As the chambers of the heart form, the cells forming the myocardium conduct the wave of depolarization faster than the remaining myocardium. Throughout development, this impulse wave moves from the venous pole to the arterial pole of the heart. The atrium acts as the interim pacemaker of the heart, but the sinus venosus soon takes over this function. The **SA node** develops during the fifth week. This node is located in the right wall of the sinus venosus, but it becomes incorporated into the wall of the right atrium with the sinus venosus at the junction of the SVC (see Fig. 13.19A and D). The SA node is located high in the right atrium, near the entrance of the **SVC**.

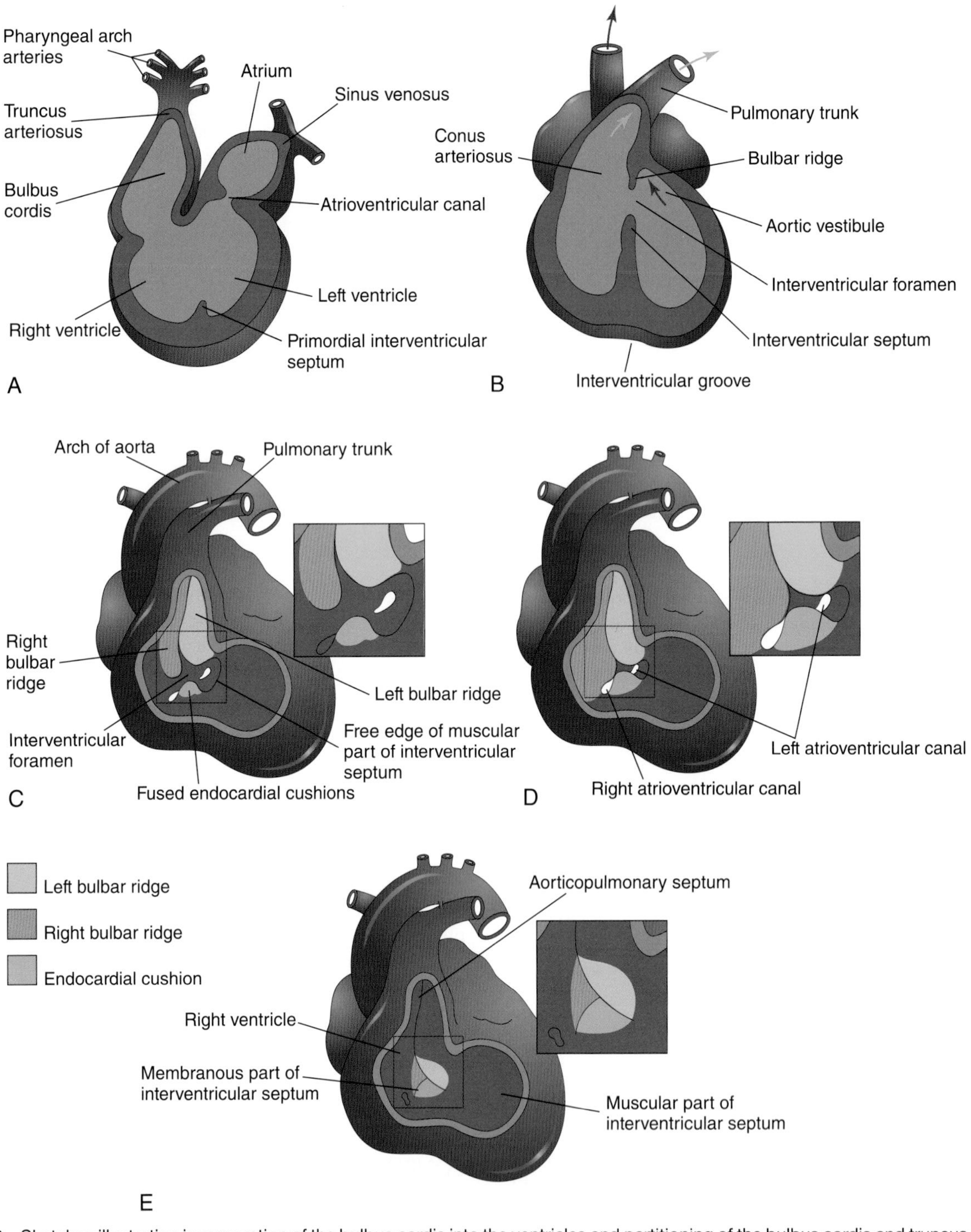

Fig. 13.18 Sketches illustrating incorporation of the bulbus cordis into the ventricles and partitioning of the bulbus cordis and truncus arteriosus into the aorta and pulmonary trunk. (A) Sagittal section at 5 weeks showing the bulbus cordis as one of the chambers of the primordial heart. (B) Schematic coronal section at 6 weeks, after the bulbus cordis has been incorporated into the ventricles to become the conus arteriosus of the right ventricle, which is the origin of the pulmonary trunk and aortic vestibule of the left ventricle. The *arrow* indicates blood flow. (C–E) Schematic drawings illustrating closure of the interventricular foramen and formation of the membranous part of the interventricular septum. The walls of the truncus arteriosus, bulbus cordis, and right ventricle have been removed. (C) At 5 weeks, showing the bulbar ridges and fused atrioventricular endocardial cushions. (D) At 6 weeks, showing how the proliferation of subendocardial tissue diminishes the interventricular foramen. (E) At 7 weeks, showing the fused bulbar ridges, the membranous part of the interventricular septum formed by extensions of tissue from the right side of the atrioventricular endocardial cushions, and closure of the interventricular foramen.

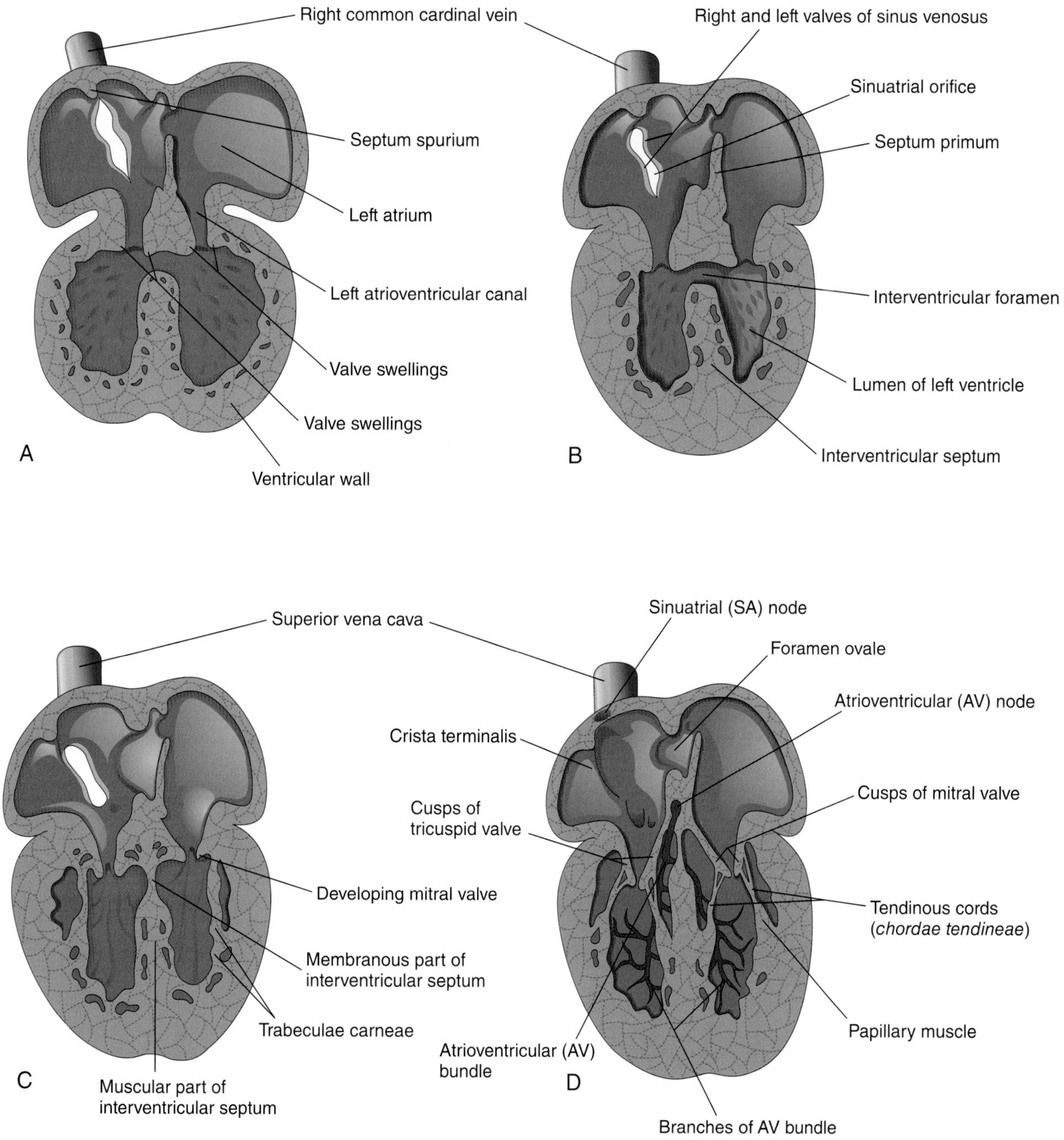

Fig. 13.19 Schematic sections of the heart illustrating successive stages in the development of the atrioventricular valves, tendinous cords (Latin *chordae tendineae*), and papillary muscles. (A) At 5 weeks. (B) At 6 weeks. (C) At 7 weeks. (D) At 20 weeks, showing the conducting system of the heart.

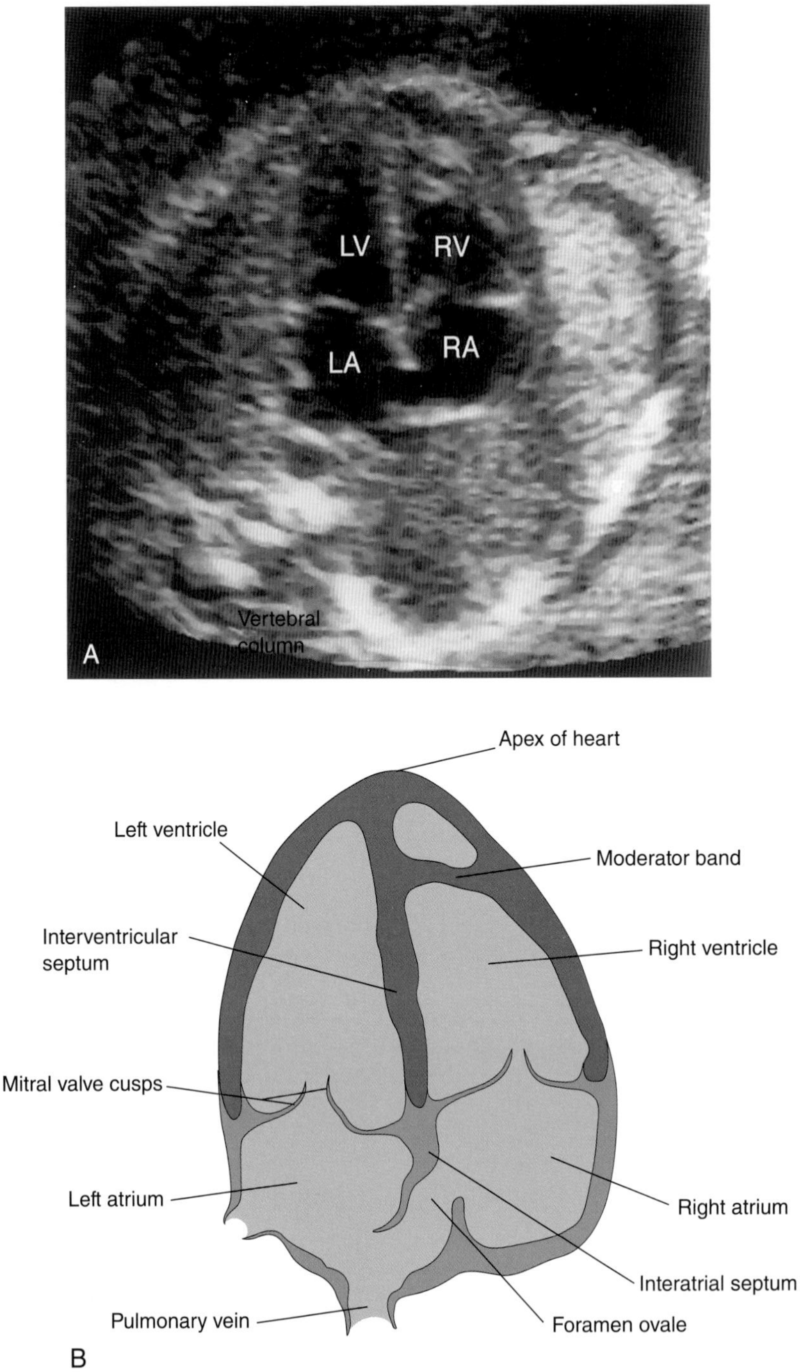

Fig. 13.20 (A) Ultrasound image showing the four-chamber view of the heart in a fetus of approximately 20 weeks' gestation. (B) Orientation sketch (Modified from the American Institute of Ultrasound in Medicine Technical Bulletin, Performance of the Basic Fetal Cardiac Ultrasound Examination). The scan was obtained across the fetal thorax. The ventricles and atria are well-formed, and two atrioventricular valves are present. The moderator band is one of the trabeculae carneae that carries part of the right branch of the atrioventricular bundle. *LA*, Left atrium; *LV*, left ventricle; *RA*, right atrium; *RV*, right ventricle. (Courtesy Dr. Wesley Lee, Division of Fetal Imaging, William Beaumont Hospital, Royal Oak, Michigan.)

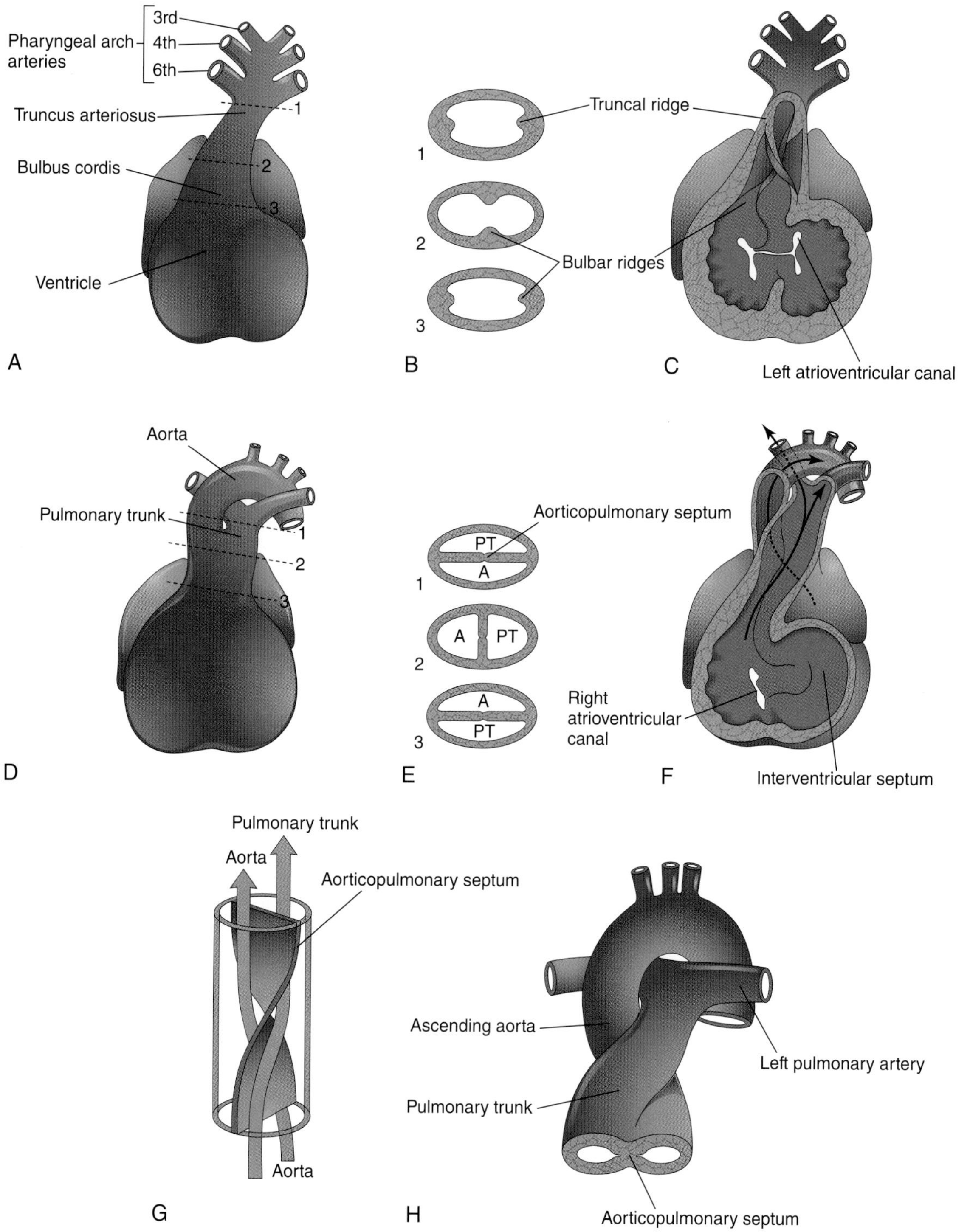

Fig. 13.21 Partitioning of the bulbus cordis and truncus arteriosus. (A) Ventral aspect of heart at 5 weeks. The *broken lines* and *arrows* indicate the levels of the sections shown in (A). (B) Transverse sections of the truncus arteriosus and bulbus cordis, illustrating the truncal and bulbar ridges. (C) The ventral wall of the heart and truncus arteriosus have been removed to demonstrate these ridges. (D) Ventral aspect of heart after the partitioning of the truncus arteriosus. The *broken lines* and *arrows* indicate the levels of the sections shown in (E). (E) Sections through the newly formed aorta *(A)* and pulmonary trunk *(PT)*, showing the aorticopulmonary septum. (F) At 6 weeks. The ventral wall of the heart and pulmonary trunk has been removed to show the aorticopulmonary septum. (G) Diagram illustrating the spiral form of the aorticopulmonary septum. (H) Drawing showing the great arteries (ascending aorta and pulmonary trunk) twisting around each other as they leave the heart.

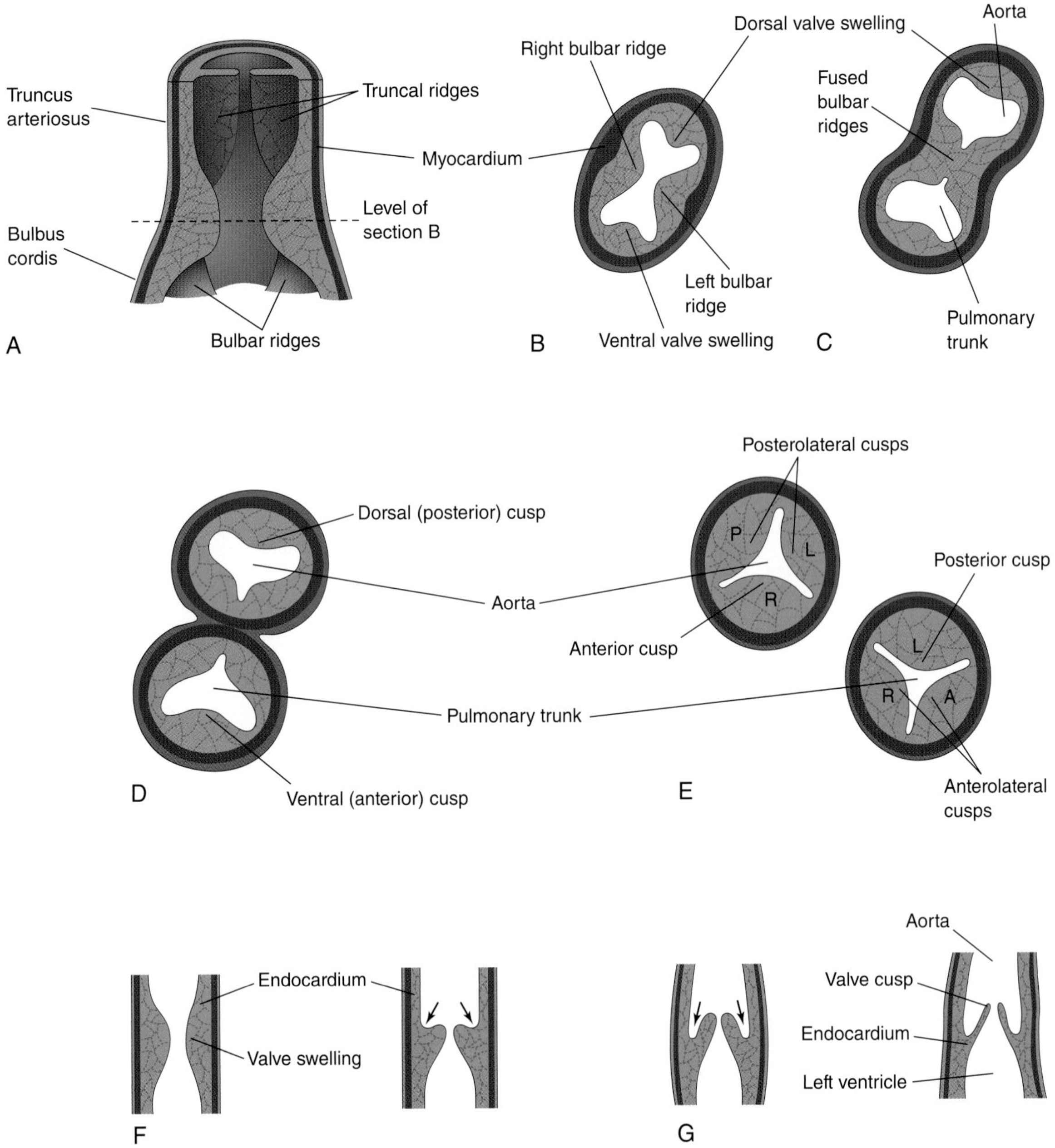

Fig. 13.22 Development of the semilunar valves of the aorta and pulmonary trunk. (A) Sketch of a section of the truncus arteriosus and bulbus cordis showing the valve swellings. (B) Transverse section of the bulbus cordis. (C) Similar section after fusion of the bulbar ridges. (D) Formation of the walls and valves of the aorta and pulmonary trunk. (E) Rotation of the vessels has established the adult relations of the valves. (F and G) Longitudinal sections of the aorticoventricular junction illustrating successive stages in the hollowing *(arrows)* and thinning of the valve swellings to form the valve cusps. *L*, Left; *P*, posterior; *R*, right.

After incorporation of the sinus venosus, cells from its left wall are found in the base of the interatrial septum just anterior to the opening of the coronary sinus. Together with cells from the AV region, they form the **AV node** and **bundle**, which are located just superior to the endocardial cushions. The fibers arising from the AV bundle pass from the atrium into the ventricle and split into the right and left **bundle branches**. These branches are distributed throughout the **ventricular myocardium** (see Fig. 13.19D).

The SA node, AV node, and AV bundle are richly supplied by nerves; however, the conducting system is well developed before these nerves enter the heart. This specialized tissue is normally the only signal pathway from the atria to the ventricles. As the four chambers of the heart develop, a band of connective tissue grows in from the epicardium (visceral layer of the serous pericardium), subsequently electrically isolating the muscle of the atria from that of the ventricles; only the AV node and bundle conduct. The connective tissue forms part of the **cardiac skeleton** (fibrous skeleton of the heart). The parasympathetic innervation of the heart is formed by neural crest cells that also play an essential role in the development of the conducting system of the heart.

Congenital Long QT Syndrome

There are three genotypes of long QT syndrome (LQTS), a congenital signaling disorder of the heart, which results in an imbalance between depolarization and repolarization and a prolonged action potential duration. The prevalence of LQTS is approximately 1:2000 with a slight preponderance in females. LQTS accounts for up to 10% of sudden deaths in young people. The symptoms of LQTS include recurrent syncope (fainting), seizures, and atrial arrhythmia, and are greatest in childhood. *The genes involved include KCNQ1, KCNH2, and SCN5A and are inherited from the parents*. Treatment includes beta-blockers, implantable cardioverter-defibrillator, and left cardiac denervation.

CORONARY BLOOD VESSELS

Knowledge of how the coronary blood vessels develop in humans is limited. Most studies have been carried out in laboratory animals; some of the findings might be evolutionary conserved. Several sources, including the proepicardium, sinus venosus, endocardium, and myocardium, have been suggested for the origin of the coronary blood vessels.

Recent observations made in human embryos of the Carnegie Collection at different stages have provided some insights into the formation of the coronary vessels. By the end of the fifth week of development, blood islands are present at the atrioventricular and interventricular grooves and in the epicardium. The precursor cells forming the coronary vessels are derived from the proepicardium and areas near the sinus venosus. Mesenchymal cells deep into the epicardium form vascular channels (vasculogenesis), which then branch, forming a network of blood vessels. By 44 days, a vascular plexus of capillaries, erythroblasts, and spindle-shaped mesenchymal cells, derived from the epicardium, penetrates the atrioventricular groove (see Fig. 13.10A) and aortic root to form the coronary ostia and coronary artery stem. During the late embryonic period and early fetal period, the tunica media and adventitia, as well as the lumen of the blood vessels, mature. The formation of venous channels (venules), evident by the sixth week, is also likely derived from the vascular plexus of the subepicardium (for details, see Tomanek, 2016).

BIRTH DEFECTS OF HEART AND GREAT VESSELS

Congenital heart defects (CHDs) are relatively common, with a frequency of 6 to 8 cases per 1000 live births, and are a leading cause of neonatal morbidity. Some CHDs are caused by single-gene or chromosomal mechanisms. Other defects result from exposure to teratogens such as the **rubella virus** (see Table 20.6); however, in many cases the cause is unknown. Most CHDs are thought to be caused by multiple factors that are genetic and environmental (i.e., **multifactorial inheritance**), each of which has a minor effect.

The molecular aspects of abnormal cardiac development are poorly understood, and gene therapy for infants with CHDs is at present a remote prospect. Imaging technology, such as real-time two-dimensional echocardiography, permits detection of fetal CHDs as early as the 16th week.

Most CHDs are well tolerated during fetal life; however, at birth, when the fetus loses contact with the maternal circulation, the impact of CHDs becomes apparent. Some types of CHDs cause very little disability; others are incompatible with extrauterine life. Because of recent advances in cardiovascular surgery, many types of CHDs can be palliated or corrected surgically, and fetal cardiac surgery may soon be possible for complex CHDs.

Dextrocardia

If the embryonic heart tube bends to the left instead of to the right (Fig. 13.23B), the heart is displaced to the right, and the heart and its vessels are reversed left to right as in a mirror image of their normal configuration. Dextrocardia is the most frequent positional defect of the heart. In **dextrocardia with situs inversus** (transposition of the abdominal viscera), such as can occur in primary ciliary dyskinesia, the incidence of accompanying cardiac defects is low. If there is no other associated vascular abnormality, the heart functions normally.

In **isolated dextrocardia**, the abnormal position of the heart is not accompanied by displacement of other viscera. This defect is usually complicated by severe cardiac defects (e.g., a single ventricle and transposition of the great vessels). *TGF-β factor Nodal is involved in the looping of the heart tube, but its role in dextrocardia is unclear*.

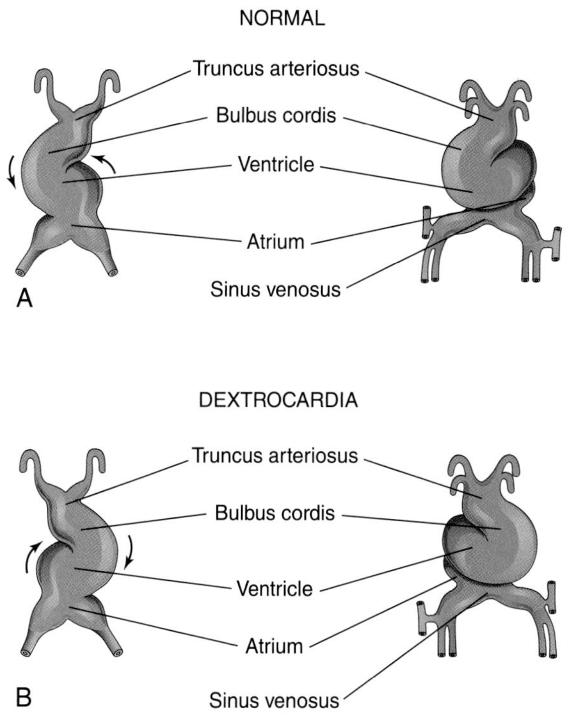

Fig. 13.23 The embryonic heart tube during the fourth week. (A) Normal looping of the tubular heart to the right. (B) Abnormal looping of the tubular heart to the left.

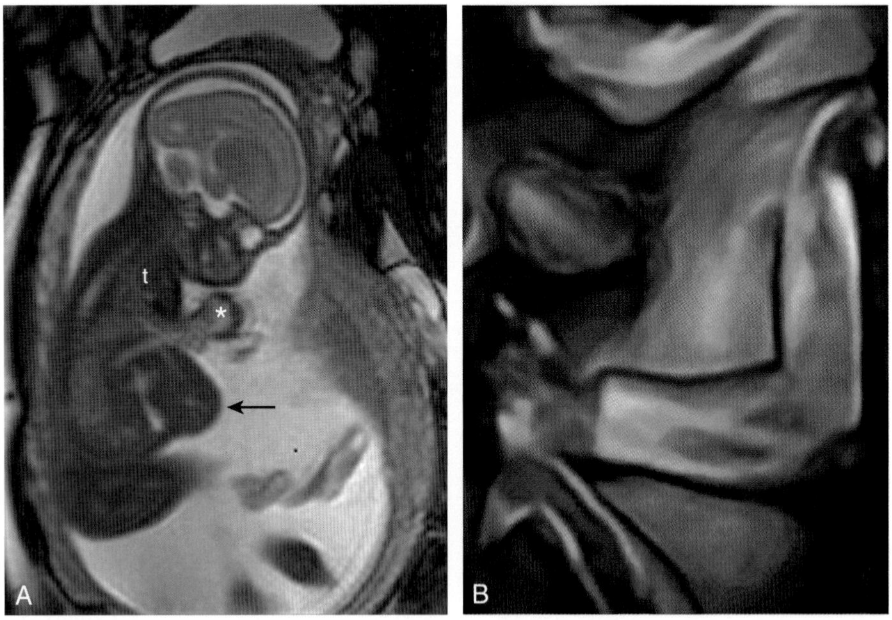

Fig. 13.24 (A) Fetal magnetic resonance image using single-shot turbo spin echo shows the heart in an ectopic position *(asterisk)* and eventration of a part of the liver at the midline *(arrow)*. Notice the small thoracic cavity *(t)*. No malformation of the central nervous system could be seen. (B) Three-dimensional reconstruction shows the heart protruding through the sternum. *Ao*, Aortic outflow tract; *LV*, left ventricle; *Po*, pulmonary outflow tract; *RV*, right ventricle. (From Leyder M, van Berkel E, Done K, et al: Ultrasound meets magnetic resonance imaging in the diagnosis of pentalogy of Cantrell with complete ectopy of the heart, *Gynecol Obstet (Sunnyvale)* 4:200, 2014.)

Ectopia Cordis

In **ectopia cordis**, an extremely rare condition (5–7:1,000,000), the heart is in an abnormal location (Fig. 13.24). In the thoracic form of ectopia cordis, the heart is partly or completely exposed to the thoracic wall. Ectopia cordis is usually associated with widely separated halves of the sternum (nonfusion) and an open pericardial sac. Death occurs in most cases during the first few days after birth, usually from infection, cardiac failure, or hypoxemia. If there are no severe cardiac defects, surgical therapy usually consists of covering the heart with skin. In some cases of ectopia cordis, the heart protrudes through the diaphragm into the abdomen.

The clinical outcome for patients with ectopia cordis has improved, and many children have survived to adulthood. The most common thoracic form of ectopia cordis results from faulty development of the sternum and pericardium because of failure of complete fusion of the lateral folds in the formation of the thoracic wall during the fourth week (see Fig. 5.1).

Atrial Septal Defects

An **atrial septal defect (ASD)** is a common CHD and occurs more frequently in females than males (see Figs. 13.25B and 13.36).

There are four clinically significant types of ASD: ostium secundum defect, endocardial cushion defect with ostium primum defect, sinus venosus defect, and common atrium. The first two types of ASD are relatively common.

Ostium secundum ASDs (see Fig. 13.26A–D) are in the area of the oval fossa and include defects of the septum primum and septum secundum. Ostium secundum ASDs are well tolerated during childhood; if left untreated, symptoms such as **pulmonary arterial hypertension** (i.e., pulmonary arterial systolic pressure ≥40 mm Hg) usually appear in the 30s or later in 10% to 20% of cases. Closure of the ASD has traditionally been carried out at open heart surgery, but more recently, endovascular catheter-based closures have been accomplished; mortality rates for either approach have been less than 1%. The defects may be multiple, and in symptomatic older children, defects of 2 cm or more in diameter are not unusual. Females with ASD outnumber males 3 to 1. Ostium secundum ASDs are one of the most common types of CHDs yet are the least severe.

Endocardial cushion defects with ostium primum ASDs are less common forms of ASDs (see Fig. 13.26E). Several cardiac defects are grouped under this heading because they result from the same developmental defect, a deficiency of the endocardial cushions and the AV septum. The septum primum does not fuse with the endocardial cushions; as a result, there is a **patent foramen primum-ostium primum defect**. Usually, there is also

Atrial Septal Defects—cont'd

a cleft in the anterior cusp of the mitral valve. In the less common complete type of endocardial cushion and AV septal defects, fusion of the endocardial cushions fails to occur. As a result, there is a large defect in the center of the heart, an **AV septal defect** (Fig. 13.27A). This type of ASD occurs in approximately 20% of persons with Down syndrome; otherwise, it is a relatively uncommon cardiac defect. It consists of a continuous interatrial and interventricular defect with markedly abnormal AV valves.

All **sinus venosus ASDs** (high ASDs) are located in the superior part of the interatrial septum close to the entry of the SVC (see Fig. 13.26F). A sinus venosus defect is a rare type of ASD. It results from incomplete absorption of the sinus venosus into the right atrium and/or abnormal development of the septum secundum. This type of ASD is commonly associated with partial anomalous pulmonary venous connections.

Common atrium is a rare cardiac defect in which the interatrial septum is absent. This defect is the result of the failure of the septum primum and septum secundum to develop (combination of ostium secundum, ostium primum, and sinus venosus defects).

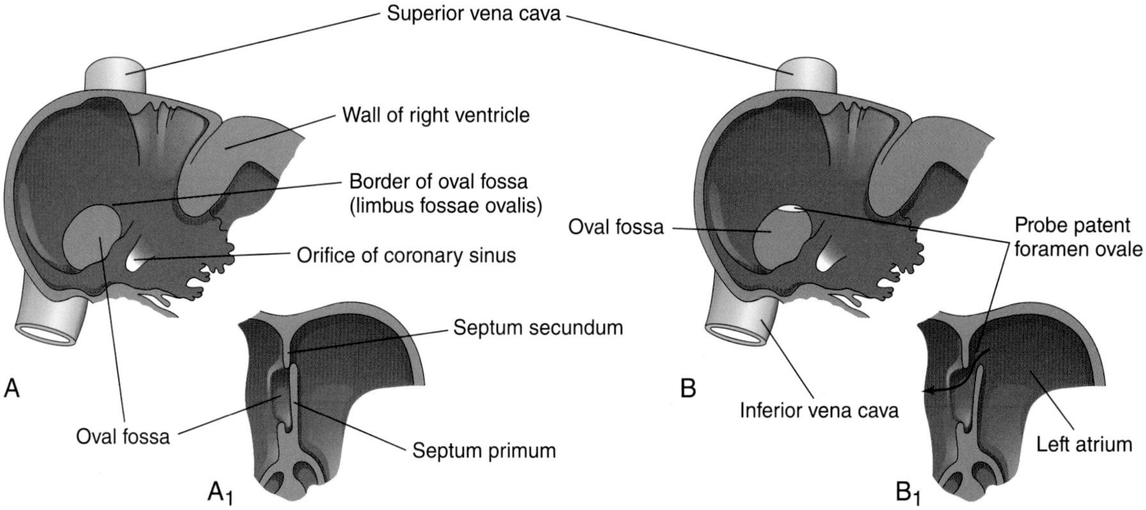

Fig. 13.25 (A) Normal postnatal appearance of the right side of the interatrial septum after adhesion of the septum primum to the septum secundum. (A_1) Sketch of a section of the interatrial septum illustrating the formation of the oval fossa in the right atrium. Note that the floor of the oval fossa is formed by the septum primum. (B and B_1) Similar views of a probe patent foramen ovale resulting from incomplete adhesion of the septum primum to the septum secundum. Some well-oxygenated blood can enter the right atrium via a patent foramen ovale; however, if the opening is small it is usually of no hemodynamic significance.

Patent Foramen Ovale

A **patent foramen ovale (PFO)**, a variant seen in approximately 25% usually results from abnormal resorption of the septum primum during the formation of the foramen secundum. If resorption occurs in abnormal locations, the septum primum is fenestrated or net like (see Fig. 13.26A). If excessive resorption of the septum primum occurs, the resulting short septum primum will not close the foramen ovale (see Fig. 13.26B). If an abnormally large foramen ovale occurs because of defective development of the septum secundum, a normal septum primum will not close the abnormal foramen ovale at birth (see Fig. 13.26C). The size of a PFO ranges from approximately 1 to 20 mm with the size increasing with age. A small isolated PFO is of no hemodynamic significance; however, if there are other defects (e.g., pulmonary stenosis or atresia), blood is shunted through the ovale into the left atrium and produces **cyanosis** (deficient oxygenation of blood). A larger PFO in adults may also be associated with migraine, cryptogenic stroke, and place individuals at higher risk of decompression sickness when scuba diving.

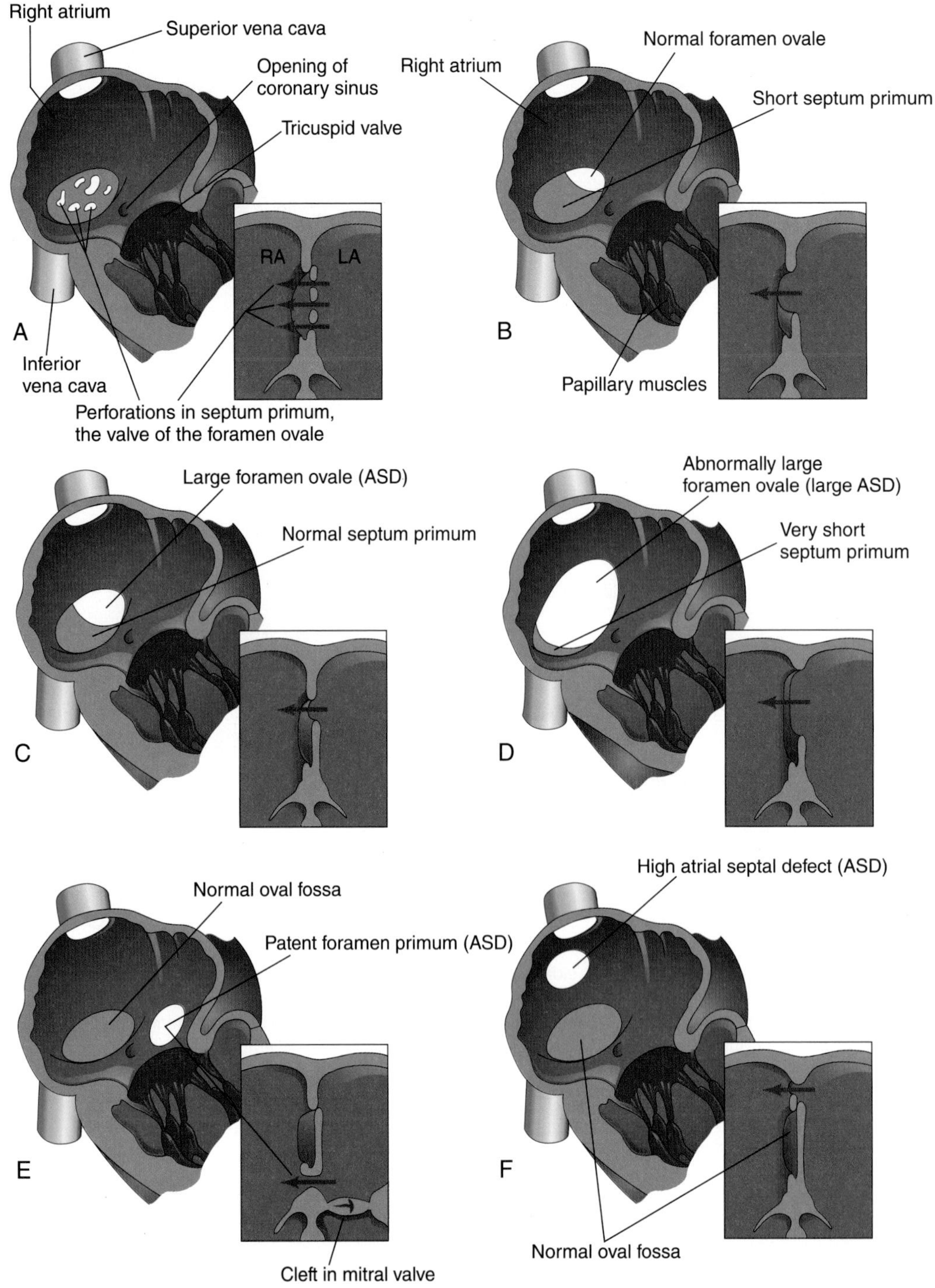

Fig. 13.26 Drawings of the right aspect of the interatrial septum. The adjacent sketches of sections of the septa illustrate various types of atrial septal defect *(ASD)*. (A) Patent foramen ovale resulting from resorption of the septum primum in abnormal locations. (B) Patent foramen ovale caused by excessive resorption of the septum primum (short flap defect). (C) Patent foramen ovale resulting from an abnormally large foramen ovale. (D) Patent foramen ovale resulting from an abnormally large foramen ovale and excessive resorption of the septum primum. (E) Endocardial cushion defect with primum-type ASD. The adjacent section shows the cleft in the anterior cusp of the mitral valve. (F) Sinus venosus ASD. The high septal defect resulted from abnormal absorption of the sinus venosus into the right atrium. In (E and F) note that the oval fossa has formed normally. *Arrows* indicate the direction of the flow of blood.

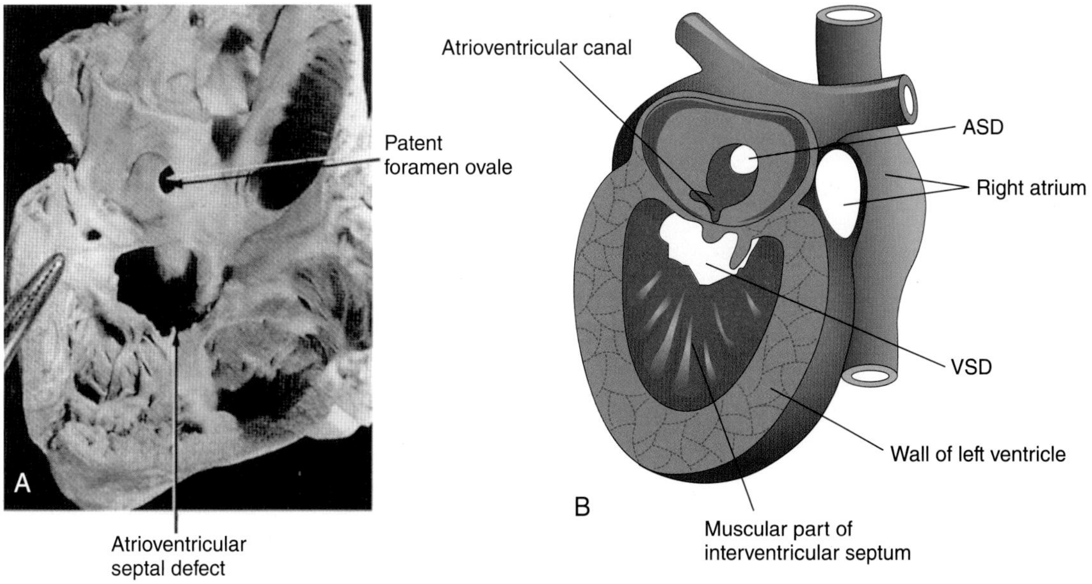

Fig. 13.27 (A) An infant's heart sectioned and viewed from the right side, showing a patent foramen ovale and an atrioventricular septal defect. (B) Schematic drawing of a heart illustrating various septal defects. *ASD*, Atrial septal defect; *VSD*, ventricular septal defect. (A, From Lev M: Autopsy diagnosis of congenitally malformed hearts, Springfield, 1953, Charles C. Thomas.)

Ventricular Septal Defects

Ventricular septal defects (VSDs) *are the most common types of CHDs*, accounting for approximately 35% of congenital heart defects (isolated VSD, 3:1000). VSDs occur more frequently in males than in females. VSDs may occur in any part of the interventricular septum (see Fig. 13.27B), but **membranous VSD** is the most common type (Fig. 13.28A; see also Fig. 13.27B). Frequently, during the first year, 30% to 50% of small VSDs close spontaneously.

Incomplete closure of the interventricular foramen results from failure of the membranous part of the interventricular septum to develop. This results from the failure of an extension of subendocardial tissue to grow from the right side of the **endocardial cushion** and fuse with the aorticopulmonary septum and the muscular part of the interventricular septum (see Fig. 13.18C–E). Large VSDs with excessive pulmonary blood flow (Fig. 13.29) and pulmonary hypertension result in **dyspnea** (difficult breathing) and cardiac failure early in infancy.

Muscular VSD is a less common type of defect and may appear anywhere in the muscular part of the interventricular septum. Sometimes there are multiple small defects, producing what is sometimes called the **"Swiss cheese" VSD**. Muscular VSDs probably occur because of excessive cavitation of myocardial tissue during the formation of the ventricular walls and the muscular part of the interventricular septum.

Absence of the interventricular septum (**single ventricle**, or common ventricle), resulting from failure of the interventricular septum to form, is extremely rare and results in a **three-chambered heart**. When there is a single ventricle, the atria empty through a single common valve or two separate AV valves into a single ventricular chamber. The aorta and pulmonary trunk arise from the ventricle. **Transposition of the great arteries (TGA**; see Fig. 13.31) or malposition of the great arteries may be present in those with a single ventricle. Most infants with a single ventricle often have a rudimentary outlet chamber. Some children die during infancy from **congestive heart failure**.

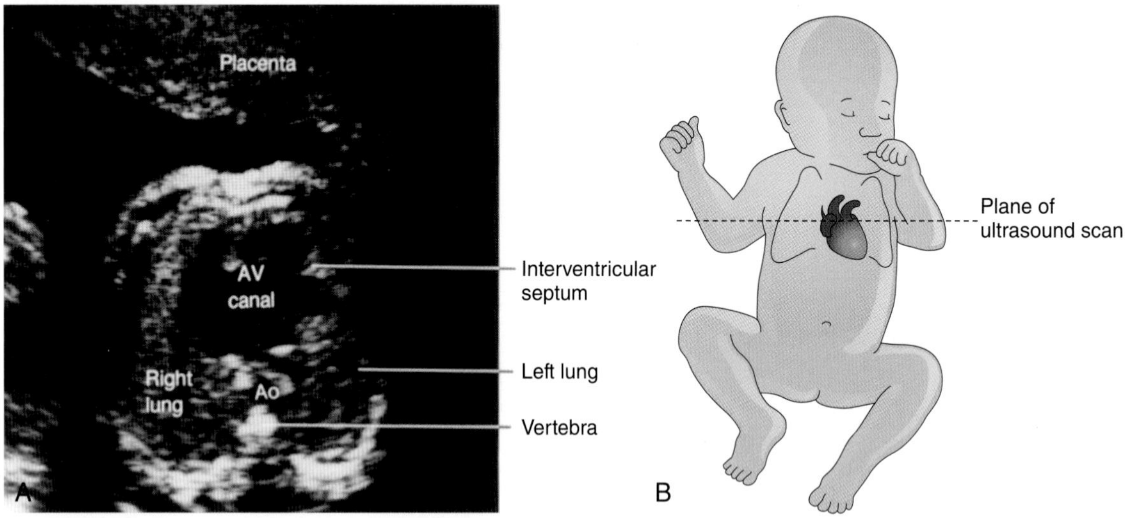

Fig. 13.28 (A) Ultrasound image of the heart of a second-trimester fetus with an atrioventricular *(AV)* canal (atrioventricular septal) defect. An atrial septal defect and a ventricular septal defect are also present. *Ao*, Aorta. (B) Orientation drawing. (A, Courtesy Dr. B. Benacerraf, Diagnostic Ultrasound Associates, P.C., Boston, Massachusetts.)

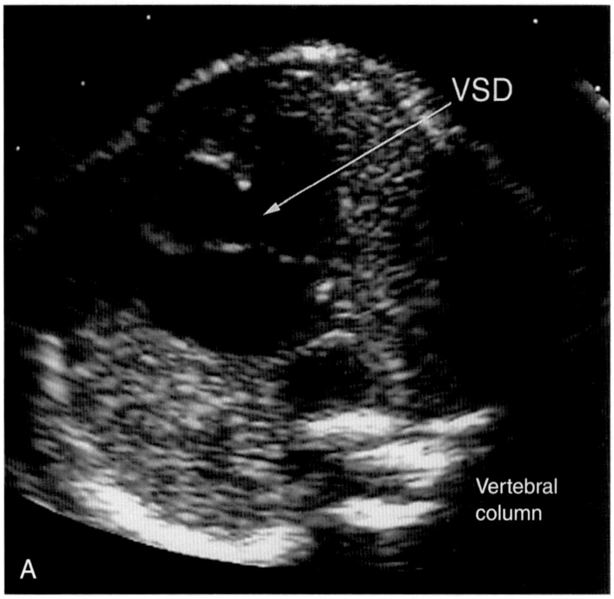

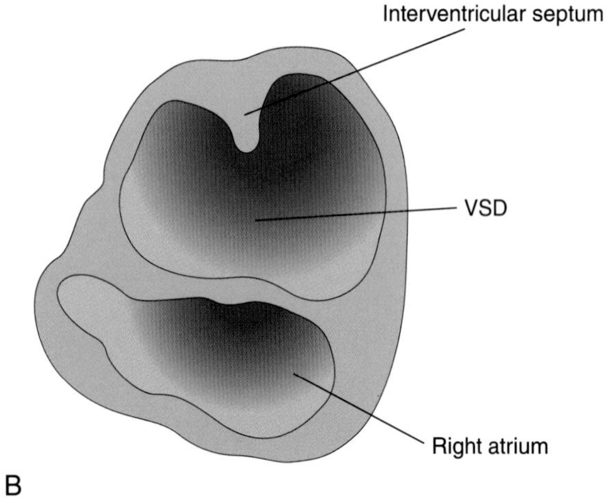

Fig. 13.29 (A) Ultrasound scan of a fetal heart at 23 weeks with an atrioventricular septal defect and a large ventricular septal defect *(VSD)*. (B) Orientation drawing. (A, Courtesy Dr. Wesley Lee, Division of Fetal Imaging, William Beaumont Hospital, Royal Oak, Michigan.)

Persistent Truncus Arteriosus

Persistent truncus arteriosus (7:100,000 live births) results from failure of the truncal ridges and the aorticopulmonary septum to develop normally and divide the truncus arteriosus into the aorta and pulmonary trunk (Fig. 13.30A and B). A **single arterial trunk**, the truncus arteriosus, arises from the heart and supplies the systemic, pulmonary, and coronary circulations. A VSD is always present with a truncus arteriosus defect; the truncus arteriosus straddles the VSD (see Fig. 13.30B).

Recent studies indicate that developmental arrest of the outflow tract, **semilunar valves**, and aortic sac in the early embryo (days 31 to 32) is involved in the pathogenesis of truncus arteriosus defects. The common type of truncus arteriosus defect is a single arterial vessel that branches to form the **pulmonary trunk** and **ascending aorta** (see Fig. 13.30A and B). In the next most common type of truncus arteriosus defect, the right and left pulmonary arteries arise close together from the dorsal wall of the truncus arteriosus (Fig. 13.30C). Less common types are illustrated in Fig. 13.30D and E.

Aorticopulmonary Septal Defect

Aorticopulmonary septal defect is a very rare condition, representing only 0.1% of all congenital heart defects, in which there is an opening **(aortic window)** between the aorta and pulmonary trunk near the aortic valve. The aorticopulmonary defect results from a localized defect in the formation of the **aorticopulmonary septum**. The presence of pulmonary and aortic valves and an intact interventricular septum distinguishes this defect from the persistent truncus arteriosus defect.

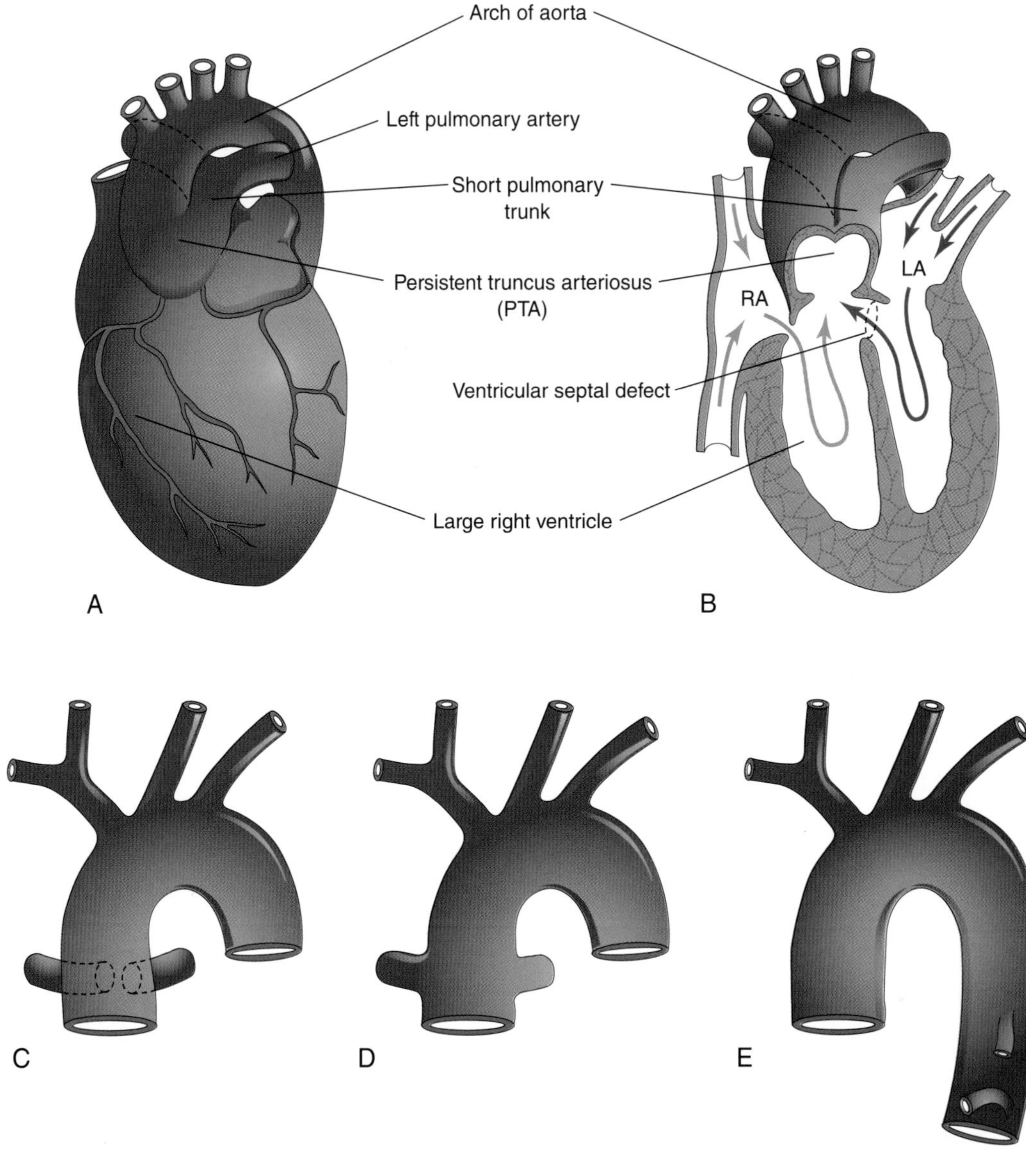

Fig. 13.30 Illustrations of common types of persistent truncus arteriosus. (A) The common trunk divides into the aorta and a short pulmonary trunk. (B) Coronal section of the heart shown in (A). Observe the circulation of blood in this heart *(arrows)* and the ventricular septal defect.*LA*, Left atrium; *RA*, right atrium. (C) The right and left pulmonary arteries arise close together from the truncus arteriosus. (D) The pulmonary arteries arise independently from the sides of the truncus arteriosus. (E) No pulmonary arteries are present; the lungs are supplied by the bronchial arteries.

Transposition of the Great Arteries

Transposition of the great arteries (TGA) is a severe congenital heart defect with an incidence of approximately 1:4,000 live births. It is the most common cause of cyanotic heart disease in neonates (Fig. 13.31) and is often associated with other cardiac defects (e.g., ASD and VSD). In typical cases, the aorta lies anterior and to the right of the pulmonary trunk and arises from the morphologic right ventricle, whereas the pulmonary trunk arises from the morphologic left ventricle. The associated ASD and VSD defects permit some interchange between the pulmonary and systemic circulations.

Because of these anatomic defects, **deoxygenated systemic venous blood** returning to the right atrium enters the right ventricle and then passes to the body through the aorta. Oxygenated pulmonary venous blood passes through the left ventricle back into the pulmonary circulation. With a patent foramen ovale and patency of the ductus arteriosus, there is some mixing of blood. However, in the absence of a patent foramen ovale, a balloon atrial septoplasty (creation of a hole between the atria) is lifesaving by permitting blood to flow from left to right while awaiting definitive surgical correction. Without surgical correction of the TGA, these infants usually die within a few months.

Many attempts have been made to explain the basis of TGA, but the **conal growth hypothesis** is favored by most investigators. According to this explanation, the **aorticopulmonary septum** fails to pursue a spiral course during the partitioning of the bulbus cordis and truncus arteriosus. This defect is thought to result from failure of the **conus arteriosus** to develop normally during the incorporation of the bulbus cordis into the ventricles. Defective migration of neural crest cells is involved. Rare variants in individual genes have been detected in some cases of children with TGA, but for most cases, the cause is unknown and may be due to polygenic inheritance.

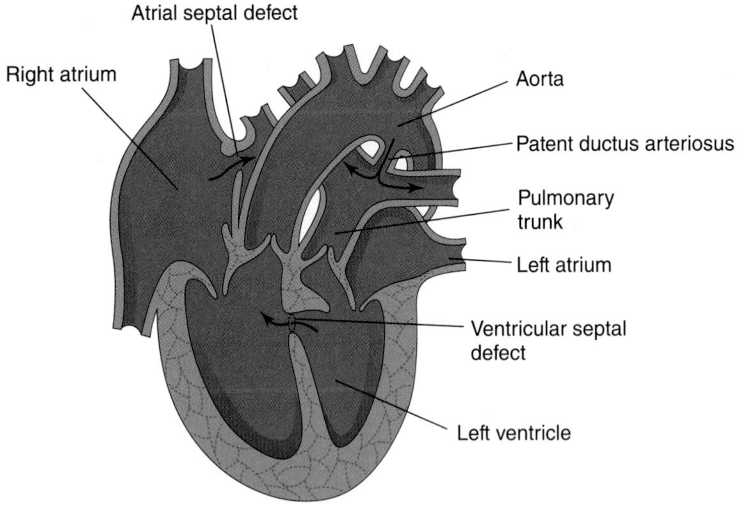

Fig. 13.31 Drawing of a heart illustrating transposition of the great arteries (TGA). The ventricular and atrial septal defects allow mixing of the arterial and venous blood. TGA is the most common single cause of cyanotic heart disease in neonates. This birth defect is often associated with other cardiac defects as shown (i.e., ventricular septal defect and atrial septal defect).

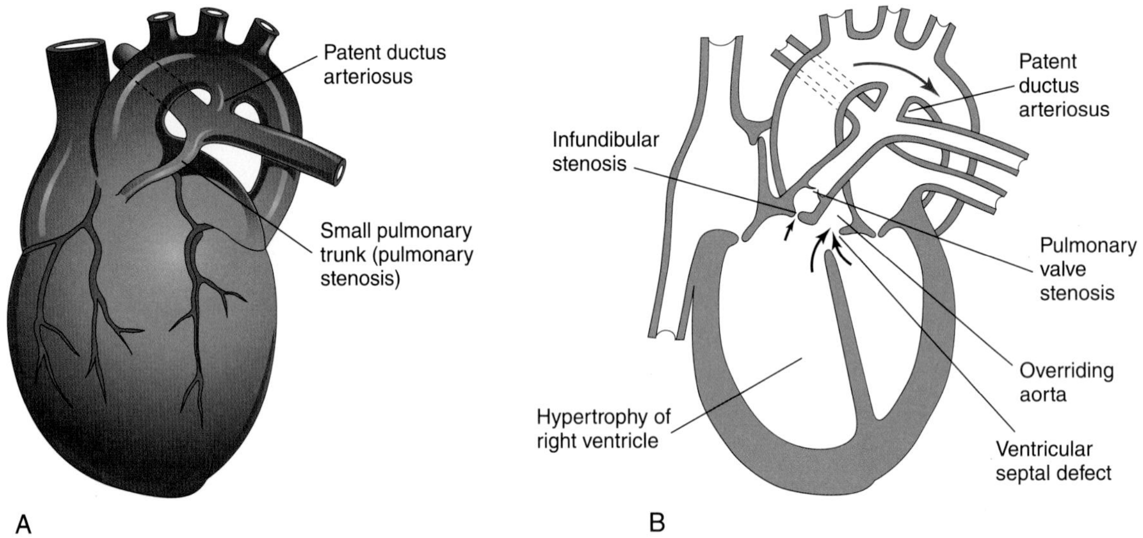

Fig. 13.32 (A) Drawing of an infant's heart showing a small pulmonary trunk (pulmonary stenosis), and a large aorta resulting from unequal partitioning of the truncus arteriosus. There is also hypertrophy of the right ventricle and a patent ductus arteriosus. (B) Frontal section of this heart illustrating the tetralogy of Fallot. Observe the four cardiac defects of this tetralogy: pulmonary valve stenosis, ventricular septal defect, overriding aorta, and hypertrophy of the right ventricle. The *arrows* indicate the flow of blood into the great vessels (aorta and pulmonary trunk).

Unequal Division of the Truncus Arteriosus

Unequal division of the truncus arteriosus results when partitioning of the truncus arteriosus superior to the valves is unequal (Figs. 13.32A and 13.33B and C). One of the great arteries is large, and the other is small. As a result, the **aorticopulmonary septum** is not aligned with the interventricular septum, and a VSD develops; of the two vessels, the one with the larger diameter usually straddles the VSD (see Fig. 13.32B).

In **pulmonary valve stenosis**, the cusps of the pulmonary valve are fused to form a dome with a narrow central opening (see Fig. 13.33D).

In **infundibular stenosis**, the conus arteriosus (infundibulum) of the right ventricle is underdeveloped. The two types of pulmonary stenosis may occur. Depending on the degree of obstruction to blood flow, there is a variable degree of hypertrophy (greater bulk) of the right ventricle (see Fig. 13.32A and B).

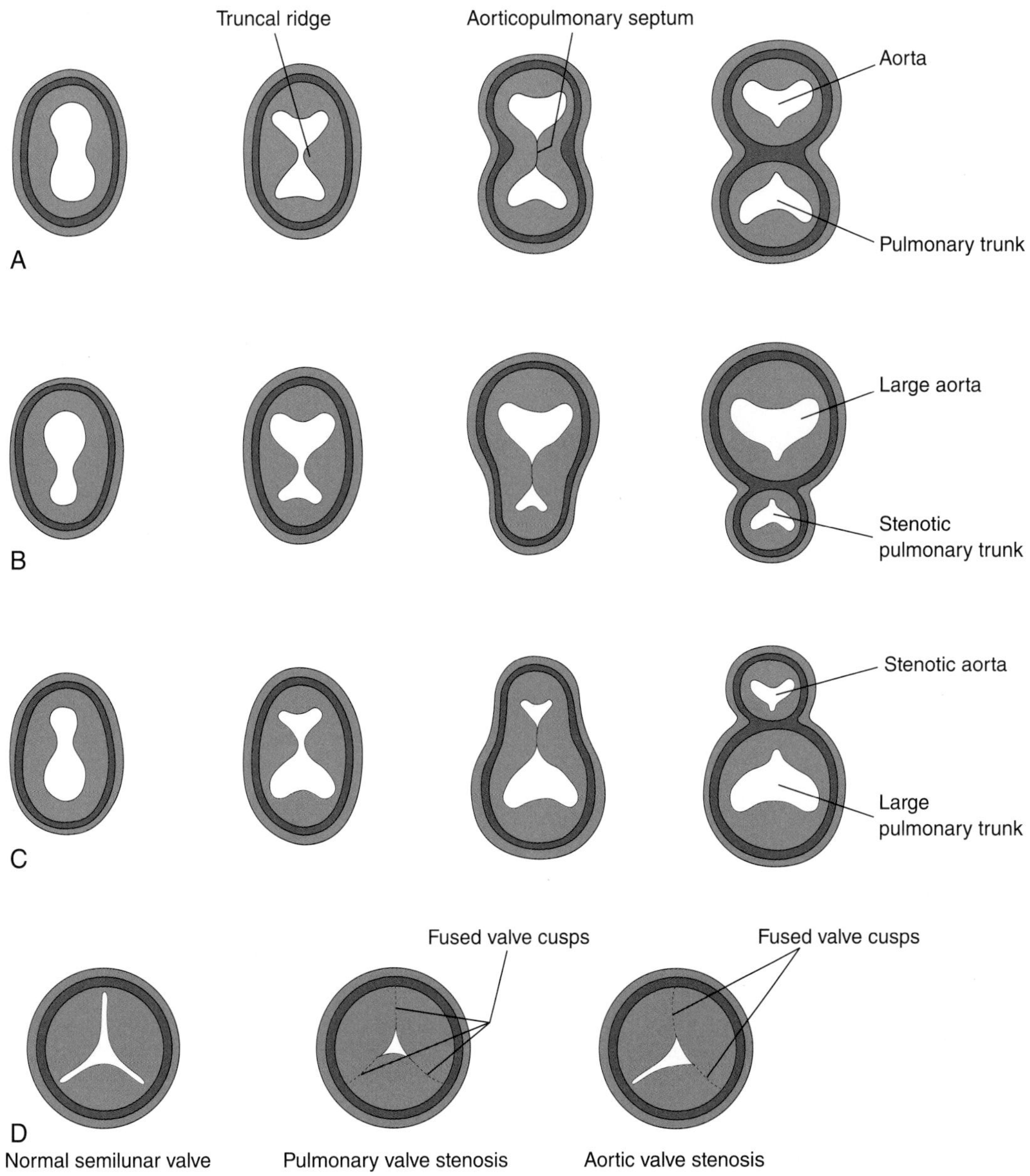

Fig. 13.33 Abnormal division of truncus arteriosus. (A–C) Sketches of transverse sections of the truncus arteriosus, illustrating normal and abnormal partitioning of the truncus arteriosus. (A) Normal. (B) Unequal partitioning of the truncus arteriosus resulting in a small pulmonary trunk. (C) Unequal partitioning resulting in a small aorta. (D) Sketches illustrating a normal semilunar valve and stenotic pulmonary and aortic valves.

Tetralogy of Fallot

Tetralogy of Fallot (3–5:10,000) is a classic group of four cardiac defects (Figs. 13.34 and 13.35; see also Fig. 13.32B) consisting of:

- Pulmonary artery stenosis (obstruction of right ventricular outflow)
- Ventricular septal defect
- Dextroposition of the aorta (overriding or straddling the aorta)
- Right ventricular hypertrophy

In these defects, the pulmonary trunk is usually small (see Fig. 13.32A), and there may be various degrees of pulmonary artery stenosis. **Cyanosis** is an obvious sign of tetralogy, but it is not usually present at birth, and in some cases, the degree of pulmonary stenosis is so mild that surgical management may be delayed for months after birth.

The tetralogy results when the division of the truncus arteriosus is unequal and the pulmonary trunk is stenotic. **Pulmonary atresia with VSD** is an extreme form of tetralogy of Fallot; the entire right ventricular output is through the aorta. Pulmonary blood flow is dependent on a patent ductus arteriosus or bronchial collateral vessels. Initial treatment may require surgical placement of a temporary shunt, but in many cases, primary surgical repair is the treatment of choice in early infancy.

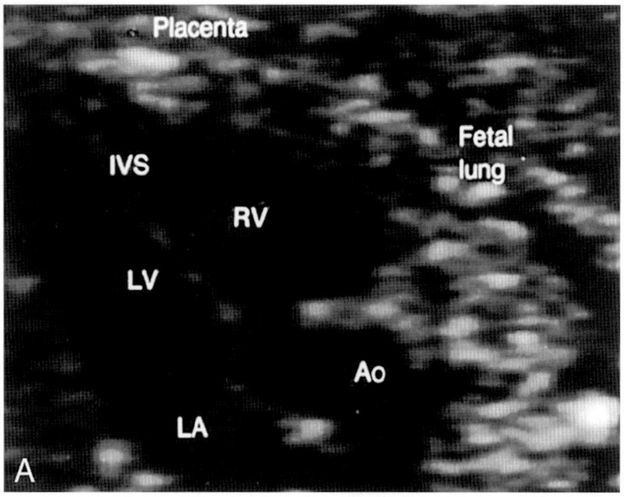

Fig. 13.34 Ultrasound image (orientation as in Fig. 13.28B) of the heart of a 20-week fetus with tetralogy of Fallot. Note that the large overriding aorta *(Ao)* straddles the interventricular septum. As a result, it receives blood from the left ventricle *(LV)* and right ventricle *(RV)*. *IVS*, Interventricular septum; *LA*, left atrium. (Courtesy Dr. B. Benacerraf, Diagnostic Ultrasound Associates, P.C., Boston, Massachusetts.)

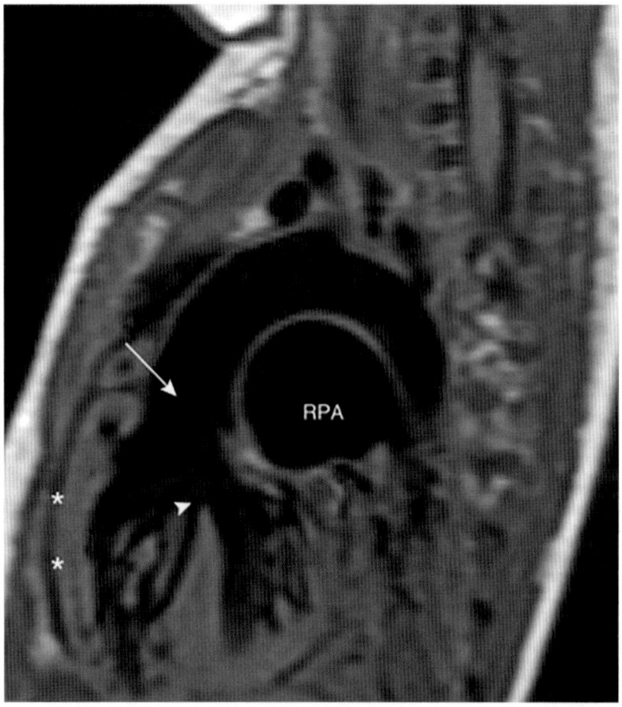

Fig. 13.35 Tetralogy of Fallot–absent pulmonary valve syndrome in a 3-day-old boy with respiratory distress. Sagittal T1-weighted magnetic resonance imaging shows features of tetralogy of Fallot with right ventricular hypertrophy *(asterisks)*, a ventricular septal defect *(arrowhead)*, and an overriding aorta *(arrow)*. The right pulmonary artery *(RPA)* is markedly dilated. (From Newman B, Towbin AJ, Chan FP: Syndromes and chromosomal anomalies. In Coley BD, editor: *Caffey's pediatric diagnostic imaging*, ed 13, Philadelphia, 2019, Elsevier.)

Aortic Stenosis and Aortic Atresia

In **aortic valve stenosis**, the edges of the valve are usually fused to form a dome with a narrow opening (see Fig. 13.33D). This defect may be congenital or develop after birth. The valvular stenosis causes extra work for the heart and results in **hypertrophy of the left ventricle** and abnormal **heart sounds (heart murmurs)**.

In subaortic stenosis, there is often a band of fibrous tissue just inferior to the aortic valve. The narrowing of the aorta results from the persistence of tissue that normally degenerates as the valve forms. **Aortic atresia** is present when obstruction of the aorta or its valve is complete.

Hypoplastic Left Heart Syndrome

The left ventricle is small and nonfunctional (Fig. 13.36); the right ventricle maintains both pulmonary and systemic circulations. The blood passes through an ASD or a dilated foramen ovale from the left to the right side of the heart, where it mixes with the systemic venous blood.

In addition to the underdeveloped left ventricle, there is atresia or stenosis of the aortic or mitral valves and hypoplasia of the ascending aorta. The incidence is approximately 3:10,000 live births.

Long-term survival through surgical palliation [cardiac transplantation or a triple staged surgery (Norwood palliation)] is possible with most children surviving into adulthood. More recently, a hybrid Norwood approach has been developed in which the first stage of the three-stage repair includes a pulmonary artery banding, stenting of the ductus arteriosus, and an atrial septostomy. This approach is less surgically complex than the classic first-stage procedure. Disturbances in the migration of neural crest cells, hemodynamic function, in apoptosis, and the proliferation of the extracellular matrix are likely responsible for the pathogenesis of many CHDs such as this syndrome. Recent studies indicate pathogenic variants (mutations) in genes and a complex mutagenic involvement in sporadic cases of hypoplastic left heart syndrome.

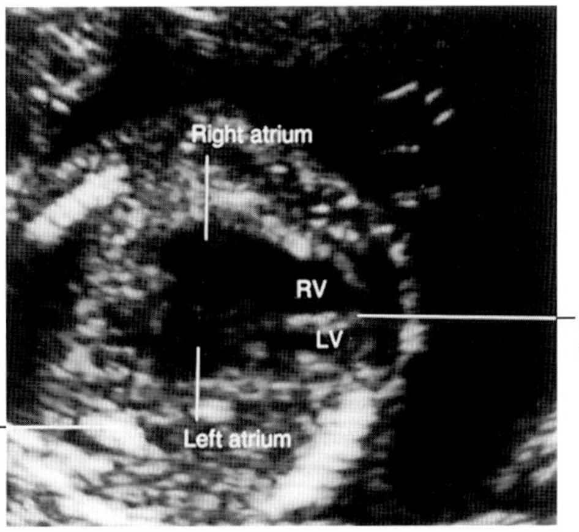

Fig. 13.36 Ultrasound image of the heart of a second-trimester fetus with a hypoplastic left heart. Note that the left ventricle *(LV)* is much smaller than the right ventricle *(RV)*. This is an oblique scan of the fetal thorax through the long axis of the ventricles. (Courtesy Dr. B. Benacerraf, Diagnostic Ultrasound Associates, P.C., Boston, Massachusetts.)

7

DERIVATIVES OF PHARYNGEAL ARCH ARTERIES

As the pharyngeal arches develop during the fourth week, they are supplied by pharyngeal arch arteries from the **aortic sac** (Fig. 13.37B). Mesodermal cells migrate from the arches to the aortic sac, connecting the pharyngeal arch arteries to the outflow tract. These arteries terminate in the dorsal aorta on the ipsilateral side. Although six pairs of arch arteries usually develop, they are not present at the same time (see Fig. 13.37B and C). By the time the sixth pair of arch arteries has formed, the first two pairs have disappeared (see Fig. 13.37C). During the eighth week, the primordial **pharyngeal arch arterial pattern** is transformed into the final fetal arterial arrangement (Fig. 13.38C).

Molecular studies indicate that the transcription factor Tbx1 regulates migration of the neural crest cells that contribute to the formation of the pharyngeal arch arteries.

DERIVATIVES OF FIRST PAIR OF PHARYNGEAL ARCH ARTERIES

Most of these arteries disappear, but remnants of them form part of the **maxillary arteries**, which supply the ears, teeth, and muscles of the eye and face. These arteries may also contribute to the formation of the **external carotid arteries** (see Fig. 13.38B).

DERIVATIVES OF SECOND PAIR OF PHARYNGEAL ARCH ARTERIES

Dorsal parts of these arteries persist and form the stems of the **stapedial arteries**; these small vessels run through the ring of the stapes, a small bone in the middle ear (see Fig. 18.16C).

DERIVATIVES OF THIRD PAIR OF PHARYNGEAL ARCH ARTERIES

Proximal parts of these arteries form the **common carotid arteries**, which supply structures in the head (see Fig. 13.38D). Distal parts of these arteries join with the dorsal **aortae** to form the **internal carotid arteries**, which supply the middle ears, orbits, brain, meninges, and pituitary gland.

DERIVATIVES OF FOURTH PAIR OF PHARYNGEAL ARCH ARTERIES

The left fourth arch artery forms **part of the arch of the aorta** (see Fig. 13.38C). The proximal part of the artery develops from the **aortic sac**, and the distal part is derived from the **left dorsal aorta**. The right fourth arch artery becomes the **proximal part of the right subclavian artery**. The distal part of the right subclavian artery forms from the **right dorsal aorta** and **right seventh intersegmental artery**.

The left subclavian artery is not derived from a pharyngeal arch artery; it is formed from the **left seventh intersegmental artery** (see Fig. 13.38A). As development proceeds, differential growth shifts the origin of the left subclavian artery cranially. Consequently, it lies close to the origin of the left common carotid artery (see Fig. 13.38D).

FATE OF FIFTH PAIR OF PHARYNGEAL ARCH ARTERIES

Approximately 50% of the time, the fifth pair of arteries consists of rudimentary vessels that soon degenerate, leaving no vascular derivatives. In the other 50% of persons, these arteries do not develop.

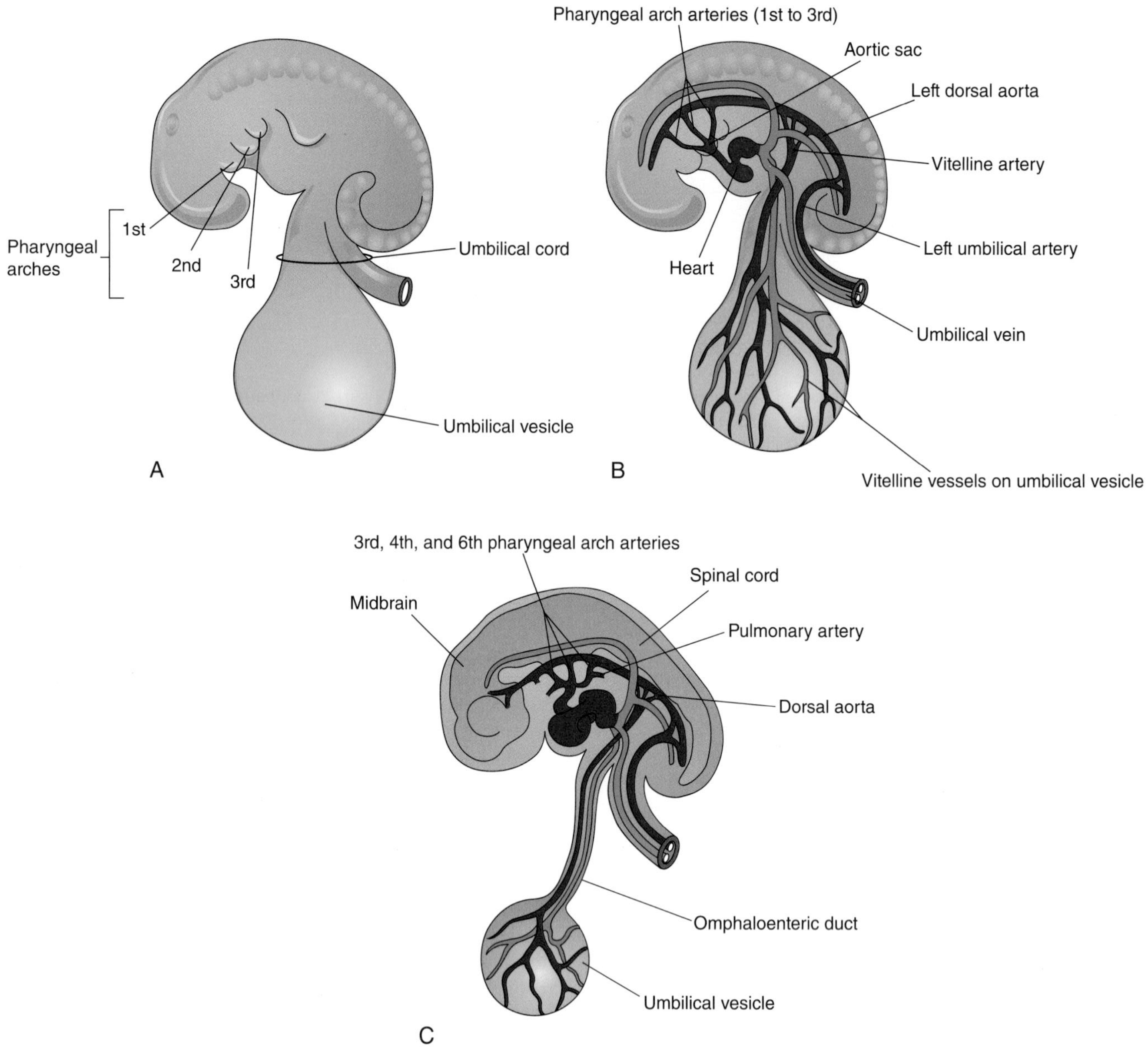

Fig. 13.37 Pharyngeal arches and pharyngeal arch arteries. (A) Left side of an embryo (approximately 26 days). (B) Schematic drawing of this embryo showing the left pharyngeal arch arteries arising from the aortic sac, running through the pharyngeal arches, and terminating in the left dorsal aorta. (C) An embryo (approximately 37 days) showing the single dorsal aorta and that most of the first two pairs of pharyngeal arch arteries have degenerated.

DERIVATIVES OF SIXTH PAIR OF PHARYNGEAL ARCH ARTERIES

The **left sixth artery** develops as follows (see Fig. 13.38B and C):

- The proximal part of the artery persists as the proximal part of the **left pulmonary artery**.
- The distal part of the artery passes from the left pulmonary artery to the dorsal aorta and forms a prenatal shunt, the **ductus arteriosus**.
- The **right sixth artery** develops as follows:
- The proximal part of the artery persists as the proximal part of the **right pulmonary artery**.
- The distal part of the artery degenerates.

The transformation of the sixth pair of arteries explains why the course of the **recurrent laryngeal nerves** differs on the two sides. These nerves supply the sixth pair of pharyngeal arches and hook around the sixth pair of arteries on their way to the developing larynx (Fig. 13.39A).

On the right, because the distal part of the right sixth artery degenerates, the right recurrent laryngeal nerve moves superiorly and hooks around the proximal part of the **right subclavian artery**, the derivative of the fourth artery (Fig. 13.39B). On the left, the left recurrent laryngeal nerve hooks around the **ductus arteriosus** formed by the distal part of the sixth artery. When this arterial shunt involutes after birth, the nerve remains around the **ligamentum arteriosum** (remnant of the ductus arteriosus) and the arch of the aorta (Fig. 13.39C).

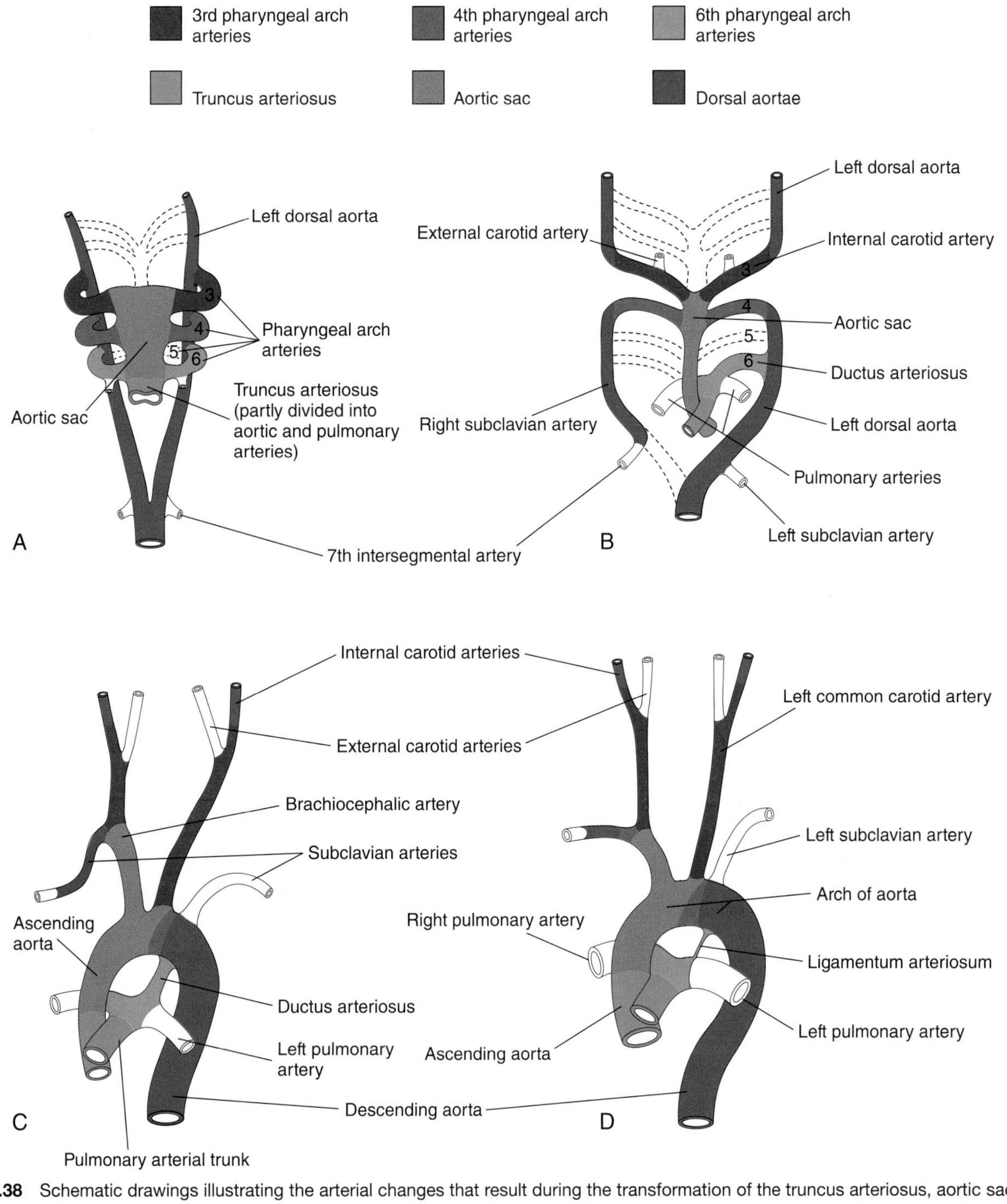

Fig. 13.38 Schematic drawings illustrating the arterial changes that result during the transformation of the truncus arteriosus, aortic sac, pharyngeal arch arteries, and dorsal aortae into the adult arterial pattern. The vessels that are not colored are not derived from these structures. (A) Pharyngeal arch arteries at 6 weeks; by this stage, the first two pairs of arteries have largely disappeared. (B) Pharyngeal arch arteries at 7 weeks; the parts of the dorsal aortae and pharyngeal arch arteries that normally disappear are indicated with *broken lines*. (C) Arterial arrangement at 8 weeks. (D) Sketch of the arterial vessels of a 6-month-old infant. Note that the ascending aorta and pulmonary arteries are considerably smaller in (C than in D). This represents the relative flow through these vessels at the different stages of development. Observe the large size of the ductus arteriosus in (C) and that it is essentially a direct continuation of the pulmonary trunk. The ductus arteriosus normally becomes functionally closed within the first few days after birth. Eventually, the ductus arteriosus becomes the ligamentum arteriosum, as shown in (D).

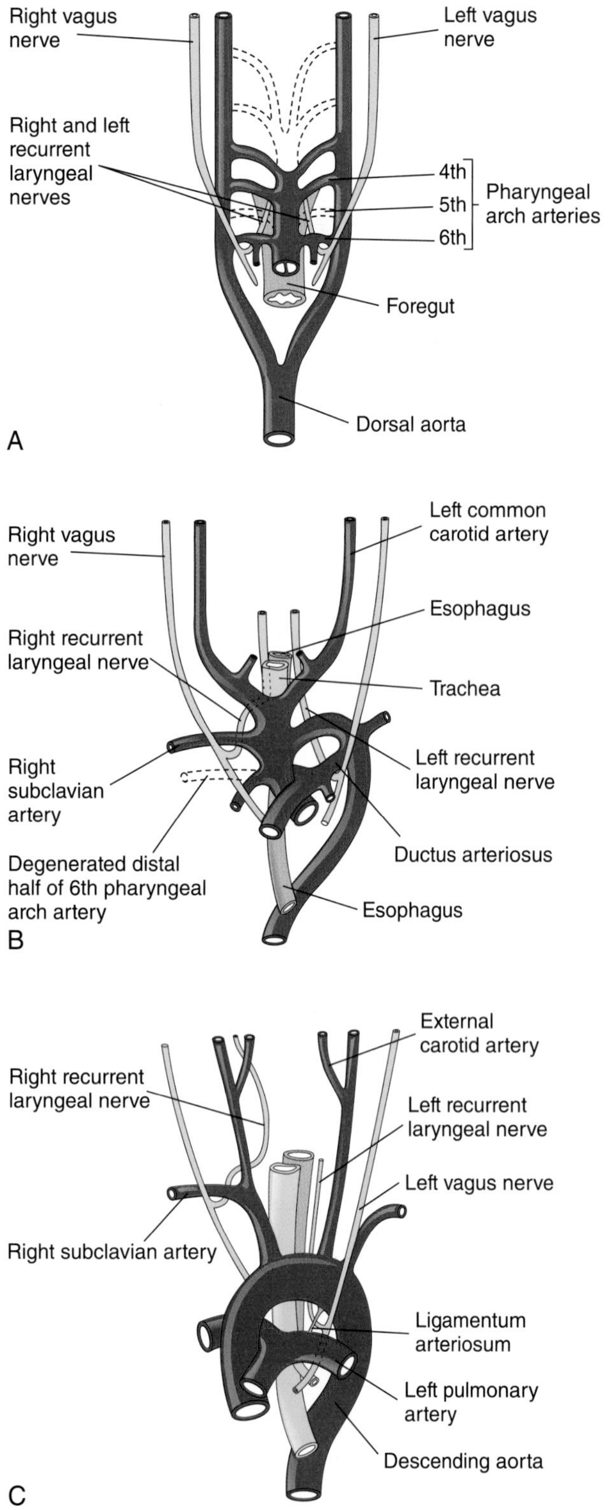

Fig. 13.39 The relation of the recurrent laryngeal nerves to the pharyngeal arch arteries. (A) At 6 weeks, showing the recurrent laryngeal nerves hooked around the sixth pair of pharyngeal arch arteries. (B) At 8 weeks, showing the right recurrent laryngeal nerve hooked around the right subclavian artery, and the left recurrent laryngeal nerve is hooked around the ductus arteriosus and the arch of the aorta. (C) After birth, showing the left recurrent nerve hooked around the ligamentum arteriosum and the arch of the aorta.

PHARYNGEAL ARCH ARTERIAL BIRTH DEFECTS

Because of the many changes involved in the transformation of the pharyngeal arch arterial system into the adult arterial pattern, arterial birth defects may occur. Most defects result from the persistence of parts of the pharyngeal arch arteries that usually disappear, or from the disappearance of parts that normally persist.

Coarctation of Aorta

Aortic coarctation (constriction) occurs in approximately 10% of children with CHDs. Coarctation is characterized by an aortic constriction of varying length (Fig. 13.40). Most coarctations occur distal to the origin of the left subclavian artery at the entrance of the ductus arteriosus (juxtaductal coarctation).

The classification into preductal and postductal coarctations is commonly used; however, in 90% of instances, the coarctation is directly opposite the ductus arteriosus. Coarctation occurs twice as often in males as in females and is associated with a mitral (bicuspid) aortic valve in 70% of cases (see Fig. 13.12E).

In **postductal coarctation**, the constriction is just distal to the ductus arteriosus (see Fig. 13.40A and B). This permits the development of collateral circulation during the fetal period (see Fig. 13.40B), thereby assisting with the passage of blood to inferior parts of the body.

In **preductal coarctation**, the constriction is proximal to the ductus arteriosus (see Fig. 13.40C). The narrowed segment may be extensive (see Fig. 13.40D); before birth, blood flows through the ductus arteriosus to the descending aorta for distribution to the lower body.

In an infant with severe **aortic coarctation**, closure of the ductus arteriosus results in **hypoperfusion** and rapid deterioration of the infant. These babies usually receive **prostaglandin E_2** in an attempt to reopen the ductus arteriosus and establish an adequate blood flow to the lower limbs. Aortic coarctation may be a feature of Turner syndrome (see Figs. 20.3 and 20.4). This and other observations suggest that genetic and/or environmental factors cause coarctation.

There are three main views about the embryologic basis of coarctation of the aorta:

- During the formation of the arch of the aorta, muscle tissue of the ductus arteriosus may be incorporated into the wall of the aorta; then, when the ductus arteriosus constricts at birth, the ductal muscle in the aorta also constricts, forming a coarctation.
- There may be abnormal involution of a small segment of the left dorsal aorta (see Fig. 13.40F). Later, this stenotic segment (area of coarctation) moves cranially with the left subclavian artery (see Fig. 13.40G).
- During fetal life, the segment of the arch of the aorta between the left subclavian artery and the ductus arteriosus is normally narrow because it carries very little blood. After the closure of the ductus arteriosus, this narrow area (isthmus) normally enlarges until it is the same diameter as the aorta. If the isthmus persists, a coarctation forms.

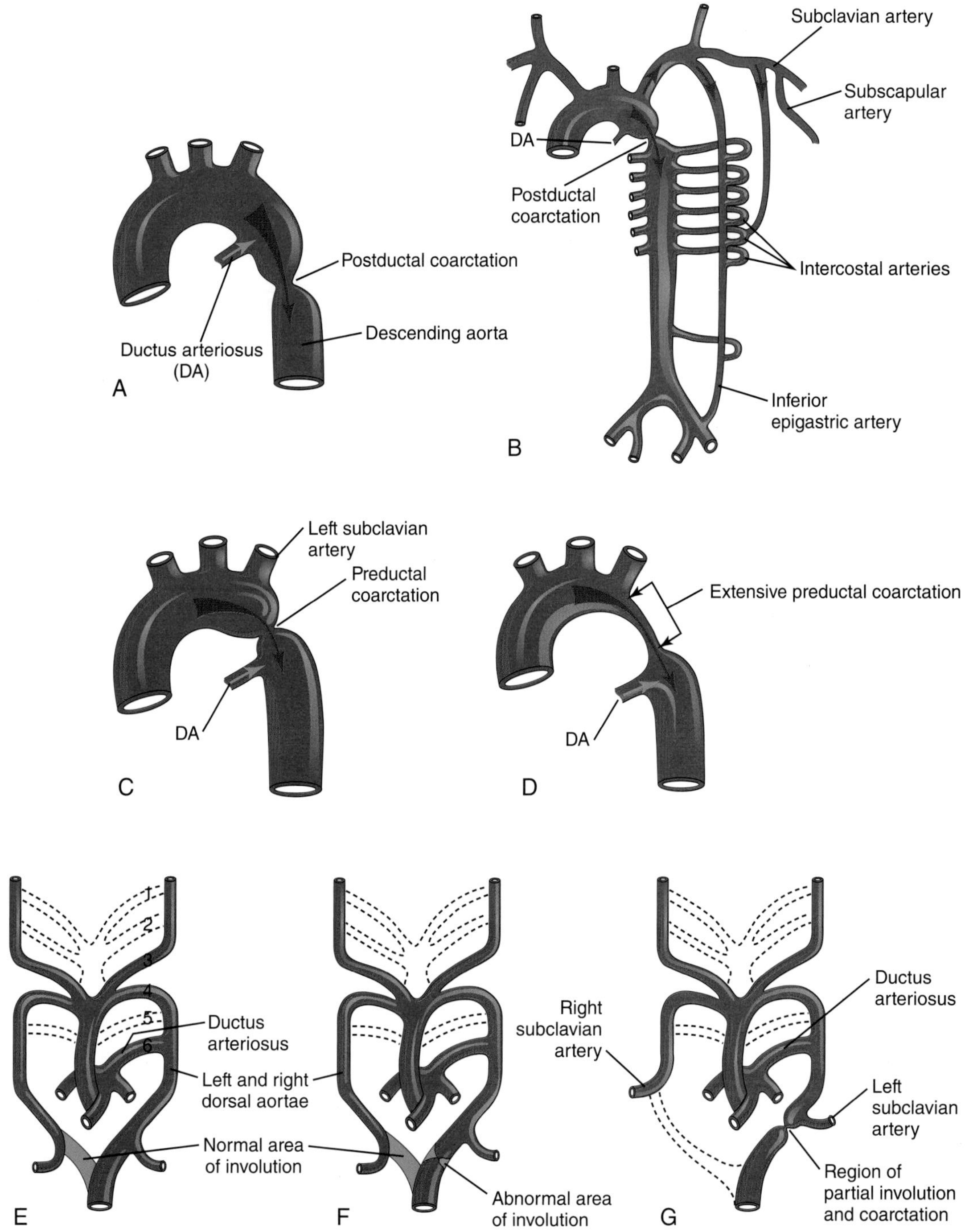

Fig. 13.40 (A) Postductal coarctation of the aorta. (B) Diagrammatic representation of the common routes of collateral circulation that develop in association with postductal coarctation of the aorta. (C and D) Preductal coarctation. (E) Sketch of the pharyngeal arch arterial pattern in a 7-week embryo, showing the areas that normally involute (see *dotted branches* of arteries). Note that the distal segment of the right dorsal aorta normally involutes as the right subclavian artery develops. (F) Abnormal involution of a small distal segment of the left dorsal aorta. (G) Later stage showing the abnormally involuted segment appearing as a coarctation of the aorta. This moves to the region of the ductus arteriosus with the left subclavian artery. These drawings (E–G) illustrate one hypothesis about the embryologic basis of coarctation of the aorta.

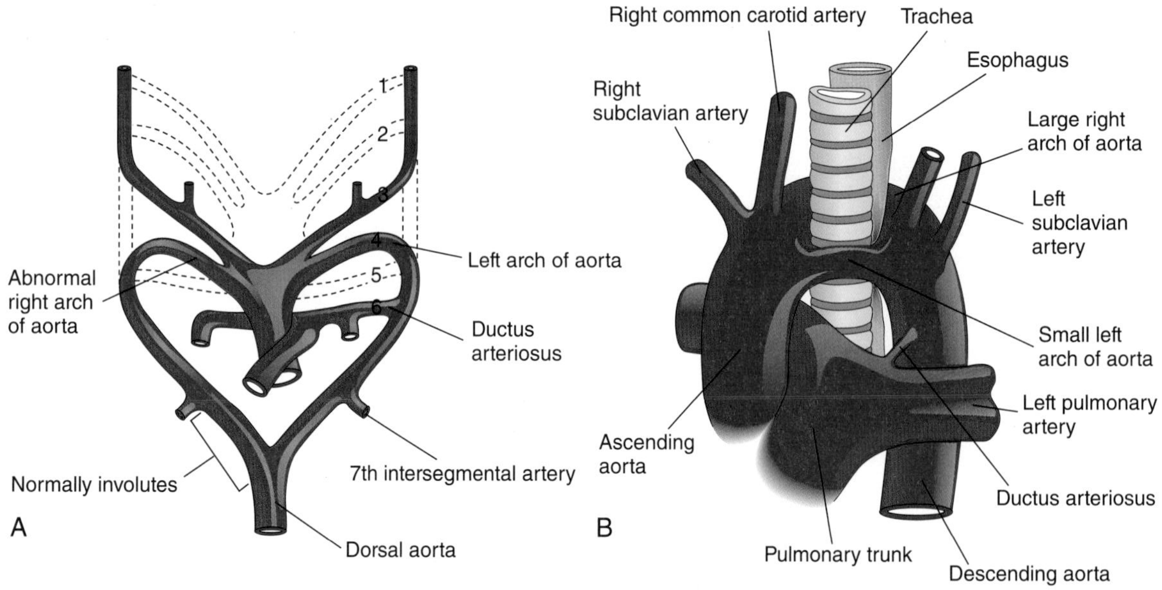

Fig. 13.41 (A) Drawing of the embryonic pharyngeal arch arteries illustrating the embryologic basis of the right and left arches of the aorta (double arch of the aorta). (B) A large right arch of the aorta and a small left arch of the aorta arise from the ascending aorta, forming a vascular ring around the trachea and esophagus. Observe that there is compression of the esophagus and trachea. The right common carotid and subclavian arteries arise separately from the large right arch of the aorta.

Double Aortic Arch

Double aortic arch is a very rare anomaly (5–7:100,000) that is characterized by a **vascular ring** around the trachea and esophagus (Fig. 13.41B). Varying degrees of compression of these structures may occur in infants. If the compression is significant, it causes wheezing respirations that are aggravated by crying, feeding, and flexion of the neck. In very severe cases, it can cause life-threatening tracheal obstruction. The vascular ring results from the failure of the distal part of the right dorsal aorta to disappear (Fig. 13.41A); as a result, right and left arches form. Usually, the right arch of the aorta is larger and passes posterior to the trachea and esophagus (see Fig. 13.41B).

Right Arch of Aorta

When the entire right dorsal aorta persists (0.1–1:1000) (Fig. 13.42A and B) and the distal part of the left dorsal aorta involutes, a right arch of the aorta results. There are two main types:

- **Right arch of the aorta without a retroesophageal component** (see Fig. 13.42B). The ductus arteriosus or ligamentum arteriosum passes from the right pulmonary artery to the right arch of the aorta. Because no vascular ring is formed, this condition is usually asymptomatic.
- **Right arch of the aorta with a retroesophageal component** (Fig. 13.42C). Originally, a small left arch of the aorta was probably involuted, leaving the right arch of the aorta posterior to the esophagus. The ductus arteriosus (ligamentum arteriosum) attaches to the distal part of the arch of the aorta and forms a ring, which may constrict the esophagus and trachea.

Anomalous Right Subclavian Artery

The right subclavian artery arises from the distal part of the arch of the aorta and passes posterior to the trachea and esophagus to supply the right upper limb (Figs. 13.43 and 13.44). A **retroesophageal right subclavian artery** occurs when the right fourth pharyngeal arch artery and the right dorsal aorta disappear cranial to the seventh intersegmental artery. As a result, the right subclavian artery forms from the right seventh intersegmental artery and the distal part of the right dorsal aorta. As development proceeds, differential growth shifts the origin of the right subclavian artery cranially until it comes to lie close to the origin of the left subclavian artery.

Although an anomalous right subclavian artery is fairly common (0.5–2:100) and always forms a vascular ring, it is rarely clinically significant because the ring is usually not tight enough to constrict the esophagus and trachea very much.

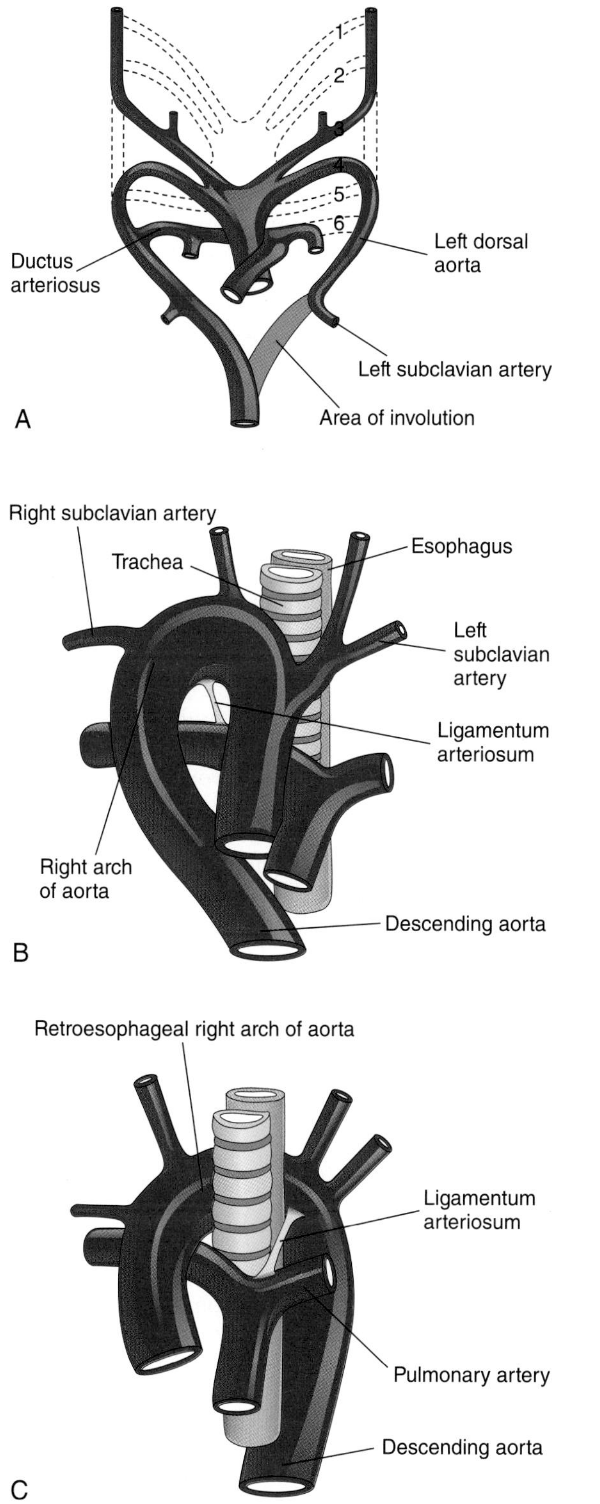

Fig. 13.42 (A) Sketch of the pharyngeal arch arteries showing the normal involution of the distal portion of the left dorsal aorta. There is also the persistence of the entire right dorsal aorta and the distal part of the right sixth pharyngeal arch artery. (B) Right pharyngeal arch artery without a retroesophageal component. (C) Right arch of the aorta with a retroesophageal component. The abnormal right arch of the aorta and the ligamentum arteriosum (postnatal remnant of the ductus arteriosus) form a ring that compresses the esophagus and trachea.

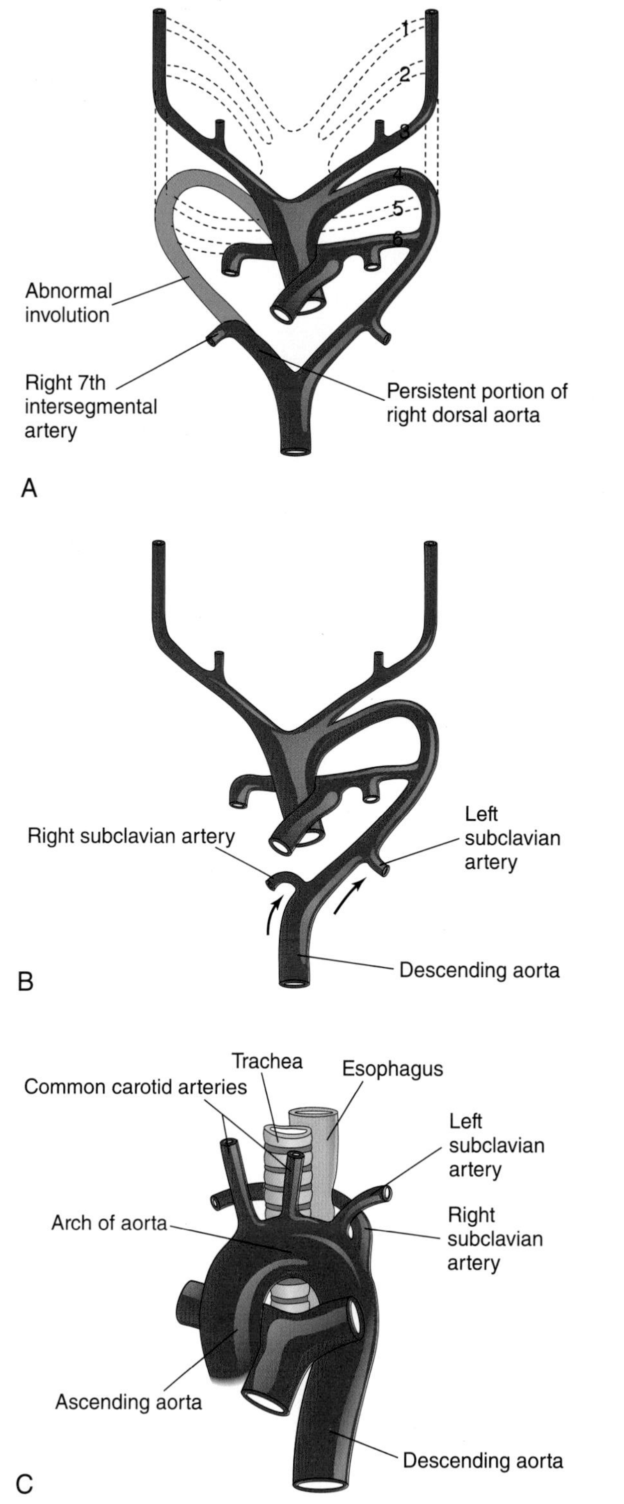

Fig. 13.43 Sketches illustrating the possible embryologic basis of the abnormal origin of the right subclavian artery. (A) The right fourth pharyngeal arch artery and the cranial part of the right dorsal aorta have involuted. As a result, the right subclavian artery forms from the right seventh intersegmental artery and the distal segment of the right dorsal aorta. (B) As the arch of the aorta forms, the right subclavian artery is carried cranially *(arrows)* with the left subclavian artery. (C) The abnormal right subclavian artery arises from the aorta and passes posterior to the trachea and esophagus.

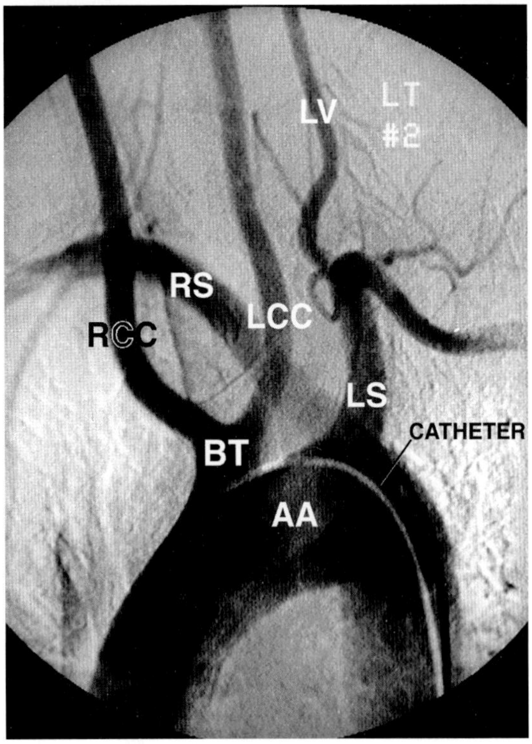

Fig. 13.44 Abnormal origin of the right subclavian artery. This left anterior oblique view of an aortic arch arteriogram shows both common carotid arteries arising from a common stem *(BT)* of the arch of the aorta. The origin of the right subclavian artery *(RS)* is distal to the separate origin of the left subclavian artery *(LS)* but is superimposed in this view. The right subclavian artery then courses cranially and to the right, posterior to the esophagus and trachea. *AA*, Arch of aorta; *BT*, brachiocephalic trunk; *LCC*, left common carotid (artery); *LT#2*, left side, number 2 view; *LV*, left vertebral artery; *RCC*, right common carotid artery. (Courtesy Dr. Gerald S. Smyser, Altru Health System, Grand Forks, North Dakota.)

FETAL AND NEONATAL CIRCULATION

14

The **fetal cardiovascular system** is designed to serve prenatal needs and permit modifications at birth that establish the neonatal circulatory pattern (Figs. 13.45 and 13.46). Good respiration in the neonatal period (1–28 days) is dependent on normal circulatory changes occurring at birth, which result in oxygenation of the blood in the lungs when fetal blood flow through the placenta ceases. In prenatal life, the lungs do not provide gas exchange, and the pulmonary vessels are vasoconstricted. The three vascular structures most important in the transitional circulation are the ductus venosus, foramen ovale, and ductus arteriosus.

FETAL CIRCULATION

Highly oxygenated (approximately 80% oxygen saturation - note: all O_2 saturation values are approximate), **nutrient-rich blood** returns under high pressure from the placenta in the **umbilical vein** (see Fig. 13.45). On approaching the liver, approximately half of the blood passes directly into the **ductus venosus**, a fetal vessel connecting the umbilical vein to the IVC (Figs. 13.47 and 13.48); consequently, this blood bypasses the liver. The other half of the blood in the umbilical vein flows into the sinusoids of the liver and enters the IVC through the **hepatic veins**.

Blood flow through the ductus venosus is regulated by a sphincter mechanism close to the umbilical vein. When the sphincter contracts, more blood is diverted to the portal vein and hepatic sinusoids and less to the ductus venosus (see Fig. 13.48). Although an anatomic sphincter in the ductus venosus has been described, its presence is not universally accepted. However, it is generally agreed that there is a physiologic sphincter that prevents overloading of the heart when venous flow in the umbilical vein is high (e.g., during uterine contractions).

After a short course in the IVC, the blood enters the right atrium of the heart. Because the IVC also contains poorly oxygenated blood from the lower limbs, abdomen, and pelvis, the blood entering the right atrium is not as well oxygenated (approximately 55% oxygen saturation) as that in the umbilical vein, but it still has high oxygen content (see Fig. 13.45). Most blood from the IVC is directed by the **crista dividens** (inferior border of the septum secundum) through the foramen ovale into the left atrium (approximately 65% oxygen saturation) (Fig. 13.49). Here it mixes with the relatively small amount of poorly oxygenated blood returning from the lungs through the pulmonary veins. The fetal lungs use oxygen from the blood instead of replenishing it. From the left atrium, the blood then passes to the left ventricle and leaves through the ascending aorta.

The arteries to the heart, neck, head, and upper limbs receive well-oxygenated blood (approximately 60% oxygen saturation) from the ascending aorta. The liver also receives well-oxygenated blood from the umbilical vein (see Figs. 13.47 and 13.48). The small amount of well-oxygenated blood from the IVC in the right atrium that does not enter the foramen ovale mixes with poorly oxygenated blood from the SVC and coronary sinus and passes into the right ventricle. This blood, which has a medium oxygen content, leaves through the pulmonary trunk.

Approximately 10% of this blood flow goes to the lungs; most blood passes through the **ductus arteriosus** into the descending aorta (approximately 50% oxygen saturation) of the fetus and returns to the placenta through the umbilical arteries (see Fig. 13.45). The ductus arteriosus protects the lungs from circulatory overloading and allows the right ventricle to strengthen in preparation for functioning at full capacity at birth. Because of the high pulmonary vascular resistance in fetal life, pulmonary blood flow is low. Approximately 10% of the blood from the ascending aorta enters the descending aorta; 65% of the blood in the descending aorta passes into the umbilical arteries (approximately 40% oxygen saturation) and is returned to the placenta for reoxygenation. The remaining 35% of the blood in the descending aorta supplies the viscera and the inferior part of the body.

TRANSITIONAL NEONATAL CIRCULATION

Important circulatory adjustments occur at birth when the circulation of fetal blood through the placenta ceases and the neonate's lungs expand and begin to function (see Fig. 13.46). As soon as the baby is born, the foramen ovale, ductus arteriosus, ductus venosus, and umbilical vessels are no longer needed. The sphincter in the ductus venosus constricts so that all blood entering the liver passes through the hepatic sinusoids. Occlusion of the placental circulation causes an immediate decrease in blood pressure in the IVC and right atrium.

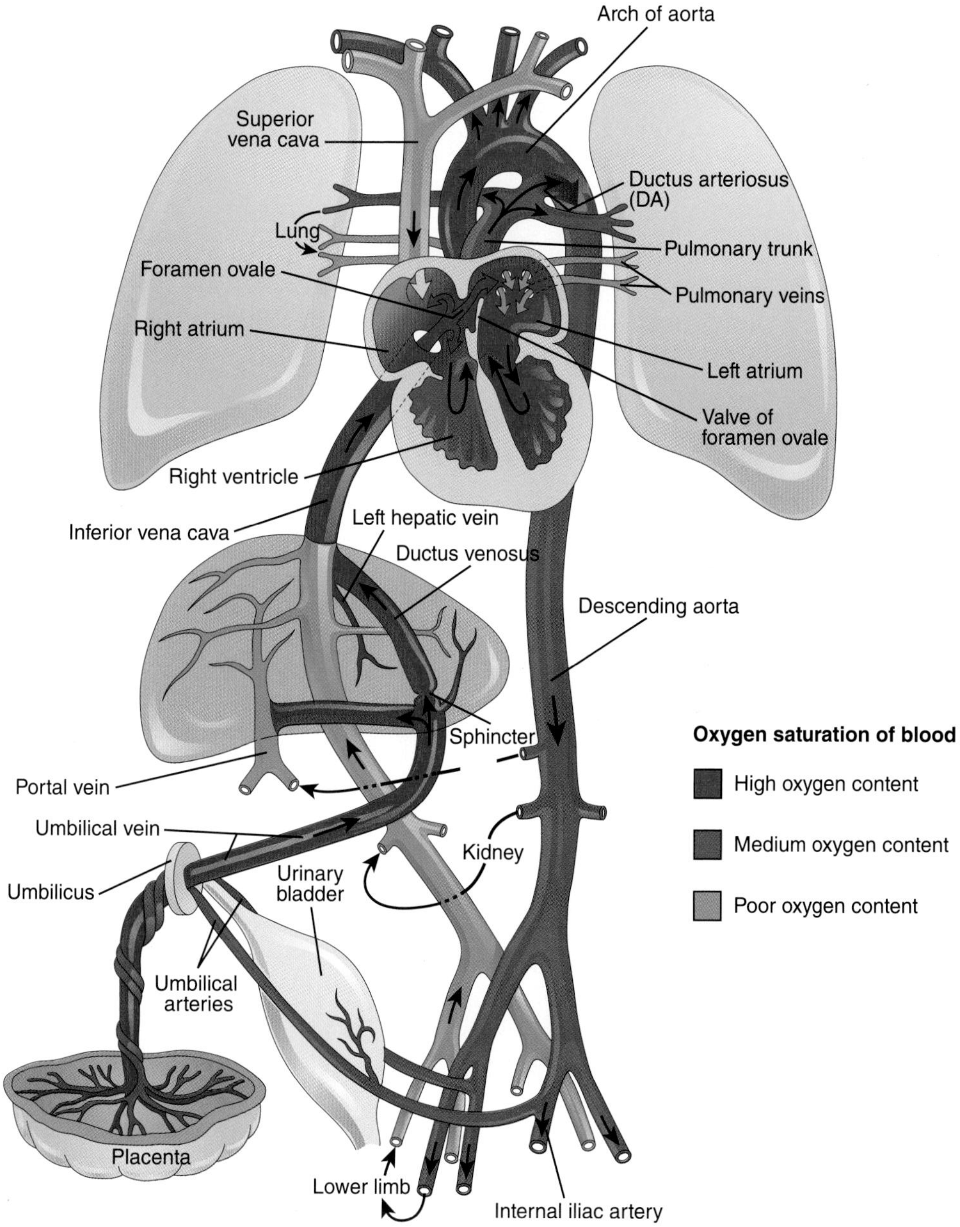

Fig. 13.45 Fetal circulation. The *colors* indicate the oxygen saturation of the blood, and the *arrows* show the course of the blood from the placenta to the heart. The organs are not drawn to scale. A small amount of highly oxygenated blood from the inferior vena cava remains in the right atrium and mixes with poorly oxygenated blood from the superior vena cava. Blood with medium oxygenation then passes into the right ventricle. Observe that three shunts permit most of the blood to bypass the liver and lungs: (1) ductus venosus, (2) foramen ovale, and (3) ductus arteriosus. The poorly oxygenated blood returns to the placenta for oxygenation and nutrients through the umbilical arteries.

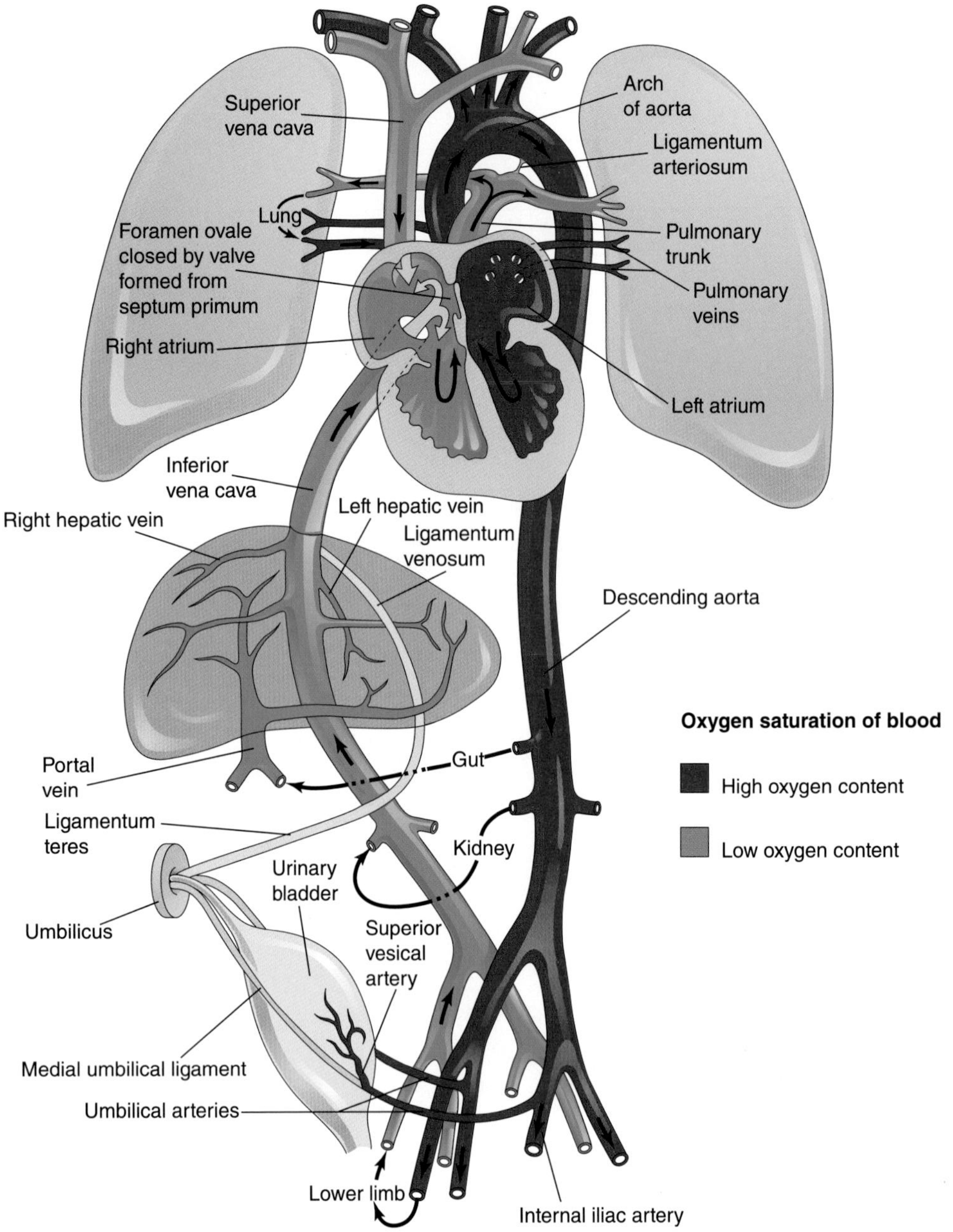

Fig. 13.46 Neonatal circulation. The adult derivatives of the fetal vessels and structures that become nonfunctional at birth are shown. The *arrows* indicate the course of the blood in the neonate. The organs are not drawn to scale. After birth, the three shunts that short-circuited the blood during fetal life cease to function, and the pulmonary and systemic circulations become separated.

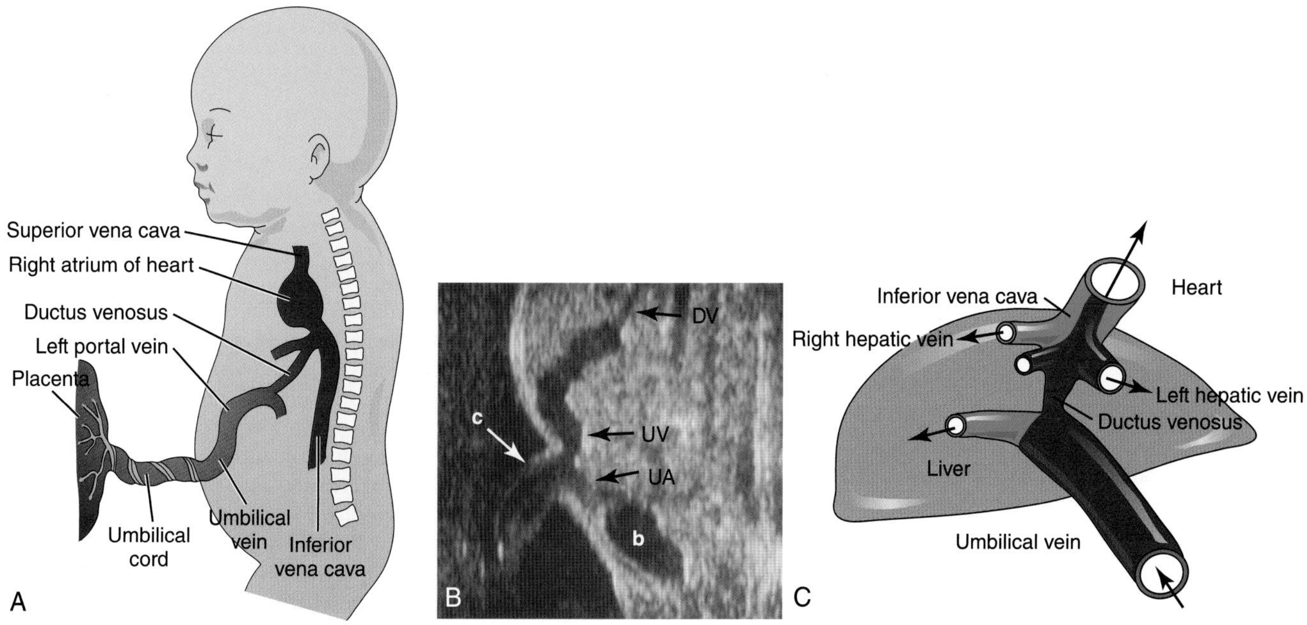

Fig. 13.47 (A) Schematic illustration of the course of the umbilical vein from the umbilical cord to the liver. (B) Ultrasound scan showing the umbilical cord and the course of its vessels in the embryo. *b*, Bladder; *c*, umbilical cord; *DV*, ductus venosus; *UA*, umbilical artery; *UV*, umbilical vein. (C) Schematic presentation of the relationship among the ductus venosus, umbilical vein, hepatic veins, and inferior vena cava. The oxygenated blood is coded with *red*. (B, From Goldstein RB: Ultrasound evaluation of the fetal abdomen. In Callen PW, editor: *Ultrasonography in obstetrics and gynecology*, ed 3, Philadelphia, 1996, Saunders; C, From Tekay A, Campbell S: Doppler ultrasonography in obstetrics. In Callen PW, editor: *Ultrasonography in obstetrics and gynecology*, ed 4, Philadelphia, 2000, Saunders.)

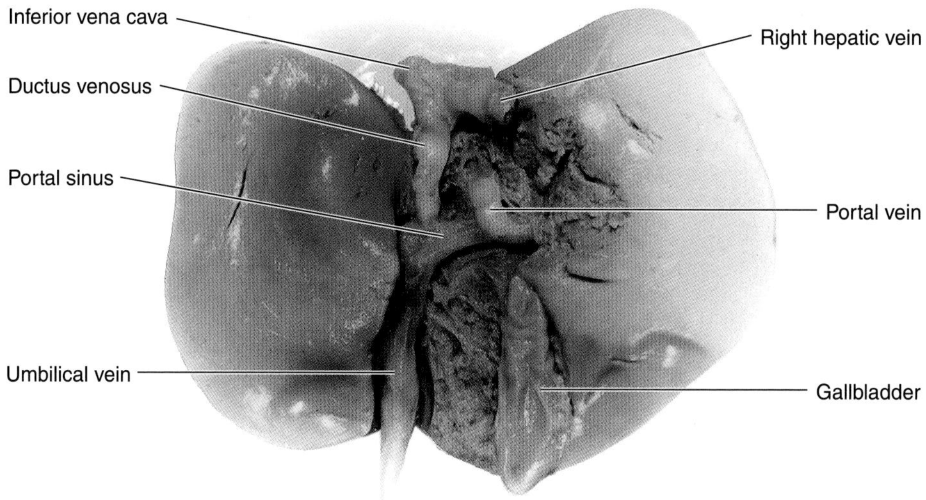

Fig. 13.48 Dissection of the visceral surface of the fetal liver. Approximately 50% of umbilical venous blood bypasses the liver and joins the inferior vena cava through the ductus venosus.

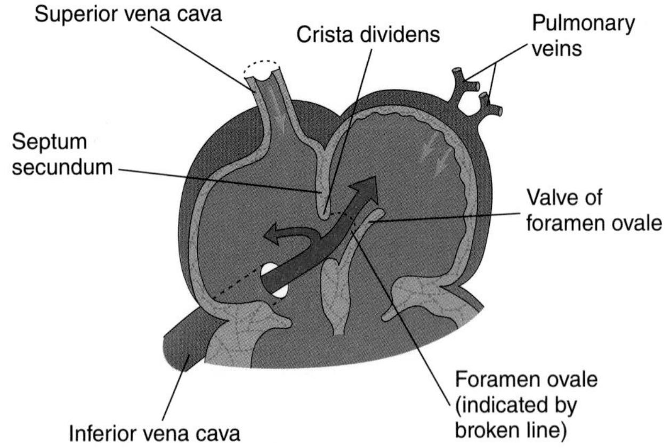

Fig. 13.49 Schematic diagram of blood flow through the fetal atria illustrating how the crista dividens (lower edge of septum secundum) separates the blood coming from the inferior vena cava into two streams. The larger stream passes through the foramen ovale into the left atrium, where it mixes with the small amount of poorly oxygenated blood coming from the lungs through the pulmonary veins. The smaller stream of blood from the inferior vena cava remains in the right atrium and mixes with poorly oxygenated blood from the superior vena cava and coronary sinus.

Aeration of the lungs at birth is associated with a:

- Dramatic decrease in pulmonary vascular resistance
- Marked increase in pulmonary blood flow
- Progressive thinning of the walls of the pulmonary arteries

The thinning of the arterial walls results mainly from stretching of the lungs at birth.

Because of increased pulmonary blood flow and loss of flow from the umbilical vein, the pressure in the left atrium is higher than that in the right atrium. The increased left atrial pressure functionally closes the **foramen ovale** by pressing the valve of the foramen against the septum secundum (see Fig. 13.46). The output from the right ventricle now flows into the pulmonary trunk. Because the pulmonary vascular resistance is lower than the systemic vascular resistance, blood flow in the ductus arteriosus reverses, passing from the descending aorta to the pulmonary trunk.

The right ventricular wall is thicker than the left ventricular wall in fetuses and neonates because the right ventricle has been working harder in utero. By the end of the first month, the left ventricular wall is thicker than the right ventricular wall because the left ventricle is now working harder. The right ventricular wall becomes thinner because of the atrophy associated with its lighter workload.

The ductus arteriosus constricts at birth, but a small amount of blood may continue to be shunted via the ductus arteriosus from the aorta to the pulmonary trunk for 24 to 48 hours in a normal full-term neonate. At the end of 24 hours, 20% of ducts are functionally closed; by 48 hours, about 80% are closed; and by 96 hours, 100% are closed. In premature neonates and those with persistent hypoxia, the ductus arteriosus may remain open much longer.

In full-term neonates, oxygen is the most important factor in controlling the closure of the ductus arteriosus; the oxygen appears to be mediated by **bradykinin**, a substance released from the lungs during initial inflation. Bradykinin has potent contractile effects on smooth muscle. The action of this substance appears to be dependent on the high oxygen content of the blood in the aorta, resulting from aeration of the lungs at birth. When the pO_2 of the blood passing through the ductus arteriosus reaches approximately 50 mm Hg, the wall of the ductus arteriosus constricts. The mechanisms by which oxygen causes ductal constriction are not well understood.

The effects of oxygen on the ductal smooth muscle may be direct or be mediated by its effects on prostaglandin E_2 secretion. *TGF-β is probably involved in the anatomic closure of the ductus arteriosus after birth.* During fetal life, the patency of the ductus arteriosus is controlled by the lower content of oxygen in the blood passing through it and by endogenously produced **prostaglandins** that act on the smooth muscle in the wall of the ductus arteriosus. The prostaglandins cause the ductus arteriosus to relax. Hypoxia and other ill-defined influences cause the local production of prostaglandin E_2 and prostacyclin I_2, which keeps the ductus arteriosus open. Inhibitors of prostaglandin synthesis, such as **indomethacin**, can cause constriction of a patent ductus arteriosus in premature neonates.

The umbilical arteries constrict at birth, preventing the loss of the neonate's blood. Because the umbilical cord is not tied for a minute or so, blood flow through the umbilical vein continues, transferring well-oxygenated fetal blood from the placenta to the neonate. *The change from the fetal to the adult pattern of blood circulation is not a sudden occurrence.* Some changes occur with the first breath; others take place over hours and days. During the transitional stage, there may be a right-to-left flow through the foramen ovale. The closure of fetal vessels and the foramen ovale is initially a functional change. Later, anatomic closure results from the proliferation of fibrous tissues.

DERIVATIVES OF FETAL VESSELS AND STRUCTURES

Because of the changes in the cardiovascular system at birth, some vessels and structures are no longer required. Over months, these fetal vessels form nonfunctional ligaments. Fetal structures, such as the foramen ovale, persist as anatomic vestiges (e.g., oval fossa; see Fig. 13.51).

UMBILICAL VEIN AND ROUND LIGAMENT OF LIVER

The umbilical vein remains patent for a considerable period and may be used for exchange transfusions of blood during the early neonatal period (first 4 weeks). These transfusions are often done to prevent brain damage and death in neonates with anemia resulting from **erythroblastosis fetalis** (hemolytic disease of the newborn). In exchange for transfusions, most of the neonate's blood is replaced with donor blood.

The umbilical vein can also be cannulated, if necessary, for the injection of contrast media or chemotherapeutic drugs. The intra-abdominal part of the umbilical vein eventually becomes the **round ligament of the liver** (ligamentum teres) (see Fig. 13.46), which passes from the umbilicus to the **porta hepatis** (fissure on the visceral surface of the liver); here it is attached to the left branch of the portal vein (Fig. 13.50).

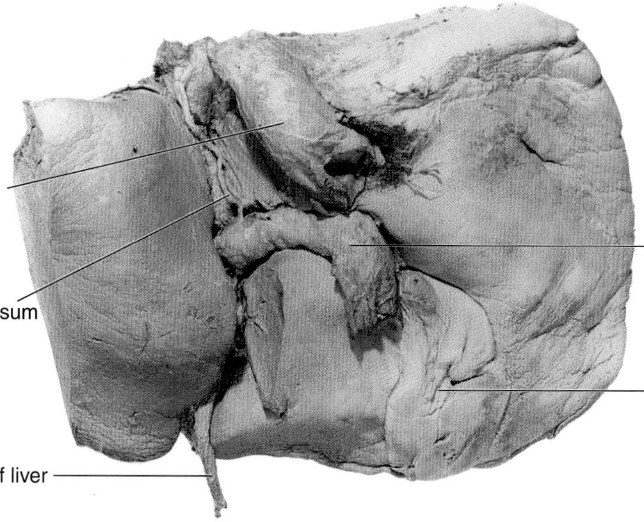

Fig. 13.50 Dissection of the visceral surface of an adult liver. Note that the umbilical vein is represented by the round ligament of the liver and the ductus venosus by the ligamentum venosum.

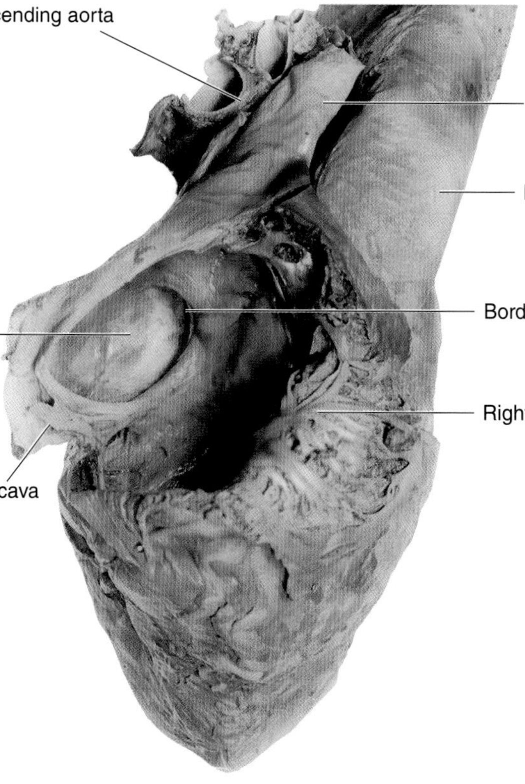

Fig. 13.51 Dissection of the right atrial aspect of the interatrial septum of an adult heart. Observe the oval fossa and the border of the oval fossa. The floor of the oval fossa is formed by the septum primum, whereas the border of the fossa is formed by the free edge of the septum secundum. Aeration of the lungs at birth is associated with a dramatic decrease in pulmonary vascular resistance and a marked increase in pulmonary flow. Because of the increased pulmonary blood flow, the pressure in the left atrium is increased above that in the right atrium. This increased left atrial pressure closes the foramen ovale by pressing the valve of the foramen ovale against the septum secundum. This forms the oval fossa.

DUCTUS VENOSUS AND LIGAMENTUM VENOSUM

The ductus venosus becomes the **ligamentum venosum**; this ligament passes through the liver from the left branch of the portal vein and attaches to the **IVC** (see Fig. 13.50).

UMBILICAL ARTERIES AND ABDOMINAL LIGAMENTS

Most of the intra-abdominal parts of the umbilical arteries become **medial umbilical ligaments** (see Fig. 13.46). The proximal parts of these vessels persist as the **superior vesical arteries**, which supply the urinary bladder.

FORAMEN OVALE AND OVAL FOSSA

The foramen ovale usually closes functionally at birth. Anatomic closure occurs by the third month and results from tissue proliferation and adhesion of the septum primum to the left margin of the septum secundum. The **septum primum** forms the floor of the oval fossa (Fig. 13.51). The inferior edge of the **septum secundum** forms a rounded fold, the border of the oval fossa (limbus fossa ovalis), which marks the former boundary of the foramen ovale.

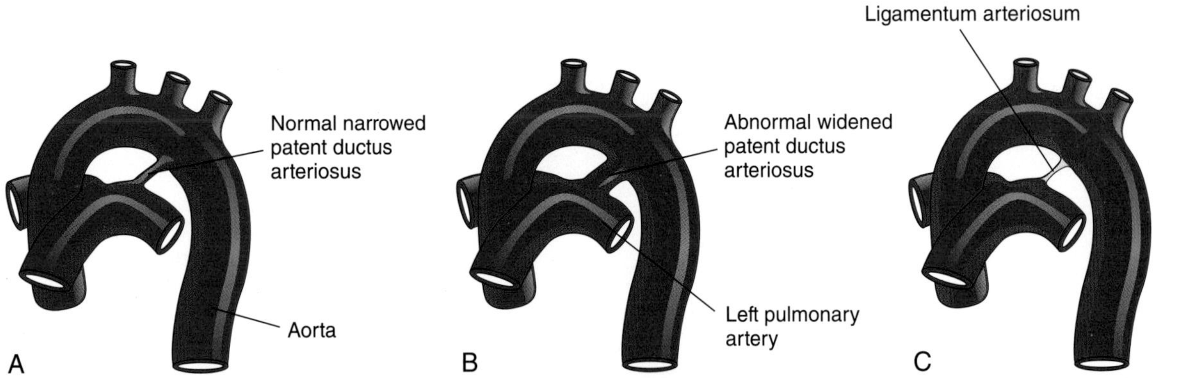

Fig. 13.52 Closure of the ductus arteriosus. (A) Ductus arteriosus of a neonate. (B) Abnormal patent ductus arteriosus in a 6-month-old infant. (C) Ligamentum arteriosum in a 6-month-old infant.

DUCTUS ARTERIOSUS AND LIGAMENTUM ARTERIOSUM

Functional closure of the ductus arteriosus in healthy term neonates is usually completed within the first few days after birth (Fig. 13.52A). Anatomic closure of the ductus arteriosus and formation of the ligamentum arteriosum normally occur by the 12th postnatal week (Fig. 13.52C). The short, thick ligamentum arteriosum extends from the left pulmonary artery to the arch of the aorta.

DEVELOPMENT OF LYMPHATIC SYSTEM

The lymphatic system begins to develop at the end of the sixth week, approximately 2 weeks after the primordia of the cardiovascular system are recognizable. Lymphatic vessels develop like that previously described for blood vessels (see Fig. 4.11) and make connections with the venous system. The early lymphatic capillaries join each other to form a network of lymphatics (Fig. 13.53A). Recent studies have shown that the precursor endothelial cells of the lymphatic vessels are derived from the cardinal veins. *Podoplanin, LYVE-1, and VEGFR3 delineate the progenitor endothelial cells. Apelin signaling, Prox1, Sox18, and COUP-TF11 appear to influence the migration and proliferation of these precursor lymphatic cells. The Rasip interacting protein 1 (Rasip1) is essential for the formation of the lymphatic valves and maintenance of the lymphatic lumen.*

DEVELOPMENT OF LYMPH SACS AND LYMPHATIC DUCTS

There are **six primary lymph sacs** present at the end of the embryonic period (see Fig. 13.53A):

- Two **jugular lymph sacs** near the junction of the subclavian veins with the anterior cardinal veins (the future internal jugular veins)
- Two **iliac lymph sacs** near the junction of the iliac veins with the posterior cardinal veins
- One **retroperitoneal lymph sac** in the root of the mesentery on the posterior abdominal wall
- One **cisterna chyli (chyle cistern)** located dorsal to the retroperitoneal lymph sac

Lymphatic vessels soon connect to the lymph sacs and pass along main veins to the head, neck, and upper limbs from the jugular lymph sacs; to the lower trunk and lower limbs from the iliac lymph sacs; and the primordial gut from the retroperitoneal lymph sac and the **cisterna chyli**. Two large channels (right and left thoracic ducts) connect the jugular lymph sacs with this cistern. Soon a large anastomosis forms between these channels (Fig. 13.53B).

Patent Ductus Arteriosus

Patent ductus arteriosus (incidence 3–8:1000 full-term live births), represents 5% to 10% of all CHD, and is two to three times more frequent in females than in males (Fig. 13.52B). The incidence is much higher in lower birth weight neonates (up to 80% in those weighing <1200g). Functional closure of the ductus arteriosus usually occurs soon after birth; however, if it remains patent, aortic blood is shunted into the pulmonary trunk. *It has been suggested that persistent patency of the ductus arteriosus may result from failure of TGF-β induction after birth.*

Patent ductus arteriosus is commonly associated with **maternal rubella infection** during early pregnancy (see Table 20.6). Preterm neonates and infants living at a high altitude may have a patent ductus arteriosus; the patency is the result of **hypoxia** (a decreased level of oxygen) and immaturity. Virtually all preterm neonates ($\leq$28 weeks) whose birth weight is less than 1750 g have a patent ductus arteriosus in the first 24 hours of postnatal life.

The embryologic basis of patent ductus arteriosus is a failure of the ductus arteriosus to involute after birth and form the ligamentum arteriosum. Failure of contraction of the muscular wall of the ductus arteriosus after birth is the primary cause of patency. There is some evidence that low oxygen content of the blood in neonates with **respiratory distress syndrome** can adversely affect the closure of the ductus arteriosus. For example, patent ductus arteriosus commonly occurs in small premature neonates with respiratory difficulties associated with a deficiency of **surfactant** (a phospholipid that reduces surface tension in alveoli in the lungs).

Patent ductus arteriosus may occur as an isolated defect or in infants with certain **chromosomal anomalies** or **cardiac defects.** Large differences between aortic and pulmonary blood pressures can cause a heavy flow of blood through the ductus arteriosus, thereby preventing normal constriction. Such pressure differences may be caused by **coarctation of the aorta** (see Fig. 13.40A–D), **TGA** (see Fig. 13.31), or **pulmonary stenosis** and **atresia** (see Fig. 13.33).

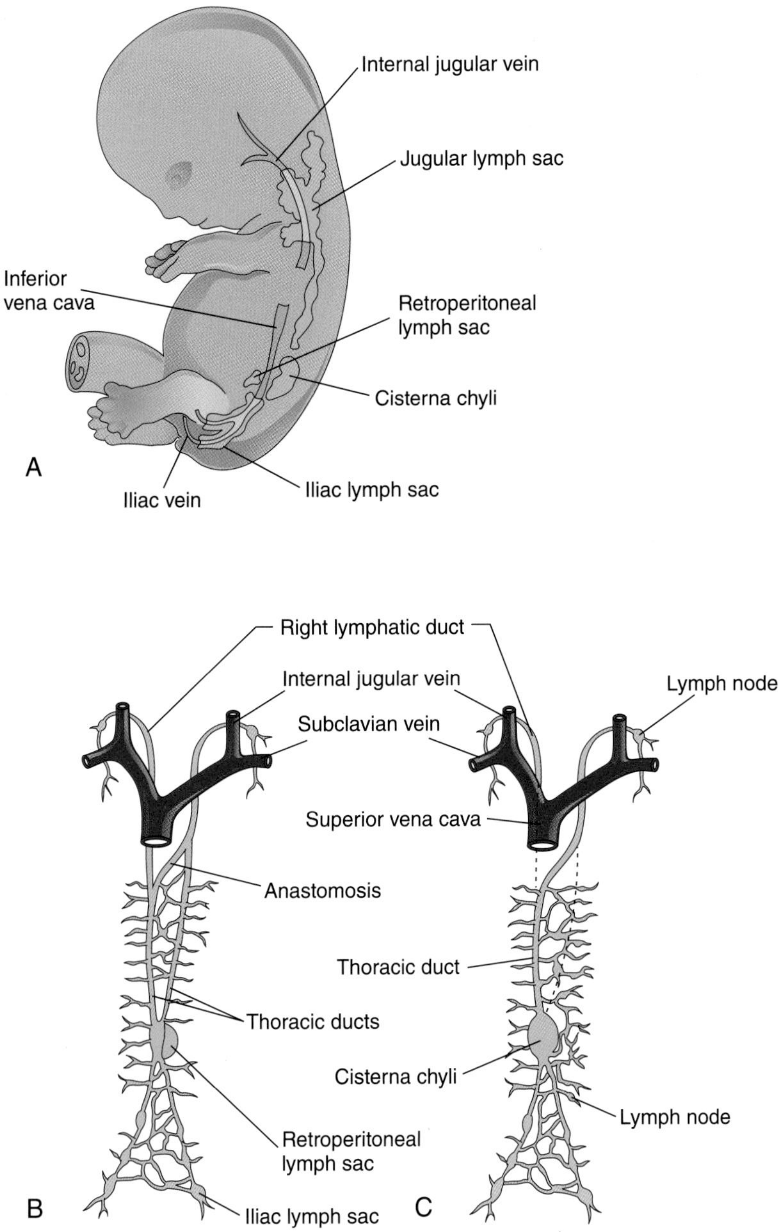

Fig. 13.53 Development of the lymphatic system. (A) Left side of a 7.5-week embryo showing the primary lymph sacs. (B) Ventral view of the lymphatic system at 9 weeks showing the paired thoracic ducts. (C) Later in the fetal period, illustrating the formation of the thoracic duct and right lymphatic duct.

DEVELOPMENT OF THORACIC DUCT

The **thoracic duct** is formed by the caudal part of the **right thoracic duct**, the anastomosis between the left and right thoracic ducts, and the cranial part of the **left thoracic duct**. As a result, there are many variations in the origin, course, and termination of the thoracic duct. The **right lymphatic duct** is derived from the cranial part of the right thoracic duct (Fig. 13.53C). The **thoracic duct** and right lymphatic duct connect with the venous system at the **venous angle** between the internal jugular vein and subclavian vein (see Fig. 13.53B).

DEVELOPMENT OF LYMPH NODES

Except for the superior part of the **cisterna chyli**, the lymph sacs are transformed into groups of lymph nodes during the early fetal period. Mesenchymal cells invade each lymph sac and break up its cavity into a network of lymphatic channels, the **primordia of the lymph sinuses**. Other mesenchymal cells give rise to the capsule and connective tissue framework of the lymph nodes. Peyer patches, lymphoid tissue found in the wall of the small intestine, begin to develop at approximately 19 weeks.

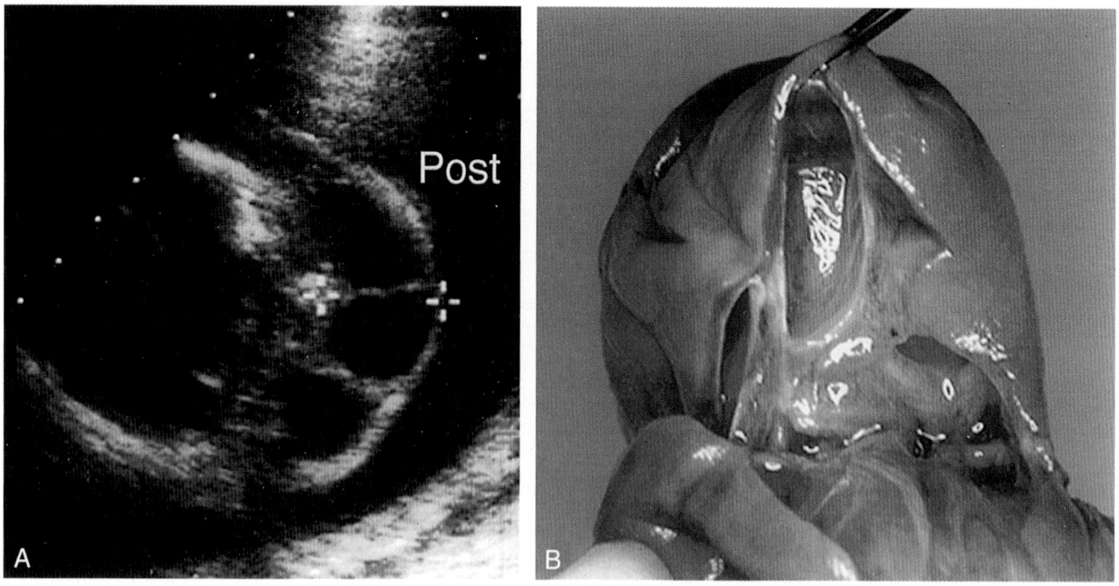

Fig. 13.54 Cystic hygroma. (A) Transverse axial sonogram of the neck of a fetus with a large cystic hygroma. (B) Photograph of a neck dissection. The hygroma was demonstrated from this cross-sectional view of the posterior fetal neck at 18.5 weeks. The lesion was characterized by multiple, septated cystic areas within the mass itself as shown in the pathology specimen. *Post*, Posterior. (Courtesy Dr. Wesley Lee, Division of Fetal Imaging, William Beaumont Hospital, Royal Oak, Michigan.)

DEVELOPMENT OF LYMPHOCYTES

The lymphocytes are derived originally from **primordial stem cells** in the umbilical vesicle mesenchyme and later from the liver and spleen. These early lymphocytes eventually enter the bone marrow, where they divide to form **lymphoblasts**. The lymphocytes that appear in lymph nodes before birth are derived from the **thymus**, a derivative of the third pair of pharyngeal pouches (see Fig. 9.7B and C). Small lymphocytes leave the thymus and circulate to other lymphoid organs. Later, some mesenchymal cells in the lymph nodes also differentiate into lymphocytes. Lymph nodules do not appear in the lymph nodes until just before and/or after birth.

DEVELOPMENT OF SPLEEN AND TONSILS

The **spleen** develops from an aggregation of mesenchymal cells in the dorsal mesogastrium (see Chapter 11). The **palatine tonsils** develop from the endoderm of the second pair of pharyngeal pouches and nearby mesenchyme. The **tubal tonsils** develop from aggregations of lymph nodules around the pharyngeal openings of the pharyngotympanic tubes. The **pharyngeal tonsils (adenoids)** develop from an aggregation of lymph **nodules** in the wall of the nasopharynx. The **lingual tonsil** develops from an aggregation of lymph nodules in the root of the tongue. Lymph nodules also develop in the mucosa of the respiratory and alimentary systems.

Anomalies of Lymphatic System

Congenital anomalies of the lymphatic system are rare. There may be a diffuse swelling of part of the body, **congenital lymphedema**. This condition may result from dilation of primordial lymphatic channels or from congenital hypoplasia of lymphatic vessels. More rarely, diffuse cystic dilation of lymphatic channels involves widespread portions of the body, such as in the thorax (congenital chylothorax).

In **cystic hygroma**, large swellings usually appear in the inferolateral part of the neck and consist of large single or multilocular, fluid-filled cavities (Fig. 13.54). Hygromas may be present at birth, but they often enlarge and become evident during infancy, especially after infection or hemorrhage. Most hygromas appear to be derived from *abnormal transformation of the jugular lymph sacs* (Fig. 13.53A). **Hygromas** are believed to arise from parts of a jugular lymph sac that are pinched off or from lymphatic spaces that fail to establish connections with the main lymphatic channels. Hygromas diagnosed in utero in the first trimester of development are associated with chromosomal abnormalities in about 50% of cases. The fetal outcome in these cases is poor.

SUMMARY OF CARDIOVASCULAR SYSTEM

- The cardiovascular system begins to develop at the end of the third week. *The primordial heart starts to beat at the beginning of the fourth week.* Mesenchymal cells derived from splanchnic mesoderm proliferate and form isolated cell clusters, which soon develop into two heart tubes that join to form the **primordial vascular system**. Splanchnic mesoderm surrounding the heart tube forms the primordial myocardium.
- The **heart primordium** consists of four chambers: the bulbus cordis, ventricle, atrium, and sinus venosus.
- The **truncus arteriosus** (primordium of the ascending aorta and pulmonary trunk) is continuous caudally with the **bulbus cordis**, which becomes part of the ventricles. As the heart grows, it bends to the right and soon acquires the general external appearance of the adult heart. The heart becomes partitioned into four chambers between the fourth and seventh weeks.

- Three systems of paired veins drain into the primordial heart: the vitelline system, which becomes the portal system; the cardinal veins, which form the **caval system**; and the umbilical veins, which involute after birth.
- As the **pharyngeal arches** form during the fourth and fifth weeks, they are penetrated by **pharyngeal arteries** that arise from the aortic sac. During the sixth to eighth weeks, the pharyngeal arch arteries are transformed into the adult arterial arrangement of the carotid, subclavian, and pulmonary arteries.
- **The critical period of heart development is from day 20 to day 50 after fertilization**. Numerous events occur during cardiac development, and deviation from the normal pattern at any time may produce one or more CHDs. Because partitioning of the primordial heart results from complex cellular and molecular processes, defects of the cardiac septa are relatively common, particularly **VSDs**. Some birth defects result from abnormal transformation of the pharyngeal arch arteries into the adult arterial pattern.
- Because the lungs are nonfunctional during prenatal life, the fetal cardiovascular system is structurally designed so that blood is oxygenated in the placenta and most of it bypasses the lungs. The modifications that establish the postnatal circulatory pattern are not abrupt but extend into infancy. Failure of these changes in the circulatory system to occur at birth results in two of the most common congenital anomalies of the heart and great vessels: **patent foramen ovale** and **patent ductus arteriosus**.
- The lymphatic system begins to develop late in the sixth week in close association with the venous system. Six primary lymph sacs develop, which later become interconnected by lymphatic vessels. Lymph nodes develop along the network of lymphatic vessels; lymph nodules do not appear until just before or after birth.

CLINICALLY ORIENTED PROBLEMS

CASE 13-1

A pediatrician detected a congenital cardiac defect in an infant, and he explained to the baby's mother that this is a common birth defect.

- What is the most common type of congenital cardiac defect?
- What percentage of congenital heart disease results from this defect?
- Discuss blood flow in infants with this defect.
- What problems would you likely encounter if the cardiac defect were large?

CASE 13-2

A female infant was born after a pregnancy complicated by a rubella infection during the first trimester. She had congenital cataracts and congenital heart disease. A radiograph of the infant's chest at 3 weeks showed generalized cardiac enlargement with some increase in pulmonary vascularity.

- What congenital cardiovascular defect is commonly associated with maternal rubella infection during early pregnancy?
- What probably caused the cardiac enlargement?

CASE 13-3

A male neonate was referred to a pediatrician because of the blue color of his skin (cyanosis). An ultrasound examination was ordered to confirm the preliminary diagnosis of tetralogy of Fallot.

- In tetralogy of Fallot, there are four cardiac defects. What are they?
- What is one of the most obvious clinical signs of tetralogy of Fallot?
- What radiographic technique might be used to confirm a tentative diagnosis of this type of congenital heart defect?
- What do you think would be the main aim of therapy in this case?

CASE 13-4

A male neonate was born after a full-term normal pregnancy. Severe generalized cyanosis was observed on the first day. A chest radiograph revealed a slightly enlarged heart with a narrow base and increased pulmonary vascularity. A clinical diagnosis of transformation of the great arteries was made.

- What radiographic technique would likely be used to verify the diagnosis?
- What would this technique reveal in the present case?
- How was the infant able to survive with this severe heart defect?

CASE 13-5

During an autopsy of a 72-year-old male who died from chronic heart failure, it was observed that his heart was very large and that the pulmonary artery and its main branches were dilated. Opening the heart revealed a very large atrial septal defect.

- What type of atrial septal defect was probably present?
- Where would the defect likely be located?
- Explain why the pulmonary artery and its main branches were dilated.
- Why might this have not been diagnosed earlier?

Discussion of these problems appears in the Appendix at the back of the book.

BIBLIOGRAPHY AND SUGGESTED READING

Anderson RH, Brown NA, Moorman AFM: Development and structures of the venous pole of the heart, *Dev Dyn* 235:2, 2006.

Ashworth M: Development of the heart *Pathology of heart disease in the fetus, infant and child: autopsy, surgical, and molecular pathology*, Cambridge, 2019, Cambridge University Press, pp 53–74. https://doi.org/10.1017/9781316337073.003.

Berman DR, Treadwell MC: Ultrasound evaluation of fetal thorax. In Norton ME, editor: *Callen's ultrasonography in obstetrics and gynecology*, ed 6, Philadelphia, 2017, Elsevier.

Bernstein E: The cardiovascular system. In Behrman RE, Kliegman RM, Jenson HB, editors: *Nelson textbook of pediatrics*, ed 17, Philadelphia, 2004, Saunders.

Borasch K, Richardson K, Plendl J: Cardiogenesis with a focus on vasculogenesis and angiogenesis, *Anat Histol Embryol* 49:643, 2020.

Bredeloux P, Pasqualin C, Bordy R, Maupoil V, Findlay I: Automatic activity arising in cardiac muscle sleeves of the pulmonary vein, *Biomolecules* 12:23, 2021.

Bubb K, du Plessis M, Hage R, Tubbs RS, Loukas M: The internal anatomy of the inferior vena cava with specific emphasis on the entrance of the renal, gonadal, and lumbar veins, *Surg Radiol Anat* 38:107, 2016.

Camp E, Munsterberg A: Ingression, migration and early differentiation of cardiac progenitors, *Front Biosci* 17:2416, 2011.

Chappell JC, Bautch VL: Vascular development: genetic mechanisms and links to vascular disease, *Curr Top Dev Biol* 90:43, 2010.

Combs MD, Yutzey KE: Heart valve development: regulatory networks in development and disease, *Circ Res* 105:408, 2009.

Conte G, Pellegrini A: On the development of the coronary arteries in human embryos, stages 13–19, *Anat Embryol (Berl)* 169:209, 1984.

Cunningham TJ, Yu MS, McKeithan WL, et al: : Id genes are essential for early heart formation, *Genes Dev* 31(13):1325–1338, 2017.

de Bakker BS, de Jong KH, Hagoort J, et al: : An interactive three-dimensional digital atlas and quantitative database of human development, *Science* 354, 2016. aag0053

Dyer LA, Kirby ML: The role of secondary heart field in cardiac development, *Dev Dyn* 336:137, 2009.

El Robrini N, Etchevers HC, Ryckebüsch L, et al: : Cardiac outflow morphogenesis depends on effects of retinoic acid signaling on multiple cell lineages, *Dev Dyn* 245:388, 2016.

Farmer D: Placental stem cells: the promise of curing diseases before birth, *Placenta* 59:113–115, 2017.

Gabriel GC, Young CB, Lo CW: Role of cilia in the pathogenesis of congenital heart disease, *Semin Cell Dev Biol* 110:2, 2021.

Gessert S, Kuhl M: The multiple phases and faces of Wnt signaling during cardiac differentiation and development, *Circ Res* 107:186, 2010.

Gloviczki P, Duncan A, Kalra M, et al: : Vascular malformations: an update, *Perspect Vasc Surg Endovasc Ther* 21:133, 2009.

Harvey RP, Meilhac SM, Buckingham M: Landmarks and lineages in the developing heart, *Circ Res* 104:1235, 2009.

He L, Lui KO, Zhou B: The formation of coronary vessels in cardiac development and disease, *Cold Spring Harb Perspect Biol* 12(5):a037168, 2020. https://doi.org/10.1101/cshperspect.a037168.

Hildreth V, Anderson RH, Henderson DJH: Autonomic innervations of the developing heart: origins and function, *Clin Anat* 22:36, 2009.

Isayama T, Kusuda S, Adams M, Berti E, Battin M, Helenius K, et al: International Network for Evaluating Outcomes of Neonates (iNeo) Investigators. International variation in the management of patent ductus arteriosus and its association with infant outcomes: a survey and linked cohort study, *J Pediatr* 244:24–29.e7, 2022. Epub Jan 4, 2022; https://doi.org/10.1016/j.jpeds.2021.12.071.

Larsen SH, Olsen M, Emmertsen K: Interventional treatment of patients with congenital heart disease: nationwide Danish experience over 39 years, *J Am Coll Cardiol* 69:2725, 2017.

Li SJ, Lee J, Hall J, Sutherland TR: The inferior vena cava: anatomical variants and acquired pathologies, *Insights Imaging* 12(1):123, 2021. https://doi.org/10.1186/s13244-021-01066-7.

Liu X, Gu X, Ma W, et al: Rasip1 controls lymphatic vessel lumen maintenance by regulating endothelial cell junctions, *Development* 145(17):dev165092, 2018. https://doi.org/10.1242/dev.165092.

Liu X, Yagi H, Saeed S, et al: : The complex genetics of hypoplastic left heart syndrome, *Nat Genet* 49(7):1152–1159, 2017.

Loukas M, Groat C, Khangura R, Owens DG, Anderson RH: The normal and abnormal anatomy of the coronary arteries, *Clin Anat* 22:114, 2009.

Loukas M, Bilinsky S, Bilinsky E, el-Sedfy A, Anderson RH: Cardiac veins: a review of the literature, *Clin Anat* 22:129, 2009.

Männer J: When does the human embryonic heart start beating? A review of contemporary and historical sources of knowledge about eh onset of blood circulation in man, *J Cardiovasc Dev Dis* 9:187, 2022.

Männer J: The anatomy of cardiac looping: a step towards the understanding of the morphogenesis of several forms of congenital cardiac malformations, *Clin Anat* 22:21, 2009.

Männer J, Yelbuz TM: Functional morphology of the cardiac jelly in the tubular heart of vertebrate embryos, *J Cardiovasc Dev Dis* 6(1):12, 2019. https://doi.org/10.3390/jcdd6010012.

Miksiunas R, Mobasheri A, Bironaite D: Homeobox genes and homeodomain proteins: new insights into cardiac development, degeneration and regeneration., *Adv Exp Med Biol* 1212:155–178, 2020.

Morris SA, Ayres NA, Espinoza J, Maskatia SA, Lee W: Sonographic evaluation of the fetal heart. In Norton ME, editor: *Callen's ultrasonography in obstetrics and gynecology,* ed 6, Philadelphia, 2017, Elsevier.

Nakano H, Nakano A: The role of metabolism in cardiac development. In Current Topics in Developmental Biology, 2024, Elsevier, pp 201-243. Heart Development and Disease. https://doi.org/10.1016/bs.ctdb.2024.01.005.

Nees SN, Chung WK: The genetics of isolated congenital heart disease, *Am J Med Genet C Semin Med Genet* 184:97, 2020.

O'Rahilly R: The timing and sequence of events in human cardiogenesis, *Acta Anat (Basel)* 79:70, 1971.

Ottaviani G, Buja LM: Update on congenital heart disease and sudden infant/perinatal death: from history to future trends, *J Clin Pathol* 70:555, 2017.

Penny DJ, Vick GW: Ventricular septal defect, *Lancet* 377:1103, 2011.

Quijada P, Trembley MA, Small EM: The role of epicardium during heart development and repair, *Circ Res* 126:377, 2020.

Ridge LA, Kewbank D, Schütz D, Stumm R, Scambler PJ, Ivins S: Dual role for CXCL12 signaling in semilunar valve development, *Cell Rep* 36(8):109610, 2021. https://doi.org/10.1016/j.celrep.2021.109610.

Sierra-Pagan JE, Garry DJ: The regulatory role of pioneer factors during cardiovascular lineage specification - a mini review, *Front Cardiovasc Med* 9:972591, 2022. https://doi.org/10.3389/fcvm.2022.972591.

Škorić-Milosavljević D, Tadros R, Bosada FM, et al: Common genetic variants contribute to risk of transposition of the great arteries, *Circ Res* 130(2):166–180, 2022. https://doi.org/10.1161/CIRCRESAHA.120.317107.

Steele RE, Sanders R, Phillips HM, Bamforth SD: PAX genes in cardiovascular development, *Int J Mol Sci* 23(14):7713, 2022. https://doi.org/10.3390/ijms23147713.

Stutt N, Song M, Wilson MD, Scott IC: Cardiac specification during gastrulation - the yellow brick road leading to tinman, *Semin Cell Dev Biol* 27:46, 2022.

Sun L, Marini D, Saini B, Schrauben E, Macgowan CK, Seed M: Understanding fetal hemodynamics using cardiovascular magnetic resonance imaging, *Fetal Diagn Ther* 47:354, 2020.

Sylva M, van den Hoff MJB, Moorman AFM: Development of the human heart, *Am J Med Genet* 164A(6):1347, 2014.

Tomanek RJ: Developmental progression of the coronary vasculature in human embryos and fetuses, *Anat Rec (Hoboken)* 299:25, 2016.

Vanover M, Wang A, Farmer D: Potential clinical applications of placental stem cells for use in fetal therapy of birth defects, *Placenta* 59:107–112, 2017.

Vollbrecht T.M., Bissell M.M., Kording F. et al.: Fetal cardiac MRI using Doppler US Gating: emerging technology and clinical implications, Radiol Cardiothorac Imaging 6(2), 2024. https://doi.org/10.1148/ryct.230182.

Yokoyama U, Ichikawa Y, Minamisawa S, Ishikawa Y: Pathology and molecular mechanisms of coarctation of the aorta and its association with the ductus arteriosus, *J Physiol Sci* 67:259, 2017.

Skeletal System 14

CHAPTER OUTLINE

As the notochord and neural tube form in the third week, the **intraembryonic mesoderm** lateral to these structures thickens to form two longitudinal columns of **paraxial mesoderm** (Fig. 14.1A and B). Toward the end of the third week, the paraxial mesoderm becomes segmented into condensed blocks—somites (see Fig. 14.1C). Externally, the somites appear as bead-like elevations along the dorsolateral surface of the embryo (see Fig. 5.6A–D). Each somite differentiates into two parts (see Fig. 14.1D and E):

- The ventromedial part is the **sclerotome**. Its cells form the vertebrae and ribs.
- The dorsolateral part is the **dermomyotome**. Cells from its myotome region form **myoblasts** (primordial muscle cells), and those from its dermatome region form the **dermis (fibroblasts)**.

DEVELOPMENT OF BONE AND CARTILAGE

At the end of the fourth week, the **sclerotome cells** form **mesenchyme**, which has a bone-forming capacity. Bones first appear as condensations of mesenchymal cells that form bone models. **Condensation** (dense cell packing) marks the beginning of selective gene activity, which precedes cell differentiation (Fig. 14.2). Most flat bones develop in mesenchyme within preexisting membranous sheaths; this type of **osteogenesis** is called **membranous (intramembranous) bone formation**. Mesenchymal models of most limb bones are transformed into cartilage bone models, which later become ossified by **endochondral bone formation**.

Proteins encoded by the Hox genes, bone morphogenetic proteins (BMP5 and BMP7), growth factor GDF5, members of the transforming growth factor-β (TGF-β) superfamily, vascular endothelial growth factor (VEGF), and other signaling molecules are endogenous regulators of chondrogenesis and skeletal development. Lineage commitment of skeletal precursor cells to chondrocytes and osteoblasts is determined by β-catenin levels. β-Catenin in the canonical Wnt signaling pathway plays a critical role in the formation of cartilage and bone (Fig. 14.3).

HISTOGENESIS OF CARTILAGE

Cartilage develops from mesenchyme during the fifth week. In areas where cartilage is programmed to develop, the mesenchyme condenses to form **chondrification centers**. The mesenchymal cells differentiate into **prechondrocytes** and then into **chondroblasts**, which secrete collagenous fibrils and ground substance (extracellular matrix). Subsequently, collagenous or elastic fibers, or both, are deposited in the intercellular substance or matrix. Three types of cartilage are distinguished according to the type of matrix that is formed:

- **Hyaline cartilage**, the most widely distributed type (e.g., synovial joints)
- **Fibrocartilage** (e.g., intervertebral discs)
- **Elastic cartilage** (e.g., auricles of the external ears)

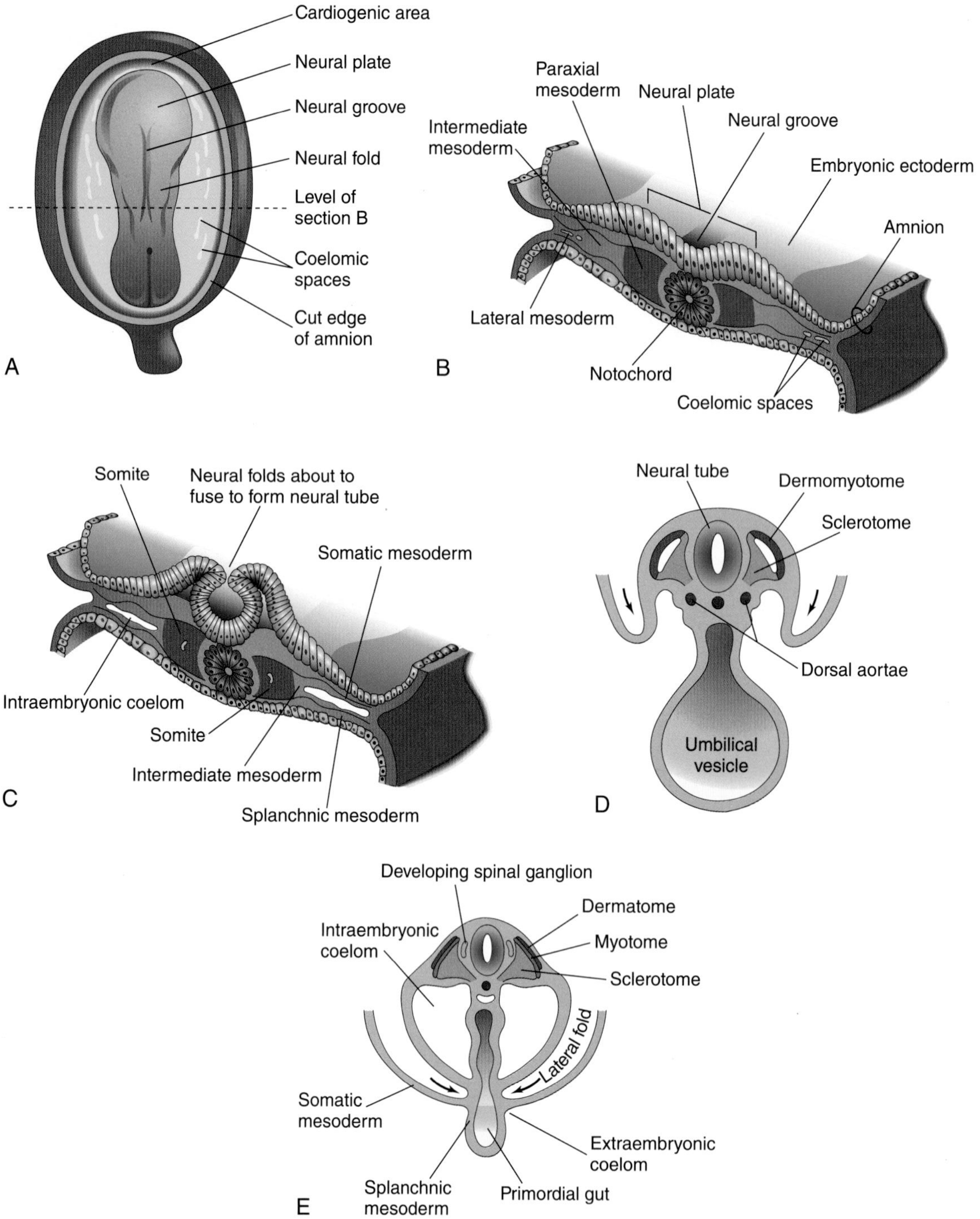

Fig. 14.1 Formation and early differentiation of somites. (A) Dorsal view of an embryo of approximately 18 days. (B) Transverse section of the embryo shown in (A) shows the paraxial mesoderm from which the somites are derived. (C) Transverse section of an embryo of approximately 22 days shows the appearance of early somites. The neural folds are about to fuse to form the neural tube. (D) Transverse section of an embryo of approximately 24 days shows the folding of the embryo in the horizontal plane *(arrows)*. The dermomyotome region of the somite gives rise to the dermatome and myotome. (E) Transverse section of an embryo of approximately 26 days shows the dermatome, myotome, and sclerotome regions of a somite.

HISTOGENESIS OF BONE

Bone primarily develops in two types of connective tissue: mesenchyme and cartilage, but it can also develop in muscle and tendon (sesamoid bones, e.g., patella). Like cartilage, bone consists of cells and an organic intercellular substance **(bone matrix)** that comprises collagen fibrils embedded in an amorphous component. Studies of the cellular and molecular events during embryonic bone formation suggest that **osteogenesis** and **chondrogenesis** are programmed early in development and are independent events under the influence of vascular changes.

INTRAMEMBRANOUS OSSIFICATION

Intramembranous ossification occurs in mesenchyme that has formed a membranous sheath (Fig. 14.4) and produces osseous tissue without prior cartilage formation. The mesenchyme condenses and becomes highly vascular. Precursor mesenchymal stem cells differentiate into **osteoblasts** (bone-forming cells) and begin to deposit **osteoid**-unmineralized matrix rich in type I collagen. Tyrosine phosphatase (SHP2), *transcription factors Foxf2, RUNX2, and Wnt signaling are key regulating factors in osteoblast differentiation.* Calcium phosphate is then deposited in **osteoid tissue** as it is organized into bone. **Bone osteoblasts** are trapped in the matrix and become **osteocytes.**

At first, new bone has no organized pattern; however, spicules of bone soon become organized and coalesce into lamellae (layers). **Concentric lamellae** develop around blood vessels, forming **osteons** (Haversian systems). Some osteoblasts remain at the periphery of the developing bone and continue to lay down lamellae, forming plates of compact

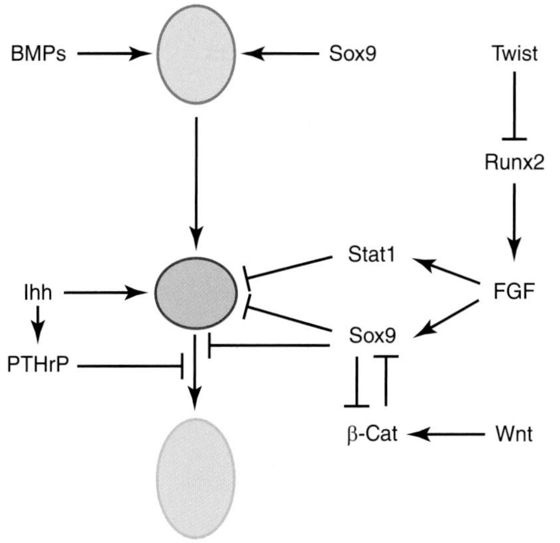

Fig. 14.2 Schematic representation of secreted molecules and transcription factors that regulate the initial differentiation, proliferation, and terminal differentiation of chondrocytes. From *top to bottom*: mesenchymal cells *(blue)*, resting and proliferating (nonhypertrophic) chondrocytes *(red)*, and hypertrophic chondrocytes *(yellow)*. Lines with *arrowheads* indicate a positive action, and lines with *bars* indicate an inhibition. *β-Cat*, β-Catenin; *BMPs*, bone morphogenic proteins; *FGF*, fibroblast growth factor; *PTHrP*, parathyroid hormone–related protein. (From Karsenty G, Kronenberg HM, Settembre C: Genetic control of bone formation. *Annu Rev Cell Dev Biol* 25:629, 2009.)

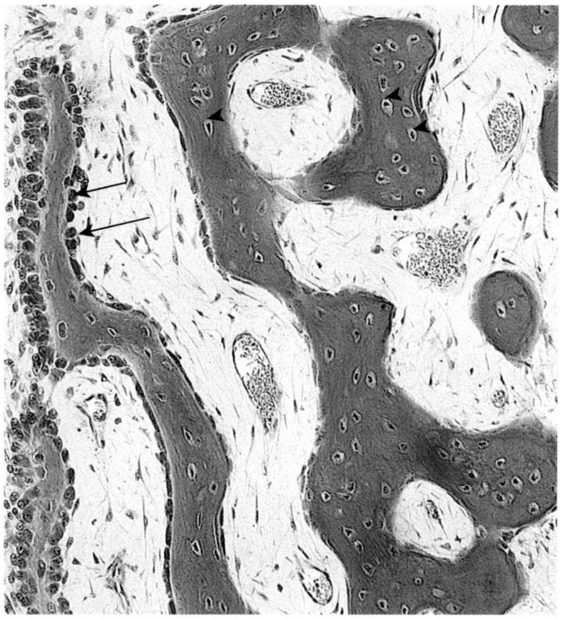

Fig. 14.4 Light micrograph of intramembranous ossification (×132). The trabeculae of bone are formed by the osteoblasts lining their surface *(arrows)*. Osteocytes are trapped in lacunae *(arrowheads)*, and primordial osteons are beginning to form. The osteons (canals) contain blood capillaries. (From Gartner LP, Hiatt JL: *Color textbook of histology*, ed 2, Philadelphia, 2001, Saunders.)

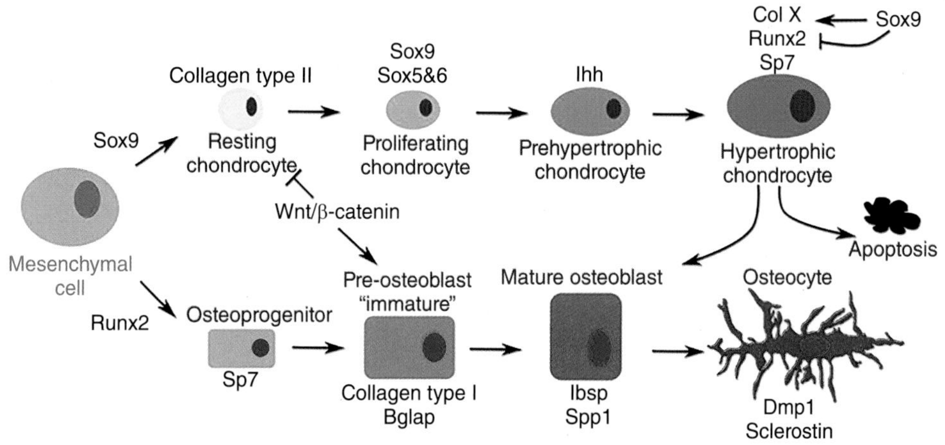

Fig. 14.3 The chondrocyte and osteoblast differentiation pathways. Simplified schematic showing the key genes that are expressed during chondrogenic and osteoblastic differentiation and the relationship between the two lineages. In hypertrophic chondrocytes, the expression of SOX9 protein persists in early hypertrophic chondrocytes where SOX9 induces the expression of *Collagen type X* and inhibits RUNX2 activity. Degradation of SOX9 protein releases inhibition of RUNX2 allowing chondrocyte-osteoblast transformation. WNT-β-CATENIN determines osteoblast versus chondrocyte fate in developing intramembranous bones. (From Galea GL, Zein MR, Allen S, Francis-West P: Making and shaping endochondral and intramembranous bones. *Dev Dyn* 250(3):414–449, 2021.)

bone on the surfaces. Between the surface plates, the intervening bone remains spiculated or spongy. This spongy environment is somewhat accentuated by the action of **osteoclast** cells that reabsorb bone. Osteoclasts are multinucleated cells with a hematopoietic origin. In the interstices of spongy bones, the mesenchyme differentiates into **bone marrow**. Hormones and cytokines regulate the remodeling of bone by the coordinated action of osteoclasts and osteoblasts.

ENDOCHONDRAL OSSIFICATION

Endochondral ossification is a type of bone formation that occurs in preexisting cartilaginous models (Fig. 14.5). In a long bone, for example, the **primary center of ossification** appears in the **diaphysis**, which forms the **shaft of a bone**. At this center of ossification, chondrocyte hypertrophy create a matrix of high-X-collagen concentration, the matrix

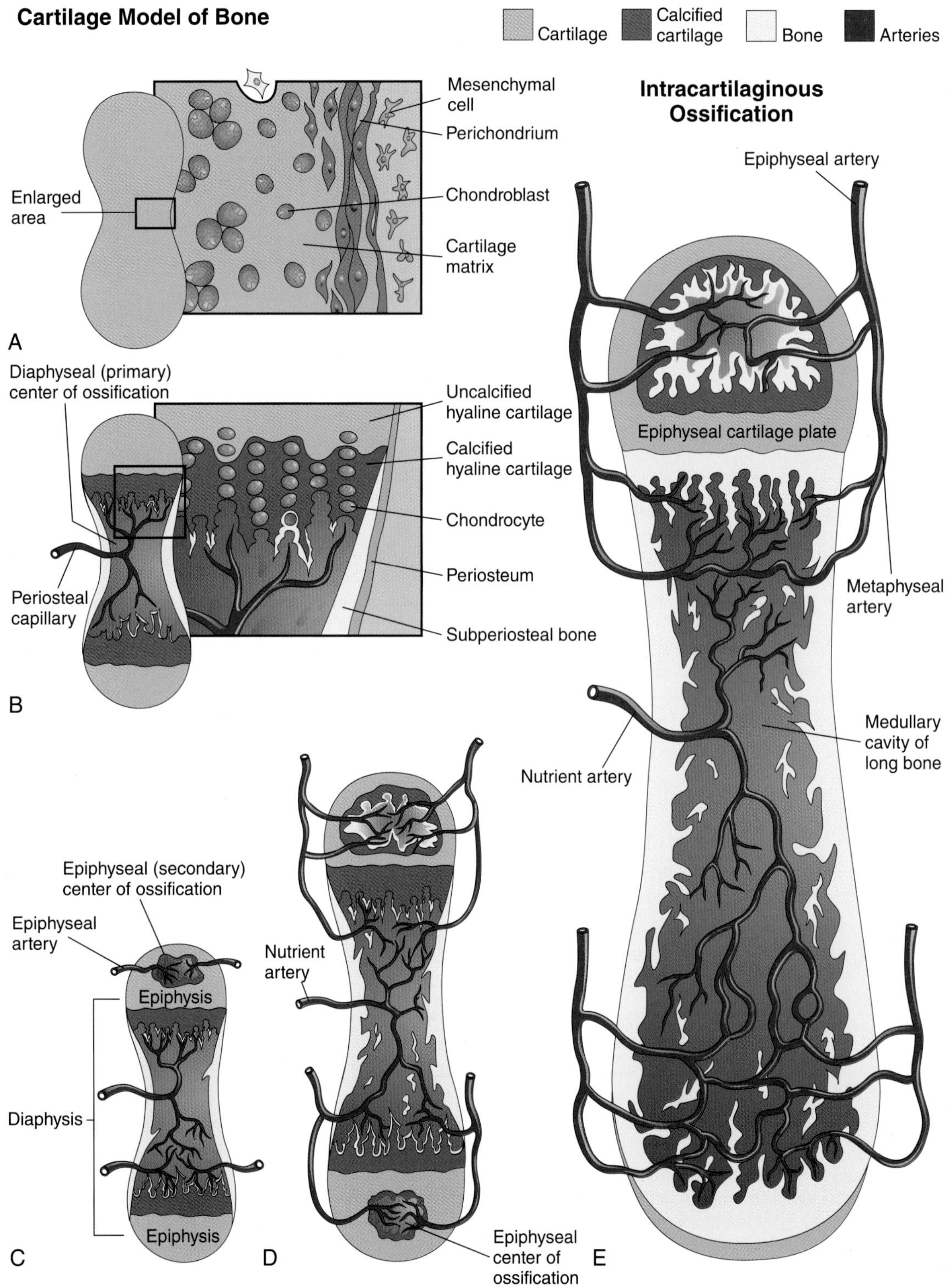

Fig. 14.5 (A–E) Schematic longitudinal sections of a 5-week embryo show endochondral ossification in a developing long bone.

becomes calcified, and the cells die. The hypertrophic chondrocytes also express VEGF, which acts as a chemotactic factor, attracting early hematopoietic progenitor cells and vascular endothelial cells.

Concurrently, a thin layer of bone is deposited under the **perichondrium** surrounding the diaphysis—the perichondrium becomes the **periosteum**. Invasion by vascular connective tissue from blood vessels surrounding the periosteum also breaks up the cartilage. **Osteoblasts** reach the developing bone from these blood vessels. This process continues toward the **epiphyses**. The spicules of bone are remodeled by the action of osteoclasts and osteoblasts. *The transcription factor SOX9 and the coactivator-associated arginine methyltransferase 1 (CARM1) regulate osteochondral ossification.*

The lengthening of long bones occurs at the **diaphyseal-epiphyseal junction** and depends on the **epiphyseal cartilage plates** (growth plates), whose chondrocytes proliferate and participate in endochondral bone formation (see Fig. 14.5E). Toward the diaphysis, the cartilage cells hypertrophy, and the matrix becomes calcified. The spicules of the bone are isolated from each other by vascular invasion from the marrow or **medullary cavity** of long bone (see Fig. 14.5E). Bone is deposited on these spicules by osteoblasts; resorption of the bone keeps the spongy bone masses relatively constant in length and enlarges the medullary cavity.

Ossification of limb bones begins at the end of the embryonic period. Thereafter, ossification makes demands on the maternal supply of calcium and phosphorus. Pregnant females are advised to maintain an adequate intake of these elements to preserve healthy bones and teeth.

At birth, the diaphyses are largely ossified, but most of the epiphyses are still cartilaginous. **Secondary ossification centers** appear in the epiphyses of most bones during the first few years after birth. The epiphyseal cartilage cells hypertrophy, and there is invasion by vascular connective tissue. Ossification spreads radially, and only the articular cartilage and the **epiphyseal cartilage plate** remain cartilaginous (see Fig. 14.5E). On completion of growth, the cartilage plate is replaced by spongy bone, the epiphyses and diaphysis are united, and no further elongation of the bone occurs.

In most bones, the epiphyses fuse with the diaphysis by the age of 20 years. Growth in the diameter of bone results from the deposition of bone at the periosteum (see Fig. 14.5B) and from resorption on the internal medullary surface. The rate of deposition and resorption is balanced to regulate the thickness of the compact bone and the size of the medullary cavity. The internal reorganization of bones continues throughout life. The development of irregular bones is similar to that of the epiphyses of long bones. Ossification begins centrally and spreads in all directions.

Rickets

Rickets, either in its hereditary or acquired form, is a bone disease in children attributable to **vitamin D deficiency**. Vitamin D is required for calcium absorption by the intestine. Rickets is a major public health concern in most parts of the world. Affected children have lower serum calcium and phosphorus levels, which impairs the formation of chondrocytes. The resulting inadequate intake **of calcium** (calcipenic rickets) and deficient intestinal absorption of phosphorus (phosphopenic rickets) affect ossification of the **epiphyseal cartilage plates** because they are not adequately mineralized, and there is a disorientation of cells at the **metaphysis**. The wrist joint and costochondral junctions are usually enlarged. The limbs are shortened and deformed, with severe bowing of the long bones in the limbs. Rickets may also delay the closure of the fontanelles of the cranial bones in infants (see Fig. 14.10A and B). Acquired rickets may also be due to restricted sunlight exposure, which results in a deficiency of vitamin D synthesis. Hereditary vitamin D–resistant rickets result from defects in vitamin D synthesis or its receptor.

DEVELOPMENT OF JOINTS

Joints begin to develop with the appearance of the joint **interzone** within the continuous cartilage bone model during the sixth week. The cells in the interzone begin to flatten and form a separation at the joint location. By the end of the eighth week, the joints resemble adult structures (Fig. 14.6). Joints are classified as **fibrous joints**, **cartilaginous joints**, and **synovial joints**. *Molecular studies show that a distinct cohort of progenitor cells expressing TGF-β receptor 2 at prospective joint sites contributes to the formation of the synovial joints and articular cartilages. Factors involved in the early formation of the interzone region include Wnt-14 and Noggin.*

FIBROUS JOINTS

During the development of fibrous joints, the **interzonal mesenchyme** between the developing bones differentiates into dense fibrous tissue (see Fig. 14.6D). For example, the sutures of the cranium are fibrous joints (see Fig. 14.10).

CARTILAGINOUS JOINTS

During the development of cartilaginous joints, the interzonal mesenchyme between the developing bones differentiates into **hyaline cartilage** (e.g., costochondral joints) or **fibrocartilage** (pubic symphysis; see Fig. 14.6C).

SYNOVIAL JOINTS

During the development of synovial joints (e.g., knee joints), the interzonal mesenchyme between the developing bones differentiates as follows (see Fig. 14.6B):

- Peripherally, the interzonal mesenchyme forms the **joint capsule** and other ligaments.
- Centrally, the mesenchyme undergoes cavitation, beginning in late embryogenesis to the postnatal period, and disappears, and the resulting space becomes the fluid-filled **joint cavity** (synovial cavity).
- Where it lines the joint capsule and articular surfaces, the mesenchyme forms the **synovial membrane**, which secretes synovial fluid and is a part of the joint capsule (fibrous capsule lined with synovial membrane).

Probably as a result of joint movements, the mesenchymal cells subsequently disappear from the surfaces of the

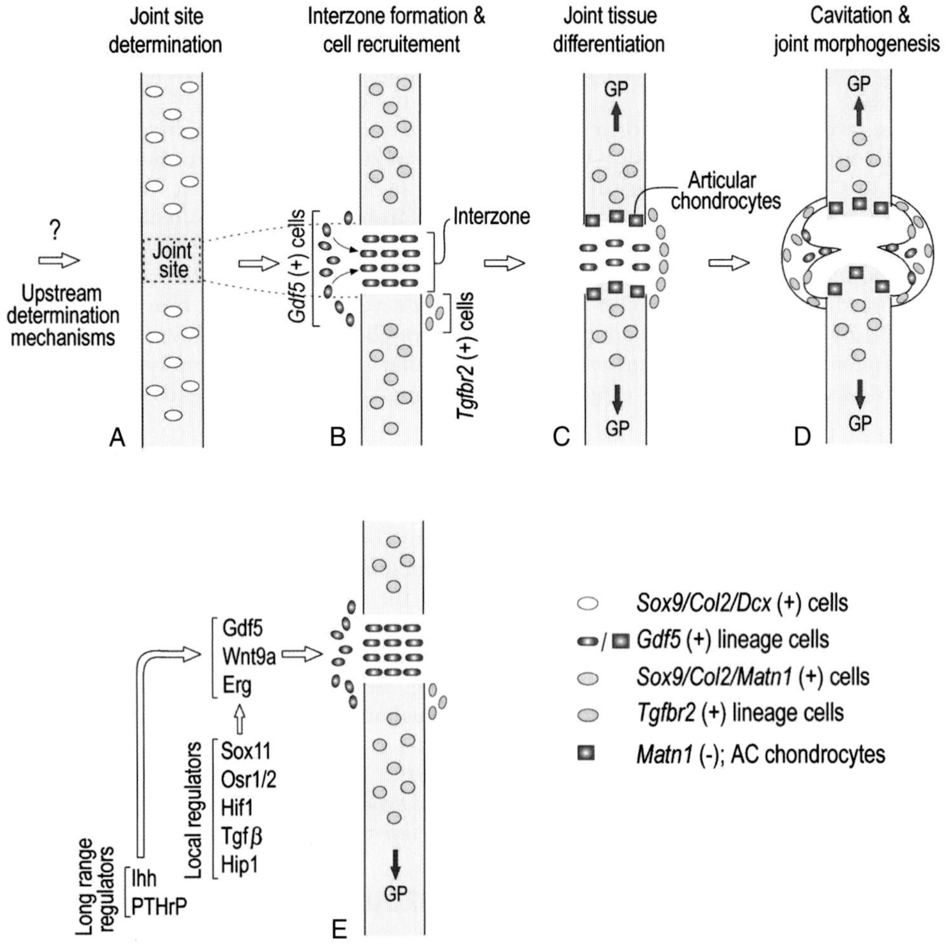

Fig. 14.6 Model of limb joint formation and morphogenesis. (A) At early developmental stages, as-yet-unknown upstream determination mechanisms would identify and prescribe the location of the joints along *Sox9/Col2/Dcx*-expressing anlagen. (B) Soon after, *Gdf5* expression would be activated along with other interzone-specific genes (see E) that would define the initial interzone mesenchymal population within the *Sox9/Col2/Matn1*-positive cartilaginous anlagen. This would be accompanied by cell immigration from the flank, and cells located dorsally and ventrally would activate *Tgfbr2* expression. (C) *Gdf5*-positive cells adjacent to their respective cartilaginous anlagen—with a *Sox9/Col2* history but negative for *matrillin-1* expression—would differentiate into articular chondrocytes. (D) Additional differentiation processes and mechanisms such as muscle movement would bring about cavitation and genesis of other joint tissues such as ligaments and other meniscus involving *Gdf5*- and *Tgfbr2*-positive and -negative cell progenies. Note that the distinct spatiotemporal steps—presented here as distinct for illustration purposes—may occur more closely and involve overlapping events. Also, the model may not entirely apply to other joints, including intervertebral and temporomandibular joints, that involve additional and/or diverse mechanisms. (E) Schematic summarizing local and long-range regulators that converge to regulate interzone gene expression at early stages of joint formation. Note that this list is not exhaustive. (From Decker RS, Koyama E, Pacifici M: Genesis and morphogenesis of limb synovial joints and articular cartilage. *Matrix Biol* 39:5, 2014.)

articular cartilages. An abnormal intrauterine environment restricting embryonic and fetal movements may interfere with limb development and cause joint fixation.

DEVELOPMENT OF AXIAL SKELETON

The axial skeleton is composed of the cranium (skull), vertebral column, ribs, and sternum. During the fourth week, cells in the **sclerotomes** surround the **neural tube** (primordium of the spinal cord) and notochord, the structure around which the primordia of the vertebrae develop (Fig. 14.7A). This positional change of the sclerotomal cells is caused by the differential growth of the surrounding structures and not by the active migration of sclerotomal cells. *The protocadherins Fat4 and Dchs 1 signaling mediate planar cell polarity and control early chondrogenesis in the developing vertebrae.* TBX6, Hox, *and* PAX *genes regulate the patterning and regional development of the vertebrae along the anterior-posterior axis.*

DEVELOPMENT OF VERTEBRAL COLUMN

During the **precartilaginous or mesenchymal stage**, mesenchymal cells from the sclerotomes are found in three main areas (see Fig. 14.7A): around the notochord, surrounding the neural tube, and in the body wall. In the frontal section of a 4-week embryo, the sclerotomes appear as paired condensations of mesenchymal cells around the notochord (see Fig. 14.7B). Each sclerotome consists of loosely arranged cells cranially and densely packed cells caudally.

Some densely packed cells move cranially, opposite the center of the **myotome** (muscle plate), where they form

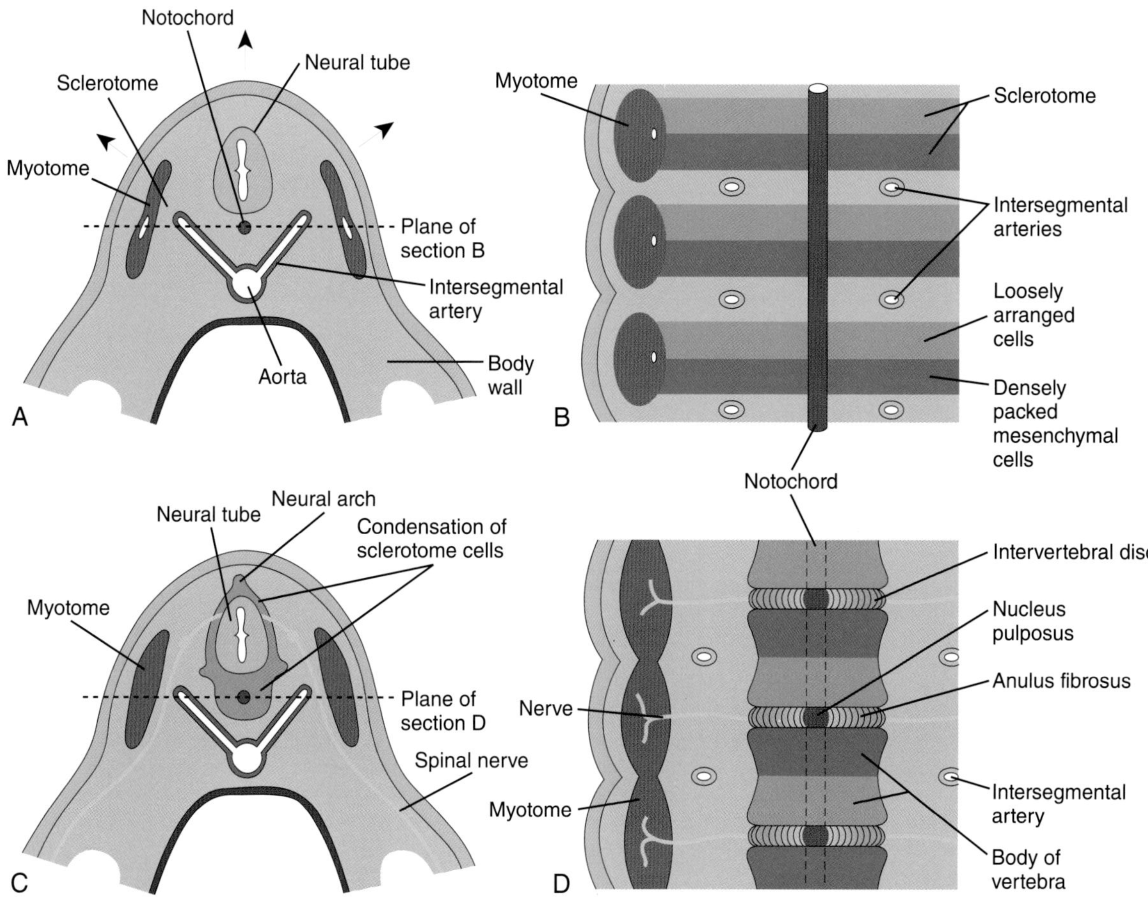

Fig. 14.7 (A) Transverse section of a 4-week embryo. The *arrows* indicate the dorsal growth of the neural tube and the simultaneous dorsolateral movement of the somite remnant, leaving behind a trail of sclerotomal cells. (B) Diagrammatic frontal section of the same embryo as in (A) shows that the condensation of sclerotomal cells around the notochord consists of a cranial area of loosely packed cells and a caudal area of densely packed cells. (C) Transverse section through a 5-week embryo shows the condensation of sclerotomal cells around the notochord and neural tube, which forms a mesenchymal vertebra. (D) Diagrammatic frontal section of the same embryo as in (C) illustrates vertebral body formation from the cranial and caudal halves of two successive sclerotomal masses. The intersegmental arteries cross the bodies of the vertebrae, and the spinal nerves lie between the vertebrae. The notochord is degenerating except in the region of the intervertebral disc, where it forms the nucleus pulposus.

the **intervertebral disc** (Fig. 14.7C and D). The remaining densely packed cells fuse with the loosely arranged cells of the immediately caudal sclerotome to form the mesenchymal **centrum**, the primordium of the body of a vertebra. Thus each centrum develops from two adjacent sclerotomes and becomes an intersegmental structure.

The nerves lie close to the intervertebral discs, and the **intersegmental arteries** lie on each side of the vertebral bodies. In the thorax, the dorsal intersegmental arteries become the **intercostal arteries**.

The notochord is involved in the patterning of the intervertebral disc. It degenerates and disappears where it is surrounded by the developing vertebral bodies. Between the vertebrae, the **notochord** expands to form the gelatinous center of the intervertebral disc, the proteoglycan, and the glycosaminoglycan-filled **nucleus pulposus** (see Fig. 14.7D). This nucleus is later surrounded by circularly arranged fibers that form the **annulus fibrosus**. The nucleus pulposus and annulus fibrosus form the avascular **intervertebral disc**. The mesenchymal cells that surround the neural tube form the **neural arch**, which is the **primordium of the vertebral arch** (see Fig. 14.7C). The mesenchymal cells in the body wall form **costal processes**, which form the ribs in the thoracic region.

Chordoma

Remnants of the notochord may persist and form a **chordoma**, an extremely rare (1:1,000,000) form of sarcoma at the base of the skull or lumbosacral region. Approximately one-third of these slow-growing malignant tumors occur at the base of the cranium and extend to the nasopharynx. Chordomas infiltrate bone and are difficult to remove. Approximately 30% of patients develop metastases. Surgical resection, when feasible, has provided long-term, disease-free survival for many patients. In some cases, local recurrence of the chordoma may occur.

CARTILAGINOUS STAGE OF VERTEBRAL DEVELOPMENT

During the sixth week, **chondrification centers** appear in each mesenchymal vertebra (Fig. 14.8A and B). The two centers in each **centrum** fuse at the end of the embryonic period to

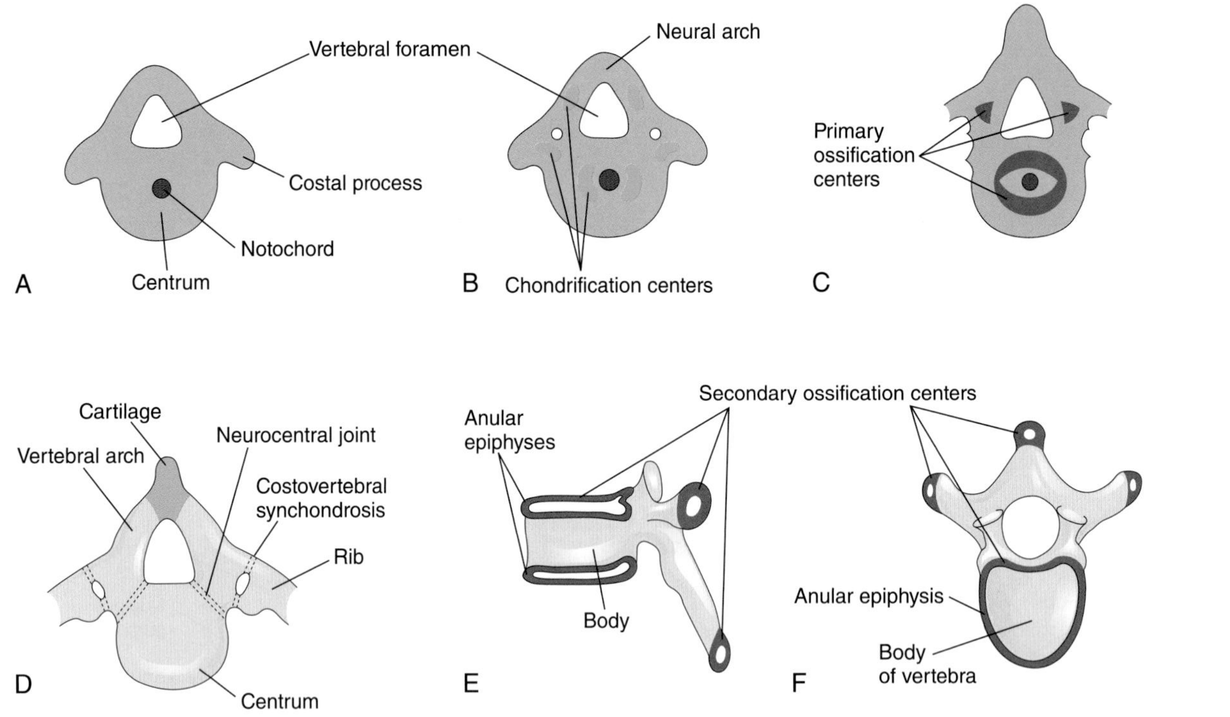

Fig. 14.8 Stages of vertebral development. (A) Mesenchymal vertebra at 5 weeks. (B) Chondrification centers in a mesenchymal vertebra at 6 weeks. The neural arch is the primordium of the vertebral arch of the vertebra. (C) Primary ossification centers in a cartilaginous vertebra at 7 weeks. (D) Thoracic vertebra at birth consists of three bony parts: vertebral arch, body of vertebra, and transverse processes. Notice the cartilage between the halves of the vertebral arch and between the arch and the centrum (neurocentral joint). (E and F) Two views of a typical thoracic vertebra at puberty show the locations of the secondary centers of ossification.

form a cartilaginous centrum. Concomitantly, the centers in the neural arches fuse with each other and the centrum. The spinous and transverse processes develop from extensions of chondrification centers in the neural arch. Chondrification spreads until a cartilaginous vertebral column is formed.

BONY STAGE OF VERTEBRAL DEVELOPMENT

Ossification of typical vertebrae begins during the seventh week and ends by the 25th year. There are two **primary ossification centers**, ventral and dorsal, for the centrum (Fig. 14.8C). These centers soon fuse to form one center. Three primary centers are present by the eighth week: one in the centrum and one in each half of the neural arch.

Ossification becomes evident in the **neural arches** during the eighth week. Each typical vertebra consists of three bony parts connected by cartilage: a vertebral arch, a body, and transverse processes (see Fig. 14.8D). The bony halves of the **vertebral arch** usually fuse during the first 3 to 5 years. The arches first unite in the lumbar region, and the union progresses cranially. The vertebral arch articulates with the **centrum** at cartilaginous **neurocentral joints**, which permit the vertebral arches to grow as the spinal cord enlarges. These joints disappear when the vertebral arch fuses with the centrum during the third to sixth years.

Five **secondary ossification centers** appear in the vertebrae after puberty:

- One for the tip of the spinous process
- One for the tip of each transverse process
- Two **anular epiphyses**, one on the superior and one on the inferior rim of the vertebral body (see Fig. 14.8E and F)

The **vertebral body** is a composite of the anular epiphyses and the mass of bone between them. The vertebral body includes the centrum, parts of the vertebral arch, and the facets of the heads of the ribs. All secondary centers unite with the rest of the vertebrae at approximately 25 years of age. Exceptions to the typical ossification of vertebrae occur in the atlas or C1 vertebra, axis or C2 vertebra, C7 vertebra, lumbar vertebrae, sacrum, and coccyx. Minor defects of the vertebrae are common but usually have little clinical importance.

Variation in the Number of Vertebrae

Most people have 7 cervical, 12 thoracic, 5 lumbar, and 5 sacral vertebrae. A few have one or two additional vertebrae or one less. To determine the number of vertebrae, it is necessary to examine the entire vertebral column because an apparent extra (or absent) vertebra in one segment of the column may be compensated for by an absent (or extra) vertebra in an adjacent segment, such as 11 thoracic vertebrae with 6 lumbar vertebrae.

The Notch signaling pathways are involved in the patterning of the vertebral column. Severe congenital birth defects, including **VACTERL syndrome** (*v*ertebral, *a*nal, *c*ardiac, *t*racheal, esophageal, *r*enal, and *l*imb birth defects) and **CHARGE syndrome** (coloboma of the eye, heart defects, including tetralogy of Fallot, patent ductus arteriosus, and ventricular or atrial septal defect, as well as scoliosis or kyphosis), are associated with pathogenic variants (mutations) of Notch-pathway genes.

DEVELOPMENT OF RIBS

Ribs develop from the mesenchymal **costal processes** of the thoracic vertebrae (see Fig. 14.8A). They become cartilaginous during the embryonic period and ossify during the fetal period. The original site of the union of the costal processes with the vertebra is replaced by **costovertebral synovial joints** (see Fig. 14.8D). Seven pairs of ribs (1–7; **true ribs**) attach through their cartilages to the sternum. Three pairs of ribs (8–10; **false ribs**) attach to the sternum through the cartilage of another rib or ribs. The last two pairs of ribs (11 and 12; **floating ribs**) do not attach to the sternum.

DEVELOPMENT OF STERNUM

A pair of vertical mesenchymal bands, the **sternal bars**, develop ventrolaterally in the body wall. **Chondrification** occurs in these bars as they move medially. By 10 weeks, they fuse craniocaudally in the median plane to form cartilaginous models of the manubrium, sternebrae (segments of the sternal body), and xiphoid process. The manubrium develops from the mesenchyme between the clavicles with contributions from neural crest cells in the region of endochondral ossification. Centers of ossification appear craniocaudally in the sternum before birth, except for the **xiphoid process**, which appears during childhood. The xiphoid process may never completely ossify.

DEVELOPMENT OF CRANIUM

The cranium (skull) develops from mesenchyme around the developing brain. The growth of the **neurocranium** (bones of the cranium enclosing the brain) is initiated from ossification centers within the **mesenchyme**, which is the primordium of the cranium. *TGF-β plays a critical role in the development of the cranium by regulating osteoblast differentiation.*

The cranium consists of two parts:

- **Neurocranium**, a bony case that encloses the brain, derived primarily from the neural crest
- **Viscerocranium**, the facial skeleton, of which the rostral portion is derived from neural crest while the posterior portion is derived from mesoderm

CARTILAGINOUS NEUROCRANIUM

Initially, the cartilaginous neurocranium **(chondrocranium)** consists of the cartilaginous base of the developing cranium, which forms by the fusion of several cartilages (Fig. 14.9A–D). Later, endochondral ossification of the chondrocranium forms the bones at the base of the cranium. The ossification pattern of these bones has a definite sequence, beginning with the **occipital** bone, body of **sphenoid**, and **ethmoid** bone.

The **parachordal cartilage**, or basal plate, forms around the cranial end of the notochord (see Fig. 14.9A) and fuses with the cartilages derived from the sclerotome regions of the occipital somites. This cartilaginous mass contributes to the **base of the occipital bone**; later, extensions grow around the cranial end of the spinal cord and form the boundaries of the **foramen magnum**, which is a large opening in the basal part of the occipital bone (see Fig. 14.9C).

The **hypophyseal cartilage** forms around the developing **pituitary gland** (hypophysis cerebri) and fuses to form the body of the sphenoid bone. The **trabeculae cranii** fuse to form the body of the ethmoid bone, and the **ala orbitalis** forms the lesser wing of the sphenoid bone.

Otic capsules develop around the **otic vesicles**, which are the primordia of the internal ears (see Fig. 18.15), and form the petrous and mastoid parts of the temporal bone. **Nasal capsules** develop around the nasal sacs and contribute to the formation of the ethmoid bone.

MEMBRANOUS NEUROCRANIUM

Intramembranous ossification occurs in the head mesenchyme at the sides and top of the brain, forming the **calvaria** (skullcap). During fetal life, the flat bones of the calvaria are separated by dense connective tissue membranes that form fibrous joints, the **sutures of calvaria** (Fig. 14.10).

Six large fibrous areas (fontanelles) are found where several sutures meet. The softness of the bones and their loose connections at the sutures enable the calvaria to change shape during birth. During **molding of the fetal cranium**, the adaptation of the fetal head to pressure in the birth canal, the frontal and occipital bones slide under the parietal bones, which is made possible by the flexion of the coronal and lambdoid sutures. Within a few days after birth, the shape of the calvaria returns to normal.

Because of the growth of the surrounding bones, the posterior and anterolateral fontanelles disappear within 2 to 3 months after birth, but they remain as sutures for several years. The posterolateral fontanelles disappear similarly by the end of the first year, and the anterior fontanelle disappears by the end of the second year. The halves of the frontal bone normally begin to fuse during the second year, and the frontal suture is usually obliterated by the eighth year. The other sutures disappear during adult life, with wide variation in timing among individuals.

CARTILAGINOUS VISCEROCRANIUM

Most mesenchyme in the head region is derived from the neural crest. **Neural crest cells** migrate into the pharyngeal arches and form the bones and connective tissue of craniofacial structures. *Transgenic studies in mice show that the frontal bones are of neural crest cell origin and the parietal bones are derived from mesenchymal. Molecular events and patterning of the bones involve the expression of a wide array of genes, including BMP/TGF-β, Wnt, FGF, Notch, Hippo, and PDFGF signaling.*

Homeobox (Hox) *genes regulate the migration and subsequent differentiation of the neural crest cells, which are crucial for the complex patterning of the head and face.* These parts of the fetal cranium are derived from the cartilaginous skeleton of the first two pairs of **pharyngeal arches** (see Fig. 9.5 and Table 9.1):

- The dorsal end of the first arch cartilage forms two middle ear bones, the malleus, and incus of the middle ear.
- The dorsal end of the second arch cartilage forms a portion of the stapes of the middle ear and the styloid process of the temporal bone. Its ventral end ossifies to form the lesser horn (cornu) of the hyoid.

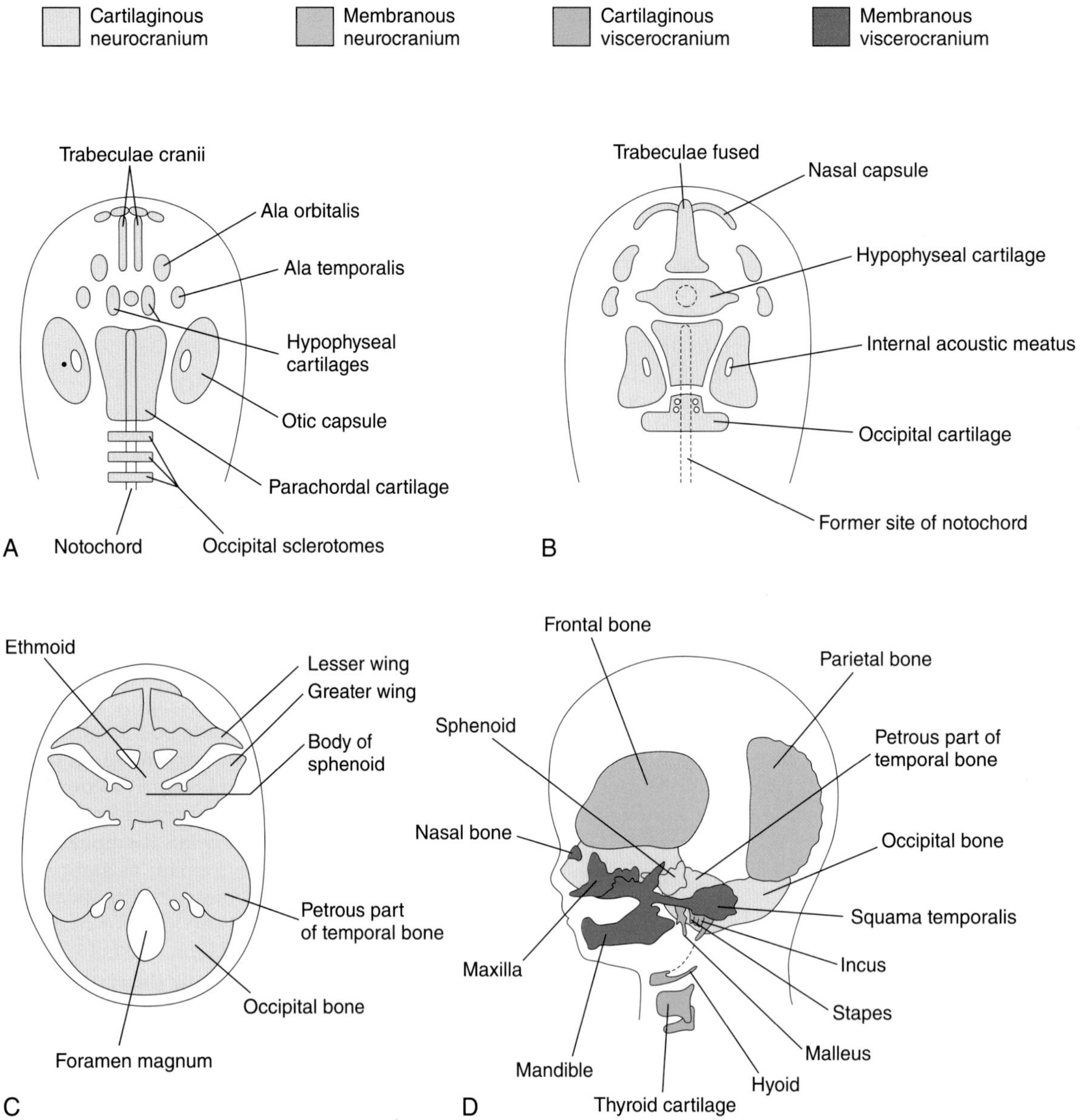

Fig. 14.9 Superior views show the developmental stages of the cranial base. (A) At 6 weeks, various cartilages begin to fuse and form the chondrocranium. (B) At 7 weeks, some of the paired cartilages have fused. (C) At 12 weeks, the cartilaginous base of the cranium is formed by the fusion of various cartilages. (D) Derivation of the bones of the fetal cranium is indicated at 20 weeks.

- The third and fourth arch cartilages form only in the ventral parts of the arches. The third arch cartilages form the greater horns of the hyoid bone and the superior cornu of the thyroid cartilage.
- The fourth arch cartilages appear to fuse to form the laryngeal cartilages, except for the epiglottis. Table 9.1).

MEMBRANOUS VISCEROCRANIUM

Intramembranous ossification occurs in the maxillary prominence of the first pharyngeal arch (see Figs. 9.4 and 9.5) and subsequently forms the **squamous temporal**, **maxillary,** and **zygomatic** bones. The **squamous temporal bones** become part of the **neurocranium** (cranial bones enclosing the brain rather than the face). The mesenchyme in the **mandibular prominence** of the first arch condenses around its cartilage and undergoes **intramembranous ossification** to form the mandible (see Fig. 9.4B). Some **endochondral ossification** occurs in the median plane of the chin and mandibular condyle.

POSTNATAL GROWTH OF CRANIUM

The neonatal cranium is large in proportion to the rest of the skeleton, and the face is relatively small compared with the calvaria. The small facial region of the cranium results from the small size of the jaws, the virtual absence of paranasal sinuses, and the underdevelopment of the facial bones.

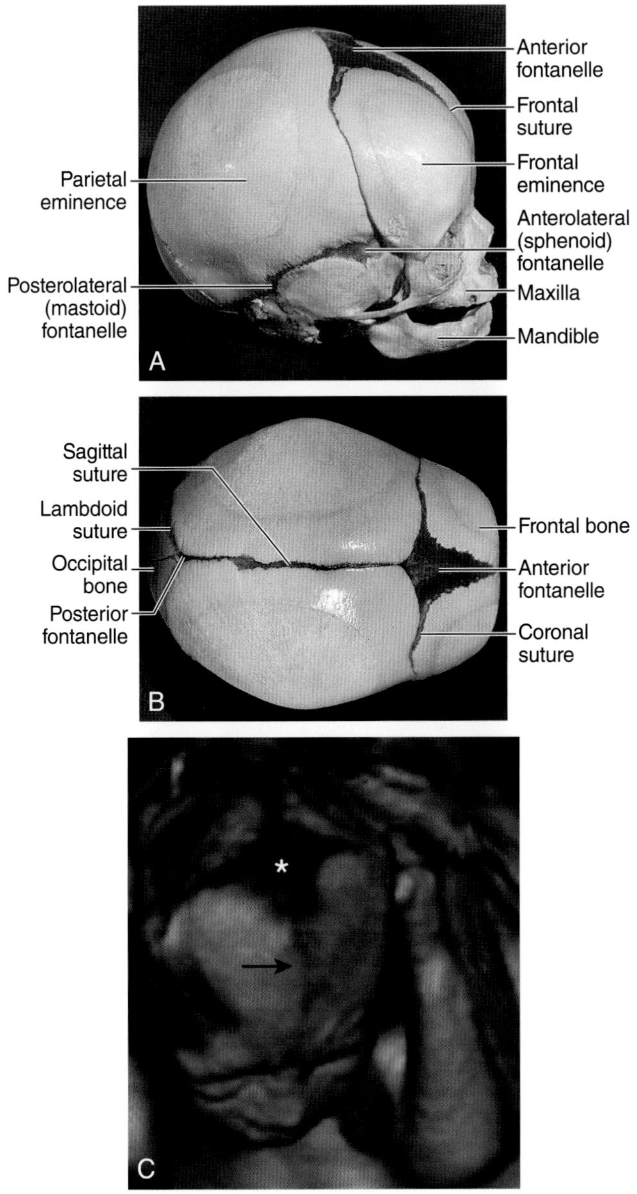

Fig. 14.10 Bones, fontanelles, and sutures of the fetal cranium (skull). (A) Lateral view. (B) Superior view. (C) In this three-dimensional ultrasound rendering of the fetal head at 22 weeks, notice the anterior fontanelle *(asterisk)* and the frontal suture *(arrow)*. The coronal and sagittal sutures are also shown. ((C) Courtesy Dr. G.J. Reid, Department of Obstetrics, Gynecology and Reproductive Sciences, University of Manitoba, Women's Hospital, Winnipeg, Manitoba, Canada.)

The fibrous sutures of the neonatal calvaria permit the brain to enlarge during infancy and childhood. The increase in size of the calvaria is greatest during the first 2 years, the period of most rapid postnatal growth of the brain. The calvaria normally increases in capacity until approximately 16 years. After this, it usually increases slightly for 3 to 4 years because of the thickening of the bones.

The rapid growth of the face and jaws coincides with the eruption of the primary (deciduous) teeth. These facial changes are more marked after the secondary (permanent) teeth erupt (see Fig. 19.14H). Concurrent enlargement of the frontal and facial regions is associated with an increase in the size of the frontal, maxillary, sphenoid, and ethmoid sinuses. The growth of the sinuses alters the shape of the face and adds resonance to the voice.

Klippel-Feil Sequence

This sequence (1:40,000) typically has a triad of features: limited range of cervical motion, short neck (brevicollis), and low posterior hairline, all of which result from congenital fusion of cervical vertebrae. This fusion is thought to result from a lack of segmentation during development, possibly from vascular disruption, and is associated with several pathogenic variants (mutations) of genes, including GDF6, GDF3, MEOX1, RIPPLY2, and MYO18B. The fusion may consist of a single (type I0), multiple continuous (type iii), or noncontinuous fused segments (type II) of cervical/thoracic vertebrae. Symptoms tend to be minimal in children but increase with age with the progression of fusion. Surgery may be required. Individuals with Klippel-Feil sequence may also have defects in other systems, including cardiovascular, renal, and gastrointestinal.

Spina Bifida

Failure of the halves of the embryonic cartilaginous neural arch to fuse results in various types of spina bifida, which are major birth defects (see Fig. 17.12). The incidence of these vertebral defects ranges from 0.04% to 0.15%; they occur more frequently in females than males. The types of spina bifida are described in Chapter 17 (see Figs. 17.14–17.17).

Accessory Ribs

Accessory ribs, which are usually rudimentary, result from the development of the costal processes of cervical or lumbar vertebrae (Fig. 14.11A). Costal processes usually form ribs only in the thoracic region. The most common (1%) accessory rib is a **lumbar rib** (see Fig. 14.11B), but it usually is clinically insignificant. A **cervical rib** occurs in 0.5% to 1% of people. This supernumerary rib is usually attached to the manubrium of the sternum (see Fig. 14.11A) or the seventh cervical vertebra and may be fused with the first rib. The pressure of a cervical rib on the brachial plexus of nerves that are located partly in the neck and axilla or on the subclavian artery often produces neurovascular symptoms (e.g., paralysis, anesthesia of the upper limb). Accessory ribs may be unilateral or bilateral.

Fused Ribs

Fusion of ribs occasionally occurs posteriorly when two or more ribs arise from a single vertebra (see Fig. 14.11C). Fused ribs are often associated with a hemivertebra (one side of a vertebra fails to develop).

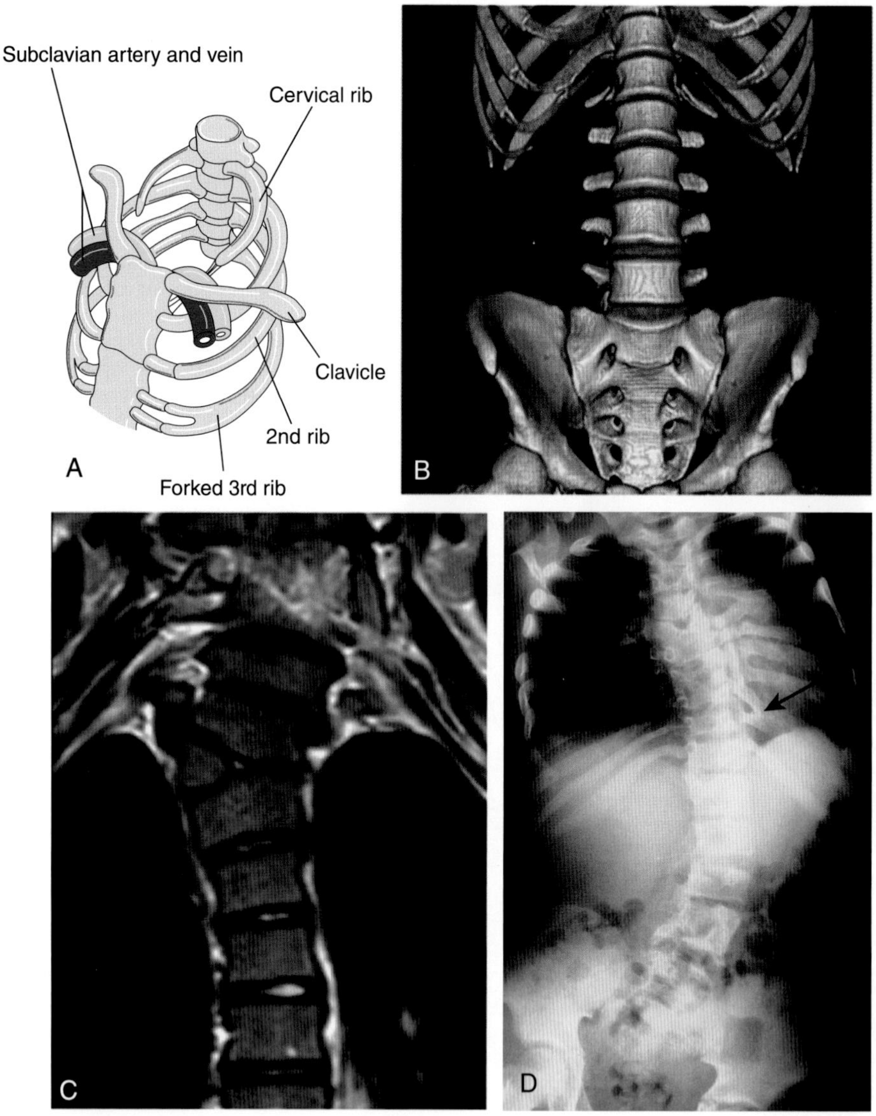

Fig. 14.11 Vertebral and rib abnormalities. (A) Cervical and forked ribs. The left cervical rib has a fibrous band that passes posterior to the subclavian vessels and attaches to the manubrium of the sternum. (B) Three-dimensional computed tomography noting lumbar ribs at L1. (C) Coronal section through the spine of a 10-year-old girl with back pain. Note the hemivertebra to the left of the right lung apex. (D) Radiograph of a child with the kyphoscoliotic deformity of the lumbar region of the vertebral column shows multiple anomalies of the vertebrae and ribs. Notice the fused ribs *(arrow)*. ((B) From Aly I, Chapman JR, Oskouian RJ, et al: Lumbar ribs: a comprehensive review, *Childs Nerv Syst* 32:781, 2016. (C) From Johal J, Loukas M, Fisahn C, et al: Hemivertebrae: a comprehensive review of embryology, imaging, classification, and management, *Childs Nerv Syst* 32:2105, 2016. (D) Courtesy Dr. Prem S. Sahni, formerly of the Department of Radiology, Children's Hospital, Winnipeg, Manitoba, Canada.)

Hemivertebra

The developing vertebral bodies have two chondrification centers that soon unite. A hemivertebra results from the *failure of one of the chondrification centers to appear* and the subsequent failure of one-half of the vertebra (unilateral) to form (see Fig. 14.11C). Hemivertebrae are often present with other congenital anomalies (facial, central nervous system, cardiovascular system, gastrointestinal, musculoskeletal, and others). Hemivertebrae are the most common cause of **congenital scoliosis** of the vertebral column (see Fig. 14.11D). Less common causes of scoliosis include **myopathic scoliosis**, resulting from weakness of the back muscles. Nonisolated cases of hemivertebra have been reported in association with genetic disorders: microdeletions, single gene defects, and several syndromes.

Spinal Dysraphism

Several conditions of the spine and associated structures fall within the term spinal dysraphism, including spinal bifida, tethered spinal cord, split cord (diastemoatomyelia), spinal cord lipoma (lipomyelomeninocele), and a dermal sinus tract. Symptoms vary in significance depending on the defect. Spinal dysraphism results from faulty closure of the neural tube caused by several mechanisms including teratogens.

Anomalies of Sternum

A concave depression of the lower sternum **(pectus excavatum)** accounts for 90% of thoracic wall defects. Males are more often affected (1 in 400–1000 live births). It is probably caused by overgrowth of the costal cartilage, which displaces the lower sternum inward. Minor sternal clefts (notch or foramen in the xiphoid process) are common and are of no clinical concern. In some cases, the sternum may protrude above the chest wall (**pectus carinatum**) giving the person a bird-like (pigeon-chest) appearance. Various sizes and forms of the **sternal foramen** occasionally occur at the junction of the third and fourth sternebrae (segments of the primordial sternum). This insignificant foramen is the result of incomplete fusion of the cartilaginous sternal bars during the embryonic period. Pectus excavatum and pectus carinatum are most likely multifactorial in origin and are associated with other structural abnormalities and genetic syndromes.

Acrania

Acrania is the complete or partial absence of the neurocranium that may be accompanied by extensive defects of the vertebral column (see Fig. 14.12). **Acrania** associated with **meroencephaly** (partial absence of the brain) occurs in approximately 1 of 10,000 births and is incompatible with life. Meroencephaly results from failure of the cranial end of the neural tube to close during the fourth week and causes failure of the neurocranium to form.

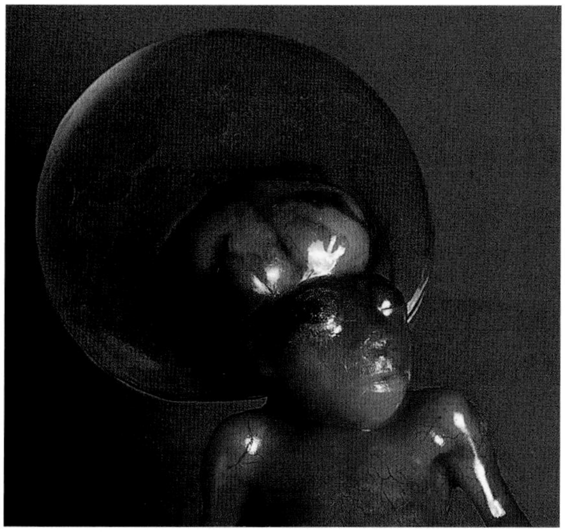

Fig. 14.12 Second-trimester fetus with holoacrania (absence of cranium or acrania). A cyst-like structure surrounds the intact fetal brain. (Courtesy A.E. Chudley, MD, Section of Genetics and Metabolism, Department of Pediatrics and Child Health, University of Manitoba, Children's Hospital, Winnipeg, Manitoba, Canada.)

Craniosynostosis

Prenatal fusion of the cranial sutures results in several birth defects. The cause of craniosynostosis is unclear. *Pathogenic variants (mutations) of the homeobox genes* MSX2, ALX4, FGFR1, FGFR2, *and* TWIST *have been implicated in the molecular mechanisms of craniosynostosis and other cranial defects*. A strong association between maternal valproic acid use during early pregnancy and infant craniosynostosis has been reported; a linkage between maternal smoking and thyroid disease has also been suggested. These birth defects are more common in males than females, and they are often associated with other skeletal defects with an incidence of 1:2500.

The type of deformed cranium produced depends on which sutures close prematurely. Suture closure prevents the growth of the bone perpendicular to the suture, causing bone growth parallel to the suture instead. If the sagittal suture closes early, the cranium becomes long, narrow, and wedge-shaped **(scaphocephaly)** (Fig. 14.13A and B). This type of cranial deformity constitutes about one-half of the cases of craniosynostosis. Another 30% of cases involve premature closure of the coronal suture, which results in a high, tower-like cranium **(brachycephaly**; see Fig. 14.13C). If the coronal suture closes prematurely on one side only, the cranium is twisted and asymmetric **(plagiocephaly)**. Premature closure of the frontal (metopic) suture results in a deformity of the frontal and orbital bones in addition to other anomalies **(trigonocephaly)** (see Fig. 14.13D).

Positional plagiocephaly is the most common cranial deformity and occurs when the neonate repeatedly rests its head in a particular position. As a result, that area of the head (most often one of the occipital bones) can become more flattened. Usually, an increase in positional changes is all that is required to restore normal shape.

Microcephaly

Neonates with microcephaly (0.2–1.0:1000) are born with normal-sized or slightly small calvaria. The **fontanelles** close during early infancy, and the other sutures close during the first year. However, this defect is not caused by premature closure of sutures. **Microcephaly** is the result of abnormal development of the central nervous system, in which the brain and neurocranium fail to grow. Infants with microcephaly have small heads and intellectual and developmental disabilities (see Fig. 17.36).

Anomalies at Craniovertebral Junction

Congenital abnormalities at the craniovertebral junction occur in approximately 1% of neonates, but they may not produce symptoms until adult life. Examples of these anomalies are **basilar invagination** (superior displacement of bone around the foramen magnum), **assimilation of the atlas** (nonsegmentation at the junction of the atlas and occipital bone), **atlantoaxial dislocation (disarrangement of atlantoaxial joint), Chiari malformation** (see Fig. 17.42A and B), and a **separate dens** (failure of the centers in the dens to fuse with the centrum of the axis).

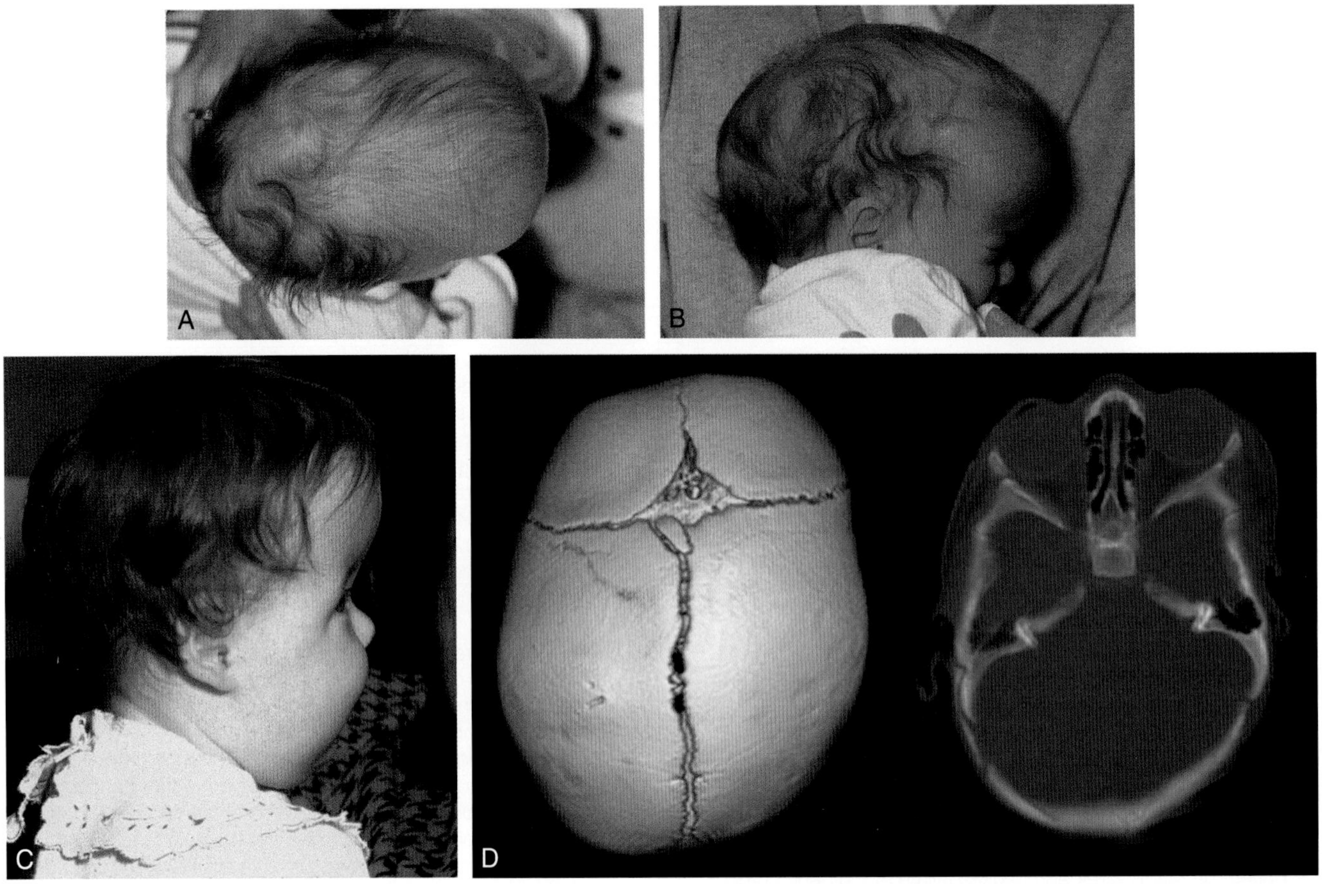

Fig. 14.13 Craniosynostosis. (A and B) The infant has scaphocephaly, a condition that results from premature closure (synostosis) of the sagittal suture. The elongated, wedge-shaped cranium is seen from above (A) and from the side (B). (C) In an infant with bilateral premature closure of the coronal suture (brachycephaly), notice the high, markedly elevated forehead. (D) Positional plagiocephaly. Top view (A) of a three-dimensional computed tomography scan (done for other reasons) showing a skull with a parallelogram shape. There is right posterior flattening and anterior displacement of the right forehead. Axial computed tomography scan (B) showing anterior displacement of the ear ipsilateral to the posterior flattening. The sutures are open. ((D) From Governale LS: Craniosynostosis. *Pediatr Neurol* 53:394, 2015.)

DEVELOPMENT OF APPENDICULAR SKELETON

The appendicular skeleton consists of the pectoral and pelvic girdles and limb bones. Mesenchymal bones form during the fifth week as condensations of mesenchyme appear in the limb buds (Fig. 14.14A–C). During the sixth week, the **mesenchymal bone models** in the limbs undergo chondrification to form **hyaline cartilage bone models** (see Fig. 14.14D and E).

The clavicle initially develops by intramembranous ossification, and it later forms growth cartilages at both ends. The models of the pectoral girdle and upper limb bones appear slightly before those of the pelvic girdle and lower limb bones. The bone models appear in a proximodistal sequence. *Patterning in the developing limbs is regulated by* Hox *genes.*

Ossification begins in the long bones by the eighth week and initially occurs in the diaphyses of the bones from **primary ossification centers** (see Fig. 14.5B–D). By 12 weeks, primary ossification centers have appeared in most bones of the limbs (Fig. 14.15A).

The clavicles begin to ossify before other bones in the body. The femurs are the next bones to show traces of ossification (see Fig. 14.15B). The first indication of the primary center of ossification in the cartilaginous model of a long bone is visible near the center of its future shaft, the diaphysis (see Fig. 14.5C). Primary centers appear at different times in different bones, but most of them appear between the 7th and 12th weeks. Virtually all primary centers of ossification are present at birth.

The **secondary ossification centers** of the bones at the knee are the first to appear in utero. The centers for the distal end of the femur and the proximal end of the tibia usually appear during the last month of intrauterine life (34–38 weeks). These centers are usually present at birth, but most secondary centers appear after birth. The part of a bone ossified from a secondary center is the **epiphysis** (see Fig. 14.5C). The bone formed from the primary center in the **diaphysis** does not fuse with that formed from the secondary centers in the epiphyses until the bone grows to its adult length. This delay enables the lengthening of the bone to continue until the final size is reached. During bone growth, the **epiphyseal cartilage plate** intervenes between

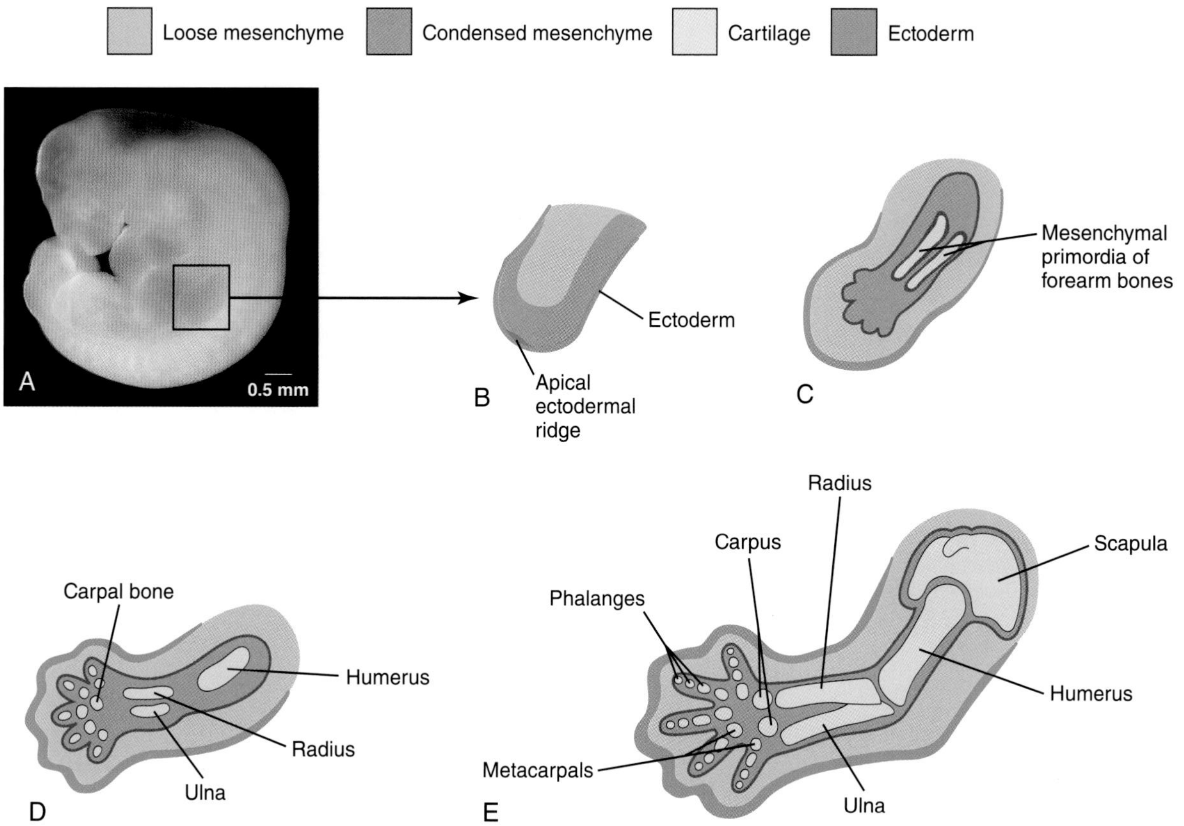

Fig. 14.14 (A) Photograph of an embryo at approximately 28 days shows the early appearance of the limb buds. (B) Longitudinal section through an upper limb bud shows the apical ectodermal ridge, which has an inductive influence on the mesenchyme. This ridge promotes the growth of the mesenchyme and imparts the ability to form specific cartilaginous elements. (C) Similar sketch of an upper limb bud at approximately 33 days shows the mesenchymal primordia of the forearm bones. The digital rays are mesenchymal condensations that undergo chondrification and ossification to form the bones of the hand. (D) Section of the upper limb at 6 weeks shows the cartilage models of the bones. (E) Later in the sixth week, the cartilaginous models of the bones of the upper limb are completed. ((A) Courtesy Dr. Brad Smith, University of Michigan, Ann Arbor, Michigan.)

the diaphysis and epiphysis (see Fig. 14.5E). The epiphyseal plate is eventually replaced by bone development on each of its two sides, diaphyseal and epiphyseal. When this occurs, the growth of the bone ceases.

Bone Age

Bone age is a good index of general maturation. Determination of the number, size, and fusion of epiphyseal centers from radiographs of the right wrist, hand, and fingers, is a commonly used method. A radiologist determines the bone age by assessing the ossification centers using two criteria:

- The time of appearance of calcified material in the diaphysis or epiphysis, or both, is specific for each diaphysis and epiphysis and for each bone and sex.
- The disappearance of the dark line representing the epiphyseal cartilage plate indicates that the epiphysis has fused with the diaphysis.

Fusion of the diaphyseal-epiphyseal centers, which occurs at specific times for each epiphysis, happens 1 to 2 years earlier in females than in males. Individual variation also occurs. Fetal ultrasonography is used for the evaluation and measurement of bones and the determination of fertilization age.

Generalized Skeletal Malformations

Achondroplasia is the most common cause of dwarfism or restricted growth (see Fig. 20.13) with disproportionate short stature. This rare defect occurs in approximately 1 of 15,000 births. The limbs become bowed and short (Fig. 14.16) because of a disturbance of the endochondral ossification during fetal life at the epiphyseal cartilage plates, particularly of the long bones. The trunk is usually short, and the head is enlarged with a bulging forehead and scooped (flat) nasal bridge.

Achondroplasia is an autosomal dominant disorder. Approximately 80% of cases arise from new pathogenic variants (mutations), and the rate increases with **paternal age**. Most cases are caused by a point mutation (G380R) in the fibroblast growth factor receptor 3 gene *(FGFR3)* that amplifies the normal inhibiting effect of endochondral ossification, specifically in the zone of chondrocyte proliferation and in mature osteoblasts. This results in shortened bones, but this does not affect the growth of bone width (periosteal bone growth).

Thanatophoric dysplasia is the most common type of lethal skeletal dysplasia, with distinct tubular bones, flattened vertebral bodies, and shortened ribs. It occurs in approximately 1 of 20,000 births. The affected infants typically die of respiratory failure, due to a small thoracic cage, within minutes or days of birth. This disorder is associated with pathogenic variants (mutations) in *FGFR3*.

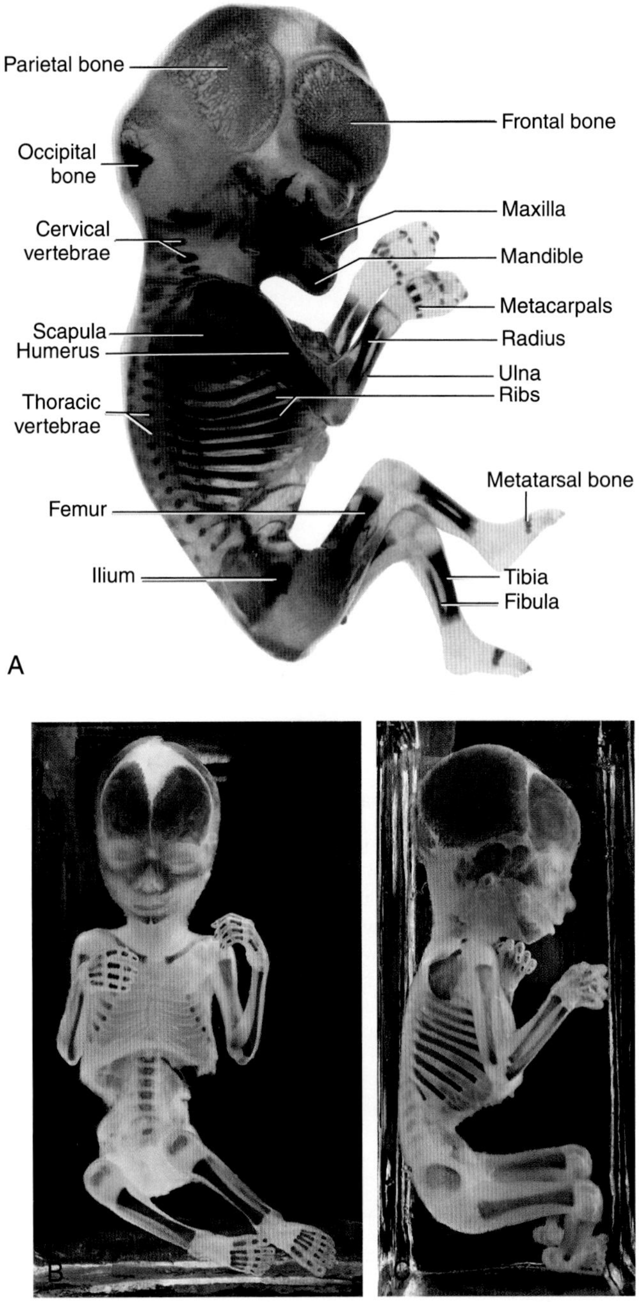

Fig. 14.15 Alizarin-stained and cleared human fetuses. (A) In a 12-week fetus, ossification has progressed from the primary centers of ossification and is endochondral in the appendicular and axial parts of the skeleton except for most of the cranial bones, which form the neurocranium. The carpus and tarsus are wholly cartilaginous at this stage, as are the epiphyses of all long bones. (B and C) Ossification in a fetus of approximately 20 weeks. ((A) Courtesy Dr. Gary Geddes, Lake Oswego, OR. (B and C) Courtesy Dr. David Bolender, Department of Cell Biology, Neurobiology, and Anatomy, Medical College of Wisconsin, Milwaukee, Wisconsin.)

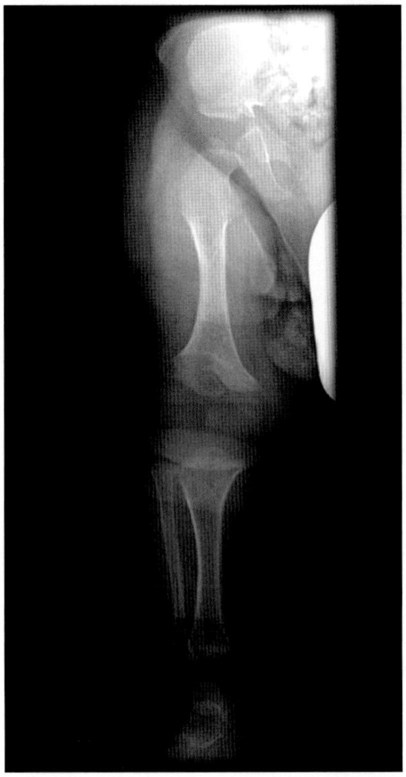

Fig. 14.16 Radiograph of the upper limb of a 2-year-old child with achondroplasia. Notice the shortened femur with metaphyseal flaring. (Courtesy Dr. Prem S. Sahni, formerly of the Department of Radiology, Children's Hospital, Winnipeg, Manitoba, Canada.)

SUMMARY OF SKELETAL SYSTEM

- The skeletal system develops from mesenchyme, which is derived from mesoderm and the neural crest. In most bones, such as the long bones in the limbs, the condensed mesenchyme undergoes **chondrification** to form cartilage models for bone formation. **Ossification** centers appear in the models by the end of the embryonic period (56 days), and the bones ossify later by **endochondral ossification**. Some bones (e.g., flat bones of the cranium) develop by intramembranous ossification.
- The vertebral column and ribs develop from mesenchymal cells derived from the sclerotomes of somites. Each vertebra is formed by the fusion of a condensation of the caudal half of one pair of **sclerotomes** with the cranial half of the subjacent pair of sclerotomes.
- The developing cranium (skull) consists of a **neurocranium** and a **viscerocranium**, each of which has membranous and cartilaginous components. The neurocranium forms the calvaria, and the viscerocranium forms the skeleton of the face.
- The appendicular skeleton develops from endochondral ossification of the cartilaginous bone models, which form from mesenchyme in the developing limbs.
- Joints are classified as fibrous joints, cartilaginous joints, and synovial joints. They develop from interzonal mesenchyme between the primordia of bones. In a **fibrous joint**, the intervening mesenchyme differentiates into dense fibrous connective tissue. In a **cartilaginous joint**, the mesenchyme between the bones differentiates into cartilage. In a **synovial joint**, a synovial cavity is formed within the intervening mesenchyme by the breakdown of the cells. Mesenchyme also gives rise to the synovial membrane, capsule, and ligaments of the joint.

CLINICALLY ORIENTED PROBLEMS

CASE 14-1

A neonate presented with a lesion in his lower back, which was thought to be a neural arch defect.

- What is the most common birth defect of the vertebral column?
- Where is the defect usually located?
- Does this birth defect usually cause symptoms (e.g., back problems)?

CASE 14-2

A young girl presented with pain in her upper limb, which worsened when she lifted heavy objects. After a radiographic examination, the physician told her parents that she had an accessory rib in her neck.

- Are accessory ribs clinically important?
- What is the embryologic basis of an accessory rib?

CASE 14-3

A mother of a girl with a "crooked spine" was told that her daughter had scoliosis.

- What vertebral defect can produce scoliosis?
- What is the embryologic basis of the vertebral defect?

CASE 14-4

A boy had a long, thin head. His mother was concerned that it might have cognitive consequences for her son.

- What is meant by the term *craniosynostosis*?
- What results from this developmental abnormality?
- Give a common example of craniosynostosis, and describe it.

CASE 14-5

A child had characteristics of Klippel-Feil syndrome.

- What are the main features of this condition?
- What vertebral anomalies are usually detected?

Discussion of these problems appears in the Appendix at the back of the book.

BIBLIOGRAPHY AND SUGGESTED READING

Andreescu N, Sharma A, Mihailescu A, Zimbru CG, David VL, Horhat R: Chest wall deformities and their possible associations with different genetic syndromes, *Eur Rev Med Pharmacol Sci* 26:5107, 2022.

Alexander PG, Tuan RS: Role of environmental factors in axial skeletal dysmorphogenesis, *Birth Defects Res C Embryo Today* 90:118, 2010.

Aly I, Chapman JR, Oskouian RJ, Loukas M, Tubbs RS: Lumbar ribs: a comprehensive review, *Child Nerv Syst* 32:781, 2016.

Ami O, Maran JC, Gabor P, et al: Three-dimensional magnetic resonance imaging of fetal head molding and brain shape changes during the second stage of labour. *PLoS One* 14(5):e0215721, 2019. https://www.doi.org.10.1371/journal/pone.0215721.

Aulehla A: Oscillatory signals controlling mesoderm patterning in vertebrate embryos, *Mech Dev* 145(Suppl), 2017.

Brewin J, Hill M, Ellis H: The prevalence of cervical ribs in a London population, *Clin Anat* 22:331, 2009.

Buckingham M: Myogenic progenitor cells and skeletal myogenesis in vertebrates, *Curr Opin Genet Dev* 16:525, 2006.

Chaturvedi A, Klionsky NB, Nadarajah U, Chaturvedi A, Meyers SP: Malformed vertebrae: a clinical and imaging review, *Insights Imaging* 9(3):343–355, 2018. https://doi.org/10.1007/s13244-018-0598-1.

Chen G, Li YP: TGF-β and BMP signaling in osteoblast, skeletal development, and bone formation, homeostasis and disease, *Bone Res* 4:16009, 2016.

Chen W, Liu J, Yuan D, Zuo Y, Liu Z, Liu S: Progress and perspectives of TBX6 gene in congenital vertebral malformations, *Oncotarget* 7:57430, 2016.

Cohen MM Jr: Perspectives on craniosynostosis: sutural biology, some well-known syndromes and some unusual syndromes, *J Craniofac Surg* 20:646, 2009.

Dahan-Oliel N, Cachecho S, Barnes D, Bedard T, Davison AM, Dieterich K: International multidisciplinary collaboration toward an annotated definition of arthrogryposis multiplex congenita, *Am J Med Genet C Semin Med Genet* 181(3):288–299, 2019. https://doi.org/10.1002/ajmg.c.31721.

Decker RS, Koyama E, Pacifici M: Genesis and morphogenesis of limb synovial joints and articular cartilage, *Matrix Biol* 39:5–10, 2014.

Dias MS, Samson T, Rizk EB, Governale LS, Richtsmeier JT: Identifying the misshapen head: craniosynostosis and related disorders, *Pediatrics* 146(3), 2020. https://doi.org/10.1542/peds.2020-015511 e2020015511

Etich J, Leßmeier L, Rehberg M, et al: Osteogenesis imperfecta-pathophysiology and therapeutic options, *Mol Cell Pediatr* 7(1):9, 2020. https://doi.org/10.1186/s40348-020-00101-9.

Galea GL, Zein MR, Allen S, Francis-West P: Making and shaping endochondral and intramembranous bones, *Dev Dyn* 250(3):414–449, 2021. https://doi.org/10.1002/dvdy.278.

Gandhi M, Rac MWF, McKinney J. Radial ray malformation. *Am J Obstet Gynecol*, 221, (6), 2019, B16-B18 https://doi.org/10.1016/j.ajog.2019.09.024.

Gartner LP, Hiatt JL: *Color atlas and textbook of histology*, ed 6, Philadelphia, 2014, Lippincott William & Wilkins.

Gentile C, Chiarelli F: Rickets in children: an update, *Biomedicines* 9(7):738, 2021. https://doi.org/10.3390/biomedicines9070738.

Governale LS: Craniosynostosis, *Pediatr Neurol* 53:394, 2015.

Hall BK: *Bones and cartilage: developmental skeletal biology*, ed 2, Philadelphia, 2015, Elsevier.

Hernandez-Andre E, Yeo L, Goncalves LF: Fetal musculoskeletal system. In Norton ME, editor: *Callen's ultrasonography in obstetrics and gynecology*, ed 6, Philadelphia, 2017, Elsevier.

Hinrichsen KV, Jacob HJ, Jacob M, Brand-Saberi B, Christ B, Grim M: Principles of ontogenesis of leg and foot in man, *Ann Anat* 176:121, 1994.

Johal J, Loukas M, Fisahn C, Chapman JR, Oskouian RJ, Tubbs RS: Hemivertebrae: a comprehensive review of embryology, imaging, classification, and management, *Childs Nerv Syst* 32:2105, 2016.

Kague E, Roy P, Asselin G: Osterix/Sp7 limits cranial bone initiation sites and is required for formation of sutures, *Dev Biol* 413:160, 2016.

Keller B, Yang T, Chen Y, et al: Interaction of TGFβ and BMP signaling pathways during chondrogenesis, *PLoS One* 6:e16421, 2011.

Kenna MA, Irace AL, Strychowsky JE, et al: Otolaryngologic manifestations of Klippel-Feil Syndrome in children, *JAMA Otolaryngol Head Neck Surg 44*:238, 2018.

Kuratani S: The neural crest and origin of the neurocranium in vertebrates. *Genesis* 56(6–7):e23213, 2018. https://doi.org/10.1002/dvg.23213.

Kuta A, Mao Y, Martin T, Ferreira de Sousa C, Whiting D, Zakaria S: Fat4-dchs1 signalling controls cell proliferation in developing vertebrae, *Development* 143:2367, 2016.

Liao J, Huang Y, Wang Q, Chen S, Zhang C, Wang D: Gene regulatory network from cranial neural crest cells to osteoblast differentiation and calvarial bone development, *Cell Mol Life Sci* 79(3):158, 2022. https://doi.org/10.1007/s00018-022-04208-2.

Lefebvre V, Bhattaram P: Vertebrate skeletogenesis, *Curr Top Dev Biol* 90:291, 2010.

Liu RE: Musculoskeletal disorders in neonates. In Martin RJ, Fanaroff AA, Walsh MC, editors: *Fanaroff and Martin's neonatal-perinatal medicine: diseases of the fetus and infant, current therapy in neonatal-perinatal medicine*, ed 10, Philadelphia, 2015, Saunders Elsevier.

Ma L, Yu X: Arthrogryposis multiplex congenita: classification, diagnosis, perioperative care, and anesthesia, *Front Med* 11:48, 2017.

Park AJ-M, Nelson SE, Mesfin A: Klippel-Feil syndrome, clinical presentation and management, *JBJS Rev* 10(2), 2022. e2100166

Pawlina W: *Histology: a text and atlas: with correlated cell and molecular biology*, ed 7, Philadelphia, 2016, Wolters Kluwer Health.

Plotkin LI, Bruzzaniti A: Molecular signaling in bone cells: regulation of cell differentiation and survival, *Adv Protein Chem Struct Biol* 116:237–281, 2019. https://doi.org/10.1016/bs.apcsb.2019.01.002.

Powel JE, Sham CE, Spiliopoulos M, Ferreira CR, Rosenthal E, Sinkovskaya ES: Genetics of non-isolated hemivertebra—a systematic review of fetal, neonatal, and infant cases, *Clin Genet* 102(3), 2022. https://doi.org/10.1111/cge.14188.

Rodríguez-Vázquez JF, Verdugo-López S, Garrido JM, Murakami G, Kim JH: Morphogenesis of the manubrium of sternum in human embryos: a new concept, *Anat Rec* 296:279, 2013.

Roth DM, Bayona F, Baddam P, Graf D. Craniofacial development: neural crest in molecular embryology. *Head Neck Pathol* 15, (1), 2021, 1–15. https://doi.org/10.1007/s12105-021-01301-z.

Stacchiotti S, Gronchi A, Fossati P, Akiyama T, Alapetite C, Baumann M: Best practices for the management of local-regional recurrent chordoma: a position paper by the Chordoma Global Consensus Group, *Ann Oncol* 28(6):1230–1242, 2017. https://doi.org/10.1093/annonc/mdx054.

Tanaka T, Takahashi A, Kobayashi Y, Saito M, Xiaolong S, Jingquan C: Foxf2 represses bone formation via Wnt2b/β-catenin signaling, *Exp Mol Med* 54:753, 2022.

Wu M, Chen G, Li YP: TGF-β and BMP signaling in osteoblast, skeletal development, and bone formation, homeostasis and disease, *Bone Res* 4:16009, 2016.

Muscular System 15

CHAPTER OUTLINE

The muscular system develops from **mesoderm**, except for the muscles of the iris of the eye, which develop from **neuroectoderm (neural crest cells)**, and the muscles of the esophagus, which are thought to develop by transdifferentiation from smooth muscle. **Myoblasts** (embryonic muscle cells) are derived from **mesenchyme**. Three types of muscle—skeletal, cardiac, and smooth—are formed during the embryonic period.

MYOD, *a member of the family of myogenic regulatory factors, activates the transcription of muscle-specific genes, and* MYOD *is considered an important regulatory gene for the induction of myogenic differentiation. The* ***induction of myogenesis*** *in stem mesenchymal cells by* MYOD *depends on the degree of mesenchymal cell differentiation.*

Most of the mesenchyme in the head is derived from the neural crest (see Fig. 4.10), particularly for tissues derived from the pharyngeal arches (see Figs. 9.1H and I and 9.2). However, the original mesenchyme in these arches gives rise to the musculature of the face and neck (see Table 9.1).

DEVELOPMENT OF SKELETAL MUSCLE

Limb and axial muscles of the trunk and head develop by **epithelial-mesenchymal transformation** from myogenic precursor cells. Studies show that myogenic precursor cells originate from the somatic mesoderm and the ventral dermomyotome of somites in response to molecular signals from nearby tissues (Figs. 15.1 and 15.2).

The first indication of **myogenesis** is the elongation of the nuclei and cell bodies of mesenchymal cells as they differentiate into myoblasts. These primordial muscle cells soon fuse to form myotubes: elongated, multinucleated, cylindrical structures.

At the molecular level, these events are preceded by activation and expression of the genes of the MYOD family of muscle-specific, basic helix-loop-helix transcription factors (including MYOD, myogenin [MYOG], MYF5, and myogenic factor 6 [MYF6], formerly called myogenic regulatory factor 4 [MRF4]) in the precursor myogenic cells. MyoD and Myf5 control gene expression synergistically

Retinoic acid enhances skeletal myogenesis by upregulating the expression of mesodermal markers and myogenic regulatory factors. It has been suggested that signaling molecules from the ventral neural tube and notochord (e.g., sonic hedgehog [SHH]) and others from the dorsal neural tube (e.g., WNTs, bone morphogenetic protein 4 [BMP4]) and from overlying ectoderm (e.g., WNTs, BMP4) regulate the beginning of myogenesis and the induction of the myotome (Fig. 15.3). *Further muscle growth in the fetus results from the ongoing fusion of myoblasts and myotubes.*

During or after the fusion of the myoblasts, **myofilaments** develop in the cytoplasm of the myotubes. Other organelles characteristic of striated muscle cells, such as **myofibrils**, also form. As the myotubes develop, they become invested with external laminae (layers), which segregate them from the surrounding connective tissue. **Fibroblasts** produce the **perimysium** and **epimysium layers** of the fibrous sheath of the muscle; the **endomysium** is formed by the external lamina and reticular fibers.

Most skeletal muscles develop before birth, and almost all remaining muscles are formed by age one. The increase in the size of a muscle after the first year results from increased fiber diameter from the formation of more myofilaments. Muscles increase in length and width to grow with the skeleton. Their ultimate size depends on the amount of muscle use. Not all embryonic muscle fibers persist; many of them fail to establish themselves as necessary units of the muscle and soon degenerate.

MYOTOMES

Each typical myotome part of a somite divides into **dorsal epaxial division** and **ventral hypaxial division**

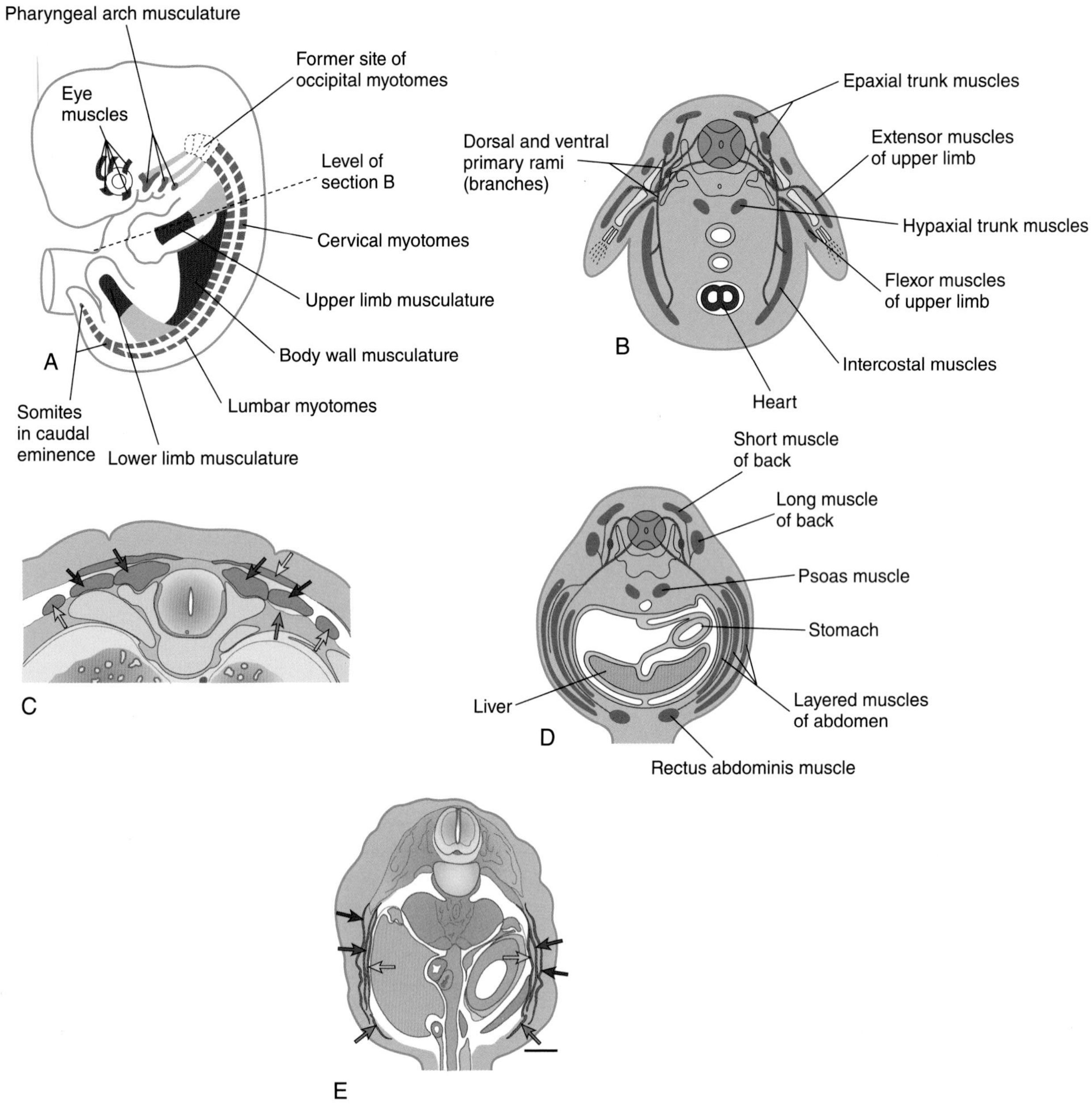

Fig. 15.1 (A) Sketch of an embryo at approximately 41 days shows the myotomes and developing muscular system. (B) Transverse section of the embryo illustrates epaxial and hypaxial derivatives of a myotome. (C) Transverse histological section stained with Azan (at approximately the level of the section in (B). *Yellow arrow*, trapezius; *blue arrows*, spinalis; *red arrows*, longissimus; *light green arrows*, iliocostalis; *dark green arrow*, levator costarum. (D) A similar section of a 7-week embryo shows the muscle layers formed from the myotomes. (E) A carmine-stained transverse histological section at the approximate position of the section in (D). *Red arrows*, external oblique; *blue arrows*, internal oblique; *purple arrows*, abdominal rectus; *green arrows*, transverse abdominal. ((C) From Mekonen HK et al: Development of the epaxial muscles in the human embryo, *Clin Anat* 29:1031, 2016. (E) From Mekonen HK et al: Development of the ventral body wall in the human embryo, *J Anat* 227:673–685, 2015.)

(see Fig. 15.1B). Every developing spinal nerve divides and sends a branch to each myotome division. The dorsal primary ramus supplies the epaxial division, and the ventral primary ramus supplies the hypaxial division. The myoblasts that form the skeletal muscles of the trunk are derived from mesenchyme in the myotome regions of the somites (see Fig. 15.1). Some muscles, such as the intercostal muscles, remain segmentally arranged like the somites, but most myoblasts migrate away from the myotome and form nonsegmented muscles.

Gene-targeting studies in the mouse embryo show that myogenic regulatory factors (MYOD, MYF6, MYF5, and MYOG) are essential for the development of the hypaxial, epaxial, abdominal, and intercostal muscles.

Myoblasts from epaxial divisions of the myotomes form the extensor muscles of the neck and vertebral column (Fig. 15.4). The embryonic extensor muscles derived from the sacral and coccygeal myotomes degenerate; their adult derivatives are the dorsal **sacrococcygeal ligaments**. Myoblasts from the hypaxial divisions of the cervical

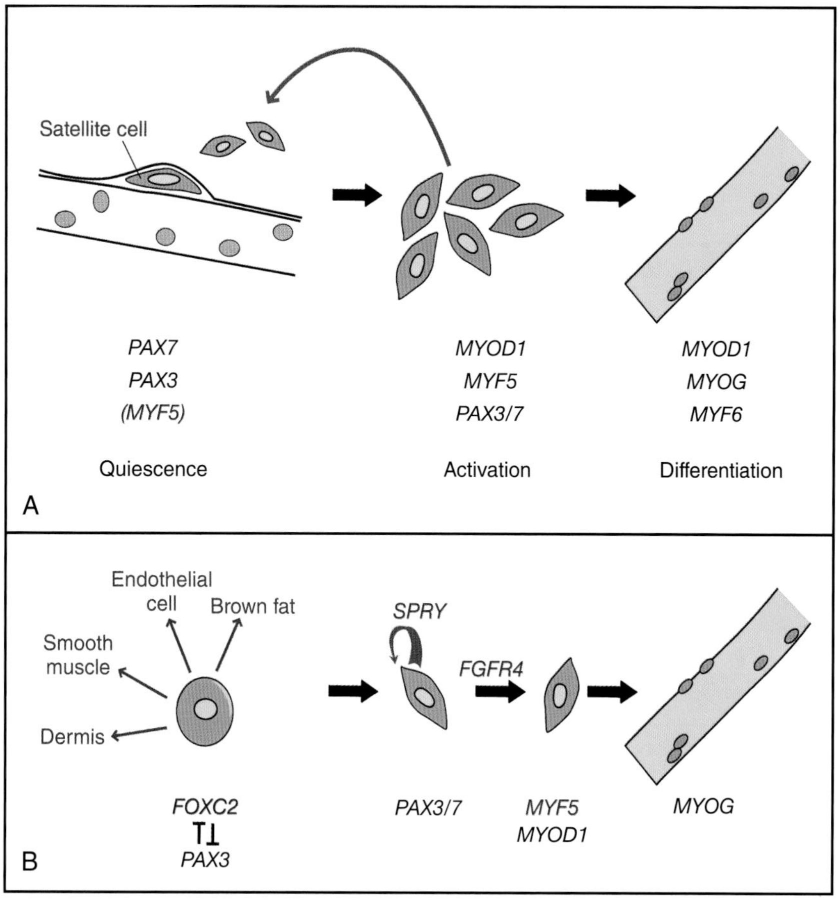

Fig. 15.2 Genetic regulation of the progression of muscle progenitor cells toward the formation of differentiated skeletal muscle. (A) Adult muscle satellite cells progress to form new muscle fibers. *MYF5* is shown in the quiescent state *(red)* to indicate that transcripts are present but not the protein. (B) During the progression of somatic cells in myogenesis, expression of *PAX3* activates target genes *(red)* that regulate various stages of this process. (From Buckingham M, Rigby PW: Gene regulatory networks and transcriptional mechanisms that control myogenesis, *Dev Cell* 28:225, 2014.)

myotomes form the scalene, prevertebral, geniohyoid, and infrahyoid muscles (see Fig. 15.4). The **thoracic myotomes** form the lateral and ventral flexor muscles of the vertebral column, and the **lumbar myotomes** form the quadratus lumborum muscle. The **sacrococcygeal myotomes** form the muscles of the pelvic diaphragm and probably the striated muscles of the anus and sex organs.

PHARYNGEAL ARCH MUSCLES

Myoblasts from the pharyngeal arches, which originate from the unsegmented paraxial mesoderm and **prechordal plate**, form the muscles of mastication, facial expression, pharynx, and larynx as described elsewhere (see Fig. 9.6 and Table 9.1). These muscles are innervated by pharyngeal arch nerves.

OCULAR MUSCLES

The origin of the extrinsic eye muscles is unclear. They may be derived from mesenchymal cells near the prechordal plate and paraxial cranial mesoderm(see Figs. 15.1 and 15.4). The mesenchyme in this area is thought to give rise to three preotic myotomes. Myoblasts differentiate from mesenchymal cells derived from these myotomes. Groups of myoblasts, each supplied by its own nerve (cranial nerve [CN] III, CN IV, or CN VI), form the extrinsic muscles of the eye.

TONGUE MUSCLES

Initially, there are four **occipital (postotic) myotomes**; the first pair disappears. Myoblasts from the remaining myotomes form the tongue muscles and are innervated by the hypoglossal nerve (CN XII).

LIMB MUSCLES

The musculature of the limbs develops from myoblasts surrounding the developing bones (see Fig. 15.1). The myoblasts form a mass of tissue on the dorsal (extensor) and ventral (flexor) aspects of the limbs. Grafting and gene-targeting studies in birds and mammals have demonstrated that the precursor myogenic cells in the limb buds originate from the somites. These cells are first located in the ventral part of the dermomyotome and are epithelial (see Fig. 14.1D). The cells then migrate into the primordium of the limb.

Molecular signals from the neural tube and notochord induce PAX3, MYOD, and MYF5 expression in the somites. In the limb bud, PAX3 regulates the expression of MET (a migratory peptide growth factor), which regulates the migration of the precursor myogenic cells.

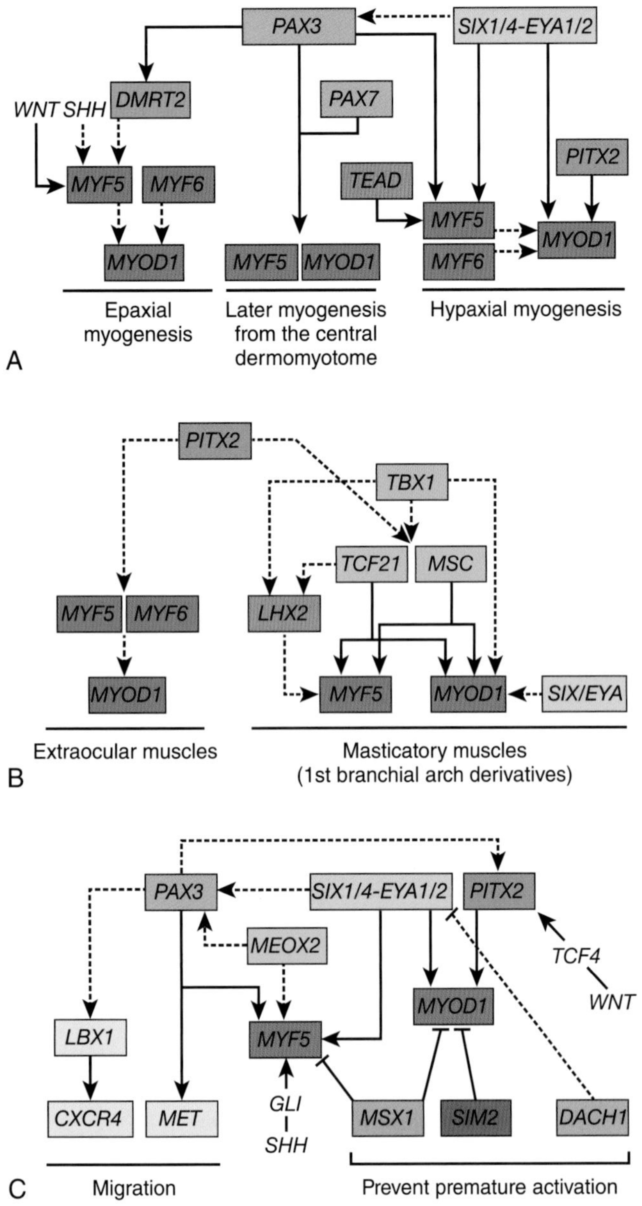

Fig. 15.3 Gene regulatory networks govern myogenesis in the trunk (A), the head (B), and cells that migrate from the hypaxial somite to the forelimb (C). (From Buckingham M, Rigby PW: Gene regulatory networks and transcriptional mechanisms that control myogenesis, *Dev Cell* 28:225, 2014.)

DEVELOPMENT OF SMOOTH MUSCLE

Smooth muscle fibers differentiate from **splanchnic mesenchyme** surrounding the endoderm of the primordial gut and its derivatives (see Fig. 15.1). The somatic mesoderm provides smooth muscle in the walls of many blood and lymphatic vessels. The muscles of the iris (sphincter and dilator pupillae) and the myoepithelial cells in mammary and sweat glands are thought to be derived from mesenchymal cells that originate from ectoderm.

The first sign of differentiation of smooth muscle is the development of elongated nuclei in spindle-shaped myoblasts. During early development, additional myoblasts continue to differentiate from mesenchymal cells but do not fuse as in skeletal muscle; they remain mononucleated.

During later development, the division of existing myoblasts gradually replaces the differentiation of new myoblasts in the production of new smooth muscle tissue. As smooth muscle cells differentiate, filamentous but nonsarcomeric contractile elements develop in their cytoplasm, and the external surface of each cell acquires a surrounding external lamina. As smooth muscle fibers develop into sheets or bundles, they receive autonomic innervation. Muscle cells and fibroblasts synthesize and lay down collagenous, elastic, and reticular fibers.

DEVELOPMENT OF CARDIAC MUSCLE

Cardiac muscle develops from the lateral splanchnic mesoderm, which gives rise to the mesenchyme surrounding the developing heart tube (see Figs. 13.1B and 13.7 C–E). **Cardiac myoblasts** differentiate from the primordial myocardium. Heart muscle is recognizable in the fourth week. It likely develops through the expression of cardiac-specific genes. *Studies suggest that PBX proteins interacting with the transcription factor HAND2 promote cardiac muscle differentiation.* Immunohistochemical studies have revealed a spatial distribution of tissue-specific antigens (myosin heavy-chain isoforms) in the embryonic heart between the fourth and eighth weeks.

Cardiac muscle fibers arise by differentiation and growth of single cells, unlike striated skeletal muscle fibers, which develop by fusion of cells. The growth of cardiac muscle fibers results from the formation of new myofilaments. The myoblasts adhere to each other as in developing skeletal muscle, but the intervening cell membranes do not disintegrate. These areas of adhesion give rise to **intercalated disks**, intercellular locations of attachment of cardiac muscles. Late in the embryonic period, special bundles of muscle cells develop from the original trabeculated myocardium that has fast-conducting gap junctions with relatively few myofibrils and relatively larger diameters than typical cardiac muscle fibers. These atypical cardiac muscle cells **(Purkinje fibers)** form the conducting system of the heart (see Figs. 13.18E and 13.19C and D).

Anomalies of Muscles

The absence of one or more skeletal muscles is more common than is generally recognized. Common examples are the sternocostal head of the pectoralis major, palmaris longus, trapezius, serratus anterior, and quadratus femoris. Usually, only a single muscle is absent on one side of the body, or only part of the muscle fails to develop. Occasionally, the same muscle or muscles may be absent on both sides of the body.

The absence of the pectoralis major (often its sternal part) is usually associated with **syndactyly** (fusion of digits). These birth defects are part of the **Poland Sequence** (or Syndrome) (1:20000) (absence of pectoralis major and minor muscles, ipsilateral breast hypoplasia, and absence of two to four ribs; Fig. 15.5). The absence of the pectoralis major is occasionally associated with the absence of the mammary gland in the breast and/or hypoplasia of the nipple. Poland Sequence is three times more common in males and typically impacts the right side.

The absence of muscles of the anterior abdominal wall may be associated with severe gastrointestinal and genitourinary defects such as **exstrophy of the bladder** (see Fig. 12.24) or prune-belly syndrome. Muscle development and muscle repair depend on the expression of muscle regulatory genes.

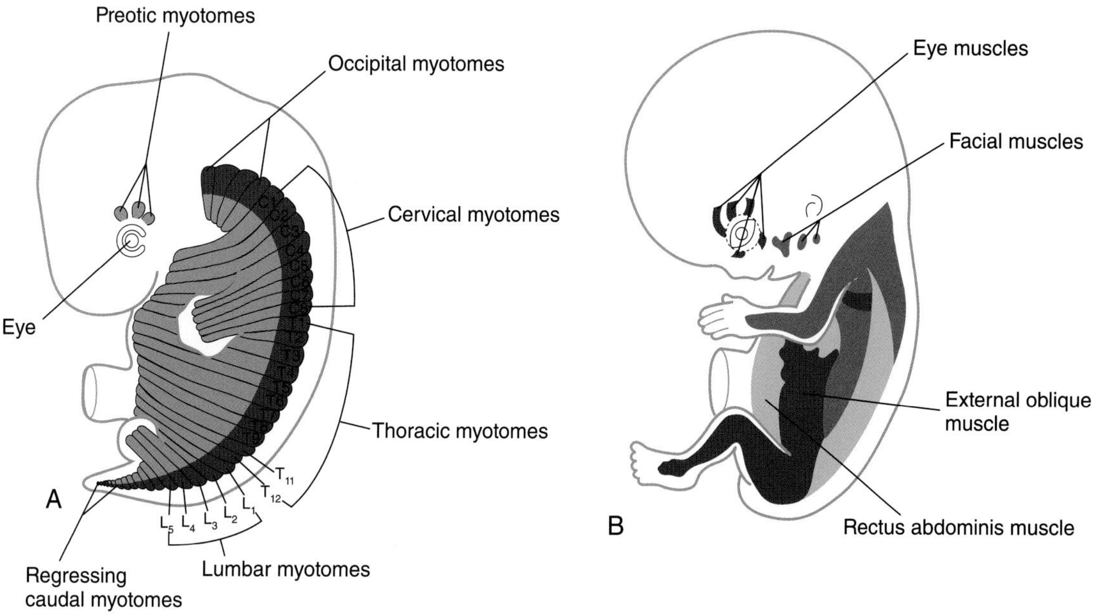

Fig. 15.4 Developing muscular system. (A) Drawing of a 6-week embryo shows the myotome regions of the somites that give rise to skeletal muscles. (B) Drawing of an 8-week embryo shows the developing trunk and limb musculature.

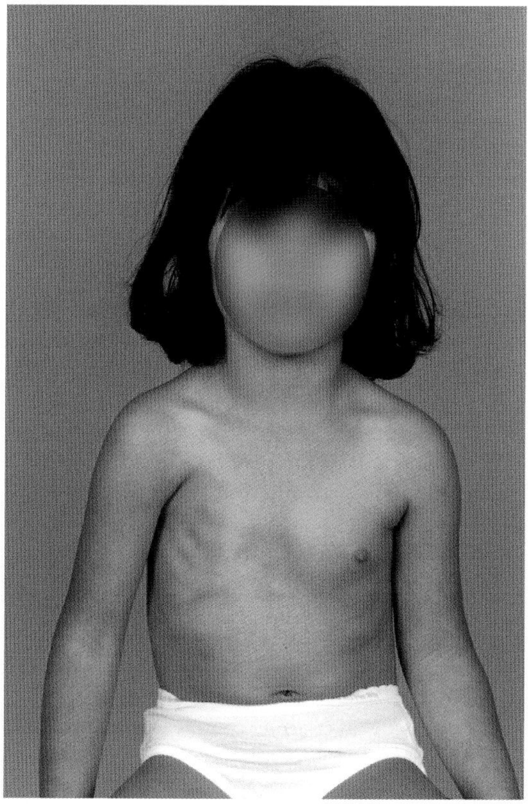

Fig. 15.5 A young girl with a severe form of Poland syndrome with the absence of the pectoralis muscles and the nipple. (From Al-Quattan MM, Kozin SH: Update on embryology of the upper limb, *J Hand Surg Am* 38:1835, 2013.)

Arthrogryposis

The term *arthrogryposis* (arthrogryposis multiplex congenita) is used clinically to describe multiple **congenital joint contractures** that affect different parts of the body (Fig. 15.6). Arthrogryposis occurs in 1 in 3000 live births. It includes more than 400 heterogeneous conditions with neurological and muscular clinical disorders. The causes of arthrogryposis are unclear. In over 30% of cases, genetic factors are involved. Neuropathic disorders and muscle and connective tissue abnormalities restrict intrauterine movement and may lead to **fetal akinesia** (absence or loss of the power of voluntary movement) and joint contractures. The involvement of contractures around certain joints and not others may offer clues to the underlying cause. For instance, **amyoplasia** typically includes bilateral flexion contractures of the wrist, the extension of the knees, and talipes equinovarus, but it spares other joints (see Fig. 16.15). Limb, nuchal translucency, cystic hygroma, and other developmental anomalies have been reported in association with arthrogryposis.

Variations in Muscles

All muscles are subject to a certain amount of variation; however, some are affected more often than others. Certain muscles are functionally vestigial (rudimentary), such as those of the external ear and scalp. Some muscles present in other primates appear in only some humans (e.g., sternalis muscle, a band sometimes found parallel to the sternum). Variations in forms, positions, and attachments of muscles are common and are usually functionally insignificant.

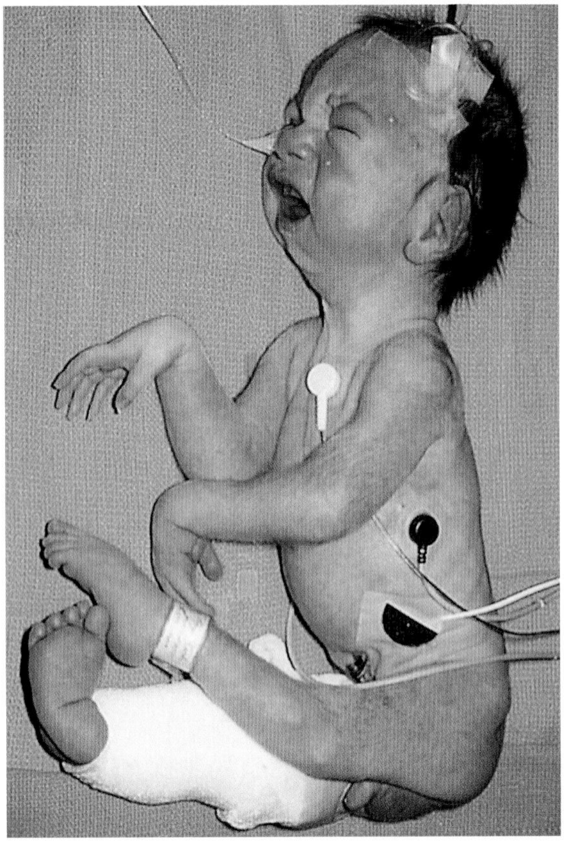

Fig. 15.6 **Neonate with multiple joint contractures due to arthrogryposis. Infants with this syndrome have stiffness of the joints associated with hypoplasia of the associated muscles.** (Courtesy Dr. A.E. Chudley, Section of Genetics and Metabolism, Department of Pediatrics and Child Health, Children's Hospital and University of Manitoba, Winnipeg, Manitoba, Canada.)

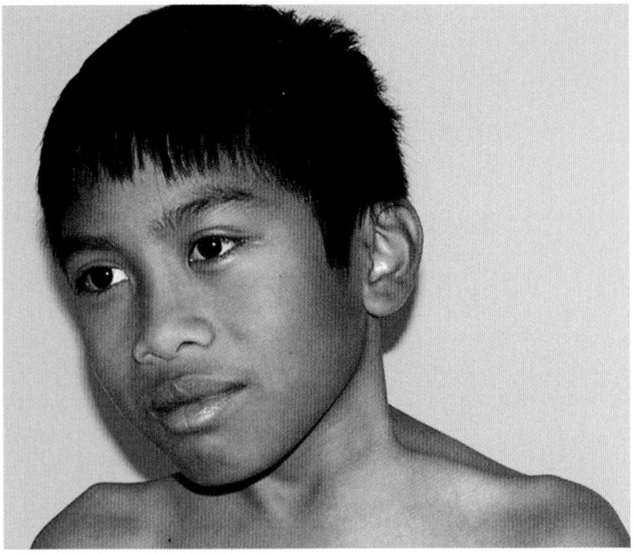

Fig. 15.7 An 11-year-old boy with untreated left congenital muscular torticollis with restricted lateral flexion to the right and limited neck rotation to the right. (From Graham J: *Smith's recognizable patterns of human deformation*, ed 3, Philadelphia, 2007, Elsevier.)

Congenital Torticollis

Some cases of torticollis (wry neck) may result from the tearing of fibers of the sternocleidomastoid muscle during childbirth. Bleeding into the muscle occurs in a localized area, forming a **hematoma**. A solid mass develops later because of **necrosis** of muscle fibers and fibrosis. Shortening of the muscle usually follows, which causes lateral bending of the head to the affected side and a slight turning of the head away from the side of the short muscle (Fig. 15.7).

Although birth trauma may be a cause of torticollis, the condition has been observed in infants delivered by cesarean section, suggesting that there are other causes, including vertebral anomalies, ocular, intrauterine crowding, and **congenital myopathy**.

Prune-Belly Syndrome

Abdominal muscle deficiency and hypotonia are signs of prune-belly syndrome (1:30,000). It occurs most commonly (95%) in males and those affected most commonly have associated **cryptorchidism** (failure of one or both testes to descend; see Fig. 12.48) and urinary tract abnormalities, such as **megaureters** (dilation of ureters). Most infants with prune-belly syndrome (95%) are male with a normal karyotype. The abdominal wall is usually so thin that the viscera (e.g., intestines) are visible and easily palpated. Prune-belly syndrome occurs sporadically and appears to be related to transient urethral obstruction in the embryo or failure of development of somatic and splanchnic mesodermal tissues.

Accessory Muscles

Accessory muscles occasionally develop. For example, an accessory soleus muscle occurs in approximately 3% of people. The primordium of the soleus muscle may undergo early splitting to form an accessory soleus. An accessory flexor muscle of the foot (quadratus plantae muscle) occasionally may develop. In some cases, accessory muscles cause clinically significant symptoms.

SUMMARY OF MUSCULAR SYSTEM

- Muscle development occurs through the formation of **myoblasts**, which undergo proliferation to form **myocytes**.
- Skeletal muscle is derived from the **myotome** regions of **somites**.
- Some head and neck muscles are derived from pharyngeal arch mesenchyme.
- The limb muscles develop from myogenic precursor cells surrounding bones in the limbs.
- Cardiac muscle and most smooth muscle are derived from splanchnic mesoderm.
- Absence or variation of some muscles is common and usually of little consequence.

CLINICALLY ORIENTED PROBLEMS

CASE 15-1

An infant with the absence of the left anterior axillary fold also had a left nipple that was much lower than usual.

- The absence of which muscle probably caused these unusual observations?
- What sequence (or syndrome) do you suspect?

- What features would you look for?
- Would the infant be likely to suffer any disability if the absence of this muscle was the only birth defect?

CASE 15-2

A medical student discovered that she had only one palmaris longus muscle.

- Is this a common occurrence?
- What is its incidence?
- Does the absence of this muscle cause a disability?

CASE 15-3

The parents of a 4-year-old girl observed that she always held her head slightly tilted to the right side and that one of her neck muscles was more prominent than the others. The clinical history revealed that her delivery had been a breech birth, one in which the buttocks presented.

- Name the muscle that was likely prominent.
- Did this muscle pull the child's head to the right side?
- What is this deformity called?
- What likely caused the muscle shortening that resulted in this condition?

CASE 15-4

A neonate had an abdominal wall defect. Failure of striated muscle to develop in the median plane of the anterior abdominal wall is associated with the formation of a severe congenital birth defect of the urinary system.

- What is this defect called?
- What is the probable embryologic basis for the failure of muscle to form in this neonate?

Discussion of these problems appears in the Appendix at the back of the book.

BIBLIOGRAPHY AND SUGGESTED READING

Applebaum M, Kalcheim C: Mechanisms of myogenic specification and patterning, *Results Probl Cell Differ* 56:77, 2015.

Aulehla A: Oscillatory signals controlling mesoderm patterning in vertebrate embryos, *Mech Dev* 145(Suppl), 2017.

Bonnet A, Dai F, Brand-Saberi B, Duprez D: Vestigial-like 2 acts downstream of MyoD activation and is associated with skeletal muscle differentiation in chick myogenesis, *Mech Dev* 127:120, 2010.

Bothe I, Tenin G, Oseni A, Dietrich S: Dynamic control of head mesoderm patterning, *Development* 138:2807, 2011.

Bouzada J, Gemmell C, Konschake M, Tubbs RS, Pechriggl E, Sañudo J: New insights into the development of the anterior abdominal wall, *Front Surg* 9:863679, 2022. https://doi.org/10.3389/fsurg.2022.863679.

Buckingham M: Myogenic progenitor cells and skeletal myogenesis in vertebrates, *Curr Opin Genet Dev* 16:525, 2006.

Buckingham M, Rigby PW: Gene regulatory networks and transcriptional mechanisms that control myogenesis, *Dev Cell* 28:225, 2014.

Gasser RF: The development of the facial muscle in man, *Am J Anat* 120:357, 1967.

Giacinti C, Giodano A: Cell cycle regulation in myogenesis. In Giordano A, Galderisi U, editors: *Cell cycle regulation and differentiation in cardiovascular and neural systems*, New York, 2010, Springer.

Hernandez-Andre E, Yeo L, Goncalves LF: Fetal musculoskeletal system. In Norton ME, editor: *Callen's ultrasonography in obstetrics and gynecology*, ed 6, Philadelphia, 2017, Elsevier.

Kablar B, Krastel K, Ying C, Tapscott SJ, Goldhamer DJ, Rudnicki MA: Myogenic determination occurs independently in somites and limb buds, *Dev Biol* 206:219, 1999.

Kablar B, Tajbakhsh S, Rudnick MA: Transdifferentiation of esophageal smooth muscle is myogenic bHLH factor-dependent, *Development* 127:1627, 2000.

Kalcheim C: Epithelial–mesenchymal transitions during neural crest and somite development, *J Clin Med* 5(1):1, 2015.

Kang SG, Kang JK: Current and future perspectives in craniosynostosis, *J Korean Neurosurg Soc* 59:247, 2016.

Kaplan SL, Coulter C, Sargent B: Physical therapy management of congenital muscular torticollis: a 2018 Evidence-Based Clinical Practice Guideline from the APTA Academy of Pediatric Physical Therapy, *Pediatr Phys Ther* 30:240–290, 2018.

Kowalczyk B, Feluś J: Arthrogryposis: an update on clinical aspects, etiology, and treatment strategies, *Arch Med Sci* 12:10, 2016.

Laquerriere A, Jaber D, Abiusi E, et al: Phenotypic spectrum and genomics of undiagnosed arthrogryposis multiplex congenita, *J Med Genet* 59(6):559–567, 2022.10.1136/jmedgenet-2020-107595

Lee JH, Protze SI, Laksman Z, Backx PH, Keller GM: Human pluripotent stem cell-derived atrial and ventricular cardiomyocytes develop from distinct mesoderm populations, *Cell Stem Cell* 21:179, 2017.

Lopes RI, Baker LA, Dénes FT: Modern management of and update on prune belly syndrome, *J Pediatr Urol* 17:548, 2021.

Ma L, Yu X: Arthrogryposis multiplex congenita: classification, diagnosis, perioperative care, and anesthesia, *Front Med* 11:48, 2017.

Martin J, Afouda BA, Hoppler S: Wnt/beta-catenin signaling regulates cardiomyogenesis via GATA transcription factors, *J Anat* 216:92, 2010.

Milanese J-S, Marcotte R, Costain WJ, Kablar B, Drouin S: Roles of skeletal muscle in development: a bioinformatics and systems biology overview. In: B Kablar, editor: *Advances in Anatomy, Embryology and Cell Biology: Roles of Skeletal Muscle in Organ Development*, Springer International Publishing, 2023, pp 21–55. https://doi.org/10.1007/978-3-031-38215-4_2.

Noden DM: Vertebrate craniofacial development—the relation between ontogenetic process and morphological outcome, *Brain Behav Evol* 38:190, 1991.

Payumo AY, McQuade LE, Walker WJ, Yamazoe S, Chen JK: Tbx16 regulates *Hox* gene activation in mesodermal progenitor cells, *Nat Chem Biol* 12:694, 2016.

Development of the Limbs 16

CHAPTER OUTLINE

15

EARLY STAGES OF LIMB DEVELOPMENT

The **upper limb buds** are visible by day 24 with the activation of a group of mesenchymal cells in the somatic lateral mesoderm (Fig. 16.1A). The **lower limb buds** appear 1 or 2 days later. Homeobox *(Hox)* genes regulate patterning in the formation of the limbs. The buds first appear as small bulges on the ventrolateral body wall (see Fig. 16.1). Each limb bud consists of a mesenchymal core covered by a layer of ectoderm. *The transcription factor TWIST 1 has been identified as the regulating factor for epithelial-mesenchymal transformation in the limb bud.*

The limb buds elongate with the proliferation of the mesenchyme. The upper limb buds appear disproportionately low on the trunk because of the early development of the cranial half of the embryo (see Fig. 16.1). The earliest stages of limb development are alike for the upper and lower limbs (see Figs. 16.1B and 16.4). Later, distinct features arise because of differences in the form and function of the hands and feet.

The upper limb buds develop opposite the caudal cervical segments, and the lower limb buds form opposite the lumbar and upper sacral segments. At the apex of each limb bud, the ectoderm thickens to form the **apical ectodermal ridge (AER)**. The AER is a specialized, multilayered epithelial structure (see Fig. 16.2), which is induced by the paracrine factor, fibroblast growth factor 10 (FGF10), from the underlying mesenchyme.

Mesenchymal cells aggregate at the posterior margin of the limb bud to form the **zone of polarizing activity**, an important signaling center in limb development. FGFs from the AER activate the zone of polarizing activity, which causes the expression of the Sonic hedgehog (SHH) genes.

Transcription factors encoded by the gene BHLHA9 (Basic Helix-Loop-Helix Family Member A9) and bone morphogenetic protein (BMP) signaling are required for its formation. From recent studies, transcription factors of the T-box family of genes have been assigned a critical role in limb development. FGF8, secreted by the AER, and BMP signaling through activation of TBX5 exert an inductive influence on the limb mesenchyme that initiates outgrowth and development of the limbs in a proximodistal axis. Retinoic acid promotes the formation of the limb bud by inhibiting FGF signaling. Transcription factors encoded by the genes BHLHA9 and SHH regulate the normal patterning of the limbs along the anterior-posterior axis. Expression of WNT7A *from the dorsal non-AER ectoderm of the limb bud and* engrailed homeobox 1 (EN1) *from the ventral aspect is involved in specifying the dorsal-ventral axis. The AER itself is maintained by inductive signals from* SHH *and* WNT7. *It has been suggested that epiprofin, a zinc finger transcription factor, regulates WNT signaling in the limb bud* (see Fig. 16.2B).

The mesenchyme adjacent to the AER consists of undifferentiated, rapidly proliferating cells, whereas mesenchymal cells proximal to it differentiate into blood vessels and cartilage bone models. The distal ends of the limb buds flatten into hand plates and foot plates (Fig. 16.3 and Fig. 16.4B and H). Studies have shown that endogenous retinoic acid is also involved in limb development and pattern formation.

By the end of the sixth week, mesenchymal tissue in the **hand plates** has condensed to form **digital rays** (see Figs. 16.3 and 16.4C) that outline the pattern of the digits (fingers) in the hand plates. During the seventh week, similar condensations of mesenchyme condense to form digital rays and digits (toes) in the footplates (see Fig. 16.4I).

At the tip of each digital ray, a part of the AER induces the development of the mesenchyme into the primordia of the **phalanges** in the digits (see Fig. 16.6C and D). The intervals between the digital rays are occupied by loose mesenchyme which soon break down, forming notches between the digital rays (Fig. 16.5; see also Fig. 16.3 and Fig. 16.4D and F). As the tissue breakdown progresses, separate digits are formed by the end of the eighth week (Fig. 16.6; see also Fig. 16.4E, F, K, and L).

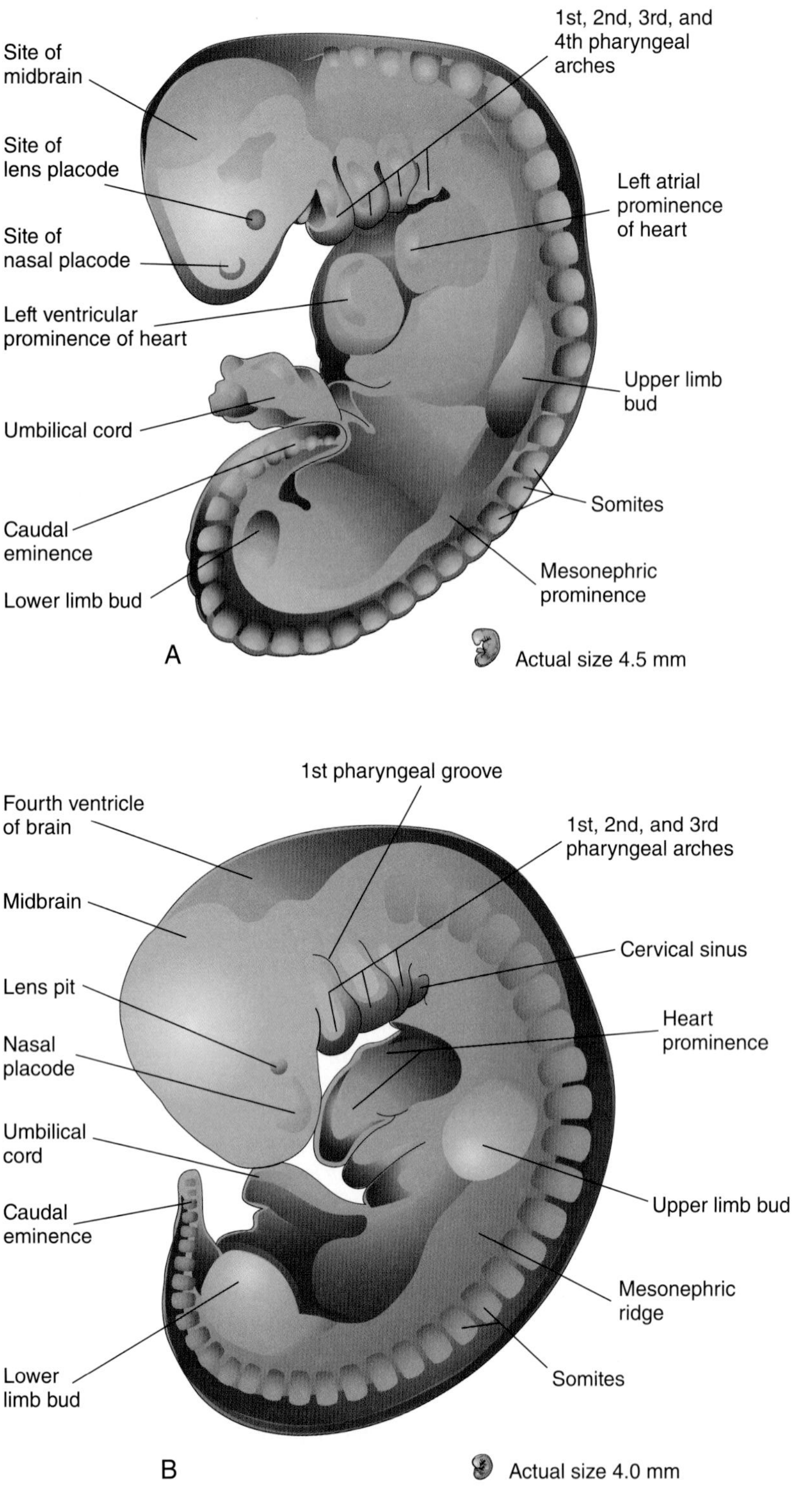

Fig. 16.1 Drawings of human embryos show the development of the limbs. (A) Lateral view of an embryo at approximately 28 days. The upper limb bud appears as a swelling or bulge on the ventrolateral body wall. The lower limb bud is much smaller than the upper limb bud. (B) Lateral view of an embryo at approximately 32 days. The upper limb buds are paddle shaped, and the lower limb buds are flipper like.(Modified from Nishimura H, Semba R, Tanimura T, Tanaka O: Prenatal development of the human with special reference to craniofacial structures: an atlas, Washington, DC, 1977, National Institutes of Health.)

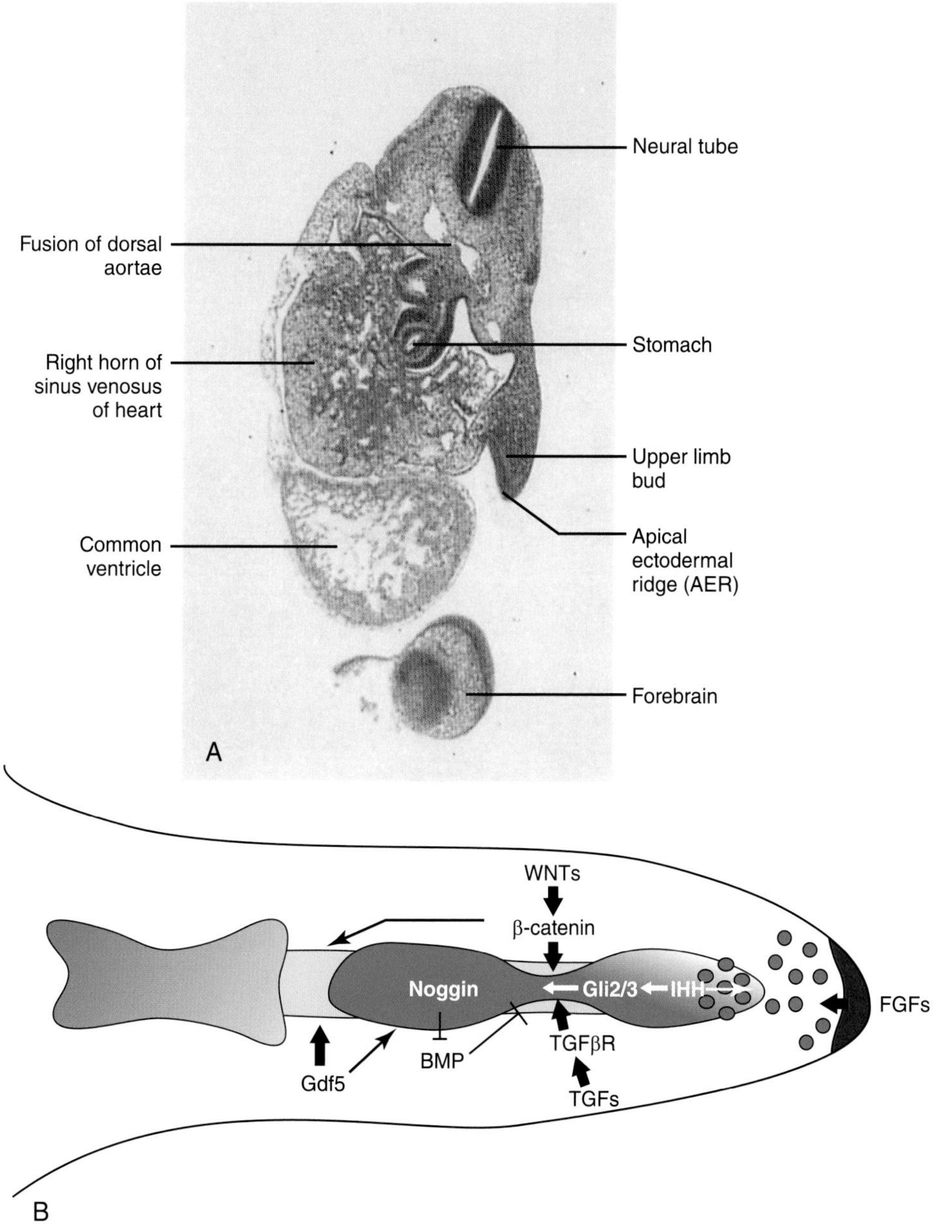

Fig. 16.2 (A) Oblique section of an embryo at approximately 28 days. Observe the paddle-like upper limb bud lateral to the embryonic heart and the *AER*. (B) Signaling pathways regulate the elongation and segmentation of the digit ray. In the AER, *FGF* signaling *(red)* maintains a small population of subridge undifferentiated mesenchymal cells, which are actively incorporated into the digital condensation *(blue)*. At the presumptive joint site, the newly differentiated chondrogenic cells dedifferentiate to interzone status under the regulation of multiple signaling pathways. *WNTs* promote chondrocyte dedifferentiation through canonical WNT signaling. *IHH* signals to the interzone region through localized expression of the transcription factors Gli2 and Gli3. Transforming growth factors signal to the interzone cells through the type II receptor. Gdf5 regulates the progression of the joint and skeletogenesis of the digit elements. *AER*, Apical epidermal ridge; *BMP*, bone morphogenetic protein; *FGF*, fibroblast growth factor; *Gdf5*, growth differentiation factor 5; *IHH*, Indian hedgehog; *TGFβR*, transforming growth factor-β receptor. (A, From Moore KL, Persaud TVN, Shiota K: *Color atlas of clinical embryology*, ed 2, Philadelphia, 2000, Saunders; B, From Hu J, He L: Patterning mechanisms controlling digit development, *J Genet Genom* 35:517–524, 2008.)

Molecular studies indicate that the earliest stages of limb patterning and digit formation involve the expression of the patched 1 gene (PTCH1), which is essential for the downstream regulation of multiple Hox genes and the SHH pathway. Gradual **apoptosis** through both the apoptosis-inducing factor and caspase-3-mediated pathways is responsible for the tissue breakdown in the interdigital regions. Antagonism between retinoic acid signaling and transforming growth factor-β (TGF-β) appears to control interdigital apoptosis and digit formation. Blockade of these cellular and molecular events could account for **syndactyly** or webbing of the fingers or toes (see Fig. 16.14C and D).

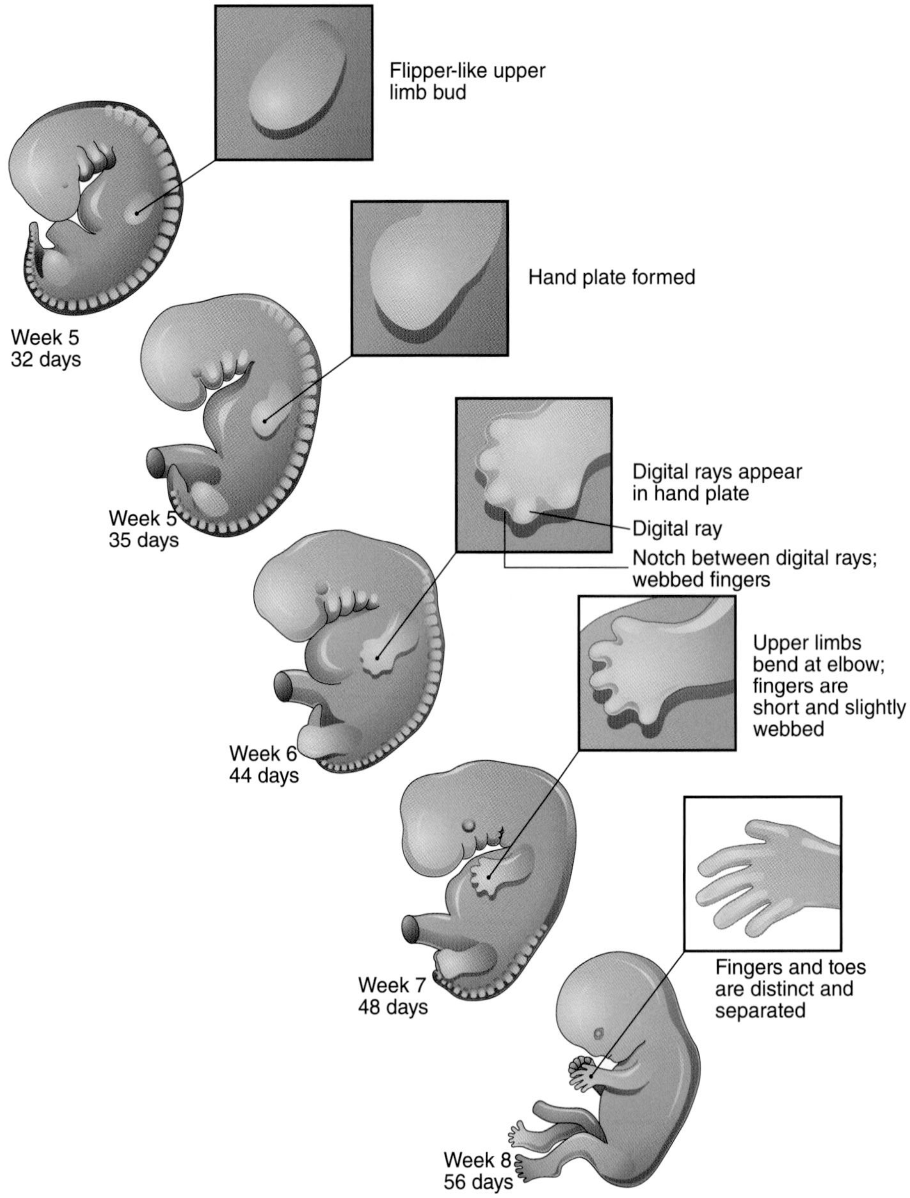

Fig. 16.3 Illustrations of development of the limbs (32–56 days). The upper limbs develop earlier than the lower limbs.

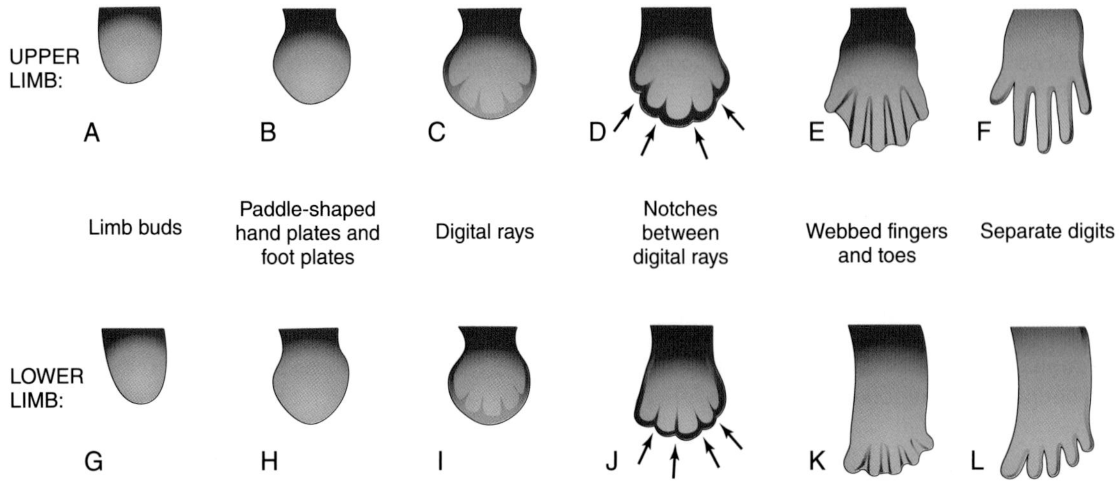

Fig. 16.4 Illustrations of limb development between the fourth and eighth weeks—hands on days 27 (A), 32 (B), 41 (C), 46 (D), 50 (E), and 52 (F); feet on days 28 (G), 36 (H), 46 (I), 49 (J), 52 (K), and 56 (L). The early stages are alike except that the development of the hands precedes that of the feet by a day or 2. The *arrows* in (D) and (J) indicate the tissue breakdown process (apoptosis) that separates the fingers and toes.

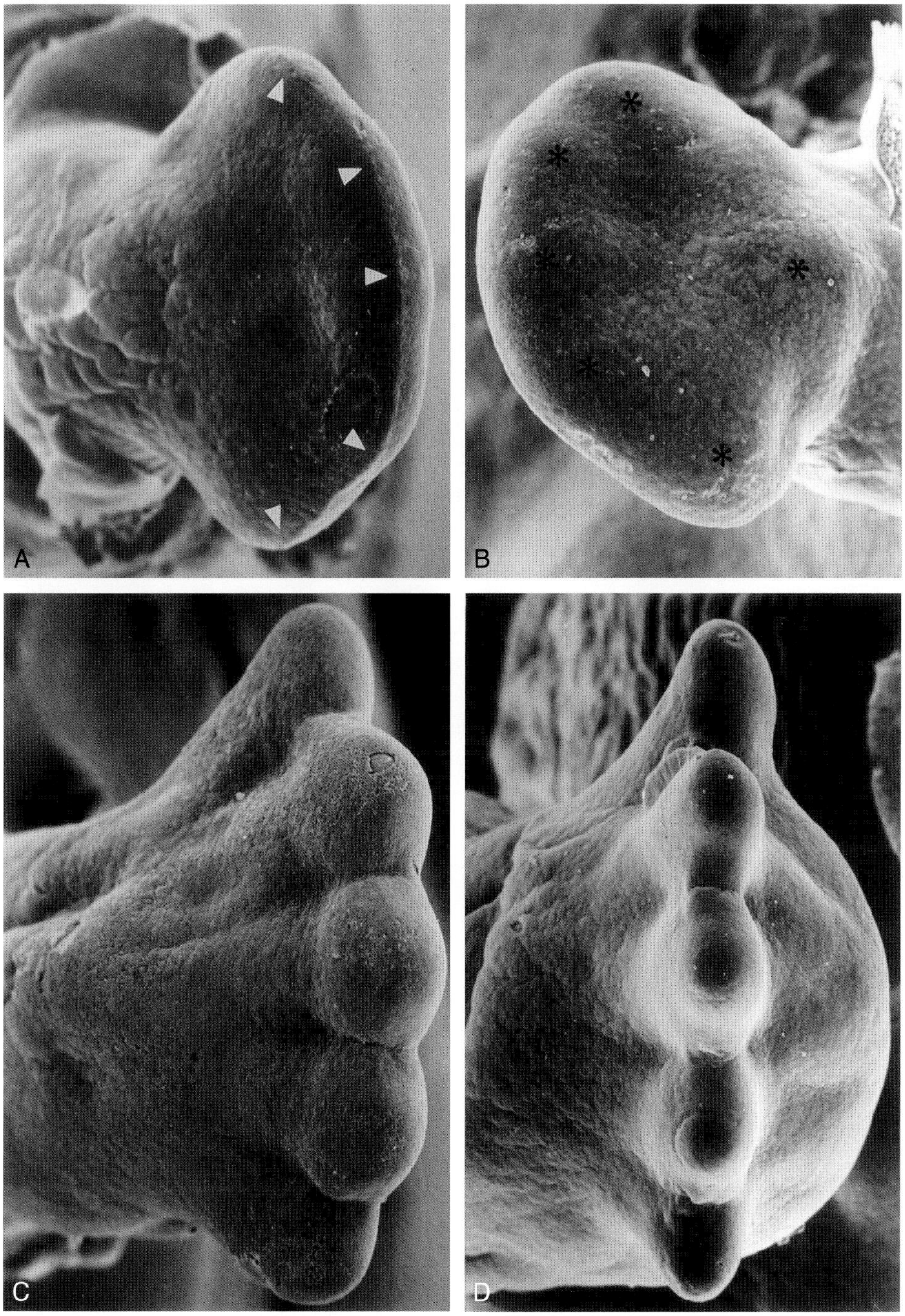

Fig. 16.5 Scanning electron micrographs show dorsal (A) and plantar (B) views of the right foot of an embryo at approximately 48 days. The toe buds (*arrowheads* in A) and the heel cushion and metatarsal tactile elevation (*asterisks* in B) have just appeared. Dorsal (C) and distal (D) views of the right foot of embryos at approximately 55 days show that the tips of the toes are separated and interdigital degeneration has begun. Notice the dorsiflexion of the metatarsus and toes (C) as well as the thickened heel cushion (D).(From Hinrichsen KV, Jacob HJ, Jacob M, et al: Principles of ontogenesis of leg and foot in man, *Ann Anat* 176:121, 1994.)

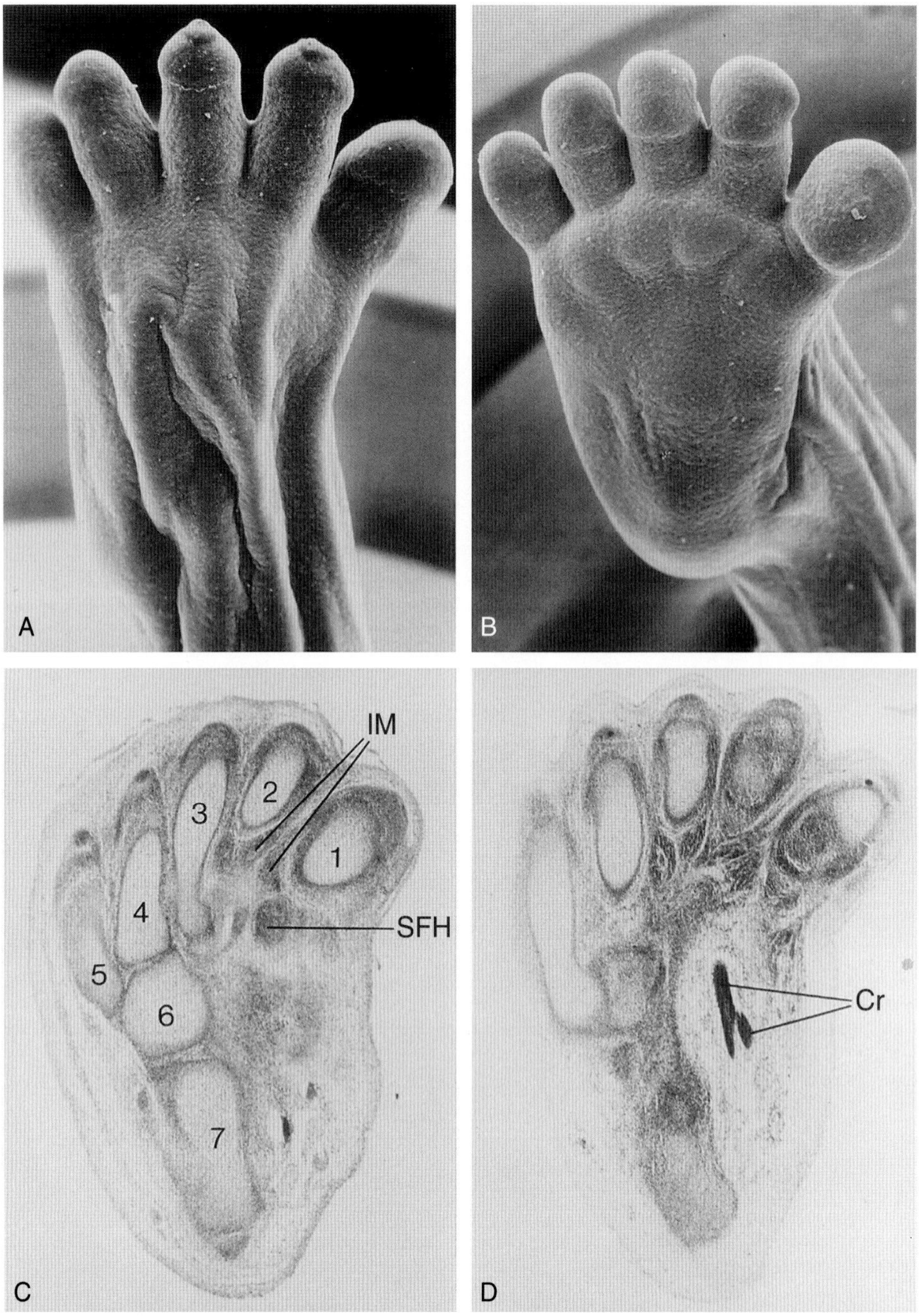

Fig. 16.6 Scanning electron micrographs show a dorsal view of the left foot (A) and a plantar view of the right foot (B) of an 8-week embryo. Although the foot is supinated, dorsiflexion is distinct. (C andD) Paraffin sections of the tarsus and metatarsus of a young fetus, stained with hematoxylin and eosin, show metatarsal cartilages *(1–5)*, cubital cartilage *(6)*, and calcaneus *(7)*. The separation between the interosseous muscles *(IM)* and the short flexor muscles of the big toe *(SFH)* is clearly seen. The plantar crossing *(Cr)* of the tendons of the long flexors of the digits and the hallux (great toe) is shown in (D).(From Hinrichsen KV, Jacob HJ, Jacob M, et al: Principles of ontogenesis of leg and foot in man, *Ann Anat* 176:121, 1994.)

15

FINAL STAGES OF LIMB DEVELOPMENT

As the limbs elongate, mesenchymal models of the bones are formed by cellular aggregations (see Fig. 16.7B). **Chondrification centers** appear in the fifth week. By the end of the sixth week, the entire limb skeleton is cartilaginous (Fig. 16.7; see Fig. 14.13D and E). **Ossification** of long bones begins in the seventh week from primary ossification centers in the diaphysis region of the long bones. **Primary ossification centers** are present in all long bones by the 12th week (see Fig. 14.14A).

From the **dermomyotome regions** of the somites, myogenic precursor cells migrate into the limb buds and later differentiate into myoblasts. *The c-Met receptor tyrosine kinase (encoded by the gene* MET*) plays an essential role in regulating this process.* As the long bones form, the myoblasts aggregate and form a large muscle mass in each limb bud (see Fig. 15.1).

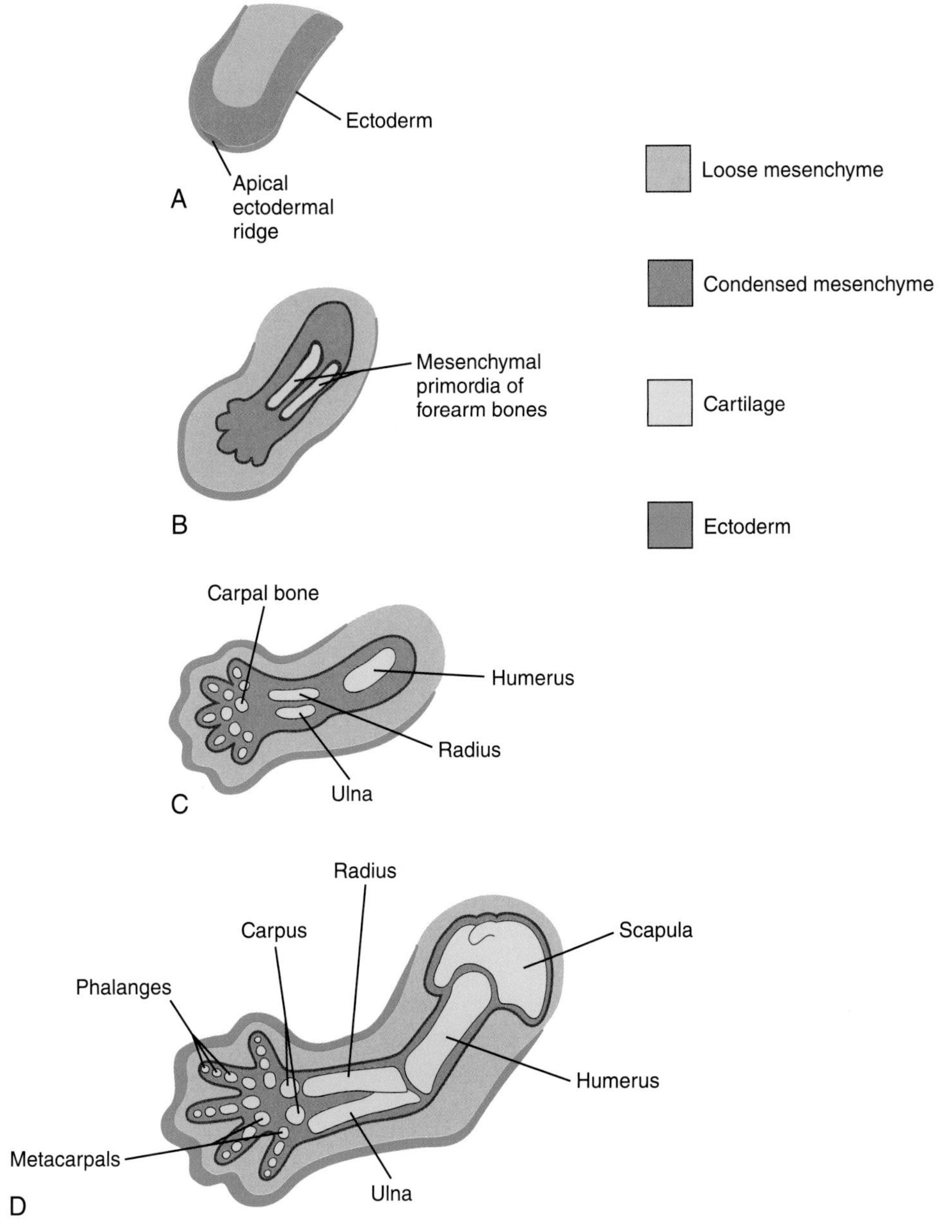

Fig. 16.7 Schematic longitudinal sections of the upper limb of a human embryo show the development of cartilaginous bones at 28 (A), 44 (B), 48 (C), and 56 (D) days.

In general, this muscle mass separates into dorsal (extensor) and ventral (flexor) components. The mesenchyme in the limb bud also gives rise to ligaments and blood vessels.

Early in the seventh week, the limbs extend ventrally. Originally, the flexor aspect of the limbs was ventral and the extensor aspect was dorsal; the preaxial and postaxial borders were cranial and caudal, respectively (see Fig. 16.10A and D). The developing upper and lower limbs rotate in opposite directions and to different degrees (Figs. 16.8 and 16.9):

- The upper limbs rotate laterally through 90 degrees on their longitudinal axis; as a result, the future elbows come to point dorsally, and the extensor muscles lie on the lateral and posterior aspects of the limb.
- The lower limbs rotate medially through almost 90 degrees; therefore the future knees come to face ventrally, and the extensor muscles lie on the anterior aspect of the limb.

Developmentally, the radius and tibia are homologous bones, as are the ulna and fibula; likewise, the thumb and great toe are homologous digits. **Synovial joints** appear at the beginning of the fetal period (ninth week), coinciding with functional differentiation of the limb muscles and their innervation.

CUTANEOUS INNERVATION OF LIMBS

15

There is a strong relationship between the growth and rotation of the limbs and their cutaneous segmental nerve supply. **Motor axons** arising from the spinal cord enter the limb buds during the fifth week and grow into the dorsal and

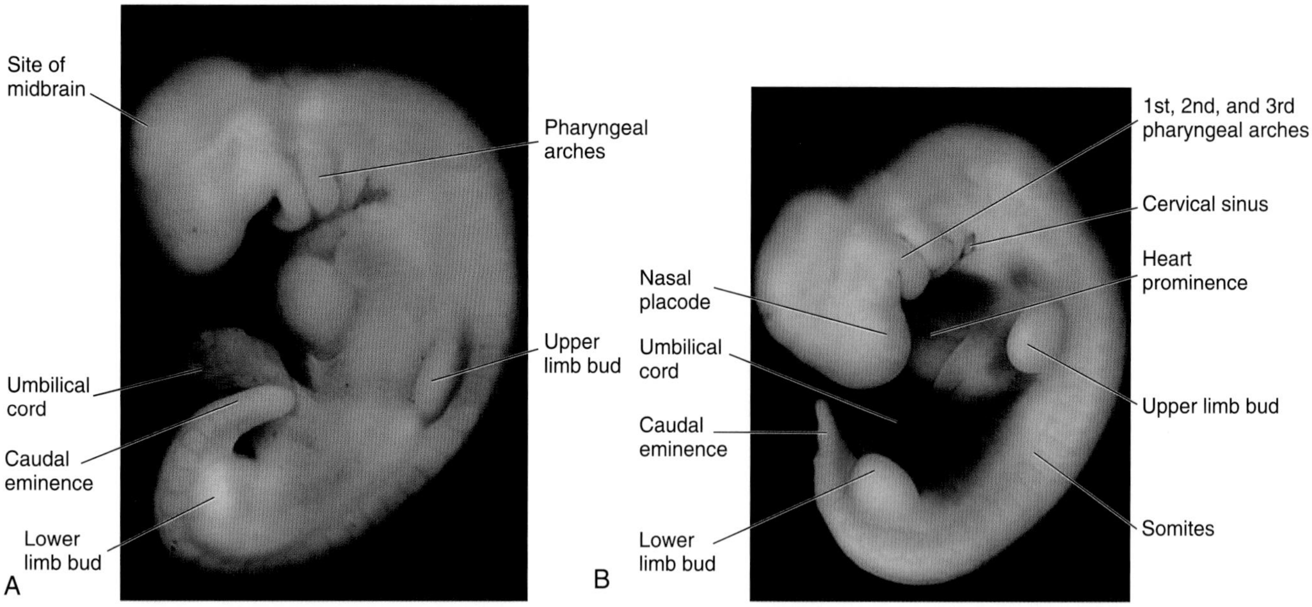

Fig. 16.8 Lateral views of embryos. (A) Lateral view of an embryo at approximately 28 days. The upper limb bud is much larger than the lower limb bud. (B) Lateral view of an embryo at approximately 32 days. The upper and lower limb buds are paddle shaped.(Modified from Nishimura H, Semba R, Tanimura T, Tanaka O: *Prenatal development of the human with special reference to craniofacial structures: an atlas*, Washington, DC, 1977, National Institutes of Health.)

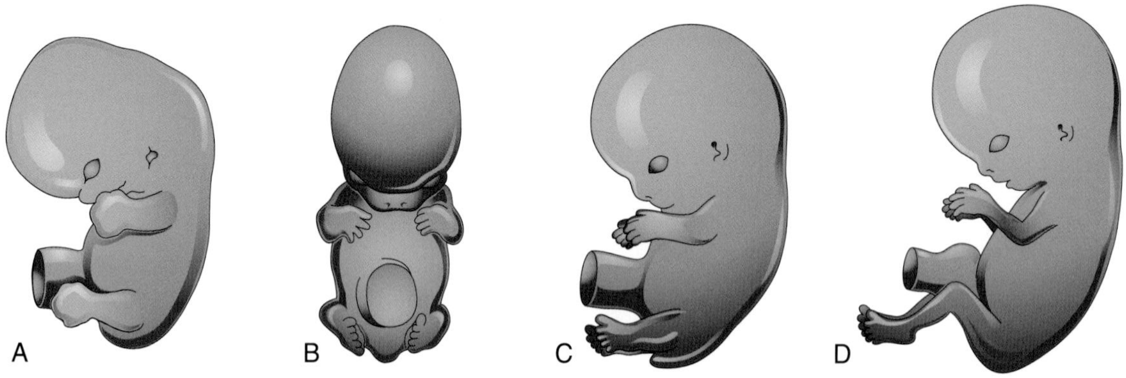

Fig. 16.9 Illustrations of positional changes of the developing limbs of embryos. (A) At approximately 48 days, the limbs extend ventrally, and the hand plates and foot plates face each other. (B) At approximately 51 days, the upper limbs are bent at the elbow, and the hands are curved over the thorax. (C) At approximately 54 days, the soles of the feet face medially. (D) At approximately 56 days (end of the embryonic stage), the elbows point caudally and the knees cranially.

ventral muscle masses. **Sensory axons** enter the limb buds after the motor axons and use them for guidance. Neural crest cells, the precursors of Schwann cells, surround the motor and sensory nerve fibers in the limbs and form the **neurolemma** (sheath of Schwann) and **myelin sheaths** (see Fig. 17.11).

During the fifth week, peripheral nerves grow from the developing brachial and lumbosacral **limb plexuses** into the mesenchyme of the limbs (Fig. 16.10B and E). The **spinal nerves** are distributed in segmental bands, supplying both the dorsal and ventral surfaces of the limbs. A **dermatome** is the area of skin supplied by a single spinal nerve and its spinal ganglion; however, cutaneous nerve areas and dermatomes show considerable overlap.

As the limbs elongate, the cutaneous distribution of the spinal nerves migrates along the limbs and no longer reaches the surface in the distal parts of the limbs. Although the original dermatomal pattern changes during the growth of the limbs, an orderly sequence of distribution can still be recognized in the adult (see Fig. 16.10C and F). In the upper limb, the areas supplied by spinal nerves C5 and C6 adjoin the areas supplied by T2, T1, and C8, but the overlap between them is minimal at the ventral axial line.

A **cutaneous nerve area** is the area of skin supplied by a peripheral nerve. If the dorsal root supplying the area is cut, the dermatomal patterns indicate that there may be a slight deficit in the area indicated. However, because there is an overlap of dermatomes, a particular area of skin is not exclusively innervated by a single segmental nerve. The limb dermatomes may be traced progressively down the lateral aspect of the upper limb and back up its medial aspect. A comparable distribution of dermatomes occurs in the lower limbs, which may be traced down the ventral aspect and then up the dorsal aspect. As the limbs descend, they carry their

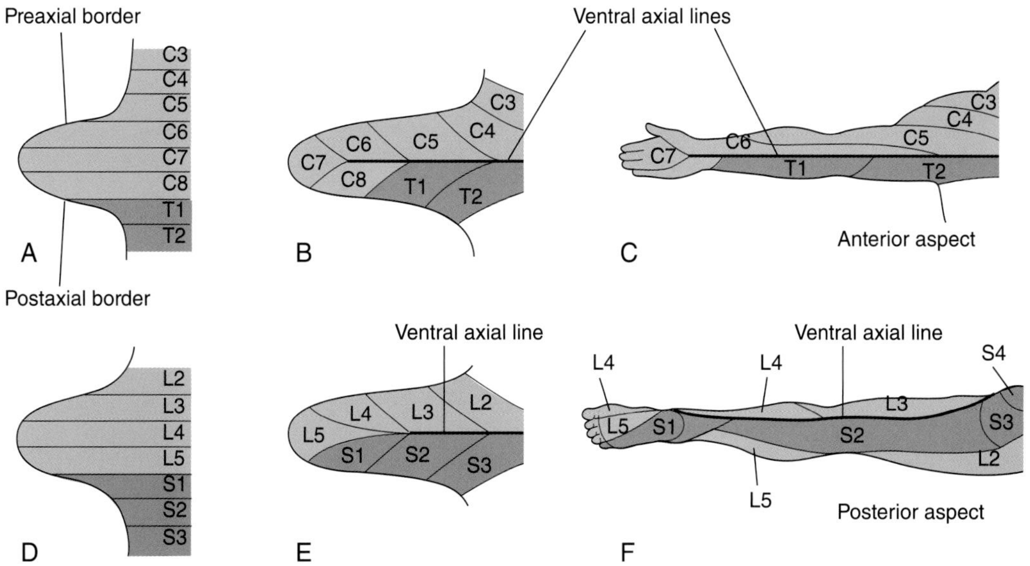

Fig. 16.10 Illustrations of development of the dermatomal patterns of the limbs. The axial lines indicate areas in which there is no sensory overlap. (A and D) Ventral aspect of the limb buds early in the fifth week. At this stage, the dermatomal patterns show the primordial segmental arrangement. (B and E) Similar views later in the fifth week show the modified arrangement of dermatomes. (C and F) The dermatomal patterns in the adult upper and lower limbs. The primordial dermatomal pattern has disappeared, but an orderly sequence of dermatomes can still be recognized. Notice in (F) that most of the original ventral surface of the lower limb lies on the back of the adult limb. This arrangement results from the medial rotation of the lower limb, which occurs toward the end of the embryonic period. In the upper limb (C), the ventral axial line extends along the anterior surface of the arm and forearm. In the lower limb (F), the ventral axial line extends along the medial side of the thigh and knee and down the posteromedial aspect of the leg to the heel.

nerves with them; this explains the oblique courses of the nerves arising from the brachial and lumbosacral plexuses.

BLOOD SUPPLY OF LIMBS

15 The limb buds are supplied by branches of the **intersegmental arteries** (Fig. 16.11A), which arise from the **dorsal aorta** and form a fine capillary network throughout the mesenchyme. The primordial vascular pattern consists of a **primary axial artery** and its branches (see Fig. 16.11B and C), which drain into a peripheral marginal sinus. Blood in the **marginal sinus** drains into a peripheral vein. The vascular patterns change as the limbs develop, chiefly through **angiogenesis**. The new vessels coalesce with other sprouts to form new vessels.

The primary axial artery becomes the **brachial artery** in the arm and the common interosseous artery in the forearm (see Fig. 16.11B), which has anterior and posterior interosseous branches. The ulnar and radial arteries are terminal branches of the brachial artery. As the digits form, the marginal sinus breaks up and the final venous pattern, represented by the basilic and cephalic veins and their tributaries, develops. In the lower limb, the primary axial artery becomes the **deep artery of the thigh** (profunda femoris artery), and the anterior and posterior **tibial arteries** in the leg.

BIRTH DEFECTS OF LIMBS

Minor birth defects involving the limbs are relatively common and can usually be corrected surgically. Although these defects are often of no serious medical consequence, they may serve as indicators of more serious defects, which may be part of a recognizable pattern.

The critical period of limb development is from 24 to 36 days after fertilization. This statement is based on clinical studies of neonates who were exposed in utero to the drug **thalidomide**, a potent human **teratogen** during the embryonic period. Many severe limb defects occurred from 1957 to 1962 as a result of maternal ingestion of thalidomide. This hypnotic drug, widely used as a sedative and antinauseant, was withdrawn from the market in December 1961. Since that time, similar limb defects have rarely been observed. Although thalidomide is now used for the treatment of leprosy and other disorders, it is ***absolutely contraindicated in females of childbearing age***.

Major limb defects appear in approximately 1 in 500 neonates. Most of these defects are caused by genetic factors. *Molecular studies have implicated pathogenic variants (mutations) in genes such as Hox, BMP, SHH, WNT7, and EN1 in some cases of limb defects.* Several unrelated birth defects of the lower limb are associated with an aberrant arterial pattern, which might be of some importance in the pathogenesis of these defects. Experimental studies indicate that thalidomide affects the formation of early blood vessels in the limb buds.

There are two main types of limb anomalies or defects:

- **Amelia**, the absence of a limb or limbs (Fig. 16.13A; see also Fig. 16.12A)
- **Meromelia**, the absence of part of a limb (see Figs. 16.12B and C and 16.13B and C); it includes hemimelia, such as the absence of the fibula in the leg, and phocomelia, in which the hands and/or feet are attached close to the body

Suppression of limb bud development during the early part of the fourth week results in amelia. Arrest or disturbance of differentiation or growth of a limb during the fifth week results in various types of meromelia.

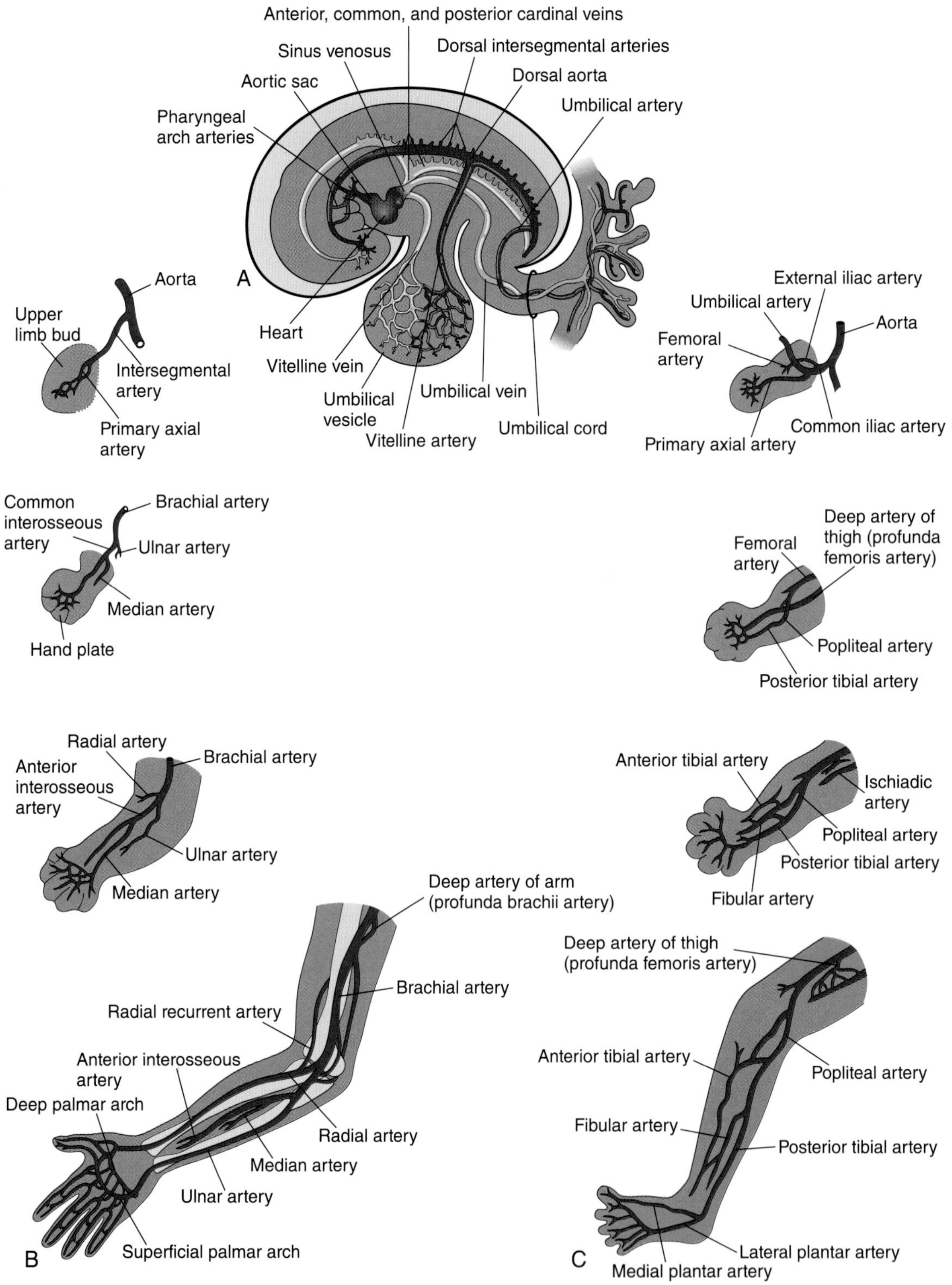

Fig. 16.11 Development of limb arteries. (A) Sketch of the primordial cardiovascular system in an embryo at approximately 26 days. (B) Development of arteries in the upper limb. (C) Development of arteries in the lower limb.

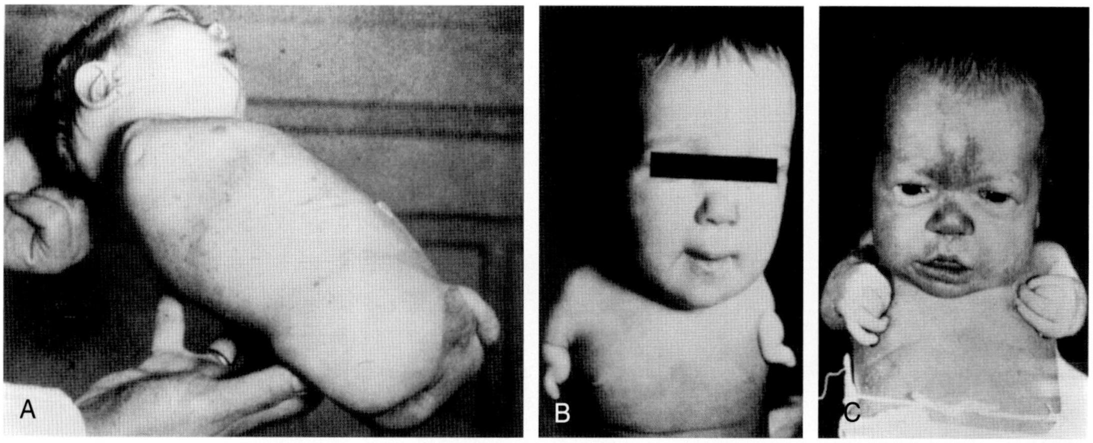

Fig. 16.12 Birth defects of limbs caused by maternal ingestion of thalidomide. (A) Quadruple amelia: absence of upper and lower limbs. (B) Meromelia of the upper limbs; the limbs are represented by rudimentary stumps. (C) Meromelia with the rudimentary upper limbs attached directly to the trunk.(From Lenz W, Knapp K: Foetal malformation due to thalidomide, *Geriatr Med Monthly* 7:253, 1962.)

Split-Hand/Foot Malformations

In severe birth defects such as bifurcate (forked) hand or cleft foot **(split-hand/foot malformations [SHFMs])**, there is the absence of one or more central digits (fingers or toes) due to the failure of development of one or more digital rays (see Fig. 16.13D and E). The hand or foot is divided into two parts that oppose and curve inward. This is a rare condition, affecting approximately 1 in 20,000 live births.

The **split-hand syndrome** is a genetically heterogeneous disease and mainly an autosomal dominant abnormality with incomplete penetrance. Possbile candidate genes include *LRP6* and *UBA2.* The malformation originates in the fifth to sixth week of development when the primordia of the hands are forming. The central part of the apical ectodermal ridge (AER) fails to develop (see Fig. 16.7), which results in a median cleft (see Fig. 16.14E).

Like other congenital anomalies, limb defects may be caused by several factors:

- Genetic factors, such as chromosomal abnormalities associated with trisomy 18 (see Fig. 20.7)
- Pathogenic variants (mutant) in genes, as in brachydactyly, abnormal shortness of the fingers, or osteogenesis imperfecta, a severe limb defect with fractures occurring before birth
- Environmental factors, such as teratogens (e.g., thalidomide, alcohol)
- A combination of genetic and environmental factors (multifactorial inheritance), as in developmental dysplasia of the hip
- Vascular disruption and ischemia (diminished blood supply), as in limb reduction defects

Experimental studies support the suggestion that mechanical influences during intrauterine development may cause some fetal limb defects. A reduced quantity of amniotic fluid **(oligohydramnios)** is commonly associated with limb deformations; however, the significance of in utero mechanical influences on congenital postural deformation is still open to question.

Radial Aplasia

In this defect (1:30,000), the radius is partially or completely absent. The hand deviates laterally, and the ulna bows with the concavity on the lateral side of the forearm. This defect results from the failure of the mesenchymal primordium of the radius to form during the fifth week of development. The absence of the radius is usually caused by genetic factors and may be associated with other abnormalities in the newborn, such as thrombocytopenia (thrombocytopenia absent radii syndrome, 0.5–1:100,000). In many cases, the absence or hypoplasia of the radius may be associated with other anomalies, including the thumb carpal bones. Such a combination of anomalies is known as a **Radial Ray Malformation**.

Polydactyly

Polydactyly is a congenital hand difference with the presence of **supernumerary digits** (more than five digits on the hands or feet) (Fig. 16.14A and B). Often, the extra digit is incompletely formed and lacks normal muscular development. If the hand is affected, the extra digit is most commonly medial (postaxial) or lateral (preaxial) rather than central. Polydactyly (2–10:1000) occurs more frequently in male infants and is associated with over 100 genetic syndromes. In the foot, the extra toe is usually on the lateral side. Polydactyly is inherited as a dominant trait.

Symbrachydactyly

Symbrachydactyly is a type of congenital upper limb undergrowth anomaly that occurs in approximately 0.6:10,000 births. It has a male-to-female (75:25) and a left-to-right (66:34) predominance. Symbrachydactyly results from a failure of the formation and differentiation of the axis of the entire limb, including the hand plate. The thumb is often found co-planar to the hand, which limits grasping and pinching (see Fig. 16.14E).

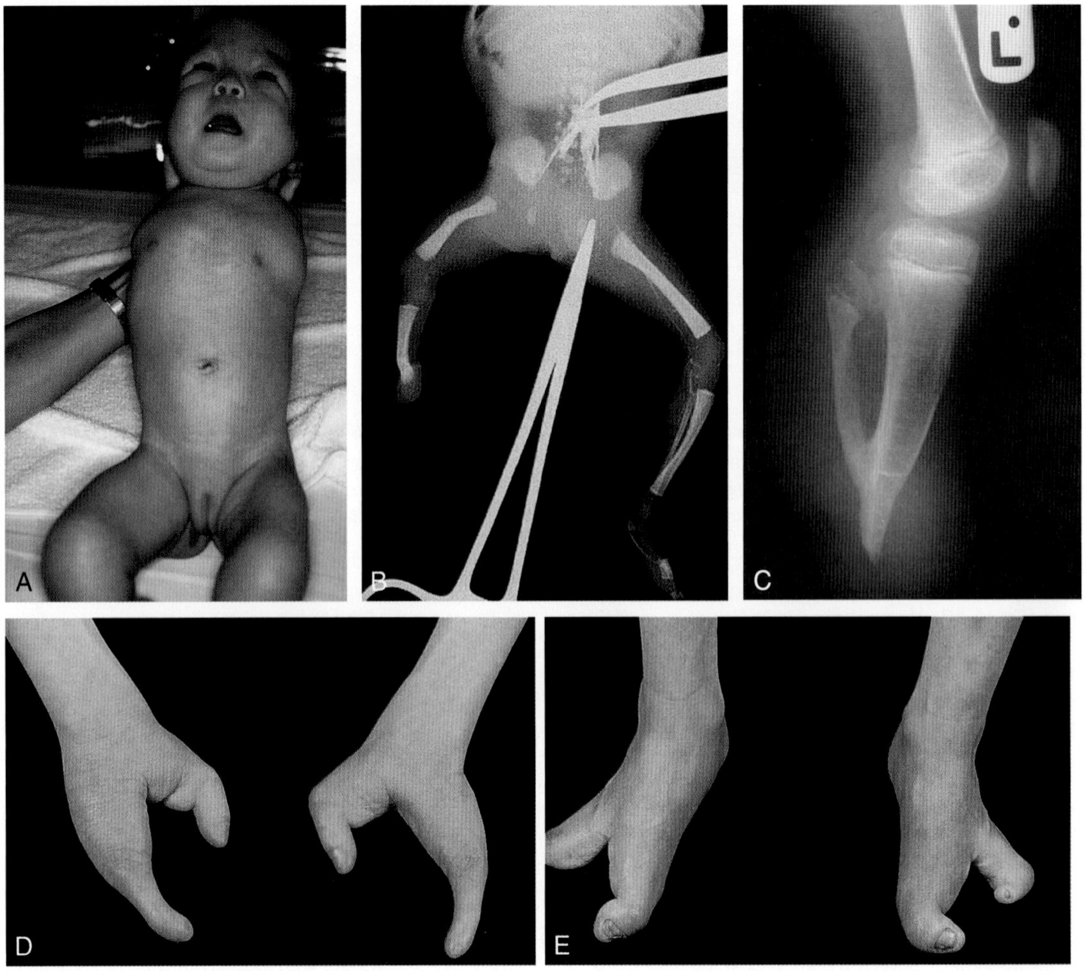

Fig. 16.13 Various types of birth defects. (A) Female neonate with amelia, complete absence of the upper limbs. (B) Radiograph of a female fetus shows the absence of the right fibula. Notice also that the right leg is shorter than the left, and the femur and tibia are bowed and hypoplastic (underdeveloped). (C) Radiograph shows partial absence and fusion of the lower ends of the tibia and fibula in a 5-year-old child. (D) Absence of the central digits of the hands results in a defect called bifurcate (forked) hand or split hand. (E) Absence of the second to fourth toes results in a bifurcate or split foot. (A, Courtesy Dr. Y. Suzuki, Achi, Japan; B, The Courtesy Dr. Joseph R. Siebert, Children's Hospital and Regional Medical Center, Seattle, Washington; C, Courtesy Dr. Prem S. Sahni, formerly of the Department of Radiology, Children's Hospital, Winnipeg, Manitoba, Canada; D and E; Courtesy A.E. Chudley, MD, Section of Genetics and Metabolism, Department of Pediatrics and Child Health, University of Manitoba, Winnipeg, Manitoba, Canada.)

Syndactyly

Syndactyly (SD) is a common birth defect of the hand or foot with an incidence of 3 to 10 in 10,000 live births. Clinically, SD is a heterogeneous anomaly, genetic in origin, and occurs more frequently in males than females. **Cutaneous syndactyly** (simple webbing between digits) is more frequent in the foot than in the hand (see Fig. 16.14C and D). Cutaneous syndactyly results from the failure of the webs to degenerate between two or more digits. **Apoptosis** is responsible for the tissue breakdown between the digits. Blockade of these cellular and molecular events is likely responsible for the defects.

Osseous syndactyly (fusion of bones, **synostosis**) occurs when the notches between the digital rays fail to develop, and as a result, separation of the digits does not occur. This defect is most frequently observed between the third and fourth fingers and between the second and third toes **(SD type I)**. It is inherited as a simple autosomal dominant trait. A case of syndactyly and polydactyly (synpolydactyly or **SD type II**), caused by pathogenic variants (mutations) of the amino-terminal, non–DNA binding part of *HoxD13*, has been reported.

Talipes Equinovarus (Clubfoot)

Talipes equinovarus is a relatively common birth defect (1–3:1000 live births) in North America, and it is the most common musculoskeletal deformation. It is characterized by multiple components that lead to an abnormal position of the foot, preventing normal weight bearing. The sole of the foot is turned medially, and the foot is inverted (Fig. 16.15). Clubfoot is bilateral in approximately 50% of cases, and it occurs approximately twice as frequently in males. It may be associated with other congenital anomalies (central nervous system, muscular, and others). Clubfoot can be diagnosed by ultrasonography between 13 and 23 weeks of gestation.

Although it is commonly stated that clubfoot results from abnormal positioning or restricted movement of the lower limbs of the fetus in utero, the evidence for this is inconclusive. Clubfoot appears to be caused by **multifactorial inheritance**, with genetic and environmental factors acting together. It may result from uneven radial and longitudinal growth and muscular imbalance. In this condition, all anatomical structures are present, so the majority of cases can be treated with casting or taping. In other cases, the deformity is flexible and is amenable to physiotherapy alone to resolve the deformation.

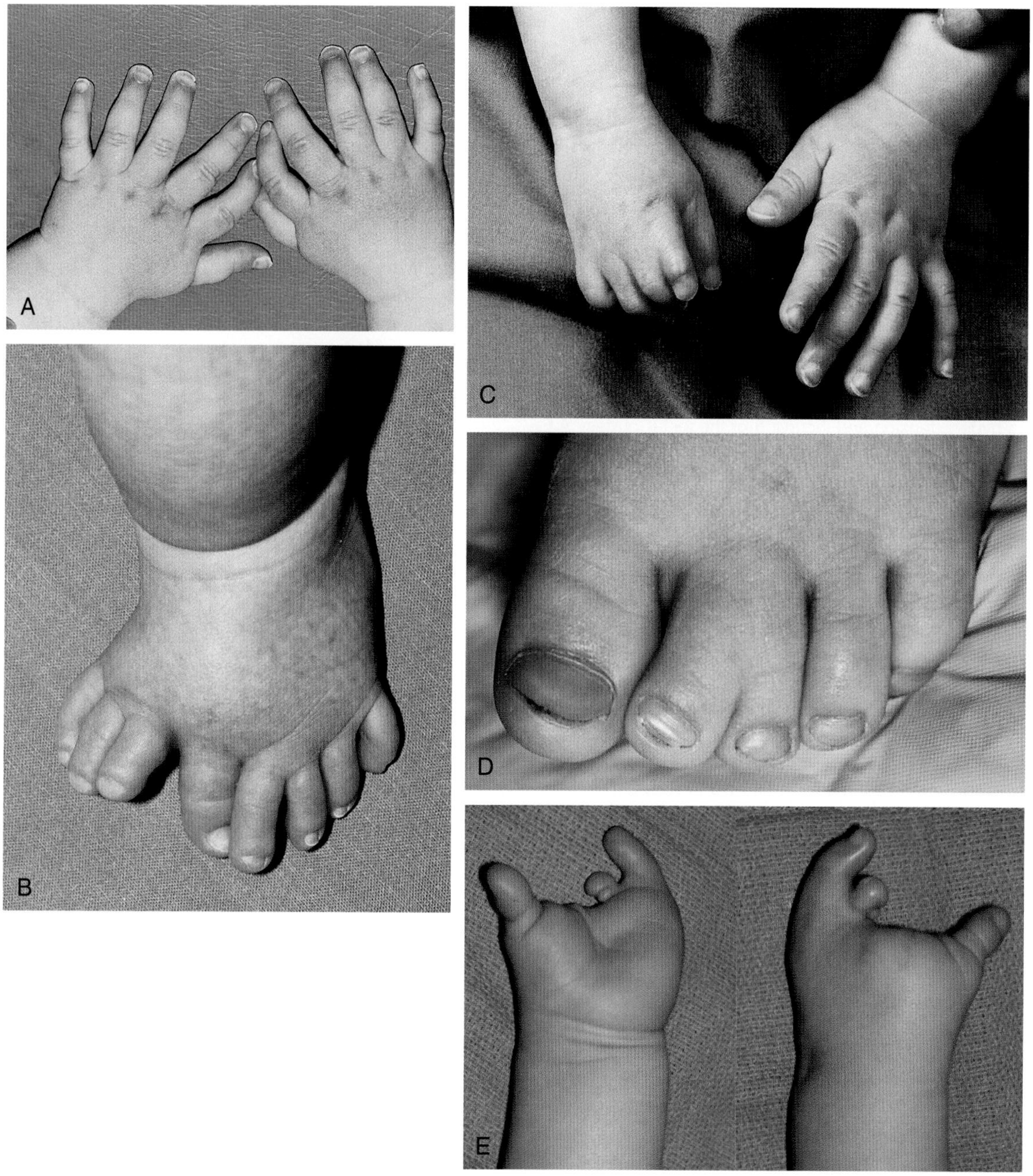

Fig. 16.14 Types of digital birth defects. Polydactyly: more than five digits on the hands (A) or feet (B). Syndactyly (webbing or fusion) of the fingers (C) or toes (D). (E) Volar and dorsal views of bidactylous hands with ulnar and radial digits and a nubbin.(A–D, Courtesy A.E. Chudley, MD, Section of Genetics and Metabolism, Department of Pediatrics and Child Health, Children's Hospital and University of Manitoba, Winnipeg, Manitoba, Canada; E, From Woodside JC, Light TR: Symbrachydactyly—diagnosis, function, and treatment, *J Hand Surg* 41:135, 2016.)

Developmental Dysplasia of the Hip

Developmental dysplasia of the hip occurs in approximately 1 in 1500 neonates, and it is more common in females than in males. The joint capsule is very relaxed at birth, and there is underdevelopment of the acetabulum of the hip bone and the head of the femur. Dislocation almost always occurs after birth. There are two causative factors:

- Abnormal development of the acetabulum occurs in approximately 15% of neonates with congenital dislocation of the hip, which is common after breech deliveries. This suggests that the breech posture during the terminal months of pregnancy may result in a shallow acetabular fossa and a displaced head of the femur.
- Generalized joint laxity is often a dominantly inherited condition that appears to be associated with congenital dislocation of the hip. It follows a multifactorial pattern of inheritance.

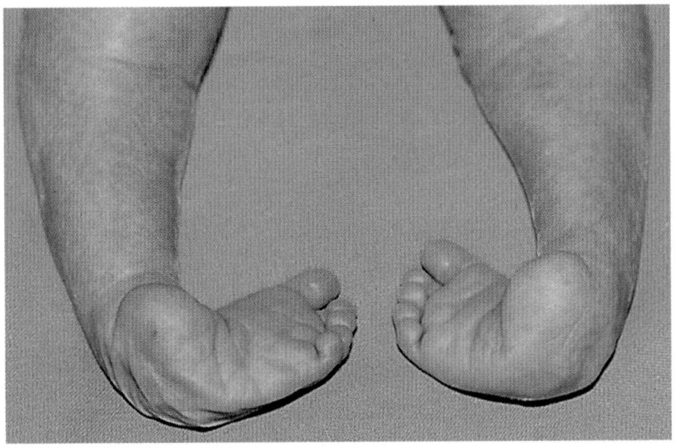

Fig. 16.15 Neonate with bilateral talipes equinovarus (clubfeet). Observe the hyperextension and incurving of the feet.(Courtesy A.E. Chudley, MD, Section of Genetics and Metabolism, Department of Pediatrics and Child Health, Children's Hospital and University of Manitoba, Winnipeg, Manitoba, Canada.)

15

SUMMARY OF LIMB DEVELOPMENT

- **Limb buds** appear toward the end of the fourth week of gestation as slight bulges of the ventrolateral body wall. The development of the upper limb buds proceeds approximately 2 days ahead of the development of the lower limb buds. The tissues of the limb buds are derived from two main sources, mesoderm and ectoderm.
- The **apical ectodermal ridge** (AER) exerts an inductive influence on the limb mesenchyme (see Fig. 16.2), promoting the growth and development of the limbs. The limb buds elongate with the proliferation of the mesenchyme within them. Apoptosis is an important mechanism in limb development; for example, in the breakdown of the tissue in the notches between the digital rays.
- Limb muscles are derived from mesenchyme (myogenic precursor cells) originating in the somites. The muscle-forming cells **(myoblasts)** form dorsal and ventral muscle masses. Nerves grow into the limb buds after the muscle masses have formed. Most blood vessels in the limb buds arise as buds from the intersegmental arteries.
- Initially, the developing limbs are directed caudally; later, they project ventrally; and finally, they rotate on their longitudinal axes. The upper and lower limbs rotate in opposite directions and to different degrees (see Fig. 16.9).
- Most birth defects of the limbs are caused by genetic factors; however, many defects probably result from an interaction of genetic and environmental factors **(multifactorial inheritance)**.

CLINICALLY ORIENTED PROBLEMS

CASE 16-1

A mother consulted her pediatrician after noticing that when her 11-month-old daughter began to stand independently, her legs seemed to be of different lengths. The pediatrician diagnosed congenital hip dysplasia.

- Are the hip joints of infants with this condition usually dislocated at birth?
- What are the probable causes of congenital dislocation of the hip?

CASE 16-2

A male infant was born with limb defects (see Fig. 16.12*). His mother said that one of her relatives had similar defects.*

- Are limb defects similar to those caused by the drug thalidomide common?
- What was the characteristic syndrome produced by thalidomide?
- Name the limb and other defects commonly associated with the thalidomide syndrome.

CASE 16-3

A neonate presented with a clubfeet. The physician explained that this is a common birth defect.

- What is the most common type of clubfoot?
- How common is it?
- Describe the feet of infants born with this birth defect, and explain the treatment.

CASE 16-4

A baby was born with syndactyly (webbing between her fingers). The doctor stated that this minor defect can be easily corrected surgically.

- Is syndactyly common?
- Does it occur more often in the hands than in the feet?
- What is the embryologic basis of syndactyly?
- What is the difference between simple and complex (osseous) syndactyly?

Discussion of these problems appears in the Appendix at the back of the book.

BIBLIOGRAPHY AND SUGGESTED READING

Ambler CA, Nowicki JL, Burke AC, Bautch VL: Assembly of trunk and limb blood vessels involves extensive migration and vasculogenesis of somite-derived angioblasts, *Dev Biol* 234:352, 2001.

Berenguer M, Duester G: Role of retinoic acid signaling, FGF signaling and *Meis* genes in control of limb development, *Biomolecules* 11:80, 2021. https://doi.org/10.3390/biom11010080.

Butterfield NC, McGlinn E, Wicking C: The molecular regulation of vertebrate limb patterning, *Curr Top Dev Biol* 90:319, 2010.

Cole P, Kaufman Y, Hatef DA, Hollier LH: Embryology of the hand and upper extremity, *J Craniofac Surg* 20:992, 2009.

Elliott AM, Evans JA, Chudley AE: Split hand foot malformation (SHFM), *Clin Genet* 68:501, 2005.

Gandhi M, Rac MWF, McKinney J: Radial ray malformation, *Am J Obstet Gynecol* 221(6):B16–B18, 2019. https://doi.org/10.1016/j.ajog.2019.09.024..

Gold NB, Westgate MN, Holmes LB: Anatomic and etiological classification of congenital limb deficiencies, *Am J Med Genet A* 155:1225, 2011.

Hall BK: *Bones and cartilage: developmental skeletal biology*, ed 2, Philadelphia, 2015, Elsevier.

Hernandez-Andre E, Yeo L, Goncalves LF: Fetal musculoskeletal system. In Norton ME, editor: *Callen's ultrasonography in obstetrics and gynecology*, ed 6, Philadelphia, 2017, Elsevier.

Hinrichsen KV, Jacob HJ, Jacob M, Brand-Saberi B, Christ B, Grim M: Principles of ontogenesis of leg and foot in man, *Ann Anat* 176:121, 1994.

Ippolito E, Gorgolinin G: Clubfoot pathology in fetus and pathogenesis. A new pathogenetic theory based on pathology, image findings, and biomechanics – a narrative review, *Ann Transl Med* 9(13):1095, 2021.

Kuitunen I, Uimonen MM, Haapanen M, Sund R, Helenius I, Ponkilainen VT: Incidence of neonatal developmental dysplasia of the hip and late detection rates based on screening strategy: a systematic review and meta-analysis, *JAMA Netw Open* 5(8):e2227638, 2022. https://doi.org/10.1001/jamanetworkopen.2022.27638.

Liu RE: Musculoskeletal disorders in neonates. In Martin RJ, Fanaroff AA, Walsh MC, editors: *Fanaroff and Martin's neonatal-perinatal medicine: diseases of the fetus and infant, current therapy in neonatal-perinatal medicine*, ed 10, Philadelphia, 2015, Saunders Elsevier.

Logan M: Finger or toe: the molecular basis of limb identity, *Development* 130:6401, 2003.

Marini JC, Forlino A, Bächinger HP: Osteogenesis imperfecta, *Nat Rev Dis Primers* 3:17052, 2017.

Mendelsohn AI, Dasen JS, Jessell TM: Divergent *Hox* coding and evasion of retinoid signaling specifies motor neurons innervating digit muscles, *Neuron* 93:792, 2017.

Montero JA, Lorda-Diez CI, Sanchez-Fernandez C, Hurle JM: Cell death in the developing vertebrate limb: A locally regulated mechanism contributing to musculoskeletal tissue morphogenesis and differentiation, *Dev Dyn* 250(9):1236–1247, 2021. https://doi.org/10.1002/dvdy.237.

Newton AH, Williams SM, Major AT, Smith CA: Cell lineage specification and signaling pathway use during development of the lateral plate mesoderm and forelimb mesenchyme, *Development* 149(18), 2022. https://doi.org/10.1242/dev.200702.

O'Rahilly R, Müller F: *Developmental stages in human embryos*, Washington, DC, 1987, Carnegie Institution of Washington.

Raines AM, Magella B, Adam M, Potter SS: Key pathways regulated by *HoxA9,10,11/HoxD9,10,11* during limb development, *BMC Dev Biol* 15:28, 2015.

Sammer DM, Chung KC: Congenital hand differences: embryology and classification, *Hand Clin* 25:151, 2009.

Sheeba CJ, Andrade RP, Palmeirim I: Getting a handle on embryo limb development: molecular interactions driving limb outgrowth and patterning, *Semin Cell Dev Biol* 49:92, 2016.

Sheeba CJ, Logan MP: The roles of T-box genes in vertebrate limb development, *Curr Top Dev Biol* 122:355, 2017.

Society for Maternal-Fetal Medicine: McKinney J, Rac MWF, Gandhi M: Congenital talipes equinovarus (clubfoot), *Am J Obstet Gynecol* 221(6):B10–B12, 2019. https://doi.org/10.1016/j.ajog.2019.09.022.

Society for Maternal-Fetal Medicine (SMFM): McKinney J, Rac MWF, Gandhi M: SMFM Fetal Anomalies consult series #2: extremities, *Am J Obstet Gynecol* 221(6):B2–B18, 2019. https://doi.org/10.1016/j.ajog.2019.09.019. Epub 2019 Sep 18. Erratum in: Am J Obstet Gynecol. 2023 Jan;228(1):125

Talamillo A, Delgado I, Nakamura T, de-Vega S, Yoshitomi Y, Unda F, et al: : Role of epiprofin, a zinc-finger transcription factor in limb development, *Dev Biol* 337:363, 2010.

Tonkin MA: Classification of congenital anomalies of the hand and upper limb, *J Hand Surg (Eur Volume)* 42:448, 2017. https://doi.org/10.1177/1753193417690965.

Towers M, Tickle C: Generation of pattern and form in the developing limb, *Int J Dev Biol* 53:805, 2009.

Van Allen MI: Structural anomalies resulting from vascular disruption, *Pediatr Clin North Am* 39:255, 1992.

Van Heest AE: Congenital disorders of the hand and upper extremity, *Pediatr Clin North Am* 43:1113, 1996.

Whitley KL, Britton JC, Pira CU, Oberg KC: LHX2 regulates *Shh* expression in the limb independent of the ZPA regulatory sequence, *FASEB J* 36(Suppl 1), 2022. https://doi.org/10.1096/fasebj.2022.36.S1.R6203.

Woodside JC, Light TR: Symbrachydactyly—diagnosis, function, and treatment, *J Hand Surg Am* 41:135, 2016.

Yamoto K, Saitsu H, Nishimura G, Kosaki R, Takayama S, Haga N, et al: Comprehensive clinical and molecular studies in split-hand/foot malformation: identification of two plausible candidate genes (LRP6 and UBA2), *Eur J Hum Genet* 27(12):1845, 2019. https://doi.org/10.1038/s41431-019-0473-7.

Zaib T, Rashid H, Khan H, Sun P: Recent advances in syndactyly: basis, current status and future perspectives, *Genes (Basel)* 13(5):771, 2022. https://doi.org/10.3390/genes13050771.

Nervous System 17

CHAPTER OUTLINE

The nervous system consists of three main regions:

- The **central nervous system (CNS)** consists of the brain and spinal cord and is protected by the cranium and vertebral column.
- The **peripheral nervous system (PNS)** includes the neurons outside the CNS as well as the cranial nerves and spinal nerves (and their associated ganglia), which connect the brain and spinal cord with peripheral structures.
- The **autonomic nervous system (ANS)** has parts in the CNS and PNS and consists of the neurons that innervate smooth muscle, cardiac muscle, glandular epithelium, and combinations of these tissues.

DEVELOPMENT OF THE NERVOUS SYSTEM

The first indications of the developing nervous system appear during the third week as the **neural plate** and **neural groove** develop on the posterior aspect of the trilaminar embryo (Fig. 17.1A). The notochord and paraxial mesenchyme induce the overlying ectoderm to differentiate into the neural plate. *This transformation (neural induction) involves the expression of intercellular proteins including members of the transforming growth factor-β (TGF) family, Wnts, sonic hedgehog (SHH), and bone morphogenic proteins (BMPs).* The formation of the neural folds, neural crest, and neural tube is illustrated in Figs. 17.1B–F and 17.2.

- The neural tube differentiates into the CNS.
- The neural crest gives rise to cells that form most of the PNS and ANS.

Neurulation (formation of the neural plate and neural tube) begins during the fourth week (22–23 days) in the region of the fourth to sixth pairs of somites (see Fig. 17.1C and D). At this stage, the cranial two-thirds of the neural plate and tube as far caudal as the fourth pair of somites represent the future brain. The caudal one-third of the plate and tube represents the future spinal cord.

Fusion of the neural folds and formation of the **neural tube** begins at the fifth somite and proceeds at multiple locations until only small areas of the tube remain open at both ends (Fig. 17.3A and B). The lumen of the neural tube becomes the **neural canal**, which communicates freely with the amniotic cavity (see Fig. 17.3C). The cranial opening **(rostral neuropore)** closes on approximately the 25th day, and the **caudal neuropore** closes on approximately the 27th day (see Fig. 17.3D).

Closure of the neuropores coincides with the establishment of vascular circulation for the neural tube. It has been reported that expression of Snx, Syndecan 4 gene (SDC4), endocytic receptor Lrp2, and Van Gogh–like 2 (VANGL2) proteins are essential for neural tube closure. The neuroprogenitor cells of the wall of the neural tube thicken to form the brain and spinal cord (Fig. 17.4). The neural canal forms the ventricular system of the brain and the central canal of the spinal cord.

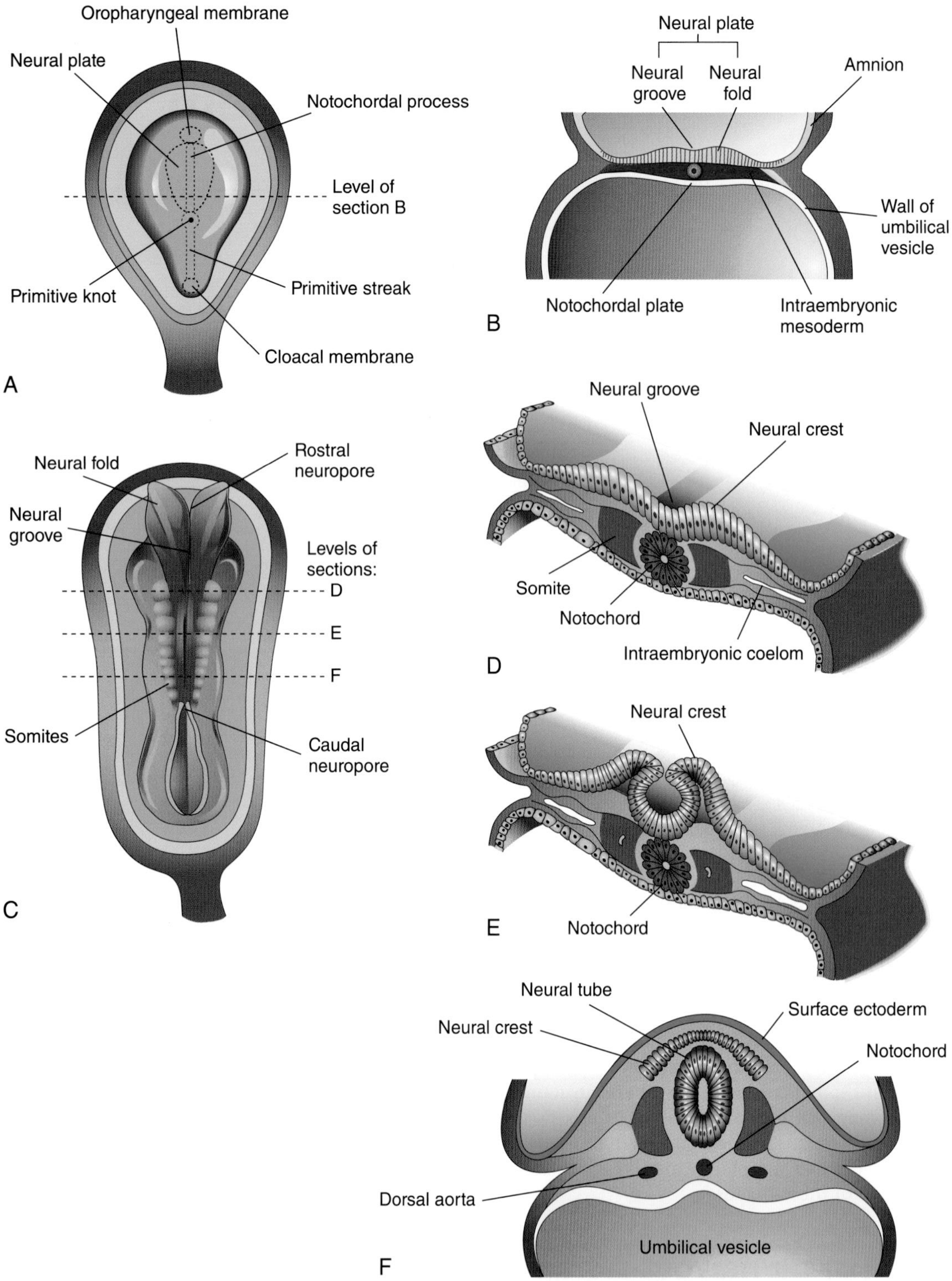

Fig. 17.1 The neural plate folds to form the neural tube. (A) Dorsal view shows an embryo of approximately 17 days that was exposed by removing the amnion. (B) Transverse section of the embryo shows the neural plate and early development of the neural groove and neural folds. (C) Dorsal view of an embryo of approximately 22 days shows that the neural folds have fused opposite the fourth to sixth somites but are spread apart at both ends. (D–F) Transverse sections of the embryo at the levels shown in (C) illustrate the formation of the neural tube and its detachment from the surface ectoderm. Some neuroectodermal cells are not included in the neural tube but remain between it and the surface ectoderm as the neural crest.

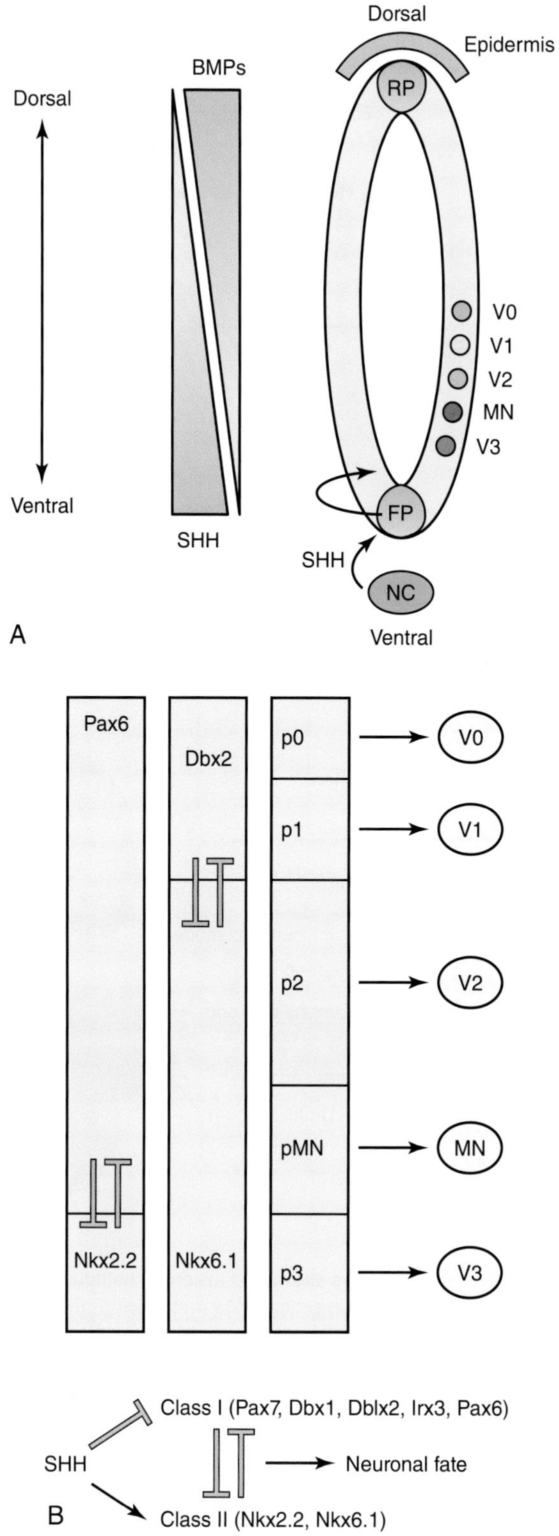

Fig. 17.2 Morphogens and transcription factors specify the fate of progenitors in the ventral neural tube. (A) Sonic hedgehog *(SHH)* is secreted by the notochord (*NC*) and the floor plate (*FP*) of the neural tube in a ventral to dorsal gradient. Similarly, bone morphogenetic proteins (*BMPs*), members of the transforming growth factor-β superfamily, are secreted by the roof plate (*RP*) of the neural tube and the overlying epidermis in a dorsal to ventral gradient. These opposing morphogen gradients determine dorsal-ventral cell fates. (B) SHH concentration gradients define the ventral expression domains of class I (repressed) and class II (activated) homeobox transcription factors. Reciprocal negative interactions assist in establishing boundaries of gene expression in the embryonic ventral spinal cord. *p*, Progenitor; *MN*, motor neuron; *V*, ventral interneuron. (A, Modified from Jessel TM: Neuronal specification in the spinal cord: inductive signals and transcription codes, *Nat Rev Genet* 1:20, 2000. B, Courtesy Dr. David Eisenstat, Manitoba Institute of Cell Biology, and Department of Human Anatomy and Cell Science, and Dr. Jeffrey T. Wigle, Department of Biochemistry and Medical Genetics, University of Manitoba, Winnipeg, Manitoba, Canada.)

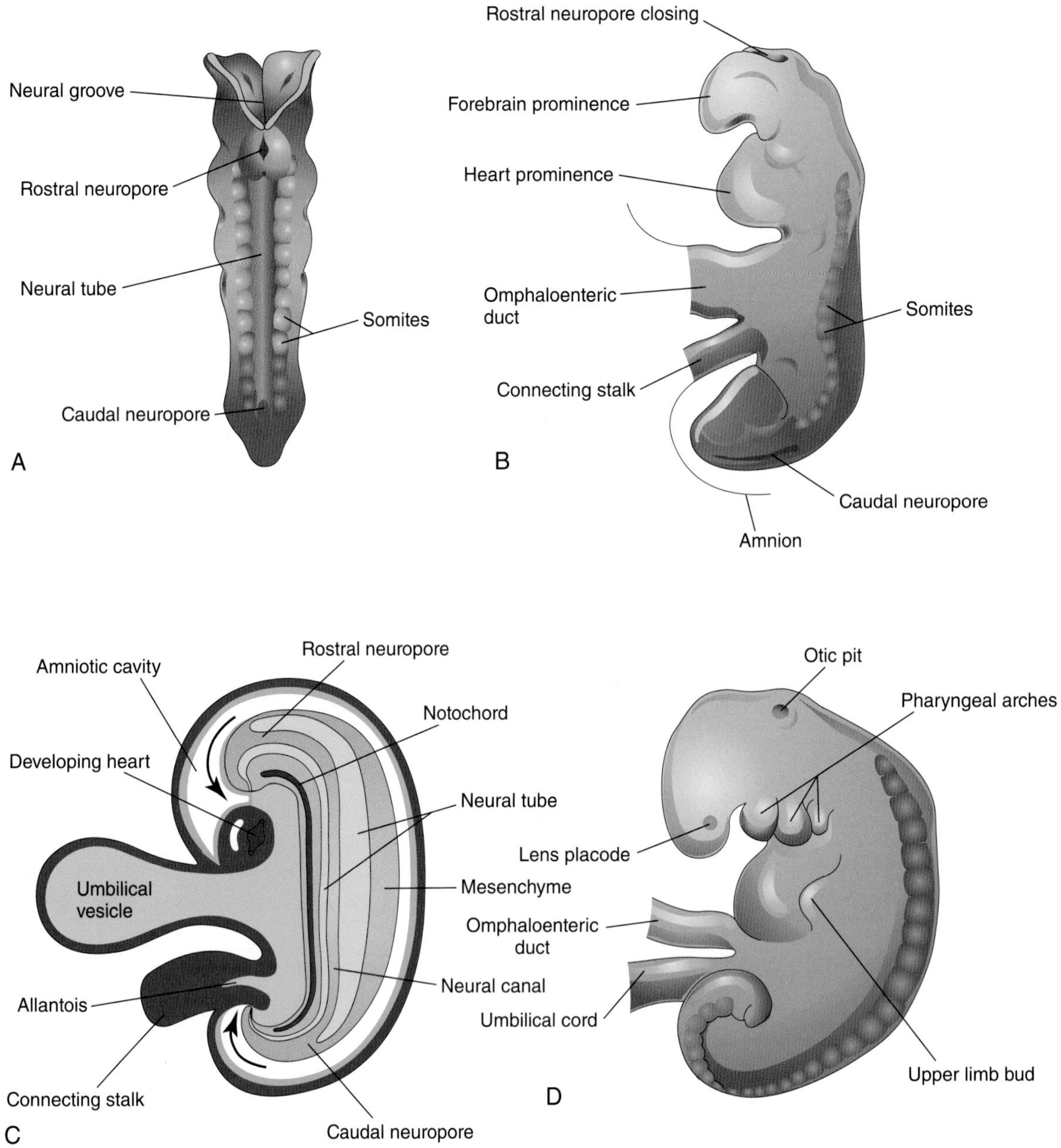

Fig. 17.3 (A) Dorsal view of an embryo of approximately 23 days shows the fusion of the neural folds, which forms the neural tube. (B) Lateral view of an embryo of approximately 24 days shows the forebrain prominence and closing of the rostral neuropore. (C) Diagrammatic sagittal section of the embryo at 23 days shows the transitory communication of the neural canal with the amniotic cavity *(arrows)*. (D) In the lateral view of an embryo of approximately 27 days, notice that the neuropores shown in (B) are closed.

DEVELOPMENT OF THE SPINAL CORD

The primordial spinal cord develops from the caudal part of the neural plate and caudal eminence. The neural tube caudal to the fourth pair of somites develops into the spinal cord (Fig. 17.5; see Figs. 17.3 and 17.4). The lateral walls of the neural tube thicken, gradually reducing the size of the neural canal until only a minute **central canal of the spinal cord** exists at 9 to 10 weeks (see Fig. 17.5C). Retinoic acid signaling is essential in the development of the spinal cord from early patterning to neurogenesis.

Initially, the wall of the neural tube is composed of a thick, pseudostratified, columnar neuroepithelium (see Fig. 17.5D). These neuroepithelial cells constitute the **ventricular zone** (ependymal layer), which gives rise to all **neurons** and **macroglial cells** (macroglia) in the spinal cord (Fig. 17.6; see Fig. 17.5E). Macroglial cells are the larger members of the neuroglial family of cells, which includes astrocytes and oligodendrocytes. Soon, a **marginal zone** composed of the outer parts of the neuroepithelial cells becomes recognizable (see Fig. 17.5E). This zone gradually becomes the **white matter of the spinal cord** as axons grow into it from nerve cell bodies in the spinal cord, spinal ganglia, and brain.

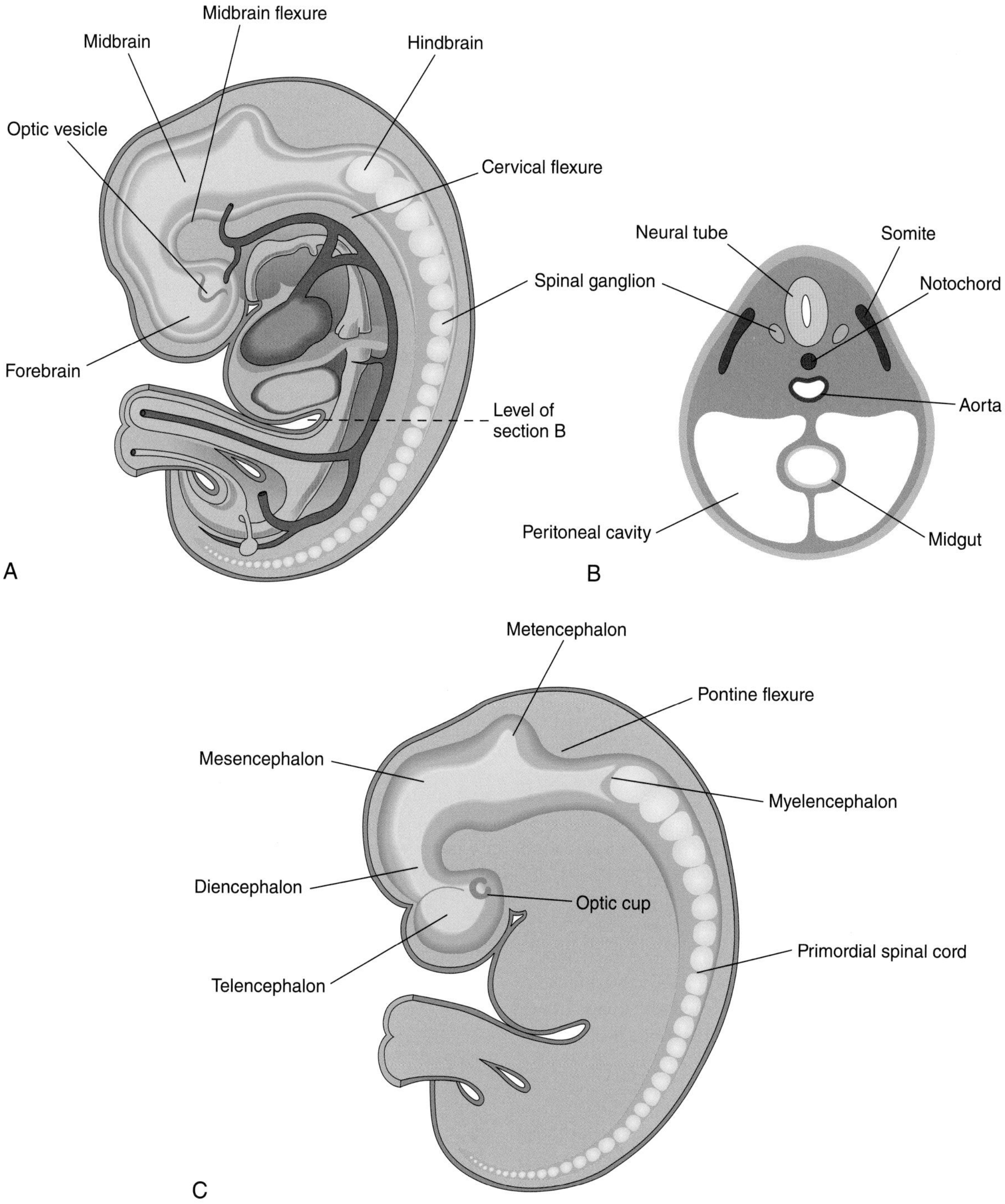

Fig. 17.4 (A) Schematic lateral view of an embryo of approximately 28 days shows the three primary brain vesicles: forebrain, midbrain, and hindbrain. Two flexures demarcate the primary divisions of the brain. (B) Transverse section of the embryo shows the neural tube that will develop into the spinal cord in this region. The spinal ganglia derived from the neural crest are also shown. (C) Schematic lateral view of the central nervous system of a 6-week embryo shows the secondary brain vesicles and the pontine flexure that occurs as the brain grows rapidly.

Nonclosure of Neural Tube

The current hypothesis is that there are multiple (possibly five) closure sites involved in the formation of the neural tube. Failure of closure of site 1 results in spina bifida cystica (see Fig. 17.15). **Meroencephaly** results from the failure of the closure of site 2 (see Fig. 17.13). **Craniorachischisis** results from the failure of sites 2, 4, and 1 to close. Site 3 nonfusion is rare.

It has been suggested that the most caudal region may have a fifth closure site from the second lumbar vertebra to the second sacral vertebra and that closure inferior to the second sacral vertebra occurs by secondary neurulation. Epidemiologic analysis of neonates with NTD supports the concept that there are multiple closures of the neural tube in humans. The **neural tube defects (NTDs)** are described later in the chapter.

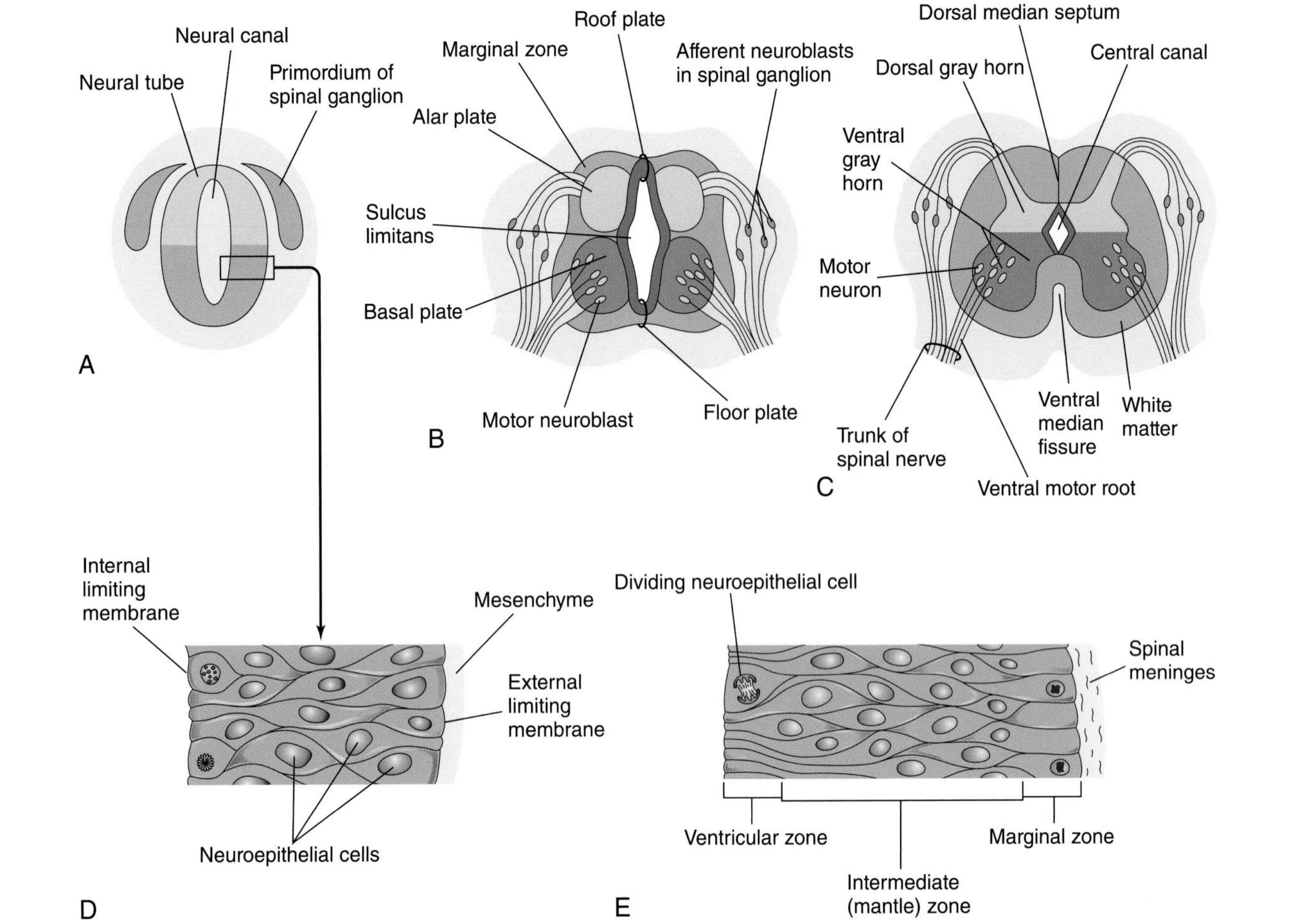

Fig. 17.5 Development of the spinal cord. (A) Transverse section of the neural tube of an embryo of approximately 23 days. (B and C) Similar sections at 6 and 9 weeks, respectively. (D) Section of the wall of the neural tube shown in (A). (E) Section of the wall of the developing spinal cord shows its three zones. Notice that the neural canal of the neural tube is converted into the central canal of the spinal cord (A–C).

Some dividing neuroepithelial cells in the ventricular zone differentiate into primordial neurons **(neuroblasts)**. These embryonic cells form an **intermediate zone** (mantle layer) between the ventricular and marginal zones. *Neuroblasts become neurons* as they develop cytoplasmic processes (see Fig. 17.6).

The supporting cells of the CNS, called **glioblasts** (spongioblasts), differentiate from neuroepithelial progenitor stem cells, mainly after neuroblast formation has ceased. The glioblasts migrate from the ventricular zone into the intermediate and marginal zones. Some glioblasts become **astroblasts** and later **astrocytes**, whereas others (oligodendrocyte progenitor cells) become **oligodendroblasts** and eventually **oligodendrocytes** (see Fig. 17.6). When the neuroepithelial cells cease producing neuroblasts and glioblasts, they differentiate into ependymal cells, which form the **ependyma** (ependymal epithelium) lining the central canal of the spinal cord. *SHH and Olig2 basic-helix-loop-helix signaling controls the proliferation, survival, and patterning of neuroepithelial progenitor cells by regulating GLI transcription factors* (see Fig. 17.2).

Microglia (microglial cells), which are scattered throughout the gray and white matter of the spinal cord, are small cells that are derived from **mesenchymal cells** (see Fig. 17.6). Microglia invade the CNS rather late in the fetal period after it has been penetrated by blood vessels. Microglia originate in the bone marrow and are part of the mononuclear phagocytic cell population.

The proliferation and differentiation of neuroepithelial cells in the developing spinal cord produce thick walls and thin roof plates and floor plates (see Fig. 17.5B). Differential thickening of the lateral walls of the spinal cord soon produces a shallow longitudinal groove on each side, the **sulcus limitans** (Fig. 17.7; see Fig. 17.5B). This groove separates the dorsal part **(alar plate)** from the ventral part **(basal plate)**. The alar and basal plates produce longitudinal bulges extending through most of the length of the developing spinal cord. This regional separation is of fundamental importance because the alar and basal plates are later associated with afferent and efferent functions, respectively.

Cell bodies in the alar plates form the **dorsal gray columns**, which extend the length of the spinal cord. In transverse sections of the cord, these columns are the **dorsal gray horns** (see Fig. 17.7). Neurons in these columns constitute afferent nuclei, and groups of them form the dorsal gray columns. As the alar plates enlarge, the **dorsal median septum** forms. Cell bodies in the basal plates form the ventral and lateral gray columns.

In transverse sections of the spinal cord, these columns are the **ventral gray horns** and **lateral gray horns**, respectively

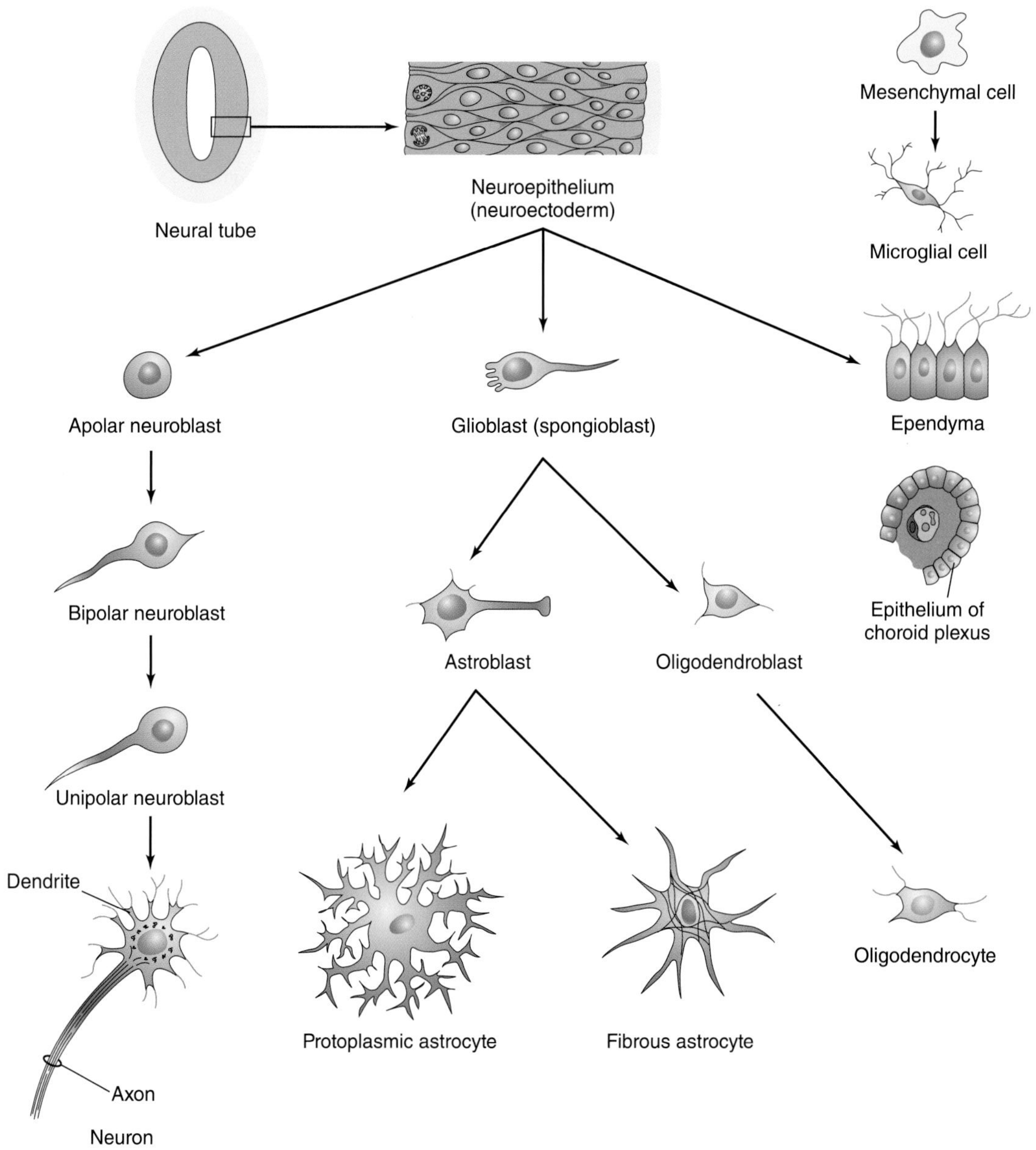

Fig. 17.6 Histogenesis of cells in the central nervous system. After further development, the multipolar neuroblast *(lower left)* becomes a nerve cell or neuron. Neuroepithelial cells give rise to all neurons and macroglial cells. Microglial cells are derived from mesenchymal cells that invade the developing nervous system with the blood vessels.

(see Fig. 17.5C). Axons of ventral horn cells grow out of the spinal cord and form the **ventral roots of the spinal nerves.** As the basal plates enlarge, they bulge ventrally on each side of the median plane. As this occurs, the **ventral median septum** forms and a deep longitudinal groove **(ventral median fissure)** develops on the ventral surface of the spinal cord (see Fig. 17.5C).

DEVELOPMENT OF SPINAL GANGLIA

The unipolar neurons in the spinal ganglia (dorsal root ganglia) are derived from **neural crest cells** (Figs. 17.8 and 17.9). The axons of cells in the spinal ganglia are at first bipolar, but the two processes soon unite in a T-shaped fashion. Both processes of spinal ganglion cells have the structural characteristics of **axons**, but the peripheral process is a dendrite in that there is conduction toward the cell body. The peripheral processes of **spinal ganglion cells** pass in the spinal nerves to sensory endings in somatic or visceral structures (see Fig. 17.8). The central processes enter the spinal cord and constitute the **dorsal roots of spinal nerves.**

DEVELOPMENT OF SPINAL MENINGES

The meninges develop from cells of the neural crest and mesenchyme between 20 and 35 days. The cells migrate to surround the neural tube and form the primordial meninges (see Fig. 17.1F).

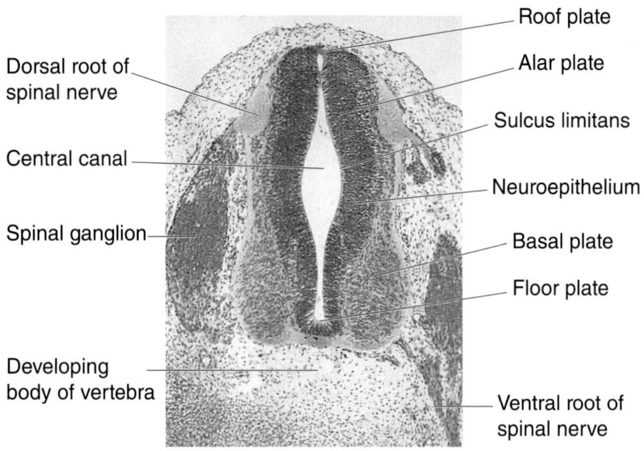

Fig. 17.7 Transverse section of an embryo (×100) at Carnegie stage 16 at approximately 40 days. The ventral root of the spinal nerve is composed of nerve fibers arising from neuroblasts in the basal plate (developing ventral horn of the spinal cord), whereas the dorsal root is formed by nerve processes arising from neuroblasts in the spinal ganglion. (From Moore KL, Persaud TVN, Shiota K: *Color atlas of clinical embryology*, ed 2, Philadelphia, 2000, Saunders.)

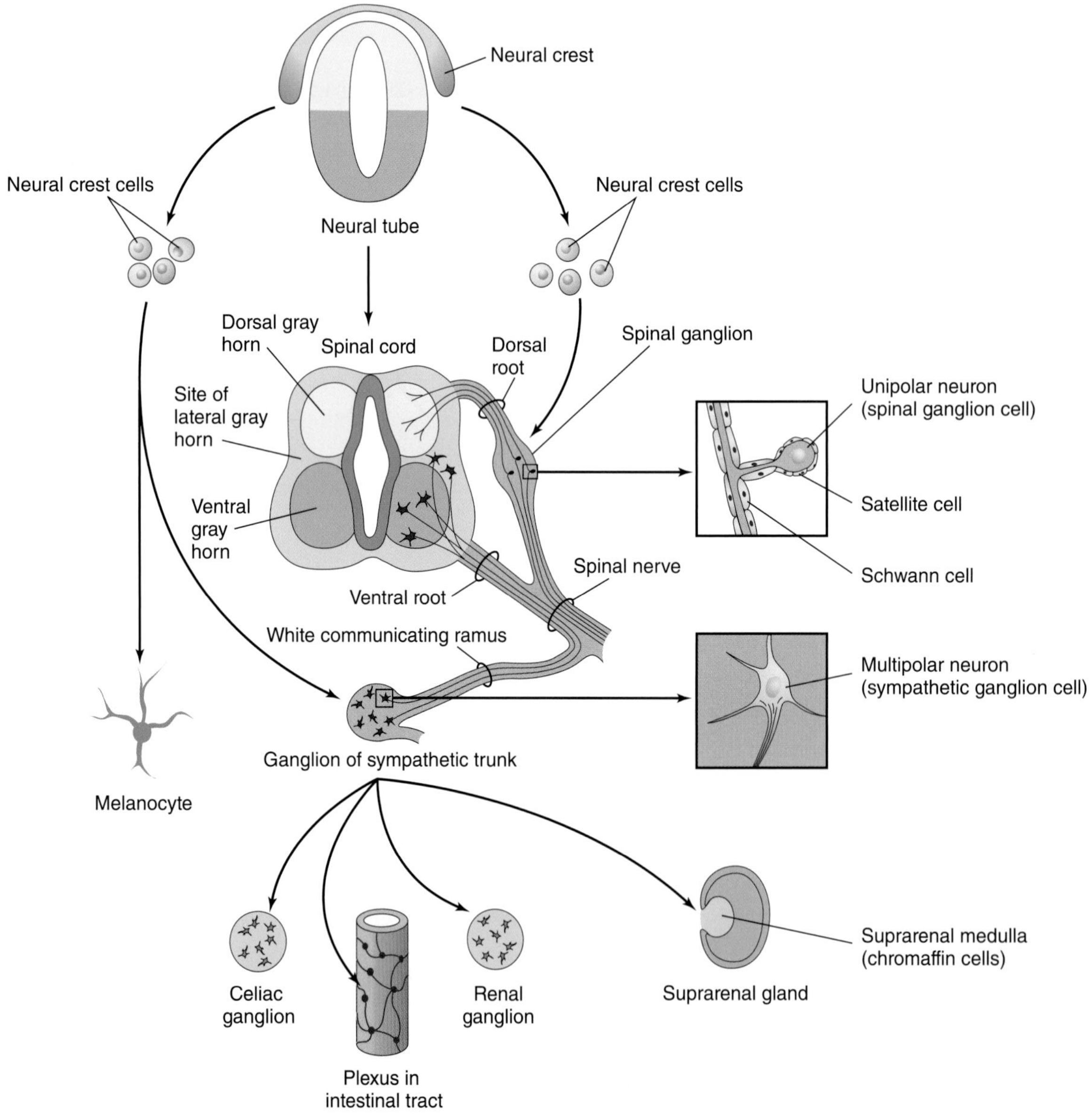

Fig. 17.8 Diagram shows some derivatives *(arrows)* of the neural crest. Neural crest cells also differentiate into the cells in the afferent ganglia of cranial nerves and many other structures (see Fig. 5.5). Formation of a spinal nerve is also illustrated.

The external layer of these membranes thickens to form the thick **dura mater** (Fig. 17.10A and B), and the internal layer, the **pia arachnoid**, is composed of the thin, delicate **pia mater** and **arachnoid mater (leptomeninges)**. Fluid-filled spaces appear within the leptomeninges that soon coalesce to form the **subarachnoid space** (see Fig. 17.12A). The origin of the pia mater and arachnoid from a single layer is indicated in the adult by **arachnoid trabeculae**, which are numerous, delicate strands of connective tissue that pass between the pia and arachnoid. **Cerebrospinal fluid (CSF)** begins to form during the fifth week (see Fig. 17.12A).

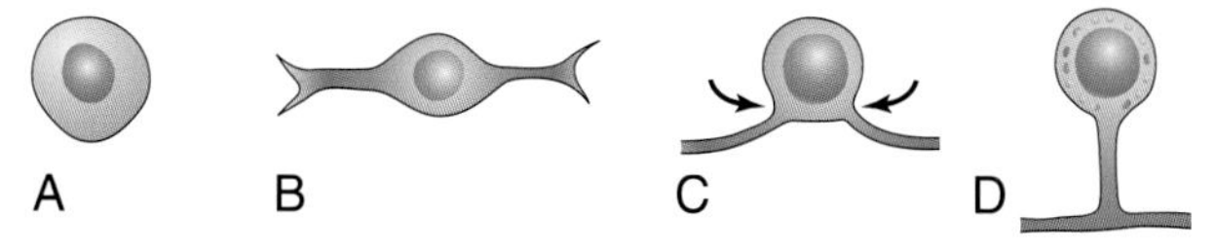

Fig. 17.9 (A–D) Diagrams show successive stages in the differentiation of a neural crest cell into a unipolar afferent neuron in a spinal ganglion. *Arrows* indicate how a unipolar neuron is formed.

POSITIONAL CHANGES OF SPINAL CORD

The spinal cord in the embryo extends the entire length of the vertebral canal (see Fig. 17.10A). The spinal nerves pass through the **intervertebral foramina** opposite their levels of origin. Because the vertebral column and dura mater grow more rapidly than the spinal cord, this positional relationship of the spinal nerves does not persist. The caudal end of the spinal cord in fetuses gradually comes to lie at relatively higher levels. In a 24-week-old fetus, it lies at the level of the first sacral vertebra (see Fig. 17.10B).

The spinal cord in neonates terminates at the level of the second or third lumbar vertebra (see Fig. 17.10C). In adults, the cord usually terminates at the inferior border of the first lumbar vertebra (see Fig. 17.10D). This is an average level because the caudal end of the spinal cord in adults may be as superior as the 12th thoracic vertebra or as inferior as the third lumbar vertebra. The **spinal nerve roots**, especially those of the lumbar and sacral segments, run obliquely from the spinal cord to the corresponding level of the vertebral column (see Fig. 17.10D). The nerve roots inferior to the end of the cord **(medullary cone)** form a bundle of spinal nerve roots called the **cauda equina**, which arises from the lumbosacral enlargement and medullary cone of the spinal cord (see Fig. 17.10D).

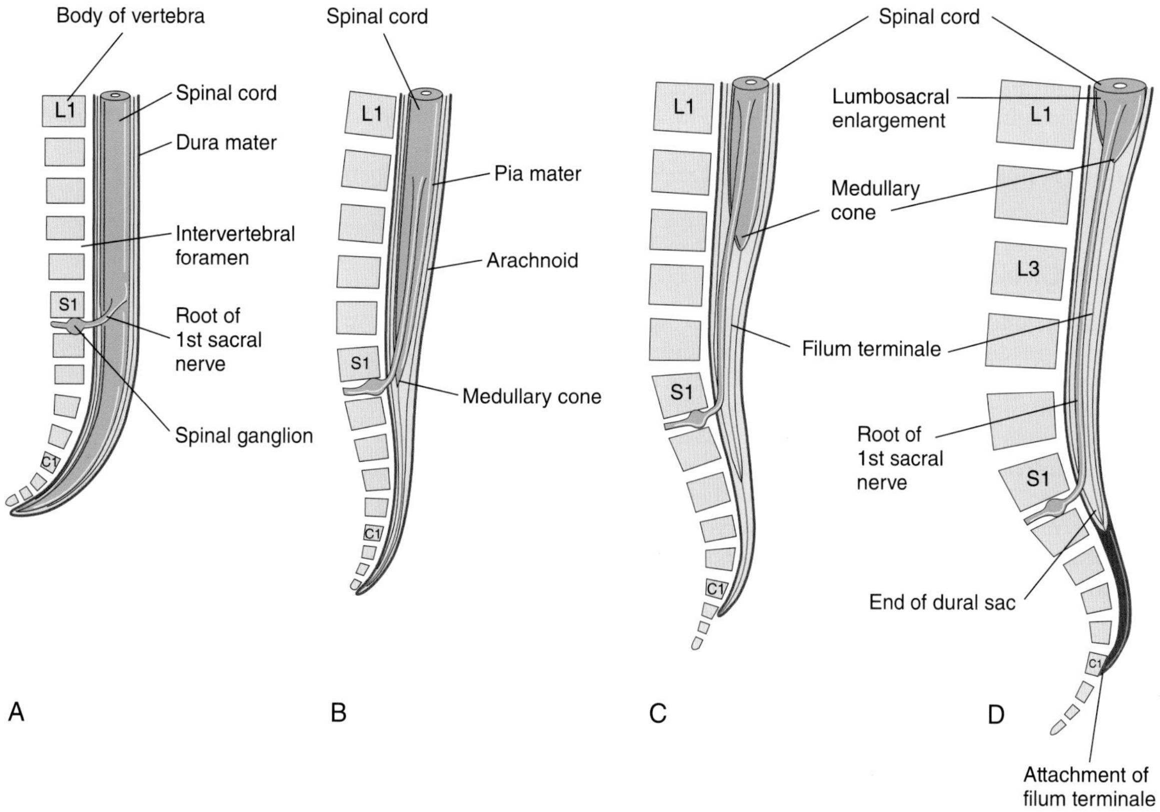

Fig. 17.10 Diagrams show the position of the caudal end of the spinal cord in relation to the vertebral column and meninges at various stages of development. The increasing inclination of the root of the first sacral nerve is also illustrated. (A) At 8 weeks. (B) At 24 weeks. (C) Neonate. (D) Adult.

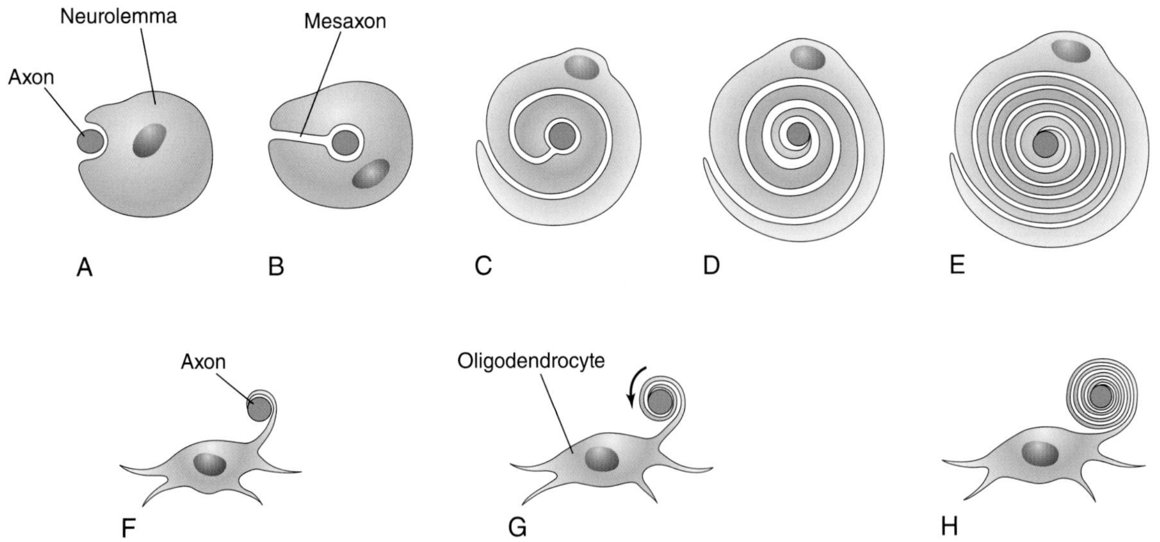

Fig. 17.11 Diagrammatic sketches illustrate the myelination of nerve fibers. (A–E) Successive stages in the myelination of an axon of a peripheral nerve fiber by the neurilemma (sheath of Schwann). The axon first indents the cell, and the cell then rotates around the axon as the mesaxon (site of invagination) elongates. The cytoplasm between the layers of the cell membrane gradually condenses. Cytoplasm remains on the inside of the sheath between the myelin and the axon. (F–H) Successive stages in the myelination of a nerve fiber in the central nervous system by an oligodendrocyte. A process of the neuroglial cell wraps itself around an axon, and the intervening layers of cytoplasm move to the body of the cell.

Although the dura mater and arachnoid mater usually end at the S2 vertebra in adults, the pia mater does not. Distal to the caudal end of the spinal cord, the pia mater forms a long fibrous thread, the **filum terminale** (terminal filum), which indicates the original level of the caudal end of the embryonic spinal cord (see Fig. 17.10C). The **filum** (Latin, "thread") extends from the medullary cone and attaches to the periosteum of the first coccygeal vertebra (see Fig. 17.10D).

MYELINATION OF NERVE FIBERS

Myelin sheaths around the nerve fibers within the spinal cord begin to form during the late fetal period and continue to form during the first postnatal year (Fig. 17.11E). *Myelin basic proteins, a family of related polypeptide isoforms, are essential in myelination;* β_1*-integrins regulate this process.* Fiber tracts become functional at approximately the time they become myelinated. Motor roots are myelinated before sensory roots. The myelin sheaths around the nerve fibers in the spinal cord are formed by **oligodendrocytes (oligodendroglial cells)**, which are types of glial cells that originate from the neuroepithelium. The plasma membranes of these cells wrap around the axon, forming several layers (see Fig. 17.11F–H). *Profilin 1 (PFN1) protein is essential in the microfilament polymerization that promotes changes to the oligodendrocyte cytoskeleton.*

The myelin sheaths around the axons of peripheral nerve fibers are formed by the plasma membranes of the **neurilemma** (sheath of Schwann cells), which are analogous to oligodendrocytes. Neurilemma cells are derived from neural crest cells that migrate peripherally and wrap themselves around the axons of somatic motor neurons and **preganglionic autonomic motor neurons** as they pass out of the CNS (see Figs. 17.8 and 17.11A–E). These cells also wrap themselves around the central and peripheral processes of somatic and visceral sensory neurons and the axons of postsynaptic autonomic motor neurons. Beginning at approximately 20 weeks, peripheral nerve fibers have a whitish appearance resulting from the deposition of myelin.

Birth Defects of Spinal Cord

Most defects result from the **failure of fusion of one or more neural arches** of the developing vertebrae during the fourth week. **NTDs** affect the tissues overlying the spinal cord: meninges, neural arches, muscles, and skin (Fig. 17.12). Defects involving the embryonic **neural arches** are referred to as **spina bifida**; subtypes of this defect are based on the degree and pattern of the NTD. The term *spina bifida* denotes nonfusion of the halves of the embryonic **neural arches**, which is common to all types of spinae bifida (see Fig. 17.12A). Severe defects also involve the spinal cord, meninges, and neurocranium (bones of the cranium enclosing the brain; see Fig. 17.13). Spina bifida ranges from clinically significant types to minor defects that are functionally unimportant (Fig. 17.14). Recent advances in fetal surgery have led to some hope for the successful closure of these defects in utero, allowing for some improvement in neurologic outcomes.

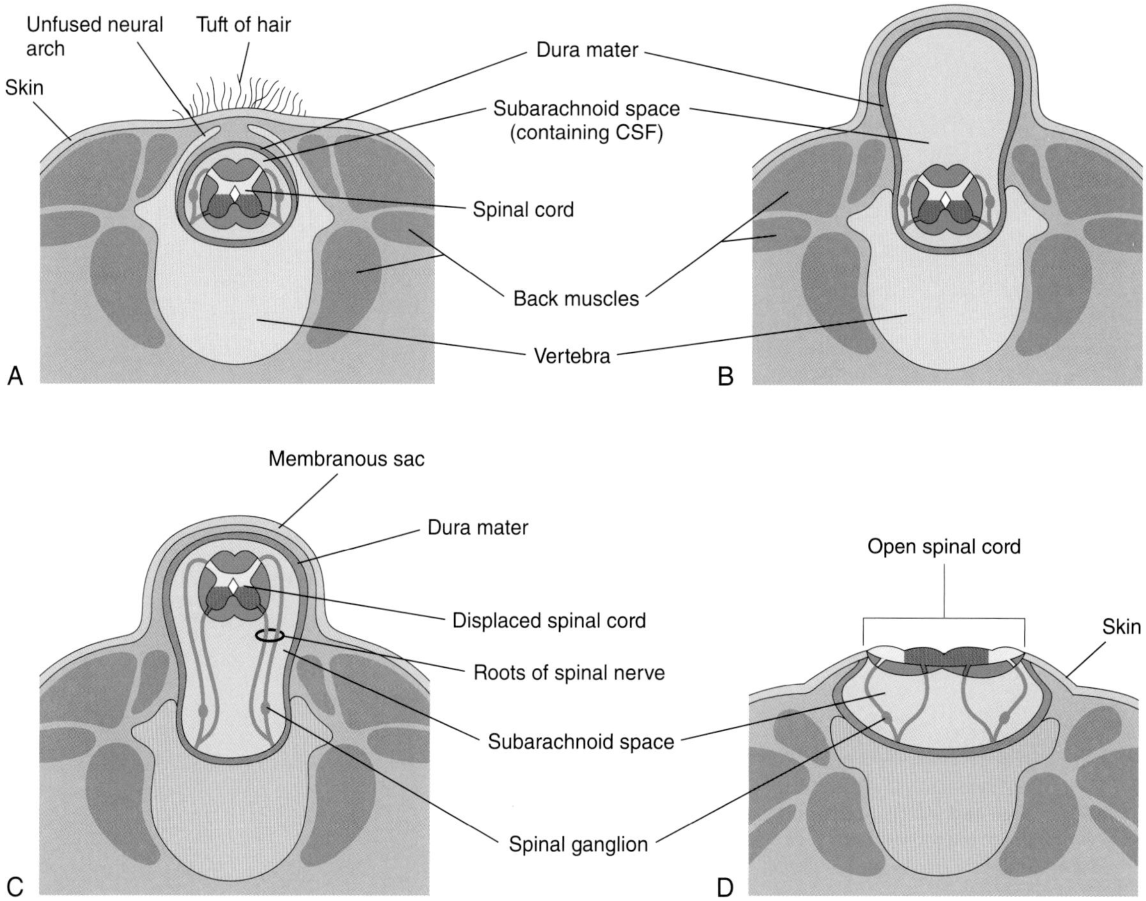

Fig. 17.12 Diagrammatic sketches illustrate various types of spina bifida and the associated defects of the vertebral arches (one or more), spinal cord, and meninges. (A) Spina bifida occulta. Observe the unfused neural arch. (B) Spina bifida with meningocele. (C) Spina bifida with meningomyelocele. (D) Spina bifida with myeloschisis. The defects illustrated in (B–D) are referred to collectively as *spina bifida cystica* because of the cyst-like sac or cyst associated with them. *CSF*, Cerebrospinal fluid.

Dermal Sinus

A dermal sinus is lined with epidermis and skin appendages extending from the skin to a deeper-lying structure, usually the spinal cord. The sinus is associated with the closure of the neural tube and the formation of the meninges in the lumbosacral region of the spinal cord. The birth defect is caused by the failure of the surface ectoderm (future skin) to detach from the neuroectoderm and meninges that envelop it. As a result, the meninges are continuous with a narrow channel that extends to a dimple in the skin of the sacral region of the back (see Fig. 17.13). The dimple indicates the region of closure of the caudal neuropore at the end of the fourth week and therefore represents the last place of separation between the surface ectoderm and the neural tube.

Spina Bifida Occulta

Spina bifida occulta is an **NTD** resulting from the failure of the halves of one or more **neural arches** to fuse in the median plane (see Fig. 17.12A). This NTD occurs in the L5 or S1 vertebra in approximately 10% of otherwise normal people. In the minor form, the only evidence of its presence may be a small dimple with a tuft of hair arising from it (see Figs. 17.12A and 17.14). The cause of the hypertrichosis (excessive hair) has not been established. An overlying lipoma dermal sinus or other birthmark may also occur. Spina bifida occulta usually produces no symptoms. A few affected infants have functionally significant defects of the underlying spinal cord and dorsal roots.

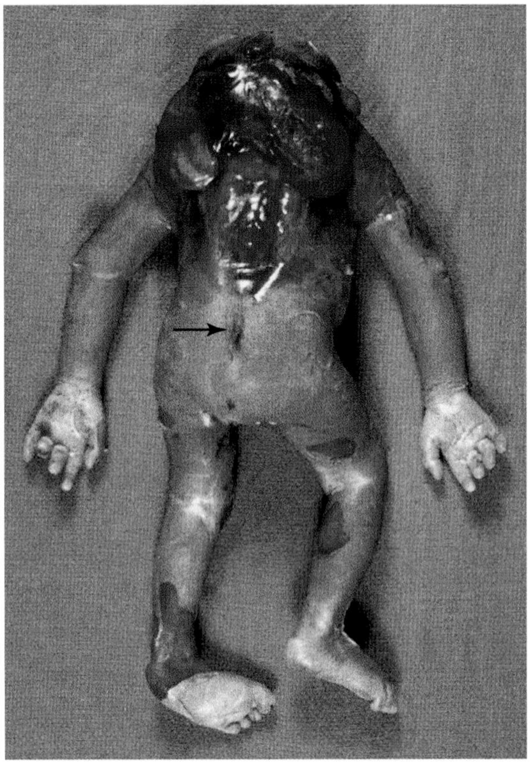

Fig. 17.13 A fetus at 20 weeks with severe neural tube defects, including acrania, cerebral regression (meroencephaly), iniencephaly (enlargement of foramen magnum), and a sacral dimple *(arrow)*. (Courtesy Dr. Marc Del Bigio, Department of Pathology (Neuropathology), University of Manitoba, Winnipeg, Manitoba, Canada.)

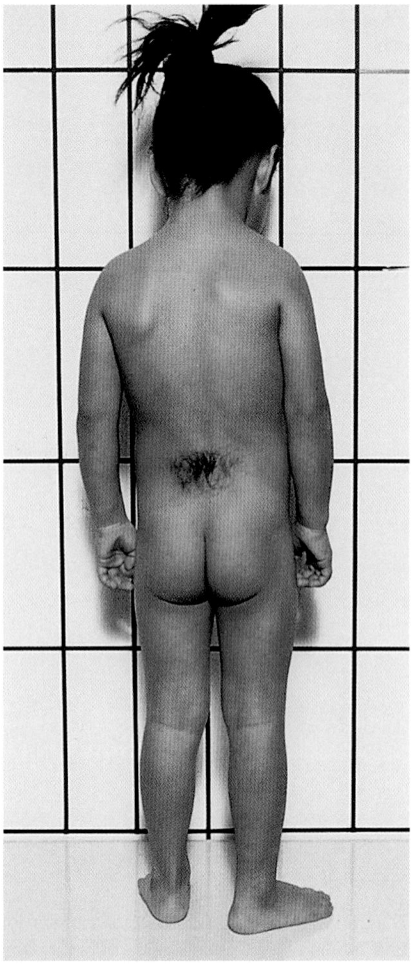

Fig. 17.14 A female child with a tuft of hair in the lumbosacral region indicating the site of a spina bifida occulta. (Courtesy A.E. Chudley, MD, Section of Genetics and Metabolism, Department of Pediatrics and Child Health, Children's Hospital and University of Manitoba, Winnipeg, Manitoba, Canada.)

Spina Bifida Cystica

Severe types of spina bifida, which involve protrusion of the spinal cord and/or meninges through defects in the vertebral arches, are referred to collectively as **spina bifida cystica** because of the **meningeal cyst** that is associated with these defects (Fig. 17.15; see Fig. 17.12B–D). This NTD occurs in approximately 1 of 5000 births and shows considerable geographic variation in incidence. When the cyst contains meninges and CSF, the defect is called **spinal bifida with meningocele**, the rarest form of spina bifida (see Fig. 17.12B). The spinal cord and spinal roots are in the normal position, but there may be spinal cord defects. Protrusion of the meninges and CSF of the spinal cord occurs through a defect in the vertebral column.

If the spinal cord or nerve roots are contained within the meningeal cyst, the defect is **spina bifida with meningomyelocele** (see Figs. 17.12C and 17.15A). Severe cases involving several vertebrae are associated with the absence of the calvaria (skullcap), the absence of most of the brain, and facial abnormalities; these severe defects are called **meroencephaly** (see Fig. 17.13 and 17.17). The defects entail drastic effects in some brain areas and lesser or no effects in others. For these neonates, death is inevitable. The term *anencephaly* for these severe defects is inappropriate because the term falsely implies that no part of the brain exists.

Spina bifida cystica shows various degrees of neurologic deficit, depending on the position and extent of the lesion. Dermatomal loss of sensation along with complete or partial skeletal muscle paralysis occurs with the lesion (see Fig. 17.15B). The level of the lesion determines the area of **anesthesia** (area of skin without sensation) and the muscles affected. **Sphincter paralysis** (bladder or anal sphincters) is common with **lumbosacral meningomyelocele** (see Figs. 17.12C and 17.15A).

Meroencephaly is strongly suspected in utero when there is a high level of **alpha-fetoprotein (AFP)** in the amniotic fluid (see Chapter 6, box titled "Alpha-Fetoprotein and Fetal Anomalies"). The level of AFP may also be elevated in maternal blood serum. Amniocentesis is usually performed on pregnant females with high levels of serum AFP for the determination of the AFP level in the amniotic fluid (see Fig. 6.13). An ultrasound scan may reveal an NTD that has resulted in spina bifida cystica. The fetal vertebral column can be detected by ultrasound at 10 to 12 weeks, and if there is a defect in the vertebral arch, a meningeal cyst may be detected in the affected area (see Figs. 17.12C and 17.15A).

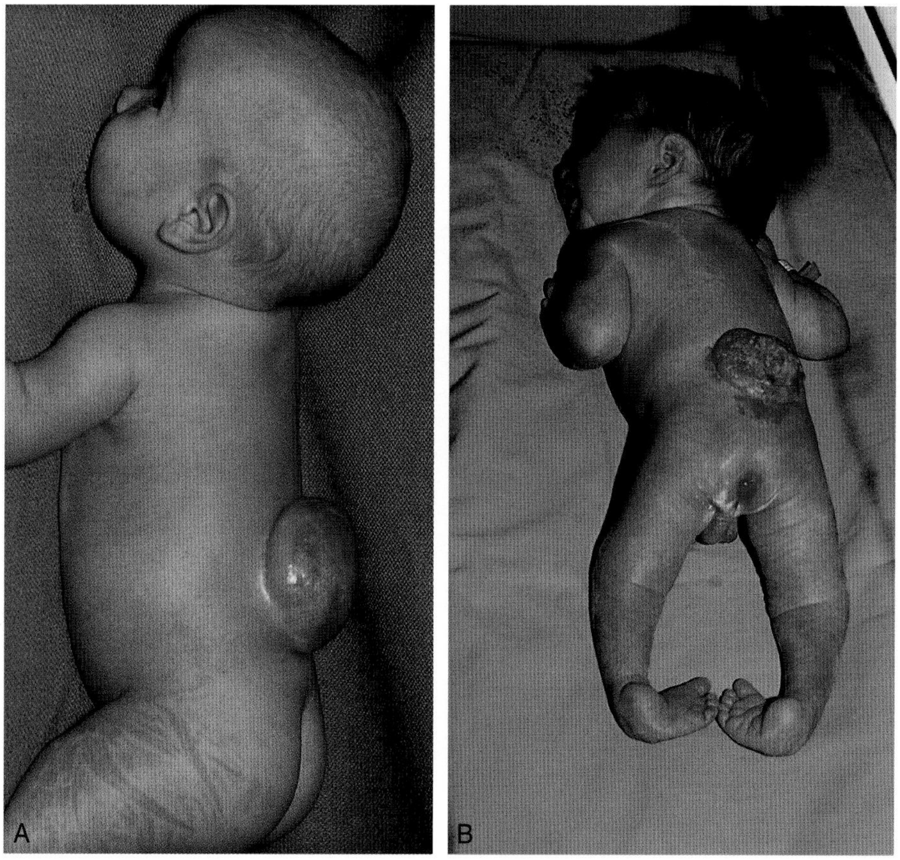

Fig. 17.15 Infants with spina bifida cystica. (A) Spina bifida with meningomyelocele in the lumbar region. (B) Spina bifida with myeloschisis in the lumbar region. Notice that the nerve involvement has affected the lower limbs of the infant. (Courtesy of the late Dr. Dwight Parkinson, Department of Surgery and Department of Human Anatomy and Cell Science, University of Manitoba, Winnipeg, Manitoba, Canada.)

Meningomyelocele (Open Spina Bifida) and Myeloschesis

Meningomyelocele is more common (0.2–0.4:1000 live births), is three to seven times more common in females, and is a more severe defect than spina bifida with meningocele (see Figs. 17.15A and 17.12B). This NTD may occur anywhere along the vertebral column; however, they are most common in the lumbar and sacral region (see Fig. 17.17). More than 90% of cases have associated hydrocephalus due to the coexistence of an **Arnold-Chiari malformation**. Some cases of meningomyelocele are associated with **craniolacunia** (defective development of the calvaria), which results in depressed, nonossified areas on the inner surfaces of the flat bones of the calvaria.

Myeloschisis is the most severe type of spina bifida (Fig. 17.16; see Figs. 17.12D and 17.15B). In this defect, the spinal cord in the affected area is open because the neural folds and overlying skin fail to fuse. As a result, the spinal cord is represented by a flattened mass of exposed nervous tissue. Myeloschisis usually results in permanent paralysis or weakness of the lower limbs.

Fetal surgery, before 26 weeks, may be an option to prevent progressive damage in menigomyelocele or myeloschisis, but does not treat existing damage to the spinal cord.

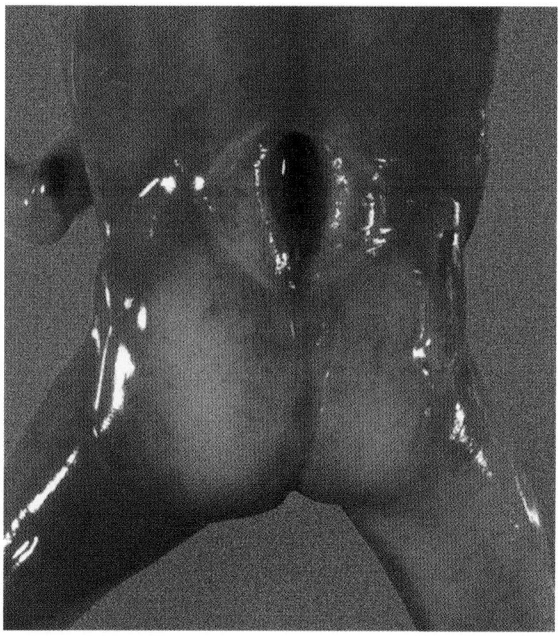

Fig. 17.16 A 19-week female fetus showing an open spinal defect in the lumbosacral region (spina bifida with myeloschisis). (Courtesy Dr. Joseph R. Siebert, Children's Hospital and Regional Medical Center, Seattle, Washington.)

Causes of Neural Tube Defects

Nutritional and environmental factors undoubtedly play a role in the production of NTDs (see Table 20.1). Gene-gene and gene-environment interactions are likely involved in most cases. Food fortification with folic acid and folic acid supplements taken before conception and continued for at least 3 months during pregnancy reduces the incidence of NTDs. In 2015 the Centers for Disease Control and Prevention urged "all women of childbearing age who can become pregnant to get 0.4 mg of folic acid every day to help reduce the risk of neural tube defects" (for more information, go https://www.cdc.gov/ncbddd/folicacid/index.html). Epidemiologic studies have also shown that low maternal B_{12} levels may significantly increase the risk of NTDs. Certain drugs (e.g., valproic acid) increase the risk of meningomyelocele. This anticonvulsant drug causes NTDs in 1% to 2% of pregnancies if taken during early pregnancy, when the neural folds are fusing (Fig. 17.17).

16

DEVELOPMENT OF BRAIN

The brain begins to develop during the third week, when the neural plate and tube are developing from the neuroectoderm (see Fig. 17.1). The **neural tube**, cranial to the fourth pair of somites, develops into the brain. Neuroprogenitor cells proliferate, migrate, and differentiate to form specific areas of the brain. Fusion of the neural folds in the cranial region and closure of the rostral neuropore form **three primary brain vesicles** from which the brain develops (Fig. 17.18):

- **Forebrain** (prosencephalon)
- **Midbrain** (mesencephalon)
- **Hindbrain** (rhombencephalon)

During the fifth week, the forebrain partly divides into two **secondary brain vesicles**, the **telencephalon** and **diencephalon**; the midbrain does not divide. The hindbrain partly divides into two vesicles, the **metencephalon** and **myelencephalon**. Consequently, there are five secondary brain vesicles (see Fig. 17.18). The development of the brain is closely involved with the surrounding meninges. Lineage tracing studies show that the meninges of the forebrain are derived from neural crest cells, and that the midbrain and hindbrain meninges originate from both neural crest and mesodermal cells. *The transcription factor FoxC1, which has been detected in all three layers of the meninges, appears to play a critical role in their formation.*

16

BRAIN FLEXURES

During the fifth week, the embryonic brain grows rapidly and bends ventrally with the head fold. The bending produces the **midbrain flexure** in the midbrain region and the **cervical flexure** at the junction of the hindbrain and spinal cord (Fig. 17.19A). Later, the development of the cortical layers and unequal growth of the brain between these flexures produce the **pontine flexure** in the opposite direction. This flexure results in thinning of the roof of the hindbrain (see Fig. 17.19C). *Early in development, a constriction-isthmic organizer is formed between the midbrain and hindbrain. It functions as a highly conserved signaling center. Wnt, Fgl, and retinoic acid expression, which occur in this region, have been implicated in the morphogenesis and patterning of the adjoining midbrain and hindbrain.*

Initially, the primordial brain has the same basic structure as the developing spinal cord; however, the brain flexures produce considerable variation in the outline of transverse sections at different levels of the brain and in the position of the gray and white matter. The **sulcus limitans** extends cranially to the junction of the midbrain and forebrain, and the alar and basal plates are recognizable only in the midbrain and hindbrain (see Figs. 17.5C and 17.19C).

HINDBRAIN

The **cervical flexure** demarcates the hindbrain from the spinal cord (see Fig. 17.19A). Later, this junction is arbitrarily defined as the level of the superior rootlet of the first cervical nerve, which is located roughly at the foramen magnum. The pontine flexure, divides the hindbrain into caudal (myelencephalon) and rostral (metencephalon) parts. The myelencephalon becomes the **medulla oblongata**, and the metencephalon becomes the **pons** and **cerebellum**. The cavity of the hindbrain becomes the **fourth ventricle** and the **central canal** in the medulla (see Fig. 17.19B and C).

MYELENCEPHALON

The caudal part of the myelencephalon resembles the spinal cord developmentally and structurally (see Fig. 17.19B). The neural canal of the neural tube forms the small central canal of the myelencephalon. Unlike those of the spinal cord, neuroblasts from the alar plates in the myelencephalon migrate into the marginal zone and form isolated areas of gray matter: the **gracile nuclei** medially and the **cuneate nuclei** laterally (see Fig. 17.19B). These nuclei are associated with correspondingly named nerve tracts that enter the medulla from the spinal cord. The ventral area of the medulla contains a pair of fiber bundles **(pyramids)** that consist of corticospinal fibers descending from the developing cerebral cortex (see Fig. 17.19B).

The rostral part of the myelencephalon (open part of the medulla) is wide and rather flat, especially opposite the pontine flexure (see Fig. 17.19C and D). The pontine flexure causes the lateral walls of the medulla to move laterally. As a result, its **roof plate** is stretched and greatly thinned (see Fig. 17.19C). The cavity of this part of the myelencephalon (part of the future fourth ventricle) becomes somewhat rhomboidal. As the walls of the medulla move laterally, the **alar plates** become lateral to the basal plates. As the positions of the plates change, the motor nuclei usually develop medial to the sensory nuclei (see Fig. 17.19C).

Neuroblasts in the **basal plates of the medulla**, like those in the spinal cord, develop into motor neurons. The neuroblasts form nuclei (groups of nerve cells) and organize into three cell columns on each side (see Fig. 17.19D). From medial to lateral, the columns are named as follows:

- **General somatic efferent**, represented by neurons of the hypoglossal nerve
- **Special visceral efferent**, represented by neurons innervating muscles derived from the pharyngeal arches (see Fig. 9.6)
- **General visceral efferent**, represented by some neurons of the vagus and glossopharyngeal nerves (see Fig. 9.6)

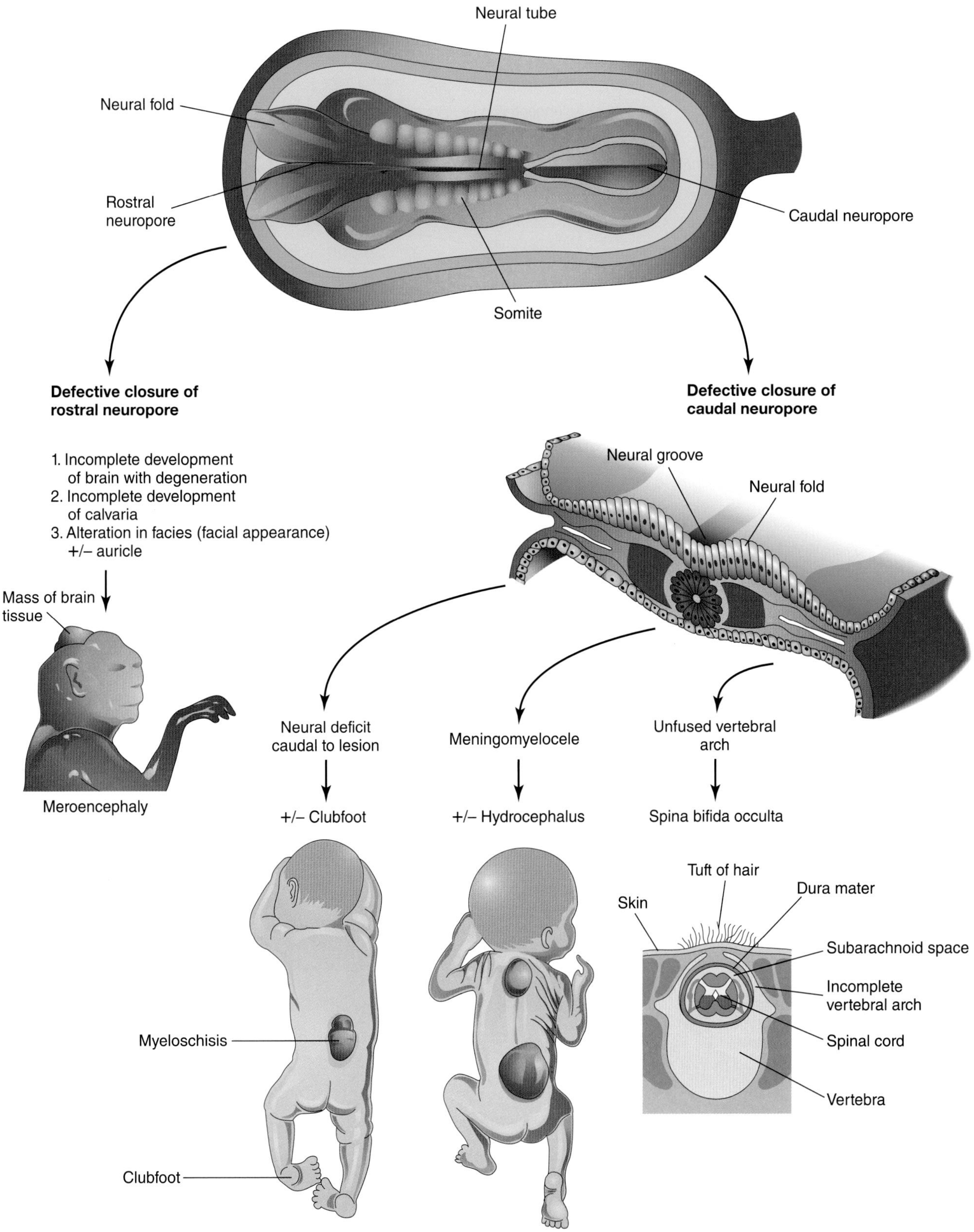

Fig. 17.17 Schematic illustration shows the embryologic basis of neural tube defects. Meroencephaly (partial absence of brain) results from defective closure of the rostral neuropore, and meningomyelocele results from defective closure of the caudal neuropore. (Modified from Jones KL: *Smith's recognizable patterns of human malformations*, ed 4, Philadelphia, 1988, Saunders.)

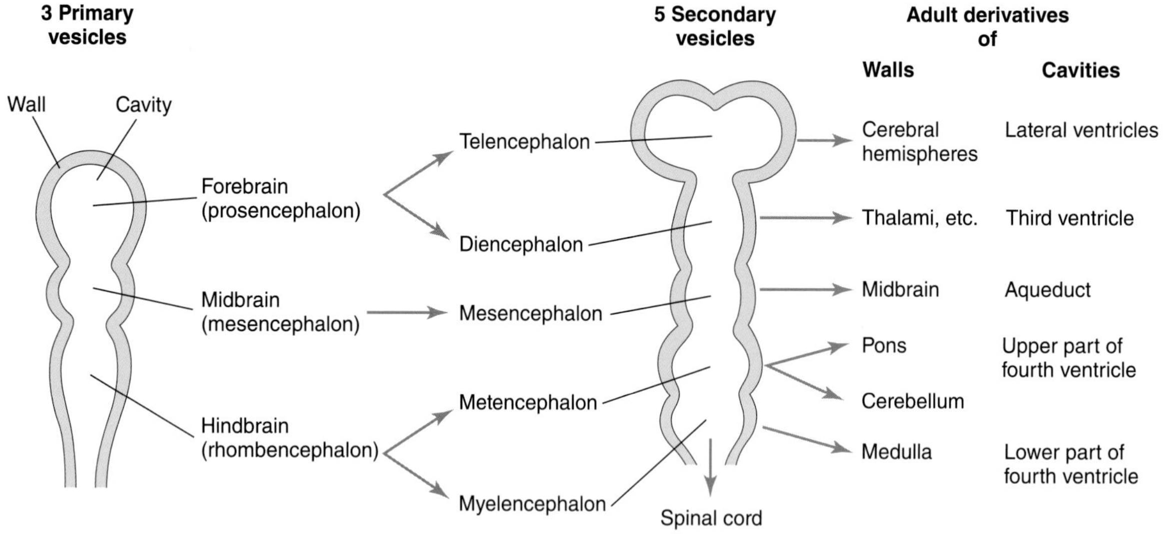

Fig. 17.18 Diagrammatic sketches of the brain vesicles indicate the adult derivatives of their walls and cavities. The rostral part of the third ventricle forms from the cavity of the telencephalon. Most of this ventricle is derived from the cavity of the diencephalon.

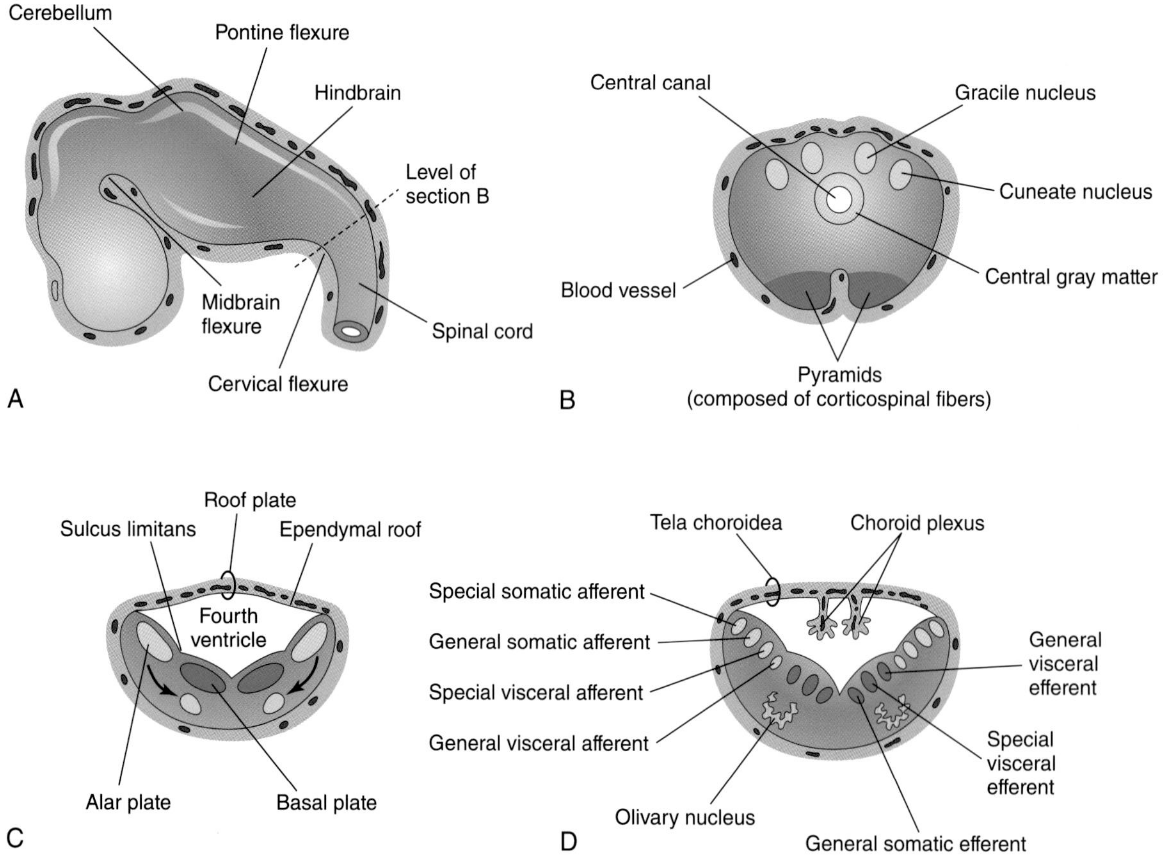

Fig. 17.19 (A) Sketch of the developing brain at the end of the fifth week of gestation shows the three primary divisions of the brain and brain flexures. (B) Transverse section of the caudal part of the myelencephalon (developing closed part of medulla). (C and D) Similar sections of the rostral part of the myelencephalon (developing open part of medulla) show the position and successive stages of differentiation of the alar and basal plates. The *arrows* in (C) show the pathway taken by neuroblasts from the alar plates to form the olivary nuclei.

Neuroblasts in the **alar plates of the medulla** form neurons that are arranged in four columns on each side. From medial to lateral, the columns are designated as follows:

- **General visceral afferent**, which receives impulses from the viscera
- **Special visceral afferent**, which receives taste fibers
- **General somatic afferent**, which receives impulses from the surface of the head
- **Special somatic afferent**, which receives impulses from the ear

Some neuroblasts from the alar plates migrate ventrally and form the neurons in the **olivary nuclei** (see Fig. 17.19C and D).

METENCEPHALON

The walls of the metencephalon form the **pons** and **cerebellum**, and the cavity of the metencephalon forms the superior part of the fourth ventricle (Fig. 17.20A). As in the rostral part of the myelencephalon, the pontine flexure causes divergence of the **lateral walls of the pons**, which spreads the gray matter in the floor of the fourth ventricle (see Fig. 17.20B). As in the myelencephalon, neuroblasts in each basal plate develop into motor nuclei and organize into three columns on each side.

The **cerebellum** develops from thickenings of **dorsal parts of the alar plates**. Initially, the **cerebellar swellings** project into the fourth ventricle (see Fig. 17.20B). As the swellings enlarge and fuse in the median plane, they overgrow the rostral half of the fourth ventricle and overlap the pons and medulla (see Fig. 17.20D). *The paired box transcription factor Pax6 plays an important role in cerebellar development.*

Some neuroblasts in the intermediate zone of the alar plates migrate to the marginal zone and differentiate into the neurons of the **cerebellar cortex**. Other neuroblasts from these plates give rise to the central nuclei, the largest of which is the **dentate nucleus** (see Fig. 17.20D). Cells from the alar plates also give rise to the **pontine nuclei**, **cochlear and vestibular nuclei**, and the **sensory nuclei of the trigeminal nerve**.

The structure of the cerebellum reflects its phylogenetic (evolutionary) development (see Fig. 17.20C and D):

- The archicerebellum **(flocculonodular lobe)**, the oldest part phylogenetically, has connections with the vestibular apparatus, especially the vestibule of the ear.

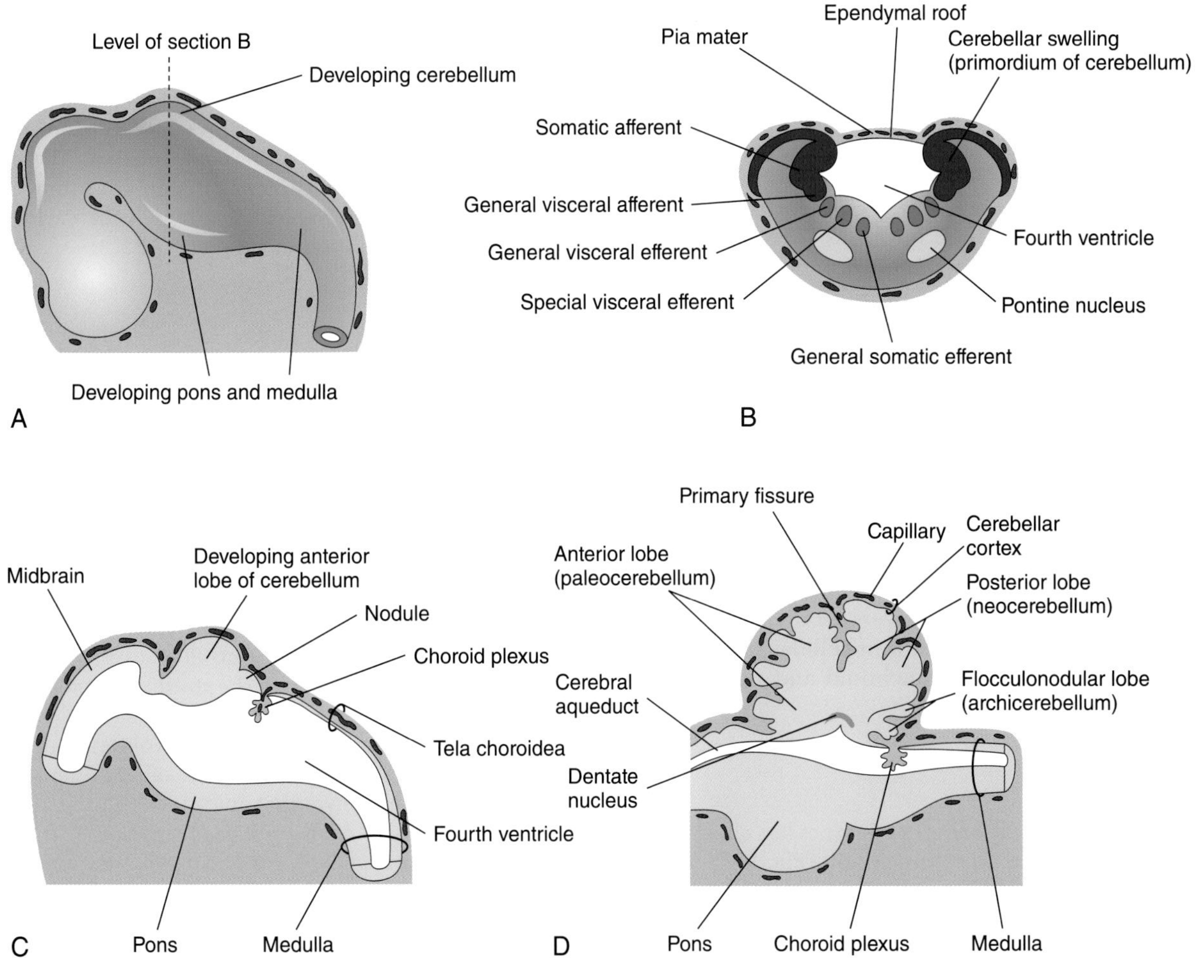

Fig. 17.20 (A) Sketch of the developing brain at the end of the fifth week. (B) Transverse section of the metencephalon (developing pons and cerebellum) shows the derivatives of the alar and basal plates. (C and D) Sagittal sections of the hindbrain at 6 and 17 weeks, respectively, show successive stages in the development of the pons and cerebellum.

- The paleocerebellum **(vermis and anterior lobe)**, of more recent development, is associated with sensory data from the limbs.
- The neocerebellum **(posterior lobe)**, the newest part phylogenetically, is concerned with selective control of limb movements.

Nerve fibers connecting the cerebral and cerebellar cortices with the spinal cord pass through the marginal layer of the ventral region of the metencephalon. This region of the brainstem, the pons, contains a robust band of nerve fibers that crosses the median plane and forms a bulky ridge on its anterior and lateral aspects (see Fig. 17.20C and D).

CHOROID PLEXUSES AND CEREBROSPINAL FLUID

16 The thin ependymal roof of the fourth ventricle is covered externally by the pia mater, which is derived from mesenchyme associated with the hindbrain (see Fig. 17.20B–D). This vascular membrane, together with the ependymal roof, forms the **tela choroidea**, the sheet of pia covering the lower part of the fourth ventricle (see Fig. 17.19D). Because of the active proliferation of the pia, the tela choroidea invaginates the fourth ventricle, where it differentiates into the **choroid plexus**, infoldings of choroidal arteries of the pia (see Figs. 17.19C and D and 17.20C and D). Similar plexuses develop in the roof of the third ventricle and the medial walls of the lateral ventricles.

The choroid plexuses secrete ventricular fluid, which becomes CSF as additions are made to it from the surfaces of the brain, spinal cord, and the pia-arachnoid layer of the meninges. Various signaling morphogens are found in CSF and the choroid plexus that are necessary for brain development. The thin roof of the fourth ventricle evaginates in three locations. These outpouchings rupture to form openings, the **median** and **lateral apertures** (foramen of Magendie and foramina of Luschka, respectively), which permit the CSF to enter the subarachnoid space from the fourth ventricle. Specific neurogenic molecules (e.g., retinoic acid) control the proliferation and differentiation of neuroprogenitor cells. The epithelial lining of the choroid plexus is derived from neuroepithelium, whereas the stroma develops from mesenchymal cells.

The main site of absorption of CSF into the venous system is through the **arachnoid villi**, which are protrusions of arachnoid mater into the **dural venous sinuses** (large venous channels between the layers of the dura mater). The arachnoid villi consist of a thin cellular layer derived from the epithelium of the arachnoid and the endothelium of the sinus.

MIDBRAIN

The midbrain **(mesencephalon)** undergoes less change than most other parts of the developing brain (Fig. 17.21A). The neural canal narrows and becomes the **cerebral aqueduct** (see Figs. 17.20D and 17.21D), a channel that connects the third and fourth ventricles.

Neuroblasts migrate from the **alar plates of the midbrain** into the **tectum** and aggregate to form four large groups of neurons, the paired **superior and inferior colliculi** (see Fig. 17.21C–E), which are concerned with visual and auditory reflexes, respectively. Neuroblasts from the **basal plates** may give rise to the red nuclei, nuclei of third and fourth cranial nerves, and reticular nuclei in the **tegmentum of the midbrain**. The **substantia nigra**, a broad layer of gray matter adjacent to the **crus cerebri** (cerebral peduncles) may also differentiate from the basal plate (see Fig. 17.21B, D, and E); however, some research indicates that the substantia nigra may derived from cells in the alar plate that migrate ventrally.

Fibers growing from the **cerebrum** (diencephalon and cerebral hemispheres) form the **crus cerebri** (cerebral peduncles) anteriorly (see Fig. 17.21B). The peduncles become progressively more prominent as more descending fiber groups (corticopontine, corticobulbar, and corticospinal) pass through the developing midbrain on their way to the brainstem and spinal cord (see Fig. 17.21C).

FOREBRAIN

As the closure of the **rostral neuropore** occurs (see Fig. 17.3B), bilateral forebrain outgrowths **(optic vesicles)** appear (see Fig. 17.4A). These vesicles are the primordia of the retinae and optic nerves (see Figs. 18.1C, F, and H and 18.11). A second pair of diverticula, the **telencephalic vesicles**, soon arise more dorsally and rostrally (see Fig. 17.21C). They are the primordia of the cerebral hemispheres, and their cavities become the **lateral ventricles** (see Fig. 17.26B).

The rostral part of the forebrain, including the primordia of the **cerebral hemispheres**, is the **telencephalon**; the caudal part of the forebrain is the **diencephalon**. The cavities of the telencephalon and diencephalon contribute to the formation of the **third ventricle**, although the cavity of the diencephalon contributes more (Fig. 17.22E).

DIENCEPHALON

Three swellings develop in the lateral walls of the third ventricle, which later become the **thalamus, hypothalamus**, and **epithalamus** (see Fig. 17.22C–E). The thalamus is separated from the epithalamus by the **epithalamic sulcus** and from the hypothalamus by the **hypothalamic sulcus** (see Fig. 17.22E). The latter sulcus is not a continuation of the **sulcus limitans** into the forebrain, and it does not, like the sulcus limitans, divide sensory and motor areas (see Fig. 17.22C).

The thalamus, a large ovoid mass of gray matter, develops rapidly on each side of the third ventricle and bulges into its cavity (see Fig. 17.22E). The thalami meet and fuse in the midline in approximately 70% to 80% of brains, forming a bridge of gray matter across the third ventricle, the interthalamic adhesion.

The hypothalamus arises by the proliferation of neuroblasts in the intermediate zone of the diencephalic walls, ventral to the hypothalamic sulci (see Fig. 17.22E). *Differential expression of Wnt/β-catenin signaling is essential for the induction, neuronal differentiation, and patterning of the hypothalamus.* Later, several nuclei concerned with endocrine activities and homeostasis develop. A pair of nuclei forms pea-sized **mammillary bodies** on the ventral surface of the hypothalamus (see Fig. 17.22C).

The **epithalamus** develops from the roof and dorsal portion of the lateral wall of the diencephalons (see

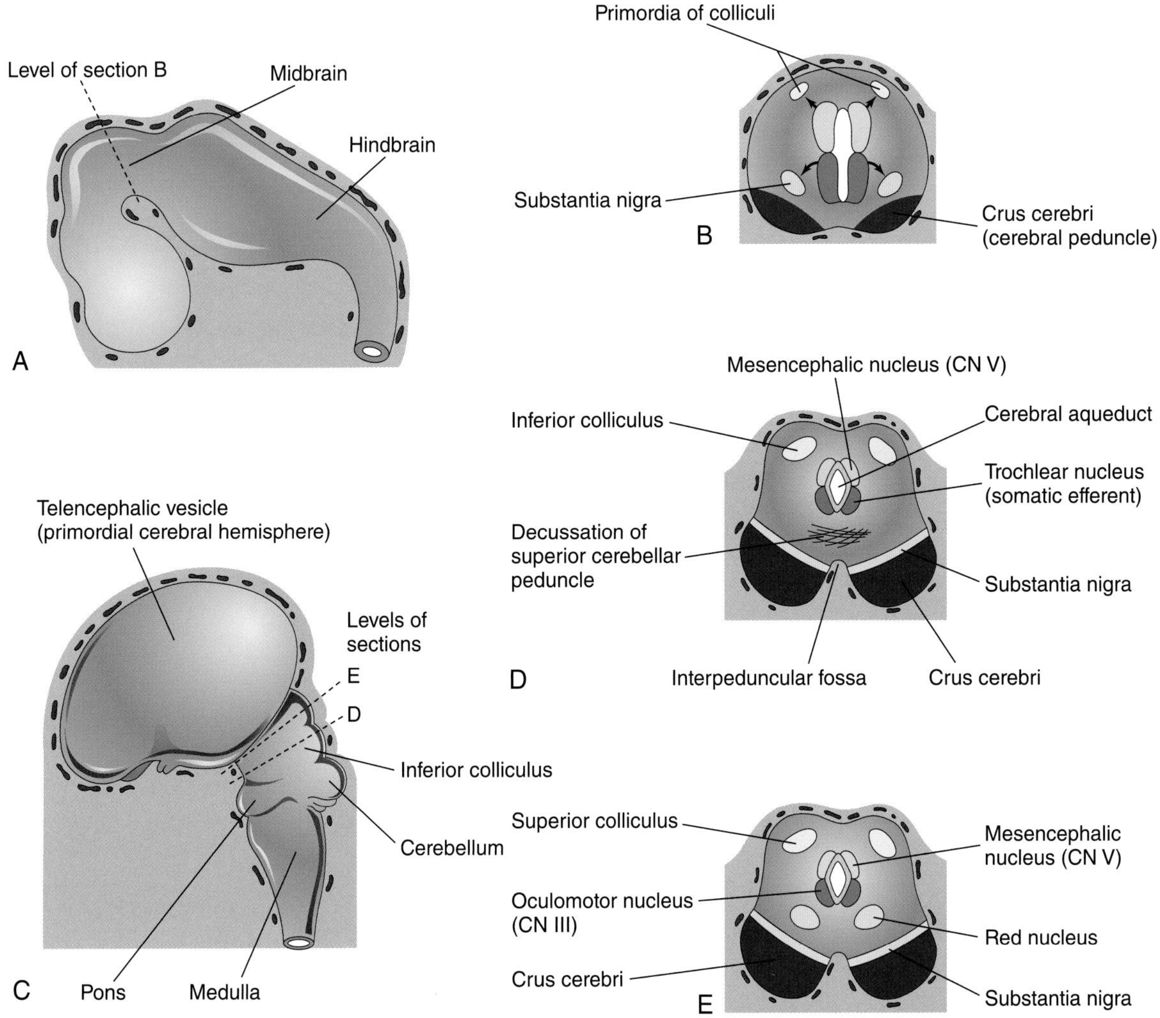

Fig. 17.21 (A) Sketch of the developing brain at the end of the fifth week. (B) Transverse section of the developing midbrain shows the early migration of cells from the basal and alar plates. (C) Sketch of the developing brain at 11 weeks. (D and E) Transverse sections of the developing midbrain at the level of the inferior and superior colliculi, respectively.

Fig. 17.22C–E). Initially, the **epithalamic swellings** are large, but later they become relatively small.

The **pineal gland** (pineal body) develops as a median diverticulum of the caudal part of the roof of the diencephalon (see Fig. 17.22D). The proliferation of cells in its walls soon converts it into a solid, cone-shaped gland.

The **pituitary gland** (hypophysis) is ectodermal in origin (Fig. 17.23 and Table 17.1). The *Notch signaling pathway has been implicated in the proliferation and differentiation of pituitary progenitor cells.* The pituitary develops from two sources:

- An upgrowth from the ectodermal roof of the stomodeum, the **hypophyseal diverticulum** (Rathke pouch)
- A downgrowth from the neuroectoderm of the diencephalon, the **neurohypophyseal diverticulum**

This double origin explains why the pituitary gland is composed of two different types of tissue:

- The **adenohypophysis** (glandular tissue), or anterior lobe, arises from the oral ectoderm.
- The **neurohypophysis** (nervous tissue), or posterior lobe, arises from the neuroectoderm.

By the third week, the hypophyseal diverticulum projects from the roof of the stomodeum and lies adjacent to the floor (ventral wall) of the diencephalon (see Fig. 17.23C). By the fifth week, the diverticulum has elongated and constricted at its attachment to the oral epithelium. By this stage, it has come into contact with the **infundibulum** (derived from the neurohypophyseal diverticulum), a ventral downgrowth of the diencephalon (see Figs. 17.23C and D and 17.23).

The stalk of the hypophyseal diverticulum passes between the chondrification centers of the developing presphenoid and basisphenoid bones of the cranium (see Fig. 17.23E). During the sixth week, the connection of the diverticulum with the oral cavity degenerates (see Fig. 17.23D and E). Cells of the anterior wall of the hypophyseal diverticulum proliferate and give rise to the **pars anterior of the pituitary gland** (see Table 17.1). Later, an extension, the **pars tuberalis**, grows around the **infundibular stem** (see Fig. 17.23E). The extensive proliferation of the anterior wall of the hypophyseal diverticulum reduces its lumen to a narrow cleft (see Fig. 17.23E). The **residual cleft** is usually not recognizable in the adult pituitary gland; however, it may be

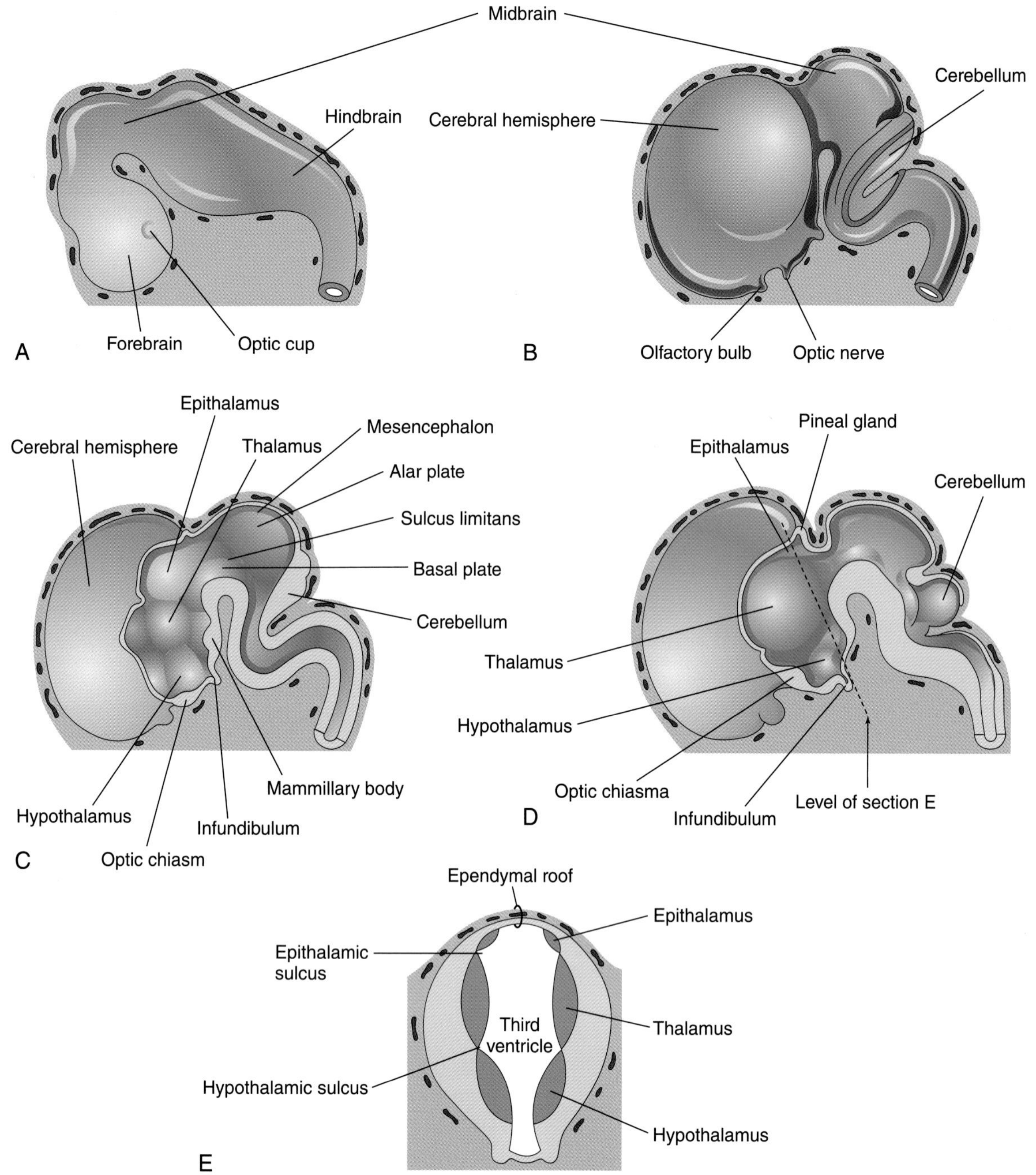

Fig. 17.22 (A) Sketch shows an external view of the brain at the end of the fifth week. (B) Similar view at 7 weeks. (C) Median section of the brain at 7 weeks shows the medial surface of the forebrain and midbrain. (D) Similar section at 8 weeks. (E) Transverse section of the diencephalon shows the epithalamus dorsally, the thalamus laterally, and the hypothalamus ventrally.

represented by a zone of cysts. Cells in the posterior wall of the hypophyseal pouch do not proliferate; they give rise to the thin, poorly defined **pars intermedia** (see Fig. 17.23F).

The part of the pituitary gland that develops from the neurohypophyseal diverticulum is the **neurohypophysis** (see Fig. 17.23B–F and Table 17.1). The **infundibulum** gives rise to the **median eminence**, **infundibular stem**, and **pars nervosa**. Initially, the walls of the infundibulum are thin, but the distal end of the infundibulum soon becomes solid as the neuroepithelial cells proliferate. These cells later differentiate into **pituicytes**, the primary cells of the posterior lobe of the pituitary gland, which are closely related to neuroglial cells. Nerve fibers grow into the pars nervosa from the hypothalamic area, to which the infundibular stem is attached (see Fig. 17.23F).

Ephrin-β2 and other signaling molecules (e.g., FGF8, BMP4, and WNT5A) from the diencephalon play an essential role in the formation of the anterior and intermediate lobes of the pituitary gland. The LIM homeobox gene LHX2 *appears to control the development of the posterior lobe.*

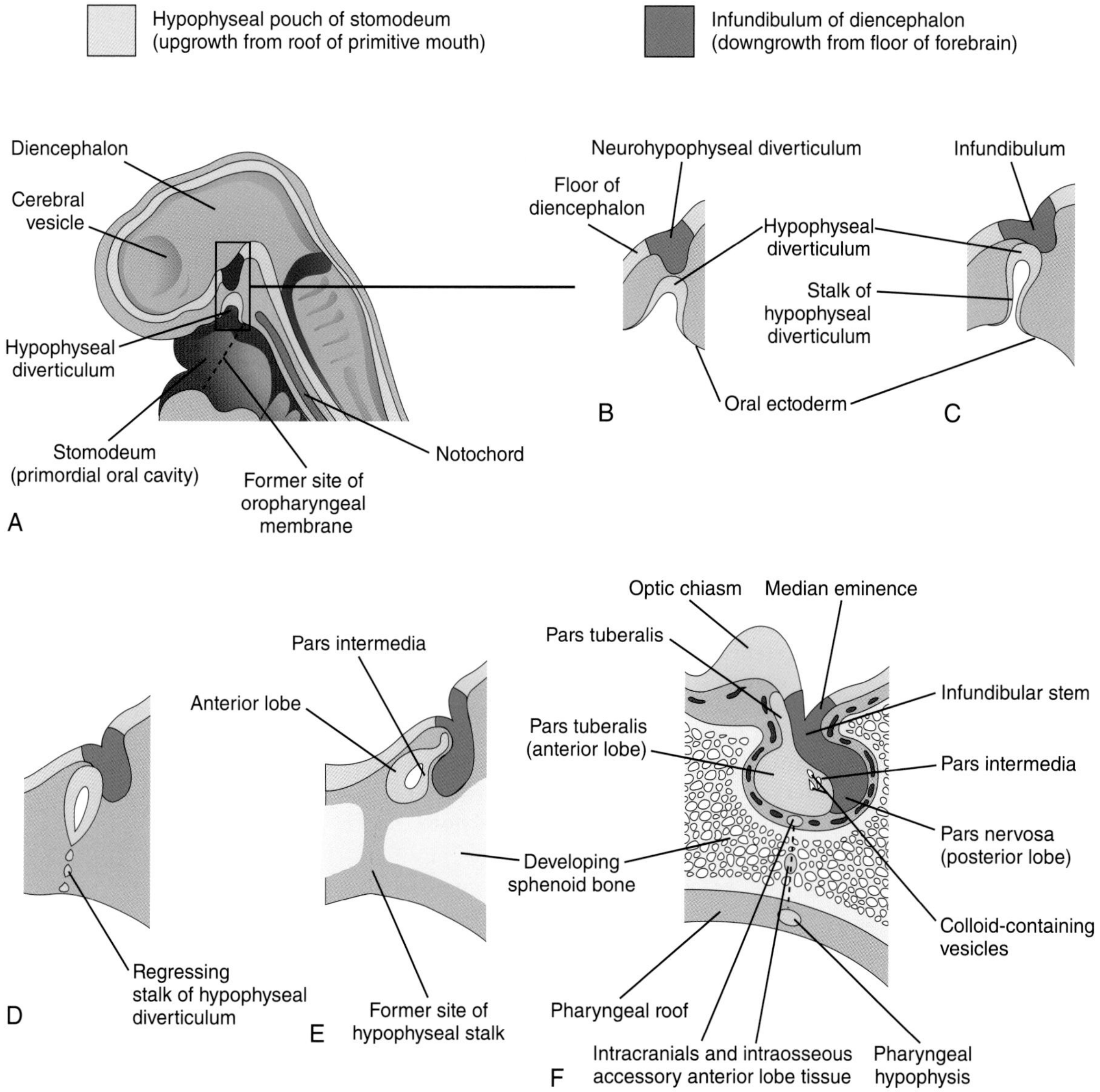

Fig. 17.23 Diagrammatic sketches illustrate the development of the pituitary gland. (A) Sagittal section of the cranial end of an embryo at approximately 36 days shows the hypophyseal diverticulum, an upgrowth from the stomodeum, and the neurohypophyseal diverticulum, a downgrowth from the forebrain. (B–D) Successive stages of the developing pituitary gland. By 8 weeks, the diverticulum loses its connection with the oral cavity and is in close contact with the infundibulum and posterior lobe (neurohypophysis) of the pituitary gland. (E and F) Sketches of later stages show proliferation of the anterior wall of the hypophyseal diverticulum to form the anterior lobe (adenohypophysis) of the pituitary gland.

Table 17.1 Pituitary Gland Derivation and Terminology

Derivation	Tissue Type	Part	Lobe
Oral Ectoderm			
Hypophyseal diverticulum from the roof of the stomodeum	Adenohypophysis (glandular tissue)	Pars anterior Pars tuberalis Pars intermedia	Anterior lobe
Neuroectoderm			
Neurohypophyseal diverticulum from the floor of the diencephalon	Neurohypophysis (nervous tissue)	Pars nervosa Infundibular stem Median eminence	Posterior lobe

Pharyngeal Hypophysis and Craniopharyngioma

A remnant of the stalk of the hypophyseal diverticulum may persist and form a **pharyngeal hypophysis** in the roof of the oropharynx (see Fig. 17.23F). Rarely, masses of anterior lobe tissue develop outside the capsule of the pituitary gland, within the sella turcica of the sphenoid bone (Fig. 17.24). A persistent hypophyseal canal is visible in radiologic images of the neonatal sphenoid bone in approximately 0.5% of cases.

Occasionally, an extremely rare (1:1,000,000), benign tumor **(craniopharyngioma)** develops in or superior to the sella turcica. Less often, these tumors form in the pharynx or basisphenoid (posterior part of the sphenoid) from remnants of the stalk of the hypophyseal diverticulum (see Fig. 17.24). These tumors arise along the path of the hypophyseal diverticulum from epithelial remnants (see Fig. 17.23D–F).

TELENCEPHALON

The telencephalon consists of a median part and two lateral diverticula, the **cerebral vesicles** (see Fig. 17.23A). These vesicles are the primordia of the **cerebral hemispheres** (see Figs. 17.22B and 17.23A). The cavity of the median portion of the telencephalon forms the extreme anterior part of the **third ventricle** (Fig. 17.25). At first, the cerebral hemispheres are in wide communication with the cavity of the third ventricle through the **interventricular foramina** (Fig. 17.26B; see Fig. 17.25).

Along the **choroid fissure**, part of the medial wall of the developing cerebral hemisphere becomes very thin (see Figs. 17.25 and 17.26A and B). Initially, this ependymal portion lies in the roof of the hemisphere and is continuous with the ependymal roof of the third ventricle (see Fig. 17.26A). The **choroid plexus of the lateral ventricle** later forms at this site (Fig. 17.27; see Fig. 17.25).

As the cerebral hemispheres expand, they cover successively the diencephalon, midbrain, and hindbrain. The hemispheres eventually meet each other in the midline, and their medial surfaces become flattened. The mesenchyme trapped in the longitudinal fissure between them gives rise to the **cerebral falx** *(falx cerebri)*, a median fold of the dura mater.

The **corpus striatum** appears during the sixth week as a prominent swelling in the floor of each cerebral hemisphere (see Fig. 17.27B). The floor of each hemisphere expands more slowly than its thin cortical walls because it contains the rather large corpus striatum, and the cerebral hemispheres become C-shaped (Fig. 17.28A and B).

The growth and curvature of the cerebral hemispheres affect the shape of the lateral ventricles, which become roughly C-shaped cavities filled with CSF. The caudal end of each hemisphere turns ventrally and then rostrally, forming the **temporal lobe** (Fig. 17.29C); in so doing, it carries the lateral ventricle (forming its **temporal horn**) and choroid fissure with it (see Fig. 17.28B and C). The thin medial wall of the hemisphere is invaginated along the choroid fissure by vascular pia mater to form the **choroid plexus of the temporal horn** (see Fig. 17.27B).

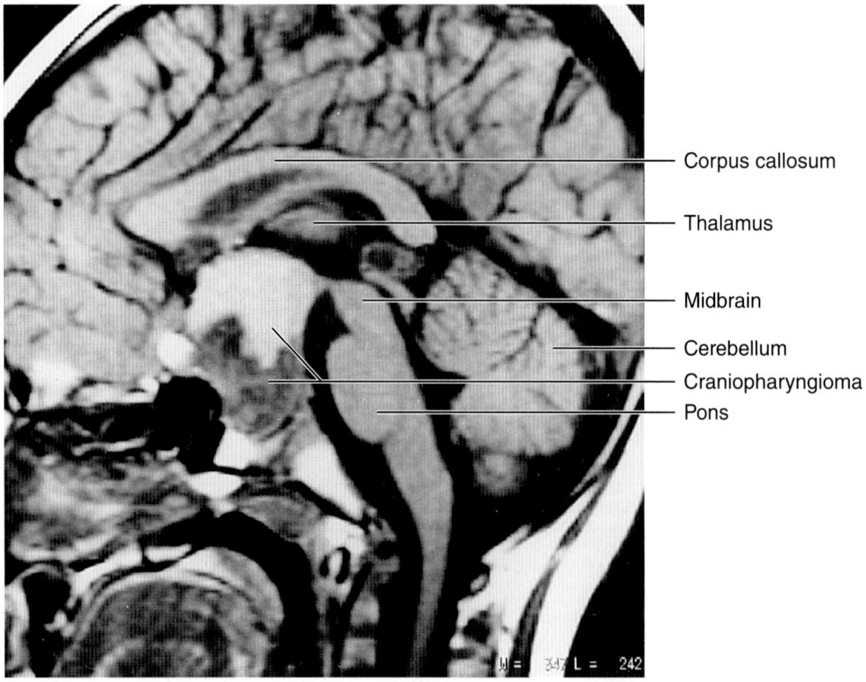

Fig. 17.24 Sagittal magnetic resonance image of the brain of a 4-year-old boy whose presenting symptoms were headaches and optic atrophy (vision loss). A large mass (4 cm) occupies an enlarged sella turcica, expanding inferiorly into the sphenoid bone and superiorly into the suprasellar cistern. A craniopharyngioma was confirmed by surgery. The inferior half of the mass is solid and appears dark, whereas the superior half is cystic and appears brighter. (Courtesy Dr. Gerald S. Smyser, Altru Health System, Grand Forks, North Dakota.)

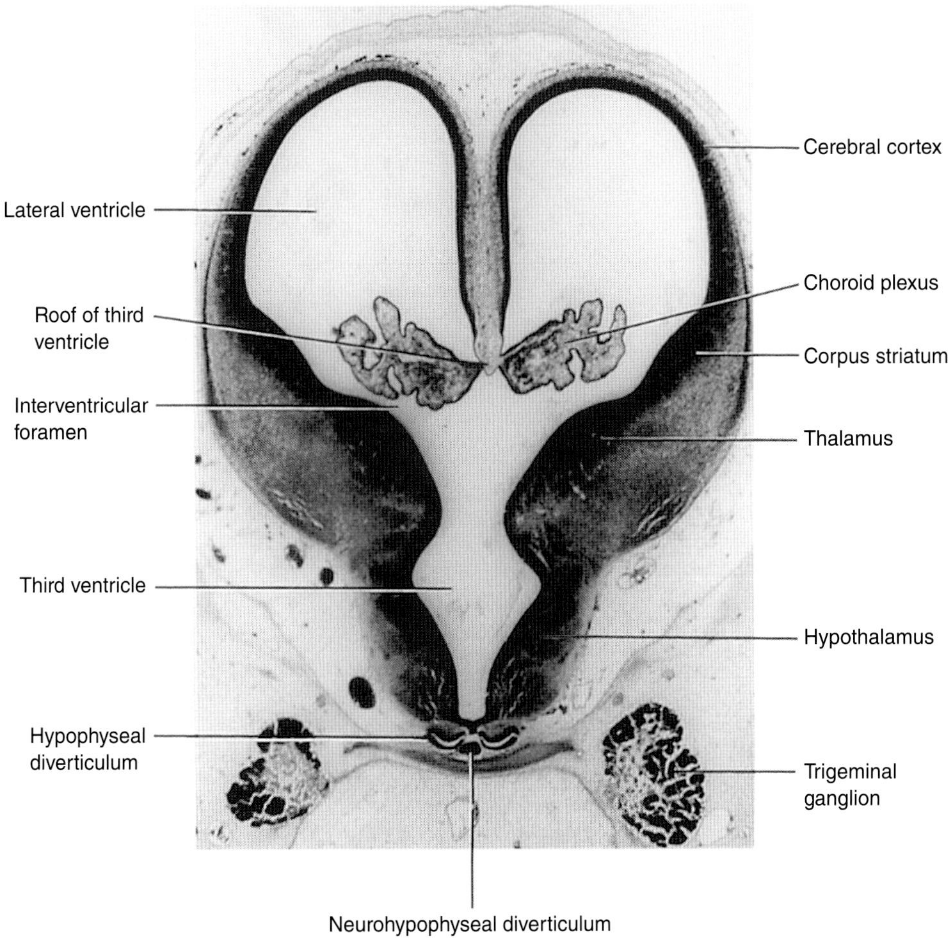

Fig. 17.25 Photomicrograph of a transverse section through the diencephalon and cerebral vesicles of a human embryo (approximately 50 days) at the level of the interventricular foramina (×20). The choroid fissure is located at the junction of the choroid plexus and the medial wall of the lateral ventricle. (Courtesy the late Professor Jean Hay, Department of Anatomy, University of Manitoba, Winnipeg, Manitoba, Canada.)

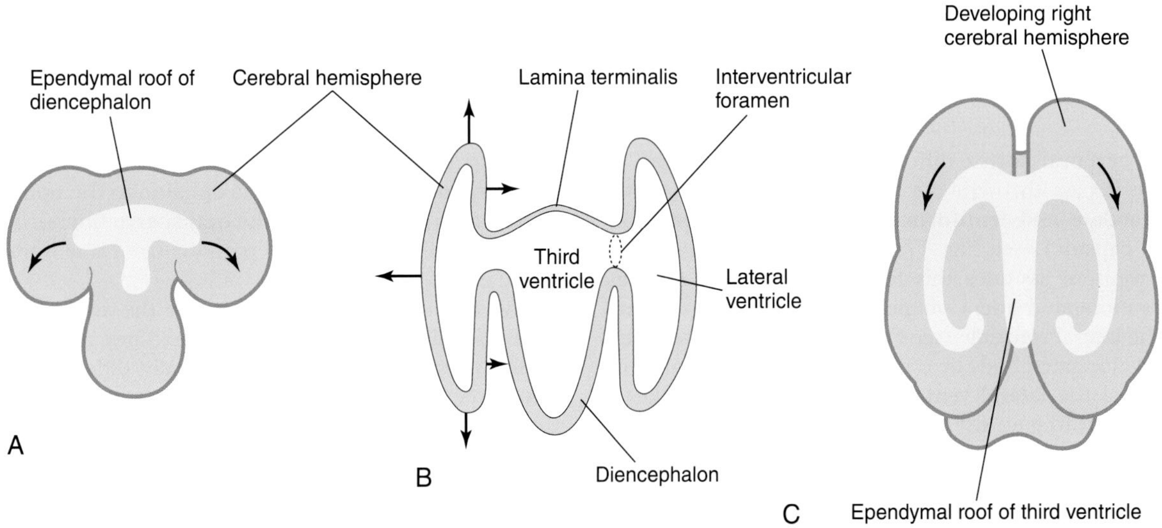

Fig. 17.26 (A) Sketch of the dorsal surface of the forebrain indicates how the ependymal roof of the diencephalon is carried out to the dorsomedial surface of the cerebral hemispheres *(arrows)*. (B) Diagrammatic section of the forebrain shows how the developing cerebral hemispheres grow from the lateral walls of the forebrain and expand in all directions until they cover the diencephalon. The *arrows* indicate some directions in which the hemispheres expand. The rostral wall of the forebrain, the lamina terminalis, is very thin. (C) Sketch of the forebrain shows how the ependymal roof is finally carried into the temporal lobes as a result of the C-shaped growth pattern of the cerebral hemispheres *(arrows)*.

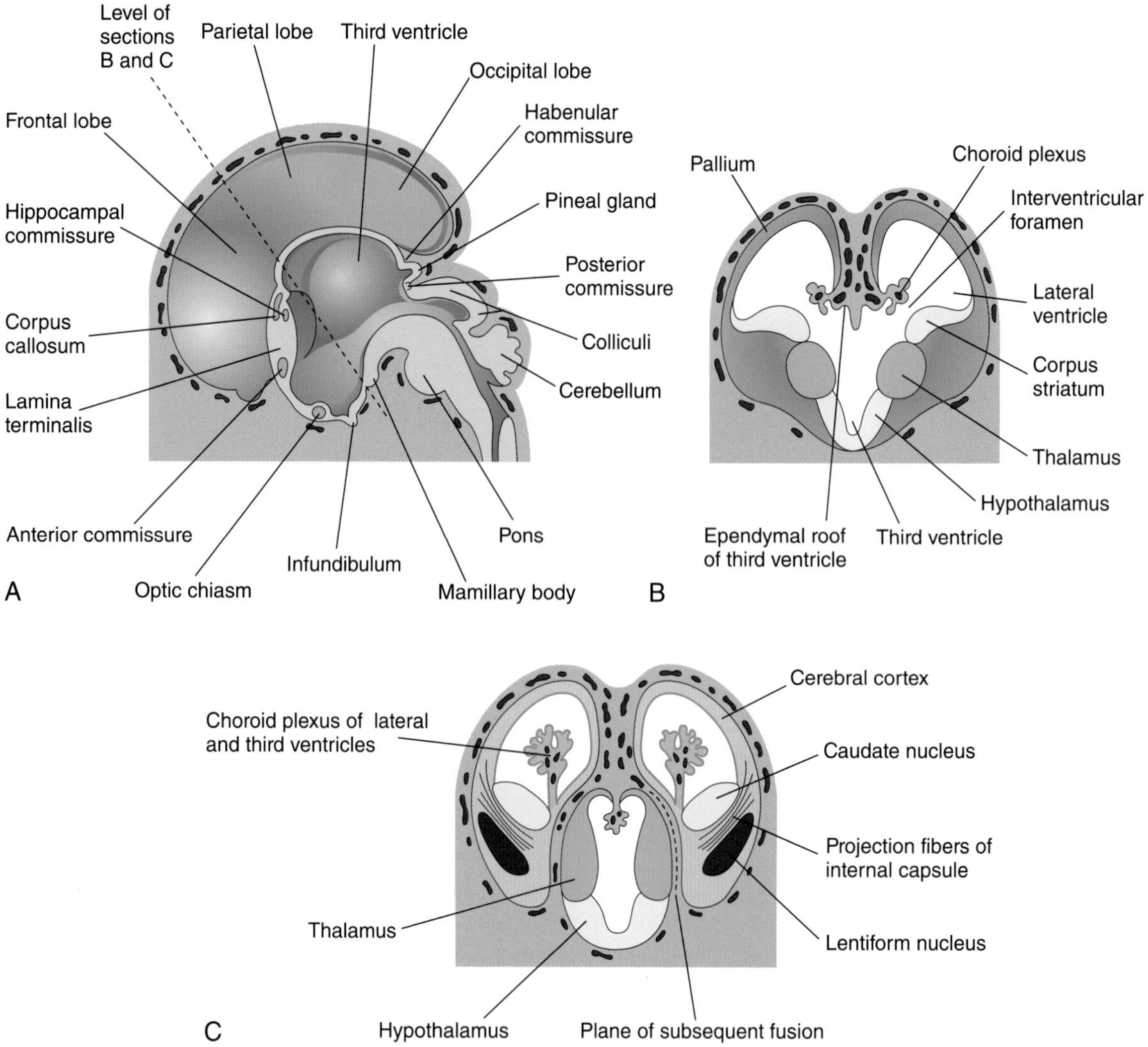

Fig. 17.27 (A) Drawing of the medial surface of the forebrain of a 10-week embryo shows the diencephalic derivatives, the main commissures, and the expanding cerebral hemispheres. (B) Transverse section of the forebrain at the level of the interventricular foramina shows the corpus striatum and choroid plexuses of the lateral ventricles. (C) Similar section at approximately 11 weeks shows the division of the corpus striatum into the caudate and lentiform nuclei by the internal capsule. The developing relationship of the cerebral hemispheres to the diencephalon is also illustrated.

As the cerebral cortex differentiates, fibers coursing to and from it pass through the **corpus striatum** and divide it into **caudate and lentiform nuclei**. This fiber pathway **(internal capsule)** (see Fig. 17.27C) becomes C-shaped as the hemisphere assumes this form. The **caudate nucleus** becomes elongated and C-shaped, conforming to the outline of the lateral ventricle (see Fig. 17.28C). Its pear-shaped head and elongated body lie on the floor of the frontal horn and body of the **lateral ventricle**, whereas its tail makes a U-shaped turn to gain the roof of the temporal or inferior horn.

CEREBRAL COMMISSURES

As the cerebral cortex develops, groups of nerve fibers (commissures) connect corresponding areas of the cerebral hemispheres with one another (see Fig. 17.27). The most important of these commissures crosses in the **lamina terminalis**, which is the rostral (anterior) end of the forebrain (see Fig. 17.26A and B and 17.27A). This lamina extends from the roof plate of the diencephalon to the **optic chiasm** (decussation or crossing of the optic nerve fibers). The lamina terminalis is the natural pathway from one hemisphere to the other.

The first commissures to form are the **anterior commissure** and **hippocampal commissure**. They are small fiber bundles that connect phylogenetically older parts of the brain (see Fig. 17.27A). The anterior commissure connects the **olfactory bulb** (rostral extremity of the olfactory tract) and related areas of one hemisphere with those of the opposite side. The hippocampal commissure connects the hippocampal formations.

The largest cerebral commissure is the corpus callosum (see Figs. 17.27A and 17.28A), which connects neocortical areas. The corpus callosum initially lies in the lamina terminalis, but fibers are added to it as the cortex enlarges, and it gradually extends beyond the lamina terminalis. The rest

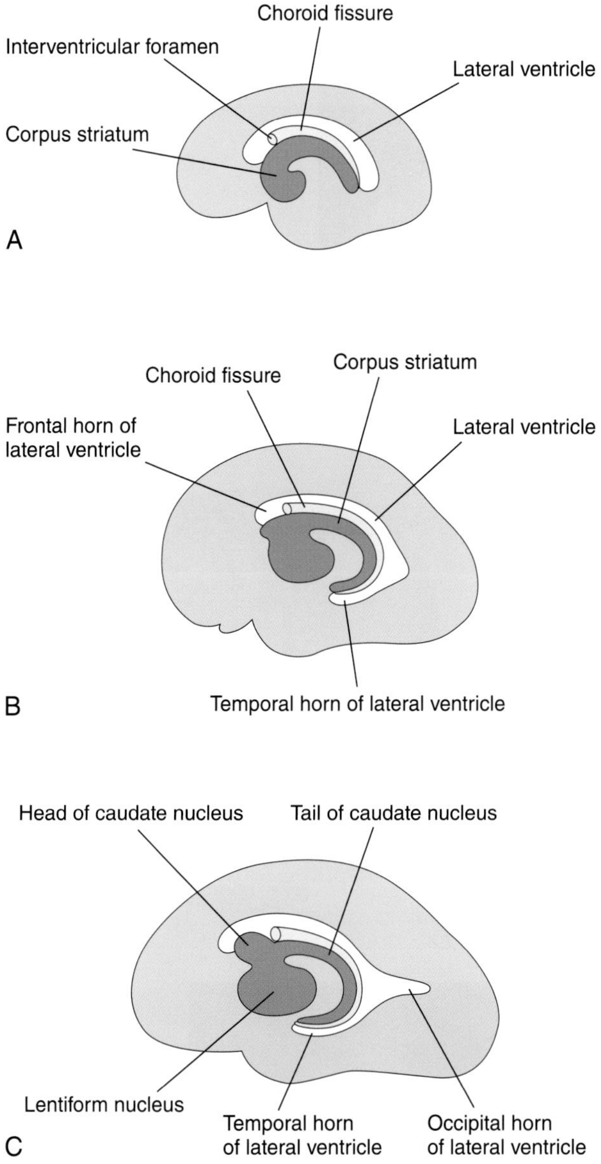

Fig. 17.28 Schematic diagrams of the medial surface of the developing right cerebral hemisphere show development of the lateral ventricle, choroid fissure, and corpus striatum. (A) At 13 weeks. (B) At 21 weeks. (C) At 32 weeks.

of the **lamina terminalis** lies between the corpus callosum and the fornix. It becomes stretched to form the **septum pellucidum**, a thin plate of brain tissue containing nerve cells and fibers.

At birth, the **corpus callosum** extends over the roof of the diencephalon. The **optic chiasm** consists of fibers from the medial halves of the retinas that cross to join the optic tract of the opposite side.

The walls of the developing cerebral hemispheres initially show three typical zones of the neural tube: ventricular, intermediate, and marginal; later a fourth one, the *subventricular zone*, appears. Cells of the intermediate zone migrate into the marginal zone and give rise to the cortical layers. The gray matter is located peripherally, and axons from its cell bodies pass centrally to form the large volume of white matter **(medullary center)**.

Initially, the surface of the cerebral hemispheres is smooth (see Fig. 17.29A); however, as growth proceeds, **sulci** (grooves) between the **gyri** (tortuous convolutions) develop (Fig. 17.30A; see Fig. 17.29B and D). The gyri are caused by infolding of the cerebral cortex. The sulci and gyri permit a considerable increase in the surface area of the cerebral cortex without requiring an extensive increase in the size of the neurocranium (see Fig. 17.30B and C). At its peak activity, neurogenesis adds approximately 100,000 cells and 400,000 new synapses per minute. As each cerebral hemisphere grows, the cortex covering the external surface of the corpus striatum grows relatively slowly and is soon overgrown (see Fig. 17.29D). This buried cortex, hidden from view in the depths of the **lateral sulcus** of the cerebral hemisphere (see Fig. 17.30A), is the **insula**.

BIRTH DEFECTS OF THE BRAIN

Because of the complexity of its embryologic history, abnormal development of the brain is common (approximately 3 of 1000 births). Most major birth defects, such as **meroencephaly** and **meningoencephalocele**, result from defective closure of the rostral neuropore (an NTD) during the fourth week (Fig. 17.31C) and involve the overlying tissues (meninges and calvaria). The factors causing NTDs are genetic, nutritional, and environmental. Birth defects of the brain can be caused by alterations in the morphogenesis or histogenesis of the nervous tissue, or they can result from developmental failures occurring in associated structures (notochord, somites, mesenchyme, and cranium).

Abnormal histogenesis of the cerebral cortex can result in **seizures** (Fig. 17.32) and various degrees of **cognitive deficiency**. Such deficiency may also result from exposure of the embryo or fetus during the 8- to 16-week period to viruses such as **cytomegalovirus, rubella virus**, or other teratogens (see Table 20.1). **Prenatal risk factors**, such as maternal infection, fetal stroke, cerebral hemorrhage, and some hereditary and genetic conditions, cause most cases of **cerebral palsy**. Preterm birth is the most common cause of cerebral palsy in North America. It appears that hypoxia during delivery is not as common a cause as was once thought.

Encephalocele

Encephalocele is a herniation of intracranial contents resulting from a defect in the cranium **(cranium bifidum)**. Encephaloceles are most common in the occipital region (Figs. 17.33 and 17.34; see Fig. 17.31A–D). The hernia may contain meninges **(meningocele)**; meninges and part of the brain **(meningoencephalocele)**; or meninges, part of the brain, and part of the ventricular system **(meningohydroencephalocele)**. Encephalocele occurs in approximately 1 of 10,000 births.

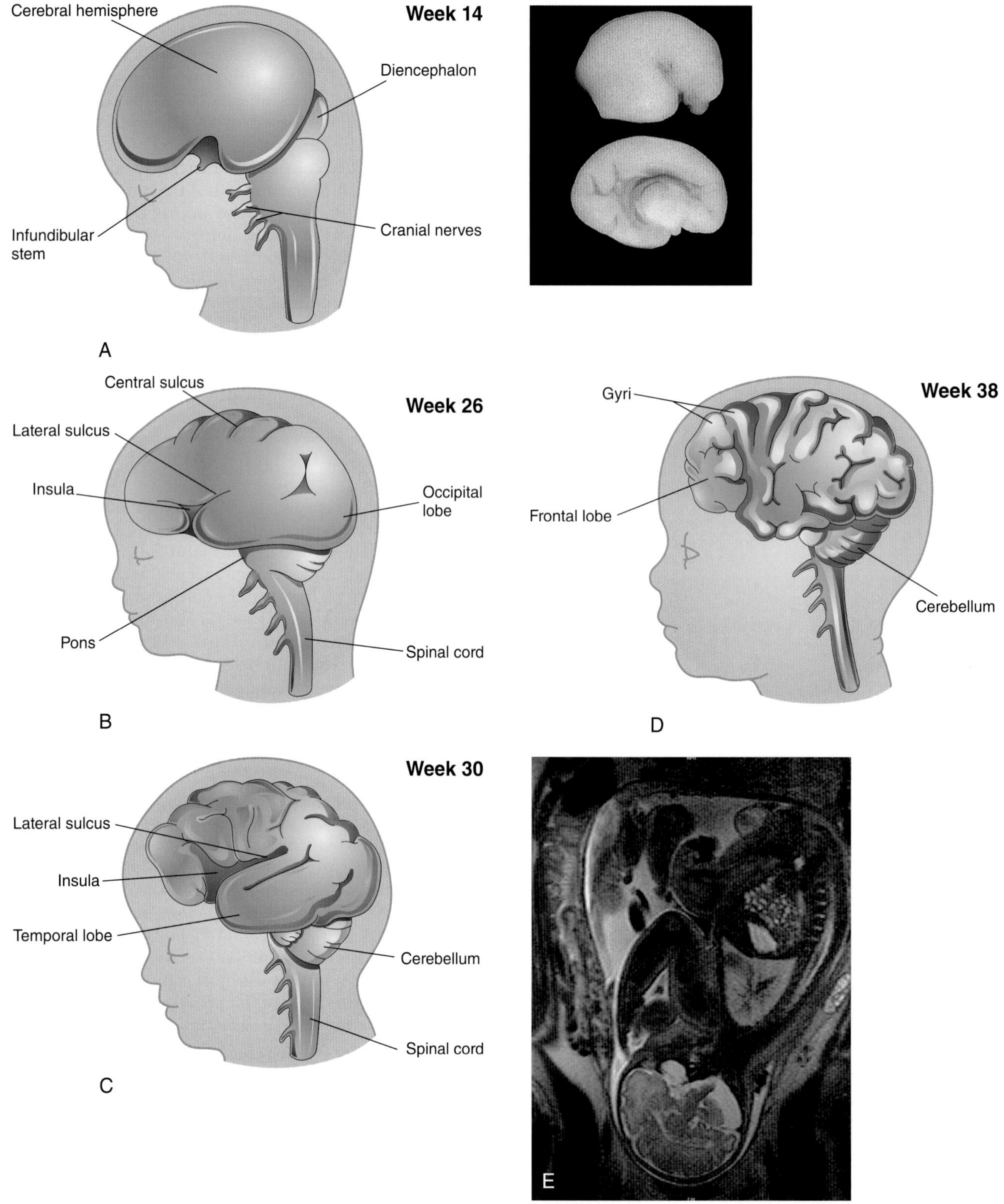

Fig. 17.29 Sketches of lateral views of the left cerebral hemisphere, diencephalon, and brainstem show successive stages in the development of the sulci and gyri in the cerebral cortex. Notice the gradual narrowing of the lateral sulcus and burying of the insula, an area of the cerebral cortex that is concealed from surface view. The surface of the cerebral hemispheres grows rapidly during the fetal period, forming many gyri (convolutions), which are separated by many sulci (grooves). (A) At 14 weeks. (B) At 26 weeks. (C) At 30 weeks. (D) At 38 weeks. (E) Magnetic resonance image of a pregnant female shows a mature fetus. Observe the brain and spinal cord. *Inset at the upper right*, The smooth lateral *(top)* and medial *(bottom)* surfaces of a human fetal brain (14 weeks). (*Inset*, Courtesy Dr. Marc Del Bigio, Department of Pathology (Neuropathology), University of Manitoba, Winnipeg, Manitoba, Canada. E, Courtesy Dr. Stuart C. Morrison, Division of Radiology (Pediatric Radiology), The Children's Hospital, Cleveland, Ohio.)

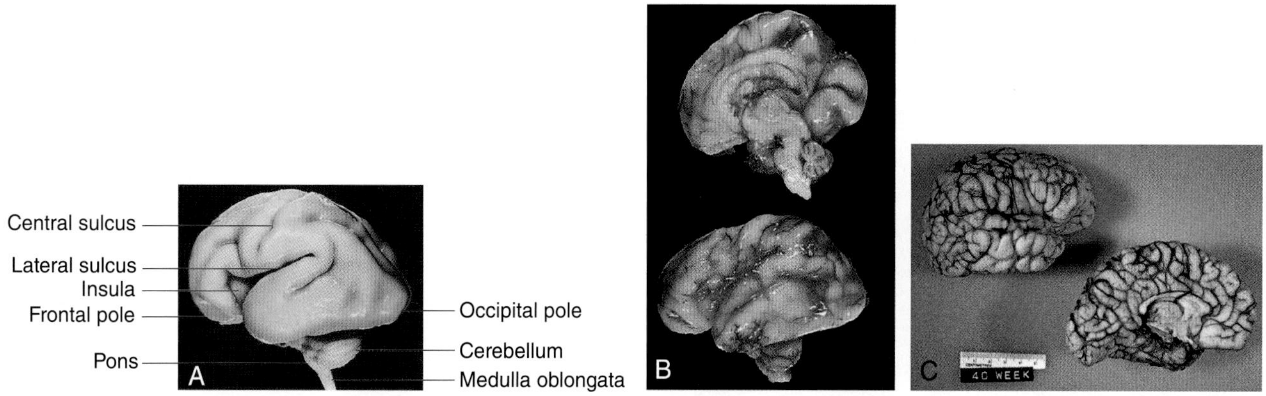

Fig. 17.30 (A) Lateral view of the brain of a fetus that died before delivery (25 weeks). (B) The medial *(top)* and lateral *(bottom)* surfaces of the fetal brain (week 25). (C) The lateral *(top)* and medial *(bottom)* surfaces of the fetal brain at week 38 (label on photo: 40 weeks from last normal menstrual period). As the brain enlarges, the gyral pattern of the cerebral hemispheres becomes more complex (compared with Fig. 17.28). (A, From Nishimura H, Semba R, Tanimura T, Tanaka O: *Prenatal development of the human with special reference to craniofacial structures: an atlas*, Bethesda, 1977, U.S. Department of Health, Education, and Welfare, National Institutes of Health. B and C, Courtesy Dr. Marc Del Bigio, Department of Pathology (Neuropathology), University of Manitoba, Winnipeg, Manitoba, Canada.)

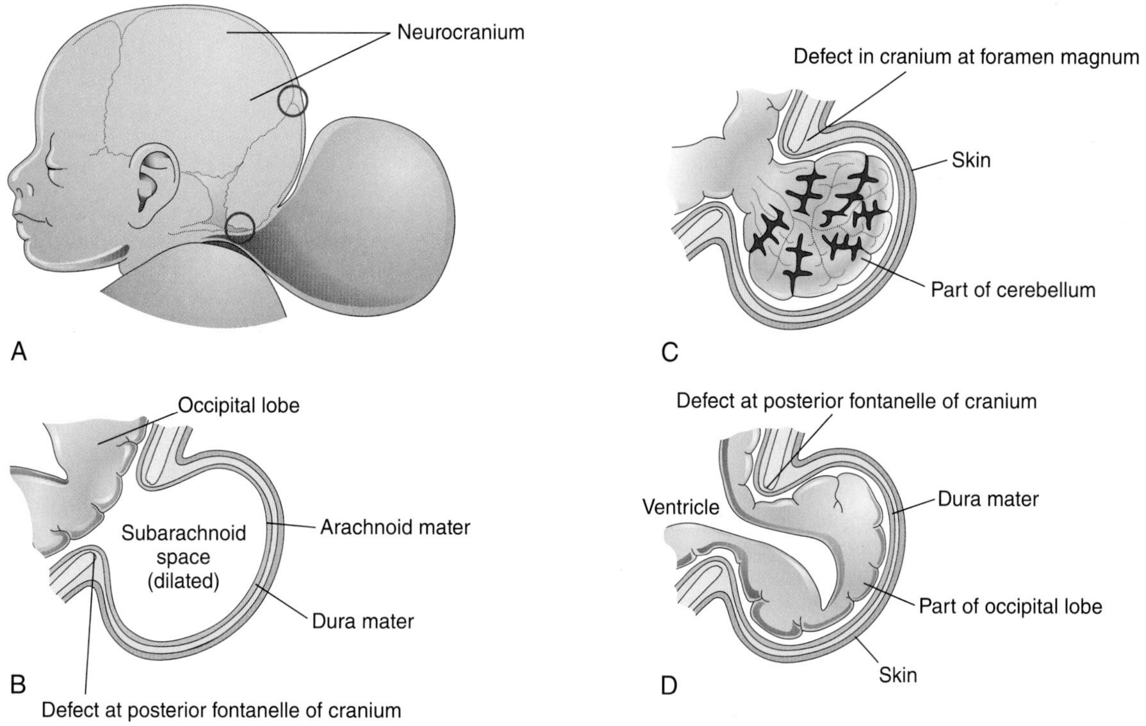

Fig. 17.31 Schematic drawings illustrate encephalocele (cranium bifidum) and various types of herniation of the brain and meninges. (A) Sketch of the head of a neonate with a large protrusion from the occipital region of the cranium. The *upper red circle* indicates a cranial defect at the posterior fontanelle (membranous interval between cranial bones). The *lower red circle* indicates a cranial defect near the foramen magnum. (B) *Meningocele* consists of a protrusion of the cranial meninges that is filled with cerebrospinal fluid. (C) *Meningoencephalocele* consists of a protrusion of part of the cerebellum that is covered by meninges and skin. (D) *Meningohydroencephalocele* consists of a protrusion of part of the occipital lobe that contains part of the posterior horn of a lateral ventricle.

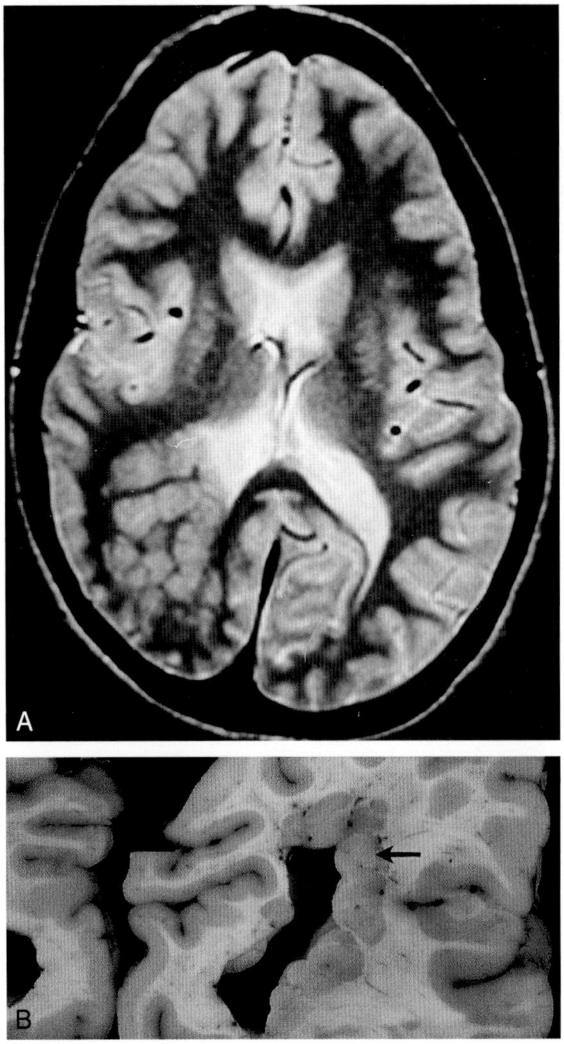

Fig. 17.32 (A) Focal heterotopic cerebral cortex. Magnetic resonance image of the brain of a 19-year-old female with seizures shows a focal heterotopic cortex of the right parietal lobe, indenting the right lateral ventricle. Notice the lack of organized cortex at the overlying surface of the brain. Heterotopic cortex is the result of an arrest of centrifugal migration of neuroblasts along the radial processes of glial cells. (B) Coronal section of an adult brain with periventricular heterotopia *(arrow)* in the parietal cerebrum. The lobulated gray matter structures along the ventricle represent cells that failed to migrate but differentiated into neurons. (A, Courtesy Dr. Gerald Smyser, Altru Health System, Grand Forks, North Dakota. B, Courtesy Dr. Marc R. Del Bigio, Department of Pathology (Neuropathology), University of Manitoba, Winnipeg, Manitoba, Canada.)

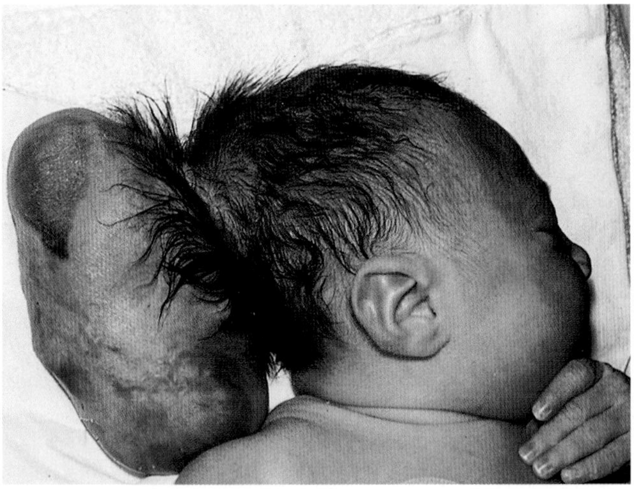

Fig. 17.33 A neonate with a large meningoencephalocele in the occipital area. (Courtesy A.E. Chudley, MD, Section of Genetics and Metabolism, Department of Pediatrics and Child Health, Children's Hospital and University of Manitoba, Winnipeg, Manitoba, Canada.)

Meroencephaly

Meroencephaly is a severe defect of the calvaria and brain that results from failure of the rostral neuropore to close during the fourth week. The forebrain, midbrain, and most of the hindbrain and calvaria are absent (Figs. 17.13 and 17.35). Most of the embryo's brain is exposed or extruding from the cranium **(exencephaly)**. Because of the abnormal structure and **vascularization** of the **embryonic exencephalic brain**, the nervous tissue undergoes degeneration. The remains of the brain appear as a spongy, vascular mass consisting mostly of hindbrain structures.

Meroencephaly is a common lethal defect, occurring in at least 1 of 1000 births. It is two to four times more common among females than males, and it is always associated with **acrania** (complete or partial absence of neurocranium). It may be associated with **rachischisis** (failure of fusion of neural arches) when defective neural tube closure is extensive (see Figs. 17.13 and 17.35). Meroencephaly is the most common serious defect seen in stillborn fetuses. Neonates with this severe NTD may survive briefly. Meroencephaly can be easily diagnosed by ultrasonography, magnetic resonance imaging (MRI) fetoscopy, and radiography because extensive parts of the brain and calvaria are absent (see Fig. 17.33).

Meroencephaly usually has a multifactorial mode of inheritance (see Figs. 20.1 and 20.23). **Polyhydramnios** is often associated with meroencephaly, possibly because the fetus lacks the neural control for swallowing amniotic fluid. As a result, the fluid does not pass into the intestines for absorption and subsequent transfer to the placenta for disposal.

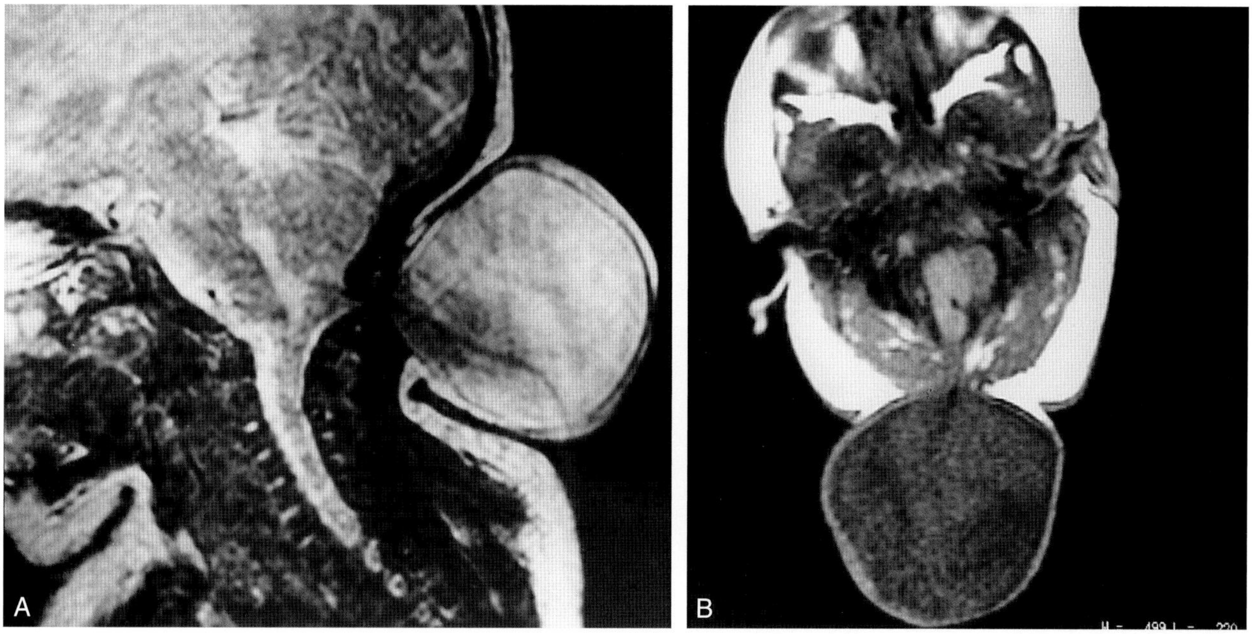

Fig. 17.34 Magnetic resonance images (MRIs) of a 1-day-old neonate show a meningocele. (A) Sagittal MRI using a sequence where the cerebrospinal fluid (CSF) appears bright. The image is blurred because of the movement of the neonate. (B) Axial image located at the cranial defect near the foramen magnum (MRI sequence so where CSF appears dark.) Compare with Fig. 17.30C. (Courtesy Dr. Gerald S. Smyser, Altru Health System, Grand Forks, North Dakota.)

Microcephaly

Microcephaly is a neurodevelopmental disorder. The calvaria and brain are small (head circumference <2 SD mean), but the face is of normal size (Fig. 17.36). These infants have severe cognitive deficits because their brain is underdeveloped. Microcephaly is the result of a **reduction in neurogenesis**. Inadequate pressure from the growing brain leads to the small size of the neurocranium. In the United States, about 25,000 infants are diagnosed annually.

Some cases appear to be genetic in origin—a heterogeneous group of disorders resulting from altered neurogenesis. Factors involved include ASPM, WDR62, and MCPH1. In autosomal recessive primary microcephaly, embryonic brain growth is reduced without affecting the structure of the brain. Exposure to large amounts of ionizing radiation, infectious agents (e.g., Zika virus, cytomegalovirus, rubella virus, *Toxoplasma gondii*), and certain drugs (e.g., maternal alcohol abuse) during the fetal period are contributing factors in some cases (see Table 20.1).

Microcephaly can be detected in utero by ultrasound scans carried out over the period of gestation. A small head may result from **premature synostosis** (osseous union) of all the cranial sutures (see Fig. 14.12D); however, the neurocranium is thin with exaggerated convolutional markings.

Agenesis of Corpus Callosum

In agenesis of corpus callosum, there is a complete or partial **absence of the corpus callosum**, which is the main neocortical commissure of the cerebral hemispheres (Fig. 17.37A and B). The condition may be asymptomatic, but seizures and cognitive deficits are common. Agenesis of the corpus callosum is associated with more than 50 human congenital syndromes.

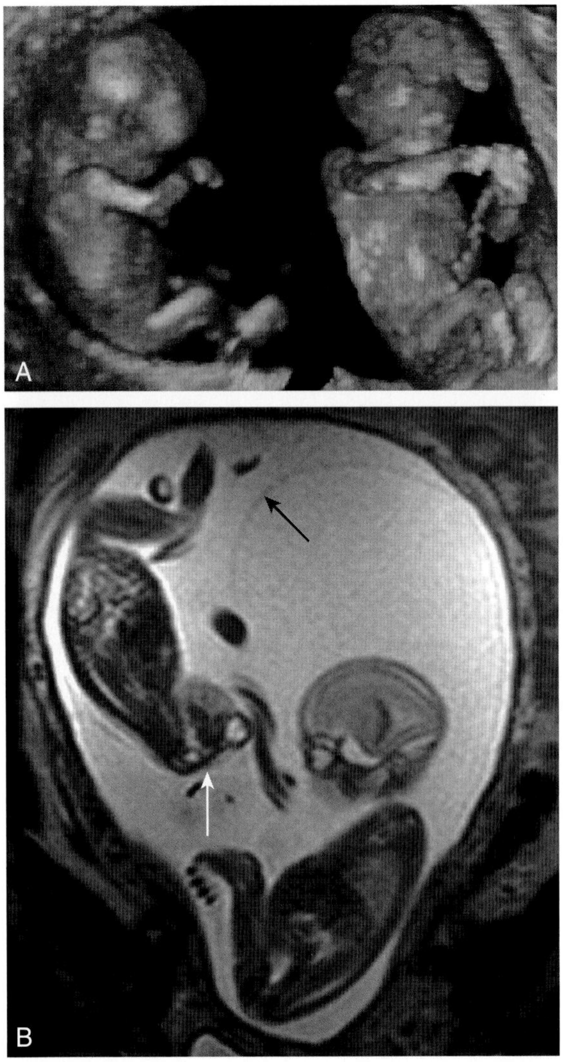

Fig. 17.35 (A) Sonogram of a normal fetus at 12 weeks *(left)* and a fetus at 14 weeks with acrania and meroencephaly *(right)*. (B) Magnetic resonance image of diamniotic-monochorionic twins, one with meroencephaly. Notice the absent calvaria *(white arrow)* of the abnormal twin and the amnion of the normal twin *(black arrow)*. (A, From Pooh RK, Pooh KH: Transvaginal 3D and Doppler ultrasonography of the fetal brain, *Semin Perinatol* 25:38, 2001. B, Courtesy Deborah Levine, MD, Director, Obstetric and Gynecologic Ultrasound, Beth Israel Deaconess Medical Center, Boston, Massachusetts.)

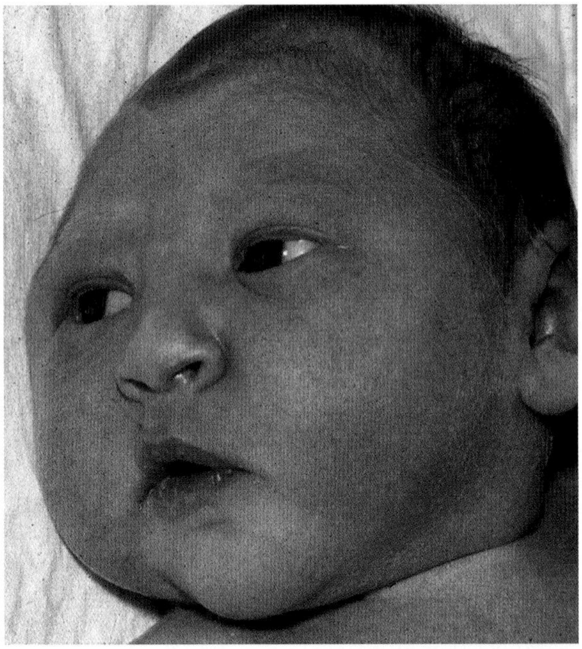

Fig. 17.36 An infant with microcephaly showing the typical normal size face and small neurocranium. This defect is usually associated with cognitive deficits. (Courtesy A.E. Chudley, MD, Section of Genetics and Metabolism, Department of Pediatrics and Child Health, Children's Hospital, University of Manitoba, Winnipeg, Manitoba, Canada.)

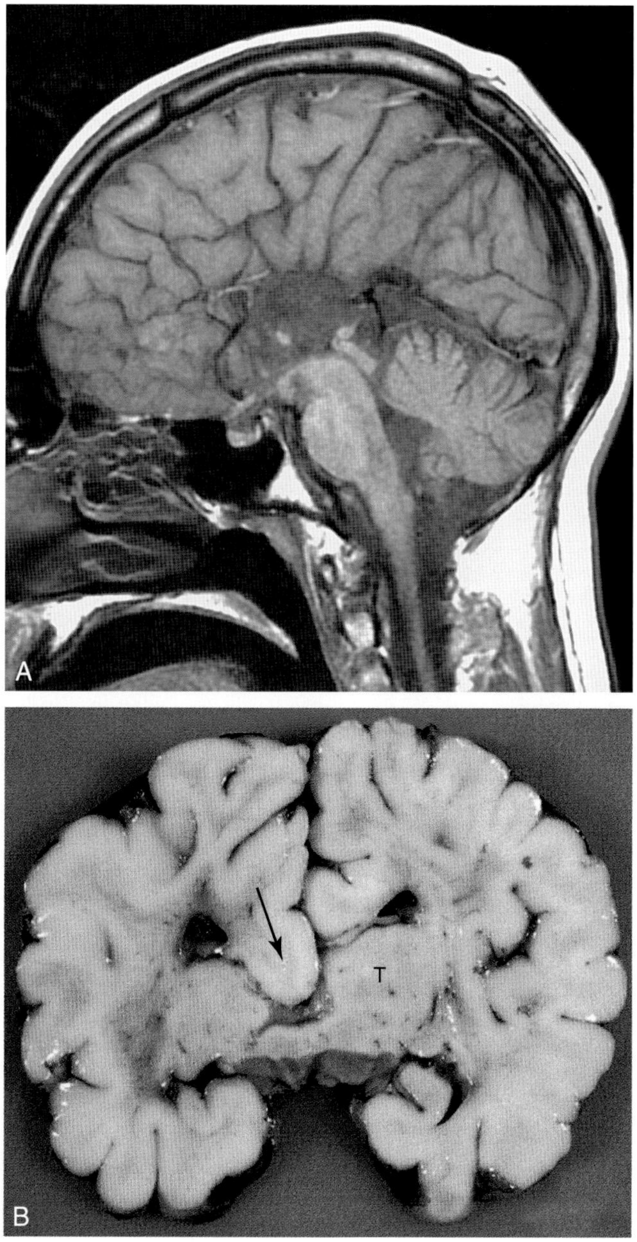

Fig. 17.37 (A) Sagittal magnetic resonance image of the brain of a 22-year-old normal-functioning man. There is complete absence of the corpus callosum. (B) A coronal slice through a child's brain shows agenesis of the corpus callosum, which would normally cross the midline to connect the two cerebral hemispheres. Notice the thalamus *(T)* and the downward displacement of the cingulum (well-marked fiber bundle) into the lateral and third ventricles *(arrow)*. (A, Courtesy Dr. Gerald S. Smyser, Altru Health System, Grand Forks, North Dakota. B, Courtesy Dr. Marc R. Del Bigio, Department of Pathology (Neuropathology), University of Manitoba, Winnipeg, Manitoba, Canada.)

Hydrocephalus

Significant **enlargement of the head** results from an imbalance between the production and absorption of CSF; as a result, there is an **excess of CSF in the ventricular system of the brain** (Fig. 17.38). Hydrocephalus results from impaired circulation and absorption of CSF and, in rare cases, from increased production of CSF by a **choroid plexus adenoma** (benign tumor). A premature infant may develop intraventricular hemorrhage leading to hydrocephalus through the obstruction of the lateral aperture (foramen of Luschka) and median aperture (foramen of Magendie). Rarely, impaired CSF circulation results from **congenital aqueductal stenosis** (Fig. 17.39; see Fig. 17.38); the **cerebral aqueduct** is narrow or consists of several minute channels. In a few cases, stenosis results from transmission of an **X-linked recessive trait**, but most cases appear to result from a fetal viral (e.g., cytomegalovirus) or *T. gondii* infection (see Table 20.1). Blood in the **subarachnoid space** may cause obliteration of the cisterns or arachnoid villi (thin, limiting membrane).

Blockage of CSF circulation results in dilation of the ventricles proximal to the obstruction, internal **accumulation of CSF**, and pressure on the cerebral hemispheres (see Fig. 17.39). This squeezes the brain between the ventricular fluid and the neurocranium. In infants, the internal pressure results in an accelerated rate of expansion of the brain and neurocranium because most of the fibrous sutures are not fused. Hydrocephalus usually refers to **obstructive or noncommunicating hydrocephalus**, in which all or part of the ventricular system is enlarged. All ventricles are enlarged if the apertures of the fourth ventricle or the subarachnoid spaces are blocked, whereas the lateral and third ventricles are dilated when only the **cerebral aqueduct** is obstructed (see Fig. 17.39). **Obstruction of an interventricular foramen** can produce dilation of one ventricle.

Hydrocephalus resulting from obliteration of the subarachnoid cisterns or malfunction of the arachnoid villi is called **nonobstructive or communicating hydrocephalus**. Although hydrocephalus may be associated with spina bifida cystica, enlargement of the head may not be obvious at birth. Hydrocephalus often produces thinning of the bones of the calvaria, prominence of the forehead, atrophy of the cerebral cortex and white matter (see Fig. 17.38B and C), and compression of the basal ganglia and diencephalon.

Holoprosencephaly

Holoprosencephaly (HPE) results from **incomplete separation of the cerebral hemispheres** and is most often associated with facial abnormalities. Genetic and environmental factors have been implicated in this severe and relatively common defect (1 in 250 fetuses and 1 in 15,000 neonates; Fig. 17.40). **Maternal diabetes** and teratogens (e.g., alcohol) can destroy embryonic cells in the median plane of the embryonic disc during the third week, producing a wide range of birth defects resulting from **defective formation of the forebrain**. In familial alobar holoprosencephaly, the forebrain is small, and the lateral ventricles often merge to form one large ventricle.

Defects in forebrain development often cause facial anomalies resulting from a reduction in tissue in the frontonasal prominence (see Figs. 9.26 and 9.27). HPE is often indicated when the eyes are abnormally close together **(hypotelorism)**. *Molecular studies have identified several holoprosencephaly related genes, including SHH.*

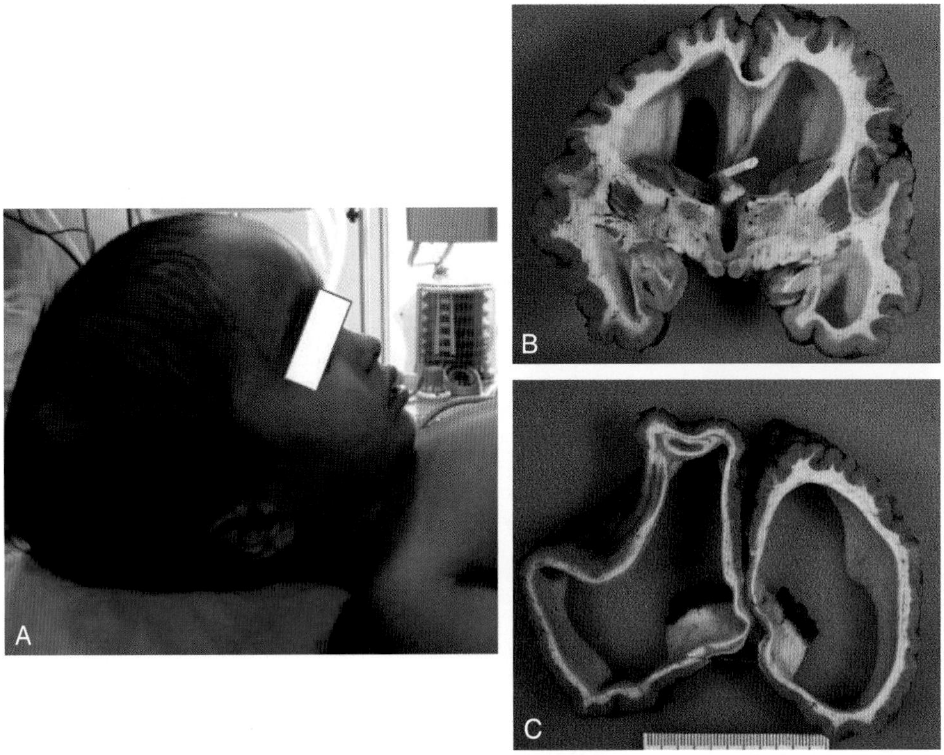

Fig. 17.38 (A) Hydrocephalus with increased head circumference in an infant. (B and C) The brain of a 10-year-old child who developed hydrocephalus in utero as a result of aqueductal stenosis. The thin white matter is well myelinated. Notice that the shunt tube in (B) which was meant to treat the hydrocephalus, lies in the frontal horn of the ventricle. (A, Rath GP: Pediatric neuroanesthesia, In Prabhakar H, editor: *Essentials of neuroanesthesia*, London, 2017, Academic Press. B and C, Courtesy Dr. Marc R. Del Bigio, Department of Pathology (Neuropathology), University of Manitoba, Winnipeg, Manitoba, Canada.)

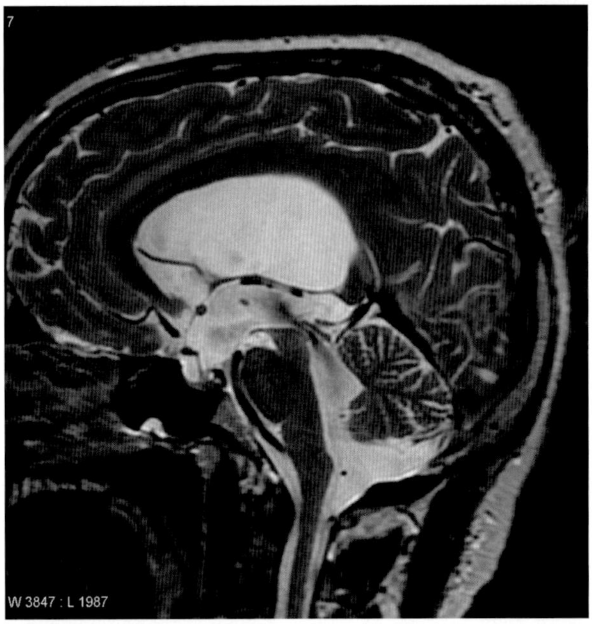

Fig. 17.39 Congenital stenosis of the cerebral aqueduct. Sagittal magnetic resonance image shows large lateral and third ventricles. The cerebrospinal fluid appears bright in this image. There is also a marked flow void within the cerebral aqueduct. (Courtesy Dr. Frank Gaillard, Radiopaedia.org.)

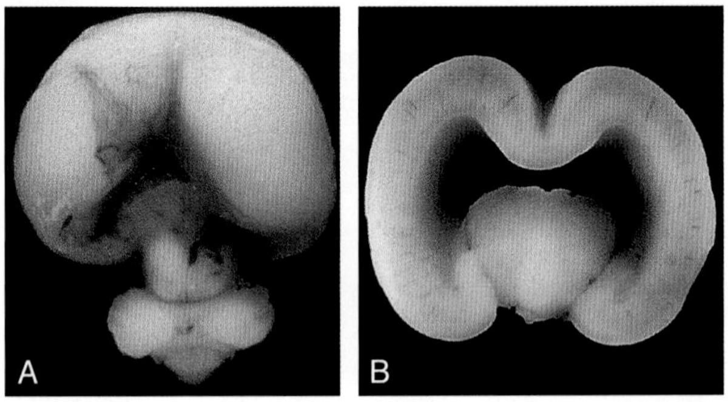

Fig. 17.40 Frontal view of an intact (A) and coronally sectioned (B) fetal brain with holoprosencephaly at 21 weeks. This defect results from the failure of cleavage of the prosencephalon (rostral neural tube) into the right and left cerebral hemispheres, telencephalon and diencephalon, and olfactory bulbs and optic tracts. (Courtesy Dr. Marc R. Del Bigio, Department of Pathology (Neuropathology), University of Manitoba, Winnipeg, Manitoba, Canada.)

Hydranencephaly

Hydranencephaly is an uncommon (1:10,000) anomaly. The **cerebral hemispheres are absent** or represented by membranous sacs with remnants of the cerebral cortex dispersed over the membranes (Fig. 17.41). The brainstem (midbrain, pons, and medulla) is relatively intact. These infants appear normal at birth, but the head grows excessively after birth because of **CSF accumulation**. A **ventriculoperitoneal shunt** is usually made to prevent further enlargement of the neurocranium. Little or no cognitive development occurs. The cause of this unusual, severe anomaly is uncertain, but evidence indicates that it may result from an early obstruction of blood flow to the areas supplied by the internal carotid arteries.

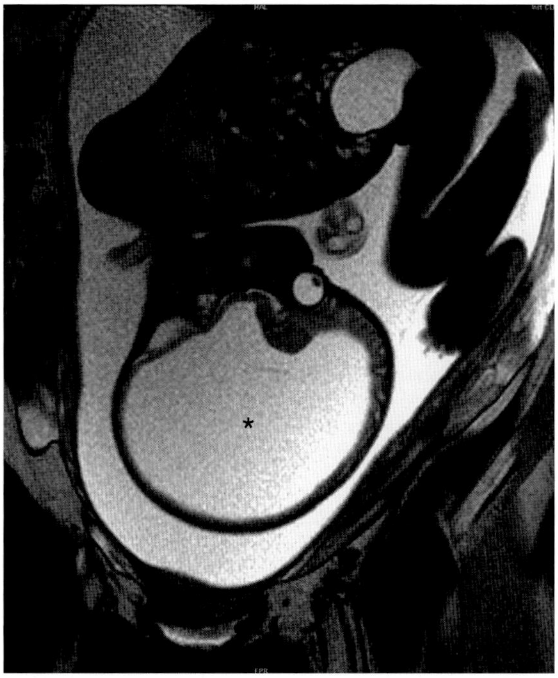

Fig. 17.41 Magnetic resonance image of a fetus with massive hydranencephaly *(asterisk)* shows excessive accumulation of cerebrospinal fluid. Notice the greatly reduced and displaced cerebral hemispheres and cerebellum. (Courtesy Dr. Stuart C. Morrison, Division of Radiology (Pediatric Radiology), The Children's Hospital, Cleveland, Ohio.)

Chiari Malformation

Chiari malformation (Fig. 17.42) is a structural defect of the cerebellum. It is characterized by a tongue-like projection of the medulla and inferior displacement of the cerebral tonsil through the foramen magnum into the vertebral canal. The posterior cranial fossa is usually abnormally small, causing pressure on the cerebellum and brainstem. The condition may lead to a type of noncommunicating hydrocephalus that obstructs the absorption and flow of CSF; as a result, the entire ventricular system is distended. Magnetic resonance imaging is now used to diagnose Chiari malformation, and as a result, more cases have been detected than before.

Several types of Chiari malformations have been described. In **Chiari type I**, the inferior part of the cerebellum herniates through the foramen magnum. This is the most common form. It is usually asymptomatic and detected in adolescence or adulthood. In **type II**, also known as **Arnold-Chiari malformation**, cerebellar tissue and the brainstem herniate through the foramen magnum, often accompanied by occipital encephalocele and lumbar myelomeningocele. In **type III**, a severe and rare form, there is herniation of the cerebellum and brainstem through the foramen magnum into the vertebral canal, which has serious neurologic consequences. In **type IV**, the most severe form, the cerebellum is absent or underdeveloped; these infants do not survive.

Cognitive Deficiency

Impairment of intelligence may result from various genetically determined conditions (e.g., Down syndrome [trisomy 21], trisomy 18 syndrome; see Table 20.1). Such defects may also result from the action of a pathogenic variant (mutation) of a gene or a chromosomal abnormality (e.g., extra chromosome 13, 17, or 21). **Chromosomal aberrations** are discussed later (see Figs. 20.1 and 20.2). Approximately 25% of cases have a demonstrable cause.

Maternal alcohol abuse is a common identifiable cause of cognitive deficits. The 8th to 16th week of development is also the period of greatest sensitivity for fetal brain damage resulting from **large doses of radiation**. By the end of the 16th week, most neuronal proliferation and cell migration to the cerebral cortex are completed.

Cell depletion of sufficient degree in the cerebral cortex results in severe cognitive deficiency as well as, disorders of protein, carbohydrate, or fat metabolism. **Maternal and fetal infections** (e.g., syphilis, rubella virus, toxoplasmosis, cytomegalovirus) and congenital **hypothyroidism** are commonly associated with cognitive deficiency.

DEVELOPMENT OF PERIPHERAL NERVOUS SYSTEM

The **peripheral nervous system (PNS)** consists of cranial, spinal, and visceral nerves and cranial, spinal, and autonomic ganglia. The PNS develops from various sources but mostly from the neural crest. All sensory cells (somatic and visceral) of the PNS are derived from **neural crest cells**. The cell bodies of these sensory cells are located outside the CNS. Studies of sectioned and 3D reconstructed human embryos showed that the cranial nerves are mostly completely formed between 26 and 32 days of development, reaching their target organs at 41 to 46 days of development. The first cranial nerve (olfactory nerve) appeared between 28 and 30 days, and the second cranial nerve (optic) developed last as an outgrowth of the brain between 44 and 48 days (*see Smit et al., 2022 for more details*).

With the exception of the cells in the spiral ganglion of the cochlea and the vestibular ganglion of the vestibulocochlear nerve (CN VIII), all peripheral sensory cells are at first bipolar. Later, the two processes unite to form a single process with peripheral and central components, resulting in a unipolar type of neuron (see Fig. 17.9D). The peripheral process terminates in a sensory ending, whereas the central process enters the spinal cord or brain (see Fig. 17.8). The sensory cells in the *ganglion* of CN VIII remain bipolar.

The cell body of each afferent neuron is closely invested by a capsule of modified Schwann cells **(satellite cells)** (see Fig. 17.8), which are derived from neural crest cells. This capsule is continuous with the **neurilemma** (sheath of Schwann) that surrounds the axons of afferent neurons. External to the satellite cells is a layer of connective tissue that is continuous with the endoneurial sheath of the nerve

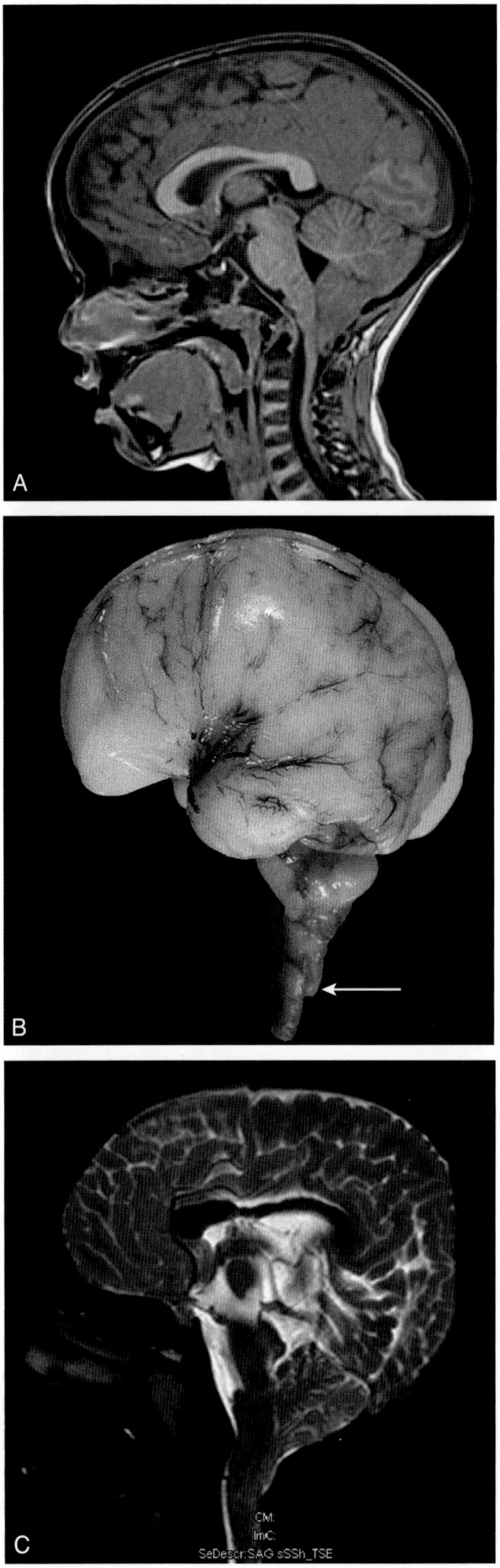

Fig. 17.42 (A) Midsagittal, T1-weighted magnetic resonance image (MRI) of a pediatric patient with Chiari I malformations and presenting with occipital headaches brought on by Valsalva maneuvers (e.g., coughing). Note the extension of the cerebellar tonsils inferior to the foramen magnum and down to the level of the odontoid process. Also, note the small cyst in the tip of the cerebellar tonsil indicative of chronic compression of this neural tissue. (B) Arnold-Chiari type II malformation in a 23-week fetus. Exposure of the hindbrain reveals cerebellar tissue *(arrow)* well below the foramen magnum. (C) Midsagittal, T2-weighted MRI of an adolescent born with myelomeningocele. By definition, these patients also have a Chiari II malformation as shown here. Note the caudal descent of the cerebellar vermis and brain stem through the foramen magnum as well as a small posterior cranial fossa/cerebellum. (A and C, Courtesy Dr. R. Shane Tubbs, Professor, Chief Scientific Officer and Vice President, Seattle Science Foundation, Seattle, Washington. B, Courtesy Dr. Marc R. Del Bigio, Department of Pathology (Neuropathology), University of Manitoba, Winnipeg, Manitoba, Canada.)

fibers. This connective tissue and the endoneurial sheath are derived from mesenchyme.

Neural crest cells in the developing brain migrate to form sensory ganglia only in relation to the trigeminal (CN V), facial (CN VII), vestibulocochlear (CN VIII), glossopharyngeal (CN IX), and vagus (CN X) nerves. Neural crest cells also differentiate into **multipolar neurons of the autonomic ganglia** (see Fig. 17.8), including ganglia of the sympathetic trunks that lie along the sides of the vertebral bodies; collateral (prevertebral) ganglia in plexuses of the thorax and abdomen (e.g., cardiac, celiac, and mesenteric plexuses); and parasympathetic (terminal) ganglia in or near the viscera (e.g., submucosal or Meissner plexus).

Cells of the **paraganglia (chromaffin cells)** are also derived from the neural crest. The term *paraganglia* includes several widely scattered groups of cells that are similar in many ways to medullary cells of the suprarenal glands. The cell groups largely lie retroperitoneally, often in association with sympathetic ganglia. The carotid and aortic bodies also have small islands of chromaffin cells associated with them. These widely scattered groups of cells constitute the **chromaffin system**.

SPINAL NERVES

Motor nerve fibers arising from the spinal cord begin to appear at the end of the fourth week (see Figs. 17.4, 17.7, and 17.8). The nerve fibers arise from cells in the **basal plates of the developing spinal cord** and emerge as a continuous series of rootlets along its ventrolateral surface. The fibers destined for a particular developing muscle group become arranged in a bundle, forming a **ventral nerve root**. The nerve fibers of the **dorsal nerve root** are formed from neural crest cells that migrate to the dorsolateral aspect of the spinal cord, where they differentiate into the cells of the **spinal ganglion** (see Figs. 17.8 and 17.9).

The central processes of **neurons in the spinal ganglion** form a single bundle that grows into the spinal cord opposite the apex of the dorsal horn of gray matter (see Fig. 17.5B and C). The distal processes of spinal ganglion cells grow toward the ventral nerve root and eventually join it to form a spinal nerve.

Immediately after being formed, a mixed spinal nerve divides into dorsal and ventral primary *rami*. The **dorsal primary ramus**, the smaller division, innervates the dorsal axial musculature (see Fig. 15.1), vertebrae, posterior intervertebral joints, and part of the skin of the back. The **ventral primary ramus**, the major division of each spinal nerve, contributes to the innervation of the limbs and ventrolateral parts of the body wall. The **major nerve plexuses** (cervical, brachial, and lumbosacral) are formed by ventral primary rami.

As the limb buds develop, the nerves from the spinal cord segments opposite to the bud elongate and grow into the limb. The nerve fibers are distributed to its muscles, which differentiate from myogenic cells that originate from the somites (see Fig. 15.1).

The skin of the developing limbs is also innervated in a segmental manner. Early in development, successive **ventral primary rami** are joined by connecting loops of nerve fibers, especially those supplying the limbs (e.g., **brachial plexus**). The dorsal division of the trunks of these plexuses supplies the extensor muscles and the extensor surface of the limbs. The ventral divisions of the trunks supply the flexor muscles and the flexor surface. The dermatomes and cutaneous innervation of the limbs were described earlier (see Fig. 16.10).

CRANIAL NERVES

Twelve pairs of cranial nerves form during the fifth and sixth weeks. They are classified into three groups, according to their embryologic origins.

SOMATIC EFFERENT CRANIAL NERVES

The trochlear (CN IV), abducent (CN VI), hypoglossal (CN XII), and the greater part of the oculomotor (CN III) nerves are homologous with the ventral roots of spinal nerves (Fig. 17.43). The cells of origin of these nerves are located in the **somatic efferent column**, which is derived from the basal plates of the brainstem. Their axons are distributed to muscles derived from the **head myotomes** (preotic and occipital; see Fig. 15.4).

The **hypoglossal nerve** (CN XII) **resembles a spinal nerve** more than do the other somatic efferent cranial nerves. CN XII develops by the fusion of the ventral root fibers of three or four occipital nerves (see Fig. 17.43A). Sensory roots, which correspond to the dorsal roots of spinal nerves, are absent. The **somatic motor fibers** originate from the **hypoglossal nucleus**, consisting of motor cells resembling those of the ventral horn of the spinal cord. These fibers leave the ventrolateral wall of the medulla in several groups, the hypoglossal nerve roots, which converge to form the common trunk of CN XII (see Fig. 17.43B). They grow rostrally and eventually innervate the muscles of the tongue, which are thought to be derived from occipital myotomes (see Fig. 15.4). With the development of the neck, the hypoglossal nerve comes to lie at a progressively higher level.

The **abducent nerve** (CN VI) arises from nerve cells in the basal plates of the metencephalon. It passes from its ventral surface to the posterior of the three preotic myotomes from which the lateral rectus muscle of the eye is thought to originate.

The **trochlear nerve** (CN IV) arises from nerve cells in the somatic efferent column in the posterior part of the

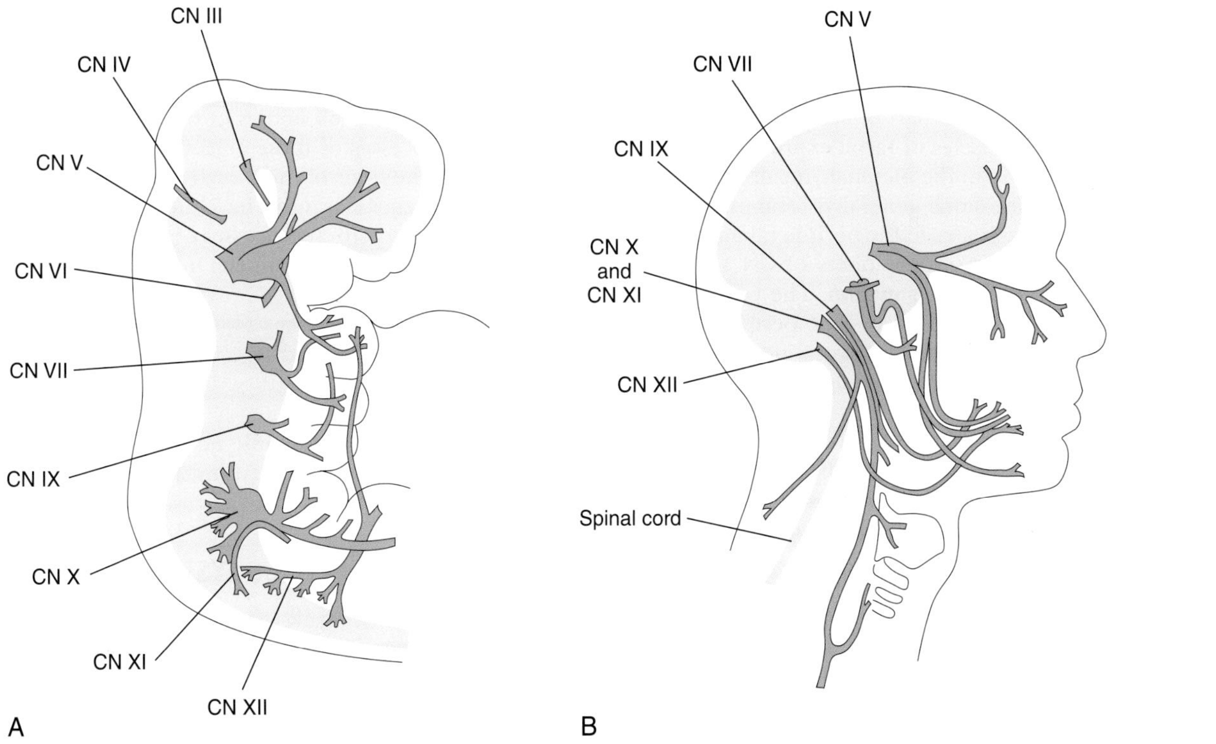

Fig. 17.43 (A) Schematic drawing of a 5-week embryo shows the distribution of most of the cranial nerves, especially those supplying the pharyngeal arches. (B) Schematic drawing of the head and neck of an adult shows the general distribution of most of the cranial nerves.

midbrain. Although it is a motor nerve, it emerges from the brainstem dorsally and passes ventrally to supply the superior oblique muscle of the eye.

The **oculomotor nerve** (CN III) supplies most muscles of the eye, including the superior, inferior, and medial recti and the inferior oblique muscles. They are derived from the first preotic myotomes.

NERVES OF PHARYNGEAL ARCHES

The trigeminal (CN V), facial (VII), glossopharyngeal (IX), and vagus (X) cranial nerves supply the embryonic pharyngeal arches. The structures that develop from these arches are, therefore, innervated by these cranial nerves (see Fig. 17.43A and see Table 9.1).

The **trigeminal nerve** (CN V) is the nerve of the first arch, but it has an ophthalmic division that is not a pharyngeal arch component. CN V is chiefly sensory and is the principal sensory nerve for the head. The large **trigeminal ganglion** lies beside the rostral end of the pons, and its cells are derived from the most anterior part of the neural crest. The central processes of cells in this ganglion form the large sensory root of CN V, which enters the lateral portion of the pons. The peripheral processes of cells in this ganglion separate into three large divisions (ophthalmic, maxillary, and mandibular nerves). Their sensory fibers supply the skin of the face and the lining of the mouth and nose (see Fig. 9.6).

The **motor fibers of CN V** arise from cells in the most anterior part of the special visceral efferent column in the metencephalon. The **motor nucleus of CN V** lies at the midlevel of the pons. The fibers leave the pons at the site of the entering sensory fibers and pass to the **muscles of mastication** and other muscles that develop in the **mandibular prominence** of the first pharyngeal arch (see Table 9.1). The mesencephalic nucleus of CN V differentiates from cells in the midbrain that extend rostrally from the metencephalon.

The **facial nerve** (CN VII) is the nerve of the second pharyngeal arch. It consists mostly of motor fibers that arise principally from a nuclear group in the special visceral efferent column in the caudal part of the pons. These fibers are distributed to the **muscles of facial expression** and to other muscles that develop in the mesenchyme of the second arch (see Table 9.1). The small general visceral efferent component of CN VII terminates in the peripheral autonomic ganglia of the head. The sensory fibers of CN VII arise from the cells of the **geniculate ganglion**. The central processes of these cells enter the pons, and the peripheral processes pass to the greater superficial petrosal nerve and, through the **chorda tympani nerve**, to the taste buds in the anterior two-thirds of the tongue.

The **glossopharyngeal nerve** (CN IX) is the nerve of the third pharyngeal arch. Its motor fibers arise from the special and, to a lesser extent, general visceral efferent columns of the anterior part of the myelencephalon. CN IX forms from several rootlets that arise from the medulla just caudal to the developing internal ear. All fibers from the special visceral efferent column are distributed to the **stylopharyngeus muscle**, which is derived from mesenchyme in the third arch (see Table 9.1). The general efferent fibers are distributed to the **otic ganglion**, from which postganglionic fibers pass to the **parotid and posterior lingual glands**. The sensory fibers of CN IX are distributed as general sensory and special visceral afferent fibers (taste fibers) to the posterior part of the tongue.

The **vagus nerve** (CN X) is formed by the fusion of the nerves of the fourth and sixth pharyngeal arches (see Table 9.1). It has large visceral efferent and visceral afferent components that are distributed to the heart, foregut and its derivatives, and a large part of the midgut. The nerve of the fourth arch becomes the **superior laryngeal nerve**, which supplies the cricothyroid muscle and constrictor muscles of the pharynx. The nerve of the sixth arch becomes the recurrent laryngeal nerve, which supplies various **laryngeal muscles**.

The **spinal accessory nerve** (CN XI) emerges as a series of rootlets from the cranial five or six cervical segments of the spinal cord (see Fig. 17.43). The fibers of the traditional cranial root are now considered to be part of CN X. The fibers of the CN X supply the sternocleidomastoid and trapezius muscles.

SPECIAL SENSORY NERVES

The **olfactory nerve** (CN I) arises from the olfactory organ. The olfactory receptor neurons differentiate from cells in the epithelial lining of the primordial nasal sac. The central processes of the **bipolar olfactory neurons** are collected into bundles to form approximately 20 **olfactory nerves**, around which the cribriform plate of the ethmoid bone develops. These unmyelinated nerve fibers end in the **olfactory bulb**.

The **optic nerve** (CN II) is formed by more than a million nerve fibers that grow into the brain from neuroblasts in the primordial retina. Because the retina develops from the evaginated wall of the forebrain, the optic nerve represents a fiber tract of the brain.

The **vestibulocochlear nerve** (CN VIII) consists of two kinds of sensory fiber in two bundles; these fibers are known as the **vestibular** and **cochlear nerves**. The vestibular nerve originates in the semicircular ducts, and the cochlear nerve proceeds from the cochlear duct, in which the **spiral organ** (of Corti) develops. The bipolar neurons of the vestibular nerve have their cell bodies in the **vestibular ganglion**. The central processes of these cells terminate in the **vestibular nuclei** on the floor of the fourth ventricle. The bipolar neurons of the cochlear nerve have their cell bodies in the **spiral ganglion**. The central processes of these cells end in the ventral and dorsal cochlear nuclei in the medulla.

DEVELOPMENT OF AUTONOMIC NERVOUS SYSTEM

16

Functionally, the **autonomic nervous system (ANS)** can be divided into sympathetic (thoracolumbar) and parasympathetic (craniosacral) parts.

SYMPATHETIC NERVOUS SYSTEM

During the fifth week, **neural crest cells** in the thoracic region migrate along each side of the spinal cord, where they form paired cellular masses (ganglia) dorsolateral to the aorta (see Fig. 17.8). All of these segmentally arranged **sympathetic ganglia** are connected in a bilateral chain by longitudinal nerve fibers. The ganglionated cords **(sympathetic**

trunks) are located on each side of the vertebral bodies. Some neural crest cells migrate ventral to the aorta and form neurons in the **preaortic ganglia**, such as the *celiac* and *mesenteric ganglia* (see Fig. 17.8). Other neural crest cells migrate to the area of the heart, lungs, and gastrointestinal tract, where they form terminal ganglia in **sympathetic organ plexuses**, located near or within these organs.

After the sympathetic trunks have formed, axons of sympathetic neurons, which are located in the **intermediolateral cell column** (lateral horn) of the thoracolumbar segments of the spinal cord, pass through the ventral root of a spinal nerve and a **white ramus communicans** (communicating branch) to a paravertebral ganglion (see Fig. 17.8). They may synapse there with neurons or ascend or descend in the sympathetic trunk to synapse at other levels. Other presynaptic fibers pass through the **paravertebral ganglia** without synapsing, forming splanchnic nerves to the viscera. The postsynaptic fibers course through a **gray communicating branch** (gray ramus communicans), passing from a sympathetic ganglion into a spinal nerve (Fig. 17.12C); the sympathetic trunks are composed of ascending and descending fibers. *BMP signaling regulates the development of the sympathetic system through SMAD4 pathways. Neurotrophin, nerve growth factor (NGF), is essential for axonal growth and elongation. It is the key signal that controls sympathetic innervation of the target organ.*

PARASYMPATHETIC NERVOUS SYSTEM

The **presynaptic parasympathetic fibers** arise from neurons in nuclei of the brainstem and in the sacral region of the spinal cord. The fibers from the brainstem leave through the oculomotor (CN III), facial (CN VII), glossopharyngeal (CN IX), and vagus (CN X) nerves. The **postsynaptic neurons** are located in peripheral ganglia or plexuses near or within the structure being innervated (e.g., pupil of the eye, salivary glands).

SUMMARY OF NERVOUS SYSTEM

- The central nervous system **(CNS)** develops from a dorsal thickening of the ectoderm **(neural plate)**, which appears around the middle of the third week. The **neural plate** is induced by the underlying notochord and paraxial mesenchyme.
- The neural plate bends to form a **neural groove** that has neural folds on each side. When the **neural folds** start to fuse to form the neural tube beginning during the fourth week, some neuroectodermal cells are not included in it but remain between the neural tube and surface ectoderm as the **neural crest**. As the neural folds are fusing to form the **neural tube**, its ends are open. The openings at each end, the **rostral** and **caudal neuropores**, communicate with the overlying amniotic cavity. Closure of the rostral neuropore occurs by the 25th day, and the caudal neuropore closes 2 days later.
- The cranial end of the neural tube forms the brain, the primordia of which are the forebrain, midbrain, and hindbrain. The **forebrain** gives rise to the **cerebral hemispheres** and **diencephalon**. The **midbrain** becomes the adult midbrain, and the **hindbrain** gives rise to the **pons**, **cerebellum**, and **medulla**. The remainder of the neural tube forms the spinal cord.
- The **neural canal**, which is the lumen of the neural tube, becomes the **ventricles of the brain** and the **central canal of the medulla and spinal cord**. The walls of the neural tube thicken by the proliferation of its neuroepithelial cells. These cells give rise to all nerve and **macroglial cells** in the CNS. The microglia differentiate from mesenchymal cells that enter the CNS with the blood vessels.
- The **pituitary gland** develops from two completely different parts (see Table 17.1): an ectodermal upgrowth from the stomodeum, the **hypophyseal diverticulum** that forms the **adenohypophysis**, and a neuroectodermal downgrowth from the diencephalon, the **neurohypophyseal diverticulum** that forms the **neurohypophysis**.
- Cells in the cranial, spinal, and autonomic ganglia are derived from **neural crest cells** that originate in the neural crest. **Schwann cells**, which myelinate the axons external to the spinal cord, also arise from neural crest cells. Similarly, most of the ANS and all chromaffin tissue, including the suprarenal medulla, develop from neural crest cells.
- Birth defects of the CNS are common (approximately 3 per 1000 births). **Neural tube defects (NTDs)** in the closure of the neural tube account for the most severe defects (e.g., spinal bifida cystica). Some birth defects are caused by genetic factors (e.g., numeric chromosomal abnormalities such as trisomy 21 [Down syndrome]). Others result from environmental factors such as infectious agents, drugs, and metabolic disease. Other CNS defects are caused by a combination of genetic and environmental factors (multifactorial inheritance).
- Major birth defects of the CNS (e.g., **meroencephaly**) are incompatible with life. Severe birth defects (e.g., spina bifida with meningomyelocele) cause functional disability (e.g., muscle paralysis in the lower limbs).
- The two main types of **hydrocephalus** are **obstructive or noncommunicating hydrocephalus** (blockage of CSF flow in the ventricular system) and **nonobstructive or communicating hydrocephalus** (blockage of CSF flow in the subarachnoid space). In most cases, congenital hydrocephalus is associated with spina bifida with meningomyelocele.
- **Cognitive deficits** may result from chromosomal abnormalities occurring during gametogenesis, metabolic disorders, maternal alcohol abuse, or infections occurring during prenatal life.

CLINICALLY ORIENTED PROBLEMS

CASE 17-1

A pregnant female developed acute polyhydramnios. After an ultrasound examination, a radiologist reported that the fetus had acrania and meroencephaly.

- How soon can meroencephaly be detected by ultrasound scanning?
- Why is polyhydramnios associated with meroencephaly?
- What other techniques can confirm the diagnosis of meroencephaly?

CASE 17-2

A male infant had a large lumbar meningomyelocele that was covered with a thin membranous sac. Within a few days, the sac ulcerated and began to leak. A marked neurologic deficit was detected inferior to the level of the sac.

- What is the embryologic basis of this defect?
- What is the basis of the neurologic deficit?
- What structures are likely to be affected?

CASE 17-3

An MRI scan of an infant with an enlarged head showed dilation of the lateral and third ventricles.

- What is this condition called?
- Where is the blockage most likely located to produce dilation of the ventricles?
- Is this condition usually recognizable before birth?
- How should this condition be treated surgically?

CASE 17-4

An infant had an abnormally small head.

- What condition is usually associated with an abnormally small head?
- Does the growth of the cranium depend on the growth of the brain?
- What environmental factors cause microencephaly?

CASE 17-5

A radiologist reported that a child's cerebral ventricles were dilated posteriorly and that the lateral ventricles were widely separated by a dilated third ventricle. Agenesis of the corpus callosum was diagnosed.

- What is the common symptom associated with agenesis of the corpus callosum?
- Are some patients asymptomatic?
- What is the basis of the dilated third ventricle?

Discussion of these problems appears in the Appendix at the back of the book.

BIBLIOGRAPHY AND SUGGESTED READING

Al-Wassia H, Bamanie H, Rahbini H, Alghamdi N, Alotaibi R, Alnagrani W: Neural tube defects from antenatal diagnosis to discharge - a tertiary academic centre experience, *Med Arch* 77(1):40–43, 2023. PMID: 36919133; PMCID: PMC10008259. https://doi.org/10.5455/medarh.2023.77.40-43.

Bell JE: The pathology of central nervous system defects in human fetuses of different gestational ages. In Persaud TVN, editor: *Advances in the study of birth defects: central nervous system and craniofacial malformations*, vol 7, New York, 1982, Alan R Liss.

Blessing M, Gllagher ER: Epidemiology, generics, and pathophysiology of craniosynostosis, *Oral Maxillofac Surg Clin N Am* 34:341, 2022.

Briscoe J: On the growth and form of the vertebrate neural tube, *Mech Dev* 145(Suppl):26–31, 2017.

Bronner ME, Simões-Costa M: The neural crest migrating into the twenty-first century, *Curr Top Dev Biol* 116:115, 2016.

Brown HM, Murray SA, Northrup H, Au KS, Niswander LA: *Snx3* is important for mammalian neural tube closure via its role in canonical and non-canonical WNT signaling, *Development* 147(22), 2020. https://doi.org/10.1242/dev.192518. dev192518.

Brown RE: Overview of CNS organization and development. In Eisenstat DD, Goldowitz D, Oberlander TF, Yager JY, editors: *Neurodevelopmental pediatrics*, Cham, 2023, Springer. https://doi.org/10.1007/978-3-031-20792-1_1.

Chinnappa K, Cárdenas A, Prieto-Colomina A, Villalba A, Márquez-Galera Á, Soler R, et al: Secondary loss of *miR-3607* reduced cortical progenitor amplification during rodent evolution, *Sci Adv* 8(2), 2022. https://doi.org/10.1126/sciadv.abj4010. eabj4010.

Dasgupta K, Jeong J: Developmental biology of the meninges, *Genesis* 57(5):e23288, 2019. https://doi.org/10.1002/dvg.23288.

Davis SW, Castinetti F, Carvalho LR, Ellsworth BS, Potok MA, Lyons RH, et al: Molecular mechanisms of pituitary organogenesis: in search of novel regulatory genes, *Mol Cell Endocrinol* 323:4, 2010.

Dawes JHP, Kelsh RN: Cell fate decisions in the neural crest, from pigment cell to neural development, *Int J Mol Sci* 22(24):13531, 2021. https://doi.org/10.3390/ijms222413531.

de Bakker BS, de Jong KH, Hagoort J, de Bree K, Besselink CT, de Kanter FE, et al: An interactive three-dimensional digital atlas and quantitative database of human development, *Science* 354, 2016. aag0053.

Ernsberger U, Rohrer H: Sympathetic tales: subdivisons of the autonomic nervous system and the impact of developmental studies, *Neural Dev* 13:20, 2018. https://doi.org/10.1186/s13064-018-0117-6.

Fenton LZ: Imaging of Congenital Malformations of the Brain, *Clin Perinatol* 49:587, 2022.

Garcia-Bonilla M, McAllister JP, Limbrick DD: Genetics and molecular pathogenesis of human hydrocephalus, *Neurol India* 69:268–274, 2021. https://digitalcommons.wustl.edu/open_access_pubs/11215.

Gibbs HC, Chang-Gonzalez A, Hwang Wonmuk: I: Midbrain-hindbrain boundary morphogenesis: at the intersection of Wnt and Fgf signaling, *Front Neuroanat* 11:64, 2017.

Gressens P, Hüppi PS: Normal and abnormal brain development. In Martin RJ, Fanaroff AA, Walsh MC, editors: *Fanaroff and Martin's neonatal-perinatal medicine: diseases of the fetus and infant,* ed 10, Philadelphia, 2014, Mosby.

Guimaraes CVA. Dahmoush HM. Fetal brain anatomy. *Neuroimag Clin N Am,* 32, (3), 2022, 663–681. https://doi.org/10.1016/j.nic.2022.04.009.

Gupta S, Sen J: Roof plate mediated morphogenesis of the forebrain: new players join the game, *Dev Biol* 413:145, 2016.

Haines DE: *Neuroanatomy atlas in clinical context. Structures, sections, and syndromes,* ed 10, Philadelphia, 2018, Wolters Kluwer.

Hata T, Kawahara T, Takayoshi R, Miyake T: Recent advances in 3D/4D ultrasound in obstetrics, *Donald Sch J Ultrasound Obstet Gynecol* 16:95, 2022.

Kahane N, Kalcheim C: Neural tube development depends on notochord-derived sonic hedgehog released into the sclerotome, *Development* 147(10):dev183996, 2020. https://doi.org/10.1242/dev.183996.

Kaplan KM, Spivak JM, Bendo JA: Embryology of the spine and associated congenital abnormalities, *Spine J* 5:564, 2005.

Kinsman SL, Johnson MV: Congenital anomalies of the central nervous system. In Kliegman RM, Johnson MV, St Geme IIIJW, Schor NF, editors: *Nelson textbook of pediatrics,* ed 20, Philadelphia, 2016, Elsevier.

Kowalczyk I, Lee C, Schuster E, Hoeren J, Trivigno V, Riedel L, et al: Neural tube closure requires the endocytic receptor Lrp2 and its functional interaction with intracellular scaffolds, *Development* 148(2):dev195008, 2021. https://doi.org/10.1242/dev.195008.

Korzh V: Development of brain ventricular system, *Cell Mol Life Sci* 75:375, 2018.

Krumlauf R, Wilkinson DG: Segmentation and patterning of the vertebrate hindbrain, *Development* 148(15):dev186460, 2021. https://doi.org/10.1242/dev.186460.

Lefcort F: Development of the autonomic nervous system: clinical implications, *Semin Neurol* 40(5):473–484, 2020. https://doi.org/10.1055/s-0040-1713926.

Mallela AN, Deng H, Gholipour A, Warfield SK, Goldschmidt E: Heterogeneous growth of the insula shapes the human brain, *Proc Natl Acad Sci U S A* 120(24), 2023:e2220200120. https://doi.org/10.1073/pnas.2220200120. Epub 2023 Jun 6. PMID: 37279278.

Martinez H, Pachón H, Kancherla V, Oakley GP: Food fortification with folic acid for prevention of spina bifida and anencephaly: The need for a paradigm shift in evidence evaluation for policy-making, *Am J Epidemiol* 190:1972, 2021.

Matsunari C, Kanahashi T, Otani H, Imai H, Yamada S, Okada T, Takakuwa T: Tentorium cerebelli formation during human embryonic and early fetal development, *Anat Rec (Hoboken)*, 2022. https://doi.org/10.1002/ar.25110. PMID: 36326822.

Moldenhauer S, Adzick NS: Fetal surgery for myelomeningocele: after the management of myelomeningocele study (MOMS), *Semin Fetal Neonatal Med* 22(6):360–366, 2017.

Muppirala AN, Limbach LE, Bradford EF, Peteresen SC: Schwann cell development: From neural crest to myelin sheath, *Wiley Interdiscip Rev Dev Biol* 10(5):e398, 2021. https://doi.org/10.1002/wdev.398.

Nakatsu T, Uwabe C, Shiota K: Neural tube closure in humans initiates at multiple sites: evidence from human embryos and implications for the pathogenesis of neural tube defects, *Anat Embryol (Berl)* 201:455, 2000.

Noden DM: Spatial integration among cells forming the cranial peripheral neurons, *J Neurobiol* 24:248, 1993.

O'Rahilly R, Müller F: *Embryonic human brain: an atlas of developmental stages,* ed 2, New York, 1999, Wiley-Liss.

Paes de Faria J, Vale-Silva R, Fässler R, Werner HB: Relvas: Pinch2 is a novel regulator of myelination in the central nervous system, *Development* 149, 2022. https://doi.org/10.1242/dev.200597.

Pilu G: Ultrasound evaluation of the fetal central nervous system. In Norton ME, editor: *Callen's ultrasonography in obstetrics and gynecology,* ed 6, Philadelphia, 2017, Elsevier.

Salvador RL, Sainz AV, Montoya FA: Evaluation of the fetal cerebellum by magnetic resonance imaging, *Radiologia* 59(5):380–390, 2017.

Scott-Solomon E, Boehm E, Kuruvilla R: The sympathetic nervous system in development and disease, *Nat Rev Neurosci* 22:685, 2021.

Smit JA, Jacobs K, Bais B, Meijer B, Seinen MN, de Bree K, et al: A three-dimensional analysis of the development of cranial nerves in human embryos, *Clin Anat* 35(5):666–672, 2022. https://doi.org/10.1002/ca.23889.

Tang W, Bronner ME: Neural crest lineage analysis: from past to future trajectory, *Development* 147(20):dev193193, 2020. https://doi.org/10.1242/dev.193193.

Tekendo-Ngongang C, Muenke M, Kruszka P, et al: Holoprosencephaly Overview. 2000 Dec 27 [Updated 2020 Mar 5]. In Adam MP, Everman DB, Mirzaa GM, editors: *GeneReviews® [Internet]*, Seattle, Washington, 1993-2022, University of Washington, Seattle.

Yeung J, Ha TJ, Swanson DJ: A novel and multivalent role of Pax6 in cerebellar development, *J Neurosci* 36:9057, 2016.

White C, Milla SS, Maloney JA, Neuberger I: Imaging of congenital spine malformations, *Clin Perinatol* 49:623, 2022.

Wiltbank AT, Steinson ER, Criswell SJ, Piller M, Kucenas S: Cd59 and inflammation regulate Schwann cell development, *Elife* 11:e76640, 2022. https://doi.org/10.7554/eLife.76640.

Development of Eyes and Ears

18

CHAPTER OUTLINE

17

DEVELOPMENT OF EYES AND RELATED STRUCTURES

The eyes are derived from four sources:

- **Neuroectoderm** of the forebrain
- **Surface ectoderm** of the head
- **Mesoderm** between the previous two layers
- **Neural crest cells**

The neuroectoderm differentiates into the retina, posterior layers of the iris, and optic nerve. The surface ectoderm forms the lens of the eye, sclera, and corneal epithelium. The mesoderm between the neuroectoderm and surface ectoderm gives rise to the fibrous and vascular coats of the eye. Three waves of neural crest cells from the prosencephalon and mesencephalon migrate into the mesenchyme and differentiate into the portion of the corneal endothelium and stroma of the cornea, ciliary body, ciliary muscles, and trabecular network. Orbital fat is derived from neural crest cells and mesenchyme.

Early eye development results from a series of highly integrated inductive signals, including OTX2, the transcription regulators PAX2, PAX6, *and other inducing factors, such as the gene* SOX2, PITX2, EFTFs, RAX, LHX2, TBX3, and FGFs.

The first evidence of eye development is the appearance of **optic grooves** in the neural folds at the cranial end of the neural plate on day 22 (Fig. 18.1A and B) *induced by RX2, PAX2, and OTX2 expression.* As the **neural folds** fuse to form the forebrain, the optic grooves evaginate from the future diencephalon to form hollow diverticula (**optic vesicles**), which project from the wall of the forebrain into the adjacent mesenchyme. The vesicles soon come in contact with the surface ectoderm (see Fig. 18.1C and D). The cavities of the optic vesicles are continuous with the cavity of the forebrain. Formation of the optic vesicles is induced by the mesenchyme adjacent to the developing brain.

As the optic vesicles grow, their distal ends expand, and their connections with the forebrain constrict to form hollow **optic stalks** (see Fig. 18.1D). Concurrently, the surface ectoderm adjacent to the vesicles thickens to form **lens placodes**, which are the primordia of the lenses (see Fig. 18.1C and D). The formation of placodes in a precursor field (preplacodal region) is induced by the optic vesicles after the surface ectoderm has been conditioned by the underlying mesenchyme. An inductive message passes from the vesicles, stimulating the surface ectodermal cells to form the **primordia of the lens**. The lens placodes invaginate as they sink deep into the surface ectoderm, forming **lens pits** (Fig. 18.2; see Fig. 18.1D). The edges of the lens pits approach each other and fuse to form spherical **lens vesicles** (see Fig. 18.1F and H), which gradually lose their connection with the surface ectoderm.

As the lens vesicles are developing, the optic vesicles invaginate to form double-walled **optic cups**, which consist of two layers that are connected to the developing brain by **optic stalks** (see Figs. 18.1E and F and 18.2). The optic cup becomes the retina, and the optic stalk becomes the optic nerve. The lens and part of the cornea develop from the ectoderm and mesoderm. The opening of each optic cup is

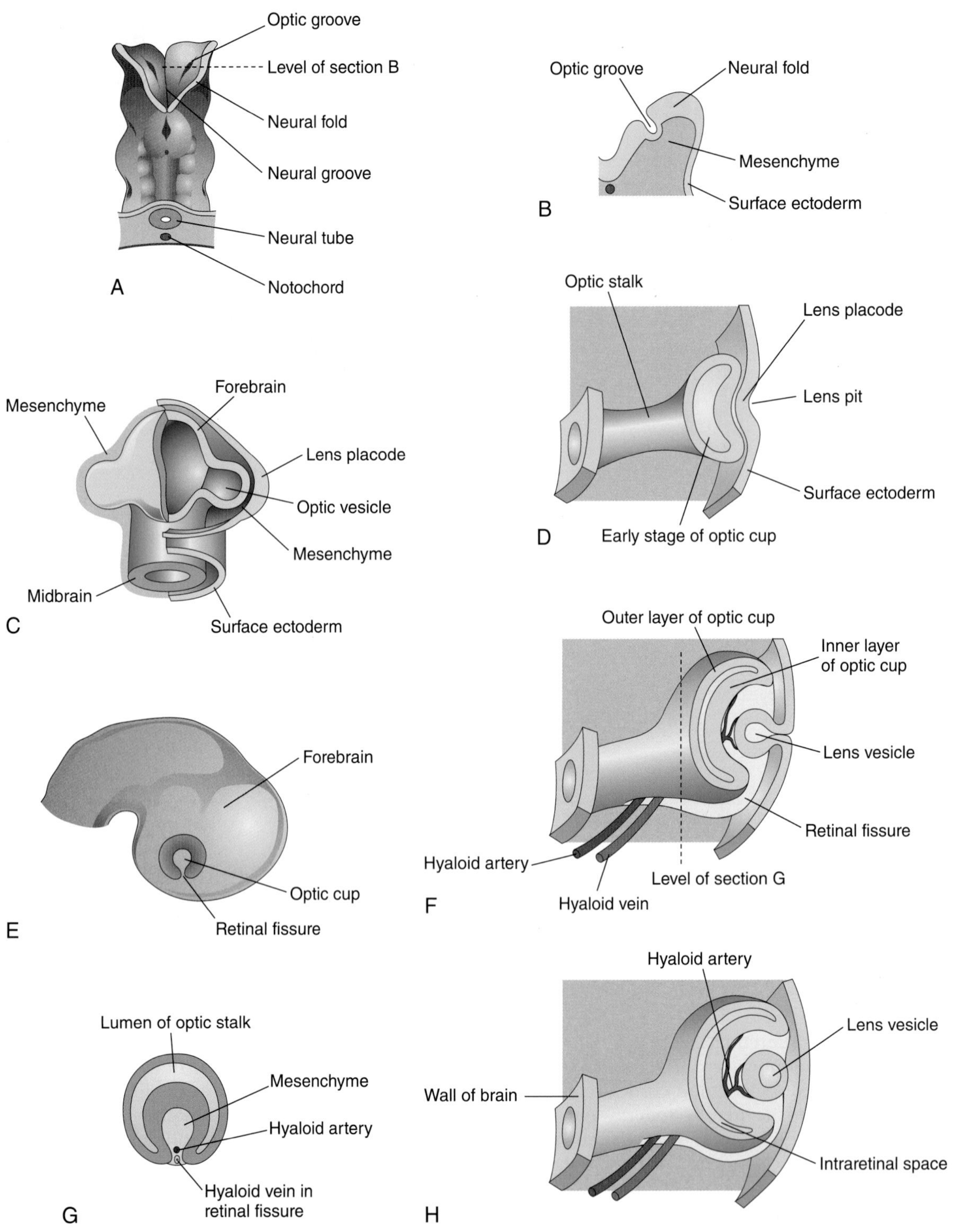

Fig. 18.1 Early stages of eye development. (A) Dorsal view of the cranial end of an embryo at approximately 22 days shows the optic grooves, which are the first indication of eye development. (B) Transverse section of a neural fold shows the optic groove in it. (C) Schematic drawing of the forebrain of an embryo at approximately 28 days shows its covering layers of mesenchyme and surface ectoderm. (D, F, and H) Schematic sections of the developing eye show the successive stages in the development of the optic cup and lens vesicle. (E) Lateral view of the brain of an embryo at approximately 32 days shows the external appearance of the optic cup. (G) Transverse section of the optic stalk shows the retinal fissure and its contents. The edges of the retinal fissure are growing together, thereby completing the optic cup and enclosing the central artery and vein of the retina in the optic stalk and cup.

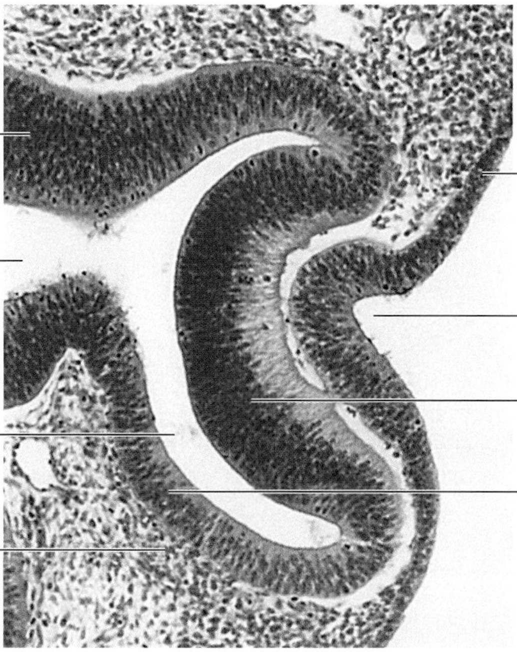

Fig. 18.2 Photomicrograph of a sagittal section of the eye of an embryo (×200) at approximately 32 days. Observe the primordium of the lens (invaginated lens placode), the walls of the optic cup (primordium of the retina), and the optic stalk (primordium of the optic nerve). (From Moore KL, Persaud TVN, Shiota K: *Color atlas of clinical embryology*, ed 2, Philadelphia, 2000, Saunders.)

large at first, but the rim of the cup infolds around the lens (Fig. 18.3A). By this time, the lens vesicles have lost their connection with the surface ectoderm and have entered the cavities of the optic cups (Fig. 18.4).

Linear grooves **(retinal fissures)** develop on the ventral surface of the optic cups and along the optic stalks (see). The center of the optic cup, where the retinal fissure is deepest, forms the **optic disc**, where the neural retina is continuous with the optic stalk (see Figs. 18.2 and 18.3C and D). The developing **axons of the ganglion cells** pass directly into the optic stalk and convert it into the optic nerve (see Fig. 18.3B and C). **Myelination** of nerve fibers begins during the latter part of fetal development and continues during the first postnatal year.

The retinal fissures contain vascular mesenchyme from which **hyaloid blood vessels** develop (see Fig. 18.3C and D). The **hyaloid artery**, a branch of the ophthalmic artery, supplies the inner layer of the optic cup, the lens vesicle, and the mesenchyme in the cavity of the optic cup (see Figs. 18.1H and 18.3C). The **hyaloid vein** returns blood from these structures. As the edges of the retinal fissure fuse, the **hyaloid vessels** are enclosed within the **primordial optic nerve** (see Fig. 18.3C–F). Distal parts of the hyaloid vessels eventually degenerate, but proximal parts of them persist as the **central artery** and **vein of the retina** (). *Bone morphogenic protein (BMP), sonic hedgehog (SHH), and fibroblast growth factor (FGF) are essential for signaling the optic vesicle and closure (PAX2) of the retinal fissure.*

RETINA

The retina develops from the walls of the optic cup, an outgrowth of the forebrain (see Fig. 18.1). The walls of the cup develop into the two layers of the retina: the outer, thin layer of the cup becomes the **pigment layer of the retina**, and the inner, thick (neural) layer differentiates into the **neural retina** (see Figs. 18.1H, 18.4, and 18.8A). *The proliferation and differentiation of retinal precursor cells are regulated by SHH, Nrl, and forkhead transcription factors. Lhx2, Six2, Pax2, Pax6, and Rax are eyelid-specific transcription factors involved in retinal neurogenesis.* By the sixth week, **melanin** appears in the retinal pigment epithelium (see Fig. 18.8A).

During the embryonic and early fetal periods, the two layers of the retina are separated by an **intraretinal space** (see Figs. 18.4 and 18.8A and B), which is derived from the cavity of the optic cup. This space gradually disappears as the two layers of the retina weakly fuse (see Figs. 18.7 and 18.8D). Because the optic cup is an outgrowth of the forebrain, the layers of the optic cup are continuous with the wall of the brain (see Fig. 18.1H).

Under the influence of the developing lens, the inner layer of the optic cup proliferates to form a thick **neuroepithelium** (see Figs. 18.2 and 18.4). Subsequently, the cells of this layer differentiate into the neural retina, the light-sensitive region of the retina. This region contains **photoreceptors** (rods and cones) and the **cell bodies of neurons** (e.g., bipolar cells, ganglion cells). *FGF signaling regulates retinal ganglion cell differentiation.*

Because the optic vesicle invaginates as it forms the optic cup, the neural retina is "inverted" light-sensitive parts of the photoreceptor cells are adjacent to the outer retinal pigment epithelium. As a result, light traverses the thickest part of the retina before reaching the photoreceptors. However, because the neural retina is essentially transparent, it does not form a barrier to light. The axons of ganglion cells in the superficial layer of the neural retina grow proximally in the wall of the optic stalk (see). As a result, the cavity of the optic stalk is gradually obliterated as the axons of the many ganglion cells form the **optic nerve** (see Fig. 18.3E and F).

The optic nerve is surrounded by three sheaths that evaginate with the optic vesicle and stalk. Consequently,

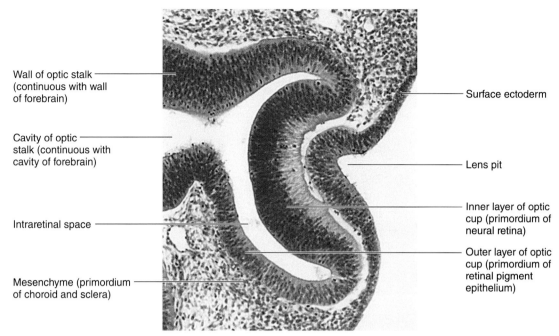

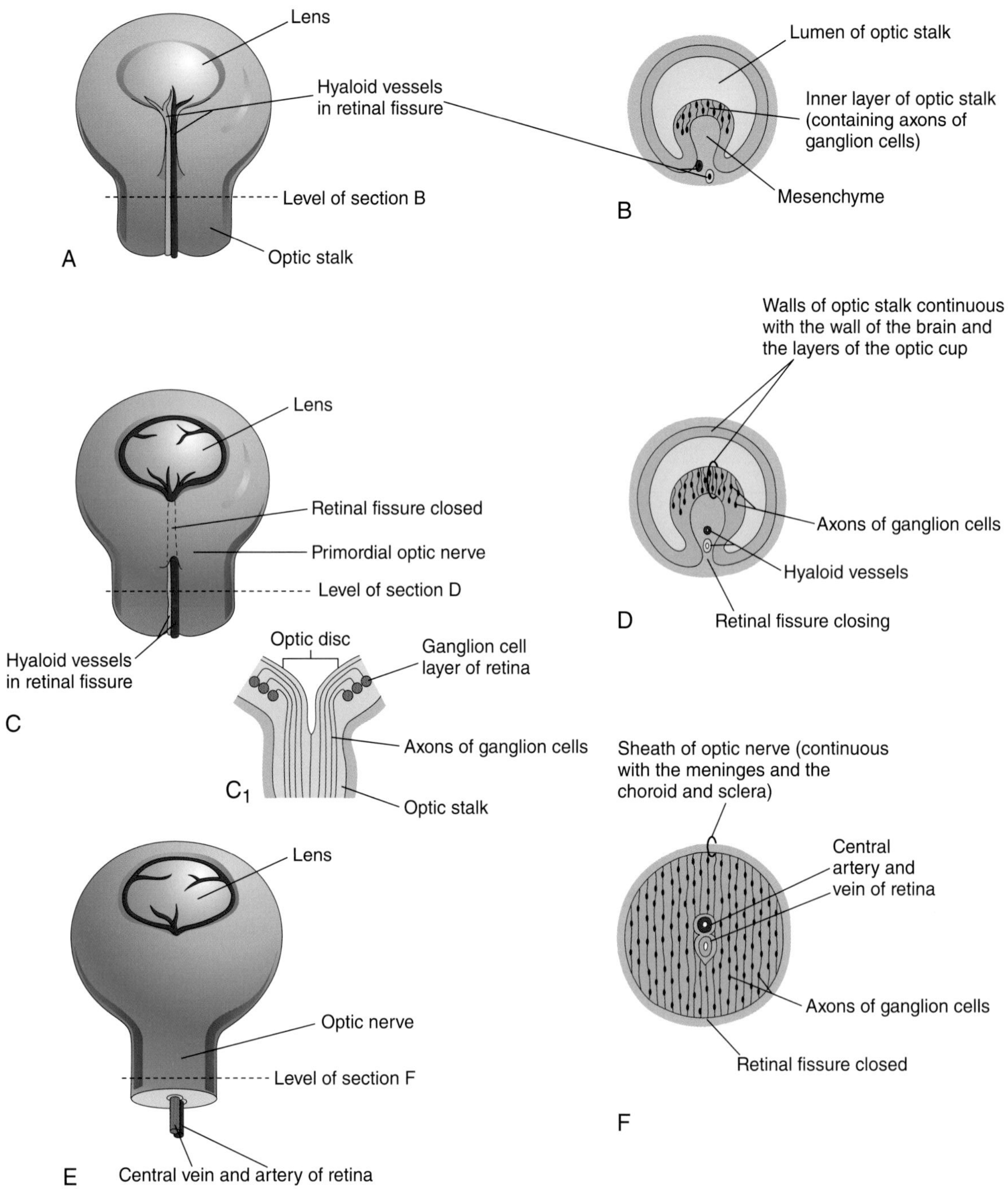

Fig. 18.3 Closure of the retinal fissure and formation of the optic nerve. (A, C, and E) Views of the inferior surface of the optic cup and stalk show progressive stages in the closure of the retinal fissure. (C_1) Schematic drawing of a longitudinal section of a part of the optic cup and stalk shows the optic disc and axons of ganglion cells of the retina growing through the optic stalk to the brain. (B, D, and F) Transverse sections of the optic stalk show successive stages in the closure of the retinal fissure and formation of the optic nerve. The lumen of the optic stalk is gradually obliterated as axons of ganglion cells accumulate in the inner layer of the optic stalk as the optic nerve forms.

they are continuous with the meninges of the brain (see Fig. 18.3F).

- The **outer dural sheath** from the dura mater is thick and fibrous and blends with the sclera.
- The **intermediate sheath** from the arachnoid mater is thin.
- The **inner sheath** from the pia mater is vascular and closely invests the optic nerve and central arterial and venous vessels of the retina as far as the optic disc.

Cerebrospinal fluid (CSF) is found in the subarachnoid space between the intermediate and inner sheaths of the optic nerve.

Myelination of the axons within the optic nerves begins in the late fetal period. During the postnatal period, after the eyes have been exposed to light for approximately 10 weeks, myelination is complete, but the process normally stops short of the **optic disc**, where the optic nerves leave the eyeballs. By 26 weeks, fetuses blink in response to bright light. Color perception begins by approximately week 34. Normal neonates

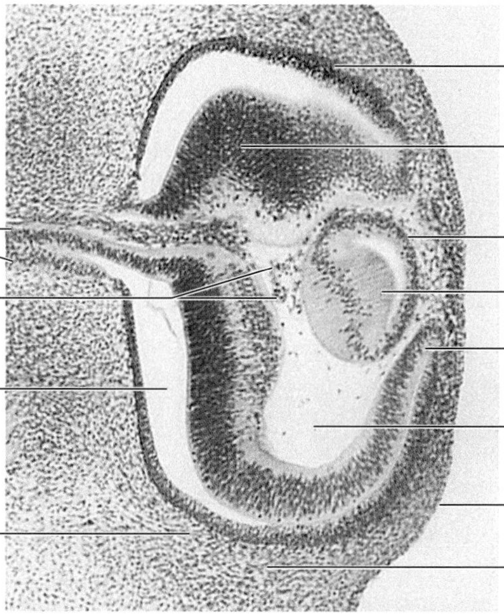

Fig. 18.4 Photomicrograph of a sagittal section of the eye of an embryo (×100) at approximately 44 days. The posterior wall of the lens vesicle forms the lens fibers. The anterior wall does not change appreciably as it becomes the anterior lens epithelium. (From Nishimura H, editor: *Atlas of human prenatal histology*, Tokyo, 1983, Igaku-Shoin.)

Birth Defects of Eyes

Coloboma

Coloboma results when there is incomplete closure of the retinal fissure, creating a gap in the eye structure. These defects can occur in any ocular structure, from the cornea to the optic nerve. The eyelid can develop such a defect, but it is caused by other mechanisms. **Retinochoroidal coloboma** is characterized by a localized gap in the retina, usually inferior to the optic disc. The defect is bilateral in most cases.

Coloboma of the iris is a defect in the inferior sector of the iris or a notch in the pupillary margin, giving the pupil a keyhole appearance (Fig. 18.5). The defect may be limited to the iris, or it may extend deeper and involve the ciliary body and retina. The coloboma may be caused by environmental factors, but a simple coloboma often is hereditary and is transmitted as an autosomal-dominant characteristic.

A complete coloboma involves defects of the iris, lens, ciliary body, choroid, retina, and optic disk.

Coloboma may be sporadic or associated with several syndromes.

Cyclopia

Cyclopia is a very rare defect (1:100,000). The eyes are partially or completely fused, forming a single **median eye** enclosed in a single orbit (Fig. 18.6). There is usually a tubular nose **(proboscis)** superior to the eye. **Cyclopia** and **synophthalmia** (fusion of the eyes) represent a spectrum of ocular defects. These severe defects are associated with other craniocerebral defects that are incompatible with life. Cyclopia appears to result from severe suppression of midline cerebral structures (**holoprosencephaly**; see Chapter 17, Fig. 17.40) that develop from the cranial part of the neural plate. Cyclopia is a hereditary condition transmitted by a recessive trait.

Microphthalmia

Congenital microphthalmia (1:10,000) is a heterogeneous group of eye defects. The eye may be very small and associated with other ocular defects, such as a facial cleft (see Fig. 9.44A) and trisomy 13 (see Fig. 20.8 and Table 20.1), or it may be normal-appearing. The affected side of the face is underdeveloped, and the orbit is small.

Severe microphthalmia results from arrested development of the eye before or shortly after the optic vesicles have formed in the fourth week. The eye is essentially underdeveloped, and the lens does not form. If the interference with development occurs before the retinal fissure closes in the sixth week, the eye is larger, but the microphthalmos is associated with gross ocular defects. When eye development is arrested in the eighth week or during the early fetal period, simple microphthalmos results (small eye with minor ocular abnormalities). Some cases of microphthalmos are inherited. The hereditary pattern may be autosomal dominant, autosomal recessive, or X-linked. Microphthalmia is associated with the pathogenic variant (mutation) of the PAX6 gene. Most cases are caused by infectious agents (e.g., rubella virus, *Toxoplasma gondii*, herpes simplex virus) that cross the placental membrane during the late embryonic and early fetal periods (see Table 20.6).

Anophthalmia

Unilateral or bilateral anophthalmia denotes the absence of the eye, which is rare (1:20,000). The eyelids form, but no eyeball develops. Because the formation of the orbit relies on stimulation from the developing eye, orbital defects are always present. This severe defect is usually accompanied by other severe craniocerebral defects. In **primary anophthalmos**, eye development is arrested early in the fourth week and results from the failure of the optic vesicle to form. In **secondary anophthalmos**, the development of the forebrain is suppressed, and the absence of the eye or eyes is one of several associated defects. Both microphthalmia and anophthalmia belong to a clinical group of heterogeneous eye anomalies that are associated with more than 90 genes.

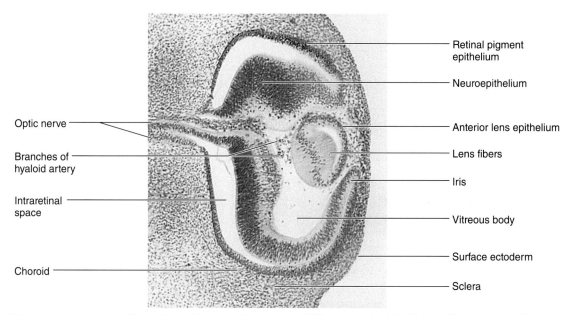

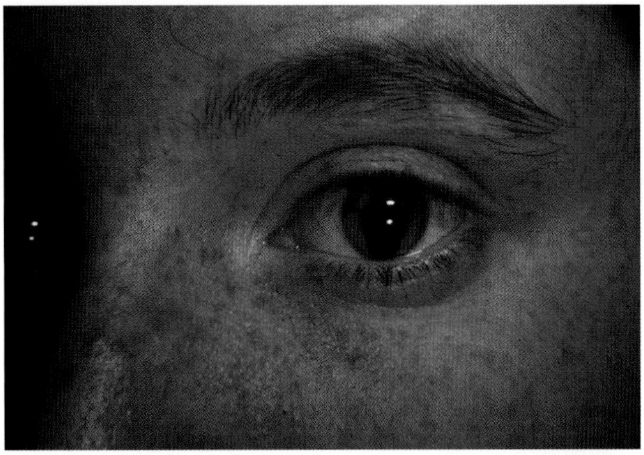

Fig. 18.5 Coloboma of the left iris. Observe the defect in the inferior part of the iris. (From Guercio J, Martyn L: Congenital malformations of the eye and orbit, *Otolaryngol Clin North Am* 40:113, 2007.)

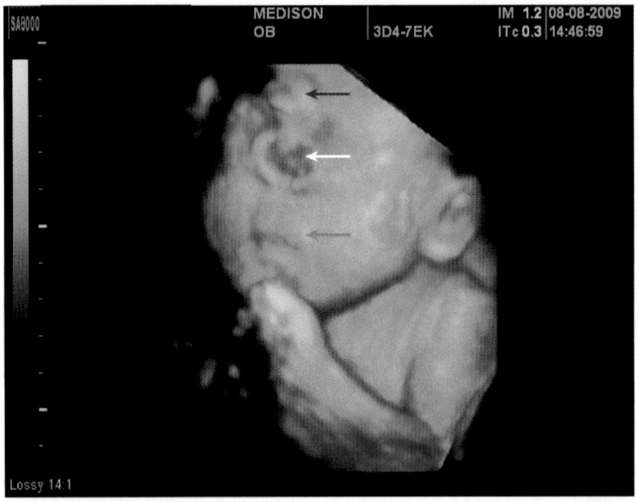

Fig. 18.6 Ultrasound image of a fetus with cyclopia (synophthalmia). Cyclopia (fusion of the eyes, shown by *white arrow*) is a severe, uncommon birth defect of the face and eyes that is associated with a proboscis (shown by *red arrow*) that represents the nose. The normal mouth is shown by the *green arrow*. (Courtesy Dr. Marcos Antonio Velasco Sanchez, Hospital General [S.S.A.] De Acapulco, Guerrero, Mexico.)

can see but not too well because they are farsighted and can focus only to about 25 cm. They respond to changes in illumination and can fixate points of contrast. Visual acuity improves rapidly over the first year of infancy to almost normal adult levels.

CILIARY BODY

The ciliary body is a wedge-shaped extension of the choroid (see Fig. 18.4). Its medial surface projects toward the lens, forming **ciliary processes** (see Fig. 18.8C and D). The pigmented portion of the ciliary epithelium is derived from the outer layer of the optic cup, which is continuous with the pigment layer of the retina (Figs. 18.7 and 18.8D). The **nonvisual retina** is the nonpigmented **ciliary epithelium**, which represents the anterior prolongation of the neural retina in which no neural elements develop (Fig. 18.9).

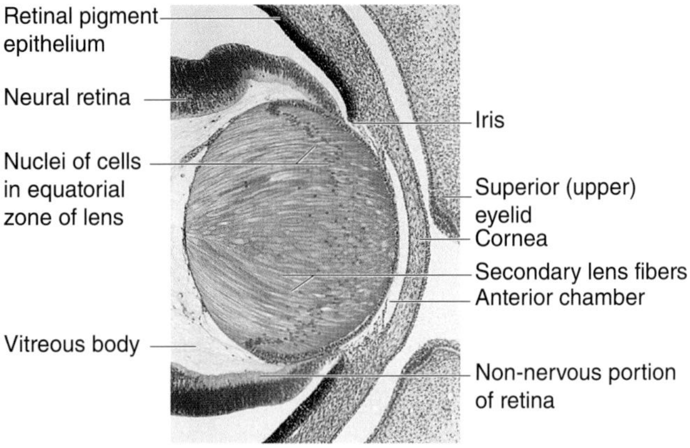

Fig. 18.7 Sagittal section of part of the developing eye of an embryo (×280) at approximately 56 days. The lens fibers have elongated and obliterated the cavity of the lens vesicle. The inner layer of the optic cup has thickened to form the primordial neural retina. The outer layer is heavily pigmented and is the primordium of the pigment layer of the retina. (From Moore KL, Persaud TVN, Shiota K: *Color atlas of clinical embryology*, ed 2, Philadelphia, 2000, Saunders.)

The **ciliary muscle** (smooth muscle of the ciliary body) is responsible for focusing the lens. The connective tissue in the ciliary body develops from mesenchyme located at the edge of the optic cup in the region between the anterior scleral condensation and the ciliary pigment epithelium.

IRIS

The iris develops from the **rim of the optic cup** (see Fig. 18.3A), which grows inward and partially covers the lens (see Figs. 18.7 and 18.8). The two layers of the optic cup remain thin in this area. The epithelium of the iris represents both layers of the optic cup; it is continuous with the double-layered epithelium of the **ciliary body** and with the retinal pigment epithelium and neural retina. The **stroma** (connective tissue framework) of the iris is derived from neural crest cells that migrate into the iris.

The **dilator pupillae** and **sphincter pupillae muscles** of the iris are derived from the neuroectoderm of the optic cup. They appear to arise from the anterior epithelial cells of the iris. These smooth muscles result from a transformation of epithelial cells into smooth muscle cells.

Color of the Iris

Iris color is typically light blue or gray in most neonates. The iris acquires its definitive color as pigmentation occurs during the first 6 to 10 months. The concentration and distribution of pigment-containing cells **(chromatophores)** in the loose vascular connective tissue of the iris determine eye color. If the **melanin** pigment is confined to the pigmented epithelium on the posterior surface of the iris, the iris appears blue. If melanin is also distributed throughout the stroma of the iris, the eye appears brown. Congenital iris heterochromia (mixed coloration) may be inherited and without any symptoms but may also be associated with other conditions including Sturge-Weber Syndrome and piebaldism (see p. 419) can result from changes to the sympathetic innervations of the eye.

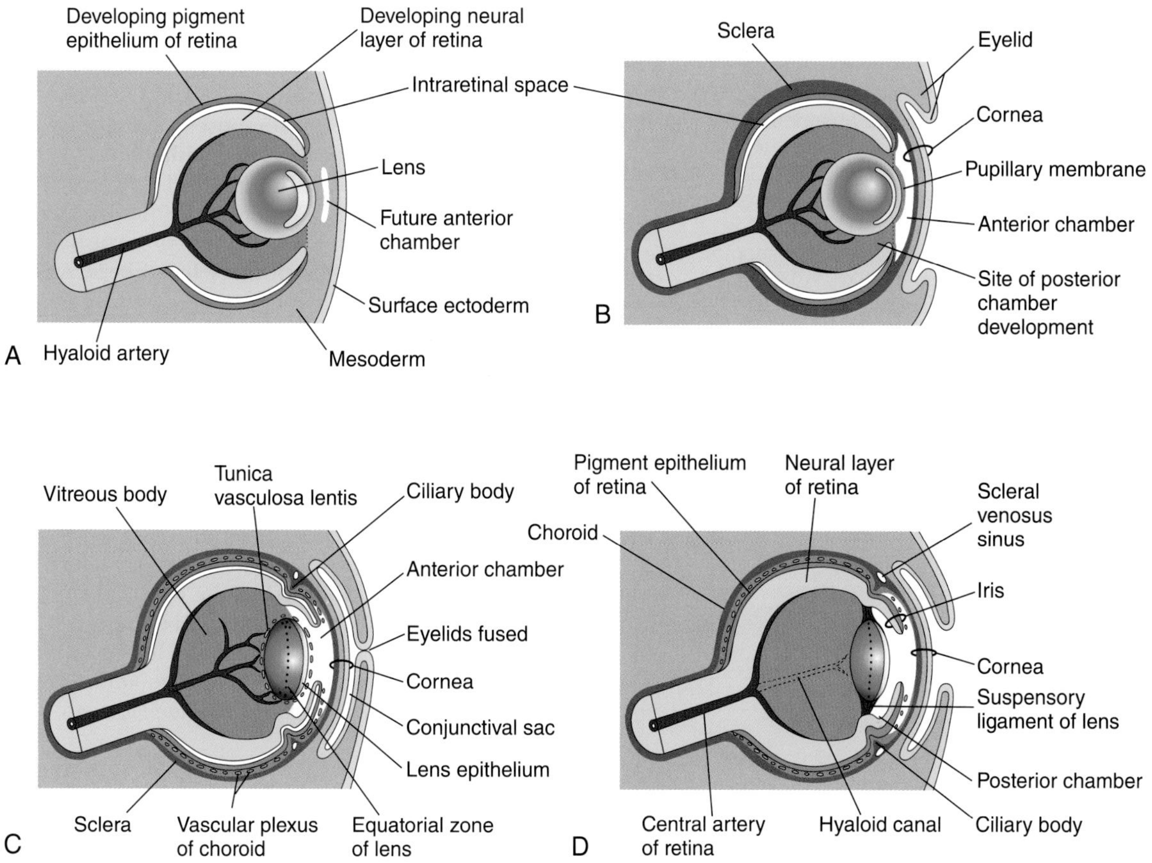

Fig. 18.8 Diagrams of sagittal sections of the eye show successive developmental stages of the lens, retina, iris, and cornea: (A) at 5 weeks, (B) at 6 weeks, (C) at 20 weeks, (D) neonate. The retina and optic nerve are formed from the optic cup and optic stalk (see Fig. 18.1D).

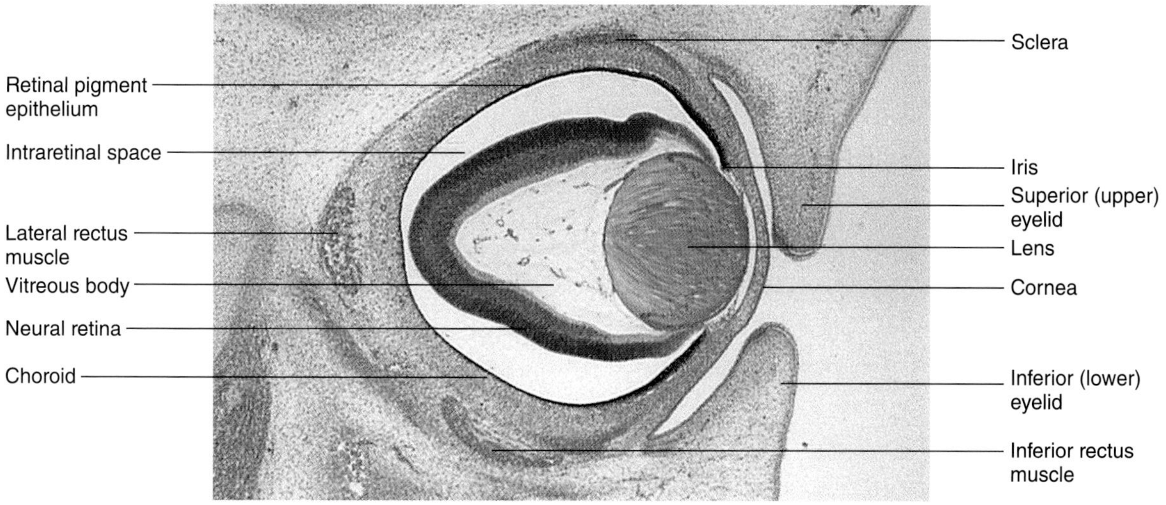

Fig. 18.9 Photomicrograph of a sagittal section of the eye of an embryo (×50) at approximately 56 days. Observe the developing neural retina and pigment layer of the retina. The large intraretinal space disappears when these two layers of the retina fuse. (From Moore KL, Persaud TVN, Shiota K: *Color atlas of clinical embryology*, ed 2, Philadelphia, 2000, Saunders.)

Congenital Aniridia

Congenital aniridia is a very rare anomaly (1-2:100,000) in which there is a partial or complete **absence of the iris**. This defect results from an arrest of development at the rim of the optic cup during the eighth week (see Fig. 18.3A). The defect may be associated with glaucoma, cataracts, and other eye abnormalities (Figs. 18.10 and 18.11). Aniridia may be familial; the trait may be transmitted in a dominant or sporadic pattern. Pathogenic variants (mutation) of *PAX6, FOXC1, and CYP1B1* genes result in aniridia.

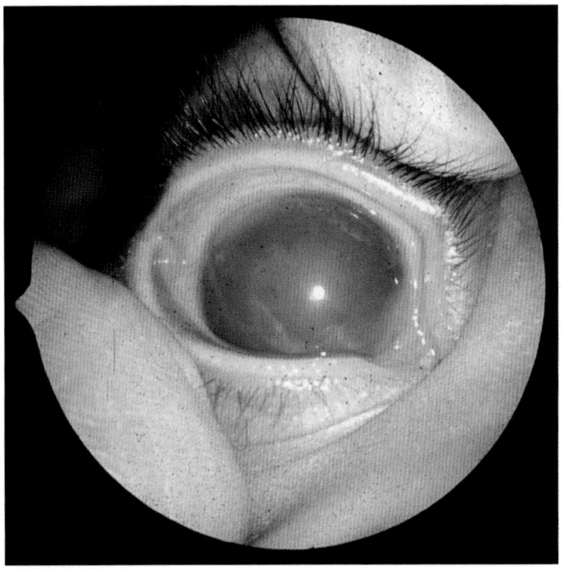

Fig. 18.10 Clouding of the cornea caused by congenital glaucoma. Clouding may also result from infection, trauma, or metabolic disorders. (From Guercio J, Martyn L: Congenital malformations of the eye and orbit, *Otolaryngol Clin North Am* 40:113, 2007.)

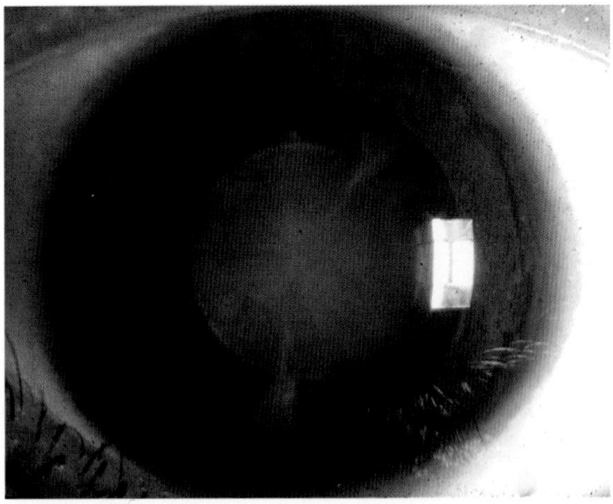

Fig. 18.11 Typical appearance of a congenital cataract that may have been caused by rubella virus infection. Cardiac defects and deafness are other birth defects commonly attributed to this infection. (From Guercio J, Martyn L: Congenital malformations of the eye and orbit, *Otolaryngol Clin North Am* 40:113, 2007.)

LENS

The lens develops from the **lens vesicle**, a derivative of the surface ectoderm (see Fig. 18.1F and H). The anterior wall of the vesicle, which is composed of cuboidal epithelium, becomes the subcapsular **lens epithelium** (see Fig. 18.8C). The nuclei of the tall columnar cells forming the posterior wall of the lens vesicle undergo dissolution (see Fig. 18.4). These cells lengthen considerably to form highly transparent epithelial cells, the **primary lens fibers**. As these fibers grow, they gradually obliterate the cavity of the lens vesicle (see Figs. 18.8A–C and 18.9). *Expression of PAX6 and SOX2 is required for the induction of the lens. The transcription factors PITX3, GATA3, and FOXE3 regulate the formation and differentiation of the lens fibers.*

The rim of the lens is called the **equatorial zone** because it is located midway between the anterior and posterior poles of the lens (see Figs. 18.8C and 18.9). The cells in the equatorial zone are cuboidal. As they elongate, they lose their nuclei and become **secondary lens fibers**. These new lens fibers are added to the external sides of the primary lens fibers. Although secondary lens fibers continue to form during adulthood and the lens increases in diameter, no new primary lens fibers are added. *Drebrin E, an actin-binding protein, regulates the morphogenesis and growth of the lens.*

The developing lens is supplied with blood by the distal part of the **hyaloid artery** (see Figs. 18.4 and 18.8). However, the lens becomes avascular in the fetal period, when this part of the hyaloid artery degenerates. Thereafter, the lens depends on diffusion from the **aqueous humor** in the **anterior chamber of the eye** (see Fig. 18.8C), which bathes its anterior surface, and from the **vitreous humor** (fluid component of vitreous body) in other parts. The developing lens is invested by a vascular mesenchymal layer, the **tunica vasculosa lentis** (see Fig. 18.8C). The anterior part of this capsule is the **pupillary membrane** (see Fig. 18.8B).

The pupillary membrane develops from the mesenchyme posterior to the cornea in continuity with the mesenchyme developing in the sclera. The part of the hyaloid artery that supplies the tunica vasculosa lentis disappears during the late fetal period (see Fig. 18.8A and D). The tunica vasculosa lentis and pupillary membrane degenerate (see Fig. 18.8C and D), but the **lens capsule** produced by the anterior lens epithelium and the lens fibers persist. This capsule represents a greatly thickened basement membrane and has a lamellar structure. The former site of the hyaloid artery is indicated by the **hyaloid canal** in the vitreous body (see Fig. 18.8D), which is usually inconspicuous in the living eye.

The **vitreous body** forms within the cavity of the optic cup (see Figs. 18.4 and 18.8C). It is composed of **vitreous humor**, which is its fluid component. The **primary vitreous humor** is derived from mesenchymal cells of neural crest origin, which secrete a **gelatinous matrix**; this surrounding substance is called the **primary vitreous body**. The primary humor is surrounded later by a gelatinous **secondary vitreous humor**, which is thought to arise from the inner layer of the optic cup. The secondary humor consists of primitive **hyalocytes** (vitreous cells), collagenous material, and traces of hyaluronic acid.

Persistent Pupillary Membrane

Remnants of the pupillary membrane, which cover the anterior surface of the lens during the embryonic period and most of the fetal period (see Fig. 18.8B), may persist as web-like strands of connective tissue or vascular arcades over the pupil in neonates, especially in premature newborns. This tissue seldom interferes with vision and tends to atrophy. Rarely, the entire pupillary membrane persists, giving rise to **congenital atresia of the pupil** (absence of a pupil opening). Surgery or laser treatment is needed in some cases to provide an adequate pupil.

Persistence of Hyaloid Artery

The distal part of the hyaloid artery normally degenerates as its proximal part becomes the central artery of the retina (see Fig. 18.8C and D). If the distal part persists, it may appear as a freely moving, nonfunctional vessel or as a worm-like structure projecting from the optic disc (see Fig. 18.3C). The **hyaloid artery remnant** sometimes may appear as a fine strand traversing the vitreous body. A remnant of the artery may also form a cyst. In unusual cases, the entire distal part of the artery persists and extends from the optic disc through the vitreous body to the lens. In most of these unusual cases, the eye is microphthalmic.

Congenital Primary Aphakia

Absence of the lens is rare and results from failure of the lens placode to form during the fourth week. Aphakia may also result from failure of lens induction by the optic vesicle. It is often associated with other eye anomalies including congenital glaucoma and microphthalmia. It is associated with defects in the FOXE3 gene.

AQUEOUS CHAMBERS

The **anterior chamber of the eye** develops from a cleft-like space that forms in the mesenchyme located between the developing lens and cornea (see Figs. 18.8A–C and 18.9). The mesenchyme superficial to this space forms the **substantia propria** (transparent connective tissue) of the cornea and the mesothelium of the anterior chamber. After the lens is established, it induces the surface ectoderm to develop into the epithelium of the cornea and conjunctiva.

The **posterior chamber of the eye** develops from a space that forms in the mesenchyme posterior to the developing iris and anterior to the developing lens. When the pupillary membrane disappears and the pupil forms (see Fig. 18.8C and D), the anterior and posterior chambers of the eye can communicate with each other through the **scleral venous sinus** (see Fig. 18.8D). This vascular structure encircling the anterior chamber of the eye is the outflow site of aqueous humor from the anterior chamber to the venous system.

Congenital Glaucoma

Congenital glaucoma is the leading cause of childhood blindness. Abnormal elevation of intraocular pressure in neonates usually results from abnormal development of the anterior angle of the anterior chamber which blocks the drainage mechanism of the aqueous humor (see Fig. 18.10). Intraocular tension rises because of an imbalance between the production of aqueous humor and its outflow. This imbalance may also result from abnormal development of the **scleral venous sinus** (see Fig. 18.8D). Congenital glaucoma (0.5–1:10,000) is **genetically heterogeneous** (includes several phenotypes that appear similar but are determined by different genotypes), but the condition may also result from a rubella infection during early pregnancy (see Table 20.6). Pathogenic variants (mutations) in the CYP1B1 gene are associated with approximately 85% of cases of congenital glaucoma. Other genes implicated in glaucoma include LTBP2, FOXC2, ANGPT1, TEXGPATCH3, GUCA1C, and CDT6.

Congenital Cataracts

In cases of congenital cataracts (1–15:10000), the lens is opaque and frequently appears grayish-white. Without treatment, blindness results. Many lens opacities are inherited; dominant transmission is more common than recessive or sex-linked transmission. More than 30 genes have been reported in association with primary cataracts. Some cataracts are caused by teratogenic agents, particularly the **rubella virus** (see Fig. 18.11 and Table 20.1), that affect early development of the lenses. The lenses are vulnerable to the rubella virus between the fourth and seventh weeks when primary lens fibers are forming. Cataracts and other ocular defects caused by the rubella virus can be completely prevented in all women of reproductive age by ensuring immunity through rubella virus vaccination.

Physical agents such as **radiation** can damage the lens and produce cataracts. Another cause (1:50,000) of cataracts is an enzymatic deficiency **(congenital galactosemia)**. These cataracts are not present at birth, but they may appear in the neonatal period. Because of the enzyme deficiency, large amounts of **galactose** from milk accumulate in the infant's blood and tissues, causing injury to the lens and resulting in cataract formation.

CORNEA

The cornea is induced by the lens vesicle. The inductive influence results in the transformation of the surface ectoderm into the transparent, multilayered, avascular cornea. The cornea is formed from three sources:

- **External corneal epithelium**, derived from surface ectoderm
- **Mesenchyme**, derived from mesoderm is continuous with the developing sclera
- **Neural crest cells** that migrate from the optic cup, corneal epithelium, and middle stromal layer of collagen-rich extracellular matrix

Edema of the Optic Disc

The retinal vessels are covered by the pia mater and lie in the extension of the subarachnoid space that surrounds the optic nerve. The relationship of the sheaths of the optic nerve to the meninges of the brain and the subarachnoid space is important clinically. An increase in CSF pressure slows venous return from the retina, causing **papilledema** (fluid accumulation) of the optic disc.

CHOROID AND SCLERA

The mesenchyme surrounding the optic cup (largely of neural crest origin) reacts to the inductive influence of the retinal pigment epithelium by differentiating into an inner vascular layer, the **choroid**, and an outer fibrous layer, the **sclera** (see Fig. 18.8C and D). The sclera develops from condensation of mesenchyme external to the choroid and is continuous with the **stroma** of the cornea. Toward the rim of the optic cup, the choroid becomes modified to form the **cores** (central masses) of the **ciliary processes** (see Fig. 18.8D), consisting chiefly of capillaries supported by delicate connective tissue. The first **choroidal blood vessels** appear during the 15th week; by the 23rd week, arteries and veins can be easily distinguished.

EYELIDS

The eyelids develop during the sixth week from two sources: mesenchyme/connective tissue derived from neural crest cells (contribute to the tarsal plate, levator muscle, orbicularis muscle, orbital septum, and tarsal muscle) and two cutaneous folds of the surface ectoderm that grow over the cornea (contribute to the conjunctiva, skin epithelium, hair follicles, and the glands) (see Fig. 18.8B and C). The fusion of the upper and lower eyelids occurs before renal function begins, protecting the developing eye from urine products in the amniotic fluid. The eyelids remain fused until the 26th to the 28th week (see Fig. 18.8C). While the eyelids are adherent, there is a closed **conjunctival sac** anterior to the cornea. As the eyelids open, the **bulbar conjunctiva** is reflected over the anterior part of the sclera and the surface epithelium of the cornea (see Fig. 18.8D). The **palpebral conjunctiva** lines the inner surface of the eyelids. *Epidermal growth factor receptor (EGFR) signaling and other related pathways regulate the formation of the eyelids.*

The **eyelashes** and **glands** in the eyelids are derived from the surface ectoderm like that described for other parts of the integument (see Fig. 19.1).

LACRIMAL GLANDS

At the superolateral angles of the orbits, the lacrimal glands develop from several solid buds from the surface ectoderm. The lacrimal ducts drain into the lacrimal sac and eventually into the **nasolacrimal duct**. The glands are small at birth and do not function fully—reflex tearing (such as from crying) does not occur until the glands develop further, at least in the 2nd month. *It has been reported that Fgf10, SOX10, TFAP2, and the noncoding RNA (miR-205) signaling pathways are essential for the development of the lacrimal gland.*

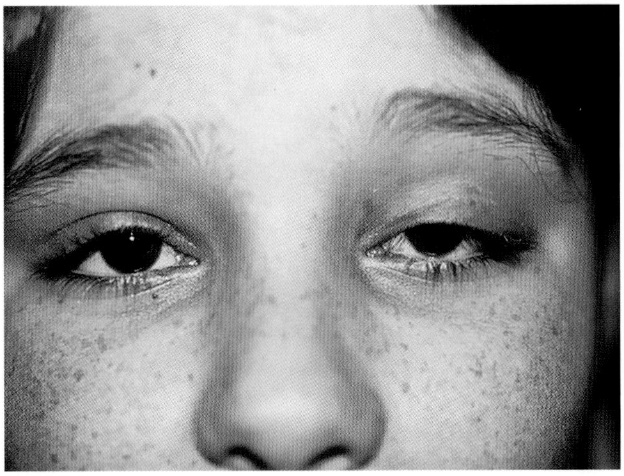

Fig. 18.12 Severe left congenital ptosis with absent skin crease (From Salmon JF, Eyelids. In *Kanski's clinical ophthalmology*, ed 9, 2020, Elsevier.)

Congenital Ptosis of Eyelid

Drooping of the superior (upper) eyelids, **ptosis**, is relatively common in neonates (Fig. 18.12). Ptosis (blepharoptosis) may result from failure of normal development of the **levator palpebrae superioris muscle.** Congenital ptosis may also result from prenatal injury or **dystrophy** (degeneration) of the superior division of the **oculomotor nerve** (CN III), which supplies this muscle. If ptosis is associated with an inability to move the eyeball superiorly, there is also a failure of the **superior rectus muscle** of the eyeball to develop normally. Congenital ptosis may be transmitted as an autosomal-dominant trait. Ptosis also is commonly associated on the affected side with the absence of sweat (anhidrosis) and a small pupil (miosis), which is known as Horner syndrome. Ptosis can affect vision if the margin of the eyelid partially or completely covers the pupil; early surgical correction is indicated.

Coloboma of the Eyelid

Large defects of the eyelid **(palpebral colobomas)** are uncommon (1:10,000). A coloboma is usually characterized by a small notch in the superior eyelid, but the defect may involve almost the entire lid. Palpebral colobomas appear to result from local developmental disturbances in the formation and growth of the eyelids. Drying and ulceration of the cornea can result from a lower eyelid coloboma.

Cryptophthalmos

Cryptophthalmos is a rare (1:20,000) autosomal recessive condition that is usually part of Fraser Syndrome (*cryptophthalmos syndrome), which includes urogenital (renal agenesis) and other anomalies*. Cryptophthalmos results from the congenital **absence of the eyelids**; as a result, skin covers the eyes. The eyeball is small and defective, and the cornea and conjunctiva usually do not develop. Fundamentally, the defect results from an absence of the **palpebral fissure** (slit) between eyelids. There is usually some degree of eyelash and eyebrow absence, and there are other eye defects. Pathogenic variants (mutations) in the FRAS1, FREM1/2, and GRIP1 genes appear to be responsible.

18

DEVELOPMENT OF EARS

The ears are composed of three parts:

- **External ear**, consisting of the auricle (pinna), external acoustic meatus (canal), and external layer of the tympanic membrane
- **Middle ear**, consisting of a chain of three small auditory ossicles and the internal layer of the tympanic membrane, which is connected to the oval window of the internal ear by the ossicles.
- **Internal ear**, consisting of the vestibulocochlear organ, which functions in hearing and balance

The external and middle parts are concerned with the transference of sound waves to the internal ears, which convert the waves into nerve impulses and register changes in equilibrium.

INTERNAL EARS

The internal ears are the first of the three parts of the ears to develop. Early in the fourth week, a thickening of the surface ectoderm, the **otic placode**, appears in a preplacodal field of precursor neurons on each side of the myelencephalon, which is the caudal part of the hindbrain (Fig. 18.13A, B, and D). *Inductive signals, including those from the paraxial mesoderm and notochord, stimulate the surface ectoderm to form the placodes* (see Fig. 4.9). *PGF signaling initiates the specification of the otic epibranchial progenitors from sensory precursors in the preplacodal region. Further development of the otic placode involves the protein-coding Pa2G4, transcription factors FoxL1/3, Wnt and Notch pathways, Pax2/8, Mcrs1, Six1, and protein-encoding Dix genes.*

Each otic placode soon invaginates and sinks deep to the surface ectoderm into the underlying mesenchyme. In so doing, it forms an **otic pit** (see Fig. 18.13C and D). The edges of the pit come together and fuse to form an **otic vesicle**, which is the primordium of the **membranous labyrinth** (Fig. 18.14; see Fig. 18.13E–G). The vesicle soon loses its connection with the surface ectoderm, and a diverticulum grows from the vesicle and elongates to form the **endolymphatic duct** and **sac** (Fig. 18.15A–E).

Two regions of the otic vesicles are recognizable (see Fig. 18.15A):

- **Dorsal utricular parts**, from which the small endolymphatic ducts, utricles, and semicircular ducts arise
- **Ventral saccular parts**, which give rise to the saccules and cochlear ducts

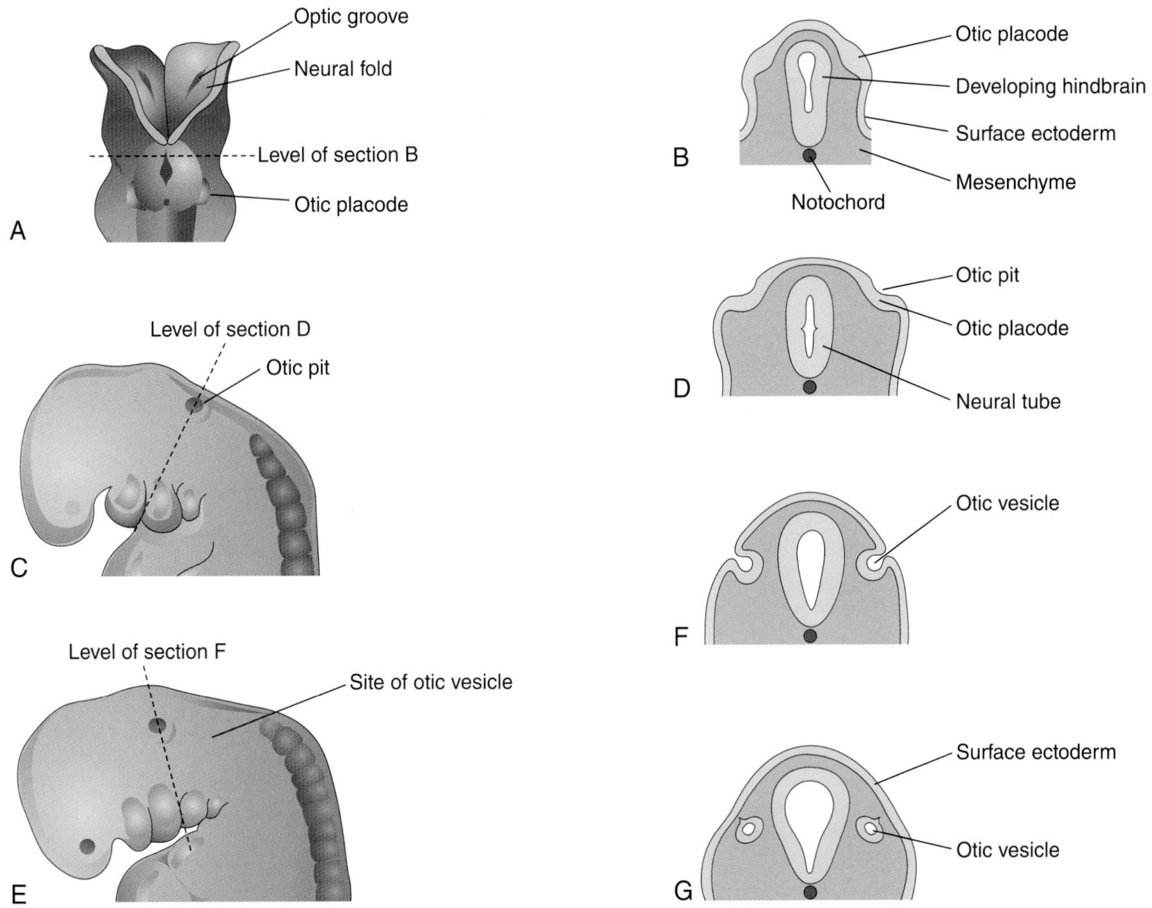

Fig. 18.13 Drawings of early development of the internal ear. (A) Dorsal view of an embryo at approximately 22 days shows the otic placodes. (B, D, F, and G) Schematic coronal sections show successive stages in the development of otic vesicles. (C and E) Lateral views of the cranial region of embryos at approximately 24 and 28 days, respectively.

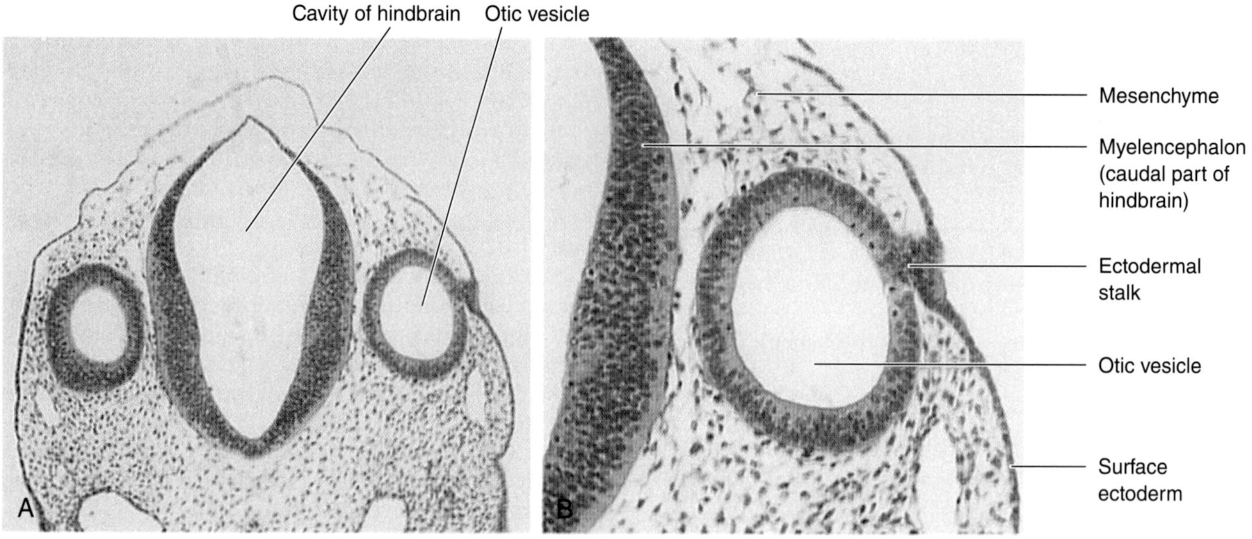

Fig. 18.14 Photomicrograph (A) of a transverse section of an embryo (×55) at approximately 26 days. The otic vesicles (primordia of the membranous labyrinths) give rise to the internal ears. Photomicrograph (B) at higher magnification of the right otic vesicle (×120). The ectodermal stalk is still attached to the remnant of the otic placode. The otic vesicle will soon lose its connection with the surface ectoderm. (From Nishimura H, editor: *Atlas of human prenatal histology*, Tokyo, 1983, Igaku-Shoin.)

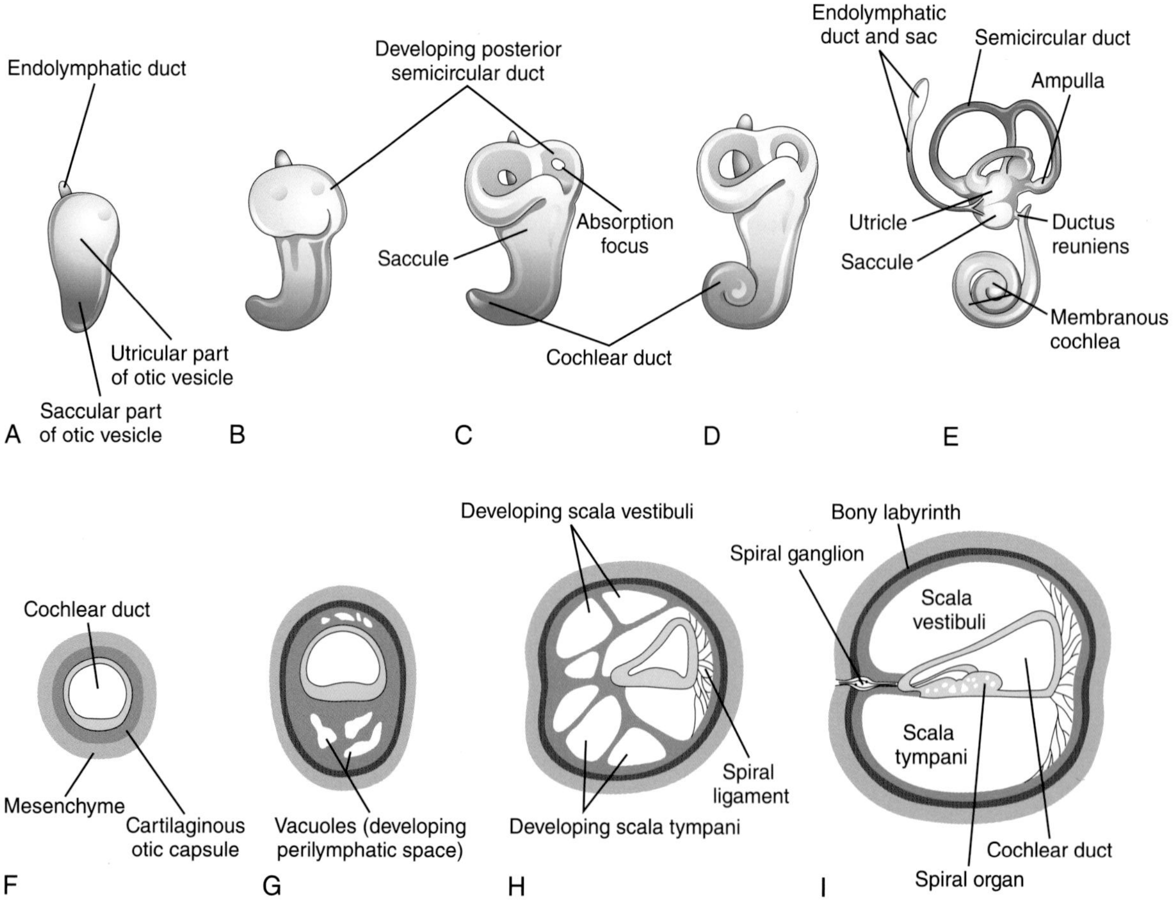

Fig. 18.15 Drawings of the otic vesicles show the development of the membranous and bony labyrinths of the internal ear. (A–E) Lateral views show successive stages in the development of the otic vesicle into the membranous labyrinth from the fifth to eighth weeks and the development of a semicircular duct. (F–I) Sections through the cochlear duct show successive stages in the development of the spiral organ and the perilymphatic space from the 8th to the 20th weeks.

Three disc-like diverticula grow out from the utricular parts of the primordial membranous labyrinths. Soon the central parts of these diverticula fuse and disappear (see Fig. 18.15B–E). The peripheral unfused parts of the diverticula become **semicircular ducts**, which are attached to the utricle and are later enclosed in the **semicircular canals of the bony labyrinth** (see Fig. 18.15I). Localized dilatations, the **ampullae**, develop at one end of each semicircular duct (see Fig. 18.15E). Specialized receptor areas **(cristae ampullares)** differentiate in the ampullae and the **utricle** and (maculae utriculi and sacculi).

The **cochlear duct** grows from the saccular part of the otic vesicle and coils to form the **membranous cochlea** (see Fig. 18.15A and C–E). The cochlea develops the final 2.5 turns by approximately week 8. *TBX1 expression in the mesenchyme surrounding the otic vesicle regulates the formation of the cochlear duct by controlling retinoic acid activity.* A connection, **(ductus reuniens)** between the cochlea with the saccule soon forms (see Fig. 18.15E). The **spiral organ** differentiates from cells in the wall of the cochlear duct (see Fig. 18.15F–I). Ganglion cells of the **vestibulocochlear nerve** (CN VIII) migrate along the coils of the membranous cochlea and form the **spiral ganglion** (see Fig. 18.15I). Nerve processes extend from this ganglion to the **spiral organ**, where they terminate on the **hair cells**. The cells in the spiral ganglion retain their embryonic bipolar condition.

Inductive influences from the otic vesicle stimulate the mesenchyme around the otic vesicle to condense and differentiate into a **cartilaginous otic capsule** (see Fig. 18.15F). *Studies indicate that expression of FGF, BMP, PRDM 16, and Sox2 signaling pathways are essential for the development of the inner ear, in particular the stereocilia cells in the cochlea.* The PAX2 *gene is required for the formation of the spiral organ of Corti and the spiral ganglion. Retinoic acid and transforming growth factor* β_1 *play a role in modulating epithelial-mesenchymal interaction in the internal ear and in directing the formation of the otic capsule or bony labyrinth.*

As the **membranous labyrinth** enlarges, vacuoles appear in the cartilaginous otic capsule and soon coalesce to form the **perilymphatic space** (see Fig. 18.15G). The membranous labyrinth is now suspended in **perilymph** (fluid similar to CSF). The perilymphatic space, which is related to the cochlear duct, develops two divisions, the **scala tympani** and **scala vestibuli** (see Fig. 18.15H and I). The cartilaginous otic capsule later ossifies to form the **bony labyrinth** of the internal ear (see Fig. 18.15I). The internal ear reaches its adult size and shape by the middle of the fetal period (20–22 weeks), and functional hearing exists at approximately 26 weeks.

MIDDLE EARS

Development of the **tubotympanic recess** (Fig. 18.16B) from the first pharyngeal pouch is described in Chapter 9. The

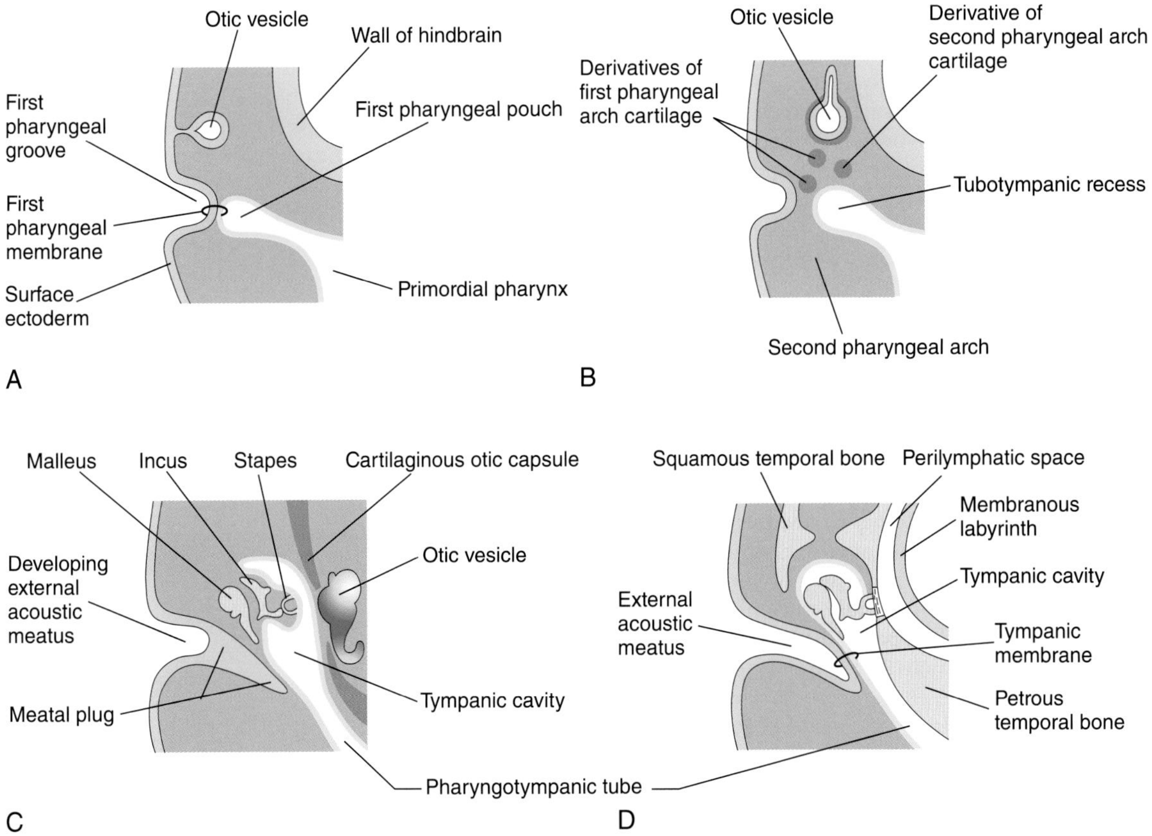

Fig. 18.16 Schematic drawings illustrate the development of the external and middle parts of the ear. Observe the relationship of these parts to the otic vesicle, the primordium of the internal ear. (A) At 4 weeks, the drawing shows the relationship of the otic vesicle to the pharyngeal apparatus. (B) At 5 weeks, the drawing shows the tubotympanic recess and pharyngeal arch cartilages. (C) Drawing of a later stage shows the tubotympanic recess (future tympanic cavity and mastoid antrum) beginning to envelop the ossicles. (D) Drawing of the final stage of ear development shows the relationship of the middle ear to the perilymphatic space and the external acoustic meatus. The tympanic membrane develops from three germ layers: surface ectoderm, mesenchyme, and endoderm of the tubotympanic recess.

proximal part of the tubotympanic recess forms the **pharyngotympanic tube** (auditory/Eustasian tube). The distal part of the recess expands and becomes the **tympanic cavity** (Fig. 18.16C), which gradually envelops the **auditory ossicles** (malleus, incus, and stapes), their tendons and ligaments, and the chorda tympani nerve. The malleus and incus are derived from the cartilage of the first pharyngeal arch. The crus, base of the foot plate, and the head of the stapes appear to be formed from neural crest, whereas the outer rim of the foot plate is derived from mesodermal cells. *Neural crest cells originating from the dorsal hindbrain migrate to specific sites on the first and second pharyngeal arches to form the three auditory ossicles (malleus, incus, and stapes). SHH, FGF, CXCL12, and BMP4 signaling control the formation of the ear ossicles.* These structures receive a more or less complete epithelial investment derived from neural crest cells of the endoderm. The neural crest cells undergo an epithelial-mesenchymal transformation. In addition to apoptosis in the middle ear, an epithelium-type organizer located at the tip of the tubotympanic recess probably plays a role in the early development of the middle ear cavity and tympanic membrane. Cavitation begins in the third month and is completed by the eighth month.

During the late fetal period, expansion of the tympanic cavity gives rise to the **mastoid antrum**, which is located in the petromastoid part of the temporal bone. The mastoid antrum is almost adult size at birth, but no mastoid cells are present in neonates. By 5 years of age, the mastoid cells are well developed and produce conical projections of the temporal bones, the **mastoid processes**. The middle ear continues to grow through puberty. The **tensor tympani muscle**, which is attached to the malleus, is derived from mesenchyme in the first pharyngeal arch and is innervated by the trigeminal nerve (CN V), the nerve of this arch. The **stapedius muscle** is derived from the second pharyngeal arch and is supplied by the facial nerve (CN VII), the nerve of this arch. *The signaling molecules fibroblast growth factor 8 (FGF8), endothelin 1 (EDN1), and T-box 1 (TBX1) are involved in middle ear development.*

EXTERNAL EARS

The **external acoustic meatus** develops from the dorsal part of the first pharyngeal groove (see Fig. 18.16A; see Fig. 9.7C). The ectodermal cells at the bottom of the meatus proliferate to form a solid epithelial plate, the **meatal plug** (see Fig. 18.16C). Late in the fetal period, the central cells of this plug degenerate, forming a cavity that becomes the internal part of the external acoustic meatus (see Fig. 18.16D). The meatus, which is relatively short at birth, attains its adult length by approximately age nine.

The primordium of the **tympanic membrane** is the first pharyngeal membrane, which forms the external surface of the tympanic membrane. In the embryo, the pharyngeal membrane separates the first pharyngeal groove from the first pharyngeal pouch (see Fig. 18.16A). As development proceeds, mesenchyme grows between the two parts of the pharyngeal membrane and differentiates into the collagenic fibers in the tympanic membrane.

The tympanic membrane develops from three sources:

- **Ectoderm** of the first pharyngeal groove
- **Endoderm** of the tubotympanic recess, a derivative of the first pharyngeal pouch

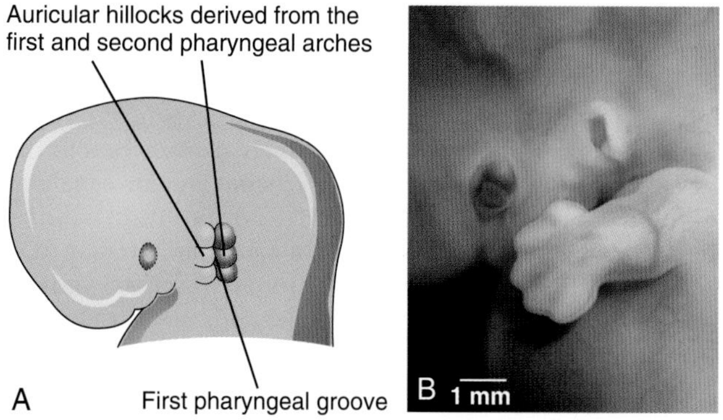

Fig. 18.17 Development of the auricle, which is the part of the external ear that is not within the head. (A) At 6 weeks, three of the auricular hillocks are located on the first pharyngeal arch and three on the second arch. (B) Photograph of a 7-week embryo shows the developing external ear. (B, Courtesy Dr. Brad Smith, University of Michigan, Ann Arbor, MI.)

- **Mesenchyme** of the first and second pharyngeal arches

The **auricle** (pinna), which projects from the side of the head, develops from mesenchymal proliferations in the first and second pharyngeal arches **(auricular hillocks)** surrounding the first pharyngeal groove (Fig. 18.17A). As the auricle grows, the contribution from the first arch is reduced, and it forms the tragus. The **lobule** (earlobe) of the auricle is the last part of the auricle to develop. The auricle reaches its adult structure by 22 weeks. *HoxA2 appears to be critical to auricle development.* The auricles begin to develop at the base of the neck (Fig. 18.17A and B). As the mandible develops, the auricles assume their normal position at the side of the head (see Fig. 18.21) due to differential growth of the head and neck.

The parts of the auricle derived from the first pharyngeal arch are supplied by the mandibular branch of the trigeminal nerve (CN V); the parts derived from the second arch are supplied by cutaneous branches of the cervical plexus, especially the lesser occipital and greater auricular nerves. The nerve of the second pharyngeal arch, the facial nerve, has few cutaneous branches; some of its fibers contribute to the sensory innervation of the skin in the mastoid region and probably in small areas on both aspects of the auricle.

SUMMARY OF EYE DEVELOPMENT

- The first indication of the eyes is the **optic grooves** in the neural folds at the cranial end of the embryo. The grooves form at the beginning of the fourth week and deepen to form hollow optic vesicles that project from the forebrain.
- The **optic vesicles** contact the surface ectoderm and induce the development of the **lens placodes**.
- As the lens placode thickens to form a **lens pit** and **lens vesicle**, the optic vesicle invaginates to form the **optic cup**. The **retina** forms from the two layers of the optic cup.
- The retina, optic nerve fibers, muscles of the iris, and epithelium of the iris and ciliary body are derived from the **neuroectoderm of the forebrain**. The sphincter and dilator muscles of the iris develop from the ectoderm at the rim of

Congenital Deafness

Because the formation of the internal ear is independent of the development of the middle and external ears, congenital impairment of hearing may be the result of maldevelopment of the sound-conducting apparatus of the middle and external ears or the neurosensory structures of the internal ear. Approximately 3 in 1000 neonates have significant hearing loss, of which there are many subtypes. Many hospitals are now providing routine screening for hearing loss before discharge to identify such neonates and institute treatment early to optimize outcomes.

Most types of congenital deafness are caused by genetic factors, and many of the genes responsible have been identified. Pathogenic variants (mutations) in the *GJB2* gene are responsible for approximately 50% of nonsyndromic recessive hearing loss. Congenital deafness may be associated with several other head and neck defects as a part of the **first arch syndrome** (see Fig. 9.14). Abnormalities of the malleus and incus, which occur frequently, are often associated with this syndrome (see Fig. 14.8D). Approximately 50% of nongenetic cases are related to infection. **Congenital cytomegalovirus (CMV) is the most common nongenetic cause of sensorineural hearing loss.** A **rubella** infection during the critical period of development of the internal ear, particularly the seventh and eighth weeks, can cause defects of the spiral organ and deafness (see Table 20.1). Other congenital infectious agents associated with hearing loss include *Toxoplasma gondii*, herpes simplex virus, and *Treponema pallidum*. **Congenital fixation of the stapes** results in conductive deafness in an otherwise normal ear. Failure of differentiation of the annular ligament, which attaches the base of the stapes to the oval window *(fenestra vestibuli)*, results in the fixation of the stapes to the bony labyrinth.

Auricular Abnormalities

Severe defects of the external ear are rare, but minor deformities are common. There is a wide variation in the shape of the auricle. Almost any minor auricular defect may occasionally be found as a usual feature in a particular family. Minor defects of the auricles may also serve as indicators of a specific pattern of congenital defects (Fig. 18.18). High-resolution computed tomography is invaluable for the evaluation and early management of children with auricular defects and significant hearing loss.

Accessory Auricle

Accessory auricles are common (5–10:1000) and may result from the development of **accessory auricular hillocks** (Fig. 18.19). The appendages usually appear anterior to the auricle, more often unilaterally than bilaterally. The appendages, which often have narrow pedicles, consist of skin, but they may contain some cartilage.

Anotia/Microtia

Anotia, the absence of the auricle, is rare (1:25,000) but is commonly associated with the first pharyngeal arch syndrome. This defect results from the failure of mesenchymal proliferation. **Microtia** (2–3:10,000) (small or rudimentary auricle) results from suppressed mesenchymal proliferation (Fig. 18.20). This defect often serves as an indicator of associated birth defects, such as atresia of the external acoustic meatus (80% of cases) and middle ear anomalies. The cause can be both genetic and environmental.

Preauricular Sinuses (Ear Pit) and Fistulas

The sinuses, located in a triangular area anterior to the auricle, are usually narrow tubes or shallow pits that have pinpoint external openings (Fig. 18.21; see Fig. 9.9E and F). Some sinuses contain a vestigial cartilaginous mass. Preauricular sinuses may be associated with internal anomalies such as deafness and kidney malformations. The embryologic basis of auricular sinuses is uncertain, but it may relate to incomplete fusion of the auricular hillocks or to abnormal mesenchymal proliferation and defective closure of the dorsal part of the first pharyngeal groove. Other auricular sinuses appear to represent ectodermal folds that are sequestered during the formation of the auricle. The preauricular sinus usually is unilateral and involves the right side, and bilateral preauricular sinuses are typically familial. Most sinuses are asymptomatic and have only minor cosmetic importance; however, they can become infected.

Auricular fistulas connecting the preauricular skin with the tympanic cavity or the tonsillar fossa (see Fig. 9.9F) are rare.

Congenital Aural Atresia

Atresia of the external acoustic meatus results from the failure of the meatal plug to canalize (Figs. 18.22 and 18.23; see Fig. 18.16C). The deep part of the meatus is usually open, but the superficial part is blocked by bone or fibrous tissue. Most cases are associated with the **first arch syndrome** (see Fig. 9.14). Abnormal development of the first and second pharyngeal arches often is involved. The auricle is also severely affected, and middle and internal ear defects sometimes occur. Atresia of the external acoustic meatus can occur bilaterally or unilaterally and usually results from the inheritance of an autosomal-dominant trait.

Complete absence of the external acoustic meatus is rare; usually, the auricle is normal (see Fig. 18.22). This defect results from the failure of inward expansion of the first pharyngeal groove and the failure of the meatal plug to disappear (see Fig. 18.16C).

Congenital Cholesteatoma

A congenital cholesteatoma is a fragment of keratinized epithelial cells that are trapped within the middle ear—it appears as a white, cyst-like structure (see Fig. 18.16C). It has been suggested that congenital cholesteatoma may originate from an epidermoid formation that normally involutes 33 weeks' gestation. Cholesteatomas can exhibit growth and invasion of neighboring bone and in most cases, are surgically excised.

the optic cup. The surface ectoderm gives rise to the **lens** and the epithelium of the lacrimal glands, eyelids, conjunctiva, and cornea. The mesenchyme gives rise to the eye muscles, except those of the iris, and to all connective and vascular tissues of the cornea, iris, ciliary body, choroid, and sclera.

- The eyes are sensitive to the teratogenic effects of **infectious agents** (e.g., cytomegalovirus). Defects of sight may result from infection of tissues and organs by certain microorganisms during the fetal period (e.g., rubella virus, *T. pallidum* [causes syphilis]).

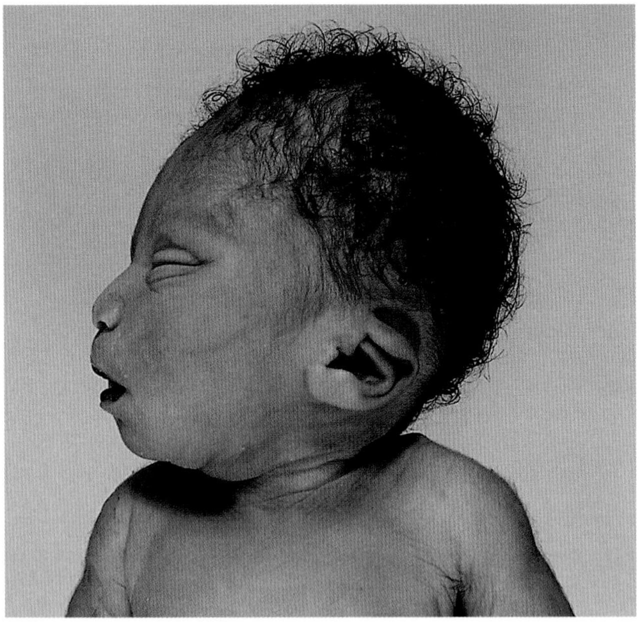

Fig. 18.18 Potter facies consists of low-set ears and a small, hooked nose associated with renal agenesis and pulmonary hypoplasia.

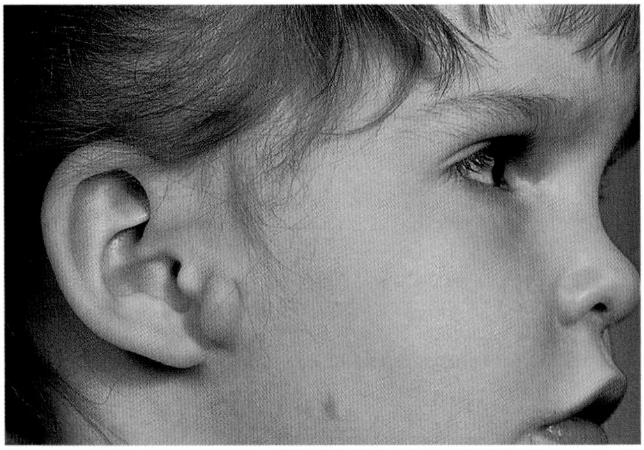

Fig. 18.19 Child with a preauricular tag or skin tag. (Courtesy Dr. A. E. Chudley, Section of Genetics and Metabolism, Department of Pediatrics and Child Health, University of Manitoba, Children's Hospital, Winnipeg, Manitoba, Canada.)

- Most ocular defects are caused by defective closure of the retinal fissure during the sixth week (e.g., coloboma of the iris).
- **Congenital cataracts** and **glaucoma** may result from intrauterine infections, but most congenital cataracts are inherited.

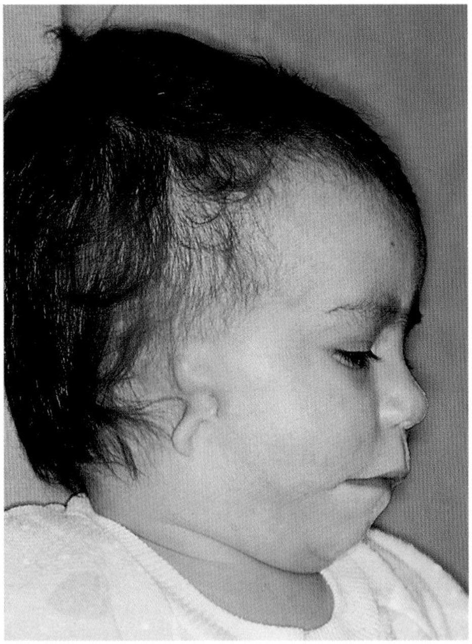

Fig. 18.20 Child with a rudimentary auricle (microtia). She also has several other birth defects. (Courtesy Dr. A. E. Chudley, Section of Genetics and Metabolism, Department of Pediatrics and Child Health, Children's Hospital, University of Manitoba, Winnipeg, Manitoba, Canada.)

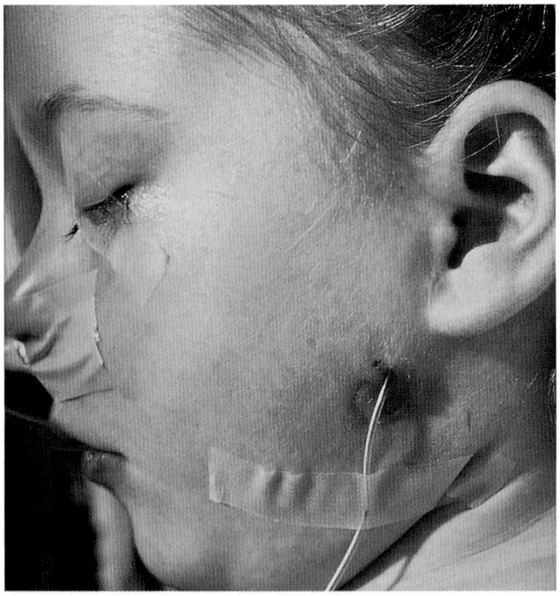

Fig. 18.21 Child with an auricular fistula related to the first pharyngeal arch. Notice the external orifice of the fistula below the auricle, the upward direction of the catheter (in the sinus tract) toward the external acoustic meatus, and the normal position of the auricle. (Courtesy Dr. Pierre Soucy, Division of Paediatric General Surgery, Children's Hospital of Eastern Ontario, Ottawa, Ontario, Canada.)

SUMMARY OF EAR DEVELOPMENT

- The **otic vesicle** develops from the surface ectoderm during the fourth week. The vesicle develops into the **membranous labyrinth** of the internal ear.
- The otic vesicle divides into a **dorsal utricular part**, which gives rise to the **utricle**, **semicircular ducts**, and **endolymphatic duct**, and a **ventral saccular part**, which gives rise to the **saccule** and **cochlear duct**. The cochlear duct gives rise to the **spiral organ**.
- The **bony labyrinth** develops from the mesenchyme adjacent to the membranous labyrinth. The epithelium lining the tympanic cavity, mastoid antrum, and

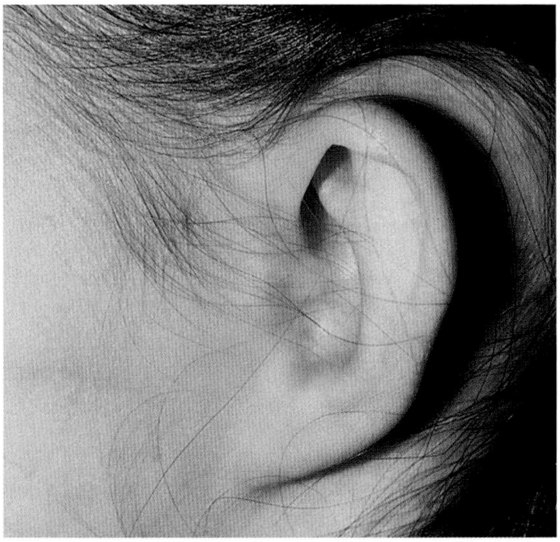

Fig. 18.22 This child has no external acoustic meatus, but the auricle is normal. Computed tomography revealed normal middle and internal ear structures. (Courtesy Dr. A. E. Chudley, Section of Genetics and Metabolism, Department of Pediatrics and Child Health, Children's Hospital, University of Manitoba, Winnipeg, Manitoba, Canada.)

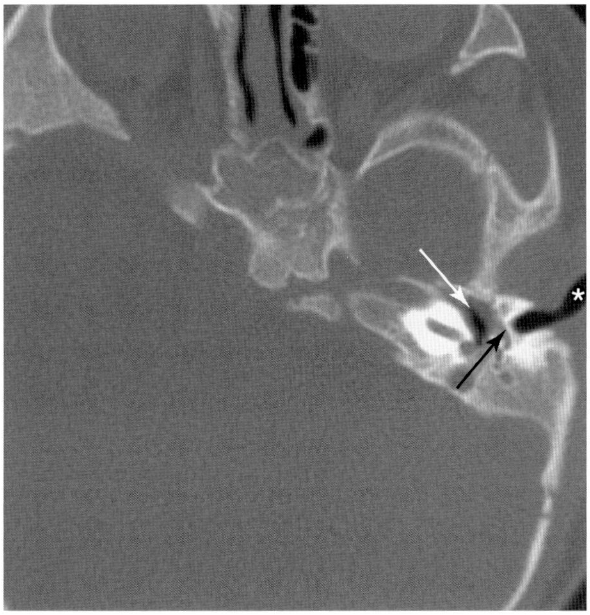

Fig. 18.23 Computed tomogram of a 9-month-old infant with atresia of the external acoustic meatus (external auditory canal; *asterisk*) shows the osseous atresia plate *(black arrow)* and the middle ear cavity *(white arrow)*. (Courtesy Dr. Gerald S. Smyser, formerly, Altru Health System, Grand Forks, ND.)

pharyngotympanic tube is derived from the endoderm of the **tubotympanic recess**, which develops from the first pharyngeal pouch.

- The auditory ossicles develop from the dorsal ends of the cartilages in the first two pharyngeal arches. The epithelium of the **external acoustic meatus** develops from the ectoderm of the first pharyngeal groove.
- The **tympanic membrane** is derived from three sources: endoderm of the first pharyngeal pouch, ectoderm of the first pharyngeal groove, and mesenchyme between the previous two layers.
- The **auricle** develops from the fusion of six **auricular hillocks**, which form from mesenchymal prominences around the margins of the first pharyngeal groove.
- **Congenital deafness** may result from abnormal development of the membranous labyrinth, bony labyrinth, or auditory ossicles. Inheritance of a recessive trait is the most common cause of congenital deafness; CMV infection is the most common nongenetic cause.
- There are many minor anomalies of the auricle; however, some of them may alert clinicians to the possible presence of associated major anomalies (e.g., defects of the middle ear). Low-set, severely malformed ears are often associated with **chromosomal abnormalities**, particularly trisomy 13 and trisomy 18.

CLINICALLY ORIENTED PROBLEMS

CASE 18-1

A fetus was born blind and deaf with congenital heart disease. The mother had a severe viral infection early in her pregnancy.

- Name the virus that was probably responsible for the birth defects.
- What is the common congenital cardiovascular lesion found in infants whose mothers have this infection early in pregnancy?
- Is the history of a rash during the first trimester an essential factor in the development of embryonic disease (embryopathy)?

CASE 18-2

An infant was born with bilateral ptosis.

- What is the probable embryologic basis of this condition?
- Are hereditary factors involved?
- Injury to what nerve can cause congenital ptosis?

CASE 18-3

An infant had multiple small calcifications in the brain, microcephaly, and microphthalmia. The mother was known to consume rare meat.

- What protozoon is likely involved?
- What is the embryologic basis of the infant's birth defects?
- What advice should the doctor give the mother concerning future pregnancies?

CASE 18-4

A female infant with intellectual disabilities had low-set, malformed ears; a prominent occiput; and rocker-bottom feet. A chromosomal abnormality was suspected.

- What is the type of chromosomal aberration?
- What is the usual cause of this abnormality?
- How long is the infant likely to survive?

CASE 18-5

An infant had partial detachment of the retina in one eye. The eye was microphthalmic, and there was persistence of the distal end of the hyaloid artery.

- What is the embryologic basis of congenital detachment of the retina?
- What is the usual fate of the hyaloid artery?

Discussion of problems appears in the Appendix at the back of the book.

BIBLIOGRAPHY AND SUGGESTED READING

Ankamreddy H, Koo H, Lee YJ, Bok J: CXCL12 is required for stirrup-shaped stapes formation during mammalian middle ear development, *Dev Dyn* 249:1117, 2020.

Anthwal N, Thompson H: The development of the mammalian outer and middle ear, *J Anat* 228, 2015. https://doi.org/10.1111/joa.12344.

Boobalan A, Thompson A, Ramakrishna P, McGaughey DM, Dong L, Shih G: Zfp503/Nlz2 is required for RPE differentiation and optic fissure closure, *Invest Ophthalmol Vis Sci* 63(12):5, 2022. https://doi.org/10.1167/iovs.63.12.5.

Box J, Chang W, Wu DK: Patterning and morphogenesis of the vertebrate ear, *Int J Dev Biol* 51:521, 2007.

Burford CM, Mason MJ: Early development of the malleus and incus in humans, *J Anat* 229:857, 2016.

Cardozo MJ, Almuedo-Castillo M, Bovolenta P: Patterning the vertebrate retina with morphogenetic signaling pathways, *Neuroscientist* 26:185, 2020. https://doi.org/10.1177/1073858419874016.

Casey MA, Lusk S, Kwan KM: Build me up optic cup: intrinsic and extrinsic mechanisms of vertebrate eye morphogenesis, *Dev Biol* 476:128, 2021.

Cho RI, Kahana A: Embryology of the orbit, *J Neurol Surg* 82:2, 2021.

Chung HA, Medina-Ruiz S, Harland RM: Sp8 regulates inner ear development, *Proc Natl Acad Sci USA* 111:632, 2014.

Barishak YR: *Embryology of the eye and its adnexa*, ed 2, Basel, 2001, Karger.

Gong Y, He X, Li Q, Bian B, Li Y, Ge L, Zeng Y, Xu H, Yin ZQ, et al: SCF/SCFR signaling plays an important role in the early morphogenesis and neurogenesis of human embryonic neural retina, *Development* 146(20):dev174409, 2019. https://doi.org/10.1242/dev.174409.

O'Rahilly R: The early development of the otic vesicle in staged human embryos, *J Embryol Exp Morphol* 11:741, 1963.

O'Rahilly R: The prenatal development of the human eye, *Exp Eye Res* 21:93, 1975.

Dash P, Rout JP, Panigrahi PK: Clinical patterns of congenital ocular anomalies in the pediatric age group (0 to 5 years) and its association with various demographic parameters, *Indian J Ophthalmol* 70:944, 2022.

Donga F, Calla M, Xia Y, Kao WW-Y: Role of EGF receptor signaling on morphogenesis of eyelid and meibomian glands, *Exp Eye Res* 163:58, 2017.

Ebeid M, Huh SH: FGF signaling: diverse roles during cochlear development, *BMB Rep* 50:487, 2017.

Ebeid M, Huh SH: PRDM16 expression and function in mammalian cochlear development, *Dev Dyn*, 2022. https://doi.org/10.1002/dvdy.480. PMID 35451126.

Farmer DT, Finley JK, Chen FY, et al: miR-205 is a critical regulator of lacrimal gland development, *Dev Biol* 427:12, 2017.

Fuhrmann S: Eye morphogenesis and patterning of the optic vesicle, *Curr Top Dev Biol 93*:61, 2010.

Gaca PJ, Lewandowicz M, Lipczynska-Lewandowska M, Simon M, Rejdak R, Wawer-Matos PA, et al: Die embryologische und fetale entwicklung der Orbita, der Augenlider und des Tränenwegsystems, *Klin Monbl Augenheilkd* 239(6):820–822, 2022. (in German). https://doi.org/10.1055/a-1835-9144.

Garg A, Zhang X: Lacrimal gland development: From signaling interactions to regenerative medicine, *Dev Dyn* 246:970–980, 2017. https://doi.org/10.1002/dvdy.24551.

Ghada MWF: Ear embryology, *Glob J Oto* 4(1):555627, 2017.

Haddad J. Jr: The ear. congenital malformations. In Kliegman RM, Stanton BF, editors: *Nelson textbook of pediatrics*, ed 19, Philadelphia, 2011, Saunders.

Harding P, Moosajee M: The molecular basis of human anophthalmia and microphthalmia, *J Dev Biol* 7(3):16, 2019. https://doi.org/10.3390/jdb7030016.

Hemkemeyer SA, Liu Z, Vollmer V, Xu Y, Lohmann B, Bähler M: The RhoGap-myosin Myo9b regulates ocular lens pit morphogenesis, *Dev Dyn*, 2022. https://doi.org/10.1002/dvdyy.522.

Hwang J, Cho J, Burm JS: Accessory auricle: classification according to location, protrusion pattern, and body shape, *Arch Plastic Surg* 45(5):411, 2018.

Jason R, Guercio BS, Martyn LJ: Congenital malformations of the eye and orbit, *Otolaryngol Clin North Am* 40:113, 2007.

Karnam S, Maddala R, Stiber JA, Rao PV: Drebrin, an actin-binding protein, is required for lens morphogenesis and growth, *Dev Dyn* 250(11):1600–1617, 2021. https://doi.org/10.1002/dvdy.353.

Kim HS, Sarrafpour S, Teng CC, Ji Liu. External disruption of ocular development in utero. *Yale J Biol Med* 97(1):41–48, 2019. https://doi.org/10.59249/rrmm8911.

Kinoshita A, Ohyama K, Tanimura S, et al: Itpr1 regulates the formation of anterior eye segment tissues derived from neural crest cells, *Development* 148, 2021. https://doi.org/10.1242/dev.188755.

Lingam G, Sen AC, Lingam V, Bhende M, Padhi TR, Xinyi S: Ocular coloboma – a comprehensive review for the clinician, *Eye* 35:2086, 2021.

Ma JY, You D, Li WY, Lu XL, Sun S, Li HW: Bone morphogenetic proteins and inner ear development, *J Zhejiang Univ Sci B* 20(2):131–145, 2019. https://doi.org/10.1631/jzus.B1800084.

Munnamalai V, Fekete DM: Wnt signaling during cochlear development, *Semin Cell Dev Biol* 24:480, 2013.

Okawa H, Morokuma S, Maehara K, et al: Eye movement activity in normal human fetuses between 24 and 39 weeks of gestation, *PLOS ONE* 12:e0178722, 2017. https://doi.org/10.1371/journal.pone.0178722.

Porter CJW, Tan SW: Congenital auricular anomalies: topographic anatomy, embryology, classification, and treatment strategies, *Plast Reconstr Surg* 115:1701, 2005.

Bauer PW, MacDonald CB, Melhem ER: Congenital inner ear malformation, *Am J Otol* 19:669, 1998.

Helwany M, Arbor TC, Tadi P: Embryology, ear. [Updated 2022 Aug 14]. In *StatPearls [Internet]*, Treasure Island, 2022, StatPearls Publishing. Available from: https://www.ncbi.nlm.nih.gov/books/NBK557588/.

Sellheyer K: Development of the choroid and related structures, *Eye* 4:255, 1990.

Shiels A, Hejtmancik JF: Molecular genetics of cataract, *Prog Mol Biol Transl Sci* 134:203, 2015.

Thompson H, Ohazama A, Sharpe PT, Tucker AS: The origin of the stapes and relationship to the otic capsule and oval window, *Dev Dynam* 241:1396, 2012.

Xia Q, Zhang D, Zhuang Y, et al: Animal model contributions to primary congenital glaucoma, *J Ophthalmol* 2022:6955461, 2022. https://doi.org/10.1155/2022/6955461.

Integumentary System 19

CHAPTER OUTLINE

The integumentary system consists of the skin and its appendages: sweat glands, nails, hairs, sebaceous glands, arrector muscles of hairs (arrector pili muscles), mammary glands, and teeth.

DEVELOPMENT OF SKIN AND APPENDAGES

The skin is a complex organ system and is the body's largest organ. The skin consists of two layers (Fig. 19.1):

- The **epidermis** is a superficial epithelial tissue that is derived from surface embryonic ectoderm.
- The **dermis** is a deep layer composed of dense irregularly arranged connective tissue that is derived from mesenchyme.

Ectodermal and mesenchymal interactions involve mutual inductive mechanisms that are mediated by a conserved set of signaling molecules, including WNT, fibroblast growth factor (FGF), transforming growth factor-β (TGF-β), and sonic hedgehog (SHH). Skin structures vary from one part of the body to another. For example, the skin of the eyelids is thin and soft and has fine hairs, whereas the skin of the eyebrows is thick and has coarse hairs. The **embryonic skin** at 4 to 5 weeks consists of a single layer of **surface ectoderm** overlying the mesoderm (see Fig. 19.1A).

EPIDERMIS

Epidermal growth occurs in stages and with increasing epidermal thickness. By 2 to 3 weeks, the primordium of the epidermis is a single layer of cuboidal undifferentiated ectodermal cells (see Fig. 19.1A). During weeks 4 to 6, these cells proliferate and form an outer layer of simple squamous epithelium, the **periderm**, and a basal layer of collagen fibers and laminin—the basement membrane zone (see Fig. 19.1B and C). The cells of the periderm continually undergo **keratinization** and **desquamation** (shedding) and they are replaced by cells arising from the **basal layer**. Keratinization of the skin begins at 19 to 20 weeks, initially with the palms, soles, head, and face. The exfoliated peridermal cells form part of **vernix caseosa** (a white, greasy substance) that covers the fetal skin (see Fig. 19.3). The vernix protects the developing skin from constant exposure to amniotic fluid, with its high content of urine, bile salts, and sloughed cells. The vernix also facilitates childbirth.

By the 8 to 11 weeks, proliferation of the basal layer forms a layer of stem cells deep to the periderm. This **stratum germinativum** (see Fig. 19.1B and D) produces new cells that are displaced into the more superficial layers. By 14 weeks, cells from the stratum germinativum have formed an **intermediate layer** that differentiates and contributes to the formation of the mature keratinized epidermis (see Fig. 19.1C). Replacement of peridermal cells continues until approximately the 21st week; thereafter, the periderm disappears, and the **stratum corneum** forms from the **stratum lucidum** (see Fig. 19.1D).

The proliferation of cells in the stratum germinativum also forms **epidermal ridges** that extend into the developing dermis (Fig. 19.2). These ridges begin to appear in embryos at 10 weeks and are permanently established by 19 weeks. Those of the hand appear approximately 1 week earlier than ridges in the feet. The epidermal ridges produce grooves on the surface of the palms and soles, including the digits. Fingerprints and footprints are already present in fetuses that are 6 months old. The pattern that develops is determined genetically and constitutes the basis for examining fingerprints in medical genetics and criminal investigations. Abnormal chromosome complements can affect the development of ridge patterns.

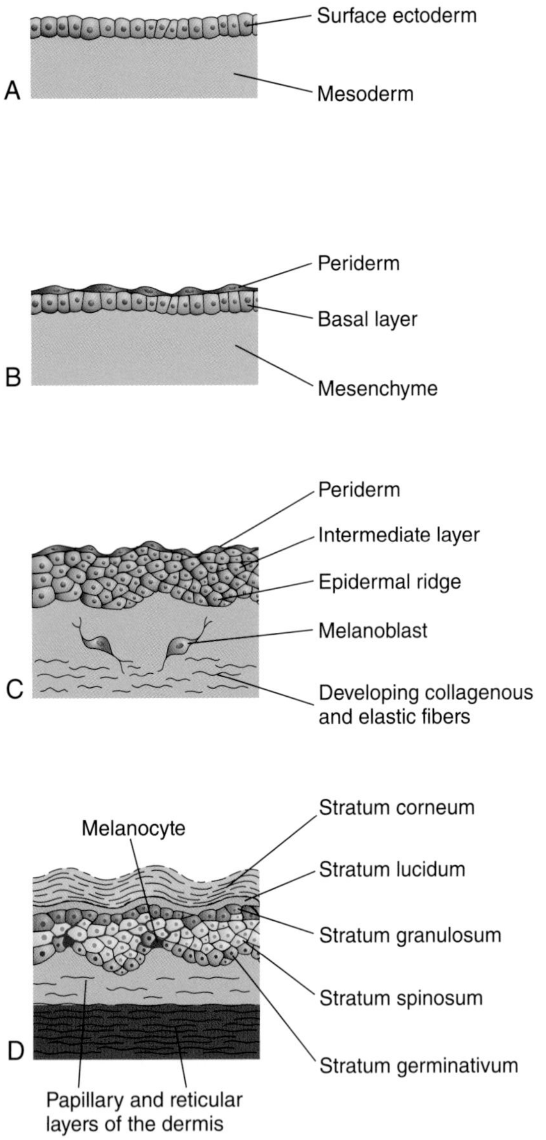

Fig. 19.1 Successive stages of skin development: (A) at 4 weeks, (B) at 7 weeks, (C) at 11 weeks, (D) neonate. Observe the melanocytes in the basal layer of the epidermis; their processes extend between the epidermal cells to supply them with melanin.

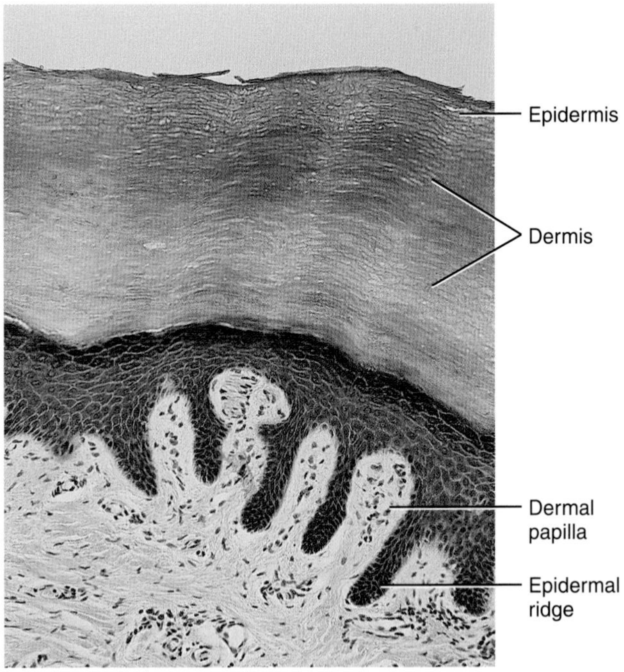

Fig. 19.2 Light micrograph of thick skin (×132). Observe the epidermis, the dermis, and the dermal papillae interdigitating with the epidermal ridges. (From Gartner LP, Hiatt JL: *Color textbook of histology*, ed 2, Philadelphia, 2001, Saunders.)

Late in the embryonic period, **neural crest cells** migrate into the mesenchyme of the developing dermis and differentiate into **melanoblasts** (see Fig. 19.1C). These cells migrate to the **dermoepidermal junction** and differentiate into **melanocytes** (pigment-producing cells); see Fig. 19.1D which form **pigment granules**. *Molecular studies indicate that Myosin X (Myo10), SOX10, MITF, DCT, KIT, and the Wnt signaling pathways are essential in this process and for melanin formation.*

Melanocytes appear in the developing skin at 40 to 50 days. In Caucasians, the cell bodies of melanocytes are usually confined to basal layers of the epidermis (see Fig. 19.1B); however, the **dendritic processes of the melanocytes** extend between the epidermal cells (see Fig. 19.1C).

Only a few melanin-containing cells are normally present in the dermis (see Fig. 19.1D). The melanocytes begin producing melanin before birth and distribute it to the epidermal cells. Melanin production is regulated by intrinsic biosynthetic pathways and enzymatic reactions involving the tyrosinase enzyme. Pigment formation can be observed prenatally in the epidermis of dark-skinned populations. The relative content of melanin inside the melanocytes accounts for the different colors of the skin.

The transformation of the surface ectoderm into the multilayered **definitive epidermis** results from continuing inductive interactions with the dermis. Skin is classified as thick or thin based on the thickness of the epidermis.

- **Thick skin** covers the palms and soles; it lacks hair follicles, arrector muscles of hairs, and sebaceous glands, but it has sweat glands.
- **Thin skin** covers most of the rest of the body; it contains hair follicles, arrector muscles of hairs, sebaceous glands, and sweat glands (Fig. 19.3).

DERMIS

The dermis develops from mesenchyme (see Fig. 19.1A and B), most of which originates from the somatic layer of lateral mesoderm; however, some of it is derived from the dermatomes of the somites (see Fig. 14.1C and E). By 11 weeks, the mesenchymal cells have begun to produce collagenous and elastic connective tissue fibers (see Figs. 19.1D and 19.3).

As the epidermal ridges form, the dermis projects into the epidermis, forming **dermal papillae**, which interdigitate with the epidermal ridges (see Fig. 19.2). **Capillary loops of blood vessels** develop in some of the papillae and provide nourishment for the epidermis (see Fig. 19.3); sensory nerve endings form in other papillae. The **developing afferent**

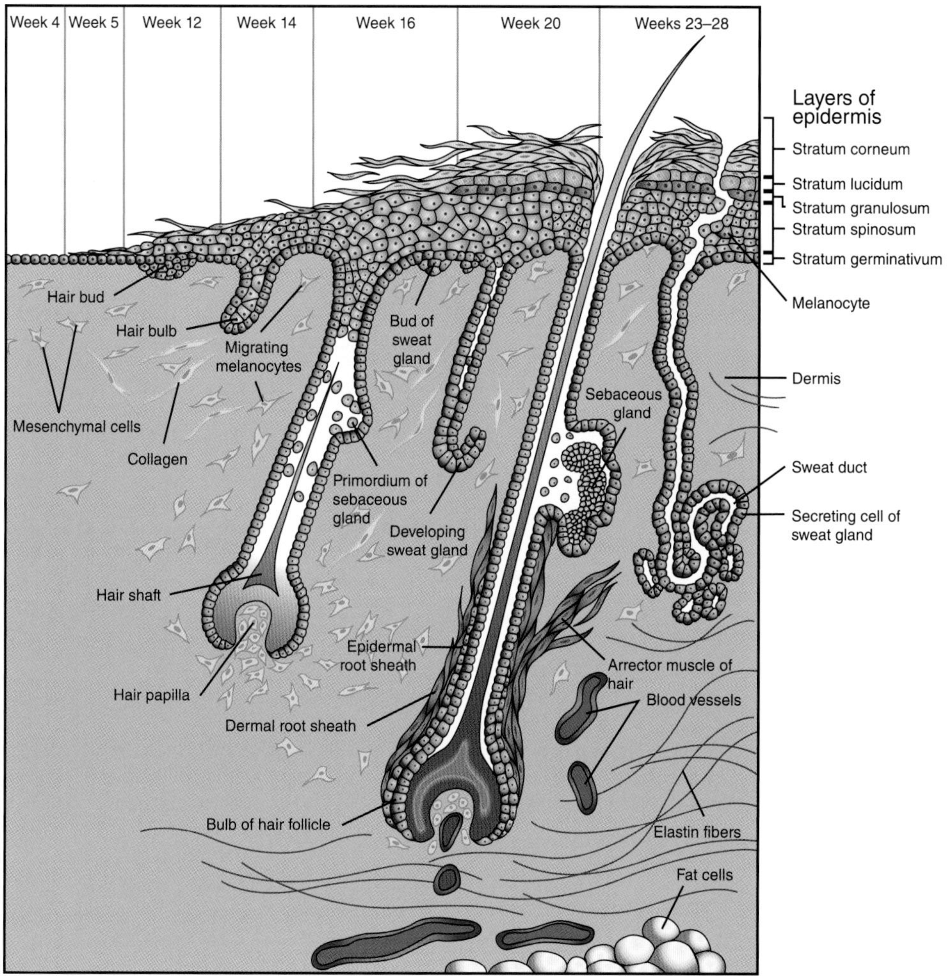

Fig. 19.3 Successive stages in the development of hairs, sebaceous glands, and arrector muscles of hair. The sebaceous gland develops as an outgrowth from the side of the hair follicle.

nerve fibers play an important role in the spatial and temporal sequence of dermal ridge formation. The development of the **dermatomal pattern** of innervation of the skin of the limbs is described elsewhere (see Fig. 16.10).

The blood vessels in the dermis begin as simple, endothelium-lined structures that differentiate from mesenchyme **(vasculogenesis)**. As the skin grows, new capillaries grow out from the primordial vessels **(angiogenesis)**. These capillary-like vessels have been observed in the dermis at the end of the fifth week. Some capillaries acquire muscular coats through the differentiation of myoblasts developing in the surrounding mesenchyme and becoming arterioles and arteries. Other capillaries, through which a return flow of blood is established, acquire muscular coats and become venules and veins. As new blood vessels form, some transitory ones disappear. By the end of the first trimester, the major vascular organization of the fetal dermis is established.

GLANDS

The glands of the skin include eccrine and apocrine sweat glands, sebaceous glands, and mammary glands. They are derived from the epidermis and grow into the dermis.

SEBACEOUS GLANDS

Sebaceous glands are derived from the epidermis. Cellular buds develop from the sides of the developing **epidermal root sheaths of hair follicles** (see Fig. 19.3). The buds invade the surrounding dermal connective tissue and branch to form the primordia of several gland alveoli and their associated ducts. The central cells of the alveoli break down, forming **sebum**, which is an oily secretion that protects the fetal skin against friction and dehydration. The secretion is released into **hair follicles** and passes to the surface of the skin, where it mixes with desquamated peridermal cells (see Fig. 19.3).

Sebaceous glands, independent of hair follicles, such as those of the glans penis and labia minora, develop as **cellular buds** from the epidermis that invade the dermis.

The Wnt/β-catenin signaling plays a critical role in the development of the skin, glands, and hair follicles and hair.

SWEAT GLANDS

Coiled, tubular **eccrine sweat glands** are located in the skin throughout most of the body. They develop as cellular buds from the epidermis that grow into the underlying mesenchyme (see Fig. 19.3). As the buds elongate, their ends

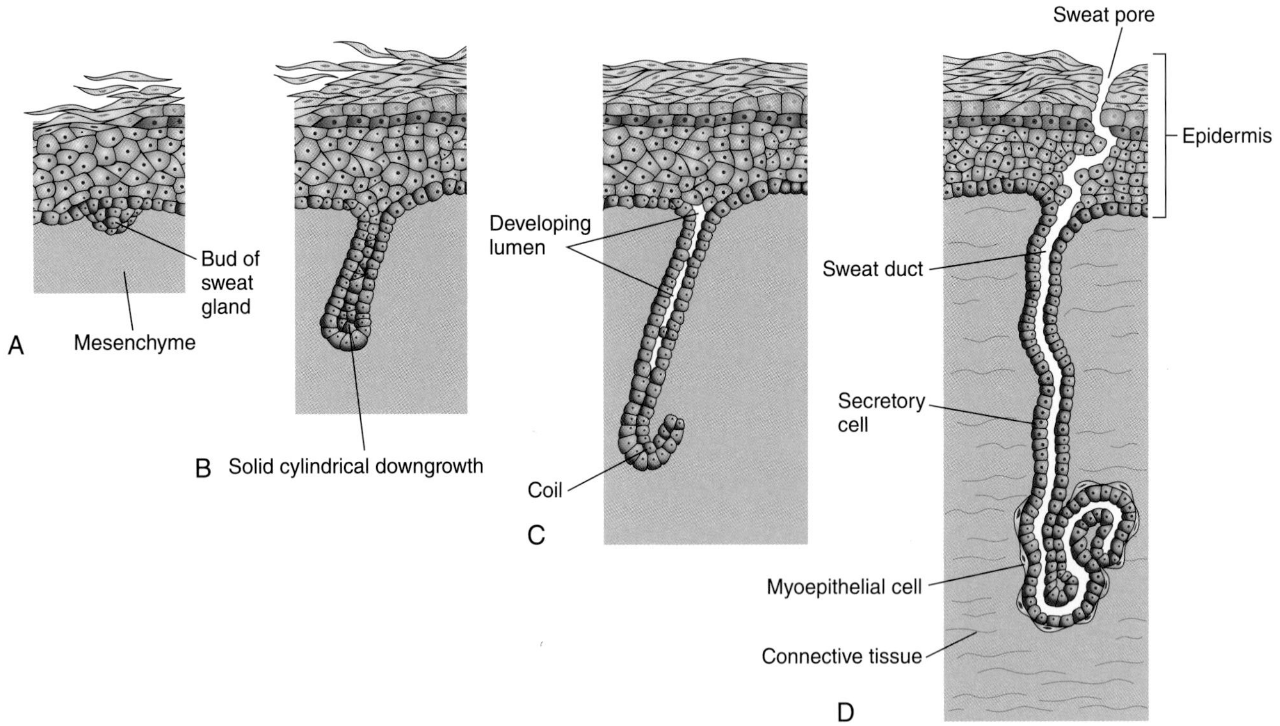

Fig. 19.4 Successive stages in the development of a sweat gland. (A and B) The cellular buds of the glands develop at approximately 20 weeks as a solid growth of epidermal cells into the mesenchyme. (C) Its terminal part coils and forms the body of the gland. The central cells degenerate to form the lumen of the gland. (D) The peripheral cells differentiate into secretory cells and contractile myoepithelial cells.

Neurocutaneous Syndromes

The central nervous system and the skin share a common ectodermal origin, and therefore genetic variations affecting such cells and cell lineages can result in the development of neurocutaneous syndromes. Such syndromes can demonstrate both neurologic and dermatologic consequences. These syndromes and their manifestations include the following:

- Tuberous sclerosis complex (TSC) (1–2:10,000)—benign tumors that can be found in almost any organ system, but most commonly the brain and skin. Almost all patients have hypomelanotic lesions and, in some cases, tumors under the fingernails or toenails (ungula tumors). The consequences of brain lesions include seizures (often the presenting symptom of TSC), behavioral issues, and other symptoms depending on the area of the brain affected.
- Sturge-Weber syndrome—this is a rare (1–2:10,000) neurocutaneous disorder with specific vascular malformations of the eye, skin, and brain. A variant in the GNAQ gene is commonly involved.
- Neurofibromatosis (NF)—there are two forms, NF1 and NF2; the former has a prevalence of 1 in 3000 and results from a defect in the *NF1* gene responsible for the formation of neurofibromin; the latter is much rare (1 in 60,000), with a genetic defect in *NF2* that results in lack of formation of merlin. NF1 includes pathognomic café-au-lait spots on the skin (by early childhood), gliomas, and peripheral nervous system neurofibromas. Management of NF1 is highly complex.

Disorders of Keratinization

Ichthyosis is a large group of relatively rare genetic skin disorders resulting from abnormal epidermal differentiation and excessive **keratinization of skin** (Fig. 19.5B). The skin is characterized by dryness and scaling, which may involve the entire surface of the body.

Harlequin ichthyosis results from a very rare keratinizing disorder that is inherited as an autosomal recessive trait with a variant of the *ABCA12* gene (prevalence 1:200,000). Infants with Harlequin ichthyosis are usually born prematurely. The skin is markedly thickened, ridged, and cracked. Affected neonates require intensive care, and even so, more than 50% die early.

A **"collodion baby,"** usually born prematurely, is covered by a thick, shiny, taut membrane that resembles collodion (a protective film) or parchment. The membranous skin cracks with the first respiratory efforts and begins to fall off in large sheets. Deficiency of transglutaminase 1 (TGM1) is the most common cause. Complete shedding may take several weeks, occasionally leaving normal-appearing skin.

Lamellar ichthyosis is an autosomal recessive disorder. A neonate with this condition may appear to be a "collodion baby" at first; however, the scaling persists. Growth of hair may be curtailed, and the development of sweat glands is often impeded. Affected infants usually suffer severely in hot weather because of their inability to sweat.

X-linked ichthyosis results from a deletion or variant of the *STS* gene, which causes a deficiency of steroid sulfatase. Most male neonates have pink or red skin with large translucent scales that shed after birth.

Epidermolytic ichthyosis or epidermolytic hyperkeratosis is an autosomal dominant condition resulting from variants of the *KRT1* and *KRT10* genes. The skin of the infant at birth may have blisters and appear to be peeling.

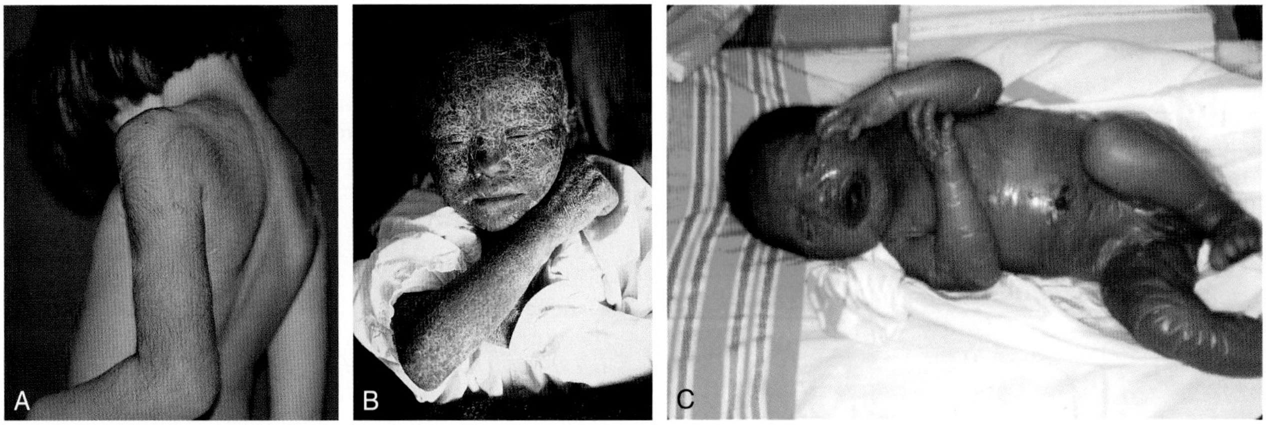

Fig. 19.5 (A) Child with congenital hypertrichosis and hyperpigmentation. Notice the excessive hairiness on the shoulders and back. (B) Child with severe keratinization of the skin (ichthyosis) from the time of birth. (C) Collodion baby. Infants with taut, shiny, cellophane-like membranes, ectropion (eversion of the eyelids), and eclabium (eversion of the lips). (A, Courtesy Dr. Mario Joao Branco Ferreira, Servico de Dermatologia, Hospital de Desterro, Lisbon, Portugal. B, Courtesy Dr. Joao Carlos Fernandes Rodrigues, Servico de Dermatologia, Hospital de Desterro, Lisbon, Portugal. C, From Craiglow, Brittany G: Ichthyosis in the newborn, *Semin Perinatol* 37(1):26–31, 2013.)

coil to form the bodies of the secretory parts of the glands (Fig. 19.4). The epithelial attachments of the developing glands to the epidermis form the **primordia of the sweat ducts**. The central cells of these ducts degenerate, forming **lumens**. The peripheral cells of the secretory parts of the glands differentiate into myoepithelial and secretory cells (see Fig. 19.4D). The **myoepithelial cells** are thought to be specialized smooth muscle cells that assist in expelling sweat from the glands. Eccrine sweat glands begin to function soon after birth.

The distribution of the large sudoriferous (producing sweat) **apocrine sweat glands** is mostly confined to the axillary, pubic, and perineal regions and the areolae surrounding the nipples. The glands develop from down growths of the stratum germinativum of the epidermis (see Fig. 19.3). As a result, the ducts of these glands do not open onto the skin surface, as do eccrine sweat glands, but into the canals of the hair follicles superficial to the entry of the sebaceous gland ducts. Secretion by apocrine sweat glands is influenced by hormones and does not begin until puberty.

Congenital Ectodermal Dysplasia

Congenital ectodermal dysplasia represents a group of more than 100 rare **hereditary disorders** involving anomalies in at least two structures derived from ectoderm. The teeth may be completely or partially absent, and the hairs and nails often are affected. **Ectrodactyly–ectodermal dysplasia–clefting syndrome** is a congenital skin condition that is transmitted as an autosomal dominant trait. It involves ectodermal and mesodermal tissues and consists of **ectodermal dysplasia** (incomplete development of epidermis and skin appendages; the skin is smooth and hairless). The **dysplasia** is associated with **hypopigmentation of skin**, scanty hair and eyebrows, absence of eyelashes, nail dystrophy, hypodontia and microdontia, **ectrodactyly** (absence of all or part of one or more fingers or toes), and cleft lip and palate. *This appears to be caused by a defect in the* TP63 *gene, which codes for a transcription factor*.

Angiomas of the Skin

Angiomas are **vascular anomalies**. Transitory or surplus primitive blood or lymphatic vessels persist in these developmental defects. Those composed of blood vessels may be mainly arterial, venous, or **cavernous angiomas**, but they are often a mixed type. Angiomas composed of lymphatics are called **cystic lymphangiomas** or **cystic hygromas** (see Fig. 13.55). True angiomas are benign tumors of endothelial cells that usually are composed of solid or hollow cords; the hollow cords contain blood.

Nevus flammeus denotes a flat, pink, or red flame-like blotch that often appears on the posterior surface of the neck. A **port-wine stain (hemangioma)** is a larger and darker angioma than a nevus flammeus and is typically anterior or lateral on the face or neck (Fig. 19.6). It is sharply demarcated when it is near the median plane, whereas the **common angioma** (pinkish red blotch) may cross the median plane. A port-wine stain in the area of distribution of the trigeminal nerve is sometimes associated with a similar type of angioma of the meninges of the brain and seizures at birth **(Sturge-Weber syndrome)**. Hemangiomas are among the most common benign neoplasms found in infants and children. When multiple, they may be associated with internal hemangiomas that affect the airways, or if in the liver, they may cause hematologic disturbances such as platelet consumption (Kasabach-Merritt syndrome).

Albinism

In **generalized (oculocutaneous) albinism**, which is an autosomal recessive condition (approximately 1:20,000), the skin, hairs, and retina lack pigment; however, the iris usually shows some pigmentation. There are eight known subtypes of albinism, which occur when the **melanocytes fail to produce melanin** because of the lack of the enzyme tyrosinase or other pigment enzymes. In localized albinism **(piebaldism)**, which is transmitted as an autosomal dominant trait, patches of skin and hair lack melanin.

MAMMARY GLANDS

Mammary glands are modified and highly specialized types of sweat glands. Gland development is similar in male and female embryos. The first evidence of mammary gland development appears in the fourth week when **mammary crests** (ridges) develop along each side of the ventral surface of the embryo. These crests extend from the axillary region (armpit) to the inguinal region (Fig. 19.7A). The crests usually disappear except for the parts at the site of the future breasts (see Fig. 19.7B).

Involution of the remaining mammary crests in the fifth week produces the **primary mammary buds** (see Fig. 19.7C). These buds are down growths of the epidermis into the underlying mesenchyme. The changes occur in response to parathyroid hormone–related peptide (PTHrP) signaling and inductive influence from the mesenchyme. Each primary mammary bud soon gives rise to several **secondary mammary buds**, which develop into **lactiferous ducts** and their branches (see Fig. 19.7D and E). *Expression of the epithelial transcription factors TBX3 and LEF1 initiates the formation of the mammary crests and buds.* **Canalization** of these buds is induced by **placental sex hormones** entering the fetal circulation. This process continues until the late fetal period, and by term, 15 to 19 lactiferous ducts are formed. The fibrous connective tissue and fat of the mammary glands develop from the surrounding mesenchyme. The structural remodeling and branching of the lactiferous ducts are controlled by hormones, including progesterone, estrogen, and prolactin.

During the late fetal period, the epidermis at the site of origin of the mammary glands becomes depressed, forming shallow **mammary pits** (see Fig. 19.7E). The nipples

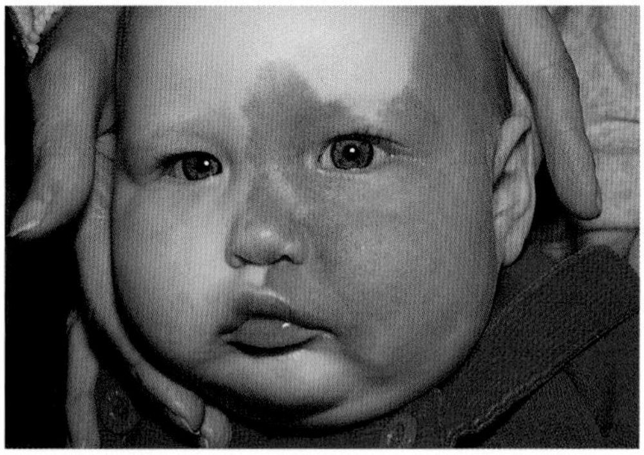

Fig. 19.6 Hemangioma (port-wine stain) in an infant. (From Anderson, D, editor: *Dorland's illustrated medical dictionary*, ed 30, Philadelphia, 2003, Saunders.)

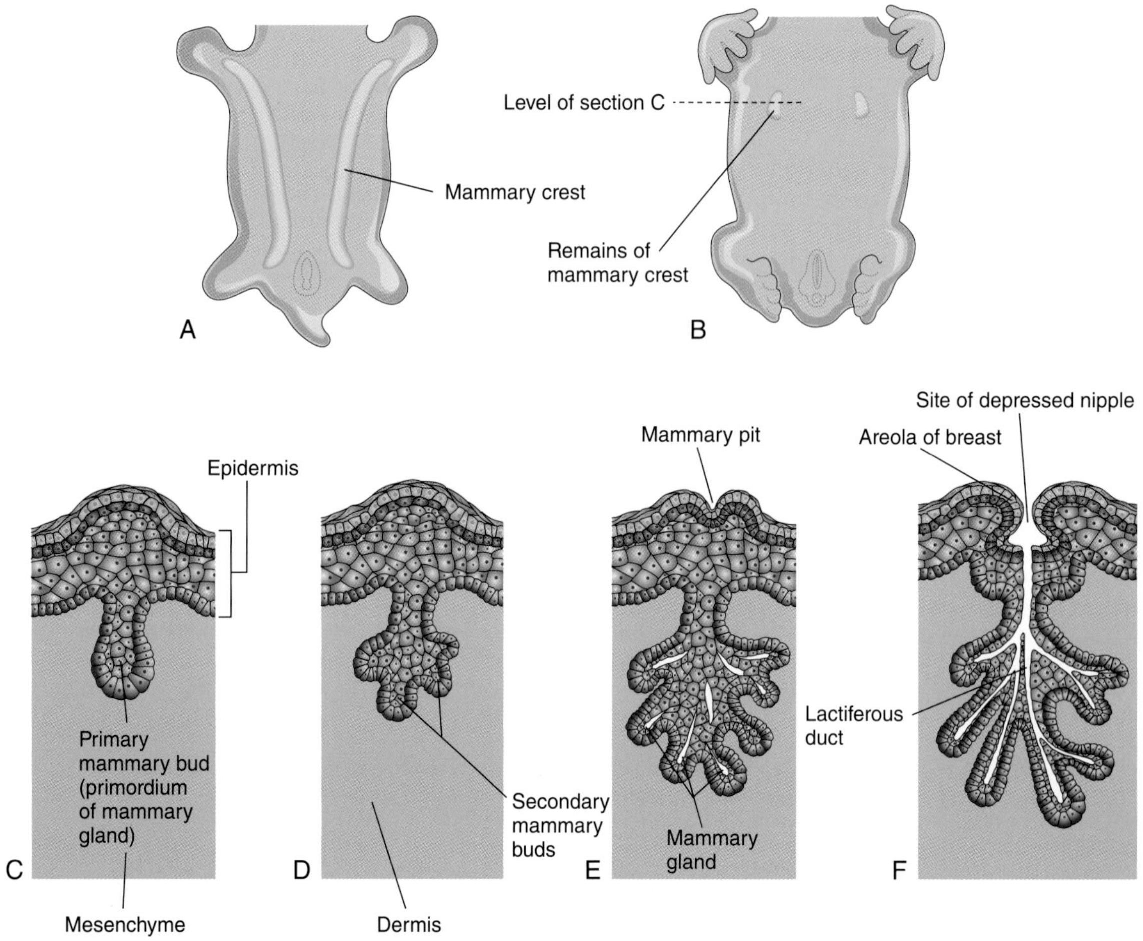

Fig. 19.7 Development of mammary glands. (A) Ventral view of an embryo of approximately 28 days shows the mammary crests. (B) Similar view at 6 weeks shows the remains of these crests. (C) Transverse section of a mammary crest at the site of a developing mammary gland. (D–F) Similar sections show successive stages of breast development between the 12th week and birth.

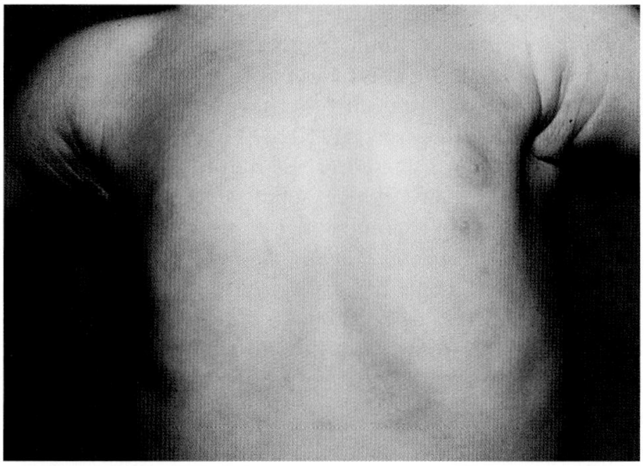

Fig. 19.8 Female infant with an extra nipple (polythelia) on the left side. (Courtesy Dr. A. E. Chudley, Section of Genetics and Metabolism, Department of Pediatrics and Child Health, Children's Hospital and University of Manitoba, Winnipeg, Manitoba, Canada.)

are poorly formed and depressed in neonates. Soon after birth, the nipples usually rise from the mammary pits because of the proliferation of the surrounding connective tissue of the **areola**, the circular area of pigmented skin around the nipples. The smooth muscle fibers of the nipples and areolae differentiate from surrounding mesenchymal cells.

The rudimentary mammary glands of male and female neonates are identical and are often enlarged. Some secretion (galactorrhea) may be produced. These transitory changes are caused by maternal hormones that pass through the placental membrane into the fetal circulation (see Fig. 7.7). The breasts of neonates contain **lactiferous ducts** but no **alveoli**. In the lactating mammary gland, these are the sites of milk secretion.

In females, the breasts enlarge rapidly during puberty, mainly because of the development of the mammary glands and the accumulation of the fibrous **stroma** (connective tissue) and fat associated with them. Full development occurs at approximately 19 years. Normally, the **lactiferous ducts** of boys remain rudimentary throughout life.

Several transcription factors, including the MYC protein, which is a basic helix-loop-helix transcription factor, are essential for the formation of the lactiferous ducts and the function of the female breast.

Gynecomastia

The rudimentary lactiferous ducts in boys normally undergo no postnatal development. **Gynecomastia** refers to the development of the rudimentary lactiferous ducts in the male mammary tissue. During mid-puberty, approximately two-thirds of boys develop various degrees of **hyperplasia** of the breasts. This subareolar hyperplasia may persist for a few months to 2 years. A decreased ratio of testosterone to estradiol is found in boys with gynecomastia. Approximately 40% of boys with **Klinefelter syndrome** have gynecomastia (see Fig. 20.12), which is associated with an XXY chromosome complement.

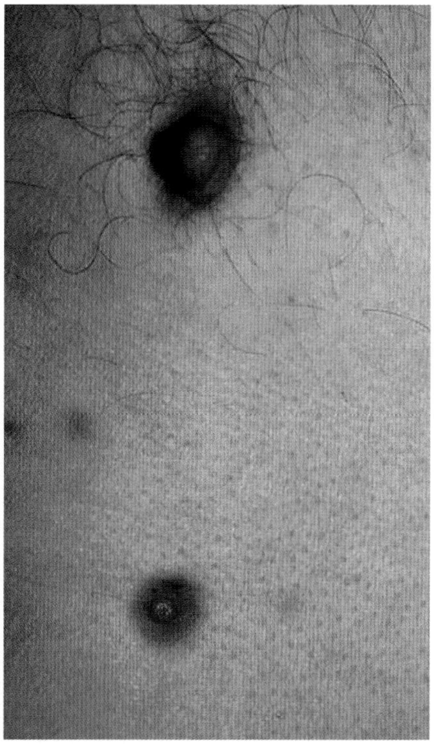

Fig. 19.9 A male with a supernumerary nipple with a surrounding areola. (Adapted from Bolognia JL, Schaffer JV, Duncan KO, Ko CJ: Developmental Anomalies. In Bolognia JL, Schaffer JV, Duncan KO, Ko CJ, editors: *Dermatology essentials*, ed 2, Elsevier, 2022.)

Absence of Nipples or Breasts

Absence of nipples (athelia) or breasts (amastia) may occur bilaterally or unilaterally. These extremely rare birth defects result from failure of development or disappearance of the mammary crests. They may also result from the failure of mammary buds to form. More common is **hypoplasia of the breast** which often is associated with **gonadal agenesis** (absence or failure of gonads to form) and **Turner syndrome** (see Fig. 20.4). **Poland syndrome** is associated with hypoplasia or absence of the breast or nipple. In these cases, there is often associated rudimentary development of muscles of the thoracic wall, usually the **pectoralis major** (see Fig. 15.5).

Supernumerary Breasts and Nipples

An extra breast **(polymastia)** or nipple **(polythelia)** occurs in approximately 0.2% to 5.6% of the female population (Fig. 19.8); it is an inheritable condition. An extra breast or nipple usually develops just inferior to the normal breast. **Supernumerary nipples** are also relatively common in males; often they are mistaken for moles (Fig. 19.9). Polythelia is often associated with other congenital defects such as renal and urinary tract anomalies. Less commonly, **supernumerary breasts or nipples** appear in the axillary or abdominal regions of females. In these positions, the nipples or breasts develop from extramammary buds that develop from remnants of the mammary crests. They usually become more obvious in women when they are pregnant. Approximately one-third of affected persons have two extra nipples or breasts. **Supernumerary mammary tissue** rarely occurs in a location other than along the course of the mammary crests (milk lines). It probably develops from tissue that was displaced from these crests.

HAIRS

Hairs begin to develop early in the fetal period (weeks 9–12), but they do not become easily recognizable until approximately the 20th week (see Fig. 19.3). Hairs are first recognizable on the eyebrows, upper lip, and chin. The **hair follicles** begin as proliferations of the stratum germinativum of the epidermis and extend into the underlying dermis. The **hair buds** become club-shaped in the 12th week, forming **hair bulbs (primordia of hair roots)** in the 14th week (see Fig. 19.3). The epithelial cells of the hair bulbs constitute the **germinal matrix**, which later produces the hair shafts.

The hair bulbs are soon invaginated by small mesenchymal **hair papillae** (Fig. 19.10; see Fig. 19.3). The peripheral cells of the developing hair follicles form **epithelial root sheaths**, and the surrounding mesenchymal cells differentiate into the **dermal root sheaths**. As cells in the **germinal matrix** proliferate, they are pushed toward the surface, where they become keratinized to form **hair shafts** (see Fig. 19.3). The hairs grow through the epidermis on the eyebrows and upper lip by the end of the 12th week.

The first hairs are called **lanugo** and are fine, soft, and lightly pigmented. Lanugo begins to appear toward the end of the 12th week and is plentiful by 17 to 20 weeks (see Fig. 19.3). These hairs help to hold the **vernix caseosa**, which covers and protects the skin of the fetus. Lanugo is replaced by coarser hairs during the perinatal period which persists over most of the body, except in the axillary and pubic regions, where it is replaced at puberty by even coarser terminal hairs. In males, similar coarse hairs also appear on the face and often on the chest and back.

Melanoblasts migrate into the hair bulbs and differentiate into melanocytes (see Fig. 19.3). The melanin produced by these cells is transferred to the hair-forming cells in the germinal matrix several weeks before birth. The relative content of melanin accounts for different hair colors. *It has been demonstrated that Sox2, within the dermal papilla cells, helps to regulate pigmentation.*

Arrector muscles of hairs, small bundles of smooth muscle fibers, differentiate from the mesenchyme surrounding the hair follicles and attach to the **dermal root sheaths of hair follicles** and the **papillary layer of the dermis**, which interdigitates with the epidermis (see Figs. 19.1D and 19.3). Contractions of the arrector muscles depress the skin over their attachment and elevate the skin around the hair shafts, causing the hairs to stand up ("goosebumps"). The arrector muscles are poorly developed in the hairs of the axillary region and in certain parts of the face. The hairs forming the eyebrows and cilia forming the eyelashes have no arrector muscles.

NAILS

Toenails and **fingernails** begin to develop at the tips of the digits at approximately 10 weeks (Fig. 19.11). Development of fingernails precedes that of toenails by approximately 4 weeks (see Table 6.1). The primordia of nails appears as

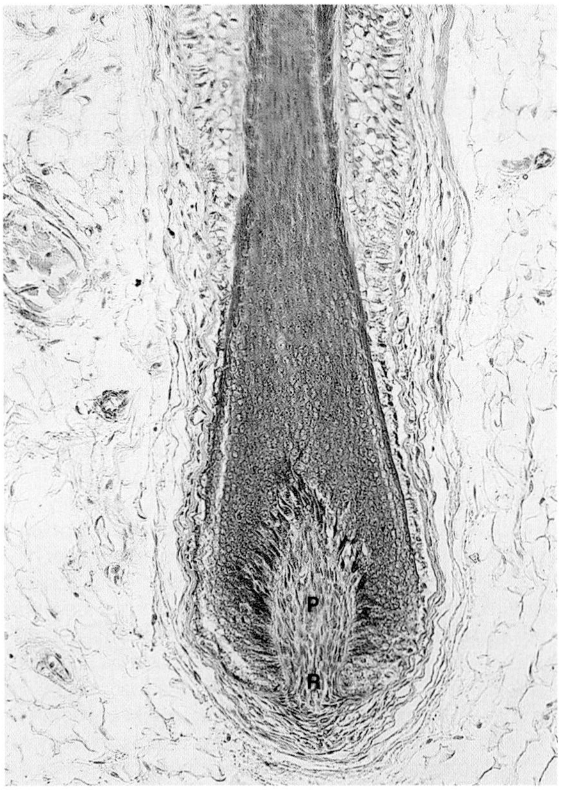

Fig. 19.10 Light micrograph of a longitudinal section of a hair follicle with its hair root *(R)* and papilla *(P)* (×132). (From Gartner LP, Hiatt JL: *Color textbook of histology*, ed 2, Philadelphia, 2001, Saunders.)

Congenital Hypotrichosis

Absence (hypotrichosis) or loss (alopecia) of hairs may occur alone or with other defects of the skin and its derivatives. These conditions may be caused by the failure of hair follicles to develop, or it may result from follicles producing poor-quality hairs. There are many types of hypotrichosis, and it may be associated with more complex syndromes.

Hypertrichosis

Excessive hairiness results from the development of **supernumerary hair follicles** or from the **persistence of lanugo hairs** that normally disappear during the perinatal period. It may be localized (e.g., on the shoulders and back) or diffuse (see Fig. 19.5A). **Localized hypertrichosis** is often associated with spina bifida occulta (see Fig. 17.14).

Pili Torti

Pili torti is a familial disorder in which the hairs are flattened and twisted and the hairs are brittle and coarse. Pili torti may occur within other genetic defects including citrullinemia and mitochondrial diseases. Other ectodermal defects (e.g., distorted fingernails) may be associated with this condition. Early onset pili torti is usually recognized at 3 months to 3 years of age.

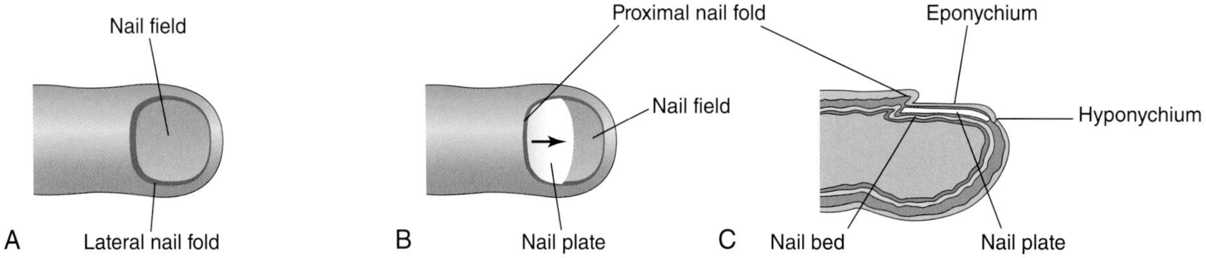

Fig. 19.11 Successive stages in the development of a fingernail. (A) The first indication of a nail is a thickening of the epidermis, the nail field, at the tip of the finger. (B) As the nail plate develops, it slowly grows toward the tip of the finger. (C) The fingernail reaches the end of the finger by 32 weeks.

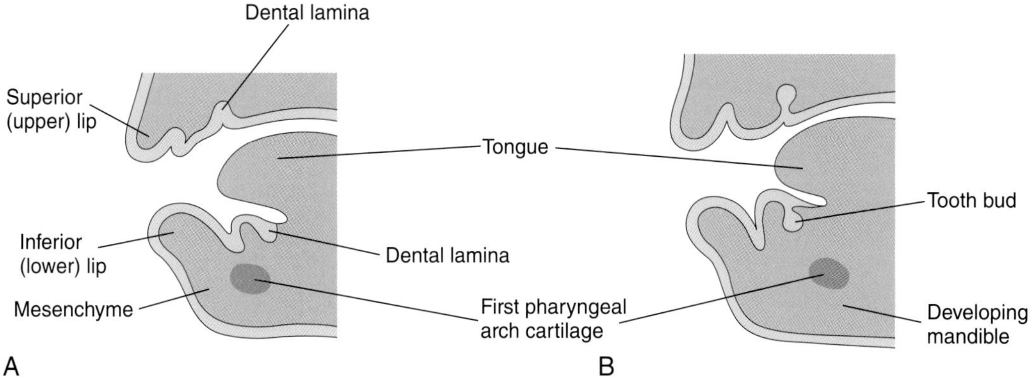

Fig. 19.12 Sketches of sagittal sections through the developing jaw illustrate the early development of the teeth. (A) Early in the sixth week, the dental laminae are present. (B) Later in the sixth week, tooth buds arise from the laminae.

Aplastic Anonychia

Congenital absence of fingernails or toenails is rare and is caused by a variant of the RSPO4 gene. Anonychia results from the failure of nail fields to form or from the failure of the proximal nail folds to form nail plates. This birth defect is permanent. **Aplastic anonychia** (defective development or absence of nails) may be associated with extremely poor development of hairs and with defects of the teeth. Anonychia may be restricted to one or more nails of the digits of the hands and feet.

thickened areas or **nail fields** of the epidermis at the tip of each digit (see Fig. 19.11A). Later, these **fields** migrate onto the dorsal surfaces of the nails, carrying their innervation from the ventral surface. The nail fields are surrounded laterally and proximally by folds of epidermis, the **nail folds** (see Fig. 19.11B). Cells from the proximal nail fold grow over the nail field and become keratinized to form the **nail plate** (see Fig. 19.11C).

At first, the developing nail is covered by a narrow band of epidermis, the **eponychium** (corneal layer of epidermis). It later degenerates, exposing the nail except at its base, where it persists as the **cuticle**. The cuticle of the nail is a thin layer of the deep surface of the **proximal nail fold** (eponychium). The skin under the free margin of the nail is the **hyponychium** (see Fig. 19.11C). The fingernails reach the fingertips by approximately 32 weeks; the toenails reach the toe tips by approximately 36 weeks. Nails that have not reached the tips of the digits at birth indicate prematurity.

TEETH

Two sets of teeth develop, the primary dentition **(deciduous teeth)** and the secondary dentition **(permanent teeth)**. Teeth develop from the oral ectoderm, mesenchyme, and neural crest cells (Fig. 19.12B). The **enamel** of teeth is derived from the ectoderm of the oral cavity; all other tissues differentiate from the surrounding mesenchyme and neural crest cells (Fig. 19.13G and H). *The molecular mechanisms and signaling pathways involve the expression and effects of many hundreds of genes, including* FGF, BMP, SHH, TNF, WNT, Satb2, Six1, and endothelin 1.

Odontogenesis (tooth development) is a characteristic atiribute of the oral epithelium (see Fig. 19.13G). Development is a continuous process involving reciprocal induction between neural crest–induced mesenchyme and the overlying oral epithelium (see Fig. 19.13A). Odontogenesis is usually divided into stages for descriptive purposes based on the appearance of the developing teeth. The first tooth buds appear in the anterior mandibular region (see Figs. 19.12B and 19.13B); later, tooth development occurs in the anterior maxillary region and then progresses posteriorly in both jaws.

Tooth development continues for years after birth (Table 19.1). The first indication of tooth development occurs early in the sixth week as a thickening of the oral epithelium (see Fig. 19.12A). These U-shaped **dental laminae** follow the curves of the primitive jaws (see Fig. 19.13A).

BUD STAGE OF TOOTH DEVELOPMENT

Each dental lamina (see Fig. 19.12A) develops 10 centers of proliferation from which **tooth buds** grow into the

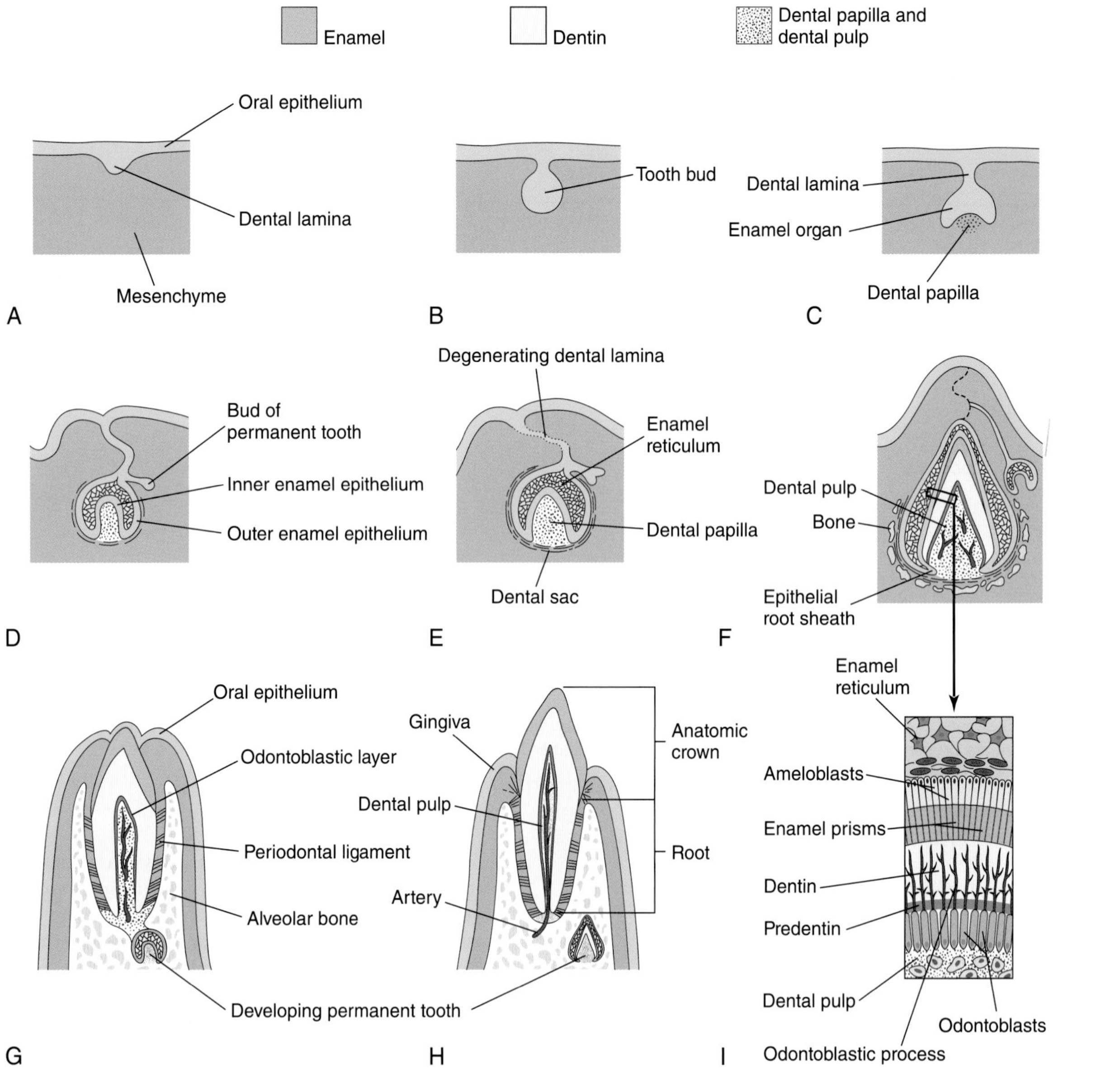

Fig. 19.13 Schematic drawings of sagittal sections illustrate successive stages in the development and eruption of an incisor tooth. (A) At 6 weeks, the dental lamina is present. (B) At 7 weeks, the tooth bud is developing from the dental lamina. (C) The cap stage of tooth development occurs at 8 weeks. (D) The early bell stage of a deciduous tooth and the bud stage of a permanent tooth are shown at 10 weeks. (E) At 14 weeks, the drawing shows the advanced bell stage of tooth development. The connection (dental lamina) of the tooth to the oral epithelium is degenerating. (F) At 28 weeks, the enamel and dentin layers can be seen. (G) At 6 months postnatally, the early stage of tooth eruption is shown. (H) At 18 months postnatally, the deciduous incisor tooth is fully erupted. The permanent incisor tooth has a well-developed crown. (I) Section through a developing tooth shows ameloblasts (enamel producers) and odontoblasts (dentin producers).

underlying mesenchyme (see Figs. 19.12B and 19.13A to C). These buds develop into **deciduous teeth** (see Table 19.1). The tooth buds for permanent teeth that have deciduous predecessors begin to appear at approximately 10 weeks from deep continuations of the dental lamina (see Fig. 19.13D). They develop lingual to the **deciduous tooth buds**.

The permanent molars have no deciduous predecessors and develop as buds from posterior extensions of the dental laminae. The tooth buds for the permanent teeth appear at different times, mostly during the fetal period (see Fig. 19.1D). The buds for the second and third permanent molars develop after birth. The deciduous teeth have well-developed crowns at birth (see Fig. 19.13H), whereas the permanent teeth remain as tooth buds (see Table 19.1).

CAP STAGE OF TOOTH DEVELOPMENT

As each tooth bud is invaginated by mesenchyme (primordium of the dental papilla and dental follicle), the buds become cap-shaped (Fig. 19.14; see Fig. 19.13C). The ectodermal part of the developing tooth, which is the **enamel organ**, a mass of ectodermal cells budded from the dental lamina, eventually produces enamel (see Fig. 19.13E and G). The internal part of each cap-shaped tooth **(dental papilla)** is the primordium of dentin and dental pulp (see Fig. 19.13E). Together, the dental papilla and enamel organ form the

Table 19.1 Eruption and Shedding of Teeth

Tooth	Eruption Time	Shedding Time
Deciduous		
Medial incisor	6–8 mo	6–7 yr
Lateral incisor	8–10 mo	7–8 yr
Canine	16–20 mo	10–12 yr
First molar	12–16 mo	9–11 yr
Second molar	20–24 mo	10–12 yr
Permanent[a]		
Medial incisor	7–8 yr	
Lateral incisor	8–9 yr	
Canine	10–12 yr	
First premolar	10–11 yr	
Second premolar	11–12 yr	
First molar	6–7 yr	
Second molar	12 yr	
Third molar	13–25 y r	

Data from Moore KL, Dalley AF, Agur AMR: *Clinically oriented anatomy*, ed 7, Baltimore, 2014, Lippincott Williams & Wilkins, 2014.
[a]The permanent teeth are not shed.

tooth bud. The outer cell layer of the enamel organ is the **outer enamel epithelium**, and the inner cell layer lining the papilla is the **inner enamel epithelium** (see Fig. 19.13D).

The central core of loosely arranged cells between the layers of enamel epithelium is the **enamel reticulum** or stellate reticulum (see Fig. 19.13E). As the enamel organ and dental papilla develop, the mesenchyme surrounding the developing tooth condenses to form the **dental sac** (dental follicle), a vascularized capsular structure (see Fig. 19.13E). The dental sac is the primordium of the **cement** and **periodontal ligament** (see Fig. 19.13G). The cement is the bone-like, mineralized connective tissue covering the root of the tooth. The periodontal ligament, which is derived from neural crest cells, is a specialized vascular connective tissue that surrounds the root of the tooth, attaching it to the alveolar bone (see Fig. 19.13G).

BELL STAGE OF TOOTH DEVELOPMENT

As the **enamel organ** differentiates, the developing tooth assumes the shape of a bell (Fig. 19.14; see Fig. 19.13D and E). The mesenchymal cells in the **dental papilla** adjacent to the internal enamel epithelium differentiate into **odontoblasts**, which produce predentin and deposit it adjacent to the epithelium (see Fig. 19.13G). Later, the **predentin** calcifies and becomes **dentin**, the second hardest tissue in the body. As the dentin thickens, the odontoblasts regress toward the center of the dental papilla; however, their finger-like cytoplasmic processes **(odontoblastic processes)** remain embedded in the dentin (Fig. 19.15; see Fig. 19.13F and I).

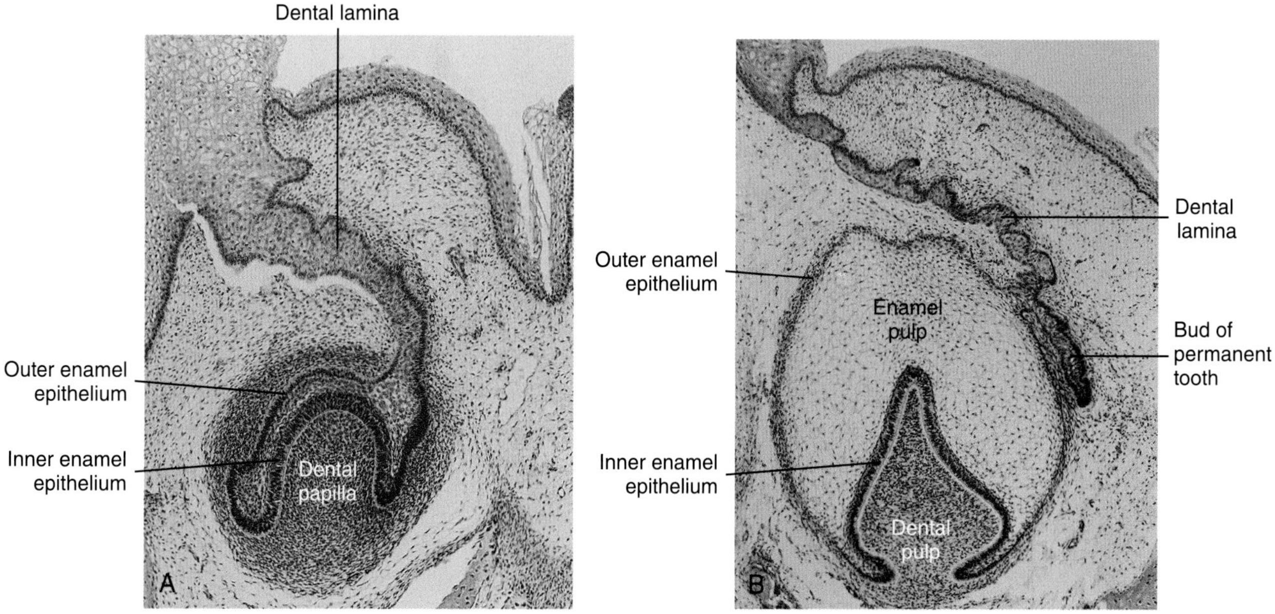

Fig. 19.14 Photomicrograph of the primordium of a lower incisor tooth. (A) A 12-week-old fetus (early bell stage). A cap-like enamel organ has formed, and the dental papilla is developing beneath it. (B) Primordium of a lower incisor tooth in a 15-week-old fetus (late bell stage). Observe the inner and outer enamel layers, the dental papilla, and the bud of the permanent tooth. (From Moore KL, Persaud TVN, Shiota K: *Color atlas of clinical embryology*, ed 2, Philadelphia, 2000, Saunders, 2000.)

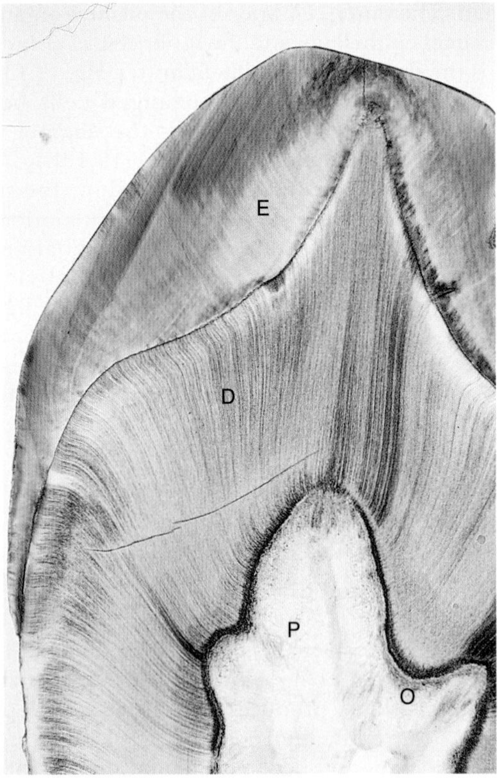

Fig. 19.15 Photomicrograph of a section of the crown and neck of a tooth (×17). Observe the enamel *(E)*, dentin *(D)*, dental pulp *(P)*, and odontoblasts *(O)*. (From Gartner LR, Hiatt JL: *Color textbook of histology*, ed 2, Philadelphia, 2001, Saunders.)

Cells of the inner enamel epithelium differentiate into **ameloblasts** (cells of the inner layer of the enamel organ) under the influence of the odontoblasts, which produce enamel in the form of prisms (rods) over the dentin (see Fig. 19.13I). As the enamel increases, the ameloblasts migrate toward the outer enamel epithelium (see Fig. 19.14A and B). Enamel is the hardest tissue in the body; it overlies and protects the dentin from being fractured (see Fig. 19.15). The color of the translucent enamel is based on the thickness and color of the underlying dentin. Enamel and dentin formation begins at the cusp (tip) of the tooth and progresses toward the future root.

The **root of the tooth** begins to develop after dentin and enamel formations are well advanced (Fig. 19.16; see Fig. 19.13H). The inner and outer enamel epithelia come together at the **neck of the tooth** (cementoenamel junction), where they form a fold, the **epithelial root sheath** (see Figs. 19.13F and 19.14). This sheath grows into the mesenchyme and initiates root formation.

The odontoblasts adjacent to the epithelial root sheath form dentin that is continuous with that of the crown of the tooth. As the dentin increases, it reduces the **pulp cavity** to a narrow **root canal** through which the vessels and nerves pass (see Fig. 19.13H). The inner cells of the dental sac differentiate into **cementoblasts**, which produce cement that is restricted to the root. Cement is deposited over the dentin of the root and meets the enamel at the **neck of the tooth,** the constricted part of the tooth, between the crown and the root (see Fig. 19.13H).

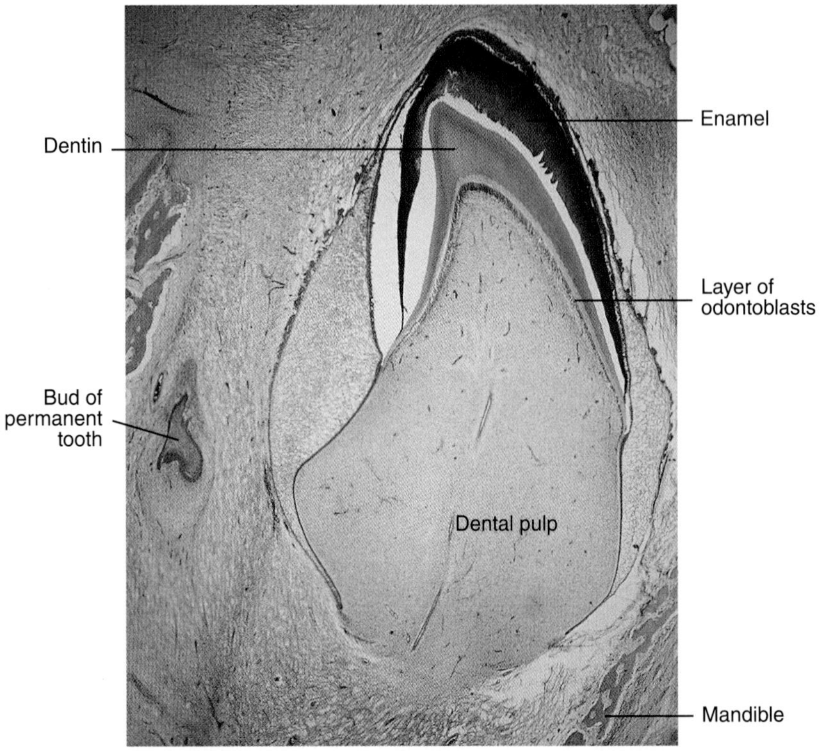

Fig. 19.16 Photomicrograph of a section of a lower incisor tooth in a mature fetus. The enamel and dentin layers and the pulp are clearly demarcated. (From Moore KL, Persaud TVN, Shiota K: *Color atlas of clinical embryology*, ed 2, Philadelphia, 2000, Saunders.)

As the teeth develop and the jaws ossify, the outer cells of the **dental sac** also become active in bone formation see (Fig. 19.13E). Each tooth soon becomes surrounded by bone, except over the crown (see Fig. 19.13G and H). The tooth is held in its **alveolus** (tooth socket) by the strong **periodontal ligament**, a derivative of the dental sac (see Fig. 19.13G and H). Some fibers of this ligament are embedded in the cement of the root; other fibers are embedded in the bony wall of the alveolus. *The shape of teeth is controlled through homebox genes (and may include MSX-1, DLX-2, and BARX-1).*

TOOTH ERUPTION

As the **deciduous teeth** develop, they begin a continuous, slow movement toward the oral cavity (see Fig. 19.13G). **Eruption** results in the emergence of the tooth from the dental follicle in the jaw to its functional position in the mouth. The **mandibular teeth** usually erupt before the **maxillary teeth**, and the teeth of females usually erupt sooner than those in males. The child's dentition contains **20 deciduous teeth**. As the root of the tooth grows, its crown gradually erupts through the **oral epithelium** (see Fig. 19.13G). The part of the oral mucosa around the erupted crown becomes the **gingiva** (see Fig. 19.13H).

The usual eruption time of the deciduous teeth is between 6 and 24 months (see Table 19.1). The mandibular medial (**central incisor**) teeth typically erupt from 6 to 8 months, but this process may not begin until 12 or 13 months in some children. Despite this, all 20 deciduous teeth are usually present by the end of the second year in healthy children. Delayed eruption of all teeth may indicate a systemic or nutritional disturbance such as **hypopituitarism** or **hypothyroidism**.

The **permanent dentition** consists of 32 teeth. The permanent teeth develop like that described for deciduous teeth. As a permanent tooth grows, the root of the corresponding deciduous tooth is gradually resorbed by **osteoclasts** (odontoclasts). Consequently, when the deciduous tooth is shed, it consists only of the crown and the uppermost part of the root. The permanent teeth usually begin to erupt during the sixth year and continue to appear until early adulthood (Fig. 19.17; see Table 19.1).

Natal Teeth

Neonates may have one or more **erupted teeth at birth**. These teeth are usually the lower incisors. One or more teeth may also erupt later in the neonatal period (up to 4 weeks); they are called **neonatal teeth**. Natal teeth are observed in 1 in 2000 neonates. This anomaly is often transmitted as an autosomal dominant trait. Only the crowns of the teeth are calcified, and their roots are usually loose. These teeth may produce maternal discomfort during breast-feeding, and the neonate's tongue may be lacerated, or the teeth may detach and be aspirated; for these reasons, natal teeth are usually extracted. Because they are prematurely erupting decidual teeth, spacers may be required to prevent overcrowding of the other teeth.

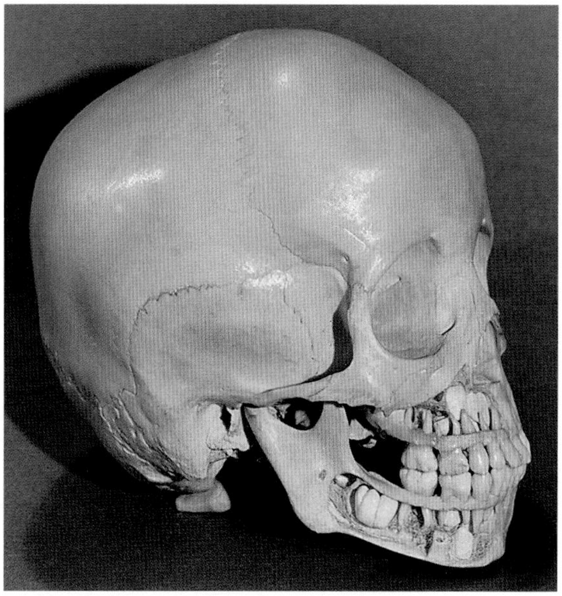

Fig. 19.17 Cranium of a 4-year-old child. Bone has been removed from the mandible and maxilla to expose the relationship of the developing permanent teeth to the erupted deciduous teeth.

Enamel Hypoplasia

Defective enamel formation causes pits and fissures in the enamel of teeth (Figs. 19.18 and 19.19A). These defects result from temporary disturbances of enamel formation. Various factors (e.g., nutritional deficiency, tetracycline therapy, infectious diseases such as measles) may injure **ameloblasts**, which produce enamel. **Rickets** occurring during the critical period of tooth development (6–12 weeks) is a common cause of enamel hypoplasia. Other factors that may cause enamel hypoplasia include infection, premature birth, and low birth weight.

The shape of the face is affected by the development of the **paranasal sinuses** (air-filled cavities in the bones of the face) and the growth of the maxilla and mandible to accommodate the teeth (see Fig. 9.26). Lengthening of the **alveolar processes** (sockets supporting the teeth) increases the length of the face during childhood.

VARIATIONS OF TOOTH SHAPE

Abnormally shaped teeth are relatively common (see Figs. 19.18 and 19.19A–E). Occasionally, there is a spherical mass of enamel**, enamel pearl**, on the root of a tooth that is separate from the enamel of the crown (see Fig. 19.18A). The pearl is formed by **aberrant groups of ameloblasts**. In other cases, the maxillary lateral incisor teeth may have a slender, tapering shape (peg-shaped incisors). A taurodont is a tooth where there is increased formation of the tooth body and

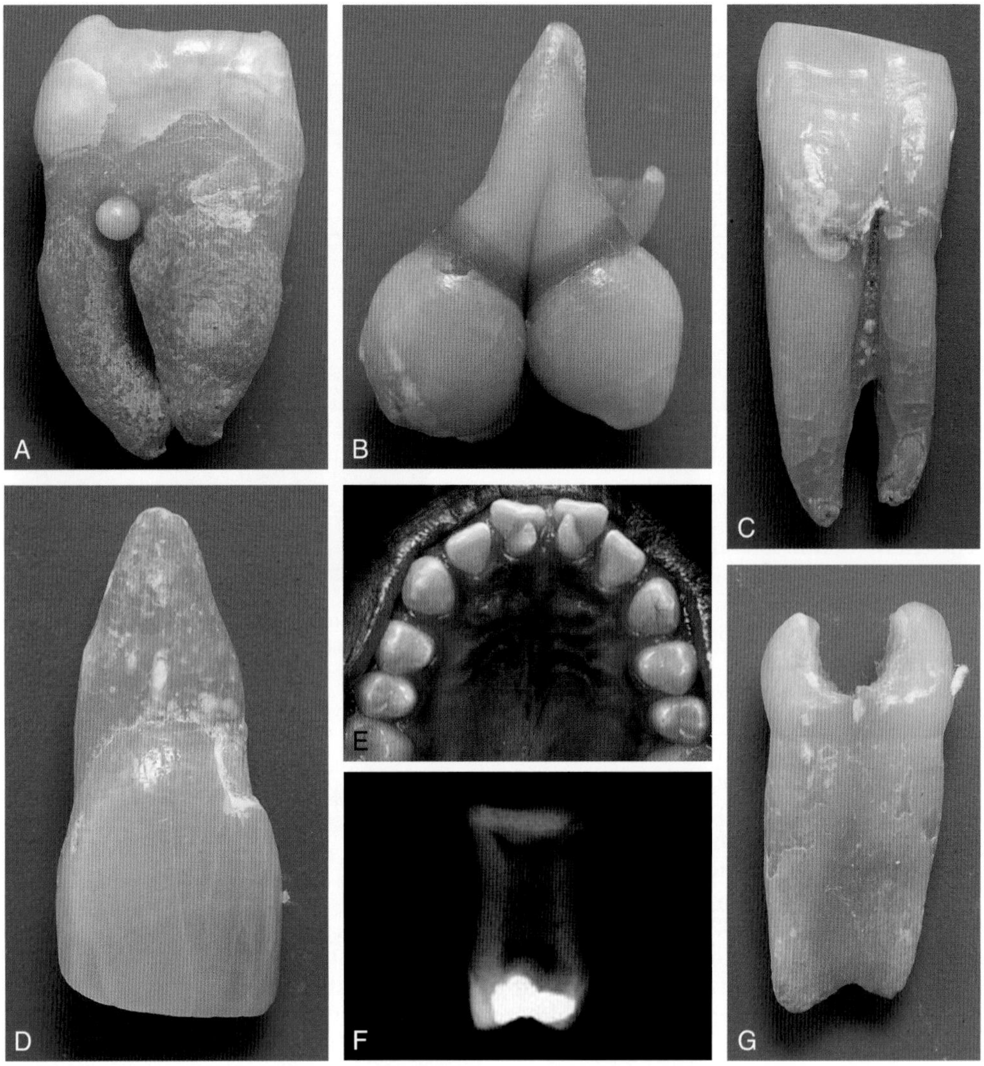

Fig. 19.18 Common anomalies of teeth. (A) Enamel pearl (with furcation [forking] of a permanent maxillary third molar). (B) Gemination and tetracycline staining (maxillary third molar). (C) Fusion of permanent mandibular central and lateral incisors. (D) Abnormally short root (microdont permanent maxillary central incisor). (E) Dens invaginatus (talon cusps on the lingual surface of the permanent maxillary central incisor). (F) Taurodont tooth (radiograph of the mesial surface of the permanent maxillary second molar). (G) Fusion (primary mandibular central and lateral incisors). (Courtesy Dr. Blaine Cleghorn, Faculty of Dentistry, Dalhousie University, Halifax, Nova Scotia, Canada.)

Numeric Abnormalities of Teeth

One or more **supernumerary teeth** (mesiodens) may develop, or the normal number of teeth may fail to form (see Fig. 19.19F). Many studies report a higher prevalence among females. Supernumerary teeth usually develop in the area of the maxillary incisors and can disrupt the position and eruption of normal teeth. The extra teeth commonly erupt posterior to the normal ones (or remain unerupted) and are asymptomatic in most cases.

In **partial anodontia**, one or more teeth are absent; this is often a familial trait. In **total anodontia**, no teeth develop; this is an extremely rare condition. It is usually associated with **ectodermal dysplasia** (congenital defect of ectodermal tissues). Occasionally, a tooth bud partially or completely divides into two separate teeth.

A partially divided tooth germ is called **germination**. The result is **macrodontia** (large teeth) with a common root canal system; small teeth **(microdontia)** also occur. If the tooth germ completely divides into two separate teeth, the result is twinning, with one additional tooth in the dentition. The fusion of two teeth results in one fewer tooth in the dentition. This condition can be differentiated radiographically from gemination by **two separate root canal systems** found with fusion.

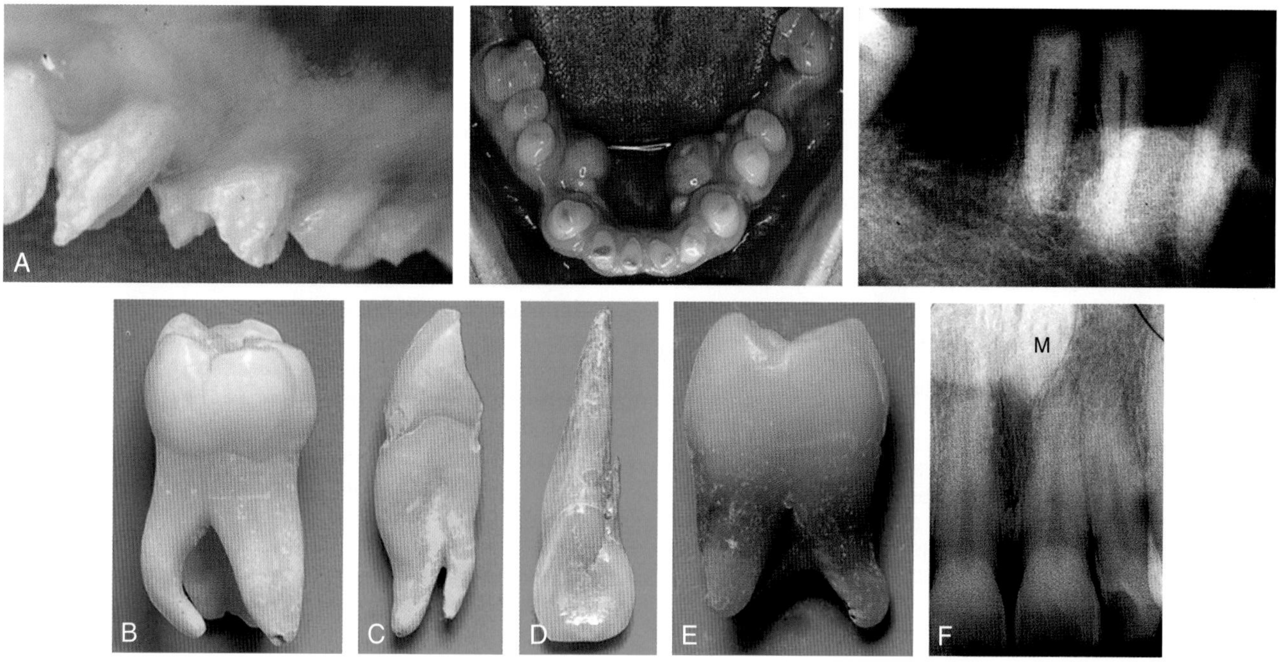

Fig. 19.19 Additional common anomalies of teeth. (A) Amelogenesis imperfecta. (B) Extra root (mandibular molar). (C) Extra root (mandibular canine). (D) Accessory root (maxillary lateral incisor). Extra roots present challenges for root canal therapy and extraction. (E) Tetracycline staining (the root of the maxillary third molar). (F) A midline supernumerary tooth (mesiodens *[M]*) located near the apex of the central incisor. The prevalence of supernumerary teeth is 1% to 3% in the general population. (A–E, Courtesy Dr. Blaine Cleghorn, Faculty of Dentistry, Dalhousie University, Halifax, Nova Scotia, Canada. F, Courtesy Dr. Steve Ahing, Faculty of Dentistry, University of Manitoba, Winnipeg, Manitoba, Canada.)

Dentigerous Cyst

A cyst may develop in a mandible, maxilla, or maxillary sinus that contains an unerupted tooth. The **dentigerous** (*tooth-bearing*) **cyst** develops because of cystic degeneration of the enamel reticulum of the enamel organ of an unerupted tooth. Most cysts are deeply situated in the jaw and are associated with misplaced or malformed secondary teeth that have failed to erupt.

Amelogenesis Imperfecta

Amelogenesis imperfecta is a complex group of at least 14 clinical entities that involve **aberrations in enamel formation** in the absence of any systemic disorder. This is an **inherited ectodermal birth defect** that primarily affects the enamel only. The enamel may be **hypoplastic**, **hypocalcified**, or **hypomature** (not fully developed). Depending on the type of amelogenesis imperfecta, the enamel may be hard or soft, pitted or smooth, and thin or normal in thickness. The incidence of amelogenesis imperfecta ranges from 1 in 700 in Sweden to 1 in 1200 in the United States. Multiple modes of inheritance patterns are involved. Variants of the genes that encode enamel, dentin, and mineralization are involved, including *AMELX*, *ENAM*, *MMP20, and KLK4*. Classification of this condition is based on clinical and radiographic findings and the mode of inheritance.

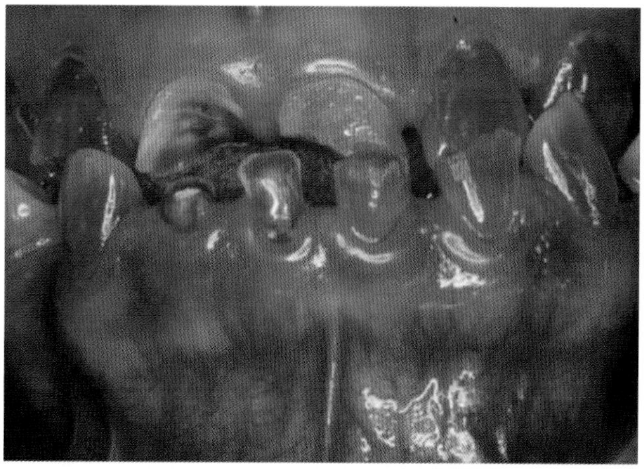

Fig. 19.20 Clinical photograph of a patient with dentinogenesis imperfecta. The teeth have an opalescent amber-colored appearance and have been very rapidly worn down. (From Hunter KD, Brierly D: Pathology of the teeth: an update. *Dig Histopath* 23(6):275–283, 2017.)

Dentinogenesis Imperfecta

This autosomal dominant disorder of the teeth is characterized clinically by translucent blue-gray to yellow-brown teeth involving primary and permanent dentition. The teeth have an opalescent sheen because the *odontoblasts fail to differentiate normally*, and poorly calcified dentin results. The enamel tends to wear down rapidly, exposing the dentin. This disorder in most cases is localized on chromosome 4q, and this condition is relatively common among white children (Fig. 19.20).

Discolored Teeth

Foreign substances incorporated into the developing enamel and dentin discolor the teeth. The hemolysis associated with **erythroblastosis fetalis** or hemolytic disease of the neonate may produce blue to black discoloration of the teeth. All **tetracyclines** are extensively incorporated into the teeth. The critical period of risk for this to occur is from approximately 14 weeks of fetal life to the 10th postnatal month for deciduous teeth and from approximately 14 weeks of fetal life to the eighth postnatal year for permanent teeth.

Tetracycline staining affects enamel and dentin because it binds to **hydroxyapatite** (the modified natural mineral structure that forms the crystal lattice of bones and teeth). The brownish-yellow discoloration (mottling) of teeth produced by tetracycline is caused by the conversion of tetracycline to a colored by-product under the action of light. The dentin is probably affected more than the enamel because it is more permeable than the enamel after tooth mineralization is complete. The enamel is completely formed on all but the third molars by approximately 8 years of age. For this reason, **tetracyclines** (broad-spectrum antibiotics) should not be administered to pregnant women or children younger than 8 years of age.

the pulp cavity with a concomitant decrease in the length of the root (see Fig. 19.18F).

Congenital syphilis affects the differentiation of the permanent teeth, resulting in incisors with central notches in their incisive edges. The molars are also affected and are called **mulberry molars** because of their characteristic features.

SUMMARY OF INTEGUMENTARY SYSTEM

- The skin and its appendages develop from ectoderm, mesenchyme, and neural crest cells. The epidermis is derived from surface ectoderm, and the dermis is derived from mesenchyme. **Melanocytes** are derived from **neural crest cells** that migrate into the epidermis.
- Cast-off cells from the epidermis mix with secretions of sebaceous glands to form the **vernix caseosa**, a whitish, greasy coating of the skin that protects the epidermis of the fetuses.
- **Hairs** develop from down growths of the epidermis into the dermis. By approximately 20 weeks, the fetus is completely covered with fine, downy hairs **(lanugo)**. These fetal hairs are shed before birth or shortly thereafter and are replaced by coarser hairs.
- Most **sebaceous glands** develop as outgrowths from the sides of hair follicles; however, some glands develop as down growths of the epidermis into the dermis. **Sweat glands** also develop from epidermal down growths into the dermis. **Mammary glands** develop similarly.
- **Birth defects of the skin** are mainly disorders of keratinization **(ichthyosis)** and pigmentation **(albinism)**. Abnormal blood vessel development results in various types of angioma.
- The absence of **mammary glands** is extremely rare, but supernumerary breasts **(polymastia)** and nipples **(polythelia)** are relatively common.
- **Teeth** develop from ectoderm, mesoderm, and neural crest cells. The **enamel** is produced by **ameloblasts**, which are derived from the oral ectoderm; all other dental tissues develop from mesenchyme, which is derived from mesoderm and neural crest cells.
- **Common birth defects of the teeth** are defective formation of enamel and dentin, abnormalities in shape, and variations in number and position.
- **Tetracyclines** are extensively incorporated into the enamel and dentin of developing teeth, producing brownish-yellow discoloration and hypoplasia of the enamel. *They should not be prescribed for pregnant women or children younger than 8 years of age.*

CLINICALLY ORIENTED PROBLEMS

CASE 19-1

A neonate had two erupted mandibular incisor teeth.

- What are these teeth called?
- How common is this anomaly?
- Are they supernumerary teeth?
- What problem or danger is associated with the presence of teeth at birth?

CASE 19-2

The deciduous teeth of an infant had a brownish-yellow color and some hypoplasia of the enamel. The mother recalled that she had been given antibiotics during the second trimester of her pregnancy.

- What is the probable cause of the infant's tooth discoloration?
- Dysfunction of what cells causes enamel hypoplasia?
- Will the secondary dentition be discolored?

CASE 19-3

An infant had a small, irregularly shaped, light red blotch on the posterior surface of the neck. It was level with the surrounding skin and blanched when light pressure was applied.

- What is this birth defect called?
- What do these observations indicate?
- Is this condition common?
- Are there other names for this skin defect?

CASE 19-4

A female neonate had a tuft of hair in the lumbosacral region of her back.

- What does this tuft of hair indicate?
- Is this condition common?
- Is this birth defect clinically important?

CASE 19-5

The skin of a male neonate had a collodion type of covering that fissured and exfoliated shortly after birth. Later, lamellar ichthyosis developed.

- Briefly describe this condition.
- Is it a common defect?
- How is it inherited?

Discussion of these problems appears in the Appendix at the back of the book.

BIBLIOGRAPHY AND SUGGESTED READING

Brâescu R, Săvinescu SD, Tatarciuc MS, Zetu IN, Giuşcâ: Căruntu I-D: Pointing on the early stages of maxillary bone and tooth development – histological findings, *Rom J Morphol Embryol* 61(1):167, 2020.

Chiego DJ Jr: *Essentials of oral histology and embryology—a clinical approach,* ed 4, Philadelphia, 2014, Mosby Elsevier.

Chiu YE: Dermatology. In Marcdante KJ, Kliegman KJ, editors: *Nelson essentials of pediatrics,* ed 7, Philadelphia, 2015, Saunders.

Coletta RD, McCoy EL, Burns V, et al: Characterization of the *Six 1* homeobox gene in normal mammary gland morphogenesis, *BMC Dev Biol* 10:4, 2010.

Duggal MS, Hosey MT, editors: *Paediatric dentistry,* ed 4, Oxford, UK, 2012, Oxford University Press.

Felipe AF, Abazari A, Hammersmith KM, Rapuano CJ, Nagra PK, Peiro BM: Corneal changes in ectrodactyly-ectodermal dysplasia-cleft lip and palate syndrome: case series and literature review, *Int Ophthalmol* 32:475, 2012.

Galli-Tsinopoulou A, Stergidou D: Polythelia: simple atavistic remnant or a suspicious clinical sign for investigation? *Pediatr Endocrinol Rev* 11:290, 2014.

Harryparsad A, Rahman L, Bunn BK: Amelogenesis imperfecta: a diagnostic and pathological review with case illustration, *SADJ* 68:404, 2013.

Inman JL, Robertson C, Mott JD, Bissell MJ: Mammary gland development: cell fate specification, stem cells and the microenvironment, *Development* 142:1028, 2015.

Kliegman RR, Stanton B, Geme J, Schor NF, Behrman RE, editors: *Nelson textbook of pediatrics,* ed 20, Philadelphia, 2016, Elsevier.

Landau Prat D, Katowitz WR, Strong A, Katowitz JA. Ocular manifestations of ectodermal dysplasia. *Orphanet J Rare Dis,* 16, (1), 2021, https://doi.org/10.1186/s13023-021-01824-2.

Lee K, Gjorevski N, Boghaert E, Radisky DC, Nelson CM: Snail1, Snail2, and E47 promote mammary epithelial branching morphogenesis, *EMBO J* 30:2662, 2011.

Little H, Kamat D, Sivaswamy L: Common neurocutaneous syndromes, *Pediatr Ann* 44(11):497, 2015.

Seppala Maisa, Fraser M, Birjandi GJ, Xavier AA, Cobourne GM: MT: Sonic hedgehog signaling and development of the dentition, *J Dev Biol* 5(2):6, 2017.

Marwaha M, Nanda KD: Ectrodactyly, ectodermal dysplasia, cleft lip, and palate (EEC syndrome), *Contemp Clin Dent* 3:205, 2012.

McDermottt KM, Liu BY, Tisty TD, Pazour GJ: Primary cilia regulate branching morphogenesis during mammary gland development, *Curr Biol* 20:731, 2010.

Moore KL, Dalley AF, Agur AMR: *Clinically oriented anatomy,* ed 8, Baltimore, 2017, Lippincott Williams & Wilkins.

Müller M, Jasmin JR, Monteil RA, Loubiere R: Embryology of the hair follicle, *Early Hum Dev* 26:59, 1999.

Nanci A: *Ten Cate's oral histology: development, structure, and function,* ed 9, St Louis, 2018, Elsevier.

Ng KJ, Lim J, Tan YN, et al: Sox2 in the dermal papilla regulates hair follicle pigmentation, *Cell Reports* 40:1, 2022.

Osborne MP, Boolbol SK: Breast anatomy and development. In Harris JR, Lippman ME, editors: *Diseases of the breast,* ed 4, Philadelphia, 2010, Lippincott Williams & Wilkins.

Paller AS, Mancini AJ: *Hurwitz clinical pediatric dermatology: a textbook of skin disorders of childhood and adolescence,* ed 4, Philadelphia, 2011, Saunders.

Papagerakis P, Mitsiadis T: Development and structure of teeth and periodontal tissues. In Rosen CJ, editor: *Primer on the metabolic bone diseases and disorders of mineral metabolism,* ed 8, New Jersey, 2013, John Wiley & Sons.

Parekh S, Harley K. Anomalies of tooth formation and eruption. R Welbury, MS Duggal, MT Hosey, *Paediatric Dentistry,* ed 5 2018, Oxford University Press: 257–276 https://doi.org/10.1093/oso/9780198789277.003.0022.

Pillaiyar T, Manickam M, Jung S-H: Recent development of signaling pathways inhibitors of melanogenesis, *Cell Signal* 40:99, 2017.

Som PM, Laitman JT, Mak K: Embryology and anatomy of the skin, its appendages, and physiologic changes in the head and neck, *Neurographics* 7:390, 2017, 2011.

Smolinski KN: Hemangiomas of infancy: clinical and biological characteristics, *Clin Pediatr (Phila)* 44:747, 2005.

Watts A, Addy MA: Tooth discolouration and staining: a review of the literature, *Br Dent J* 190:309, 2001.

Human Birth Defects

20

CHAPTER OUTLINE

Birth defects are developmental disorders (congenital anomalies) (malformations, disruptions, dysplasia, or deformations) present at birth and are the leading cause of infant mortality. They may be structural, functional, metabolic, behavioral, or hereditary. Globally, 3% to 6% of children are born annually with a serious birth defect (*National Center on Birth Defects and Developmental Disabilities*, CDC, February 2022). Neonates with isolated or multiple congenital anomalies are usually evaluated by a clinical geneticist so that a diagnosis can be determined and whether the anomaly is isolated or part of a genetic syndrome. Genetic counseling is an important part of clinical investigation and follow-up for these families.

CLASSIFICATION OF BIRTH DEFECTS

The most widely used reference guide for classifying birth defects is the *International Classification of Diseases*, but no single classification has universal acceptance. Each classification is limited by being designed for a particular purpose. Numerous attempts to classify human birth defects, especially those that result from **errors of morphogenesis** (development of form), reveal the frustration and obvious difficulties in the formulation of concrete uniform methodologies for use in medical care. Among clinicians, a practical approach for classifying birth defects that takes into consideration the time of onset of the injury, possible cause, and pathogenesis (e.g., underlying genetic mechanism) is now commonly utilized.

TERATOLOGY: STUDY OF ABNORMAL DEVELOPMENT

Teratology is the branch of embryology and pathology concerned with the etiology, developmental anatomy, and classification of malformed embryos and fetuses. *A fundamental concept in teratology is that certain stages of embryonic development are more vulnerable to disruption than others* (Fig. 20.1). Until the 1940s, it was thought that embryos were protected from environmental agents such as drugs, viruses, and chemicals by their extraembryonic or fetal membranes (amnion and chorion) and their mothers' uterine and abdominal walls.

In 1941 the first well-documented cases reported that an environmental agent **(rubella virus)** could produce severe birth defects such as cataracts (see Fig. 18.11), cardiac defects, and deafness if the rubella infection occurred during the critical period of development of the eyes, heart, and ears. In the 1950s, severe limb defects and other developmental disorders were found in infants of mothers who had been prescribed **thalidomide**, as an anti-emetic agent during early pregnancy (Fig. 20.2). These discoveries focused worldwide attention on the role of viruses and drugs as causes of human birth defects. An estimated 7% to 10% of birth defects result from the disruptive actions of drugs, viruses, and environmental toxins.

More than 10% of infant deaths worldwide (20% in North America) are attributed to birth defects. Major structural defects are observed in approximately 3% of neonates.

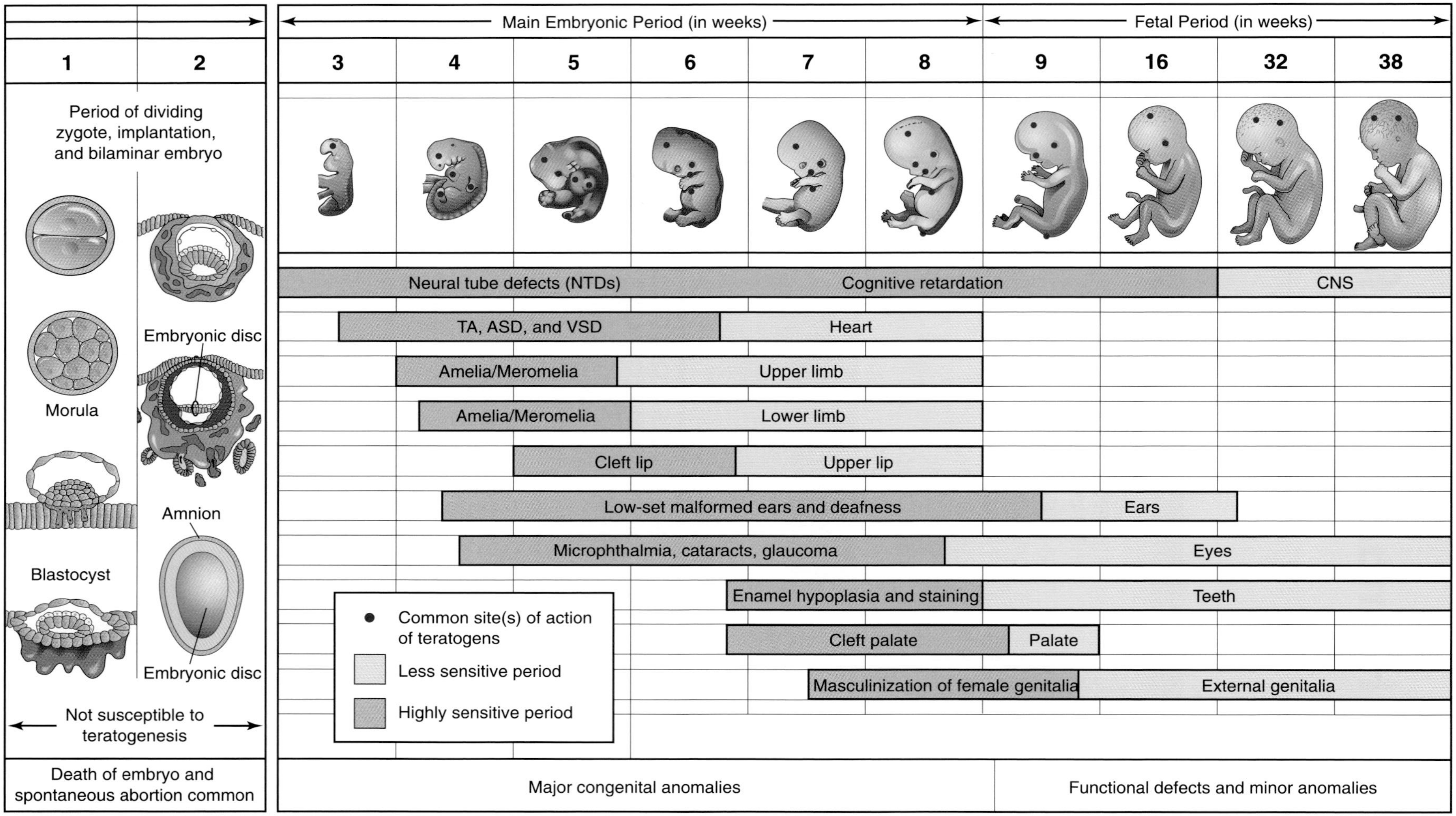

Fig. 20.1 Critical periods in human prenatal development. During the first 2 weeks of development, the embryo is usually not susceptible to teratogens; a teratogen damages all or most of the cells, resulting in the death of the embryo, or damages only a few cells, allowing the conceptus to recover and the embryo to develop without birth defects. During highly sensitive periods *(mauve)*, major birth defects may be produced (e.g., amelia, absence of limbs, neural tube defects, spina bifida cystica). During stages that are less sensitive to teratogens *(green)*, minor defects may be induced (e.g., hypoplastic thumbs). *ASD*, Atrial septal defect; *CNS*, central nervous system; *TA*, truncus arteriosus; *VSD*, ventricular septal defect.

Additional defects can be detected during infancy, and the incidence reaches approximately 6% among 2-year-old children and 8% among 5-year-old children.

The causes of birth defects are divided into three broad categories:

- **Genetic factors** such as chromosomal abnormalities
- **Environmental factors** such as drugs and viruses

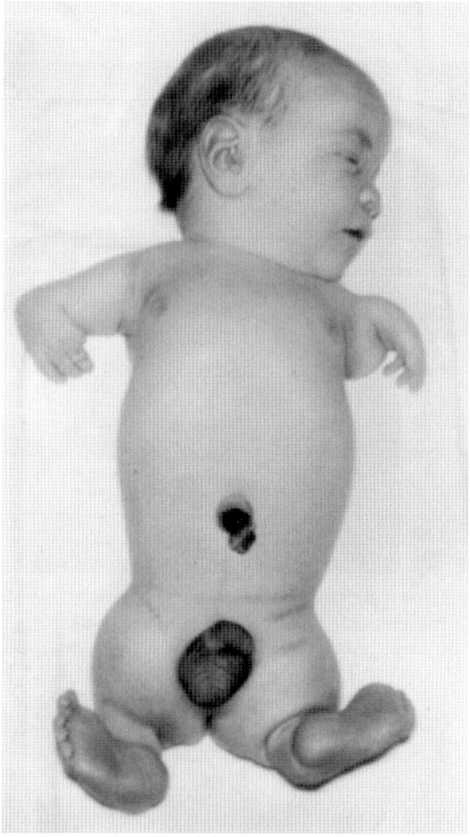

Fig. 20.2 Male neonate has typically malformed limbs (meromelia or limb reduction) resulting from thalidomide ingestion by his mother during the critical period of limb development (see Fig. 20.1). (From Moore KL: The vulnerable embryo. Causes of malformation in man. *Manit Med Rev* 43:306, 1963.)

- **Multifactorial inheritance** (genetic and environmental factors acting together)

For 50% to 60% of birth defects, the cause is unknown (Fig. 20.3). The defects may be single or involve multiple organ systems and may have major or minor clinical significance. **Single minor defects** occur in approximately 14% of neonates. Defects of the external ears, for example, are of no serious medical significance, but they may indicate the presence of associated major defects. For instance, the finding of a single umbilical artery alerts the clinician to possible cardiovascular and renal anomalies (see Fig. 7.18).

Ninety percent of infants with three or more minor defects also have one or more major defects. Of the 3% born with clinically significant defects, **multiple major defects** are found in 0.7%, and most of these infants die. **Major developmental defects** are much more common in young embryos (10%–15%), but most of them abort spontaneously during the first 6 weeks. **Chromosomal abnormalities** are detected in 50% to 60% of spontaneously aborted embryos.

BIRTH DEFECTS CAUSED BY GENETIC FACTORS

Numerically, genetic factors are the most important causes of birth defects. Aneuploidy and pathogenic variants in genes are common causes of birth defects and collectively account for up to 15% of congenital anomalies (see Fig. 20.3). Any mechanism as complex as **mitosis** or **meiosis** may occasionally results in an abnormal segregation of chromosomes (Fig. 20.5; see Figs. 2.1 and 2.2). Chromosomal aberrations occur in 6% to 7% of zygotes.

Most early abnormal zygotes never undergo normal cleavage and become blastocysts (see Figs. 2.16 and 2.17). In vitro studies of cleaving zygotes less than 5 days old have revealed a high incidence of abnormalities. More than 60% of day 2 cleaving zygotes were found to be abnormal. Many defective zygotes, blastocysts, and 3-week-old embryos abort spontaneously.

Two kinds of changes occur in chromosome complements: numeric and structural. The changes may affect the **sex chromosomes** or the **autosomes**. In some instances, both kinds of chromosomes are affected. Persons with chromosomal aberrations usually have characteristic **phenotypes**

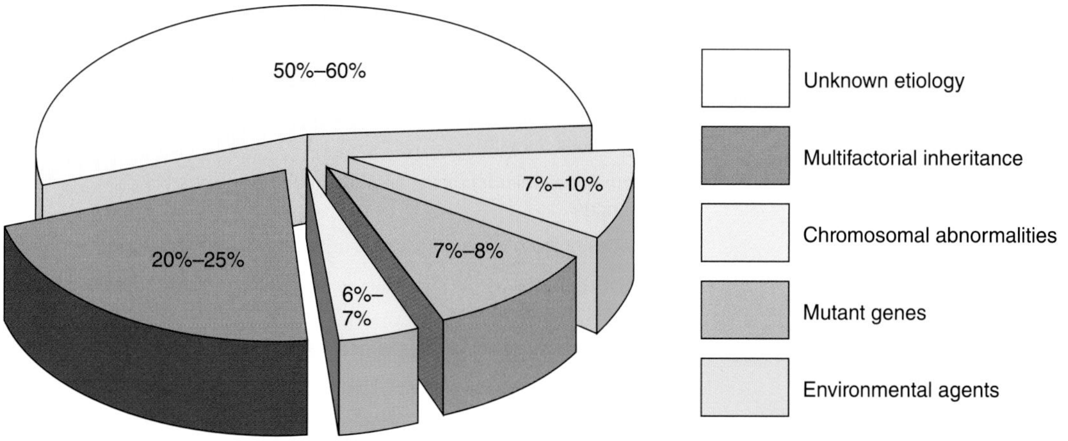

Fig. 20.3 The causes of most human birth defects are unknown, and 20% to 25% of them are caused by a combination of genetic and environmental factors (multifactorial inheritance).

(morphologic characteristics), such as the physical characteristics of infants with Down syndrome (trisomy 21) (Fig. 20.4). They often look more like other persons with the same chromosomal abnormality than their own siblings. Genetic factors initiate defects by biochemical or other means at the subcellular, cellular, or tissue level. The abnormal mechanisms initiated by the genetic factors may be identical or similar to the causal mechanisms initiated by **teratogens**, such as drugs and infections (Table 20.1).

NUMERIC CHROMOSOMAL ABNORMALITIES

In the United States, approximately 1 in 120 neonates have a chromosomal abnormality. Numeric aberrations of chromosomes (aneuploidy) usually result from **nondisjunction**, an error in cell division in which there is a failure of a chromosomal pair or two chromatids of a chromosome to disjoin during mitosis or meiosis (see Figs. 2.2 and 2.3). Other mechanisms that result in aneuploidy include reversing the

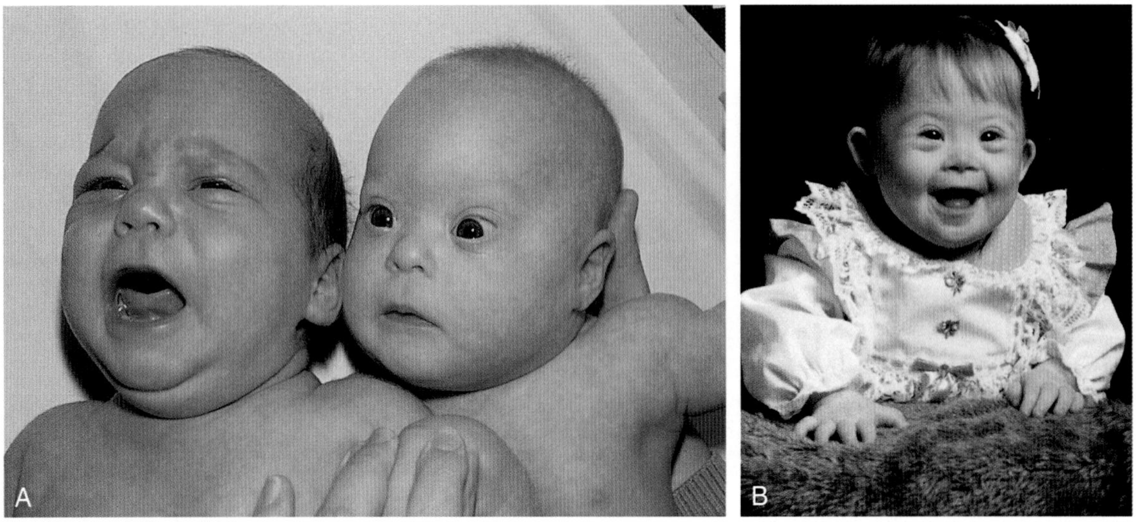

Fig. 20.4 (A) Anterior view of the faces of dizygotic male twins that are discordant for Down syndrome (trisomy 21). The smaller twin has Down syndrome and developed from a zygote that contained an extra chromosome 21. The characteristic facial features of the syndrome in this infant include upslanting palpebral fissures, epicanthal folds, and a flat nasal bridge. (B) A girl, aged 2 years 6 months, who has Down syndrome. (Courtesy Dr. A.E. Chudley, Section of Genetics and Metabolism, Department of Pediatrics and Child Health, Children's Hospital, Winnipeg, Manitoba, Canada.)

Table 20.1 Teratogens That Cause Human Birth Defects

Agents	Most Common Birth Defects
Drugs	
Alcohol	Fetal alcohol syndrome: IUGR, cognitive deficiency, microcephaly, ocular anomalies, joint abnormalities, short palpebral fissures
Androgens and high doses of progestogens	Various degrees of masculinization of female fetuses: ambiguous external genitalia resulting in labial fusion and clitoral hypertrophy
Aminopterin	IUGR; skeletal defects; CNS malformations, notably meroencephaly (most of the brain is absent)
Carbamazepine	NTD, craniofacial defects, developmental retardation
Cocaine	IUGR, prematurity, microcephaly, cerebral infarction, urogenital defects, neurobehavioral disturbances
Diethylstilbestrol	Abnormalities of the uterus and vagina, cervical erosion, and ridges
Isotretinoin (13-*cis*-retinoic acid)	Craniofacial abnormalities; NTDs such as spina bifida cystica; cardiovascular defects; cleft palate; thymic aplasia
Lithium carbonate	Various defects, usually involving the heart and great vessels
Methotrexate	Multiple defects, especially skeletal, involving the face, cranium, limbs, and vertebral column

Table 20.1 Teratogens That Cause Human Birth Defects—Cont'd

Agents	Most Common Birth Defects
Misoprostol	Limb abnormalities, ocular and cranial nerve defects, autism spectrum disorder
Phenytoin	Fetal hydantoin syndrome: IUGR, microcephaly, cognitive deficiency, ridged frontal suture, inner epicanthal folds, eyelid ptosis, broad and depressed nasal bridge, phalangeal hypoplasia
Tetracycline	Stained teeth, hypoplasia of enamel
Thalidomide	Abnormal development of limbs such as meromelia (partial absence) and amelia (complete absence); facial defects; systemic anomalies such as cardiac, kidney, and ocular defects
Trimethadione	Development delay, V-shaped eyebrows, low-set ears, cleft lip and/or palate
Valproic acid	Craniofacial anomalies, NTDs, cognitive deficiency, often hydrocephalus, heart and skeletal defects
Warfarin	Nasal hypoplasia, stippled epiphyses, hypoplastic phalanges, eye anomalies, cognitive deficiency
Chemicals	
Methylmercury	Cerebral atrophy, spasticity, seizures, cognitive deficiency
Polychlorinated biphenyls	IUGR, skin discoloration
Infections	
Cytomegalovirus	Microcephaly, chorioretinitis, sensorineural hearing loss, delayed psychomotor/cognitive development, hepatosplenomegaly, hydrocephaly, cerebral palsy, brain (periventricular) calcification
Hepatitis B virus	Preterm birth, low birth weight, fetal macrosomia
Herpes simplex virus	Skin vesicles and scarring, chorioretinitis, hepatomegaly, thrombocytopenia, petechiae, hemolytic anemia, hydranencephaly
Human parvovirus B19	Fetal anemia, nonimmune hydrops fetalis, fetal death
Rubella virus	IUGR, postnatal growth retardation, cardiac and great vessel abnormalities, microcephaly, sensorineural deafness, cataract, microphthalmos, glaucoma, pigmented retinopathy, cognitive deficiency, neonate bleeding, hepatosplenomegaly, osteopathy, tooth defects
SARS-CoV-2 virus	Spontaneous abortion, stillbirth, preterm birth, IUGR, low birth weight
Toxoplasma gondii	Microcephaly, cognitive deficiency, microphthalmia, hydrocephaly, chorioretinitis, cerebral calcifications, hearing loss, neurologic disturbance
Treponema pallidum	Hydrocephalus, congenital deafness, cognitive deficiency, abnormal teeth and bones
Venezuelan equine encephalitis virus	Microcephaly, microphthalmia, cerebral agenesis, CNS necrosis, hydrocephalus
Zika virus	Microcephaly with partial skull collapse; thin cerebral cortices; retinal mottling and macular scarring; contractures, arthrogryposis, sensorineural hearing loss, swallowing difficulties, hypertonia, neurodevelopmental problems, failure to thrive.
Varicella virus	Cutaneous scars (dermatome distribution), neurologic defects (e.g., limb paresis [incomplete paralysis]), hydrocephaly, seizures, cataracts, microphthalmia, Horner syndrome, optic atrophy, nystagmus, chorioretinitis, microcephaly, cognitive deficiency, skeletal anomalies (e.g., hypoplasia of limbs, fingers, toes), urogenital anomalies
Radiation	
High levels of ionizing radiation	Microcephaly, cognitive deficiency, skeletal anomalies, growth retardation, cataracts

CNS, Central nervous system; *IUGR*, intrauterine growth restriction; *NTD*, neural tube defect; *SARS-CoV-2*, severe acute respiratory syndrome coronavirus 2.

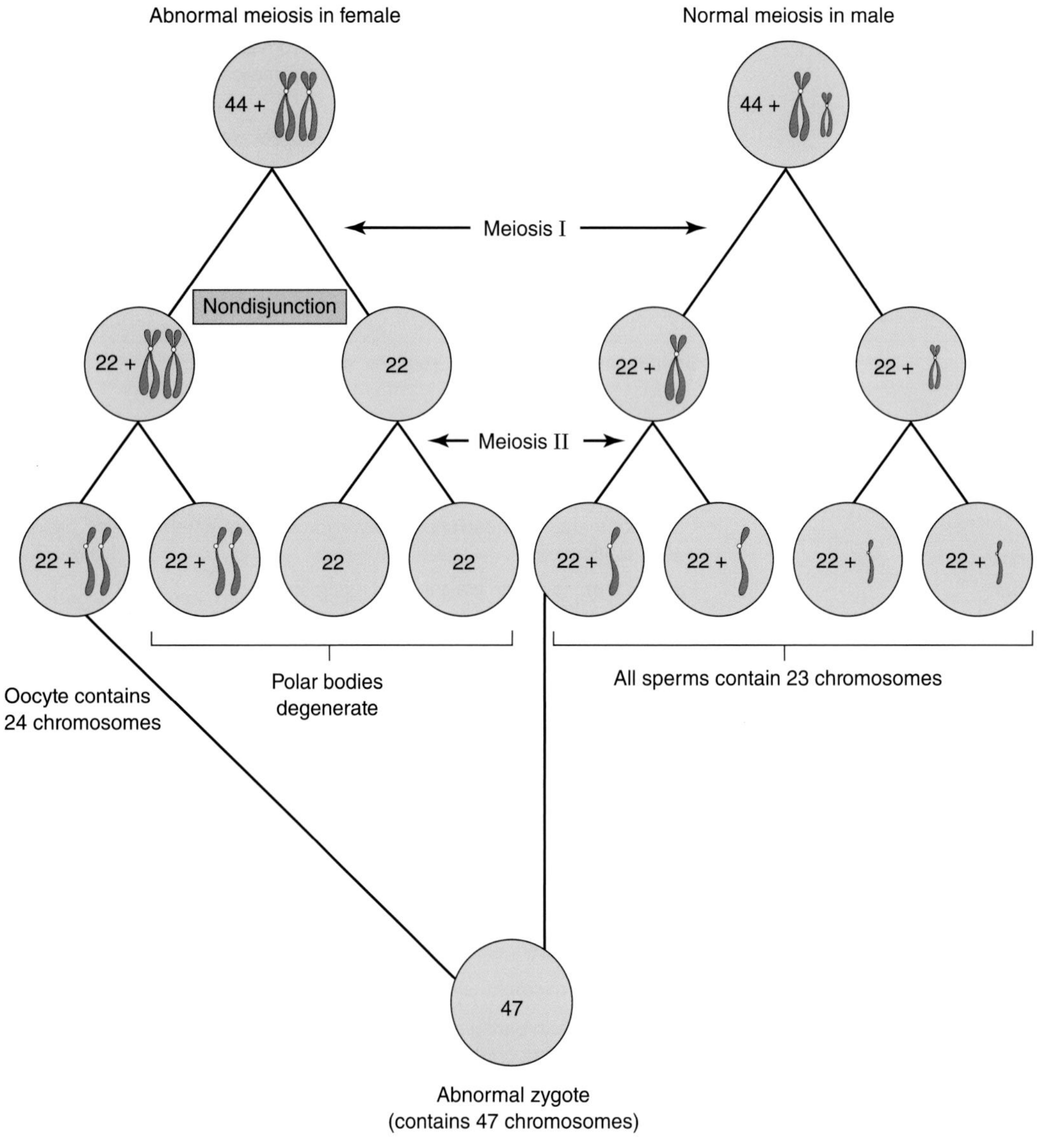

Fig. 20.5 Nondisjunction of chromosomes during the first meiotic division of a primary oocyte results in an abnormal oocyte with 24 chromosomes. Subsequent fertilization by a normal sperm produces a zygote with 47 chromosomes (aneuploidy), which is a deviation from the human diploid number of 46.

Glossary of Teratologic Terms

A birth defect is a structural abnormality of any type, but not all variations of development are defects or anomalies (marked deviation from the average or norm). **Anatomical variations are common**; for example, bones vary in their basic shape and in lesser details of surface structure. The four clinically significant types of birth defects are malformation, disruption, deformation, and dysplasia.

- **Malformation** is a morphologic defect of an organ, part of an organ, or a larger region of the body that results from an *intrinsically abnormal developmental process*. Intrinsic implies that the developmental potential of the primordium of an organ is abnormal from the beginning, such as a chromosomal abnormality of a gamete (oocyte or sperm) at fertilization. Most malformations are considered to be a defect of a **morphogenetic or developmental field** that responds as a coordinated unit to embryonic interaction and results in complex or multiple malformations.
- **Disruption** is a morphologic defect of an organ, part of an organ, or a larger region of the body that results from the *extrinsic breakdown of, or interference with, an originally normal developmental process*. Morphologic alterations after exposure to **teratogens** (e.g., drugs, chemicals, viruses) should be considered as disruptions. *Disruption cannot be inherited*, but inherited factors can predispose to and influence the development of a disruption.
- **Deformation** is an abnormal form, shape, or position of a part of the body that *results from mechanical forces*. **Intrauterine compression in utero** that results from oligohydramnios (insufficient amount of amniotic fluid) may produce an equinovarus foot or clubfoot (see Fig. 16.15). Some central nervous system (CNS) neural tube defects, such as meningomyelocele (a severe type of spina bifida), produce intrinsic functional disturbances, which cause fetal deformation (see Figs. 17.12C and 17.15A).
- **Dysplasia** is an *abnormal organization of cells in tissues* and its morphologic results. Dysplasia is the consequence of **dyshistogenesis** (abnormal tissue formation). All abnormalities relating to histogenesis are therefore classified as dysplasias, such as **congenital ectodermal dysplasia** (see Chapter 19, box titled "Congenital Ectodermal Dysplasia"). Dysplasia is causally nonspecific and often affects several organs because of the nature of the underlying cellular disturbances.

Other descriptive terms are used to describe infants with multiple defects, and the clinical terms have evolved to express causation and pathogenesis:

- A **polytopic field defect** is a pattern of defects derived from the disturbance of a single developmental field (e.g., DiGeorge anomaly).
- A **sequence** is a pattern of multiple defects derived from a single known or presumed structural defect or mechanical factor (e.g., Potter's sequence)
- A **syndrome** is a pattern of multiple defects thought to be pathogenetically related (pleiotropy) and not known to represent a single sequence or a polytopic field defect (e.g., neurofibromatosis type 1).
- An **association** is a nonrandom occurrence in two or more individuals of multiple defects not known to be a polytopic field defect, sequence, or syndrome (e.g., VATERL association [Vertebral, Anal atresia, Tracheo-Esophageal, Renal, and Limbs anomalies]).

Whereas a sequence is a pathogenetic not a causal concept, a syndrome often implies a single cause, such as trisomy 21 (Down syndrome). In both cases, the pattern of defects is known or considered to be pathogenetically related. In the case of a sequence, the primary initiating factor and cascade of secondary developmental complications are known. For example, **Potter syndrome** (sequence), which is attributed to oligohydramnios, results from renal agenesis or leakage of amniotic fluid (see Fig. 12.12C). An association, in contrast, refers to statistically, not pathogenetically or causally, related defects. One or more sequences, syndromes, or field defects may constitute an association.

Dysmorphology is an area of clinical genetics that is concerned with the observation, recognition, and interpretation of patterns of structural defects leading to a diagnosis. Recurrent patterns of birth defects enable syndrome recognition. Identifying these patterns in individuals has improved understanding of the causes and pathogenesis of these conditions.

Phenotype refers to the morphologic characteristics of a person as determined by the genotype and environment in which it is expressed.

order of meiosis I and meiosis II and premature separation of sister chromatids. As a result, the chromosomal pair or chromatids pass to one daughter cell, and the other daughter cell receives neither. Nondisjunction may occur during maternal or paternal gametogenesis.

TURNER SYNDROME

Approximately 1% of monosomy X female embryos survives; the incidence of 45,X (**Turner syndrome**) in female neonates is approximately 1 in 8000 live births. The most frequent chromosome constitution in Turner syndrome is 45,X; however, almost 50% of these people have other X chromosome anomalies identified on karyotype analysis. The phenotype of Turner syndrome is female (see Figs. 20.6–20.8). Secondary sexual characteristics do not develop completely in 90% of affected females, and hormone replacement is required.

Inactivation of Genes

During embryogenesis, one of the two X chromosomes in female somatic cells is randomly inactivated and appears as a mass of **sex chromatin**. **Inactivation of genes** on one X chromosome in somatic cells of female embryos occurs early in embryonic development. X inactivation is important clinically because it means that each cell from a carrier of an X-linked disease has the pathogenic variant (mutation) associated with the disease on the active X chromosome or on the inactivated X chromosome that is represented by sex chromatin. Skewed X inactivation in monozygotic (identical) twins is one reason given for discordance in a variety of birth defects. The genetic basis for discordance is that one twin preferentially expresses the paternal X and the other the maternal X. Certain autosomal genes can also be inactivated (silenced) due to methylation (epigenetic effects).

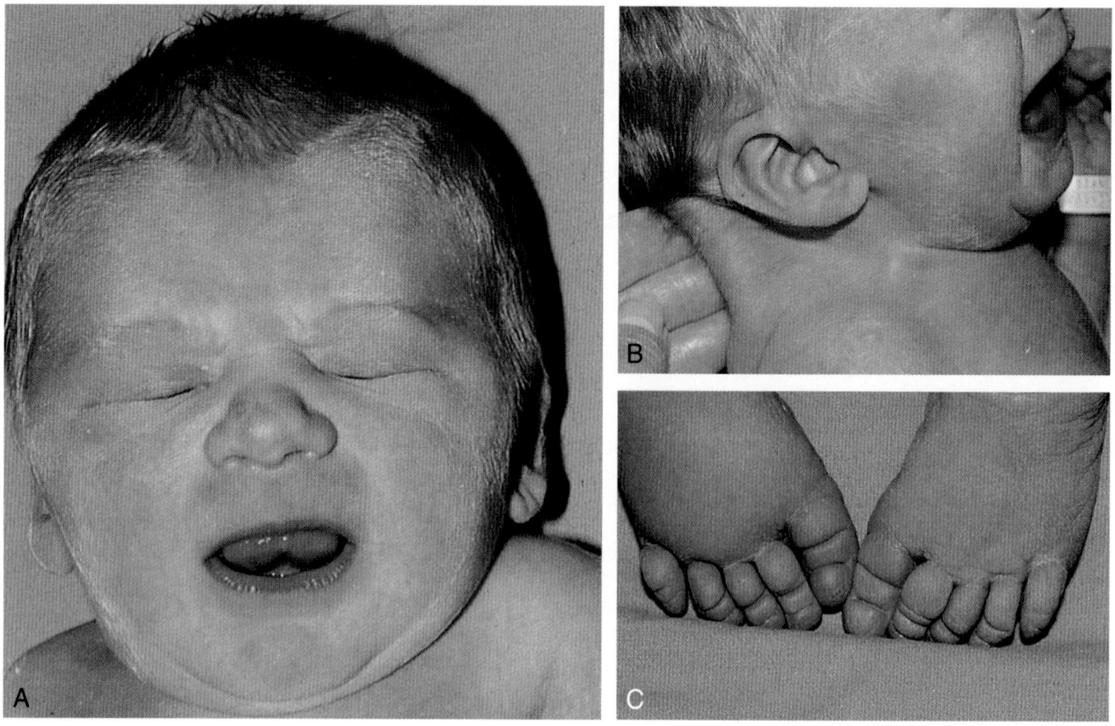

Fig. 20.6 Female infant with Turner syndrome (45,X). (A) Face of the infant. (B) Lateral view of the infant's head and neck shows a short, webbed neck and prominent ears. Infants with this syndrome have defective gonadal development (gonadal dysgenesis). (C) Lymphedema of the toes is a condition that usually leads to nail underdevelopment (hypoplasia). (Courtesy Dr. A.E. Chudley, Section of Genetics and Metabolism, Department of Pediatrics and Child Health, Children's Hospital, Winnipeg, Manitoba, Canada.)

The **monosomy X chromosome abnormality** is the most common cytogenetic abnormality observed in fetuses that abort spontaneously (see Fig. 20.8); it accounts for approximately 18% of all abortions caused by chromosomal abnormalities. The nondisjunction that causes monosomy X, when it can be traced, is in the paternal gamete (sperm) in approximately 75% of cases it is (i.e., the paternal X chromosome that is usually missing).

TRISOMY OF AUTOSOMES

Three chromosome copies in a given chromosome pair are called **trisomy**. Trisomies are the most common abnormalities of chromosome number. The usual cause of this numeric error is meiotic nondisjunction of chromosomes. Trisomy of autosomes is mainly associated with three syndromes (Table 20.2):

- Trisomy 21 or Down syndrome (see Fig. 20.4)
- Trisomy 18 or Edwards syndrome (Fig. 20.9)
- Trisomy 13 or Patau syndrome (Fig. 20.10)

Infants with trisomy 13 and trisomy 18 have multiple anomalies and severe neurodevelopmental disabilities. These life-limiting disorders have a 1-year survival rate of approximately 6% to 12%. More than one-half of trisomic embryos spontaneously abort early. Trisomy of the autosomes occurs with increasing frequency as maternal age increases. For example, trisomy 21 occurs once in approximately 1400 births among mothers between the ages of 20 and 24 years but once in approximately 25 births among mothers 45 years and older (see Fig. 20.11). The most common aneuploidy seen in older mothers is trisomy 21 (Down syndrome; see Fig. 20.4).

The Centers for Disease Control and Prevention notes that the incidence of trisomy 21 syndrome in the United States is estimated to be 1 in 700 live births. Because of the current trend of increasing maternal age, it has been estimated that children born to females older than 34 years will account for 39% of infants with trisomy 21. Translocations resulting in trisomy or mosaicism occurs in approximately 5% of the affected children. **Mosaicism**, which is a condition in which two or more cell types contain different numbers of chromosomes (normal and abnormal), can lead to a less severe phenotype or even a phenotype that is not recognized as being atiributable to the classic association. Molecular and pathophysiological studies of the different phenotypes of trisomy 21 suggest that this condition is a disorder of gene expression dysregulation.

TRISOMY OF SEX CHROMOSOMES

Trisomy of the sex chromosomes is a common disorder (Table 20.3). However, because there are no characteristic physical findings in infants or children, the disorder is not usually detected until puberty (Fig. 20.12). Diagnosis is best achieved by chromosome analysis or other molecular cytogenetic techniques.

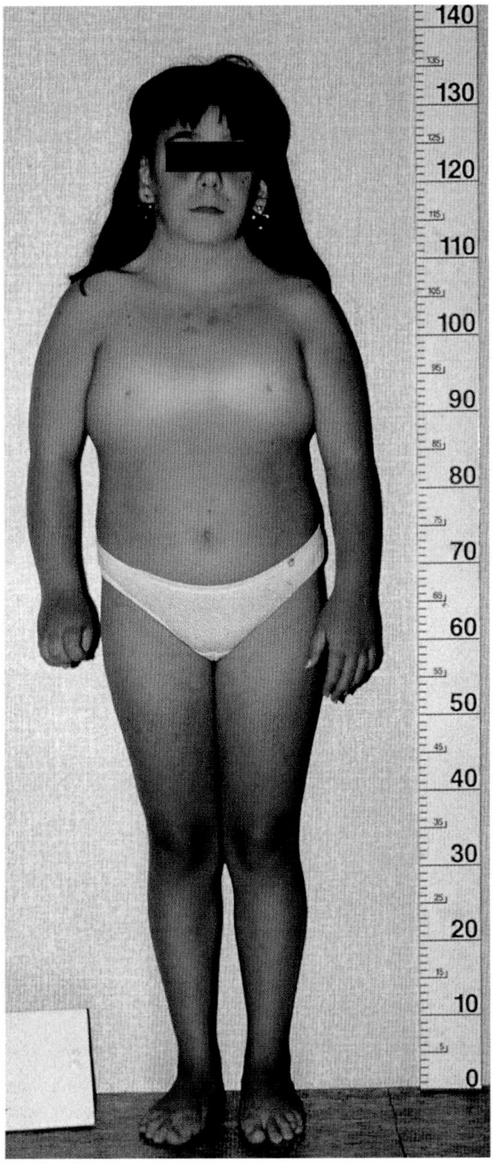

Fig. 20.7 Turner syndrome (45,X) in a 14-year-old girl. Features of the syndrome include short stature; a webbed neck; absence of sexual maturation; a broad chest with widely spaced nipples; and lymphedema swelling of the hands and feet. (Courtesy Dr. F. Antoniazzi and Dr. V. Fanos, Department of Pediatrics, University of Verona, Verona, Italy.)

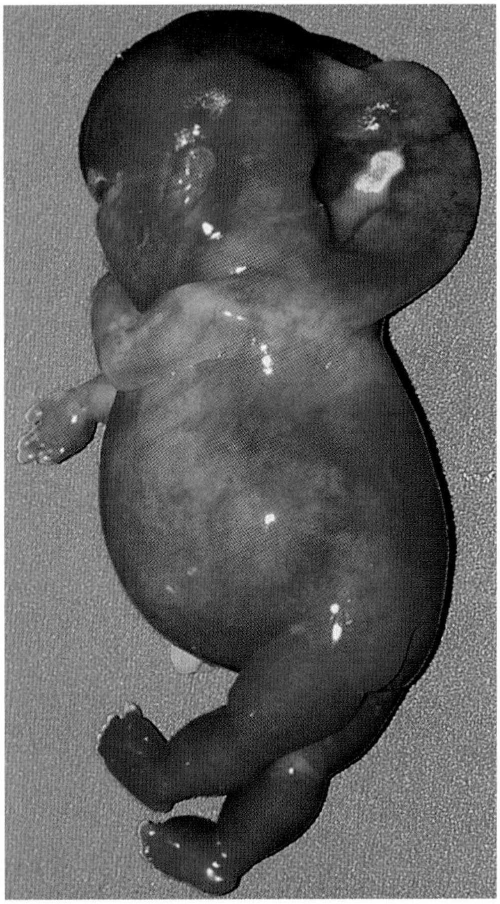

Fig. 20.8 Female fetus with Turner syndrome (45,X) at 16 weeks. Notice the excessive accumulation of watery fluid (hydrops) and the large cystic hygroma (lymphangioma) in the posterior head and cervical region. The hygroma causes the loose neck skin and webbing seen postnatally (see Fig. 20.6B). (Courtesy Dr. A.E. Chudley, Section of Genetics and Metabolism, Department of Pediatrics and Child Health, Children's Hospital, Winnipeg, Manitoba, Canada.)

Tetrasomy and Pentasomy

Persons with tetrasomy or pentasomy have cell nuclei with four or five sex chromosomes, respectively. Several chromosome complexes have been reported in females (48,XXXX and 49,XXXXX) and in males (48,XXXY, 48,XXYY, 49,XXXYY, and 49,XXXXY). The extra sex chromosomes do not accentuate sexual characteristics. However, the greater the number of sex chromosomes in males, the greater the severity of cognitive deficiency and physical impairment. The **tetrasomy X syndrome** (48,XXXX) is associated with serious cognitive deficiency and physical development. The **pentasomy X syndrome** (49,XXXXX) usually includes severe cognitive deficiency and multiple physical anomalies.

Mosaicism

A person with at least two cell lines with two or more **genotypes** is a **mosaic**. The autosomes or sex chromosomes may be involved. The defects usually are less serious than in persons with monosomy or trisomy. For instance, the features of Turner syndrome are not as evident in 45,X/46,XX **mosaic females** as in the usual 45,X females. It is also possible to have 45,X/46,XY mosaicism, where the phenotype can span the spectrum of female to male. Mosaicism usually results from nondisjunction during early cleavage of the zygote (see Fig. 2.16 and page 20). Mosaicism resulting from the **loss of a chromosome by anaphase lagging** also occurs. The chromosomes separate normally, but one of them is delayed in its migration and is eventually lost.

Table 20.2 Trisomy of Autosomes

Chromosomal Aberration and Syndrome	Incidence	Usual Clinical Manifestations
Trisomy 21 (Down syndrome)[a] (see Fig. 20.4)	1 in 800	Cognitive deficiency; brachycephaly, flat nasal bridge; upward slant to palpebral fissures; protruding tongue; transverse palmar flexion crease; clinodactyly of the fifth digit; congenital heart defects; gastrointestinal tract abnormalities
Trisomy 18 syndrome (Edwards syndrome)[b] (see Fig. 20.10)	1 in 8000	Cognitive deficiency; growth retardation; prominent occiput; short sternum; ventricular septal defect; micrognathia; low-set, malformed ears, flexed digits, hypoplastic nails; rocker bottom feet
Trisomy 13 syndrome (Patau syndrome)[b] (see Fig. 20.11)	1 in 12,000	Cognitive deficiency; severe central nervous system malformations; sloping forehead; malformed ears, scalp defects; microphthalmia; bilateral cleft lip and/or palate; polydactyly; posterior prominence of the heels

[a]The incidence of trisomy 21 at fertilization is greater than at birth; however, 75% of embryos are spontaneously aborted, and at least 20% are stillborn.
[b]Infants with this syndrome rarely survive beyond 6 months.

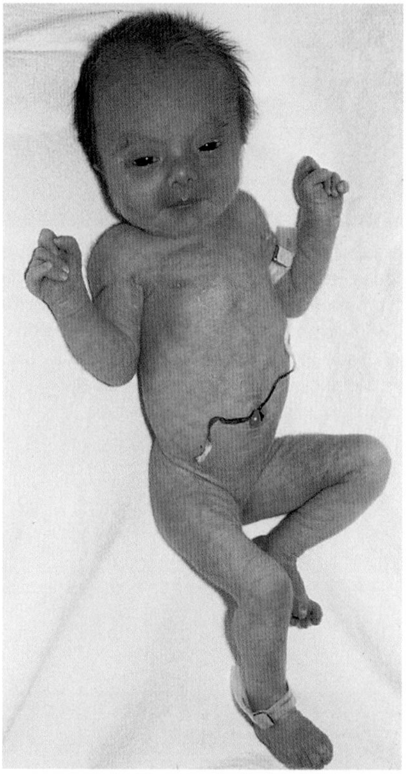

Fig. 20.9 A female neonate with the trisomy 18 syndrome has growth retardation, clenched fists with characteristic positioning of the fingers (second and fifth ones overlapping the third and fourth ones), short sternum, and narrow pelvis. (Courtesy Dr. A.E. Chudley, Section of Genetics and Metabolism, Department of Pediatrics and Child Health, Children's Hospital, Winnipeg, Manitoba, Canada.)

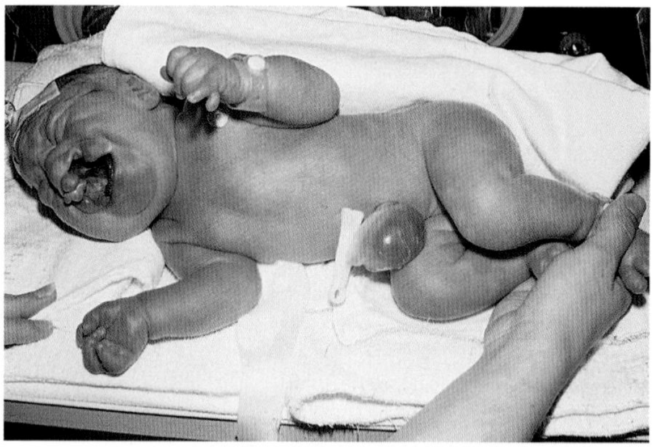

Fig. 20.10 A female neonate with trisomy 13 syndrome has a bilateral cleft lip, low-set and malformed left ear, and polydactyly (extra digits). A small omphalocele (herniation of viscera into the umbilical cord) can be seen. (Courtesy Dr. A.E. Chudley, Section of Genetics and Metabolism, Department of Pediatrics and Child Health, Children's Hospital, Winnipeg, Manitoba, Canada.)

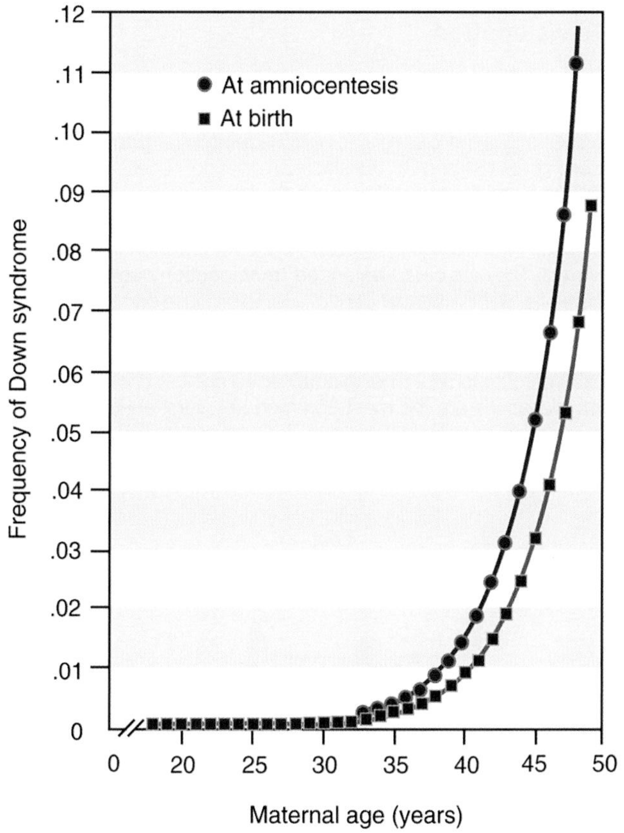

Fig. 20.11 Maternal age dependence on incidence of trisomy 21 at birth and at time of amniocentesis. (From Nussbaum RL, McInnes RR, Willard HF: The chromosomal and genomic basis of disease: disorders of the autosomes and sex chromosomes. In Nussbaum RL, McInnes RR, Willard HF, editors: *Thomson &Thomson genetics in medicine*, ed 8, Philadelphia, 2016, Elsevier.)

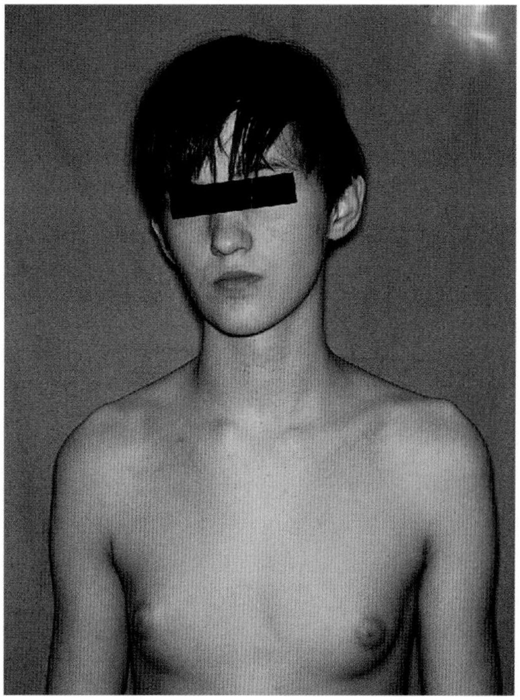

Fig. 20.12 A male adolescent with Klinefelter syndrome (XXY trisomy) has breasts. Approximately 40% of males with this syndrome have gynecomastia (development of breasts) and small testes. (Courtesy Children's Hospital, Winnipeg, Manitoba, Canada.)

Table 20.3 Trisomy of Chromosomes

Chromosome Complement[a]	Sex	Incidence[b]	Usual Characteristics
47,XXX	Female	1 in 1000	Normal in appearance; usually fertile; 15% to 25% are mildly cognitively deficient.
47,XXY	Male	1 in 1000	Klinefelter syndrome: small testes, hyalinization of seminiferous tubules; aspermatogenesis; often tall with disproportionately long lower limbs. Intelligence is less than in normal siblings. Approximately 40% of these males have gynecomastia (see Fig. 20.8).
47,XYY	Male	1 in 1000	Normal in appearance and usually tall.

[a]The numbers designate the total number of chromosomes, including the sex chromosomes shown after the comma.

[b]Data from Hook EB, Hamerton JL: The frequency of chromosome abnormalities detected in consecutive newborn studies; differences between studies; results by sex and by severity of phenotypic involvement. In Hook EB, Porter IH, editors: *Population cytogenetics: studies in humans*, New York, 1977, Academic Press. More information is provided by Nussbaum RL, McInnes RR, Willard HF: *Thompson and Thompson genetics in medicine*, ed 8, Philadelphia, 2015, Elsevier.

Triploidy and Tetraploidy

The most common type of **polyploidy** (cell nucleus containing three or more haploid sets; see Fig. 2.1) is **triploid fetus** (69 chromosomes). Triploid fetuses have severe **intrauterine growth retardation** with head–body disproportion. Although triploid fetuses are born, they do not survive very long.

Triploidy most frequently results from the fertilization of an oocyte by two sperms **(dispermy)**. Failure of one of the meiotic divisions (see Fig. 2.1), resulting in a **diploid oocyte or sperm**, may account for some cases. Triploid fetuses account for approximately 20% of chromosomally abnormal spontaneous abortions. Doubling of the diploid chromosome number from 46 to 92 **(tetraploidy)** probably occurs during the first cleavage division of the zygote (see Fig. 2.17A). Division of this abnormal zygote subsequently results in an embryo with cells containing 92 chromosomes. Tetraploid embryos abort very early, and often all that is recovered is an empty chorionic sac (blighted embryo).

STRUCTURAL CHROMOSOMAL ABNORMALITIES

Most structural chromosomal abnormalities result from **chromosome breakage**, followed by reconstitution in an abnormal combination (Fig. 20.13). The breakage may be induced by environmental factors such as viral infections, drugs, chemicals, and ionizing radiation. The type of structural abnormality depends on what happens to the broken chromosome pieces. The only two aberrations of chromosome structure that are likely to be transmitted from a parent to an embryo are structural rearrangements, such as **inversion and translocation**. Overall, structural abnormalities of chromosomes occur in about 1 in 375 neonates.

Translocation

Translocation is the transfer of a piece of one chromosome to a nonhomologous chromosome. If two nonhomologous chromosomes exchange pieces, it is called a **reciprocal translocation** (see Fig. 20.13A and G). Translocation does not necessarily cause abnormal development. For example, persons with a translocation (Robertsonian) between a number 21 chromosome and a number 14 chromosome (see Fig. 20.13G) are phenotypically normal. They are called **balanced translocation carriers**. They have a tendency, independent of age, to produce germ cells with an **abnormal translocation chromosome**. Between 3% and 4% of infants with Down syndrome have trisomy 21 due to the extra chromosome 21 being attached to another chromosome. Translocations are the most common structural abnormality of chromosomes in the general population (1:1000).

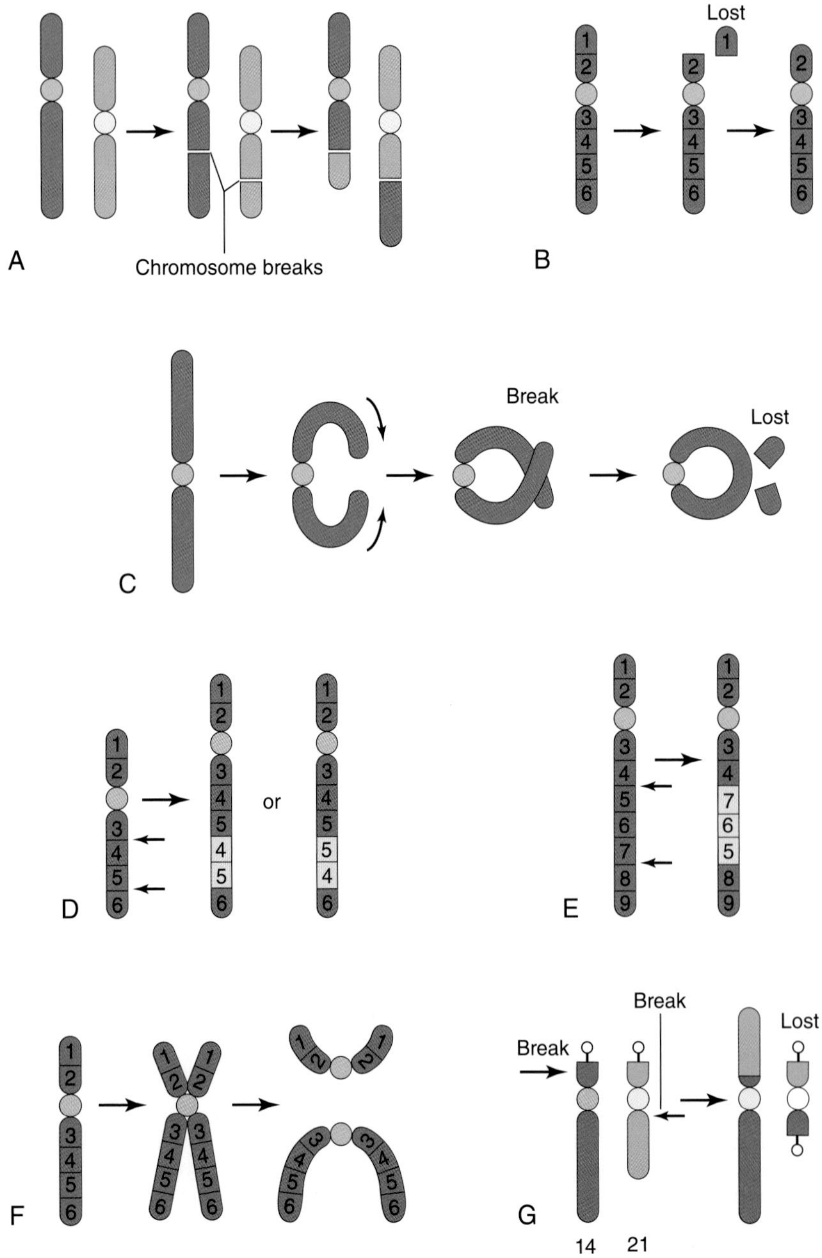

Fig. 20.13 Diagrams of structural chromosomal abnormalities. (A) Reciprocal translocation. (B) Terminal deletion. (C) Ring chromosome. (D) Duplication. (E) Paracentric inversion. (F) Isochromosome. (G) Robertsonian translocation. *Arrows* indicate how the structural abnormalities are produced. (Modified from Nussbaum RL, McInnes RR, Willard HE: *Thompson and Thompson genetics in medicine*, ed 6, Philadelphia, 2004, Saunders.)

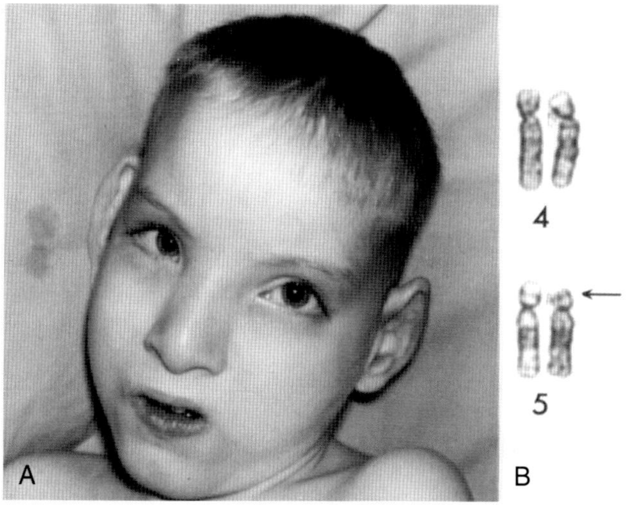

Fig. 20.14 (A) Male child with cri du chat ("cat-like cry") syndrome has microcephaly and hypertelorism (increased distance between orbits). (B) Partial karyotype of the child shows a terminal deletion of the short arm (end) of chromosome 5. The *arrow* indicates the site of the deletion. (A, From Gardner EJ: *Principles of genetics*, ed 5, New York, 1975, John Wiley & Sons. B, Cortesy the late Dr. M. Ray, Department of Human Genetics, University of Manitoba, Winnipeg, Manitoba, Canada.)

Deletion

When a chromosome breaks, part of it may be lost (see Fig. 20.13B). A partial terminal deletion from the short arm of chromosome 5 causes **cri du chat syndrome** (Fig. 20.14). Affected infants have a weak, cat-like cry; microcephaly (small neurocranium); global developmental delay; and may have congenital heart disease.

A **ring chromosome** is a type of deletion chromosome from which both ends have been lost and the broken ends have rejoined (see Fig. 20.13C). Ring chromosomes are rare, but they have been found for all chromosomes. These abnormal chromosomes have been described in persons with **45,X** (Turner syndrome), **trisomy 18** (Edwards syndrome), and other structural chromosomal abnormalities.

Inversion

Inversion is a chromosomal aberration in which a segment of a chromosome is reversed. **Paracentric inversion** is confined to a single arm of the chromosome (see Fig. 20.13E), whereas **pericentric inversion** involves both arms and includes the centromere. Carriers of pericentric inversions risk having offspring with birth defects because of unequal crossing over and malsegregation at meiosis (see Fig. 2.2).

Duplications

Some abnormalities are represented as a duplicated part of a chromosome within a chromosome (see Fig. 20.13D), attached to a chromosome, or as a separate fragment. Duplications are more common than deletions and are less harmful because there is no loss of genetic material. However, the resulting phenotype often includes cognitive impairment or birth defects. Duplication may involve part of a gene, a whole gene, or a series of genes.

Molecular Cytogenetics

Methods for merging classic cytogenetics with **DNA technology** have facilitated precise definitions of chromosome abnormalities, location, and origins, including unbalanced translocations, accessory or marker chromosomes, and **gene mapping**. One approach to chromosome identification is based on **fluorescent in situ hybridization (FISH)**, in which chromosome-specific **DNA probes** adhere to complementary regions located on specific chromosomes. This allows improved identification of chromosome location and number in metaphase spreads or interphase cells. FISH techniques applied to interphase cells may soon obviate the need to culture cells for specific chromosome analysis, as in the case of prenatal diagnosis of fetal trisomies.

Studies using **subtelomeric FISH probes** in individuals with cognitive deficiency of unknown origin, with or without birth defects, have identified **submicroscopic chromosome deletions** or duplications in 5% to 10% of these individuals. Alterations in DNA sequence copy number are identified in solid tumors and are associated with developmental abnormalities and cognitive deficiency.

Comparative genomic hybridization (CGH) can detect and map changes in specific regions of the genome. **Microarray-based CGH** (array comparative genomic hybridization), also referred to as chromosomal microarray analysis has been used to identify genomic rearrangements and changes in copy number in individuals who were previously considered to have cognitive deficiency or multiple birth defects of unknown origin despite normal test results from traditional chromosome or gene analysis. Array CGH can also identify regions of homozygosity in an individual. A chromosome **single-nucleotide polymorphism array** is a more refined genetic test that can detect very small changes in a person's chromosomes and has replaced the use of CGH in clinical practice. Noninvasive prenatal testing is available clinically in some jurisdictions for the detection of certain aneuploidies. Advances in genomic sequencing technology using whole exome sequencing and genome sequencing have further defined smaller regions of genomic rearrangements (deletions/duplications) and changes at the base-pair level that aid in the clinical diagnosis of patients with previously unexplained chromosomal and single-gene disorders. These technologies have transformed the ability to diagnose individuals with suspected genetic disorders. Genetic counseling is indicated at the pre- and post-test stage for families considering sequencing as results may be difficult to interpret, incidental findings may result (disorders unrelated to why the testing was pursued), and implications for different family members. Rapid trio-based (proband and both parents) genomic sequencing of neonates in the intensive care unit has dramatically impacted the time to diagnosis, care, and management of these babies.

Table 20.4 Contiguous Gene Syndromes

Syndrome	Clinical Features	Chromosome Findings	Parental Origin
Prader-Willi	Hypothalamic dysfunction, hypotonia, hypogonadism, hypothyroidism, extreme obesity with hyperphagia, distinct face, low bone density, short stature, small hands and feet, mild developmental delay, learning disability	del 15 q11.2–q13 (most cases)	Paternal
Angelman	Microcephaly, macrosomia, ataxia, excessive laughter, seizures, severe cognitive deficiency	del 15 q12 (most cases)	Maternal
Miller-Dieker	Type 1 lissencephaly (smooth cerebral cortex), dysmorphic face, seizures, breathing problems, severe developmental delay, cardiac defects	del 17 p13.3 (most cases) overlapping 17 p13.3 duplications (few cases)	Either parent
DiGeorge	Thymic hypoplasia, parathyroid hypoplasia, conotruncal cardiac defects, facial dysmorphism	del 22 q11 (some cases)	Either parent
Velocardiofacial (Shprintzen)	Palatal defects, hypoplastic alae nasi, long nose, conotruncal cardiac defects, speech delay, learning disorder, schizophrenia-like disorder	del 22 q11 (most cases)	Either parent
Smith-Magenis	Brachycephaly, broad nasal bridge, prominent jaw, short and broad hands, speech delay, cognitive deficiency	del 17 p11.2	Either parent
Williams	Short stature; hypercalcemia; cardiac defects, especially supravalvular aortic stenosis; characteristic elfin-like face; cognitive deficiency	del 17 q11.23 (most cases)	Either parent
Beckwith-Wiedemann	Macrosomia, macroglossia, omphalocele (some cases), hypoglycemia, hemihypertrophy, transverse earlobes	dup 11 p15 (some cases)	Paternal

Microdeletion and Microduplication

- With high-resolution chromosome banding and array-based comparative genomic hybridization (CGH), very small interstitial and terminal deletions in several chromosomal disorders can be detected. An acceptable resolution of chromosome banding on routine analysis reveals 550 bands per haploid set, whereas high-resolution chromosome banding reveals up to ~800 bands per haploid set and can typically detect deletions and duplications that are at least 5000 megabases. CGH can typically detect microdeletions and/or microduplications at a resolution of 1000 megabases. Because the deletions span several contiguous genes, these disorders and those with microduplications are referred to as contiguous gene syndromes (Table 20.4), as in these examples:
- Prader-Willi syndrome (PWS) is a sporadically occurring disorder associated with short stature, mild cognitive deficiency, obesity, hyperphagia (overeating), and hypogonadism.
- Angelman syndrome (AS) is characterized by severe cognitive deficiency, microcephaly, brachycephaly, seizures, and ataxic (jerky) movements of the limbs and trunk.
- PWS and AS are often associated with a visible deletion of bands q11–q13 on chromosome 15. The clinical phenotype is determined by the parental origin of the deleted chromosome 15. If the deletion occurs in the chromosome 15 inherited from the mother, AS occurs; if the deletion occurs in the chromosome 15 inherited from the father, the child exhibits the PWS phenotype. This suggests the phenomenon of genetic imprinting, in which differential expression of genetic material depends on the sex of the transmitting parent. One of the two parental alleles is active and the other is inactive because of epigenetic factors. Loss of expression of the active allele leads to neurodevelopmental disorders.

Isochromosomes

An **isochromosome** results when the centromere divides transversely instead of longitudinally (see Fig. 20.13E), creating a chromosome in which one arm is missing and the other is duplicated. This chromosome appears to be the most common structural abnormality of the X chromosome. Persons with this aberration often have short stature and the other features of **Turner syndrome** (see Figs. 20.6–20.8). These characteristics are related to the loss of an arm of an X chromosome.

Marfan Syndrome

This syndrome is caused by the loss of expression of FBN1 on the long arm of chromosome 15 (15q21.1), resulting in decreased levels of fibrillin-1, a major component of extracellular matrix microfibrils. The incidence of Marfan syndrome is approximately 1:5000 live births. The tissues most commonly affected are arteries (e.g., aortic dissection), perichondrium (i.e., overgrowth of long bones), and the eye (i.e., ectopia lentis).

BIRTH DEFECTS CAUSED BY PATHOGENIC VARIANTS IN GENES

Exome and genome sequencing have identified the genetic cause in numerous different single-gene disorders with birth defects (see Fig. 20.3). A **pathogenic (disease-causing) variant**, usually involving a loss or change in the function of a gene, is a permanent change in the sequence of genomic DNA. Variants can be classified as pathogenic, likely pathogenic, benign, or a variant of unknown significance. These variants are usually detected via exome and/or genome sequencing or with the use of multigene panels. Pathogenic variants can be inherited from a parent or be the result of a new change (de novo).

The **mutation rate** can be increased by several environmental agents. Defects resulting from gene mutations are inherited according to Mendelian laws; consequently, predictions can be made about the probability of their occurrence in the affected person's children and other relatives. An example of an autosomal dominant disorder that can be inherited or de novo is **achondroplasia** (Fig. 20.15), which results from a G-to-A transition mutation at nucleotide 1138 of the cDNA in the fibroblast growth factor receptor 3 gene on chromosome 4p. Other defects, such as **congenital adrenal hyperplasia** (see Fig. 20.16) and **microcephaly** (see Fig. 17.36), are attributed to autosomal recessive inheritance. Autosomal recessive disorders manifest only when pathogenic/likely pathogenic variants are present in a homozygous or compound heterozygous state. As a consequence, many carriers of these genes (heterozygotes) remain undetected.

Fragile X syndrome is the most commonly known inherited cause of intellectual disability (see Fig. 20.17) and monogenic cause of autism spectrum disorder (ASD). It is one of more than 200 X-linked disorders associated with cognitive impairment. Fragile X syndrome occurs in 1 of 4000 male and 1 in 8000 female births. ASD and attention deficit hyperactivity disorder are often seen in association with this disorder. Diagnosis of this syndrome can be confirmed by DNA studies showing the full expansion (>200 triplet repeats of CGG nucleotides) in a specific region of the *FMR1* gene. This expansion results in a loss of gene transcription. Premutations (incomplete expansion of CGG nucleotides) of *FMR1* can result in fragile X-associated tremor/ataxia syndrome (FXTAS), and fragile X-associated primary ovarian insufficiency (FXPOI) as elevation in levels of the abnormal mRNAs become cytotoxic in brain and ovaries. X-linked recessive disorders usually manifest in affected (hemizygous males) and occasionally in carrier (heterozygous) females, as in fragile X syndrome.

Several genetic disorders are caused by the **expansion of trinucleotides** (combination of three adjacent nucleotides) in specific genes. Other examples include myotonic dystrophy type 1, Huntington disease, spinobulbar atrophy (Kennedy syndrome), and Friedreich ataxia. Other genetic

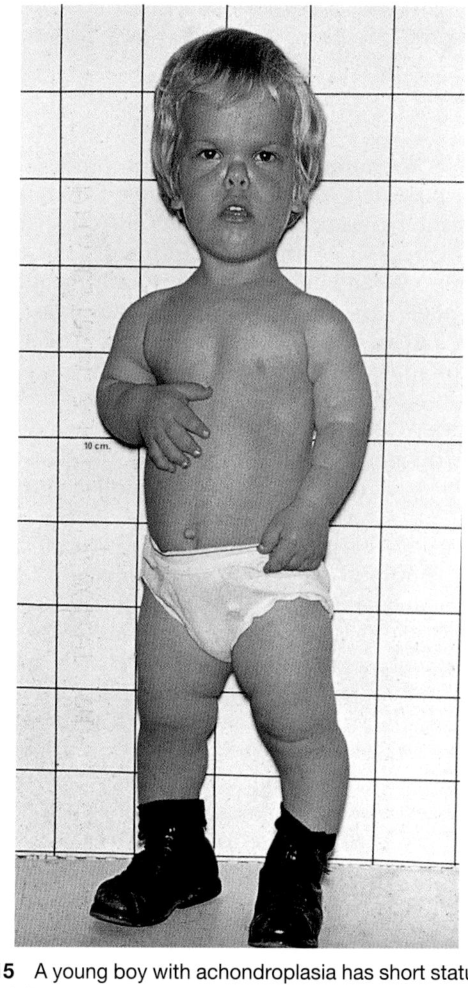

Fig. 20.15 A young boy with achondroplasia has short stature, short limbs and fingers, normal length of trunk, bowed legs, a relatively large head, a prominent forehead, and a depressed nasal bridge. (Courtesy Dr. A.E. Chudley, Section of Genetics and Metabolism, Department of Pediatrics and Child Health, Children's Hospital, Winnipeg, Manitoba, Canada.)

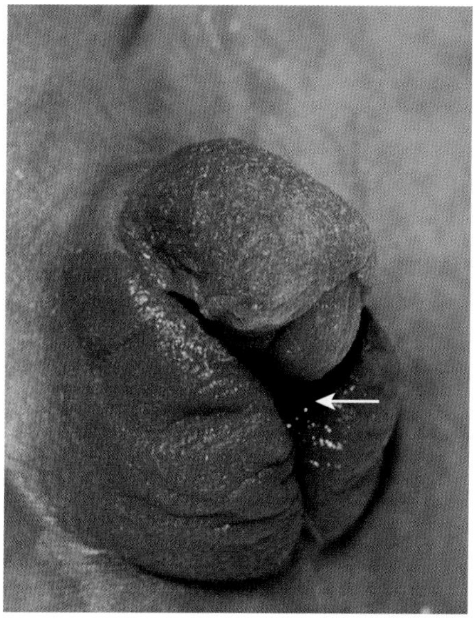

Fig. 20.16 Masculinized external genitalia of a 46,XX female infant. Observe the enlarged clitoris and fused labia majora. Virilization was caused by excessive androgens produced by the suprarenal glands during the fetal period (congenital adrenal hyperplasia). The *arrow* indicates the opening of the urogenital sinus. (Courtesy Dr. Heather Dean, Department of Pediatrics and Child Health, University of Manitoba, Winnipeg, Manitoba, Canada.)

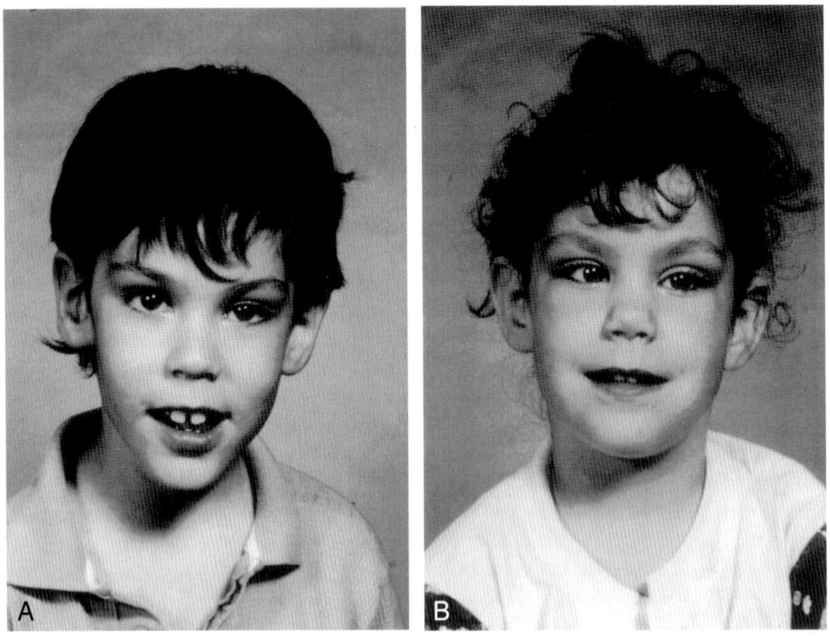

Fig. 20.17 Siblings with fragile X syndrome. (A) An 8-year-old boy has a relatively normal appearance with a long face and prominent ears. He also has significant cognitive impairment. (B) His 6-year-old sister, who also has this syndrome, has a mild learning disability and similar features of a long face and prominent ears. Notice the strabismus (crossed right eye). Although it is an X-linked disorder, female carriers sometimes express the disease. (Courtesy Dr. A.E. Chudley, Section of Genetics and Metabolism, Department of Pediatrics and Child Health, Children's Hospital, Winnipeg, Manitoba, Canada.)

disorders have been associated with the expansion of nucleotide repeats of other sizes as well including myotonic dystrophy type 2, congenital central hypoventilation syndrome, frontotemporal dementia/amyotrophic lateral sclerosis, and cleidocranial dysplasia.

The human genome comprises approximately 25,000 to 31,000 protein-coding genes per haploid set or 3 billion base pairs; the exact number remains unsettled. Because of the **Human Genome Project** and international research collaboration, many disease- and birth defect–causing mutations in genes have been and will continue to be identified. Most genes will be sequenced, and their specific function determined.

Most genes are expressed in a wide variety of cells and are involved in basic cellular metabolic functions, such as nucleic acid and protein synthesis, cytoskeleton and organelle biogenesis, and nutrient transport and other cellular mechanisms. These genes are referred to as **housekeeping genes**. The specialty genes are expressed at specific times in specific cells and define the hundreds of cell types that make up the human organism. An essential aspect of developmental biology is the regulation of gene expression. Regulation is often achieved by transcription factors that bind to regulatory or promoter elements of specific genes.

Epigenetic regulation refers to changes in phenotype or gene expression caused by mechanisms other than changes in the underlying DNA sequence. The mechanisms of epigenetic change are not entirely clear, but modifying transcriptional factors, DNA methylation, and histone modification may be key in altering developmental events. Several birth defects may be the result of altered gene expression due to environmental factors, maternal stress, or altered nutrition, rather than changes in DNA sequences.

Genomic imprinting is an epigenetic process in which the allele inherited from the mother or father is marked by methylation (imprinted), silencing the gene and allowing the expression of the nonimprinted gene from the other parent. When imprinting occurs, only the **paternal or maternal allele** (any one of a series of two or more different genes) of a gene is active in the offspring. The sex of the transmitting parent therefore influences the expression or nonexpression of certain genes (see Table 20.4).

In Prader-Willi syndrome **(PWS)** and Angelman syndrome **(AS)**, the phenotype is determined by whether a microdeletion occurs in the paternally inherited chromosome 15 (PWS) or occurs in the maternally inherited chromosome 15 (AS). In roughly 25% of cases of PWS and about 5% of AS; the condition arises from a phenomenon referred to as **uniparental disomy**. In PWS and AS, both copies of chromosome 15 (or key regions of the chromosome) originate from only one parent. PWS occurs when both are derived from the mother, and AS occurs when both are paternally derived. With uniparental isodisomy, the mechanism is thought to begin with a trisomic conceptus, followed by a loss of the extra chromosome in an early postzygotic cell division. This results in a "rescued" cell in which both chromosomes have been derived from one parent.

Uniparental disomy has involved several other chromosome pairs. Some are associated with adverse clinical outcomes involving chromosome 6 (transient neonatal diabetes mellitus) and 7 (Silver-Russell syndrome), whereas others (chromosomes 1 and 22) are not associated with abnormal phenotypic effects.

Homeobox genes are found in most eukaryote genomes examined and have highly conserved sequences and order. They were originally identified in Drosophila and are involved

Table 20.5 Human Disorders Associated With Homeobox Mutations

Syndrome	Clinical Features	Gene
Waardenburg syndrome (type I)	White forelock, lateral displacement of medial canthi of the eyes, cochlear deafness, heterochromia, tendency to facial clefting, autosomal dominant inheritance	*PAX3* (formerly *HUP2*) gene, homologous to mouse *Pax3* gene
Synpolydactyly (type II syndactyly)	Webbing and duplication of fingers, supernumerary metacarpals, autosomal dominant inheritance	*HOXD13* mutation
Holoprosencephaly (one form)	Incomplete separation of lateral cerebral ventricles, anophthalmia or cyclopia, midline facial hypoplasia or clefts, single maxillary central incisors, hypotelorism, autosomal dominant inheritance with widely variable expression	*SHH* (formerly *HPE3*) mutation, homologous to the *Drosophila* sonic hedgehog gene for segment polarity
Schizencephaly (type II)	Full-thickness cleft within the cerebral ventricles often leading to seizures, spasticity, and cognitive deficiency	Germline mutation in the *EMX2* homeobox gene, homologous to the mouse *Emx2*

in early embryonic development and specify the identity and spatial arrangements of body segments. Protein products of these genes bind to DNA and form transcriptional factors that regulate gene expression. Disorders associated with some homeobox gene mutations are described in Table 20.5.

DEVELOPMENTAL SIGNALING PATHWAYS

Normal embryogenesis is regulated by several complex signaling cascades (see Chapter 21). Mutations or alterations in any of these signaling pathways can lead to birth defects. Many pathways are cell-autonomous and alter the differentiation of only that particular cell, as seen in proteins produced by *HOXA* and *HOXD* gene clusters (in which mutations lead to a variety of limb defects). Other **transcription factors** act by influencing the pattern of gene expression of adjacent cells. These short-range signal controls can act as simple on-off switches (paracrine signals); those called **morphogens** elicit many responses in target cells depending on their level of expression (concentration).

One developmental signaling pathway is initiated by the secreted protein called **sonic hedgehog** (SHH), which sets off a chain of events resulting in activation and repression of target cells by transcription factors in the GLI family. Perturbations in the regulation of the Shh-Patched-Gli (SHH-PTCH-GLI) signaling pathway lead to several birth defects and diseases including some forms of cancer.

SHH is expressed in the notochord, the floor plate of the neural tube, the brain, and other regions, such as the zone of polarizing activity of the developing limbs and the gut. Sporadic and inherited mutations in the human *SHH* gene lead to **holoprosencephaly** (see Fig. 17.40), a midline defect of variable severity involving abnormal CNS septation, facial clefting, single central incisor, hypotelorism, or a single cyclopic eye (see Fig. 18.6). The SHH protein needs to be processed to an active form and is modified by the addition of a cholesterol moiety. Defects in cholesterol biosynthesis, such as in the autosomal recessive disorder **Smith-Lemli-Opitz syndrome** (intellectual disability, microcephaly, ptosis, small stature, bilateral two- to three-toe syndactyly and genital defects in males), share many features, particularly brain and limb defects reminiscent of SHH-related diseases (see Fig. 20.18). This suggests that signaling through SHH may play a key role in several genetic disorders.

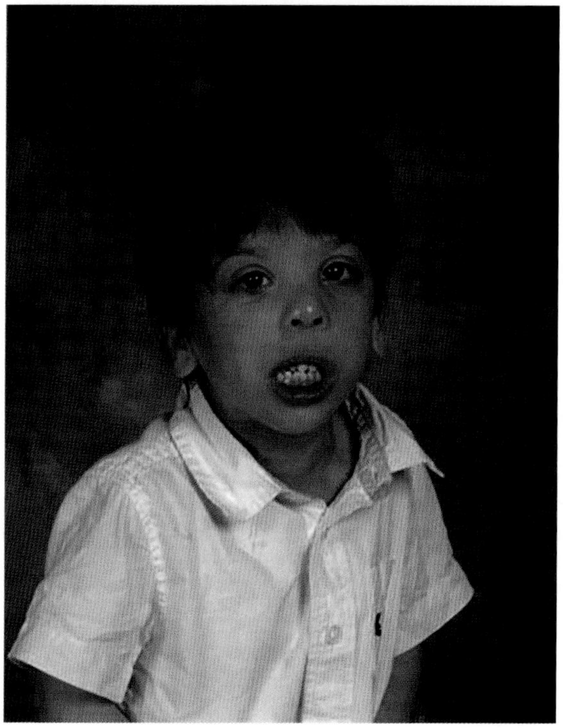

Fig. 20.18 Child with Smith-Lemli-Opitz syndrome with features that include microcephaly, low-set ears, micrognathia, and mild craniofacial dysmorphia. This child also had penoscrotal hypospadias, toe syndactyly (not shown). (From Kelly MN, Tuli SY, Tuli SS, Stern MA, Giordano BP: Brothers with Smith-Lemli-Opitz syndrome. *J Pediatr Health Care* 29(1):97–103, 2015.)

Zellweger syndrome is a severe autosomal recessive disorder (incidence in the United States: 1 in 50,000 live births) caused by defects in peroxisomal biogenesis which results in multiple anomalies including characteristic facies (high forehead, widely spaced eyes), an enlarged liver, retinal degeneration, and neurologic anomalies (see Fig. 20.19). There is no treatment for this critical metabolic condition.

There are many other "families" of disorders that involve congenital anomalies such as: ciliopathies, RASopathies, cohesionopathies, WASHopathies.

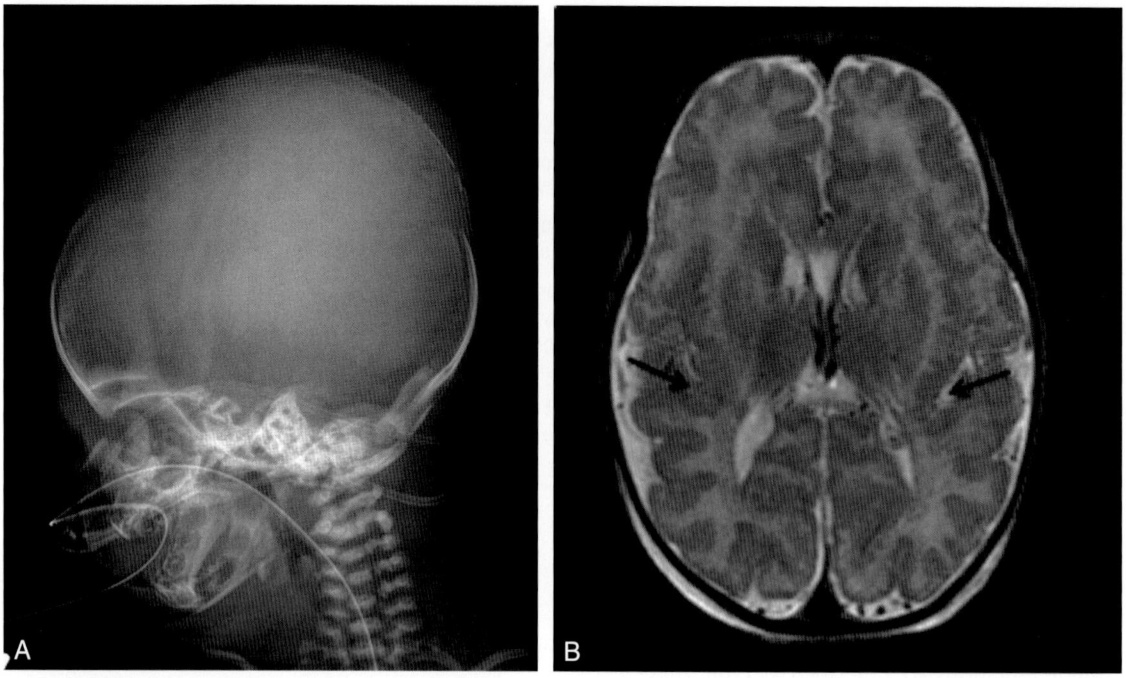

Fig. 20.19 A neonate with Zellweger syndrome (A) Lateral skull radiograph shows undermineralization of parietal bone with wide opened sutures, (B) brain magnetic resonance imaging study showed extensive perisylvian polymicrogyria (*arrows*). (Modified from Smitthimedhin A, Otero HJ: Scimitar-like ossification of patellae led to diagnosis of Zellweger syndrome in newborn: a case report. *Clin Imaging* 49:128–130, 2018.)

Three transcriptional factors encoded by *GLI* genes are in the SHH-PTCH-GLI pathway. Mutations in the *GLI3* gene have been implicated in several autosomal dominant disorders, including **Greig cephalopolysyndactyly syndrome** (deletions or point mutations); **Pallister-Hall syndrome** with hypothalamic hamartomas, central or postaxial polydactyly, and other defects of the face, brain, and limbs (frameshift or nonsense mutations); simple familial postaxial polydactyly type A and B; and preaxial polydactyly type IV (nonsense, missense, and early frameshift mutations).

A comprehensive, authoritative, and daily updated listing of all known human genetic disorders and gene loci can be found at the Online Mendelian Inheritance in Man (OMIM) website (www.ncbi.nlm.nih.gov/omim). The OMIM is authored and edited by the McKusick-Nathans Institute of Genetic Medicine at Johns Hopkins University, School of Medicine.

BIRTH DEFECTS CAUSED BY ENVIRONMENTAL FACTORS

Although the human embryo is well protected in the uterus, many environmental **teratogens** may cause developmental disruptions after maternal exposure to them (see Table 20.3). A teratogen is any agent that can produce a birth defect (congenital anomaly) or increase the incidence of a defect in the population. **Environmental factors** (e.g., infections, drugs) may simulate genetic conditions, such as when two or more children of normal parents are affected. An important principle is that not everything that is familial is genetic.

The cells, tissues, and organs of an embryo are most sensitive to teratogenic agents during periods of rapid differentiation (see Fig. 20.1). Environmental factors cause 7% to 10% of birth defects (see Fig. 20.3). Because biochemical differentiation precedes morphologic differentiation, the period during which structures are sensitive to interference by teratogens often precedes the stage of their visible development by a few days.

Teratogens do not appear to cause defects until cellular differentiation has begun; however, their early actions (e.g., during the first 2 weeks) may cause death of the embryo. The exact mechanisms by which most environmental factors, including drugs and chemicals, disrupt embryonic development and induce abnormalities remain obscure. Even the mechanisms of action of thalidomide, a well-documented teratogen, remain unclear after more than 50 years of study. More than 30 hypotheses have been postulated to explain how this drug disrupts embryonic development.

Many studies have shown that certain hereditary and environmental influences may adversely affect embryonic development by altering fundamental processes such as the intracellular compartment, surface of the cell, extracellular matrix, and fetal environment. It has been suggested that the initial cellular response may take more than one form (genetic, molecular, biochemical, or biophysical), resulting in different sequences of cellular changes (cell death, faulty cellular interaction or induction, reduced biosynthesis of substrates, impaired morphogenetic movements, and mechanical disruption). Eventually, these different types of pathologic lesions may lead to the final outcome (e.g., intrauterine death, developmental defects, fetal growth retardation, or functional disturbances) through a common pathway.

Rapid progress in molecular biology is providing more information about the genetic control of differentiation and the cascade of events involved in the expression of homeobox genes and pattern formation. It is reasonable to speculate that disruption of gene activity at any critical stage could lead to a developmental defect. This view is supported by studies that showed that exposure of mouse and amphibian embryos to excessive amounts of **retinoic acid** (a metabolite of vitamin A) altered gene expression domains and disrupted normal morphogenesis. High levels of exposure to **retinoic acid are highly teratogenic** and have been shown to disrupt developmental fields populated by cranial neural crest cells. Researchers are focusing on the molecular mechanisms of abnormal development in an attempt to understand better the pathogenesis of birth defects.

PRINCIPLES OF TERATOGENESIS

When considering the possible teratogenicity of a drug or chemical, *three important principles must be considered:*

- Critical periods of development
- Dose of the drug or chemical
- Genotype (genetic constitution) of the embryo

CRITICAL PERIODS OF HUMAN DEVELOPMENT

The embryo's stage of development when it encounters a drug or virus determines its susceptibility to the teratogen (see Fig. 20.1). The most critical period of development is when cell division, cell differentiation, and morphogenesis are at their peak.

For example, the **critical period for brain development is from 3 to 16 weeks**, but development may be disrupted after this because the brain is differentiating and growing rapidly at birth. Teratogens may produce cognitive deficiency during the embryonic and fetal periods (see Fig. 20.1).

Tooth development continues long after birth (see Table 19.1). Development of permanent teeth may be disrupted by **tetracyclines** from 14 weeks of fetal life up to 8 years after birth (see Fig. 19.20E). The **skeletal system** also has a prolonged critical period of development extending into childhood, and the growth of skeletal tissues provides a good gauge of general growth.

Environmental disturbances during the first 2 weeks after fertilization may interfere with the cleavage of the zygote and implantation of the blastocyst and may cause early death and **spontaneous abortion** of an embryo. However, disturbances during the first 2 weeks are not known to cause birth defects (see Fig. 20.1 and Fig. 20.20). Teratogens acting during the first 2 weeks kill the embryo, or their disruptive effects are compensated for by powerful regulatory properties of the early embryo. Most development during the first 4 weeks is concerned with the formation of extraembryonic structures such as the amnion, umbilical vesicle, and chorionic sac (see Fig. 3.8 and Figs. 5.1 and 5.18).

Development of the embryo is most easily disrupted when the tissues and organs are forming (Fig. 20.20; see Fig. 20.1). During this **organogenetic period** (4–8 weeks; see Fig. 1.1), teratogens may induce major birth defects. **Physiologic defects** such as minor morphologic defects of the external ears and functional disturbances such as cognitive deficiency are likely to result from disruption of development during the fetal period (ninth week to birth).

Each tissue, organ, and system of an embryo has a critical period during which its development may be disrupted (see Fig. 20.1). The type of birth defect produced depends on which parts, tissues, and organs are most susceptible at the time the teratogen is encountered. Several examples show how teratogens may affect different organ systems that are developing at the same time:

- **Thalidomide** induces limb defects and other anomalies such as cardiac and kidney defects.
- **Rubella virus** infection causes eye defects (glaucoma and cataracts), deafness, and cardiac defects.
- High levels of **ionizing radiation** produce defects in the CNS (brain and spinal cord) and eyes.

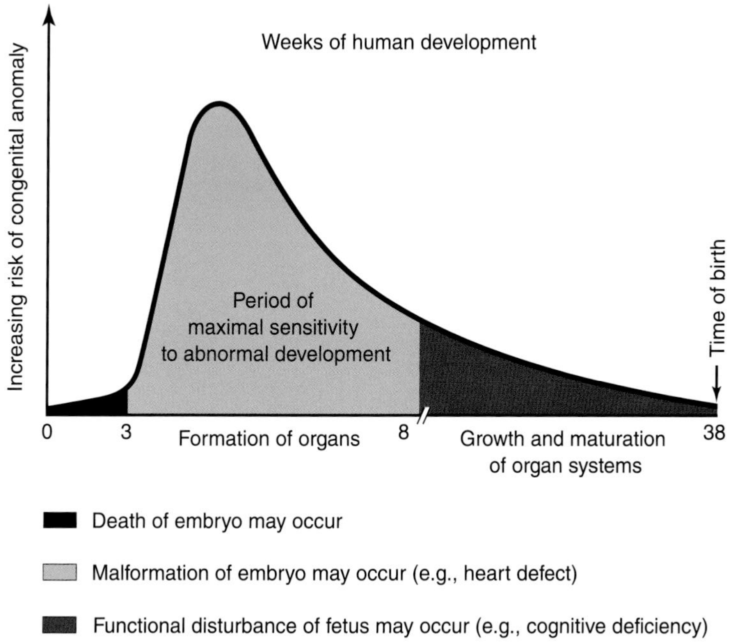

Fig. 20.20 The risk of birth defects increases during organogenesis.

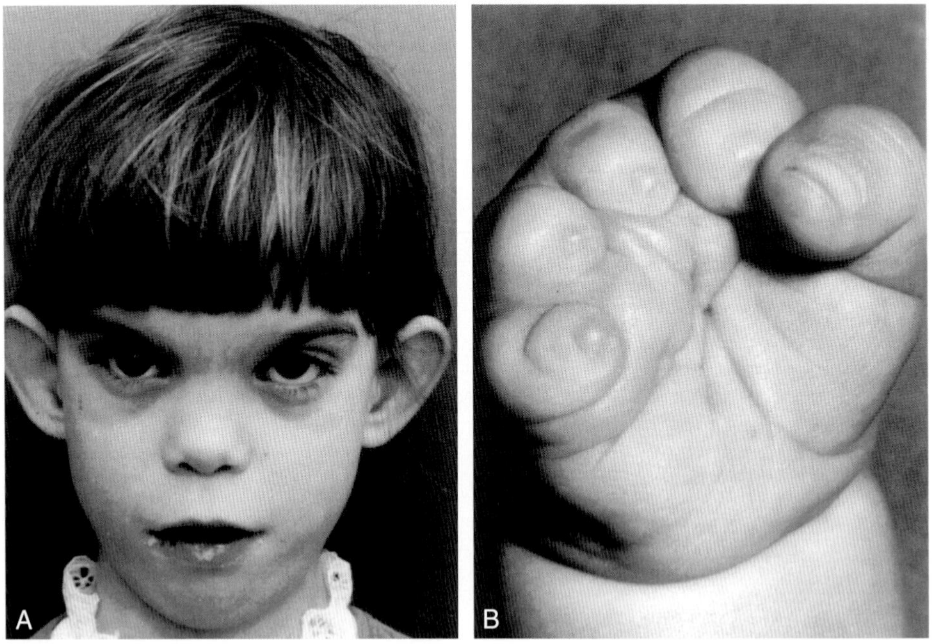

Fig. 20.21 Fetal hydantoin syndrome in a young girl. She has a learning disability due to microcephaly and cognitive deficiency. She has large ears, a wide space between the eyes (hypertelorism), epicanthal folds, and a short nose (A). Her mother has epilepsy and ingested phenytoin (Dilantin) throughout her pregnancy. (B) Right hand of a girl with severe digital hypoplasia (short fingers) born to a mother who took phenytoin (Dilantin). throughout her pregnancy. (A, Courtesy Dr. A.E. Chudley, Section of Genetics and Metabolism, Department of Pediatrics and Child Health, Children's Hospital, Winnipeg, Manitoba, Canada; B, From Chodirker BN, Chudley AE, Reed MH, Persaud TV: Possible prenatal hydantoin effect in a child born to a nonepileptic mother. *Am J Med Genet* 27:373, 1987.)

The timing of exposure is important. Early in the critical period of limb development, thalidomide causes severe defects such as meromelia, which is an absence of parts of the upper and lower limbs (see Fig. 20.2). Later in the sensitive period, thalidomide causes mild to moderate limb defects such as hypoplasia of the radius and ulna.

Embryologic timetables (see Fig. 20.1) are helpful when considering the cause of a human birth defect, but it is wrong to assume that defects always result from a single event occurring during the critical period or that it is possible to determine from these tables the exact day the defect was produced. It can only be stated that the teratogen would have had to disrupt development before the end of the critical period for the tissue, part, or organ.

DOSE OF DRUGS OR CHEMICALS

Animal research has shown that there is a dose-response relationship for teratogens, but the dose used in animals to produce defects is often at levels much higher than typical human exposures. Consequently, animal studies are not directly applicable to human pregnancies. For a drug to be considered a **human teratogen**, a dose-response relationship has to be observed, and the greater the exposure during pregnancy, the more severe the phenotypic effect.

GENOTYPE OF EMBRYO

Numerous examples in experimental animals and several suspected cases in humans show that genetic differences alter responses to a teratogen. **Phenytoin**, for example, is a well-known human teratogen (see Table 20.1). Between 5% and 10% of embryos exposed to this anticonvulsant medication develop **fetal hydantoin syndrome** (Fig. 20.21). Approximately one-third of exposed embryos, however, have only some of the birth defects, and more than one-half of the embryos are unaffected. It appears that the genotype of the embryo determines whether a teratogenic agent will disrupt its development.

HUMAN TERATOGENS

Awareness that certain agents can disrupt prenatal development offers the opportunity to prevent some birth defects. The objective of **teratogenicity testing** of drugs, chemicals, and other agents is to identify risk factors that may cause malformations during human development and alert pregnant females and their caregivers about the dangers to their embryos or fetuses.

Proof of Teratogenicity

To prove that agents are teratogens, it must be shown that the frequency of defects is increased above the spontaneous rate in pregnancies in which the mother is exposed to the agent **(prospective approach)**, or that malformed infants have a history of maternal exposure to the agent more often than normal children **(retrospective approach)**. Both types of data are difficult to obtain in an unbiased form. Case reports are not convincing unless both the agent and type of defect are so uncommon that their association in several cases can be judged not coincidental.

Drug Testing in Animals

Although testing of drugs in pregnant animals is important, the results are of limited value for predicting drug effects in human embryos. Animal experiments can suggest only that similar effects may occur in humans. If a drug or chemical produces teratogenic effects in two or more species, the probability of potential human hazard must be considered to be high, but the dose of the drug also must be considered.

DRUGS AS TERATOGENS

The use of prescription and nonprescription drugs during pregnancy is surprisingly high. Between 40% and 90% of females consume at least one nonprescription drug during pregnancy. Several studies have indicated that some pregnant females take an average of four drugs, excluding nutritional supplements, and that approximately one-half of these females take them during the highly sensitive period (see Fig. 20.1). Another report that was based on a database of prescribed drugs showed that pregnant females might be prescribed as many as 10 drugs. Despite this, less than 2% of birth defects are caused by drugs and chemicals. Only a few drugs have been positively implicated as human teratogenic agents (see Table 20.1); however, new agents continue to be identified. All medications should be avoided during the first trimester unless there is a strong medical reason for their use and then only if the drugs are recognized as reasonably safe for the embryo. Even though well-controlled studies of certain drugs (e.g., marijuana) have failed to demonstrate a teratogenic risk to embryos, they can still affect the development of the embryo (e.g., fetal decreased growth, birth weight).

Cigarette Smoking

Maternal smoking during pregnancy is a well-established cause of **intrauterine growth restriction (IUGR)**. **Low birth weight** (<2000 g) is the chief predictor of infant death. Among heavy cigarette smokers, premature delivery is twice as frequent compared with mothers who do not smoke (see Fig. 6.11).

In a population-based case-control study, there was a modest increase in the incidence of **conotruncal and atrioventricular septal heart defects** associated with maternal smoking in the first trimester. There is some evidence that maternal smoking may cause urinary tract anomalies and behavioral problems.

Nicotine constricts uterine blood vessels, decreasing uterine blood flow and lowering the supply of oxygen and nutrients available to the embryo or fetus from the maternal blood in the intervillous space of the placenta (see Figs. 7.5 and 7.7). The resulting deficiency impairs cell growth and may have an adverse effect on cognitive development. High levels of carboxyhemoglobin resulting from cigarette smoking appear in the maternal and fetal blood and may alter the capacity of the blood to transport oxygen. **Chronic fetal hypoxia** (low oxygen levels) may occur and affect fetal growth and development. Maternal smoking is also associated with smaller brain volumes in preterm infants. Moreover, there is a higher risk of sudden infant death syndrome associated with concurrent cigarette smoking and alcohol use during pregnancy.

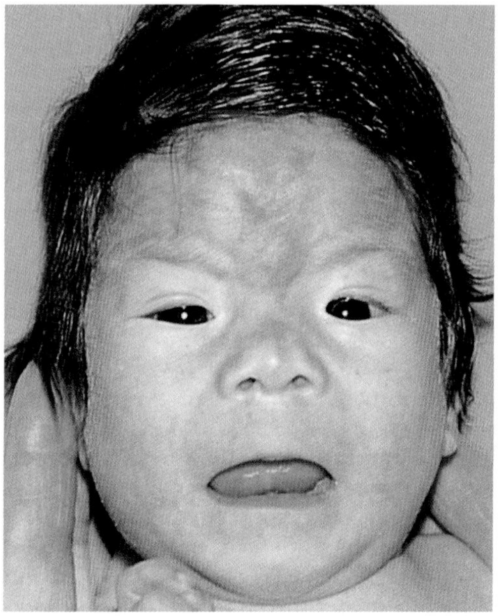

Fig. 20.22 An infant with fetal alcohol syndrome disorder has a thin upper lip, elongated and poorly formed philtrum (vertical groove in the medial part of the upper lip), short palpebral fissures, flat nasal bridge, and short nose. (Courtesy Dr. A.E. Chudley, Section of Genetics and Metabolism, Department of Pediatrics and Child Health, Children's Hospital, Winnipeg, Manitoba, Canada.)

Alcohol

Moderate and high levels of alcohol intake during early pregnancy may alter the growth and morphogenesis of the embryo or fetus. Alcohol use disorder affects 1% to 2% of females of childbearing age and it is thought to be the most common cause of cognitive deficiency. Neonates born to mothers with alcohol use disorder exhibit a specific pattern of defects, including prenatal and postnatal growth deficiency, cognitive deficiency, and other defects (Fig. 20.22 and Table 20.1).

Microcephaly (see Fig. 17.36), short palpebral fissures, epicanthal folds, maxillary hypoplasia, short nose, thin upper lip, abnormal palmar creases, joint defects, growth retardation, congenital heart disease, and multiple other birth defects and comorbidities are present in these infants. The specific pattern of defects in affected infants and children with sentinel facial features, growth impairment, and cognitive disability is called **fetal alcohol syndrome (FAS)**, with a prevalence of 1 to 2 infants per 1000 live births (see Fig. 20.22). The prevalence of FAS is related to the population studied.

Clinical experience is often necessary to make an accurate diagnosis of FAS because the physical defects in affected children can be nonspecific. Nonetheless, the overall pattern of clinical features is unique but may vary from subtle to severe.

Moderate maternal alcohol consumption (1–2 oz of alcohol per day) can result in cognitive impairment and behavioral problems. The term **fetal alcohol effects** (FAEs) was introduced after the recognition that many children exposed to alcohol in utero had no external dysmorphic features but had neurodevelopmental impairments.

The preferred term for the range of prenatal alcohol effects is **fetal alcohol spectrum disorder (FASD)**. The prevalence of FASD in the general population is 1% or higher. Because the susceptible period of brain development spans the major part of gestation (see Fig. 20.1), the safest and most prudent advice is **total abstinence from alcohol** while trying to get pregnant and during pregnancy, as there is no known safe amount or safe time.

Androgens and Progestogens

The terms **progestogens** and **progestins** are used for natural or synthetic substances that induce some or all of the biologic changes produced by **progesterone**, a hormone secreted by the corpus luteum of the ovaries that promotes and maintains a gravid endometrium (see Figs. 2.7 and 2.10D). Some of these substances have **androgenic** properties that may affect the female fetus, producing masculinization of the external genitalia (see Fig. 20.16). The incidence of birth defects varies with the hormone and the dose. Preparations that should be avoided are the progestins ethisterone and norethisterone. Progestin exposure during the critical period of development is associated with an increased prevalence of cardiovascular defects, and exposure of male fetuses during this period may double the incidence of glandular hypospadias (see Fig. 12.42).

Many females use **contraceptive hormones** (birth control pills). **Oral contraceptives** containing progestogens and estrogens taken during the early stages of an unrecognized pregnancy are suspected of being teratogenic agents, but the results of several epidemiologic studies are inconsistent. Use of oral contraceptives should be stopped as soon as pregnancy is suspected or detected because of these possible teratogenic effects.

Diethylstilbestrol (DES) a synthetic nonsteroidal estrogenic compound, is **a human teratogen**. Gross and microscopic congenital abnormalities of the uterus and vagina have been detected in females who were exposed to DES in utero. Three types of lesions were observed: vaginal adenosis, cervical erosions, and transverse vaginal ridges. Some young females between the ages of 16 and 22 years have developed **clear cell adenocarcinoma of the vagina** after a common history of exposure to DES in utero. However, the probability of cancers developing at this early age in females exposed to DES in utero appears to be relatively low (approximately 1 in 1000).

Male fetuses who were exposed to DES in utero before the 11th week of gestation had a higher incidence of genital tract anomalies, including epididymal cysts and hypoplastic testes. However, fertility in the males exposed to DES in utero seems to be unaffected. *Expression of the homeobox gene* HOXA10 *is altered after in utero exposure to DES.*

Antibiotics

Tetracycline antibiotics cross the placental membrane and are deposited in the embryo's bones and teeth at sites of active calcification (see Fig. 7.7). Tetracycline therapy during the fourth to ninth months of pregnancy may also cause tooth defects (e.g., enamel hypoplasia; see Figs. 19.9 and 19.20A), yellow to brown discoloration of the teeth (see Fig. 19.20E), and diminished growth of long bones. Because calcification of the permanent teeth begins at birth and, except for the third molars, is complete by 7 to 8 years of age, long-term tetracycline therapy during childhood can affect the permanent teeth.

Deafness has been reported in infants of mothers who have been treated with high doses of **streptomycin** and **dihydrostreptomycin** as antituberculosis agents. More than 30 cases of hearing deficit and vestibulocochlear nerve damage (cranial nerve [CN] VIII) have been reported in infants exposed to streptomycin derivatives in utero. Penicillin has been used extensively during pregnancy and appears to be harmless to the embryo and fetus.

Anticoagulants

All anticoagulants except heparin a glycosaminoglycan, (see Fig. 7.7) cross the placental membrane and may cause hemorrhage in the embryo or fetus. **Warfarin** and other coumarin derivatives act as antagonists of vitamin K. Warfarin is used for the treatment of **thromboembolic disease** and in patients with atrial fibrillation or artificial heart valves. Warfarin is a known teratogen. There are reports of infants with hypoplasia of the nasal cartilage, stippled epiphyses, and various CNS defects whose mothers took this anticoagulant during the critical period of embryonic development. The period of greatest sensitivity is between 6 and 12 weeks after fertilization. Second- and third-trimester exposure may result in cognitive deficiency, optic nerve atrophy, and microcephaly. **Heparin is not a teratogen**.

Anticonvulsants

Approximately 1 in 200 pregnant females have epilepsy and require treatment with an anticonvulsant. Of the anticonvulsant drugs available, there is strong evidence that **trimethadione** is a teratogen. The main features of the **fetal trimethadione syndrome** are prenatal and postnatal growth retardation; developmental delay; V-shaped eyebrows; low-set ears; cleft lip or palate; and cardiac, genitourinary, and limb defects. Use of this drug is contraindicated during pregnancy.

Phenytoin is a teratogen (see Fig. 20.21). **Fetal hydantoin syndrome** occurs in 5% to 10% of children of mothers treated with phenytoin or hydantoin anticonvulsants. The usual pattern of defects consists of IUGR, microcephaly (see Fig. 17.36), cognitive deficiency, ridged frontal suture, inner epicanthal folds, eyelid ptosis (see Fig. 18.13), broad depressed nasal bridge, nail and distal phalangeal hypoplasia (underdevelopment), and hernias.

Valproic acid use in pregnant females has led to a pattern of birth defects consisting of craniofacial, heart, and limb defects and postnatal cognitive developmental delay. There is also an increased risk of neural tube defects (e.g., spina bifida cystica; see Fig. 17.15). Phenobarbital is considered to be a safe antiepileptic drug for use during pregnancy. Magnesium sulfate and diazepam are also widely used for seizure prophylaxis and appear to be safe.

Antineoplastic Agents

With the exception of the folic acid antagonist **aminopterin**, few well-documented reports of teratogenic effects are available for assessment. Because the data available on the possible teratogenicity of antineoplastic drugs are inadequate, it is recommended that these drugs should be avoided, especially during the first trimester of pregnancy.

Tumor-inhibiting drugs are highly teratogenic because they inhibit mitosis in rapidly dividing cells (see Fig. 2.2). The use of **aminopterin** during the embryonic period often results in intrauterine death of embryos, and 20% to 30% of those that survive are severely malformed. **Busulfan** and **6-mercaptopurine** administered in alternating courses throughout pregnancy have produced multiple severe abnormalities, but neither drug alone appears to cause major defects (see Table 20.1).

Methotrexate, a folic acid antagonist and a derivative of aminopterin, is a potent teratogen that produces major birth defects. It is most often used as a single agent or in combination therapy for neoplastic diseases, but it is commonly used in patients with severe rheumatic diseases, including rheumatoid arthritis. Multiple skeletal, brain, and other birth defects are associated with the use of methotrexate during pregnancy.

Antihypertensive Medications

Exposure of the fetus to **angiotensin-converting enzyme inhibitors and AT1 blockers**, used as antihypertensive agents have fetotoxic potential and can cause oligohydramnios, hypoplasia of the bones of the calvaria, IUGR, renal dysfunction, and fetal death.

Insulin, Hypoglycemic Drugs, Maternal Diabetes

Insulin is not teratogenic in human embryos and it is the recommended first-line therapy for gestational diabetes mellitus when lifestyle changes have not achieved the required glycemic control. Metformin, a biguanide oral hypoglycemic drug has not been shown to be teratogenic in short-term use; there have been reports that it may slightly increase the risk of premature delivery. Glyburide is an oral hypoglycemic drug of the sulfonylurea class which has a lower level of placental transfer than other sulfonylureas and has not shown adverse fetal effects. Longer-term safety studies have not yet been published.

The incidence of birth defects (e.g., sacral agenesis) is increased two to three times among the offspring of **diabetic mothers**. Approximately 40% of perinatal deaths of diabetic infants are the result of birth defects. Females with insulin-dependent diabetes mellitus may significantly decrease their risk of having infants with birth defects by achieving good control of their disease before conception.

Retinoic Acid

Retinoic acid is a metabolite of vitamin A. **Isotretinoin** (13-*cis*-retinoic acid), which is used for treating severe cystic acne, is a potent teratogen. The critical period for exposure appears to be from the third to the fifth week. The risk of spontaneous abortion and birth defects after exposure is high. The most common major defects observed are **craniofacial dysmorphism**, microtia (see Fig. 18.21), micrognathia, cleft palate, thymic aplasia, cardiovascular defects, and neural tube defects. Postnatal longitudinal follow-up of children exposed in utero to isotretinoin revealed significant neuropsychological impairment.

Vitamin A is a valuable and necessary nutrient during pregnancy, but *high levels of vitamin A should be avoided.* An increased risk of birth defects was reported for the offspring of females who took more than 10,000 IU of vitamin A daily.

Analgesics

Aspirin (acetylsalicylic acid) and **acetaminophen** (paracetamol) are commonly used during pregnancy for the relief of fever or pain. Clinical trials suggest that large doses of analgesics may be potentially harmful to the embryo or fetus. Although epidemiologic studies indicate that aspirin is not a teratogenic agent, large doses should be avoided, especially during the first trimester.

Nonsteroidal antiinflammatory drugs used after 20 weeks may cause rare but serious defects of the fetal renal system and oligohydramnios. Use after 30 weeks may also cause premature closure of the fetal **ductus arteriosus.**

Thyroid Drugs

Potassium iodide in expectorant cough mixtures and large doses of radioactive iodine may cause **congenital goiter**. Iodides readily cross the placental membrane and interfere with thyroxin production (see Fig. 7.7). They may cause thyroid enlargement and other anomalies (arrested physical and cognitive development and dystrophy of bones and soft parts). Maternal iodine deficiency may also cause **congenital iodine deficiency** which may present with growth deficiency and intellectual disability.

Pregnant females have been advised to avoid douches or creams containing **povidone-iodine** because it is absorbed by the vagina, enters the maternal blood, and may interfere with fetal thyroid function. **Propylthiouracil** interferes with thyroxin formation in the fetus and may cause goiter. Administration of antithyroid substances for the treatment of maternal thyroid disorders may cause congenital goiter if the mother is given the substances over the amount required to control the disease.

Tranquilizers

Thalidomide is a potent teratogen, and it has been estimated that almost 12,000 neonates had defects caused by this drug. Originally intended as a tranquilizer, it has been used to treat various disorders including morning sickness. The characteristic presenting feature is **meromelia** (including phocomelia; see Fig. 20.2), but the defects range from **amelia** through intermediate stages of development to **micromelia** (see Chapter 16; Fig. 16.12).

Thalidomide also caused anomalies in other organs, such as the absence of the external and internal ears, hemangioma on the face (see Fig. 19.6), heart defects, and anomalies of the urinary and alimentary systems. The period when thalidomide caused these congenital anomalies was 20 to 36 days after fertilization. This sensitive period coincides with the critical periods for the development of the affected parts and organs (see Figs. 20.1 and 20.20).

Thalidomide is currently used for the treatment of leprosy, multiple myeloma, and several autoimmune diseases but it is **contraindicated in females of childbearing age**. The problem remains topical because of ongoing class-action suits.

Psychotropic Drugs

Lithium is the drug of choice for the long-term maintenance of patients with bipolar disorders. However, lithium has caused birth defects, mainly of the heart and great vessels, in infants whose mothers were given the drug early in pregnancy.

Although **lithium carbonate** is a known human teratogen, the US Food and Drug Administration has stated that the agent may be used during pregnancy if "in the opinion of the physician the potential benefits outweigh the possible hazards."

Benzodiazepines such as **diazepam** and **oxazepam** are frequently prescribed for pregnant females. These drugs readily cross the placental membrane (see Fig. 7.7), and their use during the first trimester of pregnancy is associated with craniofacial anomalies in neonates. **Selective serotonin reuptake inhibitors** (SSRIs) are commonly used to treat depression, mood disorders, and anxiety during pregnancy. Several reports have shown a slightly increased risk of atrial and ventricular septal defects, persistent pulmonary hypertension, impacts on brain functional networks (hyperconnectivity of the auditory network), and neurobehavioral disturbances, including autism spectrum disorder, in infants exposed to SSRIs in utero. Moreover, preterm birth and respiratory distress are associated with the use of SSRIs during pregnancy. The interference with the reuptake of the neurotransmitter serotonin (5HT), by SSRIs may be the mechanism for the effects of early fetal brain development.

Illicit Drugs

The illicit use of opioids and fentanyl, a synthetic opioid that is 50 times more potent than heroin, has alarmingly increased and often with fatal outcome.

There is no clear evidence that **marijuana** is a human teratogen, but studies indicate that its use during the first 2 months of pregnancy affects fetal growth and birth weight. Cannabinoids consumed by the pregnant mother can cross the placental barrier and directly affect the fetus. They mediate their effects primarily through G-protein coupled cannabinoid receptors, CB1 and CB2. They can adversely affect fetal growth, and cause neurological deficits and immunological impairment in the offspring. Sleep and electroencephalographic patterns in neonates exposed prenatally to marijuana were altered.

Cocaine is the most widely used illicit drug among females of childbearing age. It rapidly crosses the placenta and may induce placental abruption, spontaneous abortion, prematurity, IUGR, microcephaly, cerebral infarction, urogenital anomalies, neurobehavioral disturbances, and neurologic abnormalities.

Methadone is used during withdrawal treatment of morphine and heroin addiction. Methadone is considered to be a **behavioral teratogen**, as is **heroin**. Infants of narcotic-dependent females maintained on methadone therapy were found to have CNS dysfunction, lower birth weights, and smaller head circumferences than unexposed infants. There is also concern about the long-term postnatal developmental effects of methadone. The problem is difficult to resolve because other drugs are often used in combination with methadone, and heavy use of alcohol and cigarettes is prevalent among narcotic-dependent females. Neonatal withdrawal syndrome results when neonates are exposed to opioids in utero. The symptoms include fever, diarrhea, sleep and feeding disturbances, and hypertonia. Opioid monotherapy is commonly used to treat neonates. Maternal use of **methamphetamine**, a sympathetic nervous system stimulant, results in small-for-gestational-age fetuses with neurobehavioral problems.

ENVIRONMENTAL CHEMICALS AS TERATOGENS

There is increasing concern about the possible teratogenicity of environmental chemicals, including industrial and agricultural chemicals and air pollutants. Most of these chemicals have not been positively implicated as teratogens in humans. Systematic review and meta-analysis of epidemiological reports showed that in the United States and other populations a significant association between the occurrence of specific congenital heart defects (atrial septal defect, coarctation of the aorta, tetralogy of Fallot) in the offspring and pregnant females who were exposed to polluted air (ozone, carbon dioxide, carbon monoxide, heat particulate material).

Organic Mercury

Infants of mothers whose main diet during pregnancy consists of fish containing abnormally high levels of organic mercury acquire fetal **Minamata disease**, characterized by neurologic and behavioral disturbances resembling those of cerebral palsy. Severe brain damage, cognitive deficiency, and blindness have been detected in infants of mothers who ingested **methylmercury**-contaminated food. This organic cation is a teratogen that causes cerebral atrophy, spasticity, seizures, and cognitive deficiency. Recent studies showed that placental development and fetal growth were affected in a population with high exposure to mercury from seafood consumption.

Lead

Abundantly present in the workplace and environment, lead passes through the placental membrane (see Fig. 7.7) and accumulates in embryonic and fetal tissues. Prenatal exposure to lead is associated with increased abortions, fetal defects, IUGR, and functional deficits. Several reports have indicated that children of mothers who were exposed to subclinical levels of lead revealed neurobehavioral and psychomotor disturbances.

Polychlorinated Biphenyls

Polychlorinated biphenyls are teratogenic chemicals that produce IUGR and skin discoloration. The main dietary source of these chemicals in North America is sport fish caught in polluted waters or other wildlife in polluted areas.

INFECTIOUS AGENTS AS TERATOGENS

Throughout prenatal life, embryos and fetuses are endangered by a variety of **microorganisms**. In most cases, the assault is resisted, but in some cases, spontaneous abortion or stillbirth occurs. If they survive, fetuses are born with IUGR, birth defects, or neonatal diseases (see Table 20.1). The microorganisms cross the placental membrane and enter the embryonic and fetal bloodstream (see Fig. 7.7). There is a propensity for the CNS to be affected - some microorganisms have a variety of means to cross the main protective boundary—the fetal blood-brain barrier (BBB).

Cytomegalovirus

Cytomegalovirus (**CMV**) is a member of the herpesvirus family. As with rubella, the virus likely infects the placenta and then the fetus. Fetuses with this virus are often delivered prematurely. **CMV is the most common viral infection of the fetus**, occurring in approximately 1% of neonates. Most pregnancies end in spontaneous abortion when the infection occurs during the first trimester. It is the leading cause of congenital infection with morbidity at birth. Neonates infected during the early fetal period usually show no clinical signs and are identified through screening programs. CMV infection later in pregnancy may result in severe birth defects: developmental delay, IUGR, microphthalmia, chorioretinitis, blindness, microcephaly, cerebral calcification, cognitive deficiency, deafness, cerebral palsy, and hepatosplenomegaly (enlargement of the liver and spleen). Of particular concern are cases of asymptomatic CMV infection, which are often associated with audiologic, neurologic, and neurobehavioral disturbances in infancy (see Table 20.1). Detection of congenital CMV infection in an infant at the time of birth, or shortly thereafter, is critical for the clinical management and care of the future development of the child.

Congenital Rubella

Rubella infection is a worldwide problem that can cause severe illness, epidemics, and birth defects in pregnant females. Maternal infection with the rubella virus during the first trimester can lead to miscarriage, fetal death, or the birth of an infant with severe congenital defects. The fetus acquires the infection when the virus crosses the placental membrane (see Fig. 7.7). The overall risk of embryonic or fetal infection is approximately 20%.

The clinical features of **congenital rubella syndrome** are cataracts (see Fig. 18.12), cardiac defects, and deafness. However, other abnormalities are occasionally observed: cognitive deficiency, chorioretinitis (inflammation of the retina extending to the choroid), glaucoma (see Fig. 18.11), microphthalmia (abnormal smallness of the eye), and tooth defects (see Table 20.1).

Most infants have birth defects when the disease occurs during the first 4 to 5 weeks after fertilization. This period includes the most susceptible organogenetic periods of the eyes, internal ears, heart, and brain (see Fig. 20.1). The risk of defects from a rubella infection during the second and third trimesters is approximately 10%; however, functional defects of the CNS (e.g., cognitive deficiency) and internal ears (hearing loss) may result. Immunization with a single dose of the rubella vaccine confers life-long protection. Because of WHO Global Vaccine Action Plan fewer infants are affected nowadays.

Herpes Simplex Virus

Maternal infection with herpes simplex virus in early pregnancy increases the spontaneous abortion rate by threefold. Infection after the 20th week is associated with a higher rate of prematurity (fetus born at a gestational age of less than 37 weeks). Infection of the fetus with this virus usually occurs very late in pregnancy. Most infections are likely acquired from the mother shortly before or after delivery. The congenital defects that have been observed in neonates include cutaneous lesions, microcephaly, microphthalmia, spasticity, retinal dysplasia, and cognitive deficiency (see Table 20.1 and Fig. 17.36).

Varicella

Varicella (chickenpox) and **herpes zoster** (shingles) are caused by the same **varicella-zoster virus**, which is highly infectious. **Maternal varicella infection during the first two trimesters** causes the following birth defects: skin scarring, muscle atrophy, hypoplasia of limbs, rudimentary digits, eye and brain damage, and cognitive deficiency (see Table 20.1). There is a 20% chance of these or other defects when the infection occurs during the critical period of development (see Fig. 20.1). After 20 weeks' gestation, there is no proven teratogenic risk.

Human Immunodeficiency Virus

Human immunodeficiency virus (HIV) causes **acquired immunodeficiency syndrome**. There are conflicting reports on maternal infection with HIV and fetal outcomes. Some adverse perinatal effects included intrauterine growth retardation, infant mortality, microcephaly, and specific craniofacial features. Most cases of transmission of the virus from mother to fetus probably occur at the time of delivery. Breastfeeding increases the risk of transmitting the virus to the neonate. Preventing transmission of the virus to females and their infants is important because of the potential effects.

Zika Virus

Pregnant females infected with the Zika virus gave birth to babies with microcephaly and severe neurologic abnormalities. In 2015 the first case of Zika embryopathy was reported in Brazil, and there have been outbreaks in other countries, including the Western (Yap Island) and South Pacific (French Polynesia), South America, Central America, and the Caribbean.

Zika virus is transmitted by the *Aedes* mosquito locally to humans. In most cases, a causal relationship was established between prenatal Zika infection and the birth of babies with microcephaly and other anomalies. Transmission of the virus to the fetus is vertical. The Centers for Disease Control and Prevention (CDC) concluded from an assessment of the situation that pregnant females infected with the Zika virus, have an increased risk of spontaneous abortion and giving birth to a child of low birth weight for gestation age with microcephaly, cerebral calcification, ventriculomegaly, and ocular defects. However, the CDC did observe that many females infected with the Zika virus gave birth to healthy babies indicating that other genetic factors may be at play. There is no vaccine available for the treatment of Zika infection.

SARS-CoV-2 Virus

Late in 2019, an outbreak of a newly discovered coronavirus (severe acute respiratory syndrome coronavirus 2 [**SARS-CoV-2**]) was reported in Wuhan, China, and also in many other countries. The **coronavirus disease 2019 (COVID-19**) caused mounting deaths and devastated public health response worldwide. The World Health Organization (WHO) declared the outbreak a "Public Health Emergency of International Concern," which was quickly updated to a "pandemic." An area of special concern is the neonatal outcome of children born to mothers who had been infected with SARS-CoV-2 during pregnancy. Several studies indicated an increased risk of pregnancy complications, which included preeclampsia, miscarriage, stillbirth, preterm birth, fetal growth restriction, and possibly later neurodevelopmental problems. It was reported that SARS-CoV-2 was transmitted to the fetus in utero, not during or after birth (neonates tested positive for the virus, and coronavirus particles were found in the fetal cells of the placenta).

Toxoplasmosis

Toxoplasma gondii is an intracellular parasite that may be found in the bloodstream and tissues or reticuloendothelial cells, leukocytes, and epithelial cells.

Maternal infection is usually acquired by two routes:

- Eating raw or poorly cooked meat (usually pork or lamb) containing *Toxoplasma* cysts
- Close contact with infected domestic animals (e.g., cats) or infected soil

It is thought that the soil and garden vegetables may become contaminated with infected animal feces carrying **oocysts** (encapsulated zygotes in the life cycle of sporozoan protozoa). Oocysts can also be transported to food by flies and cockroaches.

T. gondii organism crosses the placental membrane and infects the fetus (Figs. 20.23 and 20.24; see Fig. 7.7), causing destructive changes in the brain (intracranial calcifications) and eyes (chorioretinitis) that result in cognitive deficiency, microcephaly, microphthalmia, and hydrocephaly. Fetal death may follow infection, especially during the early stages of pregnancy.

Mothers of congenitally affected infants are often unaware of having had toxoplasmosis. Because domestic and wild animals (e.g., cats, dogs, rabbits) may be infected with this parasite, pregnant females should avoid them and eat raw or poorly cooked meat from them (e.g., rabbits). Unpasteurized milk should also be avoided.

CONGENITAL SYPHILIS

The incidence of congenital syphilis is increasing, with more cases now than in the past 2 decades. From 2013 to 2018, in the United States, congenital syphilis cases increased from 362 to 1306 cases (including 128 infant deaths and stillbirths). In most cases, the fetus or infant becomes infected during pregnancy from an infected mother. Almost 40% of babies born to females with untreated syphilis may be stillborn or die from the infection. *Treponema pallidum*, the small, spiral microorganism that causes syphilis, rapidly crosses the placental membrane as early as 6 to 8 weeks of development (see Fig. 7.7). The fetus can become infected during any stage of the disease or any stage of pregnancy. Screening of pregnant females for syphilis infection and timely treatment of infected cases are recommended.

Primary maternal infections (acquired during pregnancy) usually cause serious fetal infection and birth defects. However, adequate treatment of the mother kills the microorganisms, preventing them from crossing the placental membrane and infecting the fetus.

Secondary maternal infections (acquired before pregnancy) can also result in congenital syphilis and similar fetal outcomes.

Early fetal manifestations of untreated maternal syphilis are congenital deafness, abnormal teeth and bones, hydrocephalus (excessive accumulation of cerebrospinal fluid), and cognitive deficiency (see Fig. 17.38 and Figs. 19.19 and 19.20). **Late fetal manifestations** of untreated congenital

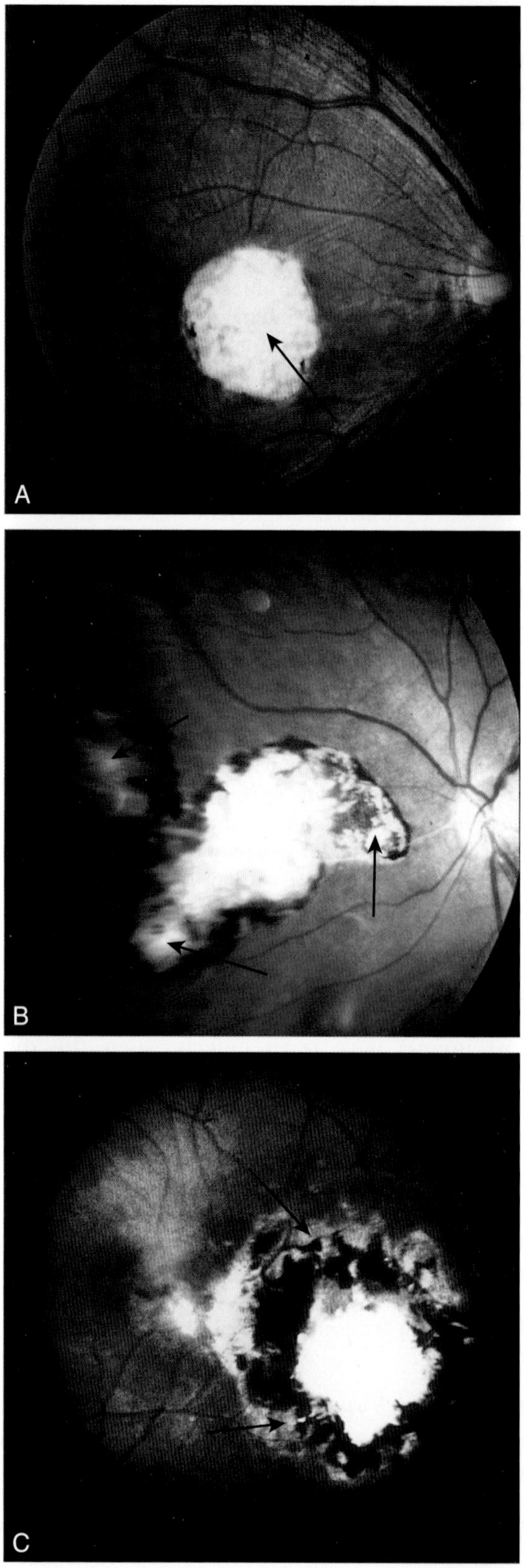

Fig. 20.23 Chorioretinitis of congenital ocular toxoplasmosis induced by *Toxoplasma* infection. (A) Necrotizing cicatricial lesion of the macula *(arrow)*. (B) Satellite lesion around and adjacent to the necrotizing cicatricial main lesion *(arrows)*. (C) Recrudescent lesion adjacent to a large necrotizing cicatricial main lesion *(arrows)*. (From Yokota K: Congenital anomalies and toxoplasmosis, *Congenit Anom [Kyoto]* 35:151, 1995.)

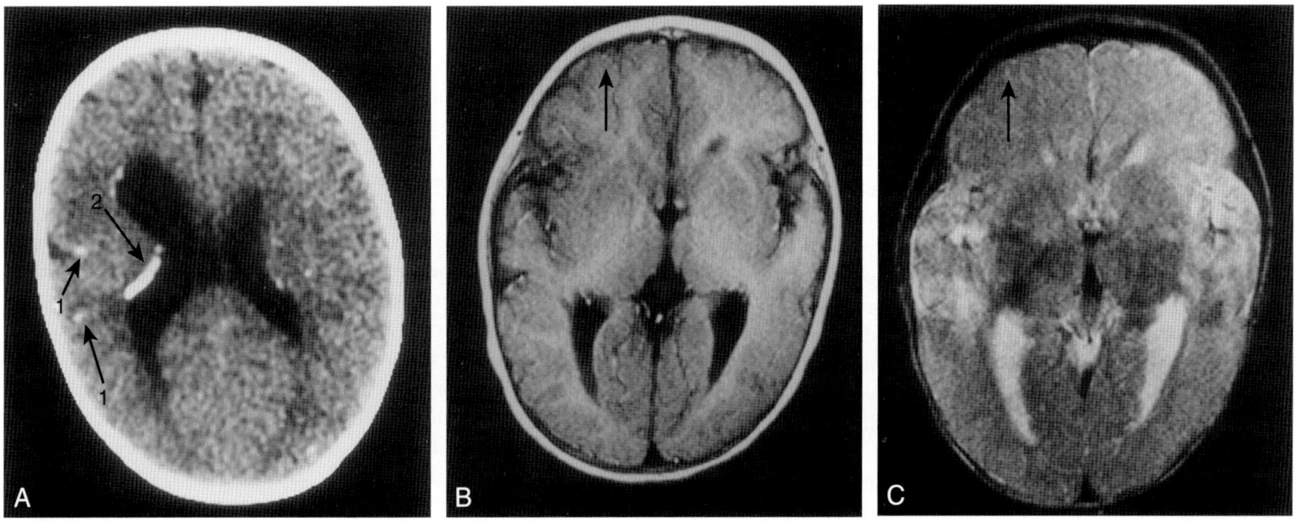

Fig. 20.24 Congenital cerebral defects induced by *Toxoplasma* infection. The diagnostic images were obtained at 2 years and 9 months of age. (A) Plain computed tomogram shows that the lateral ventricles are moderately dilated. Multiple calcified foci are apparent in the brain parenchyma *(arrows 1)* and along the ventricular wall *(arrow 2)*. (B) T1-weighted magnetic resonance image (MRI; 400/22, 0.5T) shows that the cortical gyri are widened on the left side, and the cortex is thickened in the left frontal lobe *(arrow)* compared with the corresponding structure on the right. (C) T2-weighted MRI (2500/120, 0.5T) shows abnormal hypointensity *(arrow)* of the left frontal lobe. (From Yokota K: Congenital anomalies and toxoplasmosis. *Congenit Anom [Kyoto]* 35:151, 1995.)

syphilis are destructive lesions of the palate and nasal septum, dental abnormalities (centrally notched, widely spaced, peg-shaped upper central incisors [Hutchinson teeth]), and facial defects (frontal bossing, including protuberance or swelling, saddle nose, and poorly developed maxilla).

IONIZING RADIATION AS A TERATOGEN

Exposure to high levels of ionizing radiation may injure embryonic cells, resulting in cell death, chromosome injury, cognitive deficiency, and deficient physical growth. The severity of the embryonic damage is related to the absorbed dose of radiation, the dose rate, and the stage of embryonic or fetal development when the exposure to radiation occurs.

In the past, large amounts of ionizing radiation (hundreds to several thousand rads) were given inadvertently to embryos and fetuses of pregnant females who had cancer of the cervix. In all cases, their embryos were severely malformed or died. Growth retardation, microcephaly, spina bifida cystica (see Figs. 17.15 and 17.36 and Fig. 18.12), pigment changes in the retina, cataracts, cleft palate, skeletal and visceral abnormalities, and cognitive deficiency have been observed in infants who survived after receiving high levels of ionizing radiation. Development of the CNS typically was affected. In a recent investigation of 38,009 females, maternal occupation was correlated with potential exposure to ionizing radiation. An increased risk of birth defects (hydrocephaly, anencephaly, anotia, and colon atresia) was reported.

Observations of Japanese **atomic bomb survivors** and their children suggest that 8 to 16 weeks after fertilization is the period of greatest sensitivity for radiation damage to the brain, resulting in severe cognitive deficiency. By the end of the 16th week, most neuronal proliferation is completed, after which the risk of cognitive deficiency decreases.

It is generally accepted that large doses of radiation (>25,000 millirads [mrads]) are harmful to the developing CNS. There is no conclusive proof that human birth defects have been caused by diagnostic levels of radiation (<10,000 mrads). Scattered radiation from a radiographic examination of a region of the body that is not near the uterus (e.g., thorax, sinuses, and teeth) produces a dose of only a few millirads, which is not teratogenic to the embryo or fetus. Although the risk to the embryo is minuscule from a radiation exposure of 5000 mrads or less, it is prudent to be cautious during diagnostic examinations of the pelvic region in pregnant females (radiographic examinations, especially CT scans, and medical diagnostic tests using radioisotopes) because they result in exposure of the embryo to 300 to 2500 mrads. The recommended limit of *maternal exposure of the whole body* to radiation from all sources is 500 mrad (0.005 Gray [Gy]) for the entire gestational period. **Magnetic resonance imaging** does not use ionizing radiation and poses no known risk, however, first-trimester imaging should be used in consultation with a radiologist.

ULTRASONIC WAVES

Ultrasonography is widely used during pregnancy for embryonic or fetal diagnosis and prenatal care. A review of the safety of obstetric ultrasonography indicates that there are no confirmed harmful effects on the fetus from the use of routine diagnostic ultrasound examination.

MATERNAL FACTORS AS TERATOGENS

Pregestational diabetes mellitus is a major public health problem. In the United States, more than 60 million females of reproductive age, and an estimated 4% of pregnant females worldwide have diabetes. During pregnancy, poorly controlled diabetes mellitus, is associated with an increased rate of spontaneous miscarriages and a twofold to threefold higher incidence of birth defects. **Neonates of diabetic mothers** are usually large **(macrosomia)**, with prominent fat pads over the upper back and lower jaw.

These infants are at an increased risk for brain anomalies, skeletal defects, sacral agenesis, and congenital heart defects. In addition to neonatal metabolic complications, respiratory distress syndrome, and neurodevelopmental abnormalities may occur.

Phenylketonuria (autosomal recessive inborn error of metabolism) occurs in 1 of 10,000 infants born in the United States. If untreated, females who are homozygous for **phenylalanine hydroxylase deficiency** (phenylketonuria) and those with **hyperphenylalaninemia** (abnormally high blood levels of phenylalanine) are at a higher risk for offspring with **microcephaly** (see Fig. 17.36), cardiac defects, cognitive deficiency, and IUGR. The brain damage and cognitive deficiency can be prevented if the phenylketonuric mother is placed on a phenylalanine-restricted diet before and during pregnancy.

The risk of neural tube defects (see Fig. 17.17) is greater in the offspring of mothers with low levels of **folic acid** and **vitamin B_{12}**.

Relatively, few studies are available on the effect of **paternal factors** on neonatal outcomes. A recent systematic review and meta-analysis showed that the father's age is a risk factor for the occurrence of birth defects (chromosomal, facial, urogenital, and cardiovascular) in the offspring.

MECHANICAL FACTORS AS TERATOGENS

The amniotic fluid absorbs mechanical pressures, protecting the embryo from most external trauma. A significantly reduced quantity of amniotic fluid **(oligohydramnios)** may result in mechanically induced deformation of the limbs, such as hyperextension of the knee. Congenital dislocation of the hip and clubfoot may be caused by mechanical forces, particularly in a malformed uterus. Deformations may be caused by any factor that restricts the mobility of the fetus and produces prolonged compression in an abnormal posture. Intrauterine amputations or other anomalies caused by local constriction during fetal growth may result from **amniotic bands**, which are thin strands or rings of tissue formed as a result of rupture of the amnion during early pregnancy, or vascular disruption (see Fig. 7.21).

BIRTH DEFECTS CAUSED BY MULTIFACTORIAL INHERITANCE

Multifactorial traits are often single major defects, such as cleft lip, isolated cleft palate, neural tube defects (e.g., meroencephaly, spina bifida cystica), pyloric stenosis, and congenital dislocation of the hips (see Fig. 11.4C and Figs. 17.12D, 17.15, and 17.17). Some of these defects may also occur as part of the phenotype in syndromes determined by single-gene inheritance, a chromosomal abnormality, or an environmental teratogen.

The recurrence risks used for **genetic counseling of families** having birth defects (determined by multifactorial inheritance) are empiric risks based on the frequency of the defect in the general population and different categories of relatives. In individual families, these estimates may be inaccurate because they are usually averages for the population rather than precise probabilities for the individual family.

GENETIC COUNSELING

For families who have a child with a congenital malformation, or multiple anomalies, a detailed physical examination by a clinical geneticist is an important part of the clinical workup. The genetics session typically also involves obtaining a detailed three-generation family history (often obtained by a genetic counselor) and ordering other investigations, including genetic testing, if indicated. Genetic counseling is an important component of the clinical journey for these families. Genetic counseling is a communication process designed to educate, support, and assist individuals make informed choices, adapting to a new diagnosis, or the susceptibility risk of a genetic disorder. Exome and genome sequencing are becoming clinically implemented in many jurisdictions and are frequently utilized for families with a suspected genetic disorder (including fetuses, infants, and children). The complexity of different types of results that can be generated (uninformative, pathogenic, likely pathogenic, variant of unknown significance, benign), the potential impact on extended family members, and the risk of incidental findings in addition to privacy and insurance implications justify why pre-and post-test genetic counseling is recommended for all families considering genetic sequencing.

SUMMARY OF BIRTH DEFECTS

- Birth defects are any type of structural abnormalities that are present at birth. The defect may be macroscopic or microscopic and on the surface of or within the body. The **four clinically significant types of birth defects** are malformation, disruption, deformation, and dysplasia.
- Approximately 3% of neonates have an obvious major defect. Additional defects are detected after birth; the incidence is approximately 6% among 2-year-old children and 8% among 5-year-old children. Other defects (approximately 2%) are detected later (e.g., during surgery, dissection, autopsy).
- Birth defects may be single or multiple and have minor or major clinical significance. Single minor defects occur in approximately 14% of neonates. These defects have no serious medical consequences, but they alert clinicians to the possibility of an associated major defect.
- Ninety percent of infants with multiple minor defects have one or more associated major defects. Of the 3% of neonates with a major birth defect, multiple major anomalies are found in 0.7%. Major defects are more common in early embryos (up to 15%) than they are in neonates (up to 3%).
- Some birth defects are caused by genetic factors (e.g., chromosomal abnormalities, pathogenic variants), and a few defects are caused by environmental factors (e.g., infectious agents, environmental chemicals, drugs), but most common defects result from a complex interaction between genetic and environmental factors. The cause of most birth defects is unknown (see Fig. 20.3).
- During the **first 2 weeks of development**, teratogenic agents usually kill the embryo or have no effects. During the **organogenetic period**, teratogenic agents disrupt development and may cause major birth defects. During the **fetal period**, teratogens may produce morphologic

and functional abnormalities, particularly of the brain and eyes.
- A detailed evaluation by a clinical geneticist accompanied by genetic counseling is an important consideration for babies born with congenital anomalies.

CLINICALLY ORIENTED PROBLEMS

CASE 20-1

A physician was concerned about the drugs a female said she was taking when she first sought medical advice during her pregnancy.

- What percentage of birth defects are caused by drugs, environmental chemicals, and infectious agents?
- Why may it be difficult for physicians to attribute specific birth defects to specific drugs?
- What should pregnant females know about the use of drugs during pregnancy?

CASE 20-2

During a pelvic examination, a 41-year-old female learned that she was pregnant.

- Do females this age have an increased risk of bearing fetuses with birth defects?
- If a 41-year-old female becomes pregnant, what prenatal diagnostic tests will likely be performed?
- What genetic abnormality may be detected?

CASE 20-3

A pregnant female asked her physician whether any drugs were considered safe during early pregnancy.

- Name some commonly prescribed drugs that are safe to use.
- What commonly used drugs should be avoided during pregnancy?

CASE 20-4

A 10-year-old girl contracted a rubella infection (German measles), and her mother was worried that the child might develop cataracts and heart defects.

- What did the physician tell the mother?

CASE 20-5

A pregnant female who has two cats that often "spend the night out" was told by a friend that she should avoid close contact with her cats during her pregnancy. She was also told to avoid flies and cockroaches.

- When she consulted her physician, what was she told?

Discussion of these problems appears in the Appendix at the back of the book.

BIBLIOGRAPHY AND SUGGESTED READING

Bandoli G, Chambers CD, Wells A, Palmsten K: Prenatal antidepressant use and risk of adverse neonatal outcomes, *Pediatrics* 146(1):e20192493, 2020. https://doi.org/10.1542/peds.2019-2493.

Hu CY, Huang K, Fang Y, Yang XJ, Ding K, Jiang W, Hua XG, et al: Maternal air pollution exposure and congenital heart defects in offspring: a systematic review and meta-analysis, *Chemosphere* 253:126668, 2020. ISSN 00456535. https://doi.org/10.1016/j.chemosphere.2020.126668.

Muglia LJ, Benhalima K, Tong S, Ozanne S: Maternal factors during pregnancy influencing maternal, fetal, and childhood outcomes, *BMC Med* 20:418, 2022. https://doi.org/10.1186/s12916-022-02632.

Yang P, Wang X, Liu P, Wei C, He B, Zheng J, et al: Clinical characteristics and risk assessment of newborns born to mothers with COVID-19, *J Clin Virol* 127:104356, 2020. https://doi.org/10.1016/j.jcv.2020.94356.

ACOG and SMFM: Joint statement on WHO recommendations regarding COVID-19 vaccines and pregnant individuals, Washington, DC, January 27, 2021.

Alves C, Franco RR: Prader-Willi syndrome: endocrine manifestations and management, *Arch Endocrinol Metab* 64:223, 2020.

Antonarakis SE, Skotko BG, Rafii MS, Strydom A, Pape SE, Bianchi DW, et al: Down syndrome, *Nat Rev Dis Primers* 6(1):9, 2020. https://doi.org/10.1038/s41572-019-0143-7.

Auriti C, De Rose DU, Santisi A, Martini L, Piersigilli F, Bersani I, et al: Pregnancy and viral infections: mechanisms of fetal damage, diagnosis and prevention of neonatal adverse outcomes from cytomegalovirus to SARS-CoV-2 and Zika virus, *Biochim Biophys Acta Mol Basis Dis* 1867(10):166198, 2021. https://doi.org/10.1016/j.bbadis.2021.166198.

Bandoli G, Palmsten K, Chambers C: Acetaminophen use in pregnancy: examining prevalence, timing, and indication of use in a prospective birth cohort, *Paediatr Perinat Epidemiol* 34:237, 2020.

Bekkar B, Pacheco S, Basu R, DeNicola N: Association of air pollution and heat exposure with preterm birth, low birth weight, and stillbirth in the us: a systematic review, *JAMA Netw Open* 3(6):e208243, 2020. https://doi.org/10.1001/jamanetworkopen.2020.8243.

Bowen VB, McDonald R, Grey JA, Kimball A, Torrone EA: High congenital syphilis case count among U.S. infants born in 2020, *N Engl J Med* 385:1144, 2021.

Britt WJ: Adverse outcomes of pregnancy-associated Zika virus infection, *Semin Perinatol* 42(3):155–167, 2018. https://doi.org/10.1053/j.semperi.2018.02.003.

Cook JL, Green CR, Lilley CM, et al: Fetal alcohol spectrum disorder: a guideline for diagnosis across the life span, *CMAJ* 188:191, 2016.

Chudley AE, Hagerman RJ: The fragile X syndrome, *J Pediatr* 110:821, 1987.

Freitas DA, Souza-Santos R, Carvalho LMA, Barros WB, Neves LM, Brasil P, Wakimoto MD: Congenital Zika syndrome: a systematic review, *PLoS One* 15(12):e0242367, 2020. https://doi.org/10.1371/journal.pone.0242367.

Gruhn J, Hoffmann ER: Errors of the egg: the establishment of human aneuploidy research in the maternal germline, *Annu Rev Genet* 56:369, 2022.

Kimball A, Torrone E, Miele K, Bachmann L, Thorpe P, Weinstock H, et al: Missed opportunities for prevention of congenital syphilis – United States, 2018, *MMWR Morb Mortal Wkly Rep* 69(22):661–665, 2020 Jun 5. PMC7272112

Moog U, Felbor U, Has C, Zirn B: Disorders caused by genetic mosaicism, *Dtsch Arztebl Int* 116:119, 2020.

Pietersma CS, Mulders AGMGJ, Sabanovic A, Willemsen SP, Jansen MS, Steegers EAP, Steegers-Theunissen RPM, Rousian M: The impact of maternal smoking on embryonic morphological development: the Rotterdam Periconception Cohort, *Hum Reprod* 37:696, 2022.

Rotem-Kohavi N, Williams LJ, Muller AM, Abdi H, Virji-Babul N, Bjornson BH, et al: Hub distribution of the brain functional networks of newborns prenatally exposed to maternal depression and SSRI antidepressant, *Depress Anxiety* 36:753, 2019.

Zimmerman LA, Knapp JK, Antoni S, Grant GB, Reef SE: Progress toward rubella and congenital rubella syndrome control and elimination - worldwide, 2012-2020, *MMWR Morb Mortal Wkly Rep* 71(6):196–201, 2022. https://doi.org/10.15585/mmwr.mm7106a2.

Elliott AJ, Kinney HC, Haynes RL, Dempers JD, Wright C, Fifer WP, et al: Concurrent prenatal drinking and smoking increases risk for SIDS: Safe Passage Study report, *EClinicalMedicine* 19:100247, 2020. https://doi.org/10.1016/j.eclinm.2019.100247.

Fang Y, Wang Y, Peng M, Xu J, Fan Z, Liu C, et al: Effect of paternal age on offspring birth defects: a systematic review and meta-analysis, *Aging* 12:25373, 2020.

Fu F, Li R, Yu Q, Wang D, Deng Q, Li L, et al: Application of exome sequencing for prenatal diagnosis of fetal structural anomalies: clinical experience and lessons learned from a cohort of 1618 fetuses, *Genome Med* 14(1):123, 2022. https://doi.org/10.1186/s13073-022-01130-x.

Ghazi T, Naidoo P, Naidoo RN, Chuturgoon AA: Prenatal air pollution exposure and placental DNA methylation changes: implications on fetal development and future disease susceptibility, *Cells* 10(11):3025, 2021. https://doi.org/10.3390/cells10113025.

Granja MG, Oliveira ACDR, de Figueiredo CS: SARS-CoV-2 infection in pregnant women: neuroimmune-endocrine changes at the maternal-fetal interface, *Neuroimmunomodulation* 28(1), 2021.

Grimsby J: The fragile X cognitive retardation gene (FMR1): historical perspective, phenotypes, mechanism, pathology, and epidemiology, *Clin Neuropsychol* 30(6):815, 2016.

Hadj Amor M, Dimassi S, Taj A, et al: Neuronal migration genes and a familial translocation t (3;17): candidate genes implicated in the phenotype, *BMC Med Genet* 21(1):26, 2020. https://doi.org/10.1186/s12881-020-0966-9.

Harris BS, Bishop KC, Kemeny HR, Walker JS, Rhee E, Kuller JA: Risk factors for birth defects, *Obstet Gynecol Surv* 72:123, 2017.

Jarmasz JS, Basalah DA, Chudley AE, Del Bigio MR: Human brain abnormalities associated with prenatal alcohol exposure and fetal spectrum disorder, *J Neuropathol Exp Neurol* 76(9):813–833, 2017.

Lebin LG, Novick AM: Selective serotonin reuptake inhibitors (SSRIs) in pregnancy: an updated review on risks to mother, fetus, and child, *Curr Psychiatry Rep* 24:687, 2022.

Lebov JF, Arias JF, Balmaseda A, Britt W, Cordero JF, Galvão LA, et al: International prospective observational cohort study of Zika in infants and pregnancy (ZIP study): study protocol, *BMC Pregnancy Childbirth* 19(1):282, 2019 Aug 7. https://doi.org/10.1186/s12884-019-2430-4.

Lim H, Agopian AJ, Whitehead LW: Maternal occupational exposure to ionizing radiation and major structural birth defects, *Birth Defects Res A Clin Mol Teratol* 103:243, 2015.

Luke B, Brown MB, Wantman E, Forestieri NE, Browne ML, et al: The risk of birth defects with conception by ART, *Hum Reprod* 36:116, 2021.

Mullins E, Perry A, Banerjee J, Townson J, Grozeva D, Milton R, et al: Pregnancy and neonatal outcomes in COVID-19: study protocol for a global registry of women with suspected or confirmed SARS-CoV-2 infection in pregnancy and their neonates, understanding natural history to guide treatment and prevention, *BMJ Open* 11(1):e 041247, 2021. https://doi.org/10.1136/bmjopen-2020-041247 Published 2021 Jan 29.

Naing ZW, Scott GM, Shand A, Hamilton ST, van Zuylen WJ, Basha J, et al: Congenital cytomegalovirus infection in pregnancy: a review of prevalence, clinical features, diagnosis and prevention, *Aust N Z J Obstet Gynaecol* 56:9, 2016.

Nguyen VH, Harley KG: Prenatal cannabis use and infant birth outcomes in the pregnancy Risk Assessment Monitoring System, *J Pediatr* 240:87–93, 2022. https://doi.org/10.1016/j.peds2021.08.088.

Patorno E, Huybrechts KF, Bateman BT: Lithium use in pregnancy and the risk of cardiac malformations, *N Engl J Med* 376:2245, 2017.

Popova S, Lange S, Shield K, Mihic A, Chudley AE, Mukherjee RAS, et al: Comorbidity of fetal alcohol spectrum disorder: a systematic review and meta-analysis, *Lancet* 387:978–987, 2016.

Protic DD, Aishworiya R, Salcedo-Arellano MJ, Tang SJ, Milisavljevic J, Mitrovic F, et al: Fragile X syndrome: from molecular aspect to clinical treatment, *Int J Mol Sci* 23(4):1935, 2022. https://doi.org/10.3390/ijms23041935.

Rawlinson WD, Boppana SB, Fowler KB: Congenital cytomegalovirus infection in pregnancy and the neonate: consensus recommendations for prevention, diagnosis, and therapy, *Lancet Infect Dis* 17(6):e177–e188, 2017.

Reece AS, Hulse GK: Canadian cannabis consumption and patterns of congenital anomalies: an ecological geospatial analysis, *J Addiction Med* 14(5):e195–e210, 2020. https://doi.org/10.1097/ADM.0000000000000638.

Richardson GA, Goldschmidt L, Willford J: Continued effects of prenatal cocaine use: preschool development, *Neurotoxicol Teratol* 31:325, 2009.

Briggs GG, Freeman RK, Tower CV, Forinash AB: *Briggs drugs in pregnancy and lactation. A reference guide to fetal and neonatal risk,* ed 12Philadelphia, 2021, Wolters Kluwer.

F.D.A. Drug Safety Communication: FDA recommends avoiding use of NSAIDs in pregnancy at 20 weeks or later because they can result in low amniotic fluid. October 15, 2020.

Gabbay-Benziv R, Reece EA, Wang F, Yang P: Birth defects in pregestational diabetes: defect range, glycemic threshold and pathogenesis, *World J Diabetes* 6:481, 2015.

Gomella TL, Eyal FG, Bany-Mohammed F: *Gomella's neonatology, management, procedures, on-call problems, diseases and drugs,* ed 8, Lange, 2020, Mc Graw Hill.

Jones KL, Jones MC, Campo MD: *Smith's recognizable patterns of human malformation,* ed 8, Philadelphia, 2021, Elsevier.

Levine DA: Growth and development. In Marcdante KJ, Kliegman KJ, editors: *Nelson essentials of pediatrics,* ed 7, Philadelphia, 2015, Saunders.

Levy PA, Marion RW: Human genetics and dysmorphology. In Marcdante KJ, Kliegman KJ, editors: *Nelson essentials of pediatrics,* ed 7, Philadelphia, 2015, Saunders.

Martin RJ, Fanaroff AA, Walsh MC, editors: *Fanaroff and Martin's neonatal-perinatal medicine: diseases of the fetus and infant, current therapy in neonatal-perinatal medicine,* ed 10, Philadelphia, 2015, Elsevier.

Medicode, Inc: Medicode's hospital and payer: international classification of diseases, vols 1–3, 10th revised edition, Clinical modification (ICD 10 CM), Salt Lake City, 2015, Medicode (Browser Tool: https://icd10cmtool.cdc.gov/)

Miao S, Yin J, Liu S, Zhu Q, Liao C, Jiang G. Maternal–fetal exposure to antibiotics: levels, motherto-child transmission, and potential health risks. *Environ Sci Technol* 58(9):8117–8134, 2024. https://doi.org/10.1021/acs.est.4c02018

Milewicz DM, Braverman AC, DeBacker J, Morris SA, Boileau C, Maumenee IH, et al: Marfan syndrome, *Nat Rev* 7:1, 2021.

Nussbaum RL, McInnes RR, Willard HF: *Thompson & Thompson genetics in medicine,* ed 8, Philadelphia, 2016, Elsevier.

Persaud TVN: *Environmental causes of human birth defects,* Springfield, 1990, Charles C Thomas.

Smiianov VA, Vygovskaya LA: Intrauterine infections—challenges in the perinatal period (literature review), *Wiad Lek* 70:512, 2017.

Turnpenny P, Ellard S, Cleaver R: *Emery's elements of medical genetics and genomics,* ed 16, Philadelphia, 2020, Elsevier.

Sarayani A, Albogami Y, Thai TN, Smolinski NE, Patel P, Wang Y, et al: Prenatal exposure to teratogenic medications in the era of risk evaluation and mitigation strategies, *Am J Obstet Gynecol* 227(2):263.e1–263.e38, 2022. https://doi.org/10.1016/j.ajog.2022.01.004.

Sciorio R, El Hajj N: Epigenetic risks of medically assisted reproduction, *J Clin Med* 11(8):2151, 2022. https://doi.org/10.3390/jcm11082151.

Sciorio R, Rapalini E, Esteves SC: Air quality in the clinical embryology laboratory: a mini-review, *Ther Adv Reprod Health* 15, 2021. https://doi.org/10.1177/2633494121990684.

Seppey C, Schlingemann R, Guex-Crosier Y: Suspected congenital rubella retinopathy: a spectrum of the TORCH syndrome. *Klinische Monatsblätter für Augenheilkunde* 241(04):525–528, 2024. https://doi.org/10.1055/a-2212-2526.

Seyoum Tola F: The concept of folic acid supplementation and its role in prevention of neural tube defect among pregnant women: PRISMA. *Medicine* 103(19):e38154, 2024 https://doi.org/10.1097/md.0000000000038154.

Shiota K, Uwabe C, Nishimura H: High prevalence of defective human embryos at the early postimplantation period, *Teratology* 35:309, 1987.

Shirley DT, Nataro JP: Zika virus infection, *Pediatr Clin North Am* 64:937, 2017.

Sisman J, Jaleel MA, Moreno W, Rajaram V, Collins RRJ, Savani RC, et al: Intrauterine transmission of SARS-COV-2 infection in a preterm ifant, *Pediatr Infect Dis J* 39(9):e265–e267, 2020 Sep. https://doi.org/10.1097/INF.0000000000002815.

Spranger J, Benirschke K, Hall JG, Lenz W, Lowry RB, Opitz JM, et al: Errors of morphogenesis, concepts and terms, *J Pediatr* 100:160, 1982.

Sun S, Qian H, Li C, Wang Q, Zhao A: Effect of low dose aspirin application during pregnancy on fetal congenital anomalies, *BMC Pregnancy Childbirth* 22:802, 2022. https://doi.org/10.1186/s12884-022-05142-8.

Valladares DA, Rasmussen SA: An update on teratogens for pediatric healthcare providers, *Curr Opin Pediatr* 34:565, 2022.

Venancio FA, Quilião ME, de Almeida Moura D, de Azevedo MV, de Almeida Metzker S, Mareto LK, et al: Congenital anomalies during the 2015-2018 Zika virus epidemic: a population-based cross-sectional study, *BMC Public Health* 22(1):2069, 2022 Nov 12. https://doi.org/10.1186/s12889-022-14490-1.

Wouldes TA, Lester BM: Opioid, methamphetamine, and polysubstance use: perinatal outcomes for the mother and infant. *Front Pediatr*11, 2023. https://doi.org/10.3389/fped.2023.1305508.

Zaki P, Zhu J, Mackley HB, Rosenberg JC: Pregnancy screening practices and treatment of pregnant patients among radiation oncologists: results of an international survey, *ecancermedicalscience* 15:1169, 2021. https://doi.org/10.3332/ecancer.2021.1169.

Common Signaling Pathways Used During Development

21

Jeffrey T. Wigle | David D. Eisenstat

CHAPTER OUTLINE

During the process of embryonic development, undifferentiated precursor cells differentiate and organize into the complex structures found in functional adult tissues. This intricate process requires cells to integrate many intrinsic and extrinsic cues for development to occur properly. These cues control the proliferation, differentiation, and migration of cells to determine the final size and shape of the developing organs. Disruption of these signaling pathways can result in human developmental disorders and birth defects. These key developmental signaling pathways are also frequently co-opted in adults by diseases such as cancer.

Given the diverse changes that occur during embryogenesis, it may appear that a correspondingly diverse set of signaling pathways should regulate these processes. In contrast, the differentiation of many cell types is regulated through a relatively restricted set of molecular signaling pathways:

- **Intercellular communication:** Development involves the interaction of a cell with neighboring cells directly (gap junctions) or indirectly (cell adhesion molecules).
- **Morphogens:** These diffusible molecules specify which cell type is generated at a specific anatomical location and direct the migration of cells and their processes to their final destinations. Morphogens include retinoic acid, the transforming growth factor-β (TGF-β) superfamily of proteins, including bone morphogenetic proteins (BMPs), and WNT protein families. Table 21.1 explains gene and protein nomenclature.
- **Hedgehog:** The hedgehog family of morphogen signaling pathways in human cells is localized to a structure called the primary cilium. Disruption of the components of the hedgehog pathway results in a set of diseases termed ciliopathies.
- **Receptor tyrosine kinases (RTKs):** Many growth factors signal by binding to and activating membrane-bound RTKs. These kinases are essential for the regulation of cellular proliferation, apoptosis, and migration, as well as processes such as the growth of new blood vessels and axonal processes in the nervous system.
- **Notch-Delta:** This pathway often specifies which cell fate the precursor cells adopt.
- **Transcription factors:** These evolutionarily conserved proteins activate or repress downstream genes that are essential for many cellular processes. Many transcription factors are members of the homeobox (HOX) or helix-loop-helix (HLH) families. Their activity can be regulated by all the other pathways described in this chapter.
- **Epigenetic effects:** These heritable changes in gene function do not result from a change in DNA sequence. Examples of epigenetic modifications are histone acetylation, histone methylation, microRNAs (miRNAs), and DNA methylation.
- **Stem cells:** Embryonic stem cells can give rise to all cells and tissues in the developing organism. Adult stem cells maintain tissue homeostasis in the mature organism.

Table 21.1 International Nomenclature Standards for Genes and Proteins

Gene	Human	Italic, all letters capitalized	*PAX6*
	Mouse	Italic, first letter capitalized	*Pax6*
Protein	Human	Roman, all letters capitalized	PAX6
	Mouse	Roman, all letters capitalized	PAX6

These types of stem cells and induced pluripotent stem cells (iPSC) are potential sources of cells for the regeneration and repair of injured or degenerating cells and organs. iPSC and tissue organoids derived from patient cells can be used to model developmental processes in vitro and to screen potential therapies. New advancements in spatial transcriptomics and gene editing have greatly enhanced our ability to model human diseases both in vitro and in vivo.

INTERCELLULAR COMMUNICATION

During embryonic development, cells receive signals from their external environment and communicate with neighboring cells. This communication directs the cell to undergo processes such as proliferation, differentiation, and migration. Two classes of proteins required for intercellular communication are discussed: gap junctions and cell adhesion molecules.

GAP JUNCTIONS

Gap junctions are a means for cells to directly communicate with one another; this is known as **gap junction intercellular communication** (GJIC). Although the pore size of the channels varies, only small molecules (e.g., second messengers, ions such as calcium, adenosine triphosphate [ATP]) less than 1 kDa can pass through, which excludes most proteins and nucleic acids. In the nervous and cardiac systems, gap junctions help to establish electrical cell coupling ("electrical" synapse).

Although the function of gap junctions is quite straightforward, the structure of these intercellular channels is complex and highly regulated throughout development (Fig. 21.1). Each gap junction is composed of two hemichannels known as connexons. Each hexameric connexon consists of six individual connexin subunits. An individual connexin (Cx) molecule consists of four transmembrane domains. Vertebrates have more than 20 connexin molecules. Cellular and tissue functional diversity of gap junctions depends on whether individual connexons are the same (homotypic) or different (heterotypic) and whether each connexon is made from the same (homomeric) or different (heteromeric) connexin molecules.

Early in development, GJIC is important for the rapid distribution of ions and other molecules essential for regionalization before the establishment of distinct boundaries and compartments. The importance of GJIC has been demonstrated in the developing chick hindbrain (rhombencephalon) by a combination of dye transfer and electrical coupling studies.

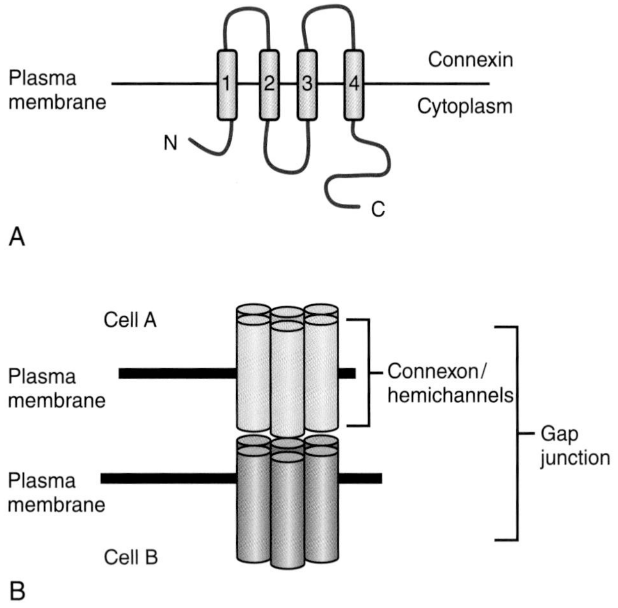

Fig. 21.1 Gap junction intercellular communication. (A) The connexin molecule consists of four transmembrane domains and two extracellular domains, and its *N*- and *C*-termini are cytoplasmic. (B) Connexons, or hemichannels, are hexameric structures consisting of six connexin subunits. A gap junction can be formed from two homophilic or heterophilic connexons. Small molecules (e.g., ions, adenosine triphosphate [ATP]) less than 1 kDa can pass through an open gap junction.

Some of the better-characterized connexins include Cx43 (heart, brain), Cx45 (heart, pancreas), Cx32 (myelin), and Cx36 (pancreas, brain). In this nomenclature system, the number following Cx refers to the molecular weight in kilodaltons (kDa) of the proteins. Mutations in Cx genes result in diseases such as hereditary peripheral neuropathy X-linked Charcot-Marie-Tooth disease (*GJB1*, formerly *CX32*). It was previously thought that connexons had to bind to a connexon on an adjacent cell to functionally signal. However, it has since been shown that unbound connexons (hemichannels) enable the exchange of ions and small molecules between the cytoplasm and the extracellular space, especially during pathophysiologic conditions. Aberrant hemichannel activation through *GJB2* (formerly *CX26*) can result in keratitis-ichthyosis-deafness syndrome.

CELL ADHESION MOLECULES

Cell adhesion molecules have large extracellular domains that interact with extracellular matrix (ECM) components or adhesion molecules on neighboring cells. These molecules often contain a transmembrane segment and a short cytoplasmic domain that regulate intracellular signaling cascades. Two classes of molecules that have important roles during embryonic development are cadherins and members of the immunoglobulin superfamily of cell adhesion molecules.

CADHERINS

Cadherins are critical for embryonic morphogenesis because they regulate the separation of cell layers (endothelial and epidermal), cell migration, cell sorting, the establishment of well-defined boundaries, synaptic connections, and the growth cones of neurons. Cadherins mediate the interaction between the cell and its extracellular milieu (neighboring cells and ECM).

Cadherins were originally classified by their site of expression. E-cadherin (epithelial cadherin) is highly expressed in epithelial cells, whereas N-cadherin (neural cadherin) is highly expressed in neural cells.

Cadherins mediate homophilic, calcium-dependent binding. A typical cadherin molecule has a large extracellular domain, a transmembrane domain, and an intracellular tail (Fig. 21.2). The extracellular domain contains five extracellular repeats (EC repeats) and four Ca^{2+}-binding sites. Cadherins form dimers that interact with cadherin dimers in adjacent cells. These complexes are found clustered in *adherens junctions*, which result in the formation of a tight barrier between epithelial or endothelial cells.

Through its intracellular domain, cadherins bind to p120 catenin, β-catenin, and α-catenin. These proteins connect the cadherin to the cytoskeleton. E-cadherin expression is lost as epithelial cells transition to mesenchymal cells (**epithelial to mesenchymal transition [EMT]**). EMT is required for the formation of neural crest cells during development, and the same process can occur in tumors that develop from epithelial cell types.

IMMUNOGLOBULIN SUPERFAMILY

There are more than 700 members of the **immunoglobulin superfamily** of cell adhesion molecules in the human genome. This large family of proteins is involved in a wide variety of cellular processes. One member of this class, the neural cell adhesion molecule (NCAM), is an abundant protein in the brain and has three isoforms that result from alternative splicing. It has a large extracellular domain that contains five immunoglobulin (Ig) repeats and two fibronectin domains (see Fig. 21.2). This region mediates the calcium-independent homophilic binding of NCAM to itself and heterophilic binding to other cell adhesion molecules (L1 and TAG1), RTKs (fibroblast growth factor receptor [FGFR]), or the ECM. Ligand binding induces intracellular signaling through the FYN and FAK intracellular kinases.

NCAM undergoes polysialylation (PSA), a unique post-translational glycosylation modification. PSA-NCAM is abundant early in neural development and becomes restricted to areas of neural plasticity and migration in adults. It is thought that PSA decreases the adhesiveness of NCAM and facilitates migration. NCAM regulates neurite outgrowth, axonal pathfinding, survival, and plasticity.

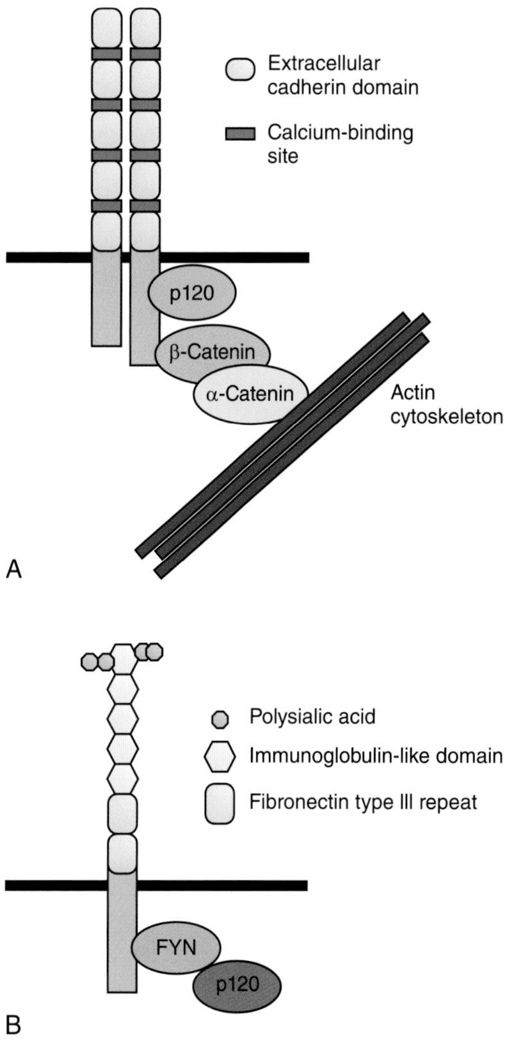

Fig. 21.2 Structure of cadherin and neural cell adhesion molecule (NCAM). (A) The cadherin extracellular domain contains four calcium-binding sites and five repeated domains called extracellular cadherin domains. Each cadherin molecule forms a homodimer. On the intracellular domain, cadherin binds directly to p120 catenin and to β-catenin, which binds to α-catenin. This complex links the cadherin molecules to the actin cytoskeleton. (B) Extracellularly, NCAM contains five immunoglobulin repeats and two fibronectin type III domains. The fifth immunoglobulin repeat is modified by polysialylation, which decreases the adhesiveness of the NCAM molecule. Intracellular signaling is transmitted by the FYN and FAK kinases.

MORPHOGENS

Extrinsic signals guide the differentiation and migration of cells during development and thereby dictate the morphology and function of developing tissues see (Chapter 5). Many of these **morphogens** are found in concentration gradients in the embryo, and different morphogens can be expressed in opposing gradients in the dorsal-ventral, anterior-posterior, proximal-distal, and medial-lateral axes. The fate of a specific cell can be determined by its location along these gradients. Cells can be attracted or repelled by morphogens depending on the particular set of receptors expressed on the cell surface.

RETINOIC ACID

The anterior (rostral, head)-posterior (caudal, tail), or anteroposterior, axis of the embryo is crucial for determining the correct location for structures such as limbs and the patterning of the nervous system. For decades, it has been clinically evident that alterations in the level of vitamin A (retinol) in the diet (excessive or insufficient amounts) can lead to the development of congenital anomalies (birth defects) (see Chapters 17 and 20).

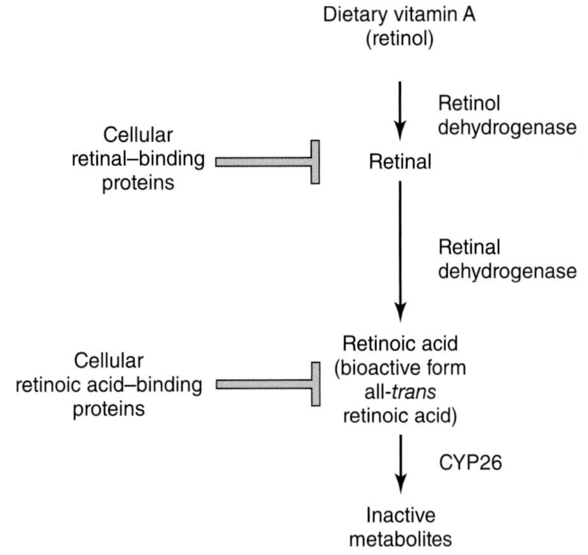

Fig. 21.3 Regulation of retinoic acid metabolism and signaling. Dietary retinol (vitamin A) is converted to retinal by the action of retinol dehydrogenases. The concentration of free retinal is controlled by the action of cellular retinal–binding proteins. Similarly, retinal is converted to retinoic acid by retinal dehydrogenases, and its free level is modulated by sequestration by cellular retinoic acid–binding proteins and degradation by CYP26. The bioactive form of retinoic acid is all-*trans* retinoic acid.

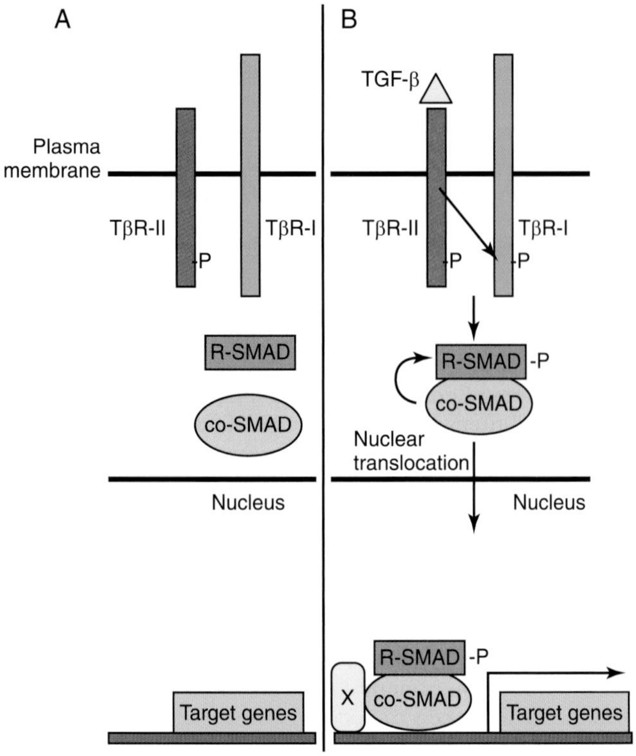

Fig. 21.4 Transforming growth factor-β *(TGF-β)*/SMAD signaling pathway. (A) The type II TGF-β receptor subunit *(TβR-II)* is constitutively active. (B) On binding of ligand to TβR-II, a type I receptor subunit is recruited to form a heterodimeric receptor complex, and the TβR-I kinase domain is transphosphorylated *(-P)*. Signaling from the activated receptor complex phosphorylates R-SMADs, which then bind to a co-SMAD, translocate from the cytoplasm to the nucleus, and activate gene transcription with cofactors *(X)*.

The bioactive form of vitamin A is **retinoic acid**, which is formed by the oxidation of retinol to retinal by retinol dehydrogenases and the subsequent oxidation of retinal by retinal aldehyde dehydrogenase. Free levels of retinoic acid can be further modulated by cellular retinoic acid–binding proteins that sequester retinoic acid. Retinoic acid also can be actively degraded into inactive metabolites by enzymes such as CYP26 (Fig. 21.3). Normally, retinoic acid *posteriorizes* the body plan. Excessive retinoic acid levels or inhibition of retinoic acid degradation lead to a truncated body axis in which structures have a more posterior nature. Insufficient retinoic acid or defects in enzymes such as retinal aldehyde dehydrogenase lead to a more anteriorized structure.

At a molecular level, retinoic acid binds to its receptors inside the cell and activates them. Retinoic acid receptors are transcription factors, and their activation regulates the expression of downstream genes. Crucial targets of retinoic acid receptors in development are the *HOX* genes. Due to their profound influence on early development, retinoids are powerful teratogens, especially during the first trimester. In the clinic, retinoids are often used for differentiation-based treatment of acute promyelocytic leukemia (using all-*trans*-retinoic acid) and neuroblastoma, a solid tumor of the developing sympathetic nervous system in children (using 13-*cis*-retinoic acid or isotretinoin).

TRANSFORMING GROWTH FACTOR-β AND BONE MORPHOGENETIC PROTEINS

Members of the TGF-β superfamily include TGF-β, BMPs, activin, and nodal. These molecules contribute to the establishment of dorsoventral patterning, cell fate decisions, and formation of specific organs, including the nervous system, kidneys, skeleton, and blood (see Chapters 5, 16, and 17).

In humans, there are three TGF-β isoforms (TGF-β_1, TGF-β_2, and TGF-β_3). Binding of these ligands to heterotetrameric (four-subunit) complexes, consisting of specific type I (inactive kinase domain) and type II TGF-β receptor subunit (TβR-II) (constitutively active) transmembrane serine-threonine kinase receptors results in intracellular signaling events (Fig. 21.4). When TGF-β ligands bind to their respective membrane-bound type II receptor, a type I receptor is recruited and transphosphorylated, and its kinase domain is activated, subsequently phosphorylating intracellular receptor–associated SMAD proteins (R-SMADs).

The SMADs are a large family of intercellular proteins that are divided into three classes: receptor-activated (R-SMADs 1–3, 5, and 8), common partner (co-SMADs such as SMAD4), and inhibitory SMADs (I-SMADs such as SMAD6 and SMAD7). R-SMAD/SMAD4 complexes translocate to the nucleus and regulate target gene transcription by interacting with other proteins or function as transcription factors by directly binding to DNA.

Inhibitory SMAD proteins block the actions of R-SMADs by several mechanisms, such as preventing phosphorylation of R-SMADs by TβR-I, induction of R-SMAD degradation, and transcriptional repression. TβR-I activation is a highly regulated process that involves membrane-anchored coreceptors and other receptor-like molecules that can sequester ligands and prevent their binding to respective TβR-II receptors. Dominant-negative forms of TβR-II have inactive kinase domains and cannot transphosphorylate TβR-I, thereby blocking downstream signaling events. The diversity of TGF-β ligand, TβR-I and TβR-II, coreceptor, ligand trap, and R-SMAD combinations contributes to particular developmental and cell-specific processes, often in combination with other signaling pathways.

HEDGEHOG AND THE PRIMARY CILIUM

The **sonic hedgehog** gene *(SHH)* was the first identified mammalian ortholog of the *Drosophila* hedgehog gene *(Hh)*. SHH and other related proteins, including desert hedgehog and Indian hedgehog, are secreted morphogens critical to early patterning, cell migration, and differentiation of many cell types and organ systems (see Chapter 5).

In *Drosophila,* cells have various thresholds for response to the secreted Hh signal. The primary receptor for SHH is Patched (PTCH in humans, PTC family in mice), a 12-transmembrane domain protein that in the absence of SHH inhibits Smoothened (SMO), a seven-transmembrane domain G protein–linked protein, and downstream signaling to the nucleus. However, in the presence of SHH, PTC/PTCH inhibition is blocked, and downstream events follow, including nuclear translocation of GLI (GLI1, GLI2, GLI3) with transcriptional activation of target genes such as *Ptc1*, *Engrailed*, and others (Fig. 21.5).

Other membrane-bound SHH coreceptors have been identified with key roles in ventral neural patterning, including BOC, GAS1, and the LDL receptor–related protein 2 (LRP2, in mammals). Individually, these coreceptors act to enhance SHH signaling. BOC and GAS1 each interact with the SHH canonical receptor PTC/PTCH to form distinct receptor complexes essential for cell proliferation mediated by SHH. The role of BOC is especially important for commissural axonal guidance during development and in medulloblastoma progression. In contrast, LRP2 promotes the internalization and subsequent degradation of PTC/PTCH on SHH binding thereby removing PTC/PTCH inhibition of SMO. Hedgehog-interacting protein is also a coreceptor, but it functions to blunt Indian hedgehog signaling by sequestering Indian hedgehog and thus preventing Indian hedgehog from binding to PTC/PTCH.

The SHH protein is modified posttranslationally by the addition of cholesterol and palmitate moieties to the *N*- and *C*-termini, respectively. These lipid modifications affect SHH's association with the cell membrane, formation of SHH multimers, and movement of SHH, altering its tissue distribution and concentration gradients. One of the best-explained activities of SHH in vertebrate development is its role in patterning the ventral neural tube (see Chapters 4 and 17). SHH is secreted at high levels by the notochord. The concentration of SHH is highest in the floor plate of the neural tube and lowest in the roof plate, where members of the TGF-β family are highly expressed. The cell fates

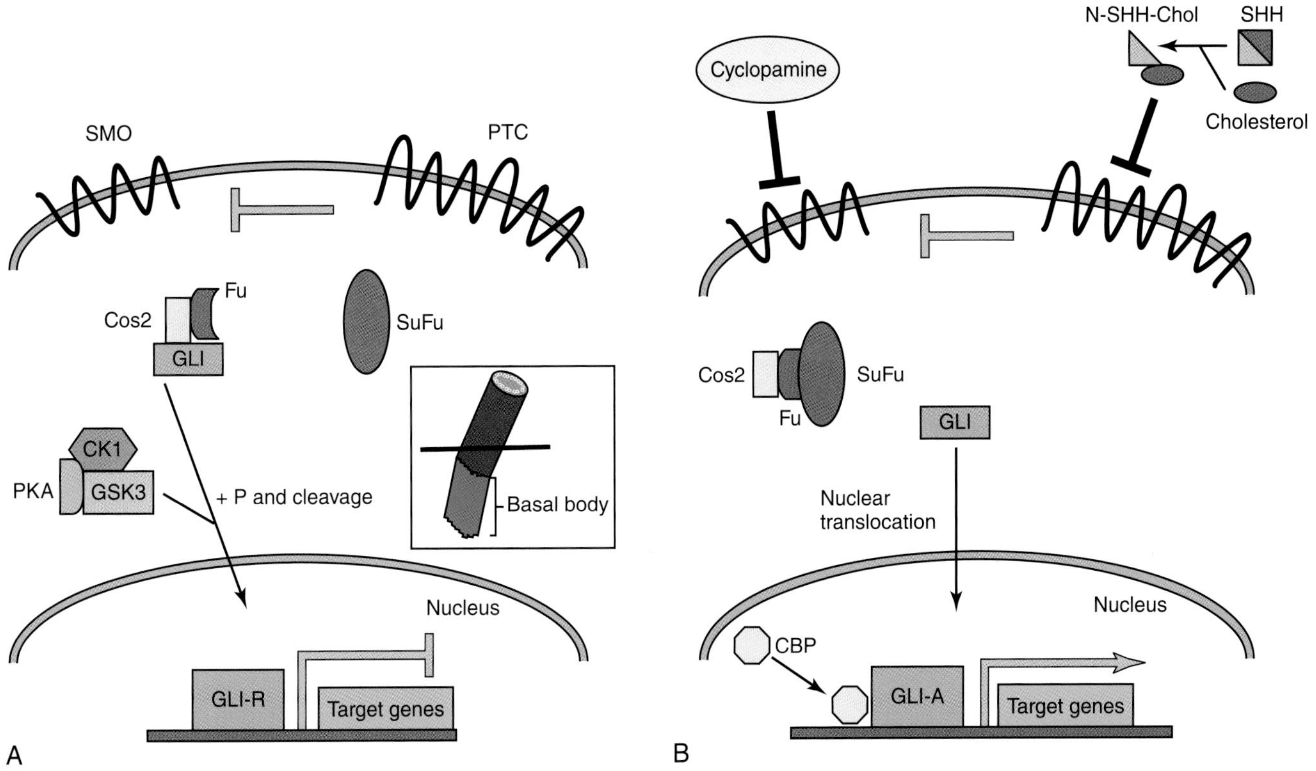

Fig. 21.5 Sonic hedgehog/Patched signaling pathway in vertebrates. (A) The Patched *(PTC)* receptor inhibits signaling from the Smoothened *(SMO)* receptor. In a complex with the kinesin-like protein Costal 2 *(Cos2)* and serine-threonine kinase Fused *(Fu)*, GLI is modified to become a transcriptional repressor *(GLI-R)*. (B) Sonic hedgehog *(SHH)* is cleaved, and cholesterol *(Chol)* is added to its *N*-terminus. This modified SHH ligand inhibits the PTC receptor, permitting SMO signaling, and activated GLI *(GLI-A)* ultimately translocates to the nucleus to activate target genes with cyclic AMP–binding protein *(CBP)*. In vertebrates, SHH signaling takes place in primary cilia *(inset)*. *CK1*, Casein kinase 1; *GSK3*, glycogen synthase kinase 3; *P*, phosphate group; *PKA*, protein kinase A; *SuFu*, suppressor of Fused.

of four ventral interneuron classes and motor neurons are determined by relative SHH concentrations and by a combinatorial code of homeobox and basic HLH (bHLH) genes.

The requirement of SHH signaling for many developmental processes is underscored by the discovery of human mutations of members of the SHH pathway and the corresponding phenotypes of genetically modified mice, in which members are inactivated (loss of function or knockout) or overexpressed (gain of function). Mutations of *SHH* and *PTCH* have been associated with holoprosencephaly, a congenital brain defect resulting in the fusion of the two cerebral hemispheres; anophthalmia or cyclopia (see Chapter 18); and dorsalization of forebrain structures. In sheep, this defect can also result from exposure to the teratogen cyclopamine, which disrupts SHH signaling (see Fig. 21.5). Some patients with severe forms of the inborn error of cholesterol synthesis, the autosomal recessive Smith-Lemli-Opitz syndrome, have holoprosencephaly (see Chapter 20).

GLI3 mutations are associated with autosomal dominant polydactyly syndromes (see Chapter 16), such as the Greig and Pallister-Hall syndromes. Gorlin syndrome, which often is caused by germline *PTCH* mutations, is a constellation of congenital malformations mostly affecting the epidermis, craniofacial structures (see Chapter 9), and the nervous system. These patients are significantly predisposed to basal cell carcinomas, especially after radiation therapy, and a few develop malignant brain tumors (medulloblastomas) during childhood. Somatic mutations of *PTCH*, *SUFU*, and *SMO* have been identified in patients with sporadic medulloblastomas not associated with Gorlin syndrome.

In vertebrates, the SHH signaling pathway is closely linked to **primary cilia** (see Fig. 21.5, inset) and their constituent intraflagellar transport (IFT) and basal body proteins. Primary cilia are sometimes referred to as nonmotile cilia. IFT proteins act upstream of the GLI activator (GLI-A) and repressor (GLI-R) proteins and are necessary for their production. Mutations involving genes encoding basal body proteins, such as *KIAA0586* (formerly *TALPID3)* and oral-facial-digital syndrome 1 *(OFD1)*, affect SHH signaling in knockout mice. A group of human cilia–related diseases called **ciliopathies** result from disruption of primary cilia function and includes rare genetic diseases and more common disorders such as autosomal recessive polycystic kidney disease. Over 40 ciliopathies have been described involving up to 200 genes. Although there may be some overlap (as with many congenital heart defects and left-right asymmetries), diseases of primary, nonmotile cilia are usually distinguished from disorders affecting motile cilia (found in sperm and epithelial cells lining the airways, ventricles of the brain, and oviducts). Manifestations of diseases affecting motile cilia include hydrocephalus, lung infections, and infertility. Table 21.2 lists some common ciliopathies involving primary and nonmotile cilia and affected organ systems.

Table 21.2 Examples of Ciliopathies Due to Defects in Primary, Nonmotile Cilia

Disease	Organ Systems Involved
Bardet-Biedl syndrome	Multisystemic
Oral-facial-digital syndromes	Multisystemic
Oculocerebrorenal syndrome of Lowe	Multisystemic
Meckel-Gruber syndrome	Brain, kidney, skeleton
Holoprosencephaly	Brain, eye
Cone-rod dystrophy	Eye
Leber congenital amaurosis	Eye
Hearing loss	Ear
Polycystic kidney disease	Kidney
Nephronophthisis	Kidney
Situs inversus	Heart, organ laterality
Greig cephalopolysyndactyly syndrome	Skeleton
Orofaciodigital syndrome	Skeleton
Ellis van Creveld syndrome	Skeleton

WNT/β-CATENIN PATHWAY

The *WNT*-encoded glycoproteins are vertebrate orthologs of the *Drosophila* gene Wingless *(Wg/DWnt)*. Similar to the other morphogens previously discussed, the 19 WNT family members control several processes during development, including the establishment of cell polarity, proliferation, apoptosis, cell fate specification, and migration. WNT signaling is very complex, and three signaling pathways have been elucidated. The classic or canonical β-catenin–dependent pathway is discussed here.

In mammals, specific WNTs bind to one of 10 Frizzled (FZD) seven-transmembrane domain cell surface receptors and bind with low-density lipoprotein receptor–related protein (LRP5/LRP6) coreceptors, thereby activating downstream intracellular signaling events (Fig. 21.6). β-Catenin plays an integral role in canonical WNT signaling. In the absence of WNT binding, in a protein complex with adenomatous polyposis coli (APC) and axin, cytoplasmic β-catenin is phosphorylated by glycogen synthase kinase 3 (GSK3) and targeted for degradation. In the presence of Wnts, GSK3 is phosphorylated by Dishevelled (DVL) and inactivated; it cannot phosphorylate β-catenin. β-Catenin is stabilized, accumulates in the cytoplasm, and translocates to the nucleus, where it activates target gene transcription in a complex with T-cell factor (TCF) transcription factors. In mammals, the many β-catenin/TCF target genes include those of vascular endothelial growth factor (*VEGF*), *MYC*, and matrix metalloproteinases (e.g., *COMP*, *DMP1*, *ECM1*).

Some noncanonical WNT signaling pathways include Frizzled receptors. However, all of these pathways are distinguished from the canonical WNT pathway by not involving β-catenin stabilization, degradation, and nuclear translocation. A well-known noncanonical Wnt signaling pathway is the WNT-cGMP/Ca^{2+} pathway. It acts through phospholipase C to increase intracellular calcium concentrations, thereby activating protein kinase C and calmodulin-dependent kinase II and resulting in myriad downstream effects.

In mammals, dysregulated WNT signaling is a prominent feature in many developmental disorders and cancer. A Frizzled gene (*FZD9*) occurs in the Williams-Beuren

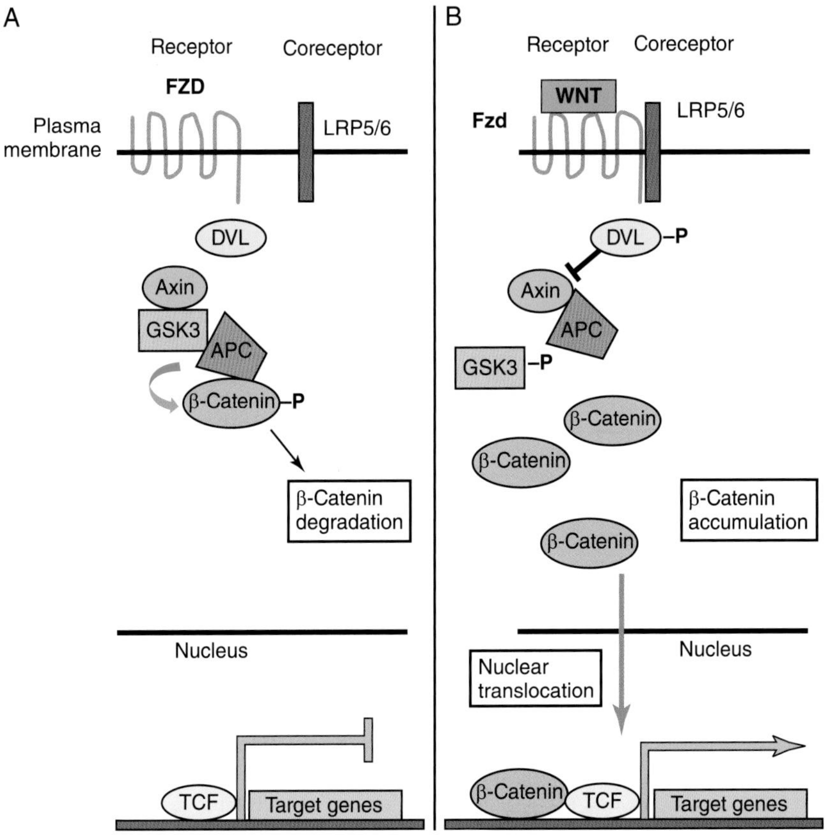

Fig. 21.6 WNT/β-catenin canonical signaling pathway in mammals. (A) In the absence of Wnt ligand binding to the Frizzled *(FZD)* receptor, β-catenin is phosphorylated *(-P)* by a multiprotein complex and targeted for degradation. Target-gene expression is repressed by T-cell factor *(TCF)*. (B) When WNT binds to the FZD receptor, lipoprotein receptor–related protein *(LRP)* coreceptors are recruited, Dishevelled *(DVL)* is phosphorylated, and β-catenin then accumulates in the cytoplasm. Some β-catenin enters the nucleus to activate target gene transcription. *APC*, Adenomatous polyposis coli; *GSK3*, glycogen synthase kinase 3.

syndrome deletion region. *LRP5* mutations are found in the osteoporosis-pseudoglioma syndrome. *Dvl2*-knockout mice have malformations of the cardiac outflow tract, abnormal somite segmentation, and neural tube defects. Similar to the SHH signaling pathway, canonical Wnt pathway mutations (in *β-catenin* [*CTNNB1*], *APC*, and *AXIN1* genes) have been described in children with medulloblastoma. Moreover, somatic *APC* mutations are common (>50%) in adults with sporadic colorectal carcinomas, and germline *APC* mutations are a feature of familial adenomatous polyposis and Turcot syndrome (multiple colorectal adenomas and increased frequency of primary brain tumors).

PROTEIN KINASES

RECEPTOR TYROSINE KINASES

COMMON FEATURES

Growth factors include insulin, epidermal growth factor, nerve growth factor, and other neurotrophins, and members of the platelet-derived growth factor family. Growth factors bind to cell surface transmembrane receptors found on target cells. These receptors are members of the RTK superfamily and have three domains: an extracellular ligand binding domain, a transmembrane domain, and an intracellular kinase domain (Fig. 21.7).

The receptors are found as monomers in their quiescent or unbound state, but on ligand binding, the receptor units dimerize. The process of dimerization brings the two intracellular kinase domains close enough that one kinase domain can phosphorylate and activate the other receptor (transphosphorylation). Transphosphorylation is required to fully activate the receptors, which initiate a series of intracellular signaling cascades. The mechanism of transphosphorylation requires both receptor subunits within a dimer to have functional kinase domains for signal transduction to occur. If there is an inactivating mutation of one receptor subunit's kinase domain, the functional consequence is to abolish signaling through a heterodimer resulting from the combination of wild-type and mutant receptor subunits (dominant-negative mode of action). A mutation in the kinase domain of the VEGF receptor 3 (VEGFR3, now called FMS-related tyrosine kinase 4 [FLT4]) results in the autosomal dominant lymphatic disorder called Milroy disease.

REGULATION OF ANGIOGENESIS BY RECEPTOR TYROSINE KINASES

Growth factors promote cellular proliferation, migration, and survival; they are antiapoptotic. Dysregulation of RTKs or their downstream signaling components is frequently found in human cancers. During embryogenesis, signaling through RTKs is crucial for normal development and affects

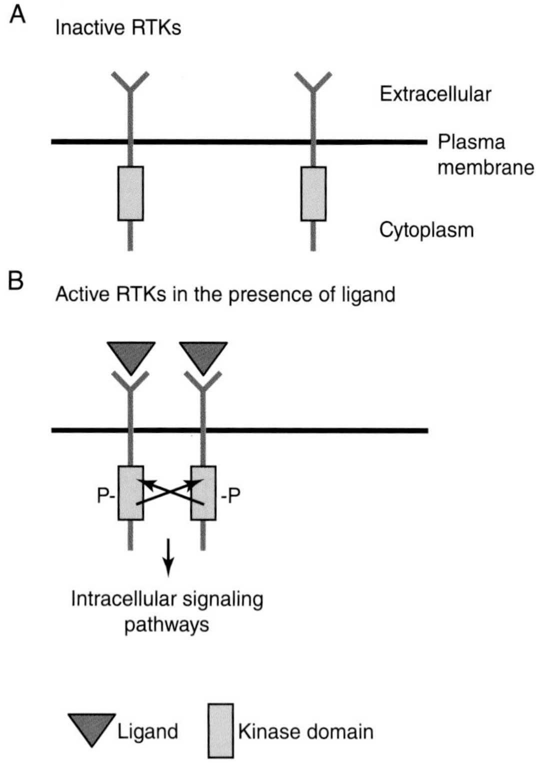

Fig. 21.7 Receptor tyrosine kinase *(RTK)* signaling. (A) In the absence of ligand, the receptors are monomers and are inactive. (B) On binding of ligand, the receptors dimerize and transphosphorylation occurs, which activates downstream signaling cascades. *P*, Phosphorylated.

many processes, such as the growth of new blood vessels (see Chapter 4), cellular migration, and neuronal axonal guidance.

Endothelial cells are derived from a progenitor cell (hemangioblast) that can give rise to the hematopoietic cell lineage and endothelial cells. The early endothelial cells proliferate and eventually coalesce to form the first primitive blood vessels. This process is called **vasculogenesis**. After the first blood vessels are formed, they undergo intensive remodeling and maturation into the mature blood vessels in a process called **angiogenesis**. The maturation process involves the recruitment of vascular smooth muscle cells to the vessels that stabilize them. Vasculogenesis and angiogenesis depend on the function of two distinct RTK classes, members of the VEGF and TIE (tyrosine kinase with immunoglobulin-like and EGF-like domains) receptor families. VEGFA is essential for endothelial and blood cell development. *VegfA*-knockout mice fail to develop blood or endothelial cells and die at early embryonic stages. Heterozygous *VegfA-knockout* mice have severe defects in their vasculature, demonstrating that *VegfA* gene dose (haploinsufficiency) is important. A related molecule, VEGFC, is crucial for the development of lymphatic endothelial cells. VEGFA signals through two receptors, VEGFR1 and VEGFR2, expressed by endothelial cells. VEGFA signals predominantly through the VEGFR2 receptor for vasculogenesis to properly occur in the embryo.

The process of angiogenic refinement depends on the function of the Angiopoietin/TIE2 signaling pathway. TIE2 (also called TEK) is an RTK that is specifically expressed by endothelial cells, and Angiopoietin 1 and Angiopoietin 2 are ligands that are expressed by the surrounding vascular smooth muscle cells. This represents a paracrine signaling system in which receptors and ligands are expressed in adjacent cells. The VEGF/VEGFR2 and Angiopoietin/TIE2 signaling pathways are co-opted by tumors to stimulate the growth of new blood vessels, which stimulates their growth and metastasis. Chromosomal recombination events involving RTKs and different partners can result in the formation of oncoproteins that drive the development of different types of cancer, such as anaplastic large cell lymphomas, acute myeloid leukemia, and 8p11 myeloproliferative syndrome. The chromosomal fusion events generate a protein that contains the intracellular kinase domain of the RTK and an oligomerization domain of another protein. These fusion proteins cluster via the oligomerization domains, resulting in RTK activation and downstream signaling. RTKs such as platelet-derived growth factor receptor, FGFR, and anaplastic lymphoma kinase are involved in chromosomal recombinations that lead to the generation of oncoproteins. This demonstrates how normal signaling pathways in developing human can be reused for disease processes such as cancer.

HIPPO SIGNALING PATHWAY

Studies in *Drosophila* identified a set of kinases in the Hippo signaling pathway that, when mutated, resulted in increased organ size during development. The human orthologs of Hippo are called mammalian STE20-like protein kinase 1 (MST1) and MST2. Activated MST1 and MST2 phosphorylate the scaffold protein Salvador homolog 1 (SAV1) and the downstream kinases large tumor suppressor homolog 1 (LATS1) and LATS2 (Fig. 21.8). Similar to MST1 and MST2, LATS1 and LATS2 are bound to scaffold proteins MOB kinase activator 1A (MOB1A) and MOB1B, which are also phosphorylated by MST1 and MST2. The MST/MOB1 complex then phosphorylates the transcriptional coactivators yes-associated protein (YAP) and transcriptional coactivator with PDZ domain (TAZ). Phosphorylated YAP and TAZ proteins are retained in the cytoplasm, ubiquitinated, and degraded by the proteasome.

When the Hippo pathway is inactive, YAP and TAZ are localized to the nucleus and bind to the TEA domain–containing sequence-specific transcription factor (TEAD), which relieves repression mediated by the vestigial-like family member 4 (VGLL4) and activation of downstream target genes. The Hippo pathway is important in relaying signals received from adjacent cells and the ECM to the nucleus. For example, culturing mesenchymal stem cells on stiff matrices results in the accumulation of YAP and TAZ in the nucleus and the differentiation of these cells into bone cells. In contrast, culturing mesenchymal stem cells on softer matrices results in activation of the Hippo pathway, decreased nuclear YAP and TAZ levels, and differentiation into adipocytes. In the developing embryo, nuclear YAP and TAZ are essential for the determination of the trophoectodermal cells of the placenta. YAP and TAZ function is required to inhibit the differentiation of human embryonic stem cells and for the generation of induced pluripotent stem cells discussed later in Stem Cells: Differentiation Versus Pluripotency section). Loss of Hippo signaling and increased YAP and TAZ nuclear localization have been implicated in several types of human cancer.

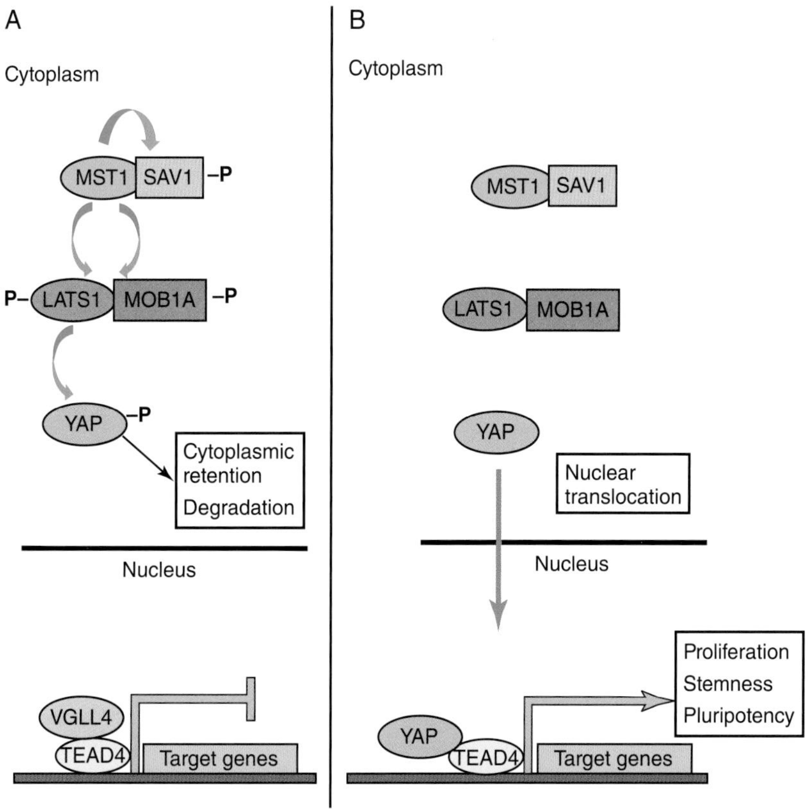

Fig. 21.8 Hippo signaling pathway in mammals. (A) Activated mammalian STE20-like protein kinase 1 *(MST1)* phosphorylates its scaffolding protein Salvador homolog 1 *(SAV1)* and the downstream kinase large tumor suppressor homolog 1 *(LATS1)* and its scaffolding protein MOB kinase activator 1 A *(MOB1A)*. On phosphorylation, LATS1 is activated and phosphorylates the yes-associated protein *(YAP)* 1 (YAP1), which results in YAP1 retention in the cytoplasm and degradation. The transcription of TEA domain–containing sequence-specific transcription factor 4 *(TEAD4)* is repressed due to the binding of the vestigial-like family member 4 *(VGLL4)* transcriptional repressor. (B) When the Hippo pathway is inactive, YAP1 translocates to the nucleus, displaces VGLL4 from TEAD4, and transcription of downstream target genes is activated, leading to increased cellular proliferation, increased "stemness," and increased pluripotency. *P*, Phosphorylated.

NOTCH-DELTA PATHWAY

The NOTCH signaling pathway is integral for cell fate determination, including maintenance of stem cell niches, proliferation, apoptosis, and differentiation. These processes are essential for all aspects of organ development through the regulation of lateral and inductive cell-cell signaling.

NOTCH proteins 1 through 4 are single transmembrane receptors that interact with membrane-bound NOTCH ligands (e.g., Delta-like ligands DLL1, DLL3, DLL4) and Serrate-like ligands (e.g., Jagged 1 [JAG1], Jagged 2 [JAG2]) on adjacent cells (Fig. 21.9). Ligand-receptor binding triggers proteolytic events; some are mediated by secretases, leading to the release of the Notch intracellular domain (NICD). When the NICD translocates to the nucleus, a series of intranuclear events induces the expression of hairy enhancer of split (HES), a helix-loop-helix (HLH) transcription factor that maintains the progenitor state by repressing proneural basic HLH genes.

The process of lateral inhibition ensures that in a population of cells with equivalent developmental potential, there are the correct numbers of two distinct cell types. In the initial cell-cell interaction, the progenitor cell responding to the NOTCH-ligand DELTA through a negative feedback mechanism reduces its own expression of DELTA, with NOTCH receptor signaling maintaining the cell as an uncommitted progenitor. However, the adjacent cell maintains DELTA expression levels with reduced Notch signaling and differentiation, mediated by, for example, proneural HLH genes. Inductive signaling with other surrounding cells expressing morphogens may overcome the cell's commitment to a neural cell fate (default state) to produce an alternative glial cell fate.

Understanding the function of the NOTCH-DELTA signaling pathway in mammalian development has been assisted by loss-of-function studies in the mouse. Evidence of *JAG1* or *NOTCH2* mutations in Alagille syndrome (arteriohepatic dysplasia), with liver, kidney, cardiovascular, ocular, and skeletal malformations, and *NOTCH3* gene mutations in the CADASIL (*c*erebral *a*utosomal *d*ominant *a*rteriopathy with *s*ubcortical *i*nfarcts and *l*eukoencephalopathy) adult vascular degenerative disease, with a tendency to early-age onset of stroke-like events, support the importance of the Notch signaling pathway in embryonic and postnatal development, respectively.

Pharmacologic manipulation of the Notch signaling pathway may be a means to treat human diseases. For example, gamma-secretase inhibitors (GSIs) have been studied

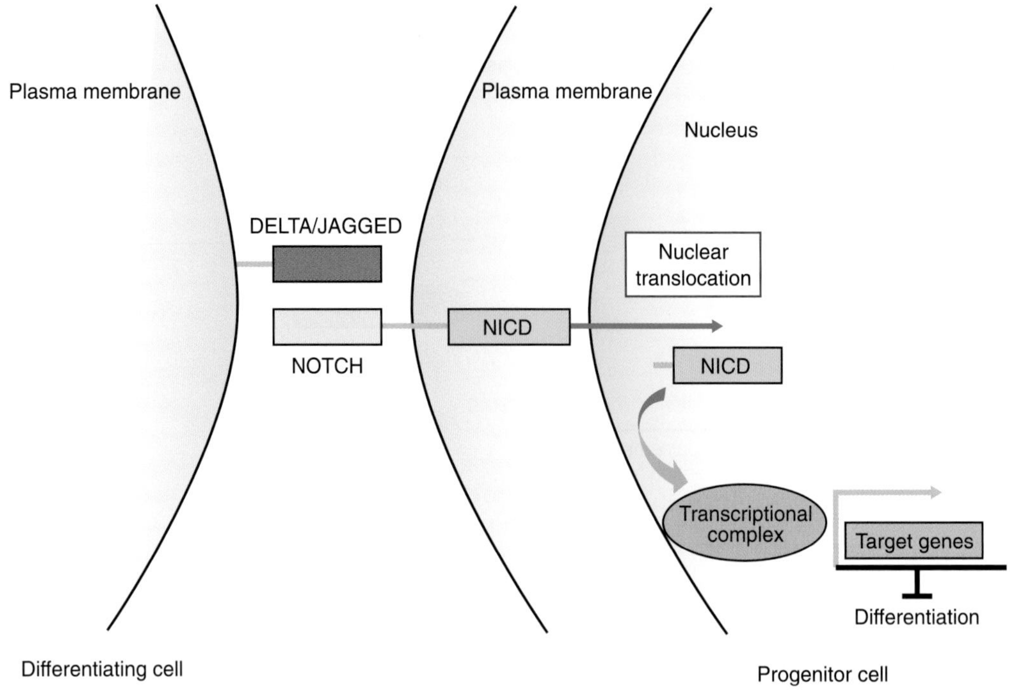

Fig. 21.9 NOTCH-DELTA signaling pathway in mammals. In progenitor cells *(right)*, activation of NOTCH signaling leads to cleavage of the NOTCH intracellular domain *(NICD)*. Proteases such as γ-secretase mediate this cleavage event. NICD translocates to the nucleus, binds to a transcriptional complex, and activates target genes, such as *HES1*, that inhibit differentiation. In differentiating cells *(left)*, NOTCH signaling is not active. *HES*, Hairy enhancer of split.

in clinical trials for such diverse disorders as Alzheimer disease, pulmonary hypertension, and cancer. For the former, gamma-secretase is also a protease required for the production of amyloid-β protein in the brain. Some of the GSIs under development are nonselective, whereas others spare the Notch signaling pathway. More recently, **ADAM** (*A Disintegrin And Metalloproteinases*) protease family members ADAM10 and ADAM17 have been implicated in organ system development and function, including the development of the brain and gastrointestinal tract. *Adam10* deficient mice have impaired Notch receptor cleavage and signaling. Also known as sheddins, ADAM10/17, which are anchored to the plasma membrane, have been considered drug targets for diverse disorders such as Alzheimer disease, inflammation, thrombosis, and cancer.

TRANSCRIPTION FACTORS

Transcription factors belong to a large class of proteins that regulate the expression of many target genes through activation or repression mechanisms. Typically, a transcription factor binds to specific nucleotide sequences in the promoter or enhancer regions of target genes and regulates the rate of transcription of its target genes by interacting with accessory proteins. Transcription factors can activate or repress target-gene transcription, depending on the cell in which they are expressed, the specific promoter, the chromatin context, and the developmental stage. Some transcription factors do not need to bind to DNA to regulate transcription but may bind to other transcription factors already bound to the promoter DNA, thereby regulating transcription. They also may bind and sequester other transcription factors from their target genes, repressing their transcription.

The transcription factor superfamily is composed of many classes of proteins. The **Forkhead** (FOX) transcription factors include more than 40 members that play diverse roles in development and disease. These proteins contain a forkhead box of 80 to 100 amino acids (winged helix) that bind specific DNA sequences. Other examples of this diverse family of proteins include the HOX (homeobox), PAX (paired homeobox), and basic HLH (bHLH) transcription factors.

HOX PROTEINS

Hox genes were first discovered in the fruit fly, *Drosophila melanogaster*. Mutations in these genes of the homeotic complex (HOM-C) lead to dramatic phenotypes (homeotic transformation), such as the *Antennapedia* gene in which legs instead of antennae sprout from the head of fruit flies. The order of the *Hox* genes along the anteroposterior axis is faithfully reproduced in their organization at the level of the chromosome. The order of the *Hox* genes along the anteroposterior axis and their chromosomal location are also conserved in humans. Defects in *HOXA1* have been shown to impair human neural development, and mutations in *HOXA13* and *HOXD13* result in limb malformations (see Chapter 16).

All of the *Hox* genes contain a 180-base pair (bp) sequence, the homeobox, which encodes a 60 amino acid homeodomain composed of three α helices. The third (recognition) helix binds to DNA sites that contain one or more TAAT or ATTA tetranucleotide-binding motifs in the promoters of their target genes. The homeodomain is the most conserved region of the protein and is highly conserved across evolution, whereas other regions of the protein are not as well conserved. Mutations in the DNA-binding region of the homeobox gene *NKX2-5* are associated with cardiac atrial-septal defects and mutations in *ARX* are associated with the central nervous system malformation syndrome lissencephaly (see Chapter 17).

PAX GENES

All *PAX* genes contain conserved bipartite DNA-binding motifs called the Pax (or paired) domain, and most PAX family members also contain a homeodomain. PAX proteins can activate and repress the transcription of target genes. The *D. melanogaster* ortholog of *Pax6*, *eyeless*, was shown to be essential for eye development because the homozygous mutant flies had no eyes. In gain-of-function experiments, ectopic expression of the eyeless led to the formation of additional eyes. In fruit flies, the *eyeless* is clearly a master regulator of eye development.

Eyeless shares a high degree of sequence conservation with its human ortholog *PAX6*. Mutant *PAX6* is associated with ocular malformations such as aniridia (absence of the iris) and Peter anomaly. In human eye diseases, the level of *PAX6* expression seems to be crucial because patients with only one functional copy (haploinsufficiency) have ocular defects, and patients without *PAX6* function are anophthalmic (see Chapter 18). This concept of haploinsufficiency is a recurring theme for many transcription factors and corresponding human malformations.

PAX3 and *PAX7* encode the homeodomain and DNA-binding domains. The human childhood cancer alveolar rhabdomyosarcoma results from a translocation that results in the formation of a chimeric protein in which PAX3 or PAX7 (including both DNA domains) is fused to the strong activating domains of the Forkhead family transcription factor FOXO1A. The autosomal dominant human disease Waardenburg syndrome type I results from mutations in the *PAX3* gene. Patients with this syndrome have hearing deficits, ocular defects (dystopia canthorum), and pigmentation abnormalities best typified by a white forelock.

BASIC HELIX-LOOP-HELIX TRANSCRIPTION FACTORS

The basic helix-loop-helix (bHLH) genes produce a class of transcription factors that determine cell fate and regulate differentiation in many different tissues during development. At a molecular level, bHLH proteins contain a basic (positively charged) DNA-binding region that is followed by two α helices that are separated by a loop. The α helices have a hydrophilic and a hydrophobic side (amphipathic). The hydrophobic side of the helix is a motif for protein-protein interactions among different members of the bHLH family. This domain is the most conserved region of the bHLH proteins across different species. The bHLH proteins often bind other bHLHs (heterodimerize) to regulate transcription. These heterodimers are composed of tissue-specific bHLH proteins bound to ubiquitously expressed bHLH proteins.

The powerful prodifferentiation effect of bHLH genes can be repressed by several mechanisms. For example, inhibitors of differentiation (Id) proteins are HLH proteins that lack the basic DNA-binding motif. When Id proteins heterodimerize with specific bHLH proteins, they prevent binding of the bHLH proteins to their target gene promoter sequences, called E-boxes. Growth factors, which tend to inhibit differentiation, increase the level of Id proteins that sequester bHLH proteins from their target promoters. Growth factors also can stimulate phosphorylation of the DNA-binding domain of bHLH proteins, which inhibits their ability to bind to DNA.

Expression of bHLH genes is crucial for the development of tissues such as muscle (myogenin *[MYOD]*) and neurons (neurogenin *[NEUROD]*) in humans (see Chapter 15). *MYOD* expression was shown to be sufficient to transdifferentiate several cell lines into muscle cells, demonstrating that it is a master regulator of muscle differentiation. Studies of knockout mice confirmed that *MyoD* and another bHLH gene, *Myf5*, were crucial for the differentiation of precursor cells into primitive muscle cells (myoblasts). Differentiation of these myoblasts into fully differentiated muscle cells is controlled by myogenin.

Mash1 (*ASCL1* in humans) and *Neurogenin1* (*NEUROD3* in humans) are proneural genes that regulate the formation of neuroblasts from the neuroepithelium (see Chapter 17). Mouse models have shown that these genes are crucial for the specification of different subpopulations of precursors in the developing central nervous system. For example, *Mash1*-knockout mice had defects in forebrain development, whereas *Neurogenin1*-knockout mice had defects in cranial sensory ganglia and ventral spinal cord neurons. Specification of these neuroblasts is regulated by other proneural genes known as *NeuroD* and *Math5* (*ATOH7* in humans). Muscle and neuronal differentiation (see Chapters 15 and 17) are controlled by a cascade of bHLH genes that function at early and late stages of cellular differentiation. Both differentiation pathways are inhibited by signaling through the Notch pathway.

EPIGENETICS

Understanding of the role of epigenetic modifications in regulating embryonic development has greatly expanded in recent years. **Epigenetics** is different from genetics in that it represents the study of heritable changes in the function of genes that cannot be explained by underlying changes in DNA sequence. This classic definition of epigenetics has expanded to include the study of modifications such as histone acetylation and phosphorylation, in which gene expression is impacted but the modifications are not necessarily inherited.

Four powerful mechanisms of epigenetic regulation are histone acetylation, histone methylation, DNA methylation, and miRNAs. These epigenetic marks (**epigenetic code**) are regulated by classes of enzymes that recognize the epigenetic marks (**readers**), add epigenetic markers to DNA or histone *(writers)*, or remove the epigenetic marks (**erasers**). Examples of epigenetic regulators are discussed subsequently and shown in Table 21.3.

Disorders of chromatin remodeling include Rett, Rubinstein-Taybi, and α-thalassemia/X-linked mental retardation syndromes and various cancers. In the laboratory, **ChIPseq** (chromatin immunoprecipitation coupled with DNA sequencing) and **RNAseq** (RNA sequencing), both

Table 21.3 Proteins Essential for the Regulation and Interpretation of Epigenetic Marks

Epigenetic Modification	Reader Protein	Writer Protein	Eraser Protein
Histone acetylation	Chromatin remodeling enzymes: SMARCA4 (formerly BRG1)	Histone acetyltransferases (HATs): E1A binding protein, 300 KD (EP300)	Histone deacetylases (HDACs): HDAC1
Histone methylation	Polycomb repressive complex: CBX2	Histone methylases (HMTs): EZH2	Histone demethylases: JARID1C
DNA methylation	MECP2	DNA methylases: DNMT1	Tet oncogene family members: methylcytosine dioxygenases (TET1)

bulk and single-cell RNAseq, are powerful high-throughput means to identify specific gene targets of transcription factors throughout the genome and assess patterns of gene expression altered during stages of development or in diseases such as cancer, including the detection of fusion gene transcripts, such as those involving FGFR and TRK receptor tyrosine kinases for which a new generation of targeted therapies are available in the clinic. Recent innovations include **ATAC-Seq** (assay for transposase-accessible chromatin with sequencing) that can be used to assess genomic regions of open and closed chromatin and modifications of ChIPseq known as **CUT & Run** (*C*leavage *U*nder *T*argets *&* *R*elease *U*sing *N*uclease) and **CUT & Tag** (*C*leavage *U*nder *T*argets and *Tag*mentation) that may be more versatile and require less cell or tissue input to assess protein-DNA interactions. Finally, **spatial transcriptomics** has revolutionized the localization of RNA transcripts far beyond in situ RNA hybridization and in situ PCR-based technologies that can assess the spatial expression of one or just a few genes in tissue sections. Current and emerging platforms will permit single-cell and single-nucleus RNAseq analysis of the whole genome in intact tissue sections obtained from model organisms or healthy and diseased tissues.

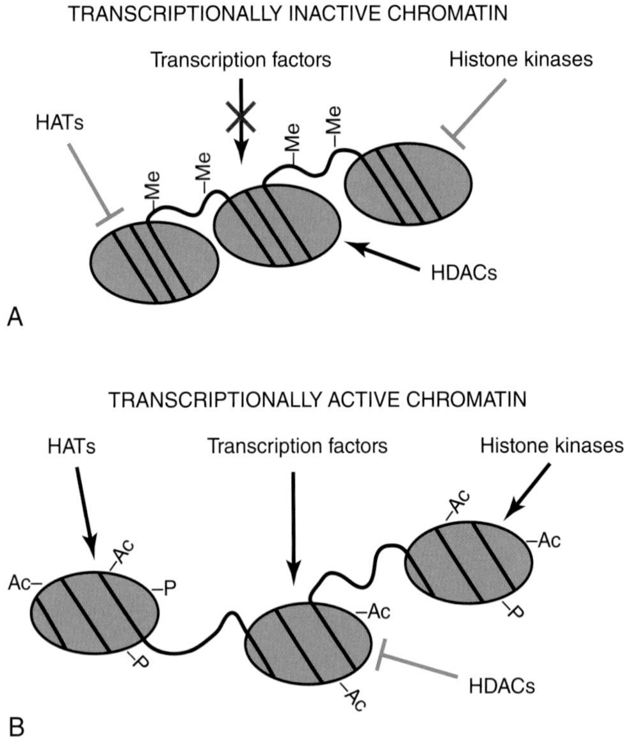

Fig. 21.10 Epigenetic modifications alter the transcriptional properties of chromatin. (A) In areas of transcriptionally inactive chromatin, the DNA is tightly bound to the histone cores. The histones are not acetylated or phosphorylated. Histone deacetylases *(HDACs)* are active, whereas histone acetyltransferases *(HATs)* and histone kinases are inactive. DNA is highly methylated *(-Me)*. (B) In areas of transcriptionally active chromatin, the DNA is not as tightly bound to the histone cores, and the DNA is unmethylated. The histone proteins are acetylated *(-Ac)* and phosphorylated *(-P)*. HDACs are inactive, whereas HATs and histone kinases are active.

HISTONES

Histones are the positively charged nuclear proteins around which genomic DNA is coiled in units of approximately 140 bp to tightly pack it in structures known as *nucleosomes* within the nucleus. Histone octamers consist of histone 2A, 2B, 3, and 4 subunits. Modification of these proteins is a common pathway by which transcription factors regulate the activity of their target promoters. Examples of histone modifications include phosphorylation, ubiquitinylation, sumoylation, acetylation, and methylation. The latter two modifications are discussed in more depth in the following sections.

HISTONE ACETYLATION

DNA is less tightly bound to acetylated histones, allowing more open access of transcription factors and other proteins to the promoters of their target genes. Histone acetylation status is controlled by genes such as histone acetyltransferases (HATs), which add acetyl groups (writers), and histone deacetylases (HDACs), which remove acetyl groups (erasers).

Transcription factors can modify histone acetylation by recruiting histone acetyltransferases or by recruiting histone deacetylases (Fig. 21.10). Reader proteins that bind to acetylated histones, such as the chromatin remodeling enzyme SMARCA4 (formerly BRG1), contain a protein structure called a *bromodomain*. Phosphorylation of histones also leads to an opening of the chromatin structure and activation of gene transcription.

HISTONE METHYLATION

Histone methyltransferases (HMTs), which are writer enzymes, catalyze the addition of a methyl group to lysine residues on histone tails. This modification is removed by histone demethylases (HDMs), which are eraser enzymes. In contrast to histone acetylation, methylation of histones can result in the addition of one, two, or three methyl groups to an individual lysine residue and the activation or repression of gene expression, depending on the particular lysine residue that is modified. For example, trimethylation of lysine 9 or lysine 27 on histone 3 (H3K9me3, H3K27me3) is associated with repressed promoters, whereas trimethylation of lysine 4 on histone 3 (H3K4me3) is associated with active promoters.

Histone methylation status is read by many different classes of proteins. Mutations of histone modification readers, writers, and erasers can lead to diseases such as neurodevelopmental disorders and cancer. The recent identification of mutations of the genes encoding histone variants H3.3 and H3.1, especially H3 K27M and H3 G34R/V, has contributed to our understanding of pediatric high-grade gliomas, especially diffuse midline gliomas incorporating diffuse intrinsic pontine gliomas.

DNA METHYLATION

In contrast to the dynamic mechanism of histone modifications, DNA methylation is used for the long-term repression of genes. Cytosine residues are rapidly methylated at GC dinucleotides after embryo implantation by DNA methyltransferases (writer enzymes). During embryonic development, pluripotency genes, which are expressed in embryonic stem cells, are repressed as the cells differentiate. Repression is maintained by methylation of these loci in differentiated cells. This methylation state is erased in the primordial germ cells to enable re-expression of pluripotency genes. DNA methylation is also used by the body for the effective repression of viral genomes that are integrated into our own. The repressive marks are not reset in the primordial germ cells and are inherited by the progeny.

In cancer, tumor suppressor genes are frequently inactivated by DNA methylation that allows uncontrolled cellular growth. Mutations in *MECP2*, which binds to methylated DNA (reader enzyme), result in the developmental disorder Rett syndrome. Several DNA demethylating agents, such as 5-azacytidine and decitabine, are being used clinically to treat various disorders, including cancer. These drugs, along with HDAC inhibitors such as valproic acid, are examples of epigenetic therapies. **DNA methylation profiling** of tumors, especially those of the central nervous system, has enabled more precise tumor diagnoses and led to the discovery of new tumor types incorporated in updated World Health Organization tumor classification systems.

MICRORNAS

MicroRNAs (miRNA or miRs) are highly conserved, short (22-nucleotide), noncoding RNAs that act posttranscriptionally to silence RNA. The biogenesis of miRNAs is complex and a highly regulated process (Fig. 21.11). After exportation to the cytoplasm, pre-miRNAs require a ribonuclease known as Dicer to become processed into mature miRNA duplexes. One miRNA strand is included in the RNA-induced silencing complex.

miRNAs target more than one-half of the genes expressed during development, and each miRNA specifically targets hundreds of genes. Although they are not considered classic epigenetic means to modify gene expression, such as DNA methylation and histone modifications, miRNAs also modify gene expression without changing the DNA sequence. The miRNAs fold over to form short hairpins, which can be distinguished from double-stranded RNA molecules.

Many diseases associated with miRNA dysregulation, including developmental syndromes and cancer, are included in the miR2Disease online database. Specific miRNAs associated with cancer are called **oncomirs**. Germline mutations of *DICER1* are associated with a familial tumor predisposition syndrome that includes several rare cancers such as pleuropulmonary blastema, cystic nephroma, and medulloepithelioma.

miRNA profiling is being developed as a prognostic biomarker for disease outcomes. Biotechnology has adopted the power of RNA interference to knock down the expression of specific RNA, and these methods are being introduced to the clinic as forms of miRNA therapy.

STEM CELLS: DIFFERENTIATION VERSUS PLURIPOTENCY

Stem cells (Fig. 21.12) have the property of self-renewal through symmetric (vertical) or asymmetric (horizontal) cell divisions. Under specific conditions in the embryo and adult, these totipotent or pluripotent cells can give rise to all of the differentiated cell types in the body. Several types of stem cell populations have been characterized: embryonic stem cells (ESCs), adult stem cells, and cancer stem cells (CSCs). ESCs, derived from the inner cell mass of the blastula, are **pluripotent** and can give rise to all differentiated cell types from the ectoderm, endoderm, and mesoderm (primary germ layers), but they do not contribute to extraembryonic tissues. ESCs express several transcription factors, such as SOX2 and OCT4, which repress differentiation.

Adult stem cells are found in relative abundance in differentiated tissues and organs that undergo rapid regeneration, such as the bone marrow, hair follicles, and the intestinal mucosal epithelium. However, there are nests of adult stem cells in many other tissues, including those that have been previously considered nonregenerative, such as the central nervous system and retina. These stem cell populations are small and located in the subventricular zone and ciliary margins, respectively. Hematopoietic stem cells derived from bone marrow, peripheral blood, and umbilical cord sources are routinely used to treat primary immunodeficiencies and various inherited metabolic disorders and as a rescue strategy after myeloablative cancer treatments.

CSCs have been under intense study since it became evident through the study of leukemias and solid tumors (e.g., colorectal cancer, malignant gliomas) that a small population of these cells, identified by various cell surface markers (e.g., CD133 in solid tumors), are often resistant to cancer treatments such as radiation or chemotherapy. Investigators are focusing their efforts on eradicating the CSC population in addition to standard therapies to produce higher cure rates.

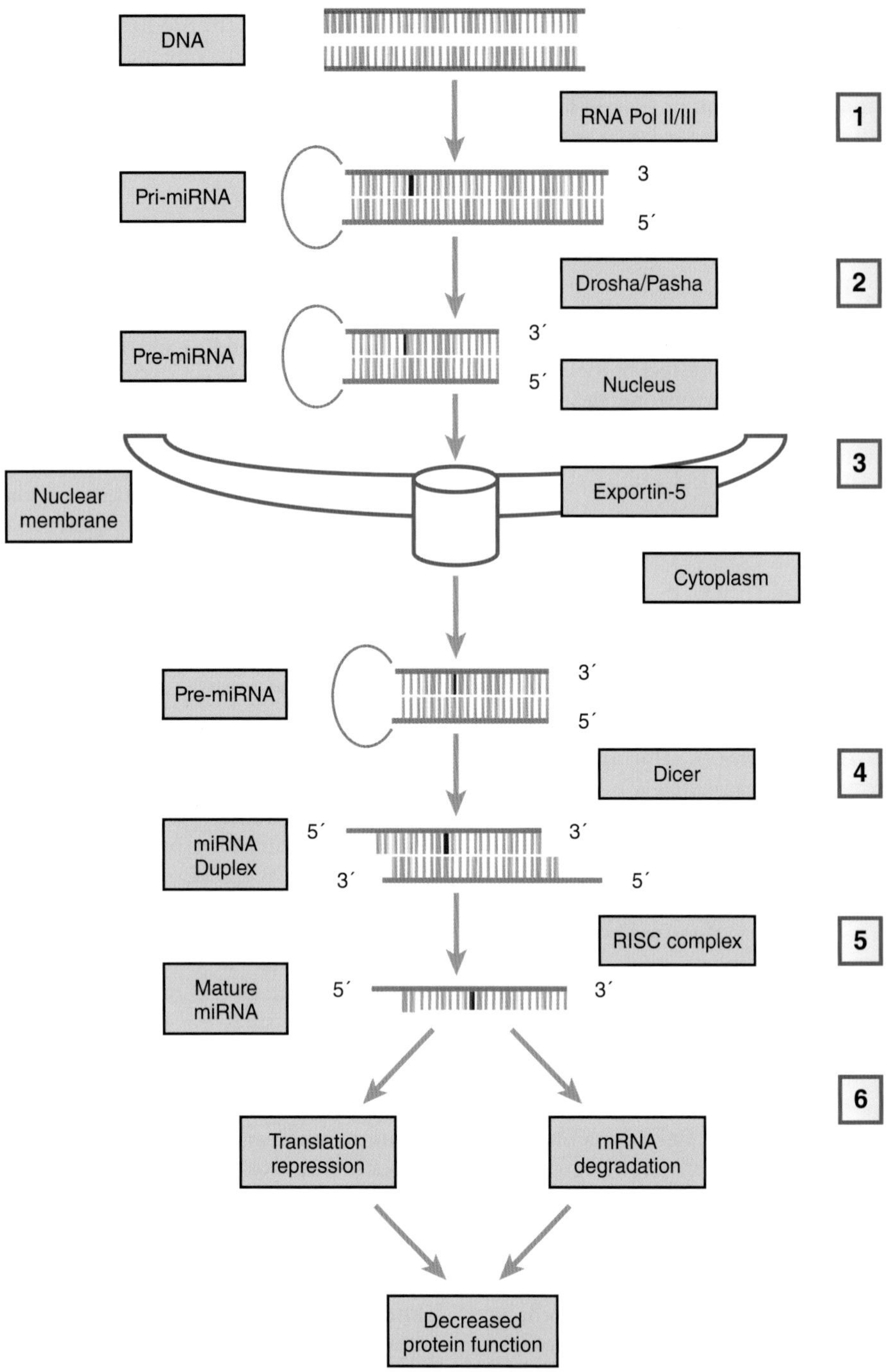

Fig. 21.11 MicroRNA (miRNA) biogenesis. Steps 1 and 2 occur in the nucleus, step 3 in the nuclear membrane, and steps 4-6 in the cytoplasm. (*1*) Through RNA polymerases II and III, DNA is converted to pri-miRNA. (*2*) Further processing by the microprocessor complex formed by the RNAse III enzyme, Drosha, and Pasha/DGCR8 cleaves pri-miRNA to pre-miRNA. (*3*) Exportin-5 facilitates the nuclear export of pre-miRNA to the cytoplasm. (*4*) Dicer, another RNAse III or endoribonuclease, processes the hairpin structure to generate miRNA duplexes. (*5*) The RISC complex enables the conversion of miRNA duplexes to mature miRNAs. (*6*) Subsequently, miRNAs can mediate either repression of translation or mRNA degradation, leading to decreased protein function. *DGCR8*, DiGeorge Syndrome Critical Region 8; *pre-miRNA*, precursor miRNA; *pri-miRNA*, primary miRNA; *RISC*, RNA-induced silencing complex.

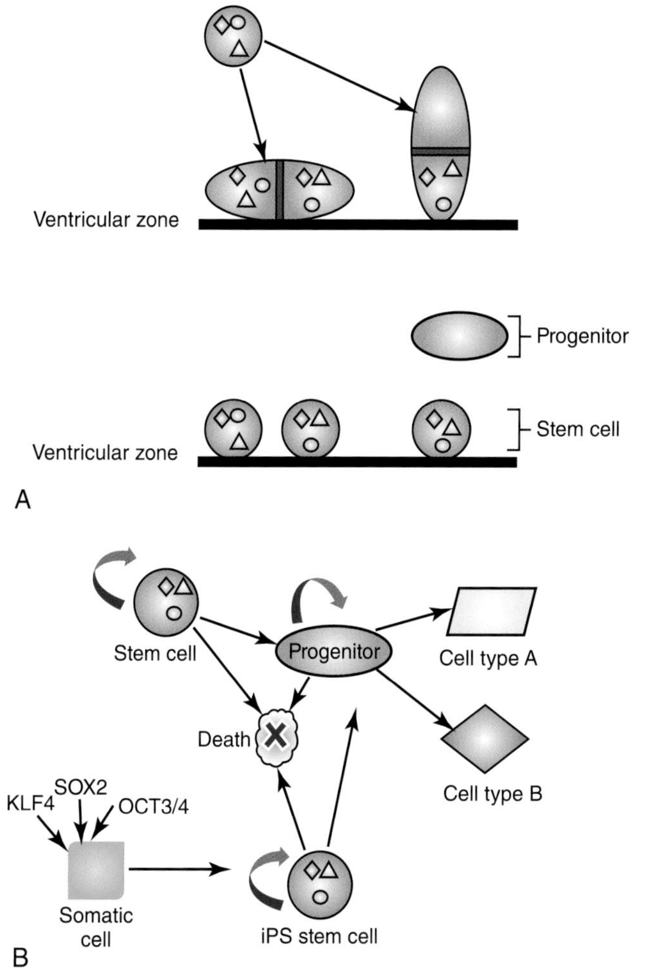

Fig. 21.12 Neural stem cells and induced pluripotent stem cells. (A) Adult or embryonic stem cells can divide symmetrically, giving rise to two equivalent daughter stem cells (vertical cell division; the plane of mitosis is perpendicular to the ventricular surface), or asymmetrically, giving rise to a daughter stem cell and a nervous system progenitor cell (horizontal cell division; the plane of mitosis is parallel to the ventricular surface). In this example, the progenitor cell does not retain the nuclear or cytoplasmic factors (colored geometric shapes) that remain in the stem cell; however, the progenitor cell expresses new proteins (e.g., receptor tyrosine kinases) in its plasma membrane. (B) Stem cells and induced pluripotent stem cells *(iPS)* have the capacity for self-renewal, cell death, and becoming progenitors. Progenitor cells have a more limited capacity for self-renewal, but they also can differentiate into various cell types or undergo cell death. Adult, differentiated somatic cells, such as skin fibroblasts, can be reprogrammed into iPS cells with the introduction of the master transcription factors SOX2, OCT3/4 (now called POU5F1), or KLF4.

The power of stem cells can be harnessed to repair degenerative disorders such as Parkinson disease and tissues severely damaged by ischemia (stroke) and trauma (spinal cord injury). Because researchers have been limited by the available sources of stem cells from embryos or adults, there has been tremendous interest in dedifferentiating adult somatic cells (e.g., epithelial cells, fibroblasts) to induce pluripotent stem cells (iPSC). Studies have identified several key master transcription factors (see Fig. 21.12B), such as *OCT4, SOX2, KLF4,* and *NANOG,* that can reprogram differentiated cells into pluripotent cells. A key step in this reprogramming event is the rewriting of the epigenetic code of the donor cells. Other studies have demonstrated the potential of **transdifferentiating** fibroblasts into neurons and cardiomyocytes in situ using tissue-specific combinations of transcription factors. These iPSCs can be manipulated using nonviral means of gene delivery, and they have the potential to treat most human diseases in which cell regeneration may restore structure and function. In addition, iPSC from human patients can be differentiated into different lineages in vitro (e.g., cardiomyocytes, neural cells, lung epithelial cells, etc.) to model the pathogenesis of human developmental disorders such as cystic fibrosis in a manner that facilitates screening with potential drug candidates. The application of the newly discovered CRISPR/*Cas* gene editing technology (see following discussion) has raised the possibility of deriving patient-specific iPSC, correcting the genetic defect in vitro, differentiating the cells into the required lineage, and then returning the corrected cells to the patient.

A recent advance in iPSC technologies has been the evolution of iPSC-derived tissue **organoids**, including heart, kidney, and specific regions of the brain. These three-dimensional (3D) structures are self-organizing and highly reproducible. Although many 3D tissue organoids have missing cell types (i.e., retinal ganglion cells in retinal organoids, microglia in cortical organoids) or an absent vasculature, tissue organoids permit the study of spatial organization and cell-cell interactions ex vivo, complementing studies using humans or intact model organisms, such as mice or zebrafish. Furthermore, tissue organoids can be used to model human disease and enable high-throughput drug compound or functional genomic screens.

GENE EDITING—THE POTENTIAL OF CRISPR/*CAS9* TECHNOLOGY

The study of embryonic development in mice has been enhanced by the development of technologies to specifically inactivate (knockout) or ectopically express genes of interest. However, these technologies have not been amenable for use in human cells or to alter gene expression in patients. This has led to the development of new approaches to specifically alter genomic DNA sequence (gene editing) in vitro and in vivo. Widespread use of early iterations of this technology, such as zinc finger nucleases or transcription activator–like effector nucleases (TALENs), was hampered by technical difficulties in the design, construction, and validation of individual reagents. In contrast, the *c*lustered *r*egularly *i*nterspaced *s*hort *p*alindromic *r*epeats (CRISPR)/*Cas9* endonuclease system is easy to use, modular in design, and highly specific and is being widely implemented. The CRISPR/*Cas9* system was discovered as a bacterial immune response to viral infections. The technology has been simplified to involve a single guide RNA that contains a 20-bp sequence that is complementary to the target genomic sequence and a double-stranded section that is bound by Cas9 and localizes the nuclease to the correct genomic location (Fig. 21.13). The guide RNA must contain a protospacer-adjacent motif sequence that is located at the 3' end of the targeting sequence that is used by Cas9 to bind DNA and cleave it. The specific double-strand break in genomic

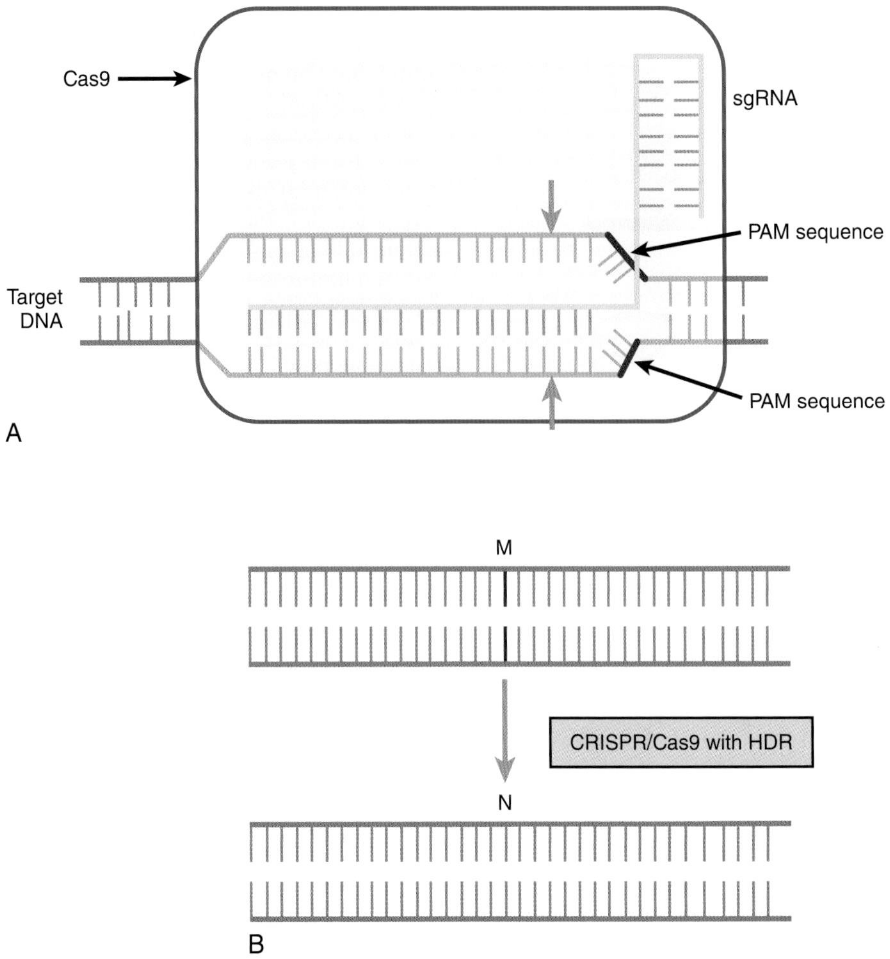

Fig. 21.13 Overview of the CRISPR/*Cas9* gene-editing system. (A) This editing system is modular and is composed of a single-stranded guide RNA *(sgRNA)* that has a region complementary to the target sequence in the genomic DNA and a stem structure that is required to localize the endonuclease Cas9, which cleaves both strands of the target DNA sequence. For DNA cleavage by Cas9 to occur, a protospacer-adjacent motif *(PAM)* sequence is required adjacent to the region to be cleaved *(blue arrows)*. (B) The resulting double-strand break can be repaired by nonhomologous end joining (NHEJ) or by homology-directed repair *(HDR)*. NHEJ results in deletions that can result in loss-of-function mutations. In contrast, HDR enables specific editing of a target sequence such as the conversion of a mutant allele *(M)* to the normal allele *(N)*.

DNA can be repaired either by nonhomologous end joining (NHEJ) or by homology-directed repair (HDR). NHEJ results in deletions that can result in missense mutations (frameshift/stop) being introduced. In contrast, HDR with the appropriate template can be used to correct genetic defects, introduce a putative disease-causing mutation, or incorporate a reporter gene into a specific locus. A nuclease related to Cas9, ***Cas12***, allows for large-scale functional genetic screens since Cas12 can effectively knockout out two different targets in a cell because it can use multiple guide RNAs encoded in a single transcript. This ability to knockout two genes in a cell allows for the identification of functional interactions between genes concerning a given cellular output such as survival or proliferation and to identify synthetic lethal interactions. The uptake of this gene-editing technology has been rapid; it has already been used to correct genetic defects in vivo in mice and ex vivo in humans and has enhanced the ability to model human developmental diseases in vitro. The therapeutic potential of this technology is very promising because it allows, for the first time, our ability to specifically alter the human genome to correct genetic defects. Genome editing using CRISPR/*Cas9* has also brought to the forefront several legal, social, and ethical concerns, given the multiple processes possible and the low cost.

SUMMARY OF COMMON SIGNALING PATHWAYS USED DURING DEVELOPMENT

- There are marked differences between the various signaling pathways, but they share many common features: ligands, membrane-bound receptors and coreceptors, intracellular signaling domains, adapters, and effector molecules.
- **Signaling pathways are co-opted at various times** during development for stem cell renewal, cell proliferation, migration, apoptosis, and differentiation.
- **Pathways have default settings** that result in the generation or maintenance of one cell fate rather than another.
- **Many genes and signaling pathways are highly conserved** throughout evolution. Orthologs of genes critical for invertebrate development (the nematode *Caenorhabditis elegans* and the fruit fly *D. melanogaster*) are found in

vertebrates, including zebrafish, mice, and humans, often as members of multigene families.

- Knowledge of gene function has been acquired by reverse genetics using model systems with loss-of-function or gain-of-function transgenic approaches and by forward genetics beginning with the description of abnormal phenotypes arising spontaneously in mice and humans and subsequent identification of the mutant gene.
- There is evidence of cross-talk among pathways. Communication among various signaling pathways facilitates our understanding of the far-reaching consequences of single gene mutations that result in malformation syndromes affecting the development of multiple organ systems or in cancers.

BIBLIOGRAPHY AND SUGGESTED READING

Alvarez-Buylla A, Ihrie RA: Sonic hedgehog signaling in the postnatal brain, *Semin Cell Dev Biol* 33:105, 2014.

Amakye D, Jagani Z, Dorsch M: Unraveling the therapeutic potential of the hedgehog pathway in cancer, *Nat Med* 19:1410, 2013.

Andersson ER, Lendahl U: Therapeutic modulation of notch signalling—are we there yet? *Nat Rev Drug Discov* 13:357, 2014.

Anzalone AV, Koblan LW, Liu DR: Genome editing with CRISPR–Cas nucleases, base editors, transposases and prime editors, *Nat Biotech* 38:824, 2020.

Aster JC: In brief: notch signalling in health and disease, *J Pathol* 232(1), 2014.

Bahubeshi A, Tischkowitz M, Foulkes WD: miRNA processing and human cancer: DICER1 cuts the mustard, *Sci Transl Med* 3, 2011. 111ps46.

Barriga EH, Mayor R: Embryonic cell-cell adhesion: a key player in collective neural crest migration, *Curr Top Dev Biol* 112:301, 2015.

Beets K, Huylebroeck D, Moya IM, et al: Robustness in angiogenesis: notch and BMP shaping waves, *Trends Genet* 29:140, 2013.

Benoit YD, Guezguez B, Boyd AL, et al: Molecular pathways: epigenetic modulation of Wnt/glycogen synthase kinase-3 signaling to target human cancer stem cells, *Clin Cancer Res* 20:5372, 2014.

Berdasco M, Esteller M: Genetic syndromes caused by mutations in epigenetic genes, *Hum Genet* 132:359, 2013.

Berindan-Neagoe I, Monroig Pdel C, Pasculli B, et al: MicroRNAome genome: a treasure for cancer diagnosis and therapy, *CA Cancer J Clin* 64:311, 2014.

Blake JA, Ziman MR: *Pax* genes: regulators of lineage specification and progenitor cell maintenance, *Development* 141:737, 2014.

Brafman D, Willert K: Wnt/β-catenin signaling during early vertebrate neural development, *Dev Neurobiol* 77:1239, 2017.

Capper D, Jones DTW, Sill M, et al: DNA methylation-based classification of central nervous system tumours, *Nature* 555(7697):469–474, 2018.

Castro DS, Guillemot F: Old and new functions of proneural factors revealed by the genome-wide characterization of their transcriptional targets, *Cell Cycle* 10:4026, 2011.

Christ A, Herzog K, Willnow TE: LRP2, an auxiliary receptor that controls sonic hedgehog signaling in development and disease, *Dev Dyn* 245:569, 2016.

Corsini NS, Knoblich JA: Human organoids: New strategies and methods for analyzing human development and disease, *Cell* 185(15):2756–2769, 2022.

Cuneo MJ, Mittag T: Oncogenic signaling of RTK fusions becomes more granular, *Mol Cell* 81:2504, 2021.

De Robertis EM: Spemann's organizer and the self-regulation of embryonic fields, *Mech Dev* 126:925, 2009.

Dekanty A, Milán M: The interplay between morphogens and tissue growth, *EMBO Rep* 12:1003, 2011.

Dhanak D, Jackson P: Development and classes of epigenetic drugs for cancer, *Biochem Biophys Res Commun* 455:58, 2014.

Doudna JA, Charpentier E: Genome editing. The new frontier of genome engineering with CRISPR-*Cas9*, *Science* 346(6213), 2014. 1258096.

Dubey A, Rose RE, Jones DR, Saint-Jeannet JP: Generating retinoic acid gradients by local degradation during craniofacial development: one cell's cue is another cell's poison, *Genesis* 56(2):e23091, 2018.

Gaarenstroom T, Hill CS: TGF-β signaling to chromatin: how smads regulate transcription during self-renewal and differentiation, *Semin Cell Dev Biol* 32:107, 2014.

Giannotta M, Trani M, Dejana E: VE-cadherin and endothelial adherens junctions: active guardians of vascular integrity, *Dev Cell* 26:441, 2013.

Goldman D: Regeneration, morphogenesis and self-organization, *Development* 141:2745, 2014.

Gier RA, Budinich KA, Evitt NH, et al: High-performance CRISPR-Cas12a genome editing for combinatorial genetic screening, *Nature Comm* 11:3455, 2020.

Guillot C, Lecuit T: Mechanics of epithelial tissue homeostasis and morphogenesis, *Science* 340:1185, 2013.

Gutierrez-Mazariegos J, Theodosiou M, Campo-Paysaa F, et al: Vitamin A: a multifunctional tool for development, *Semin Cell Dev Biol* 22:603, 2011.

Hendriks WJ, Pulido R: Protein tyrosine phosphatase variants in human hereditary disorders and disease susceptibilities, *Biochim Biophys Acta* 1832:1673, 2013.

Hori K, Sen A, Artavanis-Tsakonas S: Notch signaling at a glance, *J Cell Sci* 126(Pt 10):2135, 2013.

Imayoshi I, Kageyama R: bHLH factors in self-renewal, multipotency, and fate choice of neural progenitor cells, *Neuron* 82:9, 2014.

Inoue H, Nagata N, Kurokawa H, et al: iPS cells: a game changer for future medicine, *EMBO J* 33:409, 2014.

Izzi L, Lévesque M, Morin S, et al: Boc and gas1 each form distinct shh receptor complexes with ptch1 and are required for Shh-mediated cell proliferation, *Dev Cell* 20:788, 2011.

Jiang Q, Wang Y, Hao Y, et al: miR2Disease: a manually curated database for microRNA deregulation in human disease, *Nucleic Acids Res* 37:D98, 2009.

Kaya-Okur HS, Wu SJ, Codomo CA, et al: CUT&Tag for efficient epigenomic profiling of small samples and single cells, *Nat Commun* 10(1):1930, 2019.

Kim W, Kim M, Jho EH: Wnt/β-catenin signalling: from plasma membrane to nucleus, *Biochem J* 450:9, 2013.

Kotini M, Mayor R: Connexins in migration during development and cancer, *Dev Biol* 401:143, 2015.

Lam EW, Brosens JJ, Gomes AR, et al: Forkhead box proteins: tuning forks for transcriptional harmony, *Nat Rev Cancer* 13:482, 2013.

Lamouille S, Xu J, Derynck R: Molecular mechanisms of epithelial-mesenchymal transition, *Nat Rev Mol Cell Biol* 15:178, 2014.

Lancaster MA, Corsini NS, Wolfinger S, et al: Guided self-organization and cortical plate formation in human brain organoids, *Nat Biotechnol* 35(7):659–666, 2017.

Le Dréau G, Martí E: The multiple activities of BMPs during spinal cord development, *Cell Mol Life Sci* 70:4293, 2013.

Leung RF, George AM, Roussel EM, et al: Genetic regulation of vertebrate forebrain development by homeobox genes, *Front Neurosci* 16:843794, 2022.

Li CG, Eccles MR: PAX genes in cancer; friends or foes? *Front Genet* 3:6, 2012.

Lien WH, Fuchs E: Wnt some lose some: transcriptional governance of stem cells by Wnt/β-catenin signaling, *Genes Dev* 28:1517, 2014.

Lim J, Thiery JP: Epithelial-mesenchymal transitions: insights from development, *Development* 139:3471, 2012.

Lowe EK, Cuomo C, Voronov D, Arnone MI: Using ATAC-seq and RNA-seq to increase resolution in GRN connectivity, *Methods Cell Biol* 151:115–126, 2019.

MacGrogan D, Luxán G, de la Pompa JL: Genetic and functional genomics approaches targeting the notch pathway in cardiac development and congenital heart disease, *Brief Funct Genomics* 13:15, 2014.

Mackay A, Burford A, Carvalho D, et al: Integrated molecular meta-analysis of 1,000 pediatric high-grade and diffuse intrinsic pontine glioma, *Cancer Cell* 32(4):520, 2017.

Mallo M, Alonso CR: The regulation of *Hox* gene expression during animal development, *Development* 140:3951, 2013.

Mallo M, Wellik DM, Deschamps J: *Hox* genes and regional patterning of the vertebrate body plan, *Dev Biol* 344:7, 2010.

Manoranjan B, Venugopal C, McFarlane N, et al: Medulloblastoma stem cells: where development and cancer cross pathways, *Pediatr Res* 71(Pt 2):516, 2012.

Mašek J, Andersson ER: The developmental biology of genetic notch disorders, *Development* 144:1743, 2017.

Maze I, Noh KM, Soshnev AA, et al: Every amino acid matters: essential contributions of histone variants to mammalian development and disease, *Nat Rev Genet* 15:259, 2014.

Meijer DH, Kane MF, Mehta S, et al: Separated at birth? The functional and molecular divergence of OLIG1 and OLIG2, *Nat Rev Neurosci* 13:819, 2012.

Mo JS, Park HW, Guan KL: The hippo signaling pathway in stem cell biology and cancer, *EMBO Rep* 15:642, 2014.

Neben CL, Lo M, Jura N, Klein OD: Feedback regulation of RTK signaling in development, *Dev Biol*, 2017.

Nelson KN, Peiris MN, Meyer AN, et al: Receptor tyrosine kinases: translocation partners in hematopoietic disorders, *Trends in Mol Med* 23:59, 2017.

O'Brien P, Morin P Jr, Ouellette RJ, et al: The *Pax-5* gene: a pluripotent regulator of b-cell differentiation and cancer disease, *Cancer Res* 71:7345, 2011.

Park KM, Gerecht S: Harnessing developmental processes for vascular engineering and regeneration, *Development* 141:2760, 2014.

Pignatti E, Zeller R, Zuniga A: To BMP or not to BMP during vertebrate limb bud development, *Semin Cell Dev Biol* 32:119, 2014.

Rao A, Barkley D, França GS, Yanai I: Exploring tissue architecture using spatial transcriptomics, *Nature* 596(7871):211–220, 2021.

Reiter JF, Leroux MR: Genes and molecular pathways underpinning ciliopathies, *Nat Rev Mol Cell Biol* 18(9):533, 2017.

Rhinn M, Dollé P: Retinoic acid signalling during development, *Development* 139:843, 2012.

Roussel MF, Robinson GW: Role of MYC in medulloblastoma, *Cold Spring Harb Perspect Med* 3(11), 2013. a014308

Salma M, Andrieu-Soler C, Deleuze V, Soler E: High-throughput methods for the analysis of transcription factors and chromatin modifications: Low input, single cell and spatial genomic technologies, *Blood Cells Mol Dis* 101:102745, 2023.

Sánchez Alvarado A, Yamanaka S: Rethinking differentiation: stem cells, regeneration, and plasticity, *Cell* 157:110, 2014.

Scadden DT: Nice neighborhood: emerging concepts of the stem cell niche, *Cell* 157:41, 2014.

Schlessinger J: Receptor tyrosine kinases: legacy of the first two decades, *Cold Spring Harb Perspect Biol* 6(3), 2014. a008912

Shah N, Sukumar S: The hox genes and their roles in oncogenesis, *Nat Rev Cancer* 10:361, 2010.

Shashikant T, Ettensohn CA: Genome-wide analysis of chromatin accessibility using ATAC-seq, *Methods Cell Biol* 151:219–235, 2019.

Shearer KD, Stoney PN, Morgan PJ, et al: A vitamin for the brain, *Trends Neurosci* 35:733, 2012.

Sotomayor M, Gaudet R, Corey DP: Sorting out a promiscuous superfamily: towards cadherin connectomics, *Trends Cell Biol* 24:524, 2014.

Steffen PA, Ringrose L: What are memories made of? How polycomb and trithorax proteins mediate epigenetic memory, *Nat Rev Mol Cell Biol* 15:340, 2014.

Tee WW, Reinberg D: Chromatin features and the epigenetic regulation of pluripotency states in ESCs, *Development* 141:2376, 2014.

Thompson JA, Ziman M: Pax genes during neural development and their potential role in neuroregeneration, *Prog Neurobiol* 95:334, 2014.

Torres-Padilla ME, Chambers I: Transcription factor heterogeneity in pluripotent stem cells: a stochastic advantage, *Development* 141:2173, 2014.

Vanan MI, Underhill DA, Eisenstat DD: Targeting epigenetic pathways in the treatment of pediatric diffuse (high grade) gliomas, *Neurother* 14:274–283, 2017.

Verstraete K, Savvides SN: Extracellular assembly and activation principles of oncogenic class III receptor tyrosine kinases, *Nat Rev Cancer* 12:753, 2012.

Wilkinson G, Dennis D, Schuurmans C: Proneural genes in neocortical development, *Neuroscience* 253:256, 2013.

Willaredt MA, Tasouri E, Tucker KL: Primary cilia and forebrain development, *Mech Dev* 130:373, 2013.

Wu MY, Hill CS: Tgf-beta superfamily signaling in embryonic development and homeostasis, *Dev Cell* 16:329, 2009.

Yan F, Powell DR, Curtis DJ, Wong NC: From reads to insight: a hitchhiker's guide to ATAC-seq data analysis, *Genome Biol* 21(1):22, 2020.

Yang Y, Oliver G: Development of the mammalian lymphatic vasculature, *J Clin Invest* 124:888, 2014.

Zagozewski JL, Zhang Q, Pinto VI, et al: The role of homeobox genes in retinal development and disease, *Dev Biol* 393:195, 2014.

Discussion of Clinically Oriented Problems

APPENDIX

CHAPTER 1

1. The secondary sexual characteristics develop, reproductive functions begin, and sexual dimorphism becomes more obvious during puberty. In females, the age of presumptive puberty is after 8 years, with the process largely completed by 16 years. In males, the age of presumptive puberty is after 9 years, with the process largely completed by 18 years.
2. **Embryology** refers to the study of embryonic development; clinically, it refers to embryonic and fetal development and the study of prenatal development. **Teratology** refers to the study of abnormal embryonic and fetal development. It is concerned with birth defects and their causes. Embryologic and teratologic studies apply to clinical studies because they indicate vulnerable prenatal periods of development.
3. All of the terms refer to female sexual cells. The term ***ovum*** is imprecise because it is applied to stages from the oocyte to the implanting blastocyst. The term *ovule* is used for the oocyte of mammals (e.g., vertebral animals). A **gamete** refers to any germ cell, whether an oocyte or a sperm. The term **oocyte** is the internationally preferred term in reference to humans.

CHAPTER 2

1. Numeric changes in chromosomes arise chiefly from **nondisjunction** during mitotic or meiotic cell division. Most clinically important abnormalities in chromosome number develop during the first meiotic division. Nondisjunction is the failure of double-chromatid chromosomes to dissociate during anaphase of cell division. As a result, both chromosomes pass to the same daughter cell, and trisomy results. **Trisomy 21** (Down syndrome) is the most common numeric chromosomal disorder resulting in birth defects. This syndrome occurs approximately once in every 700 births in females 25 to 29 years of age in the United States; however, it is more common in older mothers.
2. A **morula** with an extra set of chromosomes in its cells is called a **triploid embryo**. This chromosome abnormality usually results from the fertilization of an oocyte by two sperms **(dispermy)**. A fetus could develop from a triploid morula and be born alive; however, this is unusual. Most triploid fetuses abort spontaneously; if born alive, triploid neonates die within a few days (see Fig. 20.10).
3. Blockage of the uterine tubes resulting from infection is a major cause of infertility in females. Because occlusion prevents the oocyte from contacting the sperm, fertilization cannot occur. Infertility in males usually results from defects in spermatogenesis. Nondescent of the testes is one cause of **aspermatogenesis** (failure of sperm formation); however, normally positioned testes may also not produce adequate numbers of actively motile sperm.
4. **Mosaicism** results from the nondisjunction of double-chromatid chromosomes during the early **cleavage** of a zygote rather than during gametogenesis. As a consequence, the embryo has two cell lines with different chromosome numbers. Approximately 1–2% of persons with Trisomy 21 (Down syndrome) have mosaic Trisomy 21 syndrome. They have relatively mild stigmata of the syndrome and have a lesser degree of cognitive deficits. Mosaicism can be detected before birth by cytogenetic studies after **amniocentesis** or **chorionic villus sampling**.
5. **Emergency contraception** (morning-after pills) commonly contain a progestin hormone called levonorgestrel, and if used within 5 days after unprotected sexual intercourse, they prevent pregnancy, by interfering with the function of the corpus luteum and inhibiting or delaying ovulation.
6. Many early embryos are spontaneously aborted; the overall early spontaneous abortion rate is approximately 45%. A common cause of early spontaneous abortion is the presence of **chromosomal abnormalities**, such as those resulting from nondisjunction.
7. It has been reported that one in eight women and one in ten men may be infertile. **Male infertility** may result from endocrine disorders, abnormal spermatogenesis, or blockage of a genital duct. First, Jerry's semen should be evaluated **(sperm analysis)**. The total number, motility, and morphologic characteristics of the sperms in the ejaculate are assessed in cases of male infertility. A male with fewer than 10 million sperms per milliliter of semen is likely to be sterile, especially when the specimen of semen contains immotile and morphologically abnormal sperms.

CHAPTER 3

1. Yes, a chest radiograph may be taken because the patient's uterus and ovaries would not be directly in the x-ray beam. The only radiation that the ovaries receive would be a negligible amount from scattering. Furthermore, this small amount of radiation would be highly unlikely to damage the products of conception if the patient happened to be pregnant.
2. Implantation is regulated by a delicate balance between estrogen and progesterone. The large doses of estrogen

would upset this balance. Progesterone makes the endometrium grow thicker and more vascular so that the blastocyst may become embedded and adequately nourished. When media commentators refer to the "abortion pill," they are usually referring to RU486 (mifepristone). This drug interferes with the implantation of a blastocyst by blocking the production of progesterone by the corpus luteum. Early pregnancy tests are sensitive enough to detect levels of human chorionic gonadotropin (hCG) 6 days before a missed menstrual period. The accuracy of such a test varies from approximately 76% when done 6 days before a missed period to 99% when carried out on the first day of the missed period. Early pregnancy can also be detected by **ultrasonography**.

3. More than 95% of ectopic pregnancies are in the uterine tube, and 60% of those are in the ampulla. **Endovaginal sonography** is often used to detect ectopic tubal pregnancies. The surgeon would likely perform a laparoscopic (minimally invasive) surgical procedure to remove the uterine tube containing the ectopic conceptus.
4. No, the surgery would not have produced the defect in the brain. Exposure of an embryo during the second week of development to the slight trauma that might be associated with abdominal surgery would not cause a birth defect. Furthermore, the anesthetics used during the operation would not induce a defect in the brain. Maternal exposure to teratogens during the first 2 weeks of development will not induce birth defects, but the conceptus may spontaneously abort.
5. Females older than 40 years of age have a higher risk of having a baby with a birth defect, such as Trisomy 21 (Down syndrome). Prenatal diagnosis will tell whether the embryo has severe chromosomal abnormalities that could cause its death shortly after birth. Ultrasound examination of the embryo may also be performed for the detection of certain morphologic anomalies (e.g., defects of the limbs and central nervous system). In most cases, the embryo is normal, and the pregnancy continues to full term.

CHAPTER 4

1. The hormones in contraceptive pills prevent ovulation and development of the luteal (secretory) stage of the menstrual cycle and have not been shown to increase spontaneous abortion of birth defects. Severe chromosomal abnormalities likely caused the spontaneous abortion. After discontinuing oral contraceptives, most women have a return to normal menstrual cycling in 1–3 months and most are able to get pregnant within one year.
2. A highly sensitive **radioimmune test** would likely indicate that the female was pregnant. The presence of embryonic and/or chorionic tissue in the endometrial remnants would be an absolute sign of pregnancy. By 5 days after the expected menses (approximately 5 weeks after the start of the last normal menstrual period), the embryo would be in the third week of its development. The embryo would be approximately 2 mm in diameter and could be detected with **transvaginal ultrasound techniques**.
3. The central nervous system (brain and spinal cord) begins to develop during the third embryonic week. **Meroencephaly**, in which most of the brain and calvaria are absent, may result from environmental teratogens acting during the third week of development. This severe defect of the brain occurs because of the failure of the cranial part of the neural tube to develop normally, which usually results from the nonclosure of the rostral neuropore. The physician might explain that there is no known safe amount or safe time to drink alcohol during pregnancy and that she should refrain from drinking further alcohol to minimize additional risk.
4. **Sacrococcygeal teratomas** are the most common tumor in the newborn and arise from remnants of the primitive streak. Because cells from the primitive streak are pluripotent (may affect more than one organ or tissue), the tumors contain various types of tissue derived from all three germ layers in varying stages of development. These tumors are three to four times more frequent in females than in males.
5. **Transvaginal (endovaginal) sonography** is an important technique for assessing pregnancy late in the third week and during the fourth week because the conceptus (embryo and membranes) can be visualized. It is therefore possible to determine whether the embryo is developing normally. A negative pregnancy test in the third week does not rule out an ectopic pregnancy. The serum **human chorionic gonadotrophin** (hCG) assay is the basic element of pregnancy tests and early diagnosis of an ectopic pregnancy, but because ectopic pregnancies produce hCG at a slower rate than intrauterine pregnancies, the test may be inaccurate.

CHAPTER 5

1. The physician would likely tell the patient that her baby was undergoing a critical stage of development and that it would be best for her to stop smoking. The physician would also likely tell her that heavy cigarette smoking is known to cause **intrauterine growth restriction** and **low birth rate** and that the incidence of **prematurity** increases with the number of cigarettes that are smoked. The physician would also recommend that she not consume alcohol (individuals who smoke are more likely to use alcohol) during her pregnancy because of its known teratogenic effects (see Fig. 20.22).
2. One cannot necessarily predict how a drug will affect the human embryo because human and animal embryos may differ in their response to drugs; for example, **thalidomide** is extremely teratogenic to human embryos, but it has very little effect on some experimental animals, such as rats and mice. However, drugs known to be strong **teratogens** in animals should not be used during human pregnancy, especially during the embryonic period. The germ layers form during gastrulation. All tissues and organs of the embryo develop from the three germ layers: ectoderm, mesoderm, and endoderm.
3. Information about the starting date of a pregnancy may be unreliable because it depends on the patient's recall of an event (last menses) that occurred 2 or 3 months earlier. In addition, she may have had breakthrough

bleeding at the time of her last normal menstrual period and may have thought that it was light menses. **Transvaginal** (**endovaginal**) ultrasound at 4 to 6 weeks of gestation may be carried out for estimating the probable starting date of a pregnancy and embryonic age.

4. Taking a sleeping pill may not harm the embryo, but a physician should be consulted about any medications. To cause severe limb defects, a known teratogenic drug would have to act during the critical period of limb development (24–36 days after fertilization). Teratogens interfere with the differentiation of tissues and organs, often disrupting or arresting the embryo's normal development.

CHAPTER 6

1. Physicians cannot always rely on information about the time of the last normal menstrual period provided by their patients. This is especially important in cases in which determination of fertilization age is important, for example, in **high-risk pregnancies** in which expedient induction of labor may be required. The expected date of delivery can be determined with reasonable accuracy by using **diagnostic ultrasonography** to measure the size of the fetal head and abdomen.
2. Chorionic villus sampling would likely be performed for the study of the fetal chromosomes. Also, isolation of fetal cells in maternal blood for DNA-based fetal testing may also be used. The most common chromosomal disorder detected in fetuses of females older than 40 years of age is trisomy 21 (Down syndrome). If the fetal chromosomes were normal but birth defects of the brain or limbs were suspected, **ultrasonography** would likely be performed. These methods allow one to look for **morphologic abnormalities** while scanning the entire fetus. The sex of the fetus could be determined by examining the sex chromosomes in cells obtained by chorionic villus sampling. At 10 or more weeks, the obstetric radiologist can determine fetal sex using ultrasonography.
3. There is considerable danger when uncontrolled drugs (over-the-counter drugs), such as aspirin and cough medicines, are consumed excessively or indiscriminately by pregnant females. **Withdrawal seizures** have been reported in infants born to mothers who are heavy drinkers. **Fetal alcohol syndrome** is present in some of these infants (see Fig. 20.17). The physician would likely tell the patient not to take any drugs that are not prescribed. Drugs that are most detrimental to her fetus are under legal control and are prescribed with great care.
4. Many factors (fetal, maternal, and environmental) may reduce the rate of fetal growth (intrauterine growth retardation). Examples of such factors are intrauterine infections, multiple pregnancies, and chromosomal abnormalities. Cigarette smoking, narcotic addiction, and consumption of large amounts of alcohol are also well-established causes of intrauterine growth retardation. For the general well-being of the fetus a mother consults her doctor frequently; eats a good-quality diet; and does not use illicit drugs, smoke, or drink alcohol.
5. Amniocentesis is relatively devoid of risk. The chance of inducing an abortion is estimated to be approximately 0.5% to 1.0%. Chorionic villus sampling can also be used for obtaining cells for chromosome study. In *percutaneous umbilical cord blood sampling*, a needle is inserted into the umbilical vein with the guidance of ultrasonography. Chromosome and hormone studies can be performed with the blood obtained.
6. **Alpha-fetoprotein** is produced by the yolk sac, gut, and hepatic cells of the fetus. **Neural tube defects** (spina bifida and anencephaly) are indicated by *high levels of alpha-fetoprotein*. Diagnostic studies during the second trimester for chromosomal disorders would be done to monitor the levels of alpha-fetoprotein. Further studies and confirmation could be done using ultrasonography. *Low levels of alpha-fetoprotein may indicate Trisomy 21(Down syndrome)*. Chromosome studies may also be done to check the chromosome complement of the fetal cells.

CHAPTER 7

1. **Polyhydramnios** is an excessive amount of amniotic fluid that surrounds the fetus in the amniotic sac. This condition occurs in 1% to 2% of pregnancies. When it occurs over the course of a few days, there is an associated high risk of severe fetal birth defects, especially of the central nervous system (e.g., **meroencephaly** and **spina bifida cystica**). Fetuses with gross brain defects do not ingest the usual amounts of amniotic fluid; hence, the amount of liquid increases. **Atresia** (blockage) of the esophagus is almost always accompanied by polyhydramnios because the fetus cannot swallow and absorb amniotic fluid. Twinning or a multiple pregnancy is also a predisposing cause of polyhydramnios.
2. There is a tendency for twins to "run in families." It appears unlikely that there is a genetic factor in monozygotic twinning, but a disposition to dizygotic twinning is genetically determined. The frequency of dizygotic twinning increases sharply with maternal age up to 35 years and then decreases; however, the frequency of monozygotic twinning is affected very little by the age of the mother. Determination of twin zygosity can usually be made by examining the placenta and fetal membranes. One can later determine zygosity by looking for genetically determined similarities and differences in a twin pair. Differences in DNA studies prove that twins are dizygotic.
3. A **single umbilical artery** occurs in approximately 1 of every 200 umbilical cords. This abnormality is accompanied by a 15% to 20% incidence of cardiovascular abnormalities and other anomalies. A single artery can also be associated with chromosomal anomalies (trisomy 21, trisomy 18, and trisomy 13).
4. Two zygotes were fertilized. The resulting blastocysts implanted close together, and the placentas fused. The sample of chorionic villi was obtained from the chorionic sac of the female twin. If two chorionic sacs had been observed during ultrasonography, dizygotic twinning would have been suspected.
5. **Amniotic bands** form when the amnion tears and delaminates during pregnancy. The fibrous, sticky bands surround and entangle parts of the embryo's body and produce birth defects, such as the absence of a hand or

deep grooves in a limb. This constitutes the **amniotic band syndrome** or the **amniotic band disruption complex**. An alternative causative theory for effects associated with amniotic band syndrome is developmental vascular disruption (reduced blood supply).

CHAPTER 8

1. A diagnosis of **congenital diaphragmatic hernia** (CDH) is most likely. The birth defect in the diaphragm that produces this hernia usually results from failure of the left pericardioperitoneal canal to close during the sixth week of development; consequently, herniation of the intestinal loops into the thorax occurs. This compresses the lungs, especially the left one, and results in respiratory distress. The diagnosis can be established by a radiographic or sonographic examination of the chest. The defect can also be detected prenatally using ultrasonography. Characteristically, there are air- or fluid-filled loops of the intestine in the left hemithorax of a neonate with CDH.
2. Pericardial sac defects are extremely rare and are caused by a failure in the formation of the pleuropericardial membrane that separates the pericardial cavity from the peritoneal cavity. This defect can be on one or both sides. The intestine may herniate into the pericardial sac, or, conversely, the heart may be displaced into the superior part of the peritoneal cavity.
3. **Congenital diaphragmatic hernia (CDH)** occurs in approximately 1 of every 2200 births. A neonate diagnosed with CDH would immediately be positioned with the head and thorax higher than the abdomen to facilitate inferior displacement of the abdominal organs from the thorax. After a period of preoperative stabilization, an operation is performed with a reduction of the abdominal viscera and closure of the diaphragmatic defect. Neonates with CDH may die because of severe respiratory distress from poor development of the lungs. However, most infants with this condition survive as a result of improvements in ventilator care.
4. **Gastroschisis** and epigastric hernias occur in the median plane of the epigastric region; these hernias are uncommon, occurring once in every 2000 births. The defect, usually on the right side of the umbilicus, results from the failure of the lateral body folds to fuse in this region during the fourth week of gestation. Herniation of the intestinal loops and other abdominal structures may occur through the opening.

CHAPTER 9

1. The most likely diagnosis is a cervical (branchial) sinus or **cervical cyst**. When the sinus is infected, mucoid material is intermittently discharged. The external cervical sinus is a remnant of the second pharyngeal groove, cervical sinus, or both. Normally, the groove and sinus disappear as the second pharyngeal arch grows caudally over the third and fourth arch, forming the neck. Diagnostic imaging (sonography, magnetic resonance imaging [MRI], computed tomography [CT]) is used for the diagnosis of this disorder.
2. The position of the inferior parathyroid glands varies. They develop in close association with the thymus and are carried caudally with it during its descent through the neck. If the thymus fails to descend to its usual position in the superior mediastinum, one or both inferior parathyroid glands may be located near the bifurcation of the common carotid artery. If an inferior parathyroid gland does not separate from the thymus, it may be carried into the superior mediastinum with the thymus.
3. The patient very likely has a **thyroglossal duct cyst** that arose from a small remnant of the embryonic thyroglossal duct. When complete degeneration of this duct does not occur, a cyst may form from it anywhere along the median plane of the neck between the foramen cecum of the tongue and the jugular notch in the manubrium of the sternum. A thyroglossal duct cyst may be confused with an ectopic thyroid gland, such as one that has not descended to its normal position in the neck. A thyroglossal duct cyst is usually diagnosed clinically and can be confirmed by sonography, CT, or MRI.
4. Although some people still use the colloquial term harelip, it is inaccurate. Harelip refers to hares or rabbits that *normally* have partially median split upper lips. A median cleft lip in humans is a rare defect. The two major groups of cleft lip in humans are unilateral and bilateral. Unilateral cleft lip results from the failure of the maxillary prominence on the affected side to fuse with the medial nasal prominences. Clefting of the maxilla anterior to the incisive fossa results from failure of the lateral palatine process to fuse with the median palatine process (primary palate). Between 60% and 80% of persons who have a cleft lip with or without a cleft palate are males. When both parents are normal and have had one child with a cleft lip, the chance that the next infant will have the same lip defect is approximately 4%.
5. There is substantial evidence that anticonvulsant drugs such as phenytoin or diphenylhydantoin given to females with epilepsy during pregnancy increase the incidence of cleft lip and cleft palate by twofold to threefold compared with the incidence in the general population. Multiple genes with variable expression are thought to cause orofacial clefts.

CHAPTER 10

1. The inability to pass a catheter through the esophagus into the stomach indicates **esophageal atresia**. Because this birth defect is commonly associated with tracheoesophageal fistula, the pediatrician would suspect this defect. A radiographic examination would demonstrate the atresia. The presence of this defect would be confirmed by imaging the **nasogastric tube** arrested in the proximal esophageal pouch. If necessary, a small amount of water soluable contrast agent would be injected into the tube. When a certain type of tracheoesophageal fistula is present, there would also be air in the stomach that passed to it from a connection between the esophagus and the trachea. A combined radiographic, endoscopic, and surgical approach would usually be used to detect and repair a tracheoesophageal fistula.
2. An infant with **respiratory distress syndrome** (RDS) tries to overcome the ventilatory problem by increasing the

rate and depth of respiration. Clinically, cyanosis; rapid or shallow breathing; intercostal, subcostal, and sternal retractions; and nasal flaring are prominent signs of respiratory distress. RDS is a leading cause of respiratory distress syndrome and death in live-born, premature neonates. A deficiency of pulmonary **surfactant** is associated with RDS. Glucocorticoid treatment may be given during pregnancy to accelerate fetal lung development and surfactant production. The use of nasal continuous positive airway pressure improves alveolar ventilation.

3. The most common type of **tracheoesophageal fistula** connects the trachea to the inferior part of the esophagus. This birth defect is associated with atresia of the esophagus superior to the fistula. A tracheoesophageal fistula results from incomplete division of the foregut by the tracheoesophageal septum into the esophagus and trachea.
4. In most types of tracheoesophageal fistula, air passes from the trachea through the tracheoesophageal fistula into the esophagus and stomach. **Pneumonitis** (pneumonia) resulting from the aspiration of oral and nasal secretions into the lungs is a serious complication of this birth defect. Giving the baby water or food by mouth is obviously contraindicated in such cases.

CHAPTER 11

1. The complete absence of a lumen **(duodenal atresia)** may involve the second (descending) and third (horizontal) parts of the duodenum. A vascular theory for duodenal atresia has also been proposed, in which a damaged blood supply to the duodenum may cause obstruction. The obstruction leads to distention of the stomach and proximal duodenum because the neonate swallows air, mucus, and milk. Duodenal atresia is common in infants with Trisomy (Down) syndrome, as are other severe birth defects such as annular pancreas, cardiovascular abnormalities, malrotation of the midgut, and anorectal anomalies. **Polyhydramnios** occur because the duodenal atresia prevents normal absorption of amniotic fluid from the fetal intestine distal to the obstruction. The fetus swallows amniotic fluid before birth; however, because of duodenal atresia, this fluid cannot pass along the intestine, be absorbed into the fetal circulation, and be transferred across the placental membrane into the mother's circulation, from which it would enter her urine.
2. The **omphaloenteric duct** normally undergoes complete involution by the 10th week of development, at which time the intestines return to the abdomen. In 2% to 4% of people, a remnant of the duct persists as an **ileal diverticulum** (Meckel diverticulum); however, only a small number of these defects ever become symptomatic. Remnants of the omphaloenteric duct can result in fistulas, sinus tracts, cysts, congenital bands, and mucosal remnants. In the present case, the entire duct persisted, so the diverticulum was connected to the anterior abdominal wall and umbilicus by a sinus tract. Its external opening may be confused with a **granuloma** (inflammatory lesion) of the stump of the umbilical cord.
3. The fistula was likely connected to the blind end of the rectum. The defect**, imperforate anus** with a rectovaginal fistula, results from failure of the urorectal septum to form a complete separation of the anterior and posterior parts of the urogenital sinus. Because the inferior one-third of the vagina forms from the anterior part of the urogenital sinus, it joins the rectum, which forms from the posterior part of the sinus.
4. This defect is an **omphalocele**. A small omphalocele, like the one described here, is sometimes erroneously called an umbilical cord hernia; however, it should not be confused with an umbilical hernia that occurs after birth and is covered by skin. The thin membrane covering the mass in the present case would be composed of the peritoneum and amnion. The hernia would be composed of small intestinal loops. Omphalocele occurs when the intestinal loops fail to return to the abdominal cavity from the umbilical cord during the 10th week. In the present case, because the hernia is relatively small, the intestine may have entered the abdominal cavity and then herniated later when the rectus muscles did not approach each other close enough to occlude the circular defect in the anterior abdominal wall.
5. The ileum was probably obstructed **(ileal atresia)**. Congenital atresia of the small intestine involves the ileum most frequently; the next most frequently affected region is the duodenum. The jejunum is involved least often. Some **meconium** (fetal feces) is formed from exfoliated fetal epithelium and mucus in the intestinal lumen. It is located distal to the obstructed area (atretic segment). Ileal atresia is associated with cystic fibrosis and chromosomal disorders. During surgery, the atretic ileum would probably appear as a narrow segment connecting the proximal and distal segments of the intestine. The ileal atresia could have resulted from the failure of recanalization of the lumen; however, more likely, the atresia occurred because of prenatal vascular damage—interruption of the blood supply to the ileum. Sometimes a loop of a small bowel becomes twisted, interrupting its blood supply and causing **necrosis** of the affected segment. The atretic segment of the bowel usually becomes a fibrous cord connecting the proximal and distal segments of the bowel.

CHAPTER 12

1. Duplication of the renal pelvis and the ureter results from the formation of two ureteric buds on one side of the embryo. Subsequently, the primordia of these structures fuse. Both ureters usually open into the urinary bladder. Occasionally, the extra ureter opens into the urogenital tract inferior to the bladder. This occurs when the accessory ureter is not incorporated into the base of the bladder with the other ureter; instead, the extra ureter is carried caudally with the mesonephric duct and opens with it into the caudal part of the urogenital sinus. Because this part of the urogenital sinus gives rise to the urethra and epithelium of the vagina, the ectopic (abnormally placed) ureteric orifice may be located in either of these structures, which accounts for the continual dribbling of urine into the vagina. An **ectopic ureteral orifice** that opens inferior to the bladder results in urinary incontinence because there is no urinary bladder or urethral sphincter between it and the exterior. Normally,

the oblique passage of the ureter through the wall of the bladder allows the contraction of the bladder musculature to act like a sphincter for the ureter, controlling the flow of urine from it.

2. **Accessory renal arteries** are common. Approximately 25% of kidneys receive two or more branches directly from the aorta; however, more than two is an exceptional finding. Supernumerary arteries enter either through the renal sinus or at the poles of the kidney, usually the inferior pole, and are end arteries. Accessory renal arteries, more common on the left side, represent persistent fetal renal arteries that grow out in sequence from the aorta as the kidneys "ascend" from the pelvis to the abdomen. Usually, the inferior vessels degenerate as new ones develop. Supernumerary arteries are approximately twice as common as supernumerary veins. They usually arise at the level of the kidney. The presence of a supernumerary artery is of clinical importance in other circumstances because it may cross the ureteropelvic junction and hinder urine outflow, leading to dilation of the calyces and pelvis on the same side **(hydronephrosis)**. Hydronephrotic kidneys frequently become infected **(pyelonephritis)**; infection may lead to the destruction of the kidneys.
3. **Rudimentary uterine horn pregnancies** are very rare; however, they are clinically important because it is difficult to distinguish between this type of pregnancy and a tubal pregnancy. In the present case, the uterine defect was the result of *retarded growth of the right paramesonephric duct* and incomplete fusion of this duct with its partner during the development of the uterus. Most defects resulting from incomplete fusion of the paramesonephric ducts do not cause clinical problems; however, a rudimentary horn that does not communicate with the main part of the uterus may cause pain during the menstrual period because of distention of the horn by blood. Because most rudimentary uterine horns are thicker than uterine tubes, a rudimentary horn pregnancy is likely to rupture much later than a tubal pregnancy.
4. ***Hypospadias of the glans penis*** is the term applied to a defect in which the urethral orifice is on the ventral surface of the penis near the glans penis. The ventral curving of the penis is called **chordee**. Hypospadias of the glans penis results from the failure of the urogenital folds on the ventral surface of the developing penis to fuse completely and establish communication with the terminal part of the spongy urethra within the glans penis. Hypospadias may be associated with inadequate production of androgens by the fetal testes, or there may be resistance to the hormones at the cellular level in the urogenital folds. Hypospadias is thought to have a **multifactorial** etiologic basis because close relatives of patients with hypospadias are more likely to have the defect than the general population. Moreover, recent reports associate maternal exposure to some chemical compounds, such as pesticides, and the occurrence of hypospadias in the offspring. **Glanular hypospadias**, a common defect of the urogenital tract, occurs in approximately 1 in every 300 male infants.
5. This woman has the physical and sex characteristics of a female but is genetically a male. She has a 46,XY chromosome complement and most likely has small undescended testes and no uterus. This disorder is known as **complete androgen insensitivity syndrome** (AIS). Failure of masculinization to occur in these individuals results from a resistance to the action of male sex hormones (androgens) at the cellular level in the genitalia. Competition of females with AIS in the Olympics has been controversial because it is believed that these athletes may have an endurance advantage given their higher testosterone levels.
6. The embryologic basis of an **indirect inguinal hernia** is the persistence of the processus vaginalis, a fetal outpouching of the peritoneum. This finger-like pouch evaginates the anterior abdominal wall and forms the inguinal canal. A **persistent processus vaginalis** predisposes to an indirect inguinal hernia by creating a weakness in the anterior abdominal wall and a hernial sac into which the abdominal contents may herniate if the intra-abdominal pressure becomes very high (as occurs during straining). The hernial sac would be covered by peritoneum, internal spermatic fascia, the cremaster muscle, and cremasteric fascia.

CHAPTER 13

1. **A ventricular septal defect** is the most common cardiac defect at birth. It occurs in approximately 25% of children with congenital heart disease. Most patients with a large ventricular septal defect have a massive left-to-right shunt of blood (left ventricle oxygen-rich blood mixing with oxygen-poor blood in the right ventricle). The infant may present with cyanosis and shortness of breath, pulmonary hypertension because of increased blood flow to the lungs, and congestive heart failure because the heart has to work harder to pump blood.
2. **Patent ductus arteriosus** (PDA) is the most common cardiovascular defect associated with maternal rubella infection during early pregnancy. In an infant with PDA, aortic blood is shunted into the pulmonary artery. One-half to two thirds of the left ventricular output may be shunted through the patent ductus arteriosus. This extra work for the heart results in cardiac enlargement.
3. The tetrad of cardiac defects present in **tetralogy of Fallot** are pulmonary stenosis, ventricular septal defect, overriding aorta, and right ventricular hypertrophy. Echocardiography can be used to accurately detect these vascular defects. **Cyanosis** can occur because of the shunting of unsaturated blood; however, in some infants, it may not occur ("pink tet"). The main aim of therapy is to improve the oxygenation of the blood in the infant; later, usually at 6 months of age, surgical correction of the pulmonary stenosis and closure of the ventricular septal defect occur.
4. **Echocardiography** would rapidly and accurately reveal the cardiac anatomy and details of abnormal vascular connections present in the **transposition of the great arteries. Cardiac catheterization** and MRI may be performed to verify the diagnosis. The infant was able to survive after birth because the ductus arteriosus remains open in these infants, allowing some mixing of blood between the two circulations. In other cases, there is also an **atrial septal defect** or ventricular septal defect that permits intermixing of blood. Complete

transposition of the great arteries is incompatible with life if there are no associated septal defects or a patent ductus arteriosus.

5. This would probably be a **secundum type of atrial septal defect**, located in the region of the oval fossa. This is the most common type of clinically significant atrial septal defect. Large defects, as in the present case, often extend toward the inferior vena cava. The pulmonary artery and its major branches are dilated because of this increased blood flow through the lungs and the increased pressure within the pulmonary circulation. In these cases, a considerable shunt of oxygenated blood flows from the left atrium to the right atrium. This blood, along with the normal venous return to the right atrium, enters the right ventricle and is pumped to the lungs. Large atrial septal defects may be tolerated for a long time, as in the present case, but progressive dilation of the right ventricle often leads to heart failure.

CHAPTER 14

1. The common birth defect of the vertebral column is **spina bifida occulta**. This defect of the vertebral arch of the first sacral or last lumbar vertebra, or both, occurs in approximately 10% to 20% of healthy people. The defect can also occur in cervical and thoracic vertebrae. In most cases, the spinal cord and nerves are normal, and neurologic symptoms are usually absent. Spina bifida occulta does not cause back problems in most people. Some patients may complain of pain due to a **tethered spinal cord**, in which the caudal end of the spinal cord becomes stretched and damaged because it is poorly attached.
2. A rib associated with the seventh **cervical vertebra** is clinically important because it may compress the subclavian artery or brachial plexus, or both, producing symptoms. In most cases, cervical ribs produce no symptoms. These ribs develop from the costal processes of the seventh cervical vertebra and may fuse with the first rib, resulting in compressive symptoms, as in this patient. Cervical ribs occur in 0.5% to 1% of people.
3. A **hemivertebra** can produce a lateral curvature of the vertebral column **(scoliosis)**. This birth defect of the vertebral column is composed of one-half of a body, a pedicle, and a lamina. This defect results when the mesenchymal cells from the sclerotomes on one side fail to form the primordium of one-half of a vertebra. The normal growth centers on one side of the vertebral column develop, and the imbalance causes the vertebral column to bend laterally.
4. **Craniosynostosis** indicates premature closure of one or more of the cranial sutures. This developmental abnormality results in malformations of the cranium. **Scaphocephaly**, a long, narrow cranium, results from premature closure of the sagittal suture. This type of craniosynostosis accounts for approximately 50% of cases. Brain development is normal in these infants.
5. The main features of **Klippel-Feil syndrome** are a short and webbed neck, low hairline, restricted neck movements, and fusion of one or more cervical motion segments. Other clinical features may include breathing problems, scoliosis, neurological deficits, and scapulae that are underdeveloped and elevated (Sprengel deformity). In most cases, the number of cervical vertebral bodies is less than normal. Pathogenic variants (mutation) of the *GDF6* or *GDF3* genes are associated with Klippel-Feil syndrome.

CHAPTER 15

1. The absence of the sternocostal portion of the left pectoralis major muscle is the cause of the abnormal surface features observed. The costal heads of the pectoralis major and pectoralis minor muscles are usually present. Despite the numerous and important actions of the pectoralis major muscle, the absence of all or part of this muscle usually causes no disability; however, the absence of the anterior axillary fold is striking, as is the inferior location of the nipple. The actions of other muscles associated with the shoulder joint compensate for the absence of part of the pectoralis major.
2. The **palmaris longus muscle** is a weak, superficial flexor muscle of the forearm. It is absent in some people, and this varies in different races. Approximately 13% of people lack a palmaris longus muscle on one or both sides. Its absence causes no disability. The tendon of the palmaris longus muscle is often used in tendon grafts.
3. The left **sternocleidomastoid muscle** was prominent when tensed. The left muscle is unaffected, and it does not pull the child's head to the right side. The short contracted right sternocleidomastoid muscle tethers the right mastoid process to the right clavicle and sternum, and continued growth of the left side of the neck results in tilting and rotation of the head. **Congenital torticollis** (wry neck) is a relatively common condition that may occur because of injury to the muscle during birth. Some muscle fibers mighty have been torn, resulting in bleeding into the muscle. Necrosis of some fibers occurred over several weeks, and the muscle was replaced by fibrous tissue, which shortened the muscle and pulled the girl's head to the side.
4. The absence of striated musculature in the median plane of the anterior abdominal wall of the embryo is associated with **exstrophy of the urinary bladder**. This rare but severe birth defect is caused by incomplete midline closure of the inferior part of the anterior abdominal wall and failure of mesenchymal cells to migrate from the somatic mesoderm between the surface ectoderm and the urogenital sinus during the fourth week of development. The absence of mesenchymal cells in the median plane results in the failure of striated muscles to develop. The bladder and urethra are not closed, and both are exposed to the exterior through the opening in the lower abdominal wall.

CHAPTER 16

1. **Congenital hip dysplasia**, now called **developmental dysplasia of the hip**, is a relatively common birth defect, occurring once in 1000 live births. The number of female infants with developmental dysplasia of the hip

is approximately eight times that of male infants. The hip joint is not usually dislocated at birth; however, the acetabulum is underdeveloped. Dislocation of the hip joint may not become obvious until the infant attempts to stand approximately 12 months after birth. The cause for this condition is unknown; some cases (12%–33%) are inherited, and others may be due to deforming forces acting directly on the hip joint of the fetus.

2. Severe birth defects of the limbs (amelia and meromelia), similar to those produced by thalidomide, are rare and usually have a genetic basis. The **thalidomide syndrome** consists of the absence of limbs **(amelia)**; gross defects of the limbs **(meromelia)**, such as attachment of the hands and feet to the trunk by small, irregularly shaped bones; intestinal atresia; and cardiac defects.
3. The most common type of clubfoot is **talipes equinovarus**, which occurs in approximately 1 of every 1000 neonates. In this deformation, the soles of the feet are turned medially, and the feet are sharply plantar flexed. The feet are fixed in the tiptoe position, resembling the foot of a horse (Latin *equus*, "horse"). It is most often treated with manipulation, with or without casting.
4. **Syndactyly** (fusion of digits) is the most common type of limb defect, occurring once in 2000 to 3000 live births. It varies from cutaneous webbing **(simple syndactyly)** of the digits to **synostosis** (union of the osseous phalanges—**complex syndactyly**). Syndactyly is more common in the foot than in the hand. This defect occurs when separate digital rays fail to form in the fifth week of gestation or the webbing between the developing digits fails to break down between the sixth and eighth weeks. As a consequence, separation of the digits does not occur.

CHAPTER 17

1. Ultrasound scanning of the fetus can detect the absence of the neurocranium (acrania) as early as 14 weeks (see Fig. 17.35). Fetuses with **meroencephaly** (absence of part of the brain) do not drink the usual amounts of amniotic fluid, presumably because of impairment of the neuromuscular mechanism that controls swallowing. Because fetal urine is excreted into the amniotic fluid at the usual rate, the amount of amniotic fluid increases. Normally, the fetus swallows amniotic fluid, which is absorbed by its intestines and passed to the placenta for elimination through the mother's blood and kidneys. Meroencephaly, often inaccurately called anencephaly (absence of the brain), can be detected by a plain radiograph; however, radiographs of the fetus are not usually obtained. Instead, this severe defect is diagnosed by ultrasonography or amniocentesis. An elevated level of alpha-fetoprotein in the amniotic fluid indicates an open neural tube defect, such as acrania with meroencephaly or spina bifida with myeloschisis.
2. The embryological basis for the **meningomyelocele** diagnosed in the infant is a failure of the neural tube and neural arches to fuse during the fourth week. A neurologic defect is associated with meningomyelocele because the spinal cord or nerve roots, or both, are often incorporated into the wall of the protruding sac. This damages the nerves supplying various structures. Paralysis of the lower limbs often occurs, and there may be incontinence of urine and feces resulting from paralysis of the sphincters of the anus and urinary bladder.
3. The condition is called **a noncommunicating** or obstructive **hydrocephalus.** The block is most likely in the cerebral aqueduct of the midbrain. Obstruction at this site (stenosis or atresia) interferes with or prevents the passage of ventricular fluid from the lateral and third ventricles to the fourth ventricle. In a *communicating* **hydrocephalus,** the flow of cerebrospinal fluid is blocked after exiting the ventricles. Hydrocephalus is recognized using ultrasonography in the fetal period; however, most cases are diagnosed clinically through neurological examination in the first few weeks or months after birth. Hydrocephalus can be recognized using ultrasonography of the mother's abdomen during the third trimester. Surgical treatment of hydrocephalus usually consists of shunting the excess ventricular fluid through a catheter to another part of the body (e.g., into the bloodstream or peritoneal cavity), from where it is excreted by the infant's kidneys.
4. **Microencephaly** (small brain) is usually associated with microcephaly (small calvaria). Because the growth of the cranium largely depends on the growth of the brain, an arrest in brain development can cause microcephaly. During the embryonic period, environmental exposure to agents such as certain drugs, alcohol, cytomegalovirus, *Toxoplasma gondii,* herpes simplex virus, Zika virus, and high-level radiation induces microencephaly and microcephaly. Severe mental deficiency may occur as a result of exposure of the embryo or fetus to high levels of radiation during the 8- to 16-week period of development.
5. Partial or complete **agenesis of the corpus callosum** is a rare defect and is associated with cognitive deficits in 70% of cases and seizures in 50% of patients. Some people are asymptomatic. Agenesis of the corpus callosum may occur as an isolated defect; however, it is often associated with other central nervous system anomalies, such as holoprosencephaly, which is a defect resulting from the failure of cleavage of the prosencephalon (forebrain). As in this case, a large third ventricle may be associated with agenesis of the corpus callosum. The large ventricle exists because it is able to rise over the roofs of the lateral ventricles when the corpus callosum is absent. The lateral ventricles are usually moderately enlarged.

CHAPTER 18

1. The mother had contracted **rubella** during early pregnancy because her infant had the characteristic triad of defects resulting from the infection of an embryo by the rubella virus. **Cataracts** are common when severe infections occur during the first 6 weeks of pregnancy because the lens vesicle is forming during that time. Congenital cataract is thought to result from the invasion of the embryonic fibers of the lens by the rubella virus. The most common cardiovascular lesion in infants whose mothers had rubella early in pregnancy is **patent ductus arteriosus**, which may occur alone or with other cardiac defects, such as pulmonary stenosis and septal defects. Although a history of maternal rash during the first trimester of pregnancy is helpful for diagnosing **congenital**

rubella syndrome, embryopathy (embryonic disease) can occur after a subclinical (no rash) maternal rubella infection.
2. **Congenital ptosis** (drooping of the superior eyelid) is usually caused by abnormal development or failure of the development of the levator palpebrae superioris muscle. Congenital ptosis is usually transmitted by autosomal dominant inheritance with incomplete penetrance; however, injury to the superior branch of the oculomotor nerve (CN III), which supplies the levator palpebrae superioris muscle, also can cause drooping of the upper eyelid.
3. The protozoon involved was *Toxoplasma gondii*, which is an intracellular parasite. The birth defects result from the invasion of the fetal bloodstream and developing organs by *Toxoplasma* parasites. The parasites pass across the placenta and invade the uterine villi and fetal bloodstream, then disrupt the development of the central nervous system, including the eyes, which develop from outgrowths of the brain (optic vesicles). The frequency of **congenital toxoplasmosis** varies according to the time during pregnancy when the mother was infected: 25% during the first trimester, 54% during the second trimester, and 65% during the last trimester. The physician should tell the female about *Toxoplasma* cysts in meat and advise her to cook her meat well., The physician should also tell her that *Toxoplasma* oocysts can also be found in cat feces and that it is important for her to wash her hands with antibacterial soap after handling her cat and the litter box.
4. The infant had the characteristic phenotype of **trisomy 18**: severe cognitive deficiency, low-set and malformed ears, prominent occiput, congenital heart defect, and failure to thrive. This numeric chromosomal abnormality results from nondisjunction of the number 18 chromosome pair during gametogenesis. Its incidence is approximately 1 in 8000 neonates. Almost all of the trisomy 18 fetuses abort spontaneously. Postnatal survival of these infants is poor, with 30% dying within a month of birth. The mean survival time is only 2 months. Less than 10% of these infants survive more than a year.
5. **Detachment of the retina** is a separation of the two embryonic retinal layers: the neural pigment epithelium derived from the outer layer of the optic cup and the neural retina derived from the inner layer of the cup. The intraretinal space, representing the cavity of the optic vesicle, normally disappears as the retina forms. The proximal part of the hyaloid artery normally persists as the central artery of the retina; however, the distal part of this vessel normally degenerates.

CHAPTER 19

1. **Natal teeth** occur in approximately 1 in 2000 to 3500 neonates. There are usually two teeth in the position of the mandibular medial incisors. They may be supernumerary teeth, but they are often prematurely erupted primary teeth. After it is established radiographically that they are supernumerary teeth, they are removed so that they do not interfere with the eruption of the normal primary teeth and to prevent aspiration. Natal teeth may cause maternal discomfort resulting from abrasion or biting of the nipple during nursing. They may also injure the infant's tongue, which lies between the alveolar processes of the jaws because the mandible is relatively small at birth.
2. Discoloration of the infant's teeth was likely caused by the administration of **tetracycline** to the mother during her pregnancy. Tetracyclines become incorporated into the developing enamel and dentin of the teeth and cause discoloration. **Dysfunction of ameloblasts** resulting from tetracycline therapy causes hypoplasia of the enamel (e.g., pitting). Most likely, the secondary dentition will be affected because enamel formation begins in the permanent teeth before birth (approximately 20 weeks in the incisors).
3. The birth defect of the skin is a capillary angioma or **hemangioma**. It is formed by an overgrowth of small blood vessels consisting mostly of capillaries, but there are also some arterioles and venules in it. The blotch is red because oxygen is not taken from the blood passing through it. This type of angioma is quite common, and the mother should be reassured that it has no clinical significance and requires no treatment. It will fade in a few years. Such angiomas were formerly called *nevus flammeus* (flamelike birthmarks). However, these names are sometimes applied to other types of angiomas, and to avoid confusion, it is better not to use the common names. *Nevus* is not a good term because it is derived from a Latin word meaning "mole or birthmark," which may or may not be an angioma.
4. A tuft of hair in the median plane of the back in the lumbosacral region usually indicates **spina bifida occulta**. It is the most common developmental defect of the vertebrae, and it occurs in L5 or L1, or both, in approximately 10% of people. Spina bifida occulta rarely has clinical significance, but some infants with this vertebral defect may also have a birth defect of the underlying spinal cord and nerve roots.
5. The superficial layers of the epidermis of infants with lamellar **ichthyosis**, resulting from excessive keratinization, consist of grayish-brown scales that are adherent in the center and raised at the edges. Fortunately, the condition is rare; it is inherited as an autosomal recessive trait.

CHAPTER 20

1. Between 7% and 10% of birth defects are caused by environmental factors, including drugs, environmental chemicals, and infections. It is difficult for clinicians to assign specific defects to specific drugs for several reasons:
   - The drug may be administered for the treatment of an illness that itself may cause the defect.
   - The fetal defect may cause maternal symptoms that are treated with a drug.
   - The drug may prevent the spontaneous abortion of an already malformed fetus.
   - The drug may be used with another drug that causes the birth defect.
   - Females must understand that several drugs (e.g., **alcohol, opiods, and other illicit drugs**) cause severe defects if taken during early pregnancy and that these drugs must be avoided.
2. Females older than the age of 41 years are more likely to have a child with Trisomy 21 (Down syndrome) or other

chromosomal disorders than are younger females (25–29 years). Nevertheless, females older than age 41 can have normal children. The physician caring for a pregnant 41-year-old female will recommend chorionic villi sampling, amniocentesis, or DNA-based testing of fetal cells isolated from maternal blood to determine whether the fetus has a chromosomal disorder such as trisomy 21 or trisomy 13. A 41-year-old female can have a normal baby; however, the chances of her having a child with Trisomy 21 (Down syndrome) are approximately 1 in 85 (see Table 20.2).

3. **Penicillin** has been widely used during pregnancy for decades without any suggestion of teratogenicity. Small doses of **aspirin** and other salicylates are ingested by most pregnant females, and when they are consumed as directed by a physician, the teratogenic risk is very low. Chronic consumption of large doses of aspirin during early pregnancy may be harmful. Alcohol and cigarette smoking should be discouraged, and highly addictive drugs such as opioids (e.g., fentanyl and cocaine) must be avoided.
4. The physician told the mother that there was no danger that her child would develop cataracts and cardiac defects because of the rubella infection. However, the physician also explained that cataracts often develop in *embryos* whose mothers contract the disease during early pregnancy. Cataracts occur because of the damaging effect the rubella virus has on the developing lens. The physician might have mentioned that contracting rubella before a female's childbearing years would probably confer permanent immunity to rubella infection.
5. Cats that go outside may be infected with the parasite *Toxoplasma gondii.* It is prudent to avoid contact with cats and their litter during pregnancy. Oocysts of these parasites appear in the feces of cats and can be ingested during careless handling of litter. If the female is pregnant, the parasite may cause severe fetal defects of the central nervous system, such as mental deficiency and blindness.

Index

Note: Page numbers followed by *b* indicate boxes, *f* indicate figures and *t* indicate tables.

D

G

H

O

P